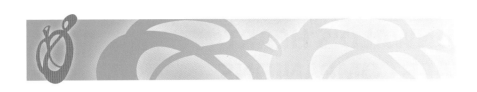

Valvular Heart Disease

A Companion to Braunwald's Heart Disease

BRAUNWALD'S HEART DISEASE COMPANIONS

Published Titles

ANTMAN
Cardiovascular Therapeutics, Fourth Edition

BLACK AND ELLIOTT
Hypertension, Second Edition

CREAGER, BECKMAN, AND LOSCALZO
Vascular Medicine, Second Edition

ISSA, MILLER, AND ZIPES
Clinical Arrhythmology and Electrophysiology, Second Edition

ISKANDRIAN AND GARCIA
Atlas of Nuclear Cardiology

KORMOS AND MILLER
Mechanical Circulatory Support

THEROUX
Acute Coronary Syndromes, Second Edition

BLUMENTHAL, FOODY, AND WONG
Preventive Cardiology

MANN
Heart Failure, Second Edition

BALLANTYNE
Clinical Lipidology

LILLY
Braunwald's Review and Assessment, Ninth Edition

TAYLOR
Atlas of Cardiovascular Computed Tomography

KRAMER
Atlas of Cardiovascular Magnetic Resonance Imaging

Upcoming Titles

BHATT
Cardiovascular Interventions

MCGUIRE
Diabetes in Cardiovascular Disease

BODEN
Chronic Coronary Syndromes

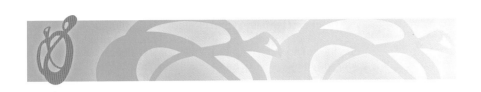

Valvular Heart Disease
A Companion to Braunwald's Heart Disease
FOURTH EDITION

Editors:

Catherine M. Otto, MD, FACC, FAHA
Professor of Medicine
Director, Heart Valve Clinic
J. Ward Kennedy-Hamilton Endowed Chair in Cardiology
Department of Medicine
University of Washington School of Medicine
Seattle, Washington

Robert O. Bonow, MD, MS, MACC, FAHA
Goldberg Distinguished Professor of Cardiology
Director, Center for Cardiovascular Innovation
Northwestern University Feinberg School of Medicine
Northwestern Memorial Hospital
Chicago, Illinois

ELSEVIER
SAUNDERS

1600 John F. Kennedy Blvd.
Ste 1800
Philadelphia, PA 19103-2899

VALVULAR HEART DISEASE, ED. 4
A COMPANION TO BRAUNWALD'S HEART DISEASE

ISBN: 978-1-4557-4860-0

Library of Congress Cataloging-in-Publication Data

Valvular heart disease (2014)
   Valvular heart disease: a companion to Braunwald's heart disease / editors, Catherine M. Otto, Robert O. Bonow.—Fourth edition.
      p. ; cm.
   Complemented by: Braunwald's heart disease / edited by Robert O. Bonow ... [et al.]. 9th ed. 2012.
   Includes bibliographical references and index.
   ISBN 978-1-4557-4860-0 (hardcover: alk. paper)
   I. Otto, Catherine M., editor of compilation. II. Bonow, Robert O., editor of compilation. III. Braunwald's heart disease. Complemented by (work): IV. Title.
   [DNLM: 1. Heart Valve Diseases. WG 260]
   RC685.V2
   616.1'25–dc23

2013022721

Executive Content Strategist: Dolores Meloni
Content Development Specialist: Joanie Milnes
Publishing Services Manager: Patricia Tannian
Project Manager: Amanda Mincher
Manager, Art and Design: Steven Stave

Printed in China

Last digit is the print number: 9 8 7 6 5 4 3 2 1

Working together
to grow libraries in
developing countries

www.elsevier.com • www.bookaid.org

David H. Adams, MD
Marie-Josée and Henry R. Kravis Professor and Chairman
Department of Cardiothoracic Surgery
The Mount Sinai Medical Center
New York, New York

Thomas M. Bashore, MD
Professor of Medicine
Clinical Chief, Division of Cardiology
Duke University Medical Center
Durham, North Carolina

Helmut Baumgartner, MD
Professor of Cardiology/Adult Congenital Heart Disease
University of Muenster
Director, Division of Adult Congenital and Valvular Heart
  Disease
Department of Cardiovascular Medicine
University Hospital Muenster
Muenster, Germany

Alan C. Braverman, MD
Alumni Endowed Professor in Cardiovascular Diseases
Department of Medicine
Washington University School of Medicine
Saint Louis, Missouri

Ben Bridgewater, MB BS, PhD, FRCS (CTh)
Consultant Cardiac Surgeon
University Hospital of South Manchester
University of Manchester
Manchester Academic Health Science Centre
NICOR, UCL
London, United Kingdom

Charles J. Bruce, MBChB, FCP (SA)
Professor of Medicine, College of Medicine
Division of Cardiovascular Diseases
Mayo Clinic
Rochester, Minnesota

Blase A. Carabello, MD
The W.A. "Tex" and Deborah Moncrief, Jr. Professor of Medicine
Vice-Chairman, Department of Medicine
Baylor College of Medicine
Medical Care Line Executive
Veteran's Affairs Medical Center
Director, Center for Heart Valve Disease
St. Luke's Episcopal Hospital
Houston, Texas

John D. Carroll, MD
Professor of Medicine
University of Colorado Denver
Director, Interventional Cardiology
Medical Director, Cardiac and Vascular Center
University of Colorado Hospital
Denver, Colorado

Javier G. Castillo, MD
Department of Cardiothoracic Surgery
The Mount Sinai Medical Center
New York, New York

John B. Chambers, MD
Professor of Clinical Cardiology
Cardiothoracic Department
Guy's and St Thomas's Hospitals
London, United Kingdom

Heidi M. Connolly, MD
Professor of Medicine
Division of Cardiovascular Diseases
Mayo Clinic
Rochester, Minnesota

Arturo Evangelista, MD
Head of Cardiac Imaging Department
Director of Aortic Diseases Unit
Hospital Universitari Vall d'Hebron
Barcelona, Spain

Elyse Foster, MD
Professor of Medicine
University of California, San Francisco
Araxe Vilensky Endowed Chair
Cardiology
San Francisco, California

Benjamin H. Freed, MD
Assistant Professor
Division of Cardiology
Northwestern University Feinberg School of Medicine
Chicago, Illinois

Mario J. Garcia, MD
Chief of Cardiology
Professor of Medicine and Radiology
Co-Director, Montefiore-Einstein Center for Heart and Vascular
  Care
Montefiore Medical Center
Bronx, New York

Brian P. Griffin, MD
The John and Rosemary Brown Endowed Chair in
  Cardiovascular Medicine
Section Head, Cardiovascular Imaging
Cleveland Clinic
Cleveland, Ohio

Howard C. Herrmann, MD
Professor of Medicine
Perelman School of Medicine of the University of Pennsylvania
Director, Cardiac Catheterization and Interventional Cardiology
Hospital of the University of Pennsylvania
Philadelphia, Pennsylvania

Bernard Iung, MD
Professor of Cardiology
Cardiology Department
Bichat Hospital
Professor of Cardiology
University Paris 7 Diderot
Paris, France

Eric V. Krieger, MD
Assistant Professor of Medicine and Cardiology
University of Washington
Seattle, Washington

Amar Krishnaswamy, MD
Interventional Cardiology
Cleveland Clinic
Cleveland, Ohio

Roberto M. Lang, MD
Professor of Medicine and Radiology
Past President of the American Society of Echocardiography
Director, Noninvasive Cardiac Imaging Laboratories
Section of Cardiology
Department of Medicine
Chicago, Illinois

Grace Lin, MD
Assistant Professor
Division of Cardiovascular Diseases
Mayo Clinic
Rochester, Minnesota

Michael J. Mack, MD
Chairman, Cardiovascular Governance Council
Baylor Healthcare System
Chairman, Research Center
The Heart Hospital Baylor Plano
Dallas, Texas

S. Chris Malaisrie, MD
Assistant Professor of Surgery
Division of Cardiac Surgery
Northwestern University Feinberg School of Medicine
Chicago, Illinois

Patrick M. McCarthy, MD
Chief, Division of Cardiac Surgery
Director, Bluhm Cardiovascular Institute
Heller-Sacks Professor of Surgery
Northwestern University Feinberg School of Medicine
Chicago, Illinois

Jordan D. Miller, PhD
Assistant Professor
Mayo Clinic College of Medicine
Departments of Surgery and Physiology
Mayo Clinic
Rochester, Minnesota

Brad Munt, MD, FRCPC, FACC
Cardiologist
St. Paul's Hospital
Vancouver, British Columbia

Rick A. Nishimura, MD
Professor of Medicine
Cardiology
Mayo Clinic
Rochester, Minnesota

Kevin D. O'Brien, MD
Professor of Medicine
University of Washington
Seattle, Washington

Patrick T. O'Gara, MD
Director of Clinical Cardiology
Brigham and Women's Hospital
Professor of Medicine
Harvard Medical School
Boston, Massachusetts

David S. Owens, MD
Assistant Professor
Division of Cardiology
University of Washington
Seattle, Washington

Donald C. Oxorn, MD
Professor of Anesthesiology
University of Washington
Adjunct Professor of Medicine
Cardiology
University of Washington
Seattle, Washington

Rajni K. Rao, MD
Department of Medicine
Division of Cardiology
University of California, San Francisco
San Francisco, California

Raphael Rosenhek, MD
Department of Cardiology
Medical University of Vienna
Vienna, Austria

Ernesto E. Salcedo, MD
Professor of Medicine
University of Colorado Denver
Director of Echocardiography
University of Colorado Hospital
Denver, Colorado

Hartzell V. Schaff, MD
Professor of Surgery
Division of Cardiovascular Surgery Mayo Clinic
Rochester, Minnesota

David M. Shavelle, MD
Director, Cardiac Catheterization Laboratory
Director, Interventional Cardiology Fellowship
Los Angeles County + University of Southern California Medical Center
Associate Clinical Professor
Cardiovascular Medicine
University of Southern California
Los Angeles, California

Karen K. Stout, MD
Director, Adult Congenital Heart Disease Program
Associate Professor of Medicine and Cardiology
Adjunct Associate Professor of Pediatrics and Cardiology
University of Washington
Seattle, Washington

Pilar Tornos, MD
Professor of Cardiology
Servei de Cardiologia
Hospital Universitary Vall d'Hebron
Barcelona, Spain

Wendy Tsang, MD, FRCP(C)
Assistant Professor, Department of Medicine
Division of Cardiology
University Health Network–Toronto General Hospital
University of Toronto
Toronto, Ontario

Alec Vahanian, MD
Cardiology Department
Bichat Hospital
Paris, France

John G. Webb, MD
MacLeod Professor of Heart Valve Intervention
University of British Columbia
Director of Cardiac Catheterization
St. Paul's Hospital
Vancouver, Canada

FOREWORD

Valvular heart disease is an important clinical problem, responsible for an estimated 20,000 deaths and 100,000 hospitalizations each year in the United States alone. In recent decades valvular disease has been caught in two important cross-currents. The first is demographic. Despite the recent decline in the prevalence of rheumatic heart disease in North America, Western Europe, and Australia, the total number of patients with valvular heart disease in these regions is rising steadily because of the increase in degenerative valvular diseases that accompanies the aging of the population. The number of patients with valvular heart disease in developing countries is rising particularly rapidly. This is because the incidence of new cases of rheumatic heart disease has not (yet) fallen to the low levels observed in developed nations, but the numbers of elderly and accompanying degenerative valve diseases are increasing. About 17 million persons worldwide suffer from valve disease.

The second important cross-current relates to the changes in the diagnosis and management of valvular heart disease. Until relatively recently, the cardiac catheterization laboratory was the principal site at which the diagnosis and functional assessment of valvular heart disease were obtained, while the management of advanced valvular disorders took place in the operating room. Now noninvasive imaging techniques—echocardiography, including three-dimensional echocardiography, as well as cardiac magnetic resonance imaging and computed tomography—all provide rich anatomic and functional information. The cardiac catheterization laboratory is increasingly becoming the site of catheter-based correction of valvular disorders. This approach began 30 years ago with balloon mitral valvuloplasty and now involves growing efforts of transcatheter insertion of prosthetic aortic valves and corrections of severe mitral regurgitation.

The editors of *Valvular Heart Disease*, Drs. Otto and Bonow, are among the world's leaders in this field. They have selected outstanding authors, each an authority in the particular area that he or she covers. They discuss in depth the cross-currents mentioned above, which makes the understanding and management of valvular heart diseases more dynamic than ever. They also cover systematically the pathogenesis, pathophysiology, clinical findings, imaging, natural history, and therapeutic options. They describe challenges involved in the care of patients who have undergone valve replacement. There are new chapters on the epidemiology of valvular heart disease, transcatheter aortic valve implantation, imaging guidance of transcatheter valve procedures, and transcatheter mitral valve replacement and repair.

This fourth edition of *Valvular Heart Disease* is a classic, the leading textbook in the field, which builds on the previous editions. We congratulate the editors and authors for their important contributions and welcome this excellent book to our growing list of *Companions to Heart Disease*.

Eugene Braunwald, MD

Douglas L. Mann, MD

Douglas P. Zipes, MD

Peter Libby, MD

PREFACE

The scientific underpinnings, clinical evaluation, and treatment of valvular heart disease continue to advance at a startling rate. In the context of this rapidly expanding knowledge base, we are pleased to present the fourth edition of *Valvular Heart Disease: A Companion to Braunwald's Heart Disease*, which we believe will be a valuable, authoritative resource for practitioners of cardiology and surgery, physicians-in-training, and students of all levels.

In keeping with the previous editions of *Valvular Heart Disease*, the fourth edition covers the breadth of the field, providing the basics of diagnosis and treatment while highlighting new, exciting advances and their potential to transform outcomes for patients with heart valve disorders. With the help of our internationally recognized authors from the United States, Canada, and Europe, we have thoroughly revised this edition to keep the content vibrant, stimulating, and up-to-date. Eleven of the 27 chapters are entirely new, including 6 chapters that cover topics not addressed in earlier editions. We have added 24 new authors, all highly accomplished and recognized in their respective disciplines. The 16 chapters that have been carried over from the previous edition have been extensively updated by their authors, and new co-authors have been added to five of these chapters. These updated chapters cover topics ranging from diagnostic imaging to management of specific rheumatic, congenital, and degenerative diseases of the aortic valve, mitral valve, and right-sided valves.

The fourth edition follows the format of the previous edition. The initial section focuses on basic principles, epidemiology, mechanisms of disease, and diagnostic methods. This is followed by a second section covering aortic valve disease and a third covering mitral valve disease. The final section discusses diverse topics including intraoperative echocardiography, right-sided valve disease, endocarditis, prosthetic valves, and management of valvular heart disease during pregnancy.

Among the many enhancements found in the fourth edition are the four new chapters that open the basic principles section. These include a chapter on the global epidemiology of valvular heart disease by Drs. John Chambers and Ben Bridgewater, two entirely new chapters on the molecular mechanisms of calcific valve disease by Dr. Jordan Miller, and a chapter on the clinical, cellular, and genetic risk factors for calcific valve disease by Drs. Kevin O'Brien and David Owens. Drs. Roberto Lang, Wendy Tsang, and Benjamin Freed have together written a superb new chapter on the three-dimensional anatomy of the mitral and aortic valves; this chapter includes insights gleaned from their experience with the three-dimensional imaging of these structures.

New chapters also cover some of the more important aspects of valve disease diagnosis and management. Drs. Elyse Foster and Rajni Rao discuss the evaluation of and treatment options for the growing number of complex patients with secondary forms of mitral regurgitation stemming from ischemic left ventricular dysfunction (ischemic mitral regurgitation) and dilated cardiomyopathy (functional mitral regurgitation). Drs. Chris Malaisrie and Patrick McCarthy, coauthors of the chapter on mitral valve surgery in the last edition, have joined forces again in the current edition to write a comprehensive, expert chapter on surgical treatment of the aortic valve and ascending aorta. Dr. David Adams, coauthor of the chapter on aortic valve surgery in the last edition, has in this edition instead joined with Dr. Javier Castillo to write a superb chapter on surgical mitral valve repair and replacement. This latter chapter is enhanced by the new chapter on the important applications of intraoperative echocardiography during mitral valve surgery by Dr. Donald Oxorn.

New and updated chapters on transcatheter valve therapeutics cover this exciting and rapidly evolving field extensively. Because of the advent of transcatheter aortic valve implantation for patients who are at high risk for surgical valve replacement, Dr. John Webb has joined Dr. Brad Munt to update this important and topical chapter. Dr. Howard Herrmann has also joined our team of authors and contributed a new chapter on current and future transcatheter approaches to mitral valve repair and replacement. The transcatheter therapeutics discussions are further enhanced by two additional new and important chapters on this subject: Dr. Michael Mack has written a new chapter on the risk assessment of patients undergoing consideration for surgical versus transcatheter valve replacement or repair, and Drs. Ernesto Salcedo and John Carroll have provided an up-to-date view of the role of imaging in guiding the delivery of transcatheter valve devices and monitoring their results. These august authors, representing their respective fields of cardiac surgery, interventional cardiology, and cardiac imaging, have played an important role in the heart valve teams at their individual institutions. The expert commentary found in their chapters embodies the concept that such a collaborative, interdisciplinary valve team provides the needed expertise to make difficult management decisions regarding patients with complex illnesses and deliver the most appropriate treatments with optimal outcomes.

This edition of *Valvular Heart Disease* includes in the print version 388 full-color figures and 162 tables; additional figures and video content are available in the online version. The chapters continue to conform to current guideline recommendations of the American College of Cardiology/American Heart Association and the European Society of Cardiology/European Association of Cardio-Thoracic Surgery.

We are indebted to all of our authors for their commitment of considerable time and effort to ensure the high quality and authoritative nature of this edition of *Valvular Heart Disease*. We are also delighted that this book remains a member of the growing family of companion texts to *Braunwald's Heart Disease: A Textbook of Cardiovascular Medicine*. As a member of the *Braunwald's* companion series, the book is also available online on the Expert Consult companion website. Figures and tables can be downloaded directly from the website for electronic slide presentations. In addition, there is a large portfolio of video content that supplements the print content of many of our chapters.

Despite the advances in diagnosis and treatments (both surgical and interventional), valvular heart disease remains a major cause of morbidity and mortality throughout the world. Rheumatic heart disease remains a scourge in developing countries, and congenital forms of aortic and mitral valve disease create a steady stream of young and middle-aged adults with aortic stenosis, aortic regurgitation, and mitral regurgitation in both developed and developing countries. The aging of the population in the United States and abroad results in an increasing number of elderly patients with degenerative forms of aortic stenosis and mitral regurgitation, who often present with age-related medical comorbidities that confound medical decision making. Unlike most other forms of cardiovascular disease, in which management decisions can be guided by the evidence base created by multiple large-scale randomized controlled clinical trials, the evidence base in valve disease is limited by a dearth of clinical trials.

In this field more than any other, expert clinical judgment and experience are the cornerstones of rational decision making and optimal patient management. We believe that the collective knowledge, experience, and expert clinical judgment of the accomplished authors of *Valvular Heart Disease* will serve as an invaluable resource for all of us who are called upon to provide care for our patients with these diseases.

Robert O. Bonow

Catherine M. Otto

ACKNOWLEDGMENTS

Sincere thanks are due to the many individuals who helped make this book a reality. In particular, we would like to express our deep appreciation to the distinguished chapter authors for their time and effort in providing excellent chapters. We also thank the publishing staff at Elsevier for their guidance and close working relationship. Finally and most important, we would like to thank our families for their constant understanding, encouragement, and support.

CONTENTS

VIDEO CONTENTS

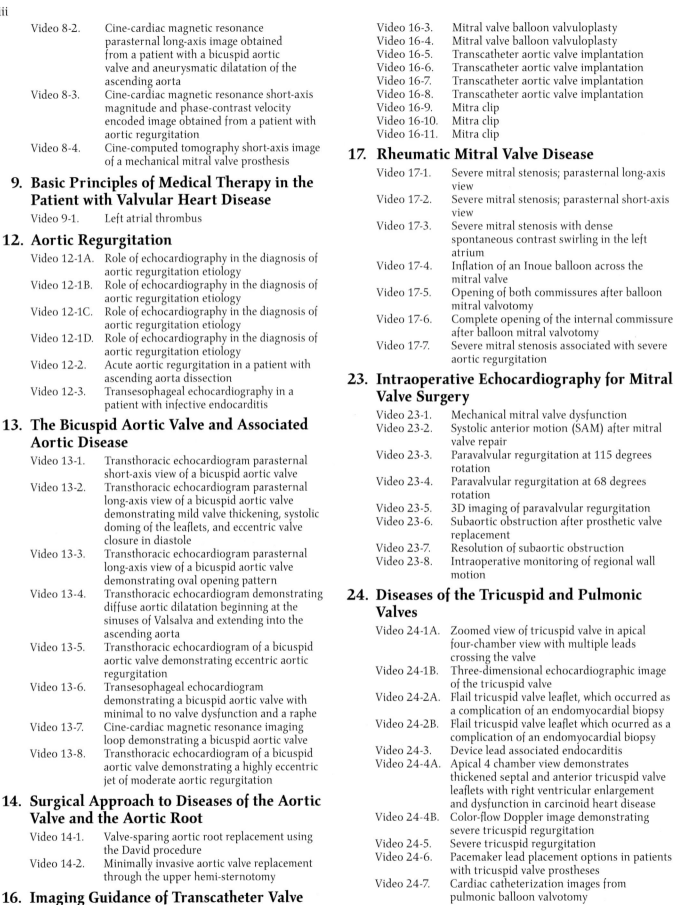

CHAPTER 1

Epidemiology of Valvular Heart Disease

John B. Chambers and Ben Bridgewater

Key Points

- Rheumatic disease is the most common cause of valve disease worldwide, especially in the young, with an estimated prevalence of 15.6 to 19.6 million.
- Endomyocardial fibrosis is an underresearched disease common in equatorial Africa.
- In industrially developed regions valve diseases of old age predominate, particularly calcific aortic stenosis and functional mitral regurgitation.
- In the United States valve disease is most common in the elderly, with a prevalence of 13% in those older than 75 years.
- Drug-induced valve disease is increasing as a result of the use of 5-HT_{2B} receptor agonists.
- Infective endocarditis is increasingly related to medical devices and intravenous drug use.
- Failure of biological replacement valves is a major burden in all regions of the world.
- Substantial variation in access to health care exists in all countries, including those that are industrially developed.
- The main global challenge is to prevent chronic rheumatic disease, which will require collaborations among social, political, and medical programs.
- Valve care in industrially developed countries needs to be organized around specialist valve clinics that refer patients, as indicated, to specialist surgeons and interventional cardiologists.

Rheumatic fever is the most common cause of valve disease in the young,[1] but it predominates in industrially underdeveloped regions. These include Africa, India, the Middle East, South America, and parts of Australia and New Zealand, China, and Russia.[1] In developed countries, the incidence of rheumatic disease declined after the second half of the 20th century, although transient local resurgences still occur.[2] This decline was predominantly the result of improvements in living conditions and health care, as follows:

- Improvements in living conditions:[3]
  - Better housing to reduce overcrowding
  - Better nutrition
- Improved access to health care
- Treatment of streptococcal throat infections
- Use of secondary prophylaxis

In addition there was a spontaneous reduction in the virulence of streptococcal serotypes, but it occurred after the incidence of rheumatic fever had already fallen.[4]

These improvements in living conditions and health care have increased longevity so that valve conditions characteristic of old age now predominate (Figure 1-1). Some 2.5% of the U.S. population has moderate or severe valve disease, but the prevalence rises after age 64 (Figure 1-2) and is 13% in those older than 75.[5] Other studies confirm this age relationship.[6,7] The contribution of old age to the world prevalence of valve disease is difficult to estimate precisely but probably now rivals that of rheumatic disease (Table 1-1). The most common valve diseases in the elderly are:

- Calcific aortic valve disease
- Aortic dilation causing aortic regurgitation
- Functional mitral regurgitation as a result of left ventricular (LV) dysfunction

At the same time there has been a rise in new diseases induced by drugs or therapeutic irradiation. There has also been an increase in endocarditis related to drug use and device implantation. Reoperation for failing biological replacement valves is common in underdeveloped countries, where mechanical prostheses are avoided because of the difficulty of organizing anticoagulation. Reoperation is also a significant load in industrially developed regions mainly as a result of improved life expectancy.

Valve disease remains underdetected,[8] and there are major variations in the provision of health care in all countries of the world, including those that are industrially developed.[9,10] This chapter reviews the causes of valve disease, describes variations in clinical care, and discusses ways in which the worldwide burden of disease could be reduced.

Causes of Valve Disease

The principal causes of valve disease and approximate prevalence are shown in Table 1-1.

Rheumatic Disease

Rheumatic fever occurs in children aged 5 to 15 years from the immune response to group A beta-hemolytic streptococcal pharyngitis. The response occurs 1 to 5 weeks after the initial infection and is caused by molecular mimicries between streptococcal M protein and human myosin and between group A carbohydrate in the streptococcus and valve tissue.

Genetically determined immune markers affect susceptibility to the initial infection and help determine the risk for development of chronic rheumatic disease.[11,12] There is some evidence for disordered signaling mechanisms and reactivation of embryologic pathways.[13] Some streptococcal serotypes (emm types

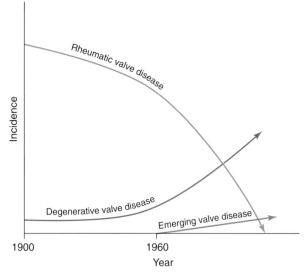

FIGURE 1-1 Diagram illustrating changes in prevalence of valve disease in industrially developed countries. *(Redrawn from Soler-Soler J, Galve E. Worldwide perspective of valve disease. Heart 2000;83:721–5.)*

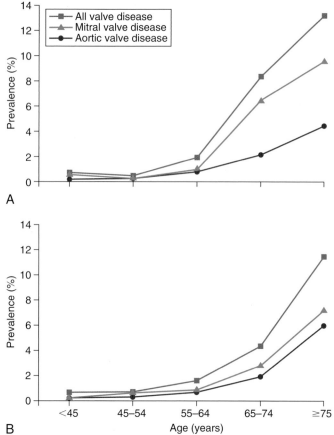

FIGURE 1-2 Effect of age on prevalence of valve disease in three pooled population-based studies. A, Graph of pooled echocardiography data available from the National Heart, Lung and Blood Institute (NHLBI) database from three population-based studies: the Coronary Artery Risk Development in Young Adults (CARDIA) Study, the Atherosclerosis Risk in Communities (ARIC) Study, and the Cardiovascular Health Study (CHS). In total there were 11,911 subjects who had undergone echocardiograms, 40% black and 59% white. These data were compared with the Olmsted county echocardiography register **(B)** in which echocardiograms were performed for clinical reasons. The population-based prevalence of all moderate or severe valve disease was 5.2%, which, when corrected for the age and sex distribution of the U.S. population at the time of the data collection in 2000, was 2.5% (95% confidence interval 2.2-2.7%). The prevalence rose after age 64 years and was 13.2% after age 74. *(Redrawn from Nkomo VT, Gardin JM, Skelton TN, et al. Burden of valvular heart diseases: a population-based study. Lancet 2006;368:1005–11.)*

3, 5, 6, 14, 18, 19, and 29) may be more likely than others to cause rheumatic fever.[11] These host and bacterial factors vary geographically.

Rheumatic fever is uncommon after one episode of pharyngitis but occurs in up to 75% of patients experiencing recurrent episodes. Cardiac involvement occurs in 10% to 40% after the first attack of rheumatic fever[13] but more frequently after multiple attacks.[14] The development of chronic rheumatic disease depends on the age at the time of the acute episodes and their severity and frequency[15] and is more likely with multiple valve involvement, failure to obtain medical help, and lack of secondary prophylaxis.[16,17] Single valve involvement and mitral stenosis are more likely in older individuals with less active carditis[14] (Figure 1-3).

There is a proliferative exudative inflammation of the collagen of the valve and annulus characterized by the presence of modified histiocytes called Aschoff bodies. The valve, annulus, and chordae are edematous and inflamed, leading to annular dilation and chordal elongation.[15] In the long term, fibrosis and calcification develop. The Jones criteria guide the diagnosis of the first episode of rheumatic fever (Table 1-2).[18] Likely rheumatic fever is defined by evidence of group A streptococcal infection (rising anti-streptolysin O (ASO) titers, positive results of culture or rapid antigen tests) and either two major criteria or one major with two minor criteria. For subsequent episodes in patients with established rheumatic disease, the World Health Organization (WHO) allows two minor criteria with evidence of a streptococcal infection including scarlet fever.

The annual incidence of acute rheumatic fever worldwide is estimated at 471,000 cases,[1] on the basis of a metaanalysis of regional reports with a median incidence from 10 to 374 cases per 100,000 population (Table 1-3).

Approximately 200,000 deaths per year occur from acute rheumatic fever or chronic rheumatic disease, mainly in children in developing countries. In Ethiopia, 20% of patients with rheumatic disease die before age 5 years, and 80% before age 25 years.[17] In underdeveloped regions, 10% to 35% of all cardiac admissions are the result of acute or chronic rheumatic disease.[4]

If one allows that 60% of patients with acute rheumatic fever experience chronic rheumatic disease, the annual incidence of new cases of chronic disease is estimated at 282,000.[1] However, there are major geographic differences, and the annual incidence in sub-Saharan Africa ranges from 1.0 to 14.6 per 1000 population.[19] The estimated annual incidence is 24 per 100,000 population in Soweto[20] but with a J-shaped age dependence, with 30 per 100,000 aged 15 to 19 years, 15 per 100,000 aged 20 to 29 years, and 53 per 100,000 older than 60 years.

The worldwide prevalence of chronic rheumatic disease is estimated at 15.6 to 19.6 million.[1] There is wide geographical variation (Figure 1-4), from approximately 0.8 to 7.9 per 1000 population in industrially underdeveloped regions[1,21-23] to only 0.3 per 1000 in developed regions.[1] However, the prevalence rises sharply if echocardiography, rather than the more usual clinical screening, is used. In a study in Cambodia and Mozambique,[8] the prevalence was 2.3 per 1000 children indicated by clinical examination, but 28.1 per 1000 when echocardiography was used. Throughout Africa the prevalence is 1.0 to 6.9 per 1000 in studies using clinical diagnosis compared with 1.4 to 14.6 per 1000 in those using echocardiography.[19] The WHO criteria use valve regurgitation to define rheumatic disease. However, valve regurgitation can be physiological or may occur for other reasons, including myxomatous degeneration. Furthermore, early rheumatic changes may not cause regurgitation. Combined criteria using any grade of regurgitation associated with at least two morphological signs give a

TABLE 1-1 Principal Causes of Valve Disease with Prevalence Where Known

CAUSE	PREVALENCE	WORLD PREVALENCE (MILLION)
1. Rheumatic disease	0.1-0.8% world[1] 3.0 Mozambique using echocardiography[8]	15.6-19.6[1]
2. Endomyocardial fibrosis	20% Coastal Mozambique[27]	—
3. Calcific aortic stenosis	0.4% U.S. pop[5] 1.7% U.S. pop aged >64[5] 2.8% U.S. pop aged ≥75[5]	12*
4. Mitral regurgitation Mitral prolapse Prolapse and regurgitation	1.7% U.S. pop[5] 7.0% U.S. pop aged >64[5] 2% U.S.[44,45] 0.2% U.S.[44,45,47]	49† ?140†
5. Endocarditis	—	—
6. Failing biological replacement valves	—	—
7. Aortic dilation	—	—
8. Congenital disease Bicuspid aortic valve Bicuspid aortic valve with severe aortic stenosis	— — 0.5-0.8%[71,72]	— 35* 4.5*
9. Systemic conditions	—	—
10. Drugs, carcinoid, irradiation	—	—

*The world population (pop) is 7 billion (7,000,000,000). The proportion aged over 60 years is about 10%[6] or 700,000,000. Assuming a prevalence of aortic stenosis of 1.74% in this age group gives a world prevalence of aortic stenosis of 12 million. The prevalence of bicuspid valve is 35 million based on a population prevalence of 0.5%.[71] In a study of patients with BAV of mean age 32 years at baseline followed for 20 years, 28 of 212 (13%) needed aortic valve replacement for severe aortic stenosis.[69,71] This finding suggests that around 4.5 million in the world could have severe aortic stenosis as a result of a bicuspid aortic valve, and the total, as a result of nonrheumatic disease, calcific stenosis in those aged >65 years and bicuspid aortic valve in those < 65 years, could be 16.5 million.
†The world population is 7 billion (7,000,000,000). The proportion aged over 60 years is about 10%[126] or 700,000,000. Using the U.S. prevalence of mitral regurgitation of 7% in those aged >64 years would suggest a world prevalence of mitral regurgitation of 140 million. Applying the U.S. prevalence of mitral prolapse associated with regurgitation of 0.2% to the world population suggests a worldwide prevalence of mitral regurgitation of 140 million. The number with rheumatic disease may be subsumed within this number.

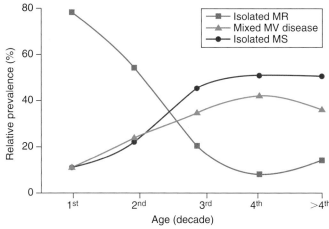

FIGURE 1-3 Time-course analysis (by decades) of the relative prevalence of isolated mitral regurgitation (MR), mixed mitral valve disease, and isolated mitral stenosis (MS). *(Redrawn from Marcus RH, Sareli P, Pocock WA, et al. The spectrum of severe rheumatic mitral valve disease in a developing country: correlations among clinical presentation, surgical pathological findings, and hemodynamic sequelae. Ann Intern Med 1994;120:177–83.)*

TABLE 1-2 Jones Criteria for Rheumatic Fever

Major criteria*	Carditis Polyarthritis Erythema marginatum Chorea Subcutaneous nodules
Minor criteria	Fever Arthralgia Elevated C-reactive protein Prolonged PR interval on electrocardiography

*Frequency of major criteria shown in parentheses.
Special Writing Group of the Committee on Rheumatic Fever and Kawasaki Disease of the Council on Cardiovascular Disease in the Young of the American Heart Association. Guidelines for the diagnosis of rheumatic fever. Jones criteria 1992 update. JAMA 1992;268:2069-2073.

TABLE 1-3 Incidence of Acute Rheumatic Fever (Cases per 100,000 Population)

Industrially developed regions	10
Eastern Europe	10.2
Middle East and North Africa	13.4
Latin America	19.6
China	21.2
South Central Asia	54
Indigenous Australia and New Zealand	374
Sub-Saharan Africa	Unknown

From Carapetis JR. Rheumatic heart disease in developing countries. N Engl J Med 2007;357:439.

prevalence approximately four times that of the WHO criteria.[24] A new World Heart Federation consensus now categorizes definite or borderline rheumatic disease through the use of a combination of regurgitant severity, transvavlular gradient and valve morphology.[25,25a]

Endomyocardial Fibrosis

Endomyocardial fibrosis (EMF) is, after rheumatic disease, the second most frequent cause of acquired heart disease in children and young adults in equatorial Africa.[26] Echocardiography of a sample of 1063 people in coastal Mozambique found a prevalence of 20% (95% confidence interval [CI] 17.4% to 22.2%).[27]

EMF begins as a febrile illness, which is followed by a latent phase of 2 to 10 years. Symptoms then reappear as LV and right ventricular (RV) thrombi and fibrosis develop, leading to RV, LV, or biventricular restrictive cardiomyopathy and encasement of the mitral or tricuspid valves. The pathology of EMF is still

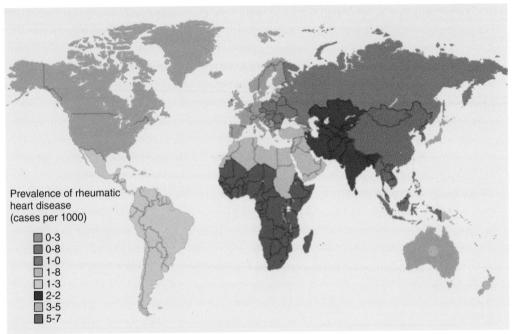

FIGURE 1-4 **World-wide prevalence of chronic rheumatic disease.** *(From Carapetis JR. Rheumatic heart disease in developing countries. N Engl J Med 2007; 357:439.)*

uncertain. There is evidence for the reactivation of embryological pathways,[13,28] and postulated etiological factors[27] that are not mutually exclusive include the following:

- Hypereosinophilia: Features are similar to those of hypereosinophilic syndromes, and the eosinophil count is transiently high in some patients with EMF
- Infection: EMF may be associated with helminths, schistosomiasis, filariasis, and malaria
- Autoimmunity
- Genetic predisposition: The incidence is high among some ethnic groups
- Dietary: Eating uncooked cassava causes an EMF-like response in African green monkeys and may be relevant in humans, especially those with protein-deficient diets
- Geochemical: Increased levels of cerium are found in the hearts of some patients with EMF living near the coast of Mozambique.

Calcific Aortic Stenosis

The incidence and severity of aortic stenosis increase with age, but the process is not a passive, degenerative one. It involves active lipid deposition, inflammation, neoangiogenesis, and calcification (see Chapter 3).[29,30] Aortic stenosis shares with other atherosclerotic processes a number of risk factors, including male gender, diabetes, dyslipidemia (low-density lipoprotein cholesterol [LDL-C] and low levels of high-density lipoprotein cholesterol [HDL-C]), lipoprotein(a), metabolic syndrome, and smoking (see Chapter 4).[31-37]

Aortic valve sclerosis is defined by valve thickening with a peak transaortic velocity on echocardiography of less than 2.5 m/s. Around 16% of patients with sclerosis progress to having stenosis within 7 years.[38] Aortic valve sclerosis is also associated with cardiovascular disease and is a marker for a higher risk of myocardial infarction,[32,39] particularly in patients with no established coronary disease[39] and those with low conventional risk profiles, such as women and patients younger than 55 years[40] (see Chapter 4).

Age-related calcification can also affect the mitral annulus but rarely causes sufficient obstruction to require surgery, except occasionally in patients with chronic renal failure.[41] If calcification is found at both the aortic valve and mitral annulus but also in the aorta, then there is a significant likelihood of associated three-vessel coronary disease.[42]

Mitral Regurgitation

The mitral valve apparatus consists of leaflets, annulus, chordae, and papillary muscles. Malfunction of one or more of these components can cause mitral regurgitation. Mitral regurgitation is categorized as "primary" if caused by intrinsic valve dysfunction and "secondary" or "functional" if because of LV dysfunction. The most common primary cause is associated with mitral prolapse.

MITRAL PROLAPSE

Mitral prolapse occurs at all ages and is associated with valve thickening, annulus dilation, and abnormal chordae.

The chordae are prone to stretching and rupture and may be deficient, particularly at the commissures or at the middle scallop of the posterior leaflet (See Chapter 18). There is either myxomatous infiltration or fibroelastic deficiency, but the degree of histological abnormality varies.[43] Myxomatous infiltration causes irregular thickening of the leaflets as seen on the echocardiogram. Prolapse associated with myxomatous degeneration has a genetic component and is more common in Marfan syndrome and Ehlers-Danlos syndrome type IV. Fibroelastic deficiency is more common in the elderly.

Methods of defining prolapse have been refined with advances in echocardiography and particularly with the realization that the mitral annulus is saddle shaped. The prevalence of prolapse, using strict criteria, is around 2%[44,45] and is associated with tricuspid prolapse in 10% of cases[46] or, more rarely, with aortic valve prolapse. Mitral regurgitation occurs in about 9% of cases with prolapse.[47] The grade of regurgitation depends on the degree of leaflet thickening and prolapse and is worse when ruptured chordae lead to flail or partially flail leaflet segments. In patients with these findings, the mean 10-year survival without heart failure is only 37%.[48]

FUNCTIONAL MITRAL REGURGITATION

The use of the terms ischemic, secondary, and functional is not fully standardized. Ischemic disease is an important cause of functional mitral regurgitation, but *ischemic regurgitation* is usually used for acute ischemic mitral regurgitation as a result of papillary muscle rupture. This condition requires emergency surgery (see Chapter 19).

Functional mitral regurgitation is chronic and primarily the result of LV dysfunction causing altered stresses on the mitral valve apparatus with restriction of the leaflets. There may also be dilation of the annulus.

The leaflet restriction may be "asymmetrical" when it affects predominantly the posterior leaflet. This type is most commonly associated with an inferoposterior myocardial infarction. It may also be "symmetrical," resulting from more generalized LV dysfunction.

The cause of LV dysfunction leading to functional mitral regurgitation reflects the causes of heart failure, which vary geographically. Important causes are ischemic disease, hypertension, and alcohol use in the West and Chagas disease and human immunodeficiency virus (HIV)[4,23] globally. In South Africa, subvalvar aneurysms below the mitral valve cause regurgitation, embolization, and rupture.[49,50] These problems may occur because of a congenital weakness of the tissue around the atrioventricular groove.

Endocarditis

The incidence of infective endocarditis is between 3 and 10 episodes per 100,000 patient-years,[51] but there are major geographical variations depending largely on the age of the population and the frequency of medical devices or intravenous (IV) drug use.[52] The incidence increases with age and is 14.5 episodes per 100,000 patient-years in those aged 70 to 80 years.[51] There is a male-to-female ratio of more than 2:1 (see Chapter 25).[51]

In the industrially underdeveloped regions, patients with endocarditis are young, about three quarters have rheumatic heart disease, and oral streptococci are the main infecting organisms.[53] The risk of endocarditis is about five times that of the general population, particularly in the presence of a murmur, for which the risk is 1 case in 1400 patient-years.[54]

However, in fully industrialized regions, most patients are older and endocarditis is increasingly associated with replacement heart valves, pacemakers,[55-57] or hemodialysis.[58] Patients with prosthetic valves have a 50 times higher risk of endocarditis than the rest of the population,[59] with early infection—within one year of implantation—usually caused by coagulase-negative staphylococci or *Staphylococcus aureus*[60] and late infection by oral commensals. Pacemakers are usually infected with *S. aureus* or coagulase-negative staphylococci.[57] In a separate, much younger, group, endocarditis is caused by intravenous drug use, with *S. aureus* as the most common infecting organism. Predisposing factors are diabetes[58] and immune deficiency including HIV.[4]

Failing Biological Valves

Biological valves have acceptable durability in older patients; failures are uncommon before 5 years in the mitral position and before 8 years in the aortic position.[60,61] However, durability is limited in younger patients, particularly those younger than 40 years old.[61,62] The main advantage of biological valves is that anticoagulation is not required. Mechanical valves are expected to have unlimited durability but require anticoagulation usually with warfarin. In general, in industrially developed regions, biological valves are implanted in the relatively older patient, typically older than 65 years, and mechanical valves are used in younger patients (see Chapter 26).

However, biological valves are implanted in younger patients[61] if anticoagulation control may be uncertain or to allow pregnancy without the potential teratogenic and bleeding complications of oral anticoagulants. This practice is common in industrially underdeveloped countries (Figure 1-5) so "redo" surgery is frequently necessary. At the Heart Institute in São Paulo, Brazil, the mean age at surgery is 49 years, and 41% of procedures are redo operations.[23] This is also a problem in developed countries because patients survive longer.[63]

In the United Kingdom, 7% of aortic valve operations are redo procedures.[64] Furthermore there is a trend toward implantation

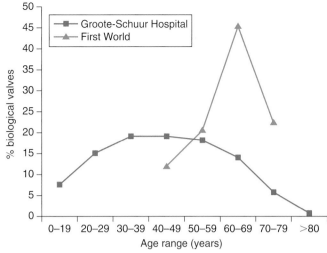

FIGURE 1-5 Diagram comparing the proportion of biological valves expressed as a percentage of total implants in an industrially developed and underdeveloped region. The *blue line* illustrates data from Groote-Schuur Hospital in Cape Town, South Africa. The *green line* illustrates data from a European center. *(Redrawn from Zilla P, Brink J, Human P, Bezuidenhout D. Prosthetic heart valves: catering for the few. Biomaterials 2008;29:385–406.)*

of younger patients with biological valves. In the United Kingdom, for patients between 56 and 60 years of age, the proportion of isolated aortic valve replacement operations using biological valves increased from 25% in 2004 to 40% in 2008. This increase results partly from the perceived longer durability of third-generation biological valves and partly from the possibility of a valve-in-valve transcatheter procedure to treat primary failure.[65]

Aortic Dilation

Secondary aortic regurgitation results from dilation of the aortic root. There may often be associated primary regurgitation as a result of a bicuspid aortic valve or arteriosclerosis. The risk factors for aortic dilation are age, weakness of the aortic wall, and the arteriosclerotic risk factors: hypertension, dyslipidemia, smoking, and diabetes. Weakness of the aortic wall as a result of medial necrosis occurs in Marfan syndrome and Ehlers-Danlos syndrome type IV.

Bicuspid aortic valve should be regarded as a general thoracic aortopathy and is associated with significant dilation of the aorta to more than 40 mm due to medial necrosis[66] in about 20% of cases,[67] in approximately one half affecting the root and in the other half the ascending aorta. Aortic dilation is more likely with associated coarctation,[68] but dissection is relatively uncommon and has a relatively high operative success probably because of the youth and underlying good health of the subjects. Prophylactic surgery is necessary in about 5% during a 20-year follow-up (see Chapter 13).[69]

Vasculitides, especially giant cell arteritis and Takayasu arteritis, may weaken the arterial wall. Other causes of aortic dilation are trauma, cocaine, and amphetamines. In contradistinction to the usual symmetrical "fusiform" dilation of a segment of aorta, a less common "saccular" aneurysm consisting of an outpouching of the aorta can result from inflammation due to syphilis.

Congenital Disease

Congenital lesions account for approximately 5% of valve operations throughout the world. Bicuspid aortic valve is the most common abnormality, affecting up to 2.0% of the population based on autopsy series[70] but 0.5% to 0.8% in larger population-based studies.[71,72] There is evidence of geographic clustering of cases,[73] which is likely as a result of genetic factors[74,75]; the risk of a bicuspid aortic valve or aortic disease is about 10% in first-degree relatives of probands.[76,77] The ratio of male to female is approximately 2:1. The valve is "anatomically" or truly bicuspid in one third of cases and "functionally" bicuspid in two thirds as a result of incomplete separation of two cusps in utero. The most common pattern, in 80% of cases, is failure of right-left separation, which is more likely to be associated with aortic dilation.[78] Failure of separation of right and noncoronary cusps is more likely to be associated with mitral prolapse.[78]

During a 20-year follow-up, 24% of patients with a bicuspid aortic valve demonstrated severe stenosis or regurgitation requiring surgery.[69] Events are far more common in those with even mild valve thickening at baseline, with surgical rates of 75% at 12 years in the presence of thickening compared with only 8% in the absence of thickening.[69] Because the young are more likely to have surgery, the frequency of bicuspid disease is around one third of unselected surgical cases.[79] However, in detailed pathological examination of surgically excised valves, the proportion of bicuspid valves in patients with aortic stenosis having surgery ranges from 67% in patients in their 40s[80] to 28% in octogenarians (Figure 1-6).[81-87]

Congenital mitral disease is uncommon. Patterns described in a series of 49 autopsy cases of congenital mitral stenosis were: dysplastic, parachute (single papillary muscle), hypoplastic associated with hypoplastic left heart, and supramitral ring.[88]

Systemic Inflammatory Conditions

Endocardial involvement is relatively common in systemic lupus erythematosus (SLE), particularly in patients with antiphospholipid antibodies.[89] However, this involvement is usually subclinical. Symptomatic significant valve disease occurs after recurrent valvulitis. Subendothelial deposition of immunoglobulins and complement occurs, causing proliferation of blood vessels, inflammation, thrombosis, and finally fibrosis.

There may be fusion of the mitral valve commissures leading to stenosis, but generalized thickening of the leaflets (30% to 70%) with regurgitation (30% to 50%) is more common.[89-91] Libman-Sacks vegetations are usually less than 10 mm in diameter, sessile, of mixed echogenicity, and rounded. They may occur anywhere, but are seen most commonly at the leaflet edges on the atrial surface of the mitral valve and, less frequently, the ventricular side of the aortic valve. The right-sided valves are rarely affected. Active vegetations have central fibrinoid degeneration with fibrosis and inflammatory infiltrate, whereas healed vegetations have central fibrosis with little or no inflammation.

Valve lesions are more common in the presence of antiphospholipid antibodies and may occur in the absence of features of SLE in the antiphospholipid syndrome.[90] Antiphospholipid antibodies cause:[91]

- Activation of endothelial cells
- Increased uptake of oxidized LDL, leading to macrophage activation
- Interference with regulatory functions of prothrombin and decreased production of proteins C and S

Rheumatoid arthritis causes an immune complex valvulitis with infiltration of plasma cells, histiocytes, lymphocytes, and eosinophils, leading to fibrosis and retraction.[91] Nodules consist of central fibrinoid necrosis surrounded by mononuclear cells, histiocytes, Langerhans and giant cells, and a border of fibrous tissue. The nodules are 4 to 12 mm in diameter and develop at the bases of the mitral or aortic valves. Occasionally there may be more generalized valvulitis. Healed valvulitis leads to leaflet fibrosis and retraction, causing regurgitation.

Ankylosing spondylitis is associated with HLA-B27–mediated chronic inflammation and proliferative endarteritis of the aortic root and left-sided valves. These conditions commonly cause:[91]

- Aortitis of the aortic root, leading to thickening and dilation and functional aortic regurgitation.
- Aortic valvulitis with thickening of the leaflets and cusp retraction.
- Downward displacement of the aortic root leading to a subaortic bulge at the base of the anterior mitral leaflet. This causes retraction of the anterior mitral leaflet with reduced coaptation.

The frequency of valve disease is uncertain because reported series are small and tend to be biased toward patients with severe disease. Aortic valve thickening has been reported in 40%, mitral valve thickening in 34%, and significant aortic dilation in 25% of cases.[91]

Carcinoid Tumors

Carcinoid tumors arise from neural crest gastrointestinal enterochromaffin cells. They are rare, occurring in 1 in 75,000 people.[92] The carcinoid syndrome develops in about half of cases as a result of hepatic spread, and carcinoid heart disease develops in 40% of patients with the syndrome.[92,93] The cardiac lesions are caused by the paraneoplastic effects of vasoactive substances, notably but not exclusively 5-hydroxytryptamine (5-HT). The drugs known to cause valve disease (Table 1-4) either are themselves or have metabolites that are agonists at 5-HT$_{2B}$ receptors. Drugs with an affinity for 5-HT$_{2A}$ and 5-HT$_{2C}$ receptors do not cause valve disease.

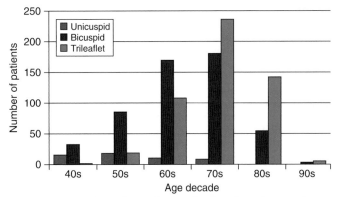

FIGURE 1-6 Numbers of cusps by decade of age in patients undergoing aortic valve surgery for aortic stenosis. Excised valves were examined in detail by a cardiac pathologist. The proportions with a bicuspid aortic valve were, by decade of age: 67% in the 40s; 57% in the 50s; 59% in the 60s; 42% in the 70s; 28% in the 80s; and 33% in the 90s. (*Data from references 81 through 87.*)

TABLE 1-4	Drugs Causing Valve Dysfunction	
AGENT	**VALVE LESION**	**PREVALENCE**
Anorexic Agents	AR, MR, TR	
Fenfluramine	AR	20% women[96] 12% men
Benfluorex		Case reports[97]
Parkinson Disease Therapy		
Pergolide	AR, MR, TR	22%[98]
Cabergoline	AR, MR, TR	34%
Migraine Therapy		
Ergotamine	AR, MR, TR	Case reports[102]
Methysergide	AR, MR	Case reports[102]
Other		
MDMA	AR, MR	28%[103]

AR, aortic regurgitation; *MR*, mitral regurgitation; *TR*, tricuspid regurgitation; *MDMA*, 3,4methylenedioxy-N-methylamphetamine or "ecstasy".

Drugs

Drug-induced lesions are similar to those found in carcinoid disease. However, in carcinoid, right-sided lesions predominate[92,93] because the vasoactive substances are inactivated within the lungs. Left-sided valves may be affected in those 5% of cases with lung metastases or a patent foramen ovale.[92,93] By contrast, drug-induced disease affects mainly the left-sided valves. Furthermore leaflet retraction is more extreme in carcinoid than in drug-induced valve disease, and there may also be fibrosis of the right ventricular outflow tract.

Interaction with the 5-HT$_{2B}$ receptor stimulates cardiac fibroblast proliferation, leading to fibrous plaques with a pearly white appearance on valves and chordae. On echocardiography this process produces:[94]

- Valve thickening
- Chordal thickening and shortening
- Restriction of movement
- Failure of coaptation
- Regurgitation

The earliest sign of valve involvement is an increase in the *tenting height* of the mitral valve, which is the distance between the point of apposition and the plane of the annulus.[94] The incidence of valve involvement has been difficult to determine exactly because of methodological problems, such as:

- Lack of blinding
- Lack of controls
- Expectation of the reporting echocardiographer
- Linkage to compensation claims (anorexic drugs)
- Small population sizes
- Failure to recognize the specific features of drug-induced valve disease
- Effect of dose and duration of therapy
- Codeterminants of valve disease, including age and hypertension

The U.S. Food and Drug Administration (FDA) approved the use of fenfluramine in 1973 as an anorexic agent for short-term use—less than 3 months. Fenfluramine is metabolized to norfenfluramine which has 5-HT$_{2B}$ activity.[6] In 1997 a report suggested that a combination of fenfluramine with the noradrenergic agonist phentermine, taken for a mean of 11 months, induced mitral regurgitation in 92% of cases and aortic regurgitation in 79%.[95] Fenfluramine and its *d*-isomer dexfenfluramine were withdrawn that year. A large observational study showed a lower, but still clinically significant, prevalence of aortic or mitral valve regurgitation in 20% of women and 12% of men undergoing fenfluramine therapy.[96] Benfluorex has been used outside the United States to treat obesity in diabetes with metabolic syndrome since 1976. It is metabolized to norfenfluramine and causes valve lesions similar to those found with fenfluramine.[97] The exact incidence is uncertain because only case reports and small case-matched studies exist. This agent was withdrawn from use in Europe in 2009. Phentermine on its own has not been shown to cause valve lesions.

Bromocriptine has only weak 5-HT$_{2B}$ effects, but pergolide and cabergoline have much stronger effects and cause valve disease when used in the relatively large doses necessary for Parkinson disease.[98] The mean cumulative cabergoline dose associated with moderate or severe valve regurgitation in one study was 4015 mg (standard deviation 3208 mg).[99] By comparison, the dose was only 2341 mg (SD 2039 mg) in patients with no or only mild valve regurgitation. There is controversy over whether valve disease can occur with the smaller doses used for microprolactinoma, typically with cumulative doses of 200 to 414 mg.[100] Studies have differed in dose, duration, and design, and there is evidence that the expectation of the echocardiographer affects the prevalence of abnormalities reported.[98] Valve dysfunction appears to be rare[100] but can occur after relatively large doses used for periods in excess of 10 years.[101]

The ergot alkaloids ergotamine, dihydroergotamine, and methysergide and their metabolite methylergonovine may also

cause endocardial fibrosis, but reports of this development have been anecdotal[102] and accurate estimates of incidence do not exist. MDMA used recreationally has been shown to induce a high incidence of valve lesions.[103]

Irradiation

Radiation-induced valve disease may be seen after high-dose high-volume mediastinal irradiation given typically for Hodgkin disease and less commonly for breast cancer. Minor valve thickening is seen in 80% of cases and may progress to asymptomatic dysfunction in 11 years and to symptoms after a further 4 years,[104] although the rate of progression is variable. One study has suggested that the effect of irradiation may be potentiated by chemotherapy,[104] but this issue is uncertain. Valve changes are more likely to affect the left-sided valves probably because of higher mechanical stresses, but the tricuspid and less commonly the pulmonic valve may also be involved.[105] The aortic and mitral valve are affected equally. The aortic valve typically shows:

- Generalized calcification and immobility similar to symptoms of age-related calcific disease
- Posterior mitral annular calcification
- Thickening extending from the mitral-aortic fibrosa over the base of the anterior mitral leaflet.

Etiology and Frequency of Disease by Valve

The etiology of valve disease is not always obvious because advanced disease with differing etiologies can look similar on echocardiography and even on surgical examination.[80] Furthermore the frequency of the various etiologies depends on numerous factors, including:

- Demographic details (e.g., country, age, socioeconomic class)
- Nature of patient group studied (e.g., unselected populations, outpatients, inpatients, surgical series, autopsies)
- Method of diagnosis (clinical examination, echocardiography, pathological examination)
- Definition of valve disease (all grades or only moderate and severe)

Thus rheumatic disease is the most common cause of valve disease in industrially underdeveloped regions, with EMF also common in equatorial Africa, whereas age-related calcific aortic valve and myxomatous mitral valve diseases are most common in industrialized regions. For example, at the Heart Institute of the University of São Paulo Medical School, the average age at surgery is 49 years, 55% of patients are female, 41% are undergoing reoperations,[23] and rheumatic disease is the most common etiology (Table 1-5).

By contrast, the Euro Heart Survey on Valvular Heart Disease recorded the etiology of moderate and severe disease presenting mainly in Western and East Europe in hospitals or in medical or surgical outpatient clinics.[106] The mean age was 65 years (SD 14), and age-related valve diseases were most common (Table 1-6), notably aortic stenosis and mitral regurgitation (Table 1-7).

In a U.S. study of 1797 men and women older than 60 years in a long-term health-care facility,[106a] 22 residents (1.2%) had mitral stenosis, 591 (33%) had mitral regurgitation, 301 (17%) had aortic stenosis, and 526 (29%) had aortic regurgitation. However, the prevalence of valve disease is far lower in population-based studies (Table 1-8).[5]

Although valve disease is more frequently diagnosed in men,[5] no gender differences were found for mitral valve disease or aortic regurgitation in the U.S. population-based studies. However, there was a trend (P = 0.06) toward a higher prevalence of aortic stenosis in men, which became statistically significant (P = 0.04) after adjustment for age (odds ratio 1.52).

TABLE 1-5 Etiology of Valve Disease at Surgery in São Paulo[23]

ETIOLOGY	PERCENTAGE OF CASES
Rheumatic disease	65
Mitral prolapse	11
Calcific aortic stenosis	10
Infective endocarditis	9
Congenital lesion	5

Compiled from Bocchi EA, Guimaraes G, Tarasoutshi F, et al. Cardiomyopathy, adult valve disease and heart failure in South America. Heart 2009;95:181–9.

TABLE 1-6 Euro Heart Survey: Frequency of Types of Valve Disease in 4910 Patients*

VALVE LESION[†]	NO. (FREQUENCY, %)
Aortic stenosis	1197 (43.1)
Mitral regurgitation	877 (31.5)
Aortic regurgitation	369 (13.3)
Mitral stenosis	336 (12.1)
Right-sided disease	42 (1.2)
Multiple valve disease	713 (20)

*Subjects were recruited as inpatients or from medical or surgical outpatient clinics between 1 April and 31 July 2001 at participating hospitals mainly in Western and East Europe. The mean age was 65 years (SD 14), and 16.8% were aged <50, 50% 50-70, 30% 70-80, and 8.3% >80 years.
[†]Aortic stenosis was defined by maximal jet velocity (V_{max}) >2.5 m/s, mitral stenosis by an orifice area <2.0 cm[2], and mitral or aortic regurgitation by the presence of ≥2/4 regurgitation).
Compiled from Iung B, Baron G, Butchart EG, et al. A prospective study of patients with valvular heart disease in Europe: the Euro Heart Survey on Valvular Heart Disease. Eur Heart J 2003;24:1231–43.

Aortic Stenosis and Regurgitation

In industrially underdeveloped regions, rheumatic disease remains the most common cause of aortic disease. In the West the frequency of chronic rheumatic disease fell after the 1950s. The proportion of aortic regurgitation of rheumatic origin dropped from 62% in 1932 through 1967[107] to 29% in 1970 through 1974[104] and 20% in 1985 through 1989.[108] In industrially developed regions and in the elderly throughout the world, aortic valve disease is predominantly the result of calcific disease (Table 1-9). About 25% of people older than 65 have aortic valve thickening, and 3% older than 75 have critical stenosis (regurgitant orifice area [ROA] <0.8 cm[2]).[1,87] In the Helsinki Ageing Study, echocardiograms were performed in 552 subjects between ages 55 and 86 years. The prevalence of at least moderate aortic stenosis (ROA ≤1.2 cm[2] and velocity ratio ≤0.35) was 4.8% in patients aged 75 to 86, and the prevalence of critical stenosis was 2.9%.[7] The prevalence of any aortic regurgitation was 29%, and that of moderate or severe regurgitation was 13%.

TABLE 1-9 Causes of Aortic Stenosis

Common	Rheumatic disease Calcific disease Bicuspid valve
Uncommon	Irradiation Drugs Congenital lesion, e.g., subaortic membrane
Rare	Ochronosis Hypercholesterolemia in children Paget disease Other congenital causes Unicuspid or quadricuspid valve Supravalvar stenosis

TABLE 1-7 Etiology of Single Left-Sided Valve Disease in the Euro Heart Survey

	AORTIC STENOSIS	AORTIC REGURGITATION	MITRAL STENOSIS	MITRAL REGURGITATION
N	1197	369	336	877
Degenerative (%)*	81.9	50.3	12.5	61.3
Rheumatic (%)	11.2	15.2	85.4	14.2
Endocarditis (%)	0.8	7.5	0.6	3.5
Inflammatory (%)	0.1	4.1	0	0.8
Congenital (%)	5.4	15.2	0.6	4.8
Ischemic (%)	0	0	0	7.3
Other (%)	0.6	7.7	0.9	8.1

*Defined as calcific aortic valve disease, mitral annulus calcification, and mitral prolapse.
Compiled from Iung B, Baron G, Butchart EG, et al. A prospective study of patients with valvular heart disease in Europe: the Euro Heart Survey on Valvular Heart Disease. Eur Heart J 2003;24:1231–43.

TABLE 1-8 Prevalence of Valve Disease in Three Pooled Population-Based Studies, Number (%)

	Age Range (yr)				
	18-44	45-54	55-64	65-74	≥75
Total participants	4351	696	1240	3879	1745
Mitral regurgitation	23 (0.5%)	1 (0.1%)	12 (1.0%)	250 (6.4%)	163 (9.3%)
Mitral stenosis	0	1 (0.1%)	3 (0.2%)	7 (0.2%)	4 (0.2%)
Aortic regurgitation	10 (0.2%)	1 (0.1%)	8 (0.7%)	37 (1.0%)	34 (2%)
Aortic stenosis	1 (0.02%)	1 (0.1%)	2 (0.2%)	50 (1.3%)	48 (2.8%)

Compiled from Nkomo VT, Gardin JM, Skelton TN, et al. Burden of valvular heart diseases: a population-based study. Lancet 2006;368:1005–11.

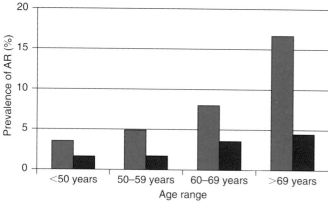

FIGURE 1-7   Effect of age on prevalence of aortic regurgitation. Mild regurgitation (1+), represented by the *blue bars*, was found in 97 (7.4%) of 1316 men and 160 (7.3%) of 2185 women. Moderate and severe regurgitation (≥2+) shown in the *red bars* was found in 38 (3.0%) men and 55 (2.5%) women. The prevalence of mild regurgitation ranged from 4.5% to 16.4% by age (*P* <0.001) and that of moderate or severe regurgitation from 1.6% to 4.55 (*P* <0.002). *(Redrawn from Lebowitz NE, Bella JN, Roman MJ, et al. Prevalence and correlates of aortic regurgitation in American Indians: the Strong Heart Study. J Am Coll Cardiol 2000;36:461–7.)*

However, the most common etiology of aortic stenosis or regurgitation before age 65 years is bicuspid aortic valve disease. This entity is found in 0.5% to 0.8% of Western populations[71,72] and in up to two thirds of all valves excised during valve replacement for aortic stenosis (see Congenital Disease and Figure 1-6). These statistics partly reflect a higher prevalence of aortic stenosis in men. As previously mentioned, there was a trend in the U.S. population-based series toward a higher prevalence of aortic stenosis in men that became statistically significant after adjustment for age.

There are a number of rare or uncommon causes of aortic stenosis, including irradiation, ochronosis, familial hypercholesterolemia, and Paget disease of the bone. Ochronosis is an inherited absence of homogentisic oxydase. Homogentisic acid accumulates in connective tissue, including the endocardium, usually causing no hemodynamic impairment. However, deposits may occasionally cause significant aortic stenosis requiring surgery.[109,110]

The frequency of aortic regurgitation increases with age (Figure 1-7).[111] Aortic regurgitation of any degree occurred in 29% and severe regurgitation in 13% of subjects in the Helsinki Ageing Study.[7] The incidence of aortic regurgitation also depends on the diameter of the aortic root and ascending aorta,[111] reflecting that it may be functional or may result from a combination of primary leaflet disease and aortic dilation. The most common causes of aortic dilation are arteriosclerosis and medial necrosis. In one study, aortic regurgitation due to syphilitic aortic dilation was found in 11% of 258 autopsies between 1932 and 1967.[107] However, the importance of syphilis declined from 1955. Rare causes of aortic regurgitation are listed in Table 1-10.

Acute aortic regurgitation occurs also as a result of endocarditis, dissection, or trauma. Over the last 30 years, infective endocarditis has increased in frequency as a cause of aortic regurgitation from about 9% to 25% of surgical cases.[112,113]

Mitral Stenosis

Rheumatic disease is the overwhelming etiology of mitral stenosis worldwide (Table 1-11) and causes isolated mitral stenosis in 40% of cases. However, the population prevalence of mitral stenosis in the United States is only 0.1%,[5] and the disorder accounts for only 10% of cases in European hospital-based series.[112,114] Although still predominantly rheumatic, mitral stenosis was labeled as degenerative in 12.5% of cases in Europe.[106] In elderly patients, particularly those with renal failure, heavy annular calcification can develop and may extend along the leaflets to cause moderate

TABLE 1-10	Causes of Aortic Regurgitation
Common	Rheumatic disease
	Calcific disease
	Aortic dilation
	Arteriosclerosis
	Marfan syndrome
	Bicuspid aortic valve
	Syphilis
	Bicuspid valve
	Endocarditis
Uncommon	Aortic dilation
	Dissection
	Ehlers-Danlos syndrome
	Sinus of Valsalva aneurysm
	Prolapse
	Irradiation
	Drugs
	Antiphospholipid syndrome
Rare	Carcinoid tumor
	Trauma
	Deceleration injury
	Instrumentation
	Aortic dilation
	Reactive arthritis
	Giant cell arteritis
	Takayasu arteritis
	Wegener granulomatosis
	Sarcoidosis
	Behçet syndrome
	Relapsing polychondritis
	Pseudoxanthoma elasticum
	Mucopolysaccharidosis types I and IV

TABLE 1-11	Causes of Mitral Stenosis
Common	Rheumatic disease
	Calcific disease
Uncommon	Irradiation
	Systemic lupus erythematosus
	Endomyocardial fibrosis
	Carcinoid tumor
Rare	Congenital lesion
	Dysplastic
	Parachute (single papillary muscle)
	Hypoplastic associated with hypoplastic left heart
	Supramitral ring
	Whipple disease
	Fabry disease
	Mucopolysaccharidosis types I and IV

obstruction, which is rarely sufficiently severe to require valve surgery. The severity may be overestimated by the difficulty in imaging the leaflet tips and by a large atrial wave augmenting the estimated mean transmitral gradient.

There are rare congenital causes, of which the most common consists of a dysplastic valve (leaflet margins thickened and rolled; chordae shortened, thickened, and matted together with fibrous tissue; papillary muscles underdeveloped; and interpapillary muscle distance reduced).

Other rare causes are SLE, Whipple disease, Fabry disease, and amyloid.[88,115-118]

Mitral Regurgitation

In industrially underdeveloped regions, rheumatic disease remains the most common cause of mitral regurgitation. In industrialized countries and in the elderly elsewhere, the etiology is predominantly functional, secondary to LV dysfunction. Mitral prolapse occurs in 2% of cases in Western populations, with significant regurgitation in about 9% of patients with prolapse.[44,45] In the

TABLE 1-12 Causes of Mitral Regurgitation

Common	Secondary (functional)
	Coronary disease
	Hypertension
	Alcohol
	Chagas disease
	Human immunodeficiency virus
	Primary
	Rheumatic disease
	Prolapse (myxomatous disease)
	Endocarditis
Uncommon	Secondary (functional)
	Idiopathic dilated myopathy
	Systolic anterior motion (hypertrophic cardiomyopathy, Friedrich ataxia, amyloid)
	Primary
	Irradiation
	Drugs
	Systemic disease: systemic lupus erythematosus, antiphospholipid syndrome, ankylosing spondylitis, rheumatoid arthritis
	Trauma: deceleration injury, instrumentation
	Endomyocardial fibrosis
Rare	Secondary (functional)
	African subvalvar aneurysm
	Hemochromatosis
	Fabry disease
	Systemic sclerosis
	Pseudoxanthoma elasticum
	Primary
	Congenital lesion: parachute anomaly, cleft valve, leaflet fenestration

TABLE 1-13 Causes of Tricuspid Stenosis

Rheumatic disease
Pacemaker
Congenital lesion:
  Tricuspid atresia
  Ebstein anomaly
Carcinoid tumor

TABLE 1-14 Causes of Tricuspid Regurgitation

Secondary	Pulmonary hypertension
	Right ventricular dysfunction cardiomyopathy infarction
Primary	Rheumatic disease
	Myxomatous degeneration
	Drugs
	Carcinoid tumor
	Endocarditis
	Trauma
	Congenital lesion (e.g., Ebstein anomaly)
	Pacemaker
	Endomyocardial fibrosis

TABLE 1-15 Causes of Pulmonic Valve Disease

Secondary (functional)	Pulmonary hypertension
	Pulmonary artery aneurysm
Primary	Congenital lesion
	Carcinoid tumor
	Endocarditis

TABLE 1-16 Causes of Multiple Valve Involvement

Rheumatic disease
Myxomatous disease
Endocarditis
Drugs
Carcinoid tumor
Irradiation

United States the population prevalence is 1.7%,[5] whereas mitral regurgitation represented 32% of a hospital-based European survey.[106] Other uncommon or rare causes are listed in Table 1-12.

Right-Sided Valve Disease

Right-sided valve disease is uncommon, occurring in 1.2% in the Euro Heart Survey.[106] It was not mentioned in U.S. population-based studies.[5]

TRICUSPID VALVE DISEASE

Tricuspid stenosis is almost always rheumatic and associated with left-sided disease (Table 1-13). Tricuspid regurgitation is commonly functional, occurring as a result of pulmonary hypertension or right ventricular myopathy or infarction. Tricuspid regurgitation associated with pacemaker electrodes is increasingly seen. This is rarely functional and is not solved by removing the electrode or changing the pacing mode. The most common mechanism is adherence of one or more leaflets to the electrode, occasionally leading to fibrous incorporation of the valve. The electrode may also perforate the leaflet. Other causes of tricuspid regurgitation are listed in Table 1-14.

PULMONIC VALVE DISEASE

Pulmonic regurgitation is commonly functional and occurs as a result of pulmonary hypertension. Either stenosis or regurgitation occurs in approximately 14% of all congenital cardiac lesions. The pulmonic valve is commonly affected in patients with carcinoid tumors. It is involved with *S. aureus* endocarditis whether community-acquired or as a result of IV drug use. Other causes are listed in Table 1-15.

Multiple Valve Disease

Multiple valve involvement is common, occurring in 20% of patients in the Euro Heart survey[106] (Table 1-16). In rheumatic disease, isolated mitral stenosis is most common, but combined aortic and mitral involvement is also frequent, with aortic regurgitation more likely to occur than stenosis. Tricuspid involvement is probably more frequent than thought because significant thickening does not occur in right-sided lesions, which therefore may be difficult to detect on echocardiography.

Variation in Care: Challenges for the Future

The management of valve disease occurs in four steps, (1) prevention, (2) detection, (3) formulation and surveillance, and (4) surgery.

Prevention

By far the greatest global challenge is to prevent chronic rheumatic disease (Table 1-17), but research is needed in the pathogenesis and pathology of all valve disease. Developmental biology may provide clues about the development of treatment strategies for EMF. Lipid lowering has not been successful in reducing the rate of progression of calcific aortic stenosis, and alternative strategies, notably to target inflammation and calcification, now need to be addressed.

TABLE 1-17 Steps to Eradicate Rheumatic Disease

- Improvement in living conditions
- Education about treatment
- Treatment of streptococcal sore throats even with a single dose of penicillin[133]
- Development of a vaccine[134]
- Identification of valve involvement by population screening echocardiography to give secondary prevention
- Agreement on criteria for identifying rheumatic involvement on echocardiography
- Research in developmental biology to modify the progression to chronic lesions
- Reclassification of rheumatic disease as notifiable to facilitate applying for funding for research and clinical care

Detection

Valve disease is underdetected. In the United States,[5] the prevalence of valve disease is 1.8% when estimated from echocardiograms performed as clinically indicated, compared with an age-corrected population prevalence of 2.5% with echocardiographic screening. Postmortem examinations show that only about 50% of aortic stenosis may be diagnosed before death,[119] and undetected or underinvestigated aortic stenosis is an important cause of perioperative and maternal deaths.[119a]

Early detection is of particular importance for rheumatic disease since the course of the illness can be modified with penicillin. However, in industrially developed regions patients with valve disease remain more likely to die than those without,[5] and it would be an advantage to detect asymptomatic moderate or severe disease to allow surveillance and optimal timing of surgery. Despite the existence of local programs, there are no national screening services anywhere in the world. There is good evidence that primary echocardiographic screening is needed in countries with a high prevalence of rheumatic disease,[8] whereas initial triage by clinical examination is likely to be more cost effective in industrialized countries.

Assessment and Surveillance

The initial management of patients with valve disease is usually conservative,[120,121] and meticulous follow-up is then vital. However, patients with valve disease are usually cared for by general cardiologists or physicians who are less skilled than specialists in diagnosing[122,123] and managing such patients.[124] In the Euro Heart Survey,[106] around half of the patients with valve disease had New York Heart Association (NYHA) functional class III or IV heart failure at the time of surgery.

There is increasing evidence that initial assessment and surveillance in a specialist valve clinic improves outcome.[125]

Surgery

Access to surgery remains variable and limited worldwide. In India, valve operations are performed at a rate of 1.8 per 100,000 population, compared with 28 per 100,000 in the Netherlands.[126] In Brazil only 11,000 operations are performed each year, and 80% of patients needing surgery remain on a waiting list.[23]

There is also variability of access to surgery in industrially developed countries. A comparison of rates of aortic valve replacement with estimated need in the United Kingdom found a variance between observed and expected, ranging between −356 and +230.[64] The causes of this variance have not been explored but may partly reflect the activity of community physicians. Twice as many men as women in the United Kingdom undergo aortic valve replacement.[64] This difference may partly be explained by a higher population prevalence of aortic stenosis in men,[5] which is probably due to the fact that bicuspid valves are approximately

twice as frequent in men. However, there may also be gender differences in care as have already been shown for the investigation and treatment of coronary disease.[127] The elderly are also at a disadvantage in this regard, and around a third with aortic stenosis are denied surgery inappropriately.[128] Development of a transcatheter aortic valve implantation program leads to an increase in conventional surgical rates[129] as clinically inappropriate perceptual barriers to referral, such as age, are lifted.

Patients may be referred to a surgeon at the correct time but receive suboptimal surgery, particularly for repairable mitral regurgitation, even though guidelines increasingly stress that they should be referred early while they are still asymptomatic.[130] The Euro Heart Survey[106] found that 50% of patients with mitral regurgitation received a replacement rather than repair, and in the United Kingdom, only about two thirds of patients with mitral valve prolapse undergo valve repair.[64] According to a 2009 UK database report, the rates of repair for degenerative mitral valve disease varied in different centers from 0 to 98%,[64] and 177 (25%) asymptomatic patients received replacement mitral valves instead of a repair. Similarly, in the United States between 2005 and 2007, the mean repair rate for 1088 surgeons was 41%, with a median of five mitral valve operations per year.[130] Individual surgeons with higher volumes have better repair rates,[130] and higher-volume units have better risk-adjusted in-hospital mortality rates.[131] These observations have led to recommended minimum procedure numbers for individual surgeons and units.[132]

REFERENCES

1. Carapetis JR. Rheumatic heart disease in developing countries. New Engl J Med 2007;357:439.
2. Veasy LG, Wiedmeier SE, Orsmond GS, et al. Resurgence of acute rheumatic fever in the Intermountain area of the United States. New Engl J Med 1987;316:421–7.
3. Gordis L. The virtual disappearance of rheumatic fever in the United States: lessons in the rise and fall of disease. Circulation 1985;72:1155–62.
4. Soler-Soler J, Galve E. Worldwide perspective of valve disease. Heart 2000;83:721–5.
5. Nkomo VT, Gardin JM, Skelton TN, et al. Burden of valvular heart diseases: a population-based study. Lancet 2006;368:1005–11.
6. Khan MA, Herzog CA, St Peter JV, et al. The prevalence of cardiac valvular insufficiency assessed by transthoracic echocardiography in obese patients treated with appetite-suppressant drugs. New Engl J Med 1998;339:713–18.
7. Lindroos M, Kupari M, Heikkala J, et al. Prevalence of aortic valve abnormalities in the elderly: an echocardiographic study of a random population sample. J Am Coll Cardiol 1993;21:1220–5.
8. Marijon E, Ou P, Celermajer S, et al. Prevalence of rheumatic heart disease detected by echocardiographic screening. New Engl J Med 2007;357:470–6.
9. d'Arcy JL, Prendergast BD, Chambers JB, et al. Valvular heart disease: the next cardiac epidemic. Heart 2011;97:91–3.
10. Dunning J, Gao H, Chambers J, et al. Aortic valve surgery—marked increases in volume and significant decreases in mechanical valve use; an analysis of 41,227 patients over 5 years from the Society for Cardiothoracic Surgery of Great Britain and Ireland National database. J Thorac Cardiovasc Surg 2011;142:776–82.
11. Mishra TK. Acute rheumatic fever and rheumatic heart disease: current scenario. J of the Indian Academy of Clinical Med 2007;8:324–30.
12. Ramaswamy R, Spina GS, Fae KC, et al. Association of mannose-binding lectin gene polymorphism but not of mannose-binding serine protease 2 with chronic severe aortic regurgitation of rheumatic etiology. Clin Vaccine immunol 2008;15:932–6.
13. Farrar EJ, Butcher JT. Valvular heart diseases in the developing world: developmental biology takes central stage. J Heart Valve Dis 2012;21:234–4.
14. Feinstein AR, Stern EK. Clinical effects of recurrent attacks of acute rheumatic fever: a prospective epidemiologic study of 105 episodes. J Chronic Dis 1967;20:13–27.
15. Marcus RH, Sareli P, Pocock WA, et al. The spectrum of severe rheumatic mitral valve disease in a developing country. Correlations among clinical presentation, surgical pathological findings, and hemodynamic sequelae. Ann Int Med 1994;120: 177–83.
16. Louw JW, Kinsley RH, Dion RA et al. Emergency heart valve replacement: an analysis of 170 patients. Ann Thorac Surg 1980;29:415–22.
17. Oli K, Asmera J. Rheumatic heart disease in Ethiopia: could it be more malignant? Ethiop Med J 2004;42:1–8.
18. Guidelines for the diagnosis of acute rheumatic fever: Jones criteria, 1992 update. Special Writing Group of the Committee of Rheumatic Fever, Endocarditis, and Kawasaki Disease of the Council on Cardiovascular Disease in the Young of the American Heart Association. JAMA 1992;268:2069–73.
19. Nkomo VT. Epidemiology and prevention of valvular heart diseases and infective endocarditis in Africa. Heart 2007;93:1510–19.
20. Sliwa K, Carrington M, Mayosi BM, et al. Incidence and characterisation of newly diagnosed rheumatic heart disease in Urban African adults: insights from the Heart of Soweto Study. Europ Heart J 2012;31:719–27.
21. Zhimin W, Yubao Z, Lei S, et al. Prevalence of chronic rheumatic heart disease in Chinese adults. Int J Cardiol 2006;107:356–9.

22. Augestad KM, Martyshova K, Martyshov S, et al. Rheumatic fever and rheumatic heart disease in Northwest Russia. Tidsskr Nor Laegeforen 1999;119:1456–9.
23. Bocchi EA, Guimaraes G, Tarasoutshi F, et al. Cardiomyopathy, adult valve disease and heart failure in South America Heart 2009;95:181–9.
24. Marijon E, Celermajer DS, Tafflet M et al. Rheumatic heart disease screening by echocardiography. The inadequacy of World Health Organization criteria for optimizing the diagnosis of subclinical disease. Circulation 2009;120:663–8.
25. Remenyi B, Wilson N, Steer A, et al. World Heart Federation criteria for echocardiographic diagnosis of rheumatic heart disease—an evidence-based guideline. Nat Rev Cardiol 2012;9:297–309.
25a. Mirabel M, Celermajer DS, Ferreira B, et al. Screening for rheumatic heart disease: evaluation of a simplified echocardiography-based approach. Eur Heart J Cardiovasc Imaging 2012;13(12):1024–9. doi: 10.1093/ehjci/jes077. Epub 2012 Apr 19. PMID: 22518053 [PubMed - in process].
26. Mayosi BM. Contemporary trends in the epidemiology and management of cardiomyopathy and pericarditis in sub-Saharan Africa. Heart 2007;93:1176–83.
27. Mocumbi AO, Yacoub S, Yacoub MH. Neglected tropical cardiomyopathies: II Endomyocardial fibrosis: Myocardial disease. Heart 2008;94:384–90.
28. Zeisberg EM, Tarnavski O, Zeisberg M, et al. Endothelial-to-mesenchymal transition contributes to cardiac fibrosis. Nature Med 2007;13:952–61
29. Otto CM, Kuusisto J, Reichenbach DD, et al. Characterization of the early lesion of "degenerative" valvular aortic stenosis: histologic and immunohistochemical studies. Circulation 1994;90:844–53.
30. Rajamannan NM, Gersh B, Bonow RO. Calcific aortic stenosis: from bench to the bedside—emerging clinical and cellular concepts. Heart 2003;89:801–5.
31. Stewart BF, Siscovick D, Lind BK, et al. Clinical factors associated with calcific aortic valve disease: Cardiovascular Health Study. J Am Coll Cardiol 1997;29:630–4.
32. Aronow WS, Ahn C, Shirani J, et al. Comparison of frequency of new coronary events in older subjects with and without valvular aortic sclerosis. Am J Cardiol 2001;88: 693–5.
33. Gotoh T, Kuroda T, Yamasawa M, et al. Correlation between lipoprotein(a) and aortic valve sclerosis assessed by echocardiography (the JMS Cardiac Echo and Cohort Study). Am J Cardiol 1995;76:928–32.
34. Briand M, Lemieux I, Dumesnil JG, et al. Metabolic syndrome negatively influences disease progression and prognosis in aortic stenosis. J Am Coll Cardiol 2006;47:2229–36.
35. Katz R, Budoff MJ, Takasu J, et al. Relationship of metabolic syndrome with incident aortic valve calcium and aortic valve calcium progression: the Multi-Ethnic Study of Atherosclerosis (MESA). Diabetes 2009;58:813–19.
36. Novaro GM, Katz R, Aviles RJ, et al. Clinical factors, but not C-reactive protein, predict progression of calcific aortic-valve disease: the Cardiovascular Health Study. J Am Coll Cardiol 2007;50:1992–8.
37. O'Brien KD. Epidemiology and genetics of calcific aortic valve disease. J Investig Med 2007;55:284–91.
38. Cosmi JE, Tunick PA, Rosenzweig BP, et al. The risk of development of aortic stenosis in patients with "benign" aortic valve thickening. Arch Int Med 2002;162:2345–7.
39. Otto CM, Lind BK, Klitzman DW, et al. Association of aortic valve sclerosis with cardiovascular mortality and morbidity in the elderly. N Engl J Med 1999;341:142–7.
40. Hsu S-Y, Hsieh I-C, Chang S-H, et al. Aortic valve sclerosis is an echocardiographic indicator of significant coronary disease in patients undergoing diagnostic coronary angiography. Int J Clin Prac 2004;59:72–7.
41. Strauman E, Meyer B, Mistell M, et al. Aortic and mitral valve disease in patients with end stage renal failure on long-term haemodialysis. Br Heart J 1992;67:236–9.
42. Jeon D, Atar S, Brasch A, et al. Association of mitral valve annulus calcification, aortic valve sclerosis and aortic root calcification with abnormal myocardial single photon emission tomography in subjects age < 65 years old. J Am Coll Cardiol 2001;38: 1988–93.
43. Pellerin D, Brecker S, Veyrat C. Degenerative mitral valve disease with emphasis on mitral valve prolapse. Heart 2002;88(Suppl IV):iv20–iv28.
44. Freed LA, Levy D, Levine RA et al. Prevalence and clinical outcome of mitral-valve prolapse. New Engl J Med 1999;341:1–7.
45. Sutton M St J, Weyman AE. Mitral valve prolapse prevalence and complications. Circulation 2002;106:1305–7.
46. Marks AR, Choong CY, Sanfilippo AJ, et al. Identification of high-risk and low-risk subgroups of patients with mitral-valve prolapse. New Engl J Med 1989;320: 1031–6.
47. Jones EC, Devereux RB, Roman MJ, et al. Prevalence and correlates of mitral regurgitation in a population-based sample (the Strong Heart Study). Am J Cardiol 2001;87:298–304.
48. Ling LH, Enriquez-Sarano M, Seward JB, et al. Clinical outcome of mitral regurgitation due to flail leaflet. New Engl J Med 1996;335:1417–23.
49. Mocumbi AOH, Ferreira MB. Neglected cardiovascular diseases in Africa. JACC 2012;55:680–7.
50. Lurie AO. Left ventricular aneurysms in the African. Brit Heart J 1960;22:181–8.
51. Habib G, Hoen B, Tornon P, et al. Guidelines on the prevention, diagnosis, and treatment of infective endocarditis. Europ Heart J 2009;30:2369–413.
52. Cabell Jr CH, Jollis JG, Peterson GE, et al. Changing patient characteristics and the effect on mortality in endocarditis. Arch Intern Med. 2002;162:90–4.
53. Koegelenberg CF, Doubell AF, Orth H, et al. Infective endocarditis in the Western Cape Province of South Africa: a three year prospective study. Quart J Med 2003;96: 217–25.
54. MacMahon SW, Hickey AJ, Wicken DE, et al. Risk of infective endocarditis in mitral prolapse with and without precordial systolic murmurs. Am J Cardiol 1987;59:105–8.
55. Tleyjeh IM, Abdel-Latif A, Rahbi H, et al. A systematic review of population-based studies of infective endocarditis. Chest 2007;132:1025–35.
56. Hill EE, Herigers P, Claus P, et al. Infective endocarditis: changing epidemiology and predictors of 6-month mortality: a prospective cohort study. Europ Heart J 2007;28: 196–203.
57. Klug D, Lacroix D, Savoye C, et al. Systemic infection related to endocarditis on pacemaker leads: clinical presentation and management. Circulation. 1997;95:2098–107.
58. Friedman ND, Kaye KS, Stout JE, et al. Healthcare-associated bloodstream infections in adults: a reason to change the accepted definition of community-acquired infections. Ann Intern Med 2002;137:791–7.
59. Oliver R, Roberts GJ, Hooper L, et al. Antibiotics for the prophylaxis of bacterial endocarditis in dentistry (review). The Cochrane Library 2008;(4):CD003813.
60. Grunkemeier GL, Li H-H, Naftel DC, et al. Long-term performance of heart valve prostheses. Current Problems in Cardiology 2000;25:73–156.
61. Rahimtoola SH. Choice of prosthetic heart valve. J Am Coll Cardiol 2010;55: 2413–26.
62. Chan V, Males T, Lapierre H, et al. Reoperation of left heart valves bioprostheses according to age at implantation. Circulation 2011;124:575–80.
63. Zilla P, Brink J, Human P, et al. Prosthetic heart valves: catering for the few. Biomaterials 2008;29:385–406.
64. Bridgewater B, Kinsman R, Walton P, et al. Demonstrating quality: the Sixth National Adult Cardiac Surgery Database Report. Henley on Thomas UK: Dendrite Clinical Systems Ltd; 2009.
65. Brown ML, Scaff HV, Lahr BD, et al. Aortic valve replacement in patients aged 50-70 years: improved outcome with mechanical versus biologic prostheses. J Thorac Cardiovasc Surg 2008;135:878–84.
66. Tadros TM, Klein MD, Shapira OM. Ascending aortic dilatation associated with bicuspid aortic valve. Pathophysiology, molecular biology, and clinical implications. Circulation 2009;119:880–90.
67. Tzemos N, Therrien J, Yip J, et al. Outcomes in adults with bicuspid aortic valves. JAMA 2008;300:1317–25.
68. Oliver JM, Alonso-Gonzalez R, Gonzalez AE, et al. Risk of aortic root or ascending aorta complications in patients with and without coarctation of the aorta. Am J Cardiol 2009;104:1001–6.
69. Michelena HI, Desjardins VA, Avierinos J-F, et al. Natural history of asymptomatic patients with normally functioning or minimally dysfunctional bicuspid aortic valve in the community. Circulation 2008;117:2776–84.
70. Roberts WC. The congenitally bicuspid aortic valve. A study of 85 autopsy cases. Am J Cardiol 1970;26:72–83.
71. Nistri S, Basso C, Marzari C, et al. Frequency of bicuspid aortic valve in conscripts by echocardiogram. Am J Cardiol 2005;96:718–21.
72. Movahed MR, Hepner AD, Ahmadi-Kashani M. Echocardiographic prevalence of bicuspid aortic valve in the population. Heart Lung Circ 2006;15:297–9.
73. Le Gal G, Bertault V, Bezon E, et al. Heterogeneous geographic distribution of patients with aortic valve stenosis: arguments for new aetiological hypothesis. Heart 2005;91:247–9.
74. Garg V, Muth AN, Ransom MK, et al. Mutations in NOTCH1 cause aortic valve disease. Nature 2005;437:270–4.
75. McBride KL, Garg V. Heredity of bicuspid aortic valve: is family screening indicated? Heart 2011;97:1193–5.
76. Huntington K, Hunter AGW, Chan K-LA. Prospective study to assess the frequency of familial clustering of congenital bicuspid aortic valve. J Am Coll Cardiol 1997;30:1809–12.
77. Cripe L, Andelfinger G, Martin LJ, et al. Bicuspid aortic valve is heritable. J Am Coll Cardiol 2004;44:138–43.
78. Schaefer BM, Lewin MB, Stout KK, et al. The bicuspid aortic valve: an integrated phenotypic classification of leaflet morphology and aortic root shape. Heart 2008;94: 1634–8.
79. Dare AJ, Veinot JP, Edwards WD, et al. New observations on the etiology of aortic valve disease: a surgical pathologic study of 236 cases from 1990. Hum Pathol 1993;24:1330–8.
80. Roberts WC, Vowels JT. Comparison of interpretations of valve structure between cardiac surgeon and cardiac pathologist among adults having isolated aortic valve replacement for aortic stenosis (± aortic regurgitation). Am J Cardiol 2009;103: 1139–45.
81. Roberts WC, Ko JM, Filardo G, et al. Valve structure and survival in quadragenarians having aortic valve replacement for aortic stenosis (± aortic regurgitation) with versus without coronary artery bypass grafting at a single US medical center (1993 to 2005). Am J Cardiol 2007;100:1683–90.
82. Roberts WC, Ko JM, Filardo G, et al. Valve structure and survival in septuagenarians having aortic valve replacement for aortic stenosis (± aortic regurgitation) with versus without coronary artery bypass grafting at a single US medical center (1993 to 2005). Am J Cardiol 2007;100:1157–65.
83. Roberts WC, Ko JM, Filardo G, et al. Valve structure and survival in sexagenarians having aortic valve replacement for aortic stenosis (± aortic regurgitation) with versus without coronary artery bypass grafting at a single US medical center (1993 to 2005). Am J Cardiol 2007;100:1286–92.
84. Roberts WC, Ko JM. Frequency by decades of unicuspid, bicuspid, and tricuspid aortic valves in adults having isolated aortic valve replacement for aortic stenosis with or without associated aortic regurgitation. Circulation 2005;111:920–5.
85. Roberts WC, Ko JM, Filardo G, et al. Valve structure and survival in quinqagenarians having aortic valve replacement for aortic stenosis (± regurgitation) with versus without coronary artery bypass grafting at a single US medical center 1993-2005. Am J Cardiol 2007;100:1584–91.
86. Roberts WC, Ko JM, Matter GJ. Aortic valve replacement for aortic stenosis in nonagenarians. Am J Cardiol 2006;989:1251–3.
87. Roberts WC, Ko JM, Garner WL, et al. Valve structure and survival in octogenarians having aortic valve replacement for aortic stenosis (± regurgitation) with versus without coronary artery bypass grafting at a single US medical center 1993-2005. Am J Cardiol 2007;100:489–95.
88. Ruckman RN, Van Praagh R. Anatomic types of congenital mitral stenosis: Report of 49 autopsy cases with consideration of diagnosis and surgical implications. Am J Cardiol 1978;42:592–601.

EPIDEMIOLOGY OF VALVULAR HEART DISEASE

89. Roldan CA, Shively BK, Lau CC, et al. Systemic lupus erythematosus valve disease by transesophageal echocardiography and the role of antiphospholipid antibodies. J Am Coll Cardiol 1992;20:1127–34.
90. Asherson RA, Cervera R. Antiphospholipid antibodies and the heart. Lesson sand pitfalls for the cardiologist. Circulation 1991;84:920–3.
91. Roldan CA. Valvular and coronary heart disease in systemic inflammatory diseases. Heart 2008;94:1089–101.
92. Fox DJ, Khattar RS. Carcinoid heart disease: presentation, diagnosis, and management. Heart 2004;90:1224–8
93. Gustaffson BI, Hauso O, Drozdov I, et al. Carcinoid heart disease. Int J Cardiol 2008;129:318–24.
94. Lancellotti P, Livadariu E, Markov M, et al. Cabergoline and the risk of valvular lesions in endocrine disease. European Journal of Endocrinology 2008;159:1–5.
95. Connolly HM, Crary JL, McGoon MD, et al. Valvular heart disease associated with fenfluramine-phentermine. N Engl J Med 1997;337:581–8.
96. Dahl CF, Allen MR, Urie PM, et al. Valvular regurgitation and surgery associated with fenfluramine use: an analysis of 5743 individuals. BMC Med 2008;6:34.
97. Le Ven F, Tribouilloy C, Habib G, et al. Valvular heart disease associated with benfluorex therapy: results from the French multicentre registry. Europ J Echo 2011;12:265–71.
98. Antonini A, Poewe W. Fibrotic heart-valve reactions to dopamine-agonist treatment in Parkinson disease. Lancet Neurol 2007;6:826–9.
99. Zanettini R, Antonini A, Gatto G, et al. Valvular heart disease and the use of dopamine agonists for parkinson disease. New Engl J Med 2007;356:39–46.
100. Sherlock M, Toogood AA, Steeds R. Dopamine agonist therapy for hyperprolactinaemia and cardiac valve dysfunction; a lot done but much more to do. Heart 2009;95:522–3.
101. Gu H, Luck S, Carroll P, et al. Cardiac valve disease and low-dose dopamine agonist therapy: an artefact of reporting bias? Clin Endocrinol 2011;74:608–10.
102. Redfield MM, Nicholson WJ, Edwards WD, et al. Valve disease associated with ergot alkaloid use. Echocardiographic and pathologic correlations. Ann Intern Med 1992;117:50–2.
103. Droogmans S, Cosyns B, D'Haenen H, et al. Possible association between 3,4-met hylenedioxymethamphetamine abuse and valvular heart disease. Am J Cardiol 2007;100:1442–5.
104. Carlson RG, Mayfield WR, Normann S, et al. Radiation-associated valvular disease. Chest 1991;99:538–45.
105. Veinot JP, Edwards WD. Pathology of radiation-induced heart disease: a surgical and autopsy study of 27 cases. Human Pathology 1996;27:766–73.
106. Iung B, Baron G, Butchart EG, et al. A prospective study of patients with valvular heart disease in Europe: the Euro Heart Survey on Valvular Heart Disease. Europ Heart J 2003;24:1231–43.
106a. Aranow WS, Ahn C, Kronzon I. Prevalence of echocardiographic findings in 554 men and in 1,243 women aged > 60 years in a long-term health care facility. Am J Cardiol 1997;79:379–80.
107. Barondess JA, Sande M. Some changing aspects of aortic regurgitation. Arch Intern Med 1969;124:600–5.
108. Acar J, Michel PL, Dorent R, et al. Evolution des étiologies des valvulopathies operées en France sur un période de 20 ans. Arch Mal du Coeur 1992;85:411–5.
109. Gould L, Reddy CVR, DePalma D, et al. Cardiac manifestations of ochronosis, J Thorac Cardiovasc Surg 1976;72:788–91.
110. Hungaishi M, Taguchi J, Ikari Y, et al. Aortic valve stenosis in alkaptonuria. Circulation 1998;98:1148–9.
111. Lebowitz NE, Bella JN, Roman MJ, et al. Prevalence and correlates of aortic regurgitation in American Indians: The Strong Heart Study. J Am Coll Cardiol 2000;36:461–7.
112. Olson LJ, Subramanian R, Edwards WD. Surgical pathology of pure aortic insufficiency: a study of 225 cases. Mayo Clin Proc 1984;59:835–41.
113. Loire R, Mann J. Insuffisance aortic et maladie aortique dégénerative. Ann Cardiol Angiol 1990;39:327–31.

114. Horstkotte D, Loogen F. The natural history of aortic valve stenosis. Eur Heart J 1988;9(Suppl E):57–64.
115. John RM, Hunter D, Swanton RH. Echocardiographic abnormalities in type IV mucopolysaccharidosis. Arch Dis Child 1990;65:746–9.
116. McAllister HA, Fenoglio JJ. Cardiac involvement in Whipple disease. Circulation 1975;52:152–6.
117. Edwards JN, Edwards WD, Steckelberg JM, et al. Mitral stenosis associated with valvular tophi. Mayo Clin Proc 1984;59:509–12.
118. Matula G, Karpman LS, Frank S, Stinson E. Mitral obstruction from staphylococcal endocarditis corrected surgically. JAMA 1975;233:58–9.
119. Andersen JA, Hansen BF, Lynborg K. Isolated valvular aortic stenosis. Clinicopathological findings in an autopsy material of elderly patients. Acta Med Scand 1975;197:61–4.
119a. 2001 Report of the National Confidential Enquiry into Perioperative Deaths. London: NCEPOD; 2001. p. 66–9.
120. Bonow RO, Carabello BA, Chatterjee K, et al. American College of Cardiology/American Heart Association Task Force on Practice Guidelines. 2008 focused update incorporated into the ACC/AHA 2006 guidelines for the management of patients with valvular heart disease: a report of the American College of Cardiology/American Heart Association Task Force on Practice Guidelines (Writing Committee to revise the 1998 guidelines for the management of patients with valvular heart disease). Endorsed by the Society of Cardiovascular Anesthesiologists, Society for Cardiovascular Angiography and Interventions, and Society of Thoracic Surgeons. J Am Coll Cardiol 2008;52: e1–e142.
121. Vahanian A, Baumgartner H, Bax J, et al. Guidelines on the management of valvular heart disease. Eur Heart J 2007;28:230–68.
122. Fink JC, Schmid CH, Selker HP. A decision aid for referring patients with systolic murmurs for echocardiography. J Gen Int Med 1994;9:479–84.
123. Mangione S, Nieman LZ. Cardiac auscultatory skills of internal medicine and family practice trainees. A comparison of diagnostic proficiency. JAMA 1997;278:717–22.
124. Taggu W, Topham A, Hart L et al. A cardiac sonographer led follow up clinic for heart valve disease. Int J Cardiol. 2009;132:240–3.
125. Chambers J, Ray S, Prendergast B, et al. Specialist valve clinics: recommendations from the British Heart Valve Society working group on improving quality in the delivery of care for patients with heart valve disease. Heart 10.1136/heartjnl-2013-303754.
126. Takkenberg JJM, Rajamannan NM, Rosenhek R, et al. The need for a global perspective on heart valve disease epidemiology. The SHVD working group on epidemiology of heart valve disease founding statement. J Heart Valve Dis 2008;17:135–9.
127. Raine RA, Crayford TJB, Chan KL, et al. Gender differences in the investigation and treatment of patients with acute myocardial ischaemia and infarction in England. Int J Health Mechanics 1999;15:136–46.
128. Iung B. Management of the elderly patient with aortic stenosis. Heart 2008;94:519–24.
129. Grant SW, Devbhandari MP, Grayson AD et al. What is the impact of providing a Transcatheter Aortic Valve Implantation (TAVI) service on conventional aortic valve surgical activity, patient risk factors and outcomes in the first two years? Heart 2010;96:1633–7.
130. Bolling SF, Li S, O'Brien SM, et al. Predictors of mitral valve repair: clinical and surgeon factors. Ann Thorac Surg 2010;90:1904–11.
131. Gammie JS, O'Brien SM, Griffith BP, et al. Influence of hospital procedural volume on care process and mortality for patients undergoing elective surgery for mitral regurgitation. Circulation. 2007;115:881–7.
132. Bridgewater B, Hooper T, Munsch C, et al. Mitral repair best practice proposed standards. Heart 2006;92:939–44.
133. Arguedas A, Mohs E. Prevention of rheumatic fever in Costa Rica. J Pediatr 1992;121:569–72.
134. Guilherme L, Fae KC, Hiha F, et al. Towards a vaccine against rheumatic fever. Clin Dev Immunol 2006;13:125–32.

CHAPTER 2

Three-Dimensional Anatomy of the Aortic and Mitral Valves

Wendy Tsang, Benjamin H. Freed, and Roberto M. Lang

Key Points

- The mitral valve is a complicated three-dimensional (3D) structure made up of multiple, distinct anatomic components including the annulus, commissures, leaflets, chordae tendinae, papillary mucscles, and left ventricle. Optimal interaction of these different elements is crucial for the valve's functional integrity.
- The mitral annulus is a fibromuscular ring to which the anterior and posterior mitral valve leaflets attach. The normal mitral valve annulus has a 3D saddle shape with its "lowest points" at the level of both commissures.
- The annulus is a dynamic structure that undergoes 3D deformation in its circumference, excursion, curvature, shape, and size for proper function, which in turn makes it susceptible to ventricular remodeling.
- 3D echocardiography provides a considerable amount of mechanistic insight into the complex annular alterations that occur in different disease processes, such as degenerative and ischemic mitral valve disease, and the conformational changes that occur to both the mitral and aortic annuli with mitral valve repair.
- The leaflet segmentation scheme proposed by Carpentier is the most widely used, dividing the posterior leaflet into three scallops with three apposing anterior segments.
- The aortic valve is a part of the aortic root complex, which is composed of the sinuses of Valsalva, the fibrous interleaflet triangles, and the valvular leaflets themselves.
- Approximately two thirds of the circumference of the lower part of the aortic root is connected to the septum, and the remaining third is connected via a fibrous continuity known as the aortic-mitral curtain to the mitral valve.
- The aortic valve leaflets are attached in a semilunar fashion throughout the entire length of the aortic root, with the highest point of attachment at the level of the sinotubular junction and the lowest in the ventricular myocardium below the anatomic ventriculoarterial junction.
- The surgical definition of aortic annulus describes a semilunar crownlike structure demarcated by the hinges of the aortic valve leaflets, whereas the imaging definition refers to the virtual or projected ring that connects the three most basal insertion points of the leaflets.
- The aortic annulus and the left ventricular outflow tract are elliptical rather than circular structures.
- The aortic annulus changes dynamically during the cardiac cycle. It is largest in the first third of systole and smallest during isovolumic relaxation

Advances in 3D echocardiography technology have ushered its use into mainstream clinical practice.[1] 3D echocardiography offers a realistic, multiplanar image of both valves and their spatial relationships with adjacent structures, providing anatomic and functional insight that has furthered our understanding of normal spatial relationships and the anatomic and functional abnormalities that develop in patients with valvular heart disease.

Mitral Valve Anatomy

The mitral valve is a complicated 3D structure composed of multiple, distinct anatomical components. Optimal interaction of these different elements comprising the annulus, commissures, leaflets, chordae tendinae, papillary muscles, and left ventricle is crucial for its functional integrity.

Mitral Annulus

The mitral annulus is a fibromuscular ring to which the anterior and posterior mitral valve leaflets attach. The normal mitral valve annulus has a 3D saddle shape with its "lowest points" at the level of both commissures. This allows proper leaflet apposition during systole and minimizes leaflet stress.[2] The annulus can be divided into the anterior and posterior annulus based on the insertion of the corresponding leaflets. The anterior portion of the annulus attaches to the right and left fibrous trigones. The right trigone is a fibrous area situated between the membranous septum, the mitral valve, the tricuspid valve, and the noncoronary cusp at the aortic annulus. The left trigone is a fibrous area located at the nadir of the left coronary cusp of the aortic annulus and the left border of the aortic-mitral curtain. The aortic-mitral curtain is the fibrous tissue between the anterior mitral valve leaflet, the left and noncoronary cusps of the aortic valve, and the left and right trigone.[3]

The posterior portion of the annulus is less developed owing to the discontinuity of the fibrous skeleton of the heart in this region. This difference explains why the posterior portion of the mitral annulus is more prone to pathologic dilation and the anterior portion is relatively resistant.[4] The annulus is a dynamic structure that undergoes 3D deformation in its circumference, excursion, curvature, shape, and size for proper function, which makes it susceptible to ventricular remodeling.[5-9]

Mitral Valve Leaflets

The mitral valve has an anterior and a posterior leaflet (Figure 2-1). The atrial, or smooth, surface is free of any attachments whereas the ventricular, or rough, surface connects to the papillary muscles via the chordae tendinae. The posterior leaflet, which is quadrangular, is attached to approximately three fifths of the annular circumference. The anterior leaflet has a semicircular shape and is attached to approximately two fifths of the annular circumference.[10] Although the posterior leaflet attaches to a larger portion of the annular circumference, it is shorter than the anterior leaflet.

There are two major terminology classifications for the segmental anatomy of the mitral leaflets, which help with the description of the localization of specific mitral valve lesions. The leaflet segmentation scheme proposed by Carpentier[11] is the most widely

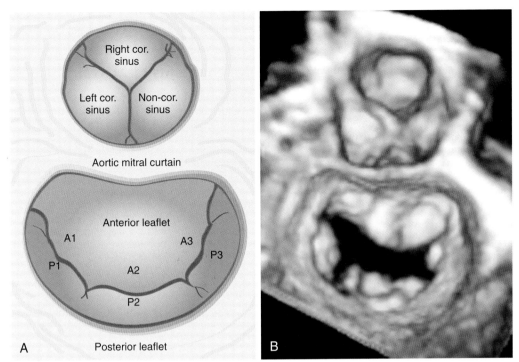

FIGURE 2-1 **Anatomic relationship of the aortic and mitral valves. A,** Schematic diagram and **B,** *en face* three-dimensional echocardiographic zoom-mode image of the mitral valve from the left atrial, or the surgeon's, perspective depicting typical anatomic relationships. In this view, the aortic valve occupies the 12 o'clock position. The aortic mitral curtain separates the anterior leaflet from the aortic valve. *A1* to *A3,* Anterior leaflet segments; *cor.,* coronary; *P1* to *P3,* posterior leaflet segments.

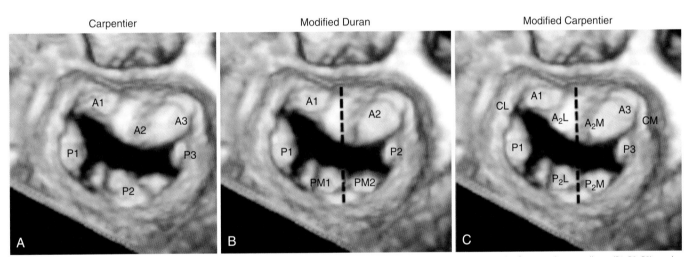

FIGURE 2-2 **Classification of mitral valve segmental anatomy. A,** The Carpentier system divides the posterior leaflet into three scallops *(P1, P2, P3)* on the basis of leaflet indentation. The anterior leaflet is then divided and classified into three segments on the basis of their relationship to the posterior leaflet *(A1, A2, A3).* **B,** The Duran system divides the leaflet on the basis of the chordal insertion of the papillary muscles. Thus the anterior leaflet is divided into two segments *(A1, A2)* and the posterior into four segments *(P1, PM1, P2, PM2).* Segments A1, P1 and PM1 attach to the anterolateral papillary muscle, and segments A2, P2, and PM2 to the posteromedial papillary muscle. **C,** The modified Carpentier system divides A2 and P2 into lateral *(A₂L, P₂L)* and medial *(A₂M, P₂M)* segments, allowing grouping of leaflet segments according to papillary muscle attachment. Thus, segments A1, A₂L, P1, and P2L are attached to the anterolateral papillary muscle, and A3, A₂M, P3, and P₂M to the posteromedial papillary muscle.

used. In this scheme, the posterior leaflet has two well-defined indentations dividing it into three separate sections or "scallops." The anterolateral scallop is defined as P1, the middle scallop as P2, and the posteromedial scallop as P3. The anterior leaflet typically has a smoother surface and is devoid of indentations. The segment of the anterior leaflet opposing P1 is designated A1 (anterior segment), the segment opposite to P2 is A2 (middle segment), and the segment opposite to P3 is A3 (posterior segment) (Figure 2-2).

The modified Duran nomenclature is based on the chordal insertion of the papillary muscles.[12] In this classification,

the posterior leaflet is divided into P1, PM₁, PM₂, and P2 and the anterior leaflet is divided into A1 and A2. If a line were drawn directly down the center of the mitral valve, then P1, PM₁, and A1 would be grouped together because they all attach to the anterolateral papillary muscle, and P2, PM₂, and A2 would be grouped together because they attach to the posteromedial papillary muscle (see Figure 2-2).

A final proposed classification is the modified Carpentier classification, which is a combination of both the Carpentier and the modified Duran nomenclature.[13] This classification scheme divides A2 and P2 into medial (M) and lateral (L) segments, grouping P1, P$_2$L, A1, and A$_2$L because they are attached to the anterolateral papillary muscle and P$_2$M, P3, A$_2$M, and A3 because they are attached to the posteromedial papillary muscle. This last terminology converts the well-known Carpentier leaflet segmentation into anatomically relevant groupings (see Figure 2-2).

Mitral Valve Commissures

During systole, the margins of the two mitral leaflets oppose each other for several millimeters to ensure valve competency against normal left ventricular (LV) end-systolic pressure.[14,15] The distinct area where the anterior and posterior leaflets appose each other during systole is known as the commissure. Carpentier divides the commissures into anterolateral and posteromedial commissures.[11] The amount of tissue in the commissures varies from several millimeters of leaflet tissue to distinct leaflet segments.

Mitral Valve Chordae

The chordae tendinae are responsible for determining the position and tension on the anterior and posterior leaflets at LV end-systole. The chordae are fibrous extensions originating from the heads of the papillary muscles and infrequently from the inferolateral ventricular wall. They are named according to their insertion site on the mitral leaflets. Marginal or primary chordae insert on the free margins of the mitral leaflets and prevent marginal prolapse. Intermediate or secondary "strut" chordae insert on the ventricular surfaces of the leaflets, preventing billowing while reducing tension on the leaflet tissues.[16,17] These chords may also play a role in determining dynamic ventricular shape and function through their contribution to ventricle-valve continuity.[18,19] Basal or tertiary chordae insert on the posterior leaflet base and mitral annulus. Their specific function is unclear.

Papillary Muscles

The two papillary muscles—the anterolateral and the posteromedial—originate from the area between the apical and middle thirds of the LV free wall. The anterolateral papillary muscle has an anterior head and a posterior head, whereas the posteromedial papillary muscle usually has anterior, intermediate, and posterior heads.[20] The anterolateral papillary muscle has a dual blood supply from both the left anterior descending and left circumflex arteries, and the posteromedial papillary muscle receives its single blood supply from the right coronary artery when the right coronary is dominant, which is the situation in 90% of individuals. When the left coronary is dominant, the posteromedial papillary muscle is supplied by the left circumflex. Because the papillary muscles connect directly to the left ventricle, any geometric alteration of the ventricle can change the axial relationship of the chordae and leaflets, resulting in poor leaflet coaptation.

Mitral Valve Apparatus Quantification

In addition to its ability to provide detailed and multidimensional images of the mitral valve, 3D echocardiography also provides accurate and reproducible quantification of mitral valve geometry and dynamics throughout the cardiac cycle. With the advent of 3D imaging, new parameters of annular, coaptation, leaflet, and subvalvular geometry are easily obtained.[3,10] These measurements have generated new insights into the mechanics of the mitral valve. A detailed description of the most commonly used parameters is shown in Figures 2-3 and 2-4.

3D echocardiography provides a considerable amount of mechanistic insight into the complex annular alterations that occur in different disease processes, such as degenerative and ischemic mitral valve diseases and the conformational changes that occur to both the mitral and aortic annuli with mitral valve

repair. These new insights can potentially lead to improved surgical techniques that could eventually lead to better patient outcomes.

Mechanisms of Mitral Valve Dysfunction

Diseases that affect the mitral valve are best described by defining the *etiology* of the disease, the specific *lesions* caused by the disease, and the *dysfunction* it creates on the mitral valve apparatus. This "pathophysiologic triad," first described by Carpentier et al[21] in the early 1980s, is still extremely useful today in characterizing different types of mitral valve disorders.

Mitral valve disease is due to either primary (direct) or secondary (indirect) causes. Examples of diseases that directly affect the mitral valve are congenital malformations, rheumatic disease, valvular tumors, and degenerative diseases. Diseases that indirectly affect the mitral valve include ischemic and nonischemic dilated cardiomyopathy, hypertrophic cardiomyopathy, and myocardial infiltrative diseases.

No matter what the etiology of the mitral valve disease, each disease process frequently results in one or more lesions. For example, dilated cardiomyopathy can result in mitral annular dilation in what is commonly referred to as functional mitral regurgitation (MR). Degenerative diseases such as Barlow disease and fibroelastic deficiency result in multiple types of lesions, including excess myxomatous leaflet tissue, chordal elongation, thinning, and rupture. Rheumatic heart disease results in commissural fusion, leaflet thickening, and chordal agglutination. Myocardial infarction can lead to lesions such as papillary muscle displacement, leaflet tethering, and mitral annulus dilation.

These lesions, in turn, lead to mitral valve dysfunction. Instead of classifying this dysfunction as simply mitral stenosis (MS) or MR, Carpentier[11] developed a classification scheme to aid in the surgical strategy on the basis of the type of leaflet motion (Table 2-1). Patients with mitral annular dilation or leaflet perforation usually have normal leaflet motion and are categorized as having type I dysfunction. Type II dysfunction consists of prolapse (free edge of one or both leaflets overriding the plane of the annulus during valve closure) and flail (excessive motion of the leaflet margin above the plane of the annulus) due to excessive and redundant leaflet tissue and chordal rupture, respectively (Figure 2-5). Leaflet restriction during valve closure due to fusion of various components of the mitral valve apparatus is defined as type IIIa dysfunction, whereas leaflet restriction during valve opening resulting from leaflet tethering, is defined as type IIIb dysfunction.

It is important to emphasize that the different components of the pathophysiologic triad are not mutually exclusive and can be clinically combined in different ways. For example, the typical lesions seen in type IIIa dysfunction can also occur in conjunction with the lesions of type II dysfunction. Type IIIb dysfunction is the result of ventricular remodeling, with the primary lesion being leaflet tethering due to papillary muscle displacement as occurs in ischemic MR. Associated annular dilation is a common finding in patients with chronic degenerative MR, but the classification of dysfunction should differentiate the primary lesion causing the regurgitation (i.e., chordal rupture) from secondary lesions (i.e., annular dilation).

Degenerative Mitral Valve Disease

Mitral valve prolapse is now recognized as the most common cause of MR in developed countries.[22] It results primarily from two distinctive types of degenerative diseases, Barlow disease and fibroelastic deficiency (Table 2-2). There is considerable overlap between these two entities, and it is difficult to reliably distinguish them on the basis of either the gross or histologic appearance of the valve. Some valves may represent a forme fruste of Barlow disease and demonstrate myxoid infiltration on subsequent histologic examination.[6]

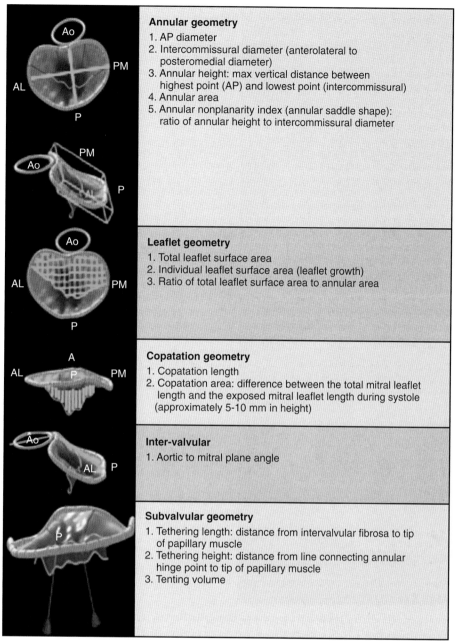

Annular geometry
1. AP diameter
2. Intercommissural diameter (anterolateral to posteromedial diameter)
3. Annular height: max vertical distance between highest point (AP) and lowest point (intercommissural)
4. Annular area
5. Annular nonplanarity index (annular saddle shape): ratio of annular height to intercommissural diameter

Leaflet geometry
1. Total leaflet surface area
2. Individual leaflet surface area (leaflet growth)
3. Ratio of total leaflet surface area to annular area

Copatation geometry
1. Copatation length
2. Copatation area: difference between the total mitral leaflet length and the exposed mitral leaflet length during systole (approximately 5-10 mm in height)

Inter-valvular
1. Aortic to mitral plane angle

Subvalvular geometry
1. Tethering length: distance from intervalvular fibrosa to tip of papillary muscle
2. Tethering height: distance from line connecting annular hinge point to tip of papillary muscle
3. Tenting volume

FIGURE 2-3 Volumetric reconstruction of the mitral valve. 3D echocardiography–based software provides measurements of mitral annular, leaflet, coaptation line, intervalvular relationships, and subvalvular geometry. *A,* Anterior; *AL,* anterolateral; *Ao,* aortic valve; *P,* posterior; *PM,* posteromedial.

BARLOW DISEASE

Barlow disease results from an excess of myxomatous tissue, which is an abnormal accumulation of mucopolysaccharides in one or both of the leaflets and many or few of the chordae.[23] This myxoid infiltration results in thick, bulky, redundant, billowing leaflets and elongated chordae, which often lead to bileaflet, multisegmental prolapse (Figure 2-6). Barlow disease is usually diagnosed in young adulthood, and patients are typically monitored for many decades with well-preserved LV size until criteria for surgery are met in the fourth or fifth decade of life.

FIBROELASTIC DEFICIENCY

In contrast, fibroelastic deficiency results from acute loss of mechanical integrity due to abnormalities of connective tissue structure and/or function.[23] It usually leads to either a localized or unisegmental prolapse due to elongated chordae or flail leaflet due to ruptured chordae (see Figure 2-6). Patients most

commonly present in the sixth decade of life with a relatively short history of MR. This entity is the most common form of organic mitral valve disease for which mitral valve repair surgery is required. There is considerable overlap between these two entities and it is difficult to reliably distinguish them based on either the gross or histologic appearance of the valve. Some valves may represent a forme fruste of Barlow disease and will demonstrate myxoid infiltration on subsequent histological examination.[6]

Ischemic Mitral Regurgitation

Ischemic MR is a pathophysiologic outcome of ventricular remodeling arising from ischemic heart disease. The adverse changes that occur in the ventricle after an ischemic event commonly result in type IIIB dysfunction of the mitral valve with leaflet restriction during systole.[11] Ischemic MR occurs in approximately 20% to 25% of patients with myocardial infarction even in the era

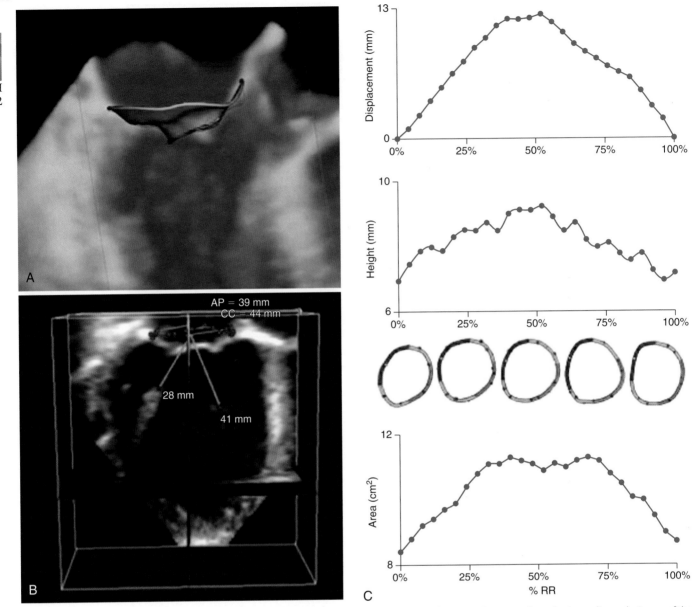

FIGURE 2-4 Functional anatomy of the mitral annulus during the cardiac cycle. A, Three-dimensional transesophageal echocardiography image of the mitral valve with a three-dimensional mitral valve model of the annulus, leaflets, and coaptation line imposed on the image. **B,** three-dimensional transesophageal echocardiographic dataset of the mitral valve with a three-dimensional mitral valve model of the mitral annulus and papillary muscles superimposed on the image. **C,** Results from specialized three-dimensional echocardiographic software tracking mitral annular displacement, height, and area during systole. *AP,* Anteroposterior; *CC,* inter-commisural; *RR,* R-R interval.

TABLE 2-1   Carpentier Functional Classification for Mitral Valve Dysfunction

	TYPE 1	TYPE 2	TYPE IIIA	TYPE IIIB
Motion of leaflet margin	Normal	Prolapse or flail	Restricted leaflet opening	Restricted leaflet closure
Associated disease processes	Chronic atrial fibrillation Bacterial endocarditis	Degenerative disease (Barlow disease or fibroelastic deficiency)	Rheumatic disease	Myocardial infarction Dilated cardiomyopathy
Associated lesions	Annular dilation Leaflet perforation	Leaflet thickening Leaflet billowing Leaflet elongation Chordal thickening Chordal rupture	Commissure fusion Leaflet thickening Chordal thickening	Papillary displacement Chordae tethering Annular dilation

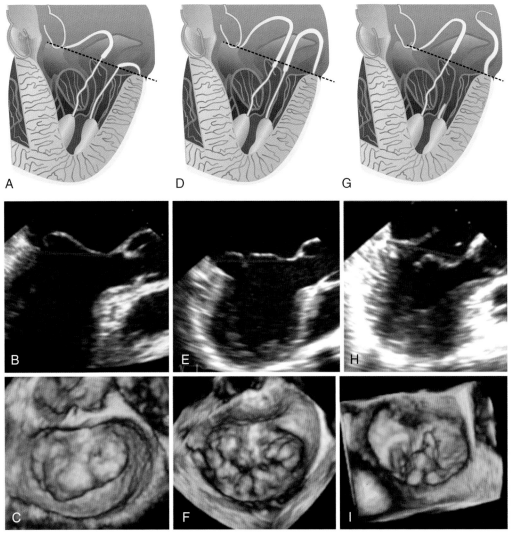

FIGURE 2-5 Myxomatous disease with mitral valve prolapse. A, Schematic demonstrating anterior leaflet prolapse. **B,** Imaging from two-dimensional transesophageal echocardiography. **C,** three-dimensional transesophageal echocardiographic image of the mitral valve with anterior leaflet prolapse as viewed *en face* from the left atrium. Leaflet prolapse is diagnosed when the free edge of the leaflet overrides the plane of the mitral annulus during systole. **D,** Schematic demonstrating bileaflet billowing of the mitral valve due to chordae elongation. **E,** Images of bileaflet mitral valve billowing from two-dimensional transesophageal echocardiography and **F,** three-dimensional transesophageal echocardiography as viewed *en face* from the left atrium. Leaflet billowing is diagnosed when there is systolic excursion of the leaflet body into the left atrium as a result of excess leaflet tissue, with the leaflet free edge remaining below the plane of the mitral annulus. **G,** Schematic demonstrating anterior mitral leaflet prolapse and posterior mitral leaflet flail due to chordal rupture. **H,** A two-dimensional transesophageal echocardiographic example of P2 flail segment. **I,** Corresponding three-dimensional transesophageal echocardiographic *en face* image as viewed from the left atrium. The *dashed black* and *solid red lines* in parts **A** to **H** represents the mitral annular plane.

of reperfusion, and these patients have significantly worse outcomes irrespective of the severity of MR.[24] The resultant volume overload caused by MR worsens myocardial contractility, which in turn worsens LV dysfunction, eventually leading to heart failure and death.[25-28]

MECHANISM OF ISCHEMIC MITRAL REGURGITATION

Classically, ischemic MR was thought to develop as a result of posteromedial papillary muscle dysfunction, given this muscle's dependence on a single blood supply. In the last decade, however, multiple studies have shown that papillary muscle dysfunction is not responsible for ischemic MR. In fact, a wide spectrum of geometric distortions secondary to LV remodeling result in this type of valve dysfunction.

As mentioned earlier, the mitral valve is dynamic and changes from a saddle shape (hyperbolic paraboloid) during systole to a flatter configuration during diastole. During systole, competing forces act on the mitral valve leaflets. Increased LV pressure acts to push the leaflets toward the left atrium while tethering forces

from the chordae act to pull the leaflets in the direction of the left ventricle. The saddle shape morphology is believed to balance these forces by optimizing leaflet curvature, and, thus, minimizing mitral leaflet stress.[2] In the setting of a myocardial infarction and resultant LV remodeling, an outward and apical displacement of the posteromedial papillary muscle occurs, which tethers the mitral valve leaflets into the left ventricle, restricting their ability to coapt effectively at the level of the mitral annulus.[29] Furthermore, the mitral annulus dilates, making leaflet coaptation even more difficult (Figures 2-7 and 2-8).[30]

Although the terms ischemic MR and functional MR have been used interchangeably, they have distinctly different meanings. Unlike ischemic MR, in which displacement of the posteromedial papillary muscle predominates, functional MR is a result of bilateral papillary muscle displacement (symmetric tethering) typically caused by dilated cardiomyopathy. The direction of the MR jet can help in differentiating the two types of valvular dysfunction. The ischemic MR jet is usually eccentric and directed toward the posterior "restricted" leaflet, whereas the functional MR jet is commonly directed centrally, toward the roof of the left atrium.

TABLE 2-2	Key Differences Between Barlow Disease and Fibroelastic Deficiency	
DIFFERENTIATING CHARACTERISTICS	BARLOW DISEASE	FIBROELASTIC DEFICIENCY
Pathology	Excess of myxomatous tissue	Impaired production of connective tissue
Typical age at diagnosis	Younger (<40 years)	Older (>60 years)
Duration of disease	Years to decades	Days to months
Physical findings	Midsystolic click and late systolic murmur	Holosystolic murmur
Leaflet involvement	Multisegmental	Unisegmental
Leaflet lesions	Leaflet billowing and thickening	Thin leaflets with a thickened involved segment
Chordae lesions	Chordal thickening and elongation	Chordal elongation and chordal rupture
Carpentier classification	Type II	Type II
Type of dysfunction	Bileaflet prolapse	Prolapse and/or flail
Complexity of valve repair	More complex	Less complex

3D echocardiography has provided further insights into the pathophysiology of both functional MR and ischemic MR (Figure 2-9). For example, several investigators using 3D echocardiography showed that increased sphericity of the left ventricle, rather than contractile dysfunction, contributes more significantly to bilateral papillary displacement and, in turn, functional MR.[31,32] A later study has shown that anteroapical myocardial infarctions that extend to the inferior apex can also cause ischemic MR.[33] This finding suggests that inferior myocardial infarctions are not solely responsible for ischemic MR but that this entity can develop even when the myocardium immediately underlying the posteromedial papillary muscle is not directly involved.

As 3D echocardiography technology continues to develop and dynamic visualization of the mitral valve continues to evolve, an increasing number of studies have focused on the quantitative analysis of the morpho-anatomy of ischemic MR. Currently, the three main areas of clinical research are mitral leaflet tethering, mitral annular geometric change, and compensatory leaflet growth.

MITRAL LEAFLET TETHERING IN ISCHEMIC MITRAL REGURGITATION. Mitral leaflet tethering is a major contributing factor to the development of ischemic MR. Two-dimensional (2D) echocardiography has been extensively used to calculate the mitral valve leaflet tenting area and leaflet tenting length; however, studies have shown that the asymmetry of these single-plane measurements is commonly inaccurate when compared

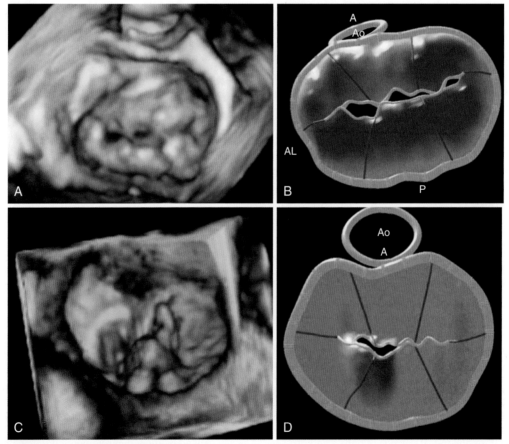

FIGURE 2-6 Barlow disease and fibroelastic deficiency. A, *En face* three-dimensional transesophageal echocardiographic image of a mitral valve as viewed from the left atrium, demonstrating bileaflet prolapse in a patient with Barlow disease. **B,** The corresponding parametric map, in which the color gradations towards orange indicate the distance of the leaflet from the mitral annular plane toward the left atrium. **C,** *En face* three-dimensional transesophageal echocardiographic image of a mitral valve as viewed from the left atrium, demonstrating a flail P2 segment due to fibroelastic deficiency. **D,** The corresponding parametric map demonstrates the abnormal P2 segment. *A,* anterior; *AL,* anterolateral; *Ao,* aortic valve; *P,* posterior.

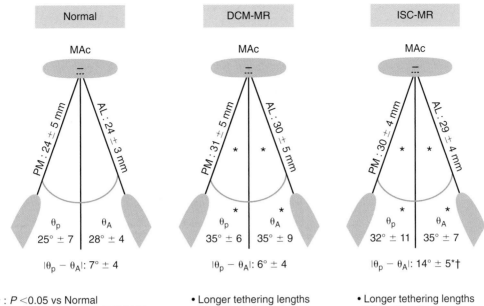

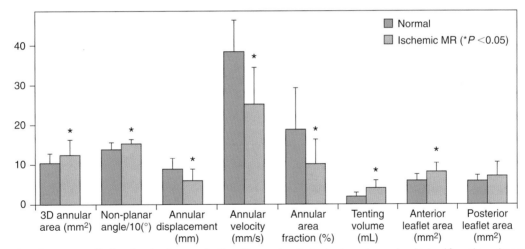

FIGURE 2-7 Papillary muscle orientation in secondary forms of mitral regurgitation. The papillary muscles in patients with mitral regurgitation (MR) secondary to dilated cardiomyopathy (DCM) or ischemia (ISC) are longer than those in patients with normal mitral valves. The increase in papillary muscle length is symmetric in patients with dilated cardiomyopathy, but in patients with ischemic mitral regurgitation, the increase in papillary muscle length is asymmetric with a greater increase in the posteromedial (PM) than the anterolateral (AL) papillary muscle. θP and θA are the angles between the left ventricular long-axis and the line connecting the mitral annular center (MAC) to the tip of the posteromedial and anterolateral papillary muscles respectively. *$P < 0.05$

FIGURE 2-8 Functional anatomy of ischemic mitral regurgitation. Changes in mitral valve dynamics can be obtained from three-dimensional transesophageal echocardiography data using specialized software. Compared with normal mitral valves, patients with ischemic mitral regurgitation have larger, flatter annuli with lower displacement, velocity, and pulsatility. Also, there is greater tenting volume owing mostly to increased anterior mitral leaflet area.

with intraoperative findings.[34] 3D echocardiography overcomes this limitation by providing more accurate and reproducible measurements (see Figure 2-9).

In studies examining leaflet tethering, patients with severe MR were shown to have significantly longer tenting lengths and larger volume than control patients.[7] Furthermore, the leaflet site where peak tenting occurred was different in each subject; this finding suggests that different chordae are involved in the disease process.

MITRAL VALVE ANNULUS IN ISCHEMIC MITRAL REGURGITATION. Conformational changes of the mitral valve annulus also contribute to the development of ischemic MR. Multiple studies have shown that the annulus dilates and flattens, becoming essentially adynamic throughout the cardiac cycle.[7,29] In addition, there are more subtle anatomic changes, such as greater dilation in the anteroposterior dimension and greater overall dilation and flattening in anterior than in inferior infarcts.[7,35] Studies of the dynamic changes in mitral valve annular surface area and

annular longitudinal displacement throughout the cardiac cycle have also demonstrated that the mitral annular surface area is larger and the annular pulsatility and displacement lower in patients with ischemic MR.[36] As the mitral annulus enlarges, it loses its motility, becoming progressively unable to modify its shape throughout the cardiac cycle (see Figure 2-8).

LEAFLET GROWTH IN ISCHEMIC MITRAL REGURGITATION. One of the most intriguing findings is that, although leaflet tethering and annular geometric changes drive the development of ischemic MR, leaflet growth occurs in an attempt to compensate for the decrease in leaflet coaptation.[37] In one of the earliest studies to examine this phenomenon, Chaput et al[38] found that leaflet area increased by 35% in patients with LV dysfunction. In fact, 2 months after a myocardial infarction, area and thickness were shown to be significantly larger in tethered leaflets than in nontethered leaflets.[39] Studies using molecular histopathology showed that this leaflet growth might be due to an increase in

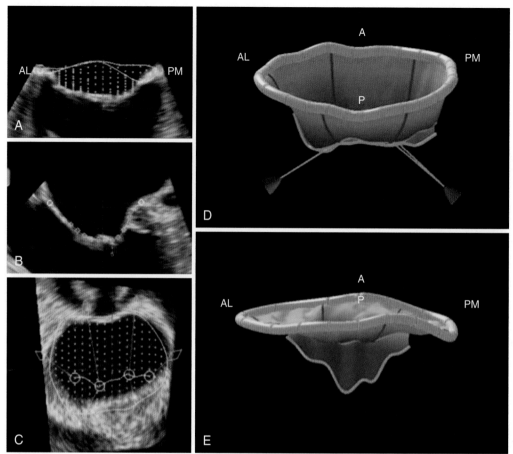

FIGURE 2-9 **Parametric models of ischemic mitral regurgitation and the normal mitral valve. A** to **C,** From a three-dimensional transesophageal echocardiography dataset, three-dimensional morphologic analysis of the mitral valve can be performed. First, the mitral annulus, leaflet shape, and papillary muscles are manually traced in multiple parallel planes. **D,** Then the results are interpolated to create a parametric model, which is a color-coded, three-dimensional, surface-rendered image of the mitral valve. This is an example of a parametric mitral valve model from a patient with ischemic cardiomyopathy, depicting a funnel-shaped deformity (loss of saddle shape), displacement of the coaptation zone, and increase in annulus-to-papillary muscle tethering length (*red structure* represents papillary muscle). **E,** For comparison, the parametric model of a normal mitral valve. *A,* Anterior; *AL,* anterolateral; *P,* posterior; *PM,* posteromedial.

alpha-smooth muscle actin in tethered leaflets, indicating endothelial-mesenchymal transdifferentiation.

A 2012 3D echocardiography study examined the interaction between leaflet tethering, annular dilation and flattening, and leaflet elongation.[40] The researchers measured multiple variables, including tenting length and volume, total leaflet area, total annular area, coaptation length, and area. They demonstrated that mitral leaflet coaptation decreases in proportion with the increased displacement of the papillary muscles, despite the presence of a compensatory increase in total leaflet area (see Figure 2-7). In addition, the ratio of total leaflet area to total annular area required to ensure proper coaptation in midsystole was lower in patients with severe MR than in patients with only mild MR. Indeed, coaptation area was the strongest determinant of MR severity. The question as to why sufficient leaflet growth develops in some patients but not in others remains unknown.[4]

TREATMENT OF ISCHEMIC MITRAL REGURGITATION

The most commonly used surgical technique for ameliorating ischemic MR is an undersized complete mitral valve annuloplasty ring. By reducing annular size, this procedure attempts to increase leaflet coaptation, and, therefore, decrease MR. Unfortunately, many patients undergoing ring annuloplasty for ischemic MR often have persistent or recurrent MR.[41,42] This is because, though the annuloplasty ring shifts the posterior annulus and leaflet anteriorly, the anterior annulus remains fixed at the aortic root, further exacerbating the apical tethering of the chordae.[43,44] Recurrence

of MR after ring annuloplasty is associated with continued LV remodeling and poor patient outcomes.[42]

Multiple studies using 3D echocardiography after mitral valve ring annuloplasty have shown that although this procedure reduces mitral annular size, it also reduces pulsatility and motion of the entire valve because of the inherent rigid structure of the ring.[36] Newer annuloplasty rings are therefore in production that better conform to the natural 3D dynamics of the mitral valve annulus.[45] As well, some surgeons use incomplete mitral annuloplasty rings. Quantification of the mitral valve annular height and intercommissural diameter by 3D echocardiography is helpful in assessing the suitability of different customized prosthesis and/or repair strategies aimed at restoring or maintaining the saddle-shape of the annulus. Despite this, annuloplasty rings, in general, do not address the tethering component and may not be completely sufficient in decreasing MR.

Mitral Stenosis

Although the prevalence of rheumatic mitral valve disease has significantly diminished in the United States, it is still a major cause of MS and MR worldwide.[46] Other causes of MS include congenital, inflammatory, infiltrative, and carcinoid heart diseases, but these are much less common. These diseases result in lesions such as commissure fusion, leaflet thickening, and chordae fusion, which lead to mitral valve leaflet restriction primarily during systole.[47] According to the Carpentier classification scheme of mitral valve dysfunction, this constitutes a type IIIA dysfunction.[11]

Percutaneous mitral valvuloplasty is the preferred treatment for selected patients with MS.[48] Appropriate indications for this type of treatment depend on accurate measurements of the mitral valve area (MVA), and successful outcomes depend on the detailed assessment of the valve morphology and the subvalvular apparatus. Echocardiography plays an important role by confirming the diagnosis, evaluating the mitral valve apparatus and its associated structures, and assessing the severity of MS.

3D echocardiography has many advantages over 2D echocardiography in examining the mitral valve anatomy.[49] The echocardiographic Wilkins score, which includes leaflet thickening, leaflet mobility, valve calcification, and involvement of the subvalvular apparatus, was developed in order to predict which patients would benefit most from balloon mitral valvotomy. With 3D echocardiography and its ability to visualize the mitral valve from both the left atrial and left ventricular perspectives, the morphologic assessment of the mitral valve becomes more accurate (Figure 2-10). The interobserver and intraobserver variability of the 3D echocardiography Wilkins score has been shown to be far superior to that of the 2D echocardiography assessment.[50]

There are several ways to quantitatively measure the severity of MS. Planimetry is the best method because it provides a direct method for measuring the mitral valve area independent of loading conditions and associated cardiac conditions.[51] The major limitation of 2D-derived planimetry in MS is that there is no assurance that the selected view used for planimetry is the smallest and most perpendicular (*en face*) view of the mitral valve orifice.

3D echocardiography overcomes this limitation by providing the narrowest orifice cross-section of the mitral valve funnel orifice, thereby achieving a much more accurate assessment of the mitral valve area (Figure 2-11). Multiple studies have shown the superiority of 3D echocardiography in the examination of patients with rheumatic MS.[50,52,53] The accuracy of 3D echocardiography planimetry has been proven to be superior to that of the invasive Gorlin method for measuring mitral valve area.[52] Also, 3D echocardiography planimetry provides a more accurate assessment of the mitral valve area before and after valvotomy than 2D echocardiography planimetry, 2D echocardiography pressure half-time, and the Gorlin method.[53]

Aortic Valve Anatomy

The aortic valve is a part of the aortic root complex, which is composed of the sinuses of Valsalva, the fibrous interleaflet triangles, and the valvular leaflets themselves.[54-56] The basal attachments of the aortic valve leaflets delineate the start of the aortic root from the left ventricle, while the sinotubular ridge separates the aortic root from the ascending aorta. Along the anterior margin of the aortic root lies the subpulmonary infundibulum and along the posterior margin, the orifice of the mitral valve and the muscular interventricular septum. Overall, approximately two thirds of the circumference of the lower part of the aortic root is connected to the septum and the remaining third is connected via a fibrous continuity known as the *aortic-mitral curtain* to the mitral valve (Figure 2-12).

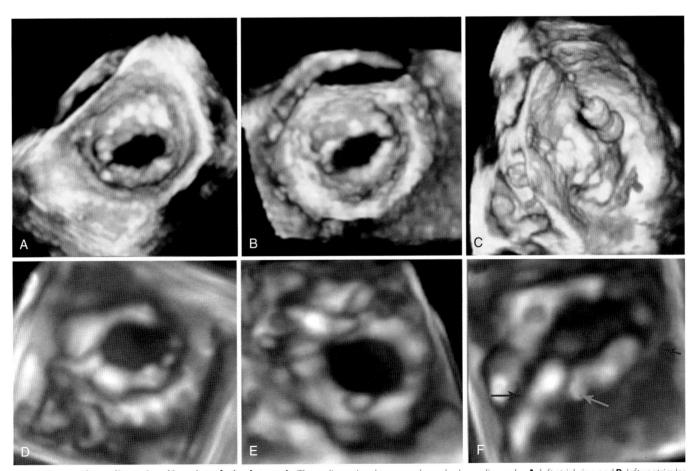

FIGURE 2-10   Three-dimensional imaging of mitral stenosis. Three-dimensional transesophageal echocardiography; **A,** left atrial view and **B,** left ventricular view of a stenotic mitral valve in diastole. **C,** three-dimensional echocardiography–guided balloon mitral valvotomy in the patient with mitral stenosis. Three-dimensional transesophageal echocardiographic zoomed postvalvotomy views of the mitral valve from the **D,** left atrial and **E,** left ventricular perspectives confirm splitting of the commissure. **F,** 3D transesophageal echocardiographic zoomed postvalvotomy view of the mitral valve from the left ventricular perspective demonstrating not only splitting of the commissures *(red arrows)* but also a leaflet tear *(green arrow)*.

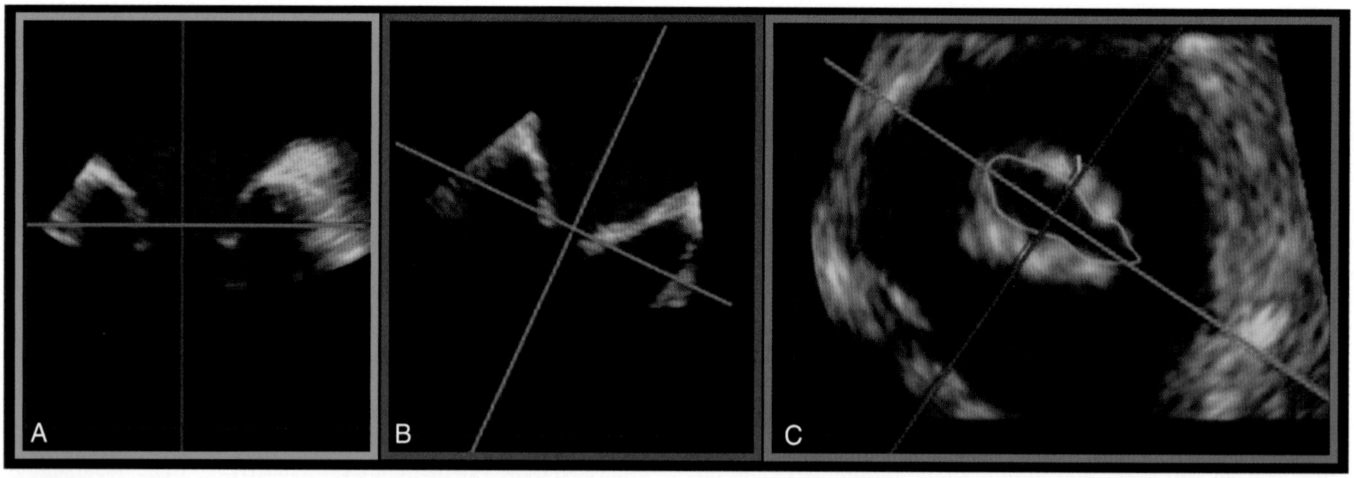

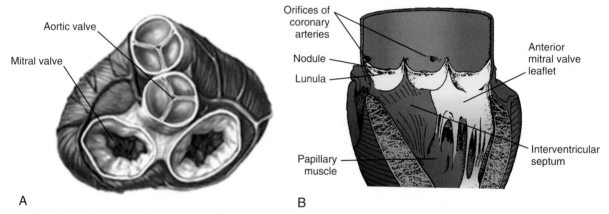

FIGURE 2-11   Mitral valve area in mitral stenosis. A and **B,** From a zoomed three-dimensional transesophageal echocardiography acquisition of the mitral valve, multiplanar analysis can be used to identify the largest mitral valve orifice area during diastole, which can then be directly traced *en face* to obtain the mitral annular area **(C)**. Each *colored line (red, blue, green)* represents a cut-plane through the 3D dataset.

FIGURE 2-12   Relation of the aortic valve to other cardiac structures. A, Superior view of the heart demonstrating the relationship of the aortic and mitral valves and the continuity of the fibrous aortic-mitral curtain. **B,** Open section of the left ventricular outflow tract, aortic valve, and aortic root, showing the relationship of the aortic valve leaflets with the anterior mitral valve leaflet and the septum.

The aortic valve is composed of three leaflets, which are attached in a semilunar fashion throughout the entire length of the aortic root with the highest point of attachment at the level of the sinotubular junction and the lowest in the ventricular myocardium below the anatomic ventriculoarterial junction. The free edge of each cusp curves up from the commissures and is slightly thickened at the tip or midpoint, which is also known as the *node of Arantius*. Each leaflet is identified by its relationship to the coronary arteries. Thus, the right and left coronary leaflets lie below the takeoffs of the right and left coronary arteries, respectively, whereas the noncoronary cusp is not associated with any coronary artery but is adjacent to the interatrial septum. Marked variability exists for all aspects of the leaflets, including height, width, and surface area. The aortic valve area (AVA) is the area between the leaflets during LV systole. It must be noted that the shape of the area between the leaflets during systole varies and may be stellate, circular, triangular, or an intermediate form of these variants.[57]

Beyond defining the start of the aortic root, the insertion sites of the aortic valve leaflets also define the sinuses of Valsalva and the aortic annulus. The sinuses of Valsalva are areas of expansion of the aortic root wall, with the inferior margin located at the leaflet insertion points and the superior margin at the sinotubular junction. Each sinus is separated from the others at its base by the interleaflet triangle.[58] Absence of any of these interleaflet triangles results in a loss of the coronet shape of the leaflet insertion

points and a more ringlike shape, which is associated with valvular stenosis.[58]

The definition of the aortic annulus with respect to the aortic valve leaflet insertion points is more complex as a result of leaflet attachment along the entire root. Because of this anatomy, the surgical definition of *aortic annulus* is a semilunar crownlike structure demarcated by the hinges of the aortic valve leaflets, whereas the imaging definition is the virtual or projected ring that connects the three most basal insertion points of the leaflets. It is now recognized that the aortic annulus, when defined as the virtual ring that connects the three most basal insertion points of the leaflets, is not circular but elliptical.[59] Normal reported adult aortic annular area measurements by planimetry using 3D echocardiography images is 4.0 ± 0.8 cm^2.[60] In comparison with 2D echocardiography measurements, these 3D measurements have been shown to have superior reproducibility, with the variability originating from suboptimal cut-plane selection.[61]

Aortic Valve Physiology

With normal function, the aortic leaflets move toward the sinuses of Valsalva during LV systole and coapt at the level of the aortic annulus during LV diastole to prevent regurgitation. While the aortic leaflets are open, they do not occlude the coronary artery orifices because the sinuses of Valsalva provide a space behind the open leaflets that separates the leaflets from the ostium.[56] The sinuses also form vortices during early systole, ensuring that when blood flows through the aortic root, at the level of the sinotubular junction, the sinotubular ridge directs some blood into the space between the leaflets and the wall of the sinuses.[62] These vortices play a role not only in preventing the leaflets from striking the aortic wall during valve opening but also in promoting valve closure. Owing to the importance of these eddy flows in the sinuses, the curvature of the sinuses of Valsalva is central to determining the distribution of stress on the valve leaflets.[63] Although blood flow contributes to the opening and closing of the aortic valve, the actual motion of the aortic leaflets does not completely parallel the blood flow pattern because the leaflets open prior to any forward blood flow into the aorta and close prior to cessation of forward blood flow.[57,64-67] Overall, 3D echocardiography is improving our knowledge of the interaction between the anatomy and physiology of the aortic root. This issue is important, given the increasing use of valve-sparing aortic root replacement techniques and the development of aortic valve repair techniques.[68-70]

The mitral and aortic valves are anatomically linked through a shared fibrous border called the aortic-mitral curtain, suggesting that the functions of the aortic and mitral valves are linked or coupled (Figure 2-13).[71] Indeed, studies of this valvular coupling in normal human hearts have demonstrated that the mitral annular area is minimal when the aortic projected area is maximal, and vice versa.[72] Thus, mitral annular contraction may facilitate aortic annular expansion, leading to improved blood flow through the aortic valve during LV ejection. Conversely, aortic annular contraction may facilitate mitral annular expansion, thereby improving blood flow through the mitral valve.

3D echocardiography quantification of this coupling has been used to examine not only how the mitral valve annulus changes after annuloplasty ring repair but also how this geometric alteration affects the annular function of the aortic valve.[73] It has been shown that after mitral valve repair, the aortic valve annulus has reduced pulsatility and motion throughout the cardiac cycle because of the rigid structure of the mitral annuloplasty ring. These changes in aortic valve geometry are likely due to the aortic-mitral curtain. When this coupling was studied in patients with isolated aortic stenosis (AS) undergoing surgical aortic valve replacement, it was found that this coupling remains abnormal after valve replacement, resulting in reduced mitral annular area. This phenomenon is also likely due to changes in the aortic-mitral curtain.[74] Clinically, this valvular coupling is observed by noting decreased MR severity following aortic valve replacement.[75,76]

Left Ventricular Outflow Tract

Like the aortic annulus, the LV outflow tract cross-section is not circular but elliptical.[20] The 2D echocardiographic parasternal

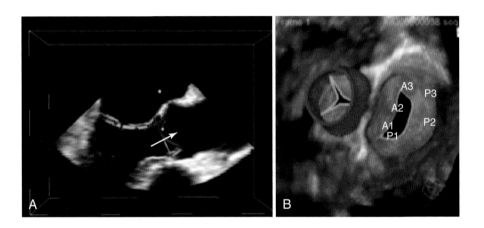

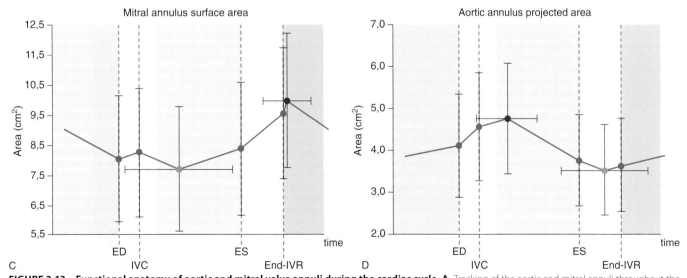

FIGURE 2-13 Functional anatomy of aortic and mitral valve annuli during the cardiac cycle. A, Tracking of the aortic and mitral annuli throughout the cardiac cycle using a three-dimensional transesophageal echocardiography data set. The *white arrow* represents blood flow through the aortic valve. **B,** When viewed from the left atrium, the fibrous continuity linking the aortic and mitral valves can be appreciated. *A1* to *A3,* Anterior leaflet segments; *P1* to *P3,* posterior leaflet segments. **C,** Graph showing that the mitral annular area is smallest during early systole and largest during early diastole. **D,** In contrast, the projected aortic annular area is largest in early systole and smallest in early diastole. *IVC,* isovolumic contraction; *IVR,* isovolumic relaxation; *ED,* end-diastole; *ES,* end-systole.

long-axis view of the aortic valve and root often underestimates the area of the LV outflow tract area because it presumes a circular shape. 3D echocardiography enables multiplane imaging of aortic valve (e.g., simultaneous displays of the valve in both long and short axis), demonstrating the true morphology of the LV outflow tract (Figure 2-14). As well, 3D echocardiography often confirms normal and abnormal findings when structures visualized in one plane can be examined in real time by checking a second orthogonal plane.

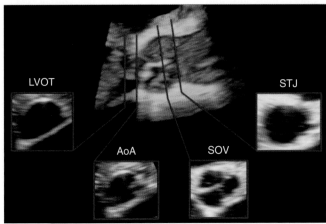

FIGURE 2-14   Three-dimensional imaging of the aortic valve. From a wide-angle, multi-beat transesophageal echocardiographic acquisition of the aortic root, with multiplanar analysis, exact *en face* images of the left ventricular outflow tract (LVOT), the aortic annulus (AoA), the sinus of Valsalva (SOV), and the sinotubular junction (STJ) can be obtained.

Three-Dimensional Assessment of the Aortic Valve

3D echocardiography has improved the anatomic assessment of the aortic valve. Through-plane motion of the aortic annulus throughout the cardiac cycle due to active longitudinal excursion of the LV base often hampers adequate visualization of the true aortic valve opening orifice and morphology throughout the cardiac cycle. With 3D echocardiography, irrespective of the actual spatial orientation of the aortic root, the true *en face* cut plane of the aortic annulus is contained within the 3D data set. Thus, with the use of multiplanar analysis, accurate measurements of the aortic annulus can be easily obtained from 3D datasets (Figure 2-15). Moreover, the 3D *en face* views allow comprehensive visualization of the entire aortic valve complex in motion. 3D echocardiography also provides additional information on the spatial relationship with surrounding structures, such as the LV outflow tract and mitral annulus.

With early-generation 3D TEE probes, adequate structural assessment of the aortic valve was possible in 81% of patients with mixed aortic valve pathology.[77] In comparison with 2D echocardiography, 3D echocardiography more accurately identifies abnormal aortic leaflet morphology, especially bicuspid and quadricuspid aortic valves.[78-82] As well, 3D echocardiography has been proven useful for the assessment of leaflet masses such as Lambl excrescences and aortic valve papillary fibroelastomas.[83-85]

3D echocardiography can accurately quantitate aortic root structures. The entire aortic root can be captured in a single 3D dataset, and, with the use of multiplanar analysis, accurate planimetry and dimensions of the aortic valve, the LV outflow tract, the sinuses of Valsalva, and the sinotubular junction can be

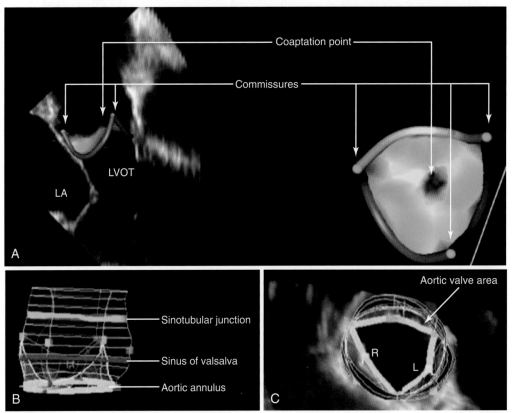

FIGURE 2-15   Three-dimensional functional anatomy of the aortic valve. A, Using specialized software and a data set from three-dimensional transesophageal echocardiography, the aortic valve complex can be tracked throughout the cardiac cycle. In the generated three-dimensional model, the leaflet commissures and coaptation point can be visualized. **B,** Also from the three-dimensional data set, a reconstructed aortic root model can be obtained from which areas at the sinotubular junction, sinus of Valsalva, and aortic annulus can be obtained throughout the cardiac cycle. **C,** *En face* view of the aortic valve area as visualized from the aorta. *L,* Left; *LA,* left atrium; *LVOT,* left ventricular outflow tract; *R,* right.

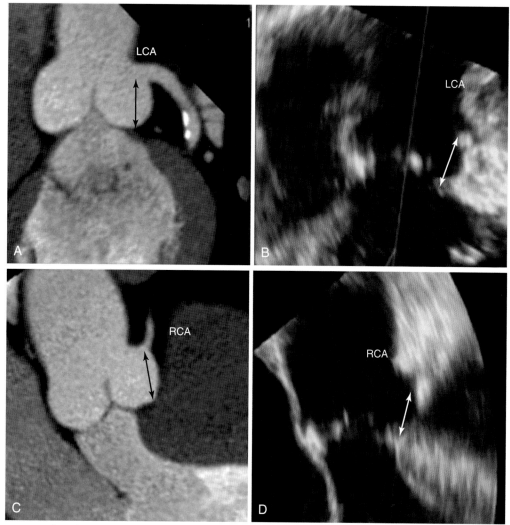

FIGURE 2-16   Assessment of aortic cusp anatomy. Images demonstrating measurement of the left coronary artery (LCA; *arrows*) obtained from **A,** multislice computed tomography with contrast and **B,** three-dimensional transesophageal echocardiography using wide-angle, multibeat acquisition. Images demonstrating measurement of the right coronary artery (RCA; *arrows*) obtained from **C,** multislice computed tomography with contrast and **D,** three-dimensional transesophageal echocardiography using wide-angle, multibeat acquisition. *(Modified from Otani K, Takeuchi M, Kaku K, et al. Assessment of the aortic root using real-time 3D transesophageal echocardiography. Circ J 2010;74:2649–2657.)*

obtained. The reason is that multiplanar analysis can be used on the 3D data sets to visualize any desired longitudinal or oblique plane. It allows exact parallel alignment of the cut plane to the structure in question, which is sometimes impossible to obtain in the 2D short-axis view and in a heart in a horizontal position or with aortic root pathology. In addition, multiplanar analysis allows assessment of supravalvular and subvalvular anatomy within the 3D volume to evaluate the presence of serial aortic outflow tract stenoses. Finally, variation in the aortic cusp dimensions and distance from the projected aortic annulus to the coronary artery ostia can be accurately measured from 3D data sets (Figure 2-16).[60] Accurate aortic annular dimensions and distances from the aortic annulus to the coronary ostium are important measurements to obtain before transcatheter aortic valve implantation to avoid complications such as improper valve sizing and obstruction of the coronary ostium.

Dynamic quantitation of aortic root structures using 3D echocardiography datasets is also possible. With available software, changes in the projected aortic annular area throughout the cardiac cycle have been evaluated, demonstrating that it is largest in the first third of systole and smallest during isovolumic relaxation.[72] Other measurements that can be obtained throughout the cardiac cycle from specialized software include true aortic annular area, sinus of Valsalva area, sinotubular area, leaflet

height, leaflet commissural distances, leaflet intercommissural distances, and leaflet coaptation length.

Like the concept of leaflet mobility in classifying MR, aortic cusp mobility forms the basis of a functional classification system for aortic regurgitation (AR). One of the first classifications of AR used to guide surgical repair was described in 1997.[86] However, this classification system was limited because it did not address AR secondary to aortic root pathology or aortic cusp perforation.[69] This classification was refined in 2005 to include assessment of the aortic root (Table 2-3).[87] With use of this classification system in one study, the needed repair techniques were properly predicted in the majority of patients with low rates of reoperation for recurrence of AR.[88] 3D echocardiography can improve the classification of AR through its ability to assess leaflet mobility as well as to quantify dynamic changes in cusp size and shape throughout the cardiac cycle.[60,72]

Conclusion

The growing scientific literature on 3D echocardiography and its increasing utilization in clinical practice is evidence of its rapid technologic development.[8] However, conventional 3D imaging of valves is still limited by its less than optimal frame rates and the significant time commitment required to acquire, manipulate,

TABLE 2-3	Functional Classification of Aortic Regurgitation and Repair Strategies	
TYPE OF AORTIC REGURGITATION	**MECHANISM OF AORTIC REGURGITATION**	**TYPE(S) OF AORTIC VALVE REPAIR**
1A	Dilated sinotubular junction Normal cusp mobility	Sinotubular junction remodeling, subcommissural annuloplasty
1B	Dilated sinuses of Valsalva Normal cusp mobility	Valve-sparing aortic root replacement
1C	Dilated ventriculoaortic junction Normal cusp mobility	Subcommissural annuloplasty, sinotubular junction annuloplasty
1D	Aortic cusp perforation Normal cusp mobility	Aortic cusp repair, autologous or bovine pericardium
II	Aortic cusp prolapse Excessive cusp mobility	Cusp prolapse repair with subcommissural annuloplasty; Focal prolapse: plication, triangular resection Generalized prolapse: free margin resuspension
III	Restricted cusp mobility Thickening, fibrosis, calcification	Cusp repair with subcommissural annuloplasty Shaving, decalcification, patch

interpret, and analyze its data sets. Further improvement in temporal and spatial resolution and feasibility of color Doppler imaging acquisition in a single cardiac cycle will facilitate the seamless integration of 3D echocardiography into the clinical workflow.

Additional technologic challenges include (1) the lack of automation of most analytical programs, (2) the inability to integrate quantitative software into the ultrasound equipment and clinical reporting systems, (3) the large storage requirements of 3D data-sets, and (4) the high cost of the equipment. As these issues are progressively addressed, it is likely that 3D transthoracic and transesophageal methods of echocardiography will become invaluable additions to the diagnosis and management of valvular heart disease and the overall field of cardiovascular imaging.

REFERENCES

1. Lang RM, Mor-Avi V, Sugeng L, et al. Three-dimensional echocardiography: the benefits of the additional dimension. J Am Coll Cardiol 2006;48:2053–69.
2. Salgo IS, Gorman JH, 3rd, Gorman RC, et al. Effect of annular shape on leaflet curvature in reducing mitral leaflet stress. Circulation 2002;106:711–7.
3. Berdajs D, Zund G, Camenisch C, et al. Annulus fibrosus of the mitral valve: reality or myth. J Cardiac Surg 2007;22:406–9.
4. Lang RM, Adams DH. 3D Echocardiographic quantification in functional mitral regurgitation. JACC Cardiovasc Imaging 2012;5:346–7.
5. Levine RA, Handschumacher MD, Sanfilippo AJ, et al. Three-dimensional echocardiographic reconstruction of the mitral valve, with implications for the diagnosis of mitral valve prolapse. Circulation 1989;80:589–98.
6. Adams DH, Anyanwu AC, Sugeng L, et al. Degenerative mitral valve regurgitation: surgical reconstruction. Curr Cardiol Rep 2008;10:226–32.
7. Watanabe N, Ogasawara Y, Yamaura Y, et al. Mitral annulus flattens in ischemic mitral regurgitation: geometric differences between inferior and anterior myocardial infarction: a real-time 3-dimensional echocardiographic study. Circulation 2005;112 (Suppl I):I458–I462.
8. Lang RM, Mor-Avi V, Dent JM, et al. Three-dimensional echocardiography: is it ready for everyday clinical use? JACC Cardiovasc Imaging 2009;2:114–7.
9. Gorman JH, 3rd, Gupta KB, Streicher JT, et al. Dynamic three-dimensional imaging of the mitral valve and left ventricle by rapid sonomicrometry array localization. J Thorac Cardiovasc Surg 1996;112:712–26.
10. O'Gara P, Sugeng L, Lang R, et al. The role of imaging in chronic degenerative mitral regurgitation. JACC Cardiovasc Imaging. 2008;1:221–37.
11. Carpentier A. Cardiac valve surgery—the "French correction." J Thorac Cardiovasc Surg 1983;86323–337.
12. Kumar N, Kumar M, Duran CM. A revised terminology for recording surgical findings of the mitral valve. J Heart Valve Dis 1995;4:70–5; discussion 76–7.
13. Shah P. Intraoperative echocardiography for mitral valve disease. In: Otto CM, Bonow RO, editors. Valvular Heart Disease. 3rd ed. Philadelphia: Saunders Elsevier; 2009. p. 322–33.
14. Muresian H. The clinical anatomy of the mitral valve. Clin Anat 2009;22:85–98.
15. Yamauchi T, Taniguchi K, Kuki S, et al. Evaluation of the mitral valve leaflet morphology after mitral valve reconstruction with a concept "coaptation length index." J Cardiac Surg 2004;19:535–8.
16. Timek TA, Nielsen SL, Green GR, et al. Influence of anterior mitral leaflet second-order chordae on leaflet dynamics and valve competence. Ann Thorac Surg 2001;72:535–40; discussion 541.
17. Messas E, Bel A, Szymanski C, et al. Relief of mitral leaflet tethering following chronic myocardial infarction by chordal cutting diminishes left ventricular remodeling. Circ Cardiovasc Imaging 2010;3:679–86.
18. Rodriguez F, Langer F, Harrington KB, et al. Effect of cutting second-order chordae on in-vivo anterior mitral leaflet compound curvature. J Heart Valve Dis 2005;14:592–601; discussion 601–2.
19. Rodriguez F, Langer F, Harrington KB, et al. Importance of mitral valve second-order chordae for left ventricular geometry, wall thickening mechanics, and global systolic function. Circulation 2004;110(Suppl II):II115–II122.
20. Dreyfus GD, Bahrami T, Alayle N, et al. Repair of anterior leaflet prolapse by papillary muscle repositioning: a new surgical option. Ann Thorac Surg 2001;71:1464–70.
21. Carpentier A, Adams DH, Filsoufi S. Pathophysiology, preoperative valve analysis, and surgical indications. In: Carpentier A, Adams DH, Filsoufi S, editors. Carpentier's Reconstructive Valve Surgery. Maryland, Heights, Missouri: Saunders-Elsevier; 2012. p. 43–53.
22. Griffin BP. Myxomatous mitral valve disease. In: Otto CM, Bonow RO, editors. Valvular Heart Disease. 3rd ed. Philadelphia: Saunders Elsevier; 2009. p. 243–59.
23. Anyanwu AC, Adams DH. Etiologic classification of degenerative mitral valve disease: Barlow's disease and fibroelastic deficiency. Sem Thorac Cardiovasc Surg 2007;19:90–6.
24. Beeri R, Otsuji Y, Schwammenthal E, et al. Ischemic mitral regurgitation. In: Ottto CM, Bonow RO, editors. Valvular heart disease. 3rd ed. Philadelphia: Saunders Elsevier; 2009. p. 260–73.
25. Lamas GA, Mitchell GF, Flaker GC, et al. Clinical significance of mitral regurgitation after acute myocardial infarction. Survival and Ventricular Enlargement Investigators. Circulation 1997;96:827–33.
26. Bursi F, Enriquez-Sarano M, Nkomo VT, et al. Heart failure and death after myocardial infarction in the community: the emerging role of mitral regurgitation. Circulation 2005;111:295–301.
27. Grigioni F, Detaint D, Avierinos JF, et al. Contribution of ischemic mitral regurgitation to congestive heart failure after myocardial infarction. J Am Coll Cardiol 2005;45:260–7.
28. Grigioni F, Enriquez-Sarano M, Zehr KJ, et al. Ischemic mitral regurgitation: long-term outcome and prognostic implications with quantitative Doppler assessment. Circulation 2001;103:1759–64.
29. Otsuji Y, Levine RA, Takeuchi M, et al. Mechanism of ischemic mitral regurgitation. J Cardiol 2008;51:145–56.
30. Grewal J, Suri R, Mankad S, et al. Mitral annular dynamics in myxomatous valve disease: new insights with real-time 3-dimensional echocardiography. Circulation 2010;121: 1423–31.
31. Dent JM, Spotnitz WD, Nolan SP, et al. Mechanism of mitral leaflet excursion. Am J Physiol 1995;269(suppl):H2100–2108.
32. Otsuji Y, Handschumacher MD, Schwammenthal E, et al. Insights from three-dimensional echocardiography into the mechanism of functional mitral regurgitation: direct in vivo demonstration of altered leaflet tethering geometry. Circulation 1997;96:1999–2008.
33. Yosefy C, Beeri R, Guerrero JL, et al. Mitral regurgitation after anteroapical infarction: new mechanistic insights. Circulation, 2011;123:1529–36.
34. Daimon M, Shiota T, Gillinov AM, et al. Percutaneous mitral valve repair for chronic ischemic mitral regurgitation: a real-time three-dimensional echocardiographic study in an ovine model. Circulation 2005;111:2183–9.
35. Vergnat M, Jassar AS, Jackson BM, et al. Ischemic mitral regurgitation: a quantitative three-dimensional echocardiographic analysis. Ann Thorac Surg 2011;91:157–64.
36. Veronesi F, Corsi C, Sugeng L, et al. Quantification of mitral apparatus dynamics in functional and ischemic mitral regurgitation using real-time 3-dimensional echocardiography. J Am Soc Echocardiogr 2008;21:347–54.
37. Lang RM, Tsang W, Weinert L, et al. Valvular heart disease: the value of 3-dimensional echocardiography. J Am Coll Cardiol 2011;58:1933–44.
38. Chaput M, Handschumacher MD, Tournoux F, et al. Mitral leaflet adaptation to ventricular remodeling: occurrence and adequacy in patients with functional mitral regurgitation. Circulation 2008;118:845–52.
39. Dal-Bianco JP, Aikawa E, Bischoff J, et al. Active adaptation of the tethered mitral valve: insights into a compensatory mechanism for functional mitral regurgitation. Circulation 2009;120:334–42.
40. Saito K, Okura H, Watanabe N, et al. Influence of chronic tethering of the mitral valve on mitral leaflet size and coaptation in functional mitral regurgitation. JACC Cardiovasc Imaging 2012;5:337–45.
41. Liel-Cohen N, Otsuji Y, Vlahakes GJ et al. Functional ischemic mitral regurgitation can persist despite annular ring annuloplasty: mechanistic insights (abstract). Circulation 1997;96:I–540.
42. Hung J, Handschumacher MD, Rudski L, et al. Persistence of ischemic mitral regurgitation despite annular ring reduction: mechanistic insights from 3D echocardiography (abstract). Circulation 1999;100:I–73.

43. Kuwahara E, Otsuji Y, Iguro Y, et al. Mechanism of recurrent/persistent ischemic/functional mitral regurgitation in the chronic phase after surgical annuloplasty: importance of augmented posterior leaflet tethering. Circulation 2006;114(suppl I): I529–I534.

44. Green GR, Dagum P, Glasson JR, et al. Restricted posterior leaflet motion after mitral ring annuloplasty. Ann Thorac Surg 1999;68:2100–6.

45. Jensen MO, Jensen H, Levine RA, et al. Saddle-shaped mitral valve annuloplasty rings improve leaflet coaptation geometry. J Thorac Cardiovasc Surg 2011;142:697–703.

46. Steer AC, Carapetis JR. Prevention and treatment of rheumatic heart disease in the developing world. Nature Rev Cardiol 2009;6:689–98.

47. Iung B, Vahanian A. Rheumatic mitral valve disease. In: Otto CM, Bonow RO, editors. Valvular heart disease. 3rd ed. Philadelphia: Saunders Elsevier; 2009. p. 221–42.

48. Bonow RO, Carabello BA, Kanu C, et al. ACC/AHA 2006 guidelines for the management of patients with valvular heart disease: a report of the American College of Cardiology/American Heart Association Task Force on Practice Guidelines (writing committee to revise the 1998 Guidelines for the Management of Patients With Valvular Heart Disease). Developed in collaboration with the Society of Cardiovascular Anesthesiologists. Endorsed by the Society for Cardiovascular Angiography and Interventions and the Society of Thoracic Surgeons. Circulation 2006;114:e84–231.

49. Mannaerts HF, Kamp O, Visser CA. Should mitral valve area assessment in patients with mitral stenosis be based on anatomical or on functional evaluation? A plea for 3D echocardiography as the new clinical standard. Eur Heart J 2004;25:2073–174.

50. Zamorano J, Cordeiro P, Sugeng L, et al. Real-time three-dimensional echocardiography for rheumatic mitral valve stenosis evaluation: an accurate and novel approach. J Am Coll Cardiol 2004;43:2091–6.

51. Baumgartner H, Hung J, Bermejo J, et al. Echocardiographic assessment of valve stenosis: EAE/ASE recommendations for clinical practice. J Am Soc Echocardiogr 2009; 22:1–23.

52. Perez de Isla L, Casanova C, Almeria C, et al. Which method should be the reference method to evaluate the severity of rheumatic mitral stenosis? Gorlin's method versus 3D-echo. Eur J Echocardiogr 2007;8:470–3.

53. Zamorano J, Perez de Isla L, Sugeng L, et al. Non-invasive assessment of mitral valve area during percutaneous balloon mitral valvuloplasty: role of real-time 3D echocardiography. Eur Heart J 2004;25:2086–91.

54. Piazza N, de Jaegere P, Schultz C, et al. Anatomy of the aortic valvar complex and its implications for transcatheter implantation of the aortic valve. Circ Cardiovasc Interv 2008;1:74–81.

55. Anderson RH. Clinical anatomy of the aortic root. Heart 2000;84:670–3.

56. Underwood MJ, El Khoury G, Deronck D, et al. The aortic root: structure, function, and surgical reconstruction. Heart. 2000;83:376–40.

57. Handke M, Heinrichs G, Beyersdorf F, et al. In vivo analysis of aortic valve dynamics by transesophageal 3-dimensional echocardiography with high temporal resolution. J Thorac Cardiovasc Surg 2003;125:1412–9.

58. Sutton JP, 3rd, Ho SY, Anderson RH. The forgotten interleaflet triangles: a review of the surgical anatomy of the aortic valve. Ann Thorac Surg 1995;59:419–27.

59. Messika-Zeitoun D, Serfaty JM, Brochet E, et al. Multimodal assessment of the aortic annulus diameter: implications for transcatheter aortic valve implantation. J Am Coll Cardiol 2010;55:186–94.

60. Otani K, Takeuchi M, Kaku K, et al. Assessment of the aortic root using real-time 3D transesophageal echocardiography. Circ J 2010;74:2649–57.

61. Kasprzak JD, Nosir YF, Dall'Agata A, et al. Quantification of the aortic valve area in three-dimensional echocardiographic data sets: analysis of orifice overestimation resulting from suboptimal cut-plane selection. Am Heart J 1998;135:995–1003.

62. Thubrikar M, Nolan SP, Bosher LP, et al. The cyclic changes and structure of the base of the aortic valve. Am Heart J 1980;99:217–24.

63. Thubrikar MJ, Nolan SP, Aouad J, et al. Stress sharing between the sinus and leaflets of canine aortic valve. Ann Thorac Surg 1986;42:434–40.

64. Thubrikar M, Bosher LP, Nolan SP. The mechanism of opening of the aortic valve. J Thorac Cardiovasc Surg 1979;77:863–70.

65. Van Steenhoven AA, Verlaan CW, Veenstra PC, et al. In vivo cinematographic analysis of behavior of the aortic valve. Am J Physiol 1981;240:H286–92.

66. Higashidate M, Tamiya K, Beppu T, et al. Regulation of the aortic valve opening. In vivo dynamic measurement of aortic valve orifice area. J Thorac Cardiovasc Surg 1995;110: 496–503.

67. Handke M, Jahnke C, Heinrichs G, et al. New three-dimensional echocardiographic system using digital radiofrequency data–visualization and quantitative analysis of aortic valve dynamics with high resolution: methods, feasibility, and initial clinical experience. Circulation 2003;107:2876–9.

68. Urbanski PP, Zhan X, Hijazi H, et al. Valve-sparing aortic root repair without down-sizing of the annulus. J Thorac Cardiovasc Surg 2012;143:294–302.

69. Augoustides JG, Szeto WY, Bavaria JE. Advances in aortic valve repair: focus on functional approach, clinical outcomes, and central role of echocardiography. J Cardiothor Vasc An 2010;24:1016–20.

70. Aicher D, Fries R, Rodionycheva S, et al. Aortic valve repair leads to a low incidence of valve-related complications. Eur J Cardiothorac Surg 2010;37:127–32.

71. Lansac E, Lim KH, Shomura Y, et al. Dynamic balance of the aortomitral junction. J Thorac Cardiovasc Surg 2002;123:911–8.

72. Veronesi F, Corsi C, Sugeng L, et al. A study of functional anatomy of aortic-mitral valve coupling using 3D matrix transesophageal echocardiography. Circ Cardiovasc Imaging 2009;2:24–31.

73. Veronesi F, Caiani EG, Sugeng L, et al. Effect of mitral valve repair on mitral-aortic coupling: a real-time three-dimensional transesophageal echocardiography study. J Am Soc Echocardiogr 2012;25:54–531.

74. Tsang W. Changes in aortic-mitral coupling in severe aortic stenosis (abstract). J Am Coll Cardiol 2011;57:2057.

75. Vanden Eynden F, Bouchard D, El-Hamamsy I, et al. Effect of aortic valve replacement for aortic stenosis on severity of mitral regurgitation. Ann Thorac Surg 2007;83: 1279–84.

76. Ruel M, Kapila V, Price J, et al. Natural history and predictors of outcome in patients with concomitant functional mitral regurgitation at the time of aortic valve replacement. Circulation 2006;114(Suppl I):I541–I546.

77. Kasprzak JD, Salustri A, Roelandt JR, et al. Three-dimensional echocardiography of the aortic valve: feasibility, clinical potential, and limitations. Echocardiogr 1998;15:127–38.

78. Armen TA, Vandse R, Bickle K, et al. Three-dimensional echocardiographic evaluation of an incidental quadricuspid aortic valve. Eur J Echocardiogr 2008;9:318–20.

79. Burri MV, Nanda NC, Singh A, et al. Live/real time three-dimensional transthoracic echocardiographic identification of quadricuspid aortic valve. Echocardiogr 2007;24: 653–5.

80. Singh P, Dutta R, Nanda NC. Live/real time three-dimensional transthoracic echocardiographic assessment of bicuspid aortic valve morphology. Echocardiography 2009;26: 478–80.

81. Unsworth B, Malik I, Mikhail GW. Recognising bicuspid aortic stenosis in patients referred for transcatheter aortic valve implantation: routine screening with three-dimensional transoesophageal echocardiography. Heart 2010;96:645.

82. Xiao Z, Meng W, Zhang E. Quadricuspid aortic valve by using intraoperative transesophageal echocardiography. Cardiovasc Ultrasoun 2010;8:36.

83. Dichtl W, Muller LC, Pachinger O, et al. Images in cardiovascular medicine. Improved preoperative assessment of papillary fibroelastoma by dynamic three-dimensional echocardiography. Circulation 2002;106:1300.

84. Kelpis TG, Ninios VN, Economopoulos VA, et al. Aortic valve papillary fibroelastoma: a three-dimensional transesophageal echocardiographic appearance. Ann Thorac Surg 2010;89:2043.

85. Samal AK, Nanda N, Thakur AC, et al. Three-dimensional echocardiographic assessment of Lambl's excrescences on the aortic valve. Echocardiogr 1999;16:437–41.

86. Haydar HS, He GW, Hovaguimian H, et al. Valve repair for aortic insufficiency: surgical classification and techniques. Eur J Cardiothorac Surg 1997;11:258–65.

87. El Khoury G, Glineur D, Rubay J, et al. Functional classification of aortic root/valve abnormalities and their correlation with etiologies and surgical procedures. Curr Opin Cardiol 2005;20:115–21.

88. Boodhwani M, de Kerchove L, Glineur D, et al. Repair-oriented classification of aortic insufficiency: impact on surgical techniques and clinical outcomes. J Thorac Cardiovasc Surg 2009;137:286–94.

CH 2

THREE-DIMENSIONAL ANATOMY OF THE AORTIC AND MITRAL VALVES

CHAPTER 3

Cellular and Molecular Basis of Calcific Aortic Valve Disease

Jordan D. Miller

Key Points

- Initiation and progression of fibrocalcific aortic valve disease is an active process.
- Calcification in stenotic valves is often associated with increases in osteogenic signaling and the presence of osteoblast-like and osteoclast-like cells, but can also occur in the absence of bone-related cells.
- Fibrosis in stenotic valves is associated with increases in transforming growth factor-β signaling and matrix remodeling protein activity.
- There is a complex interplay between aortic valve interstitial cell biology and matrix stiffness and remodeling.
- Insights from genetically altered mouse models suggests that initiation and progression of fibrocalcific valve disease constitute a complex process that will likely require targeting of multiple pathways to slow progression of disease.

General Concepts and Histologic Changes

General Concepts

Fibrocalcific aortic valve disease was once thought to be a degenerative disease characterized by the passive accumulation of calcium in the valve cusp. Landmark studies over the past decade, however, demonstrated that osteoblast and osteoclast markers are frequently on cells in valves from patients with this disease, and subsets of patients have evidence of bone matrix in the calcified regions of the valve.[1] Collectively, these observations suggest that aortic valve calcification and expansion of calcified deposits constitute an active process similar to that observed in bone. The ensuing sections focus on cellular and molecular mechanisms regulating the formation and activity of osteoblast-like cells in the calcifying aortic valve and propose potential therapeutic strategies to slow or reverse progression of calcific valve disease.

Key Histologic Changes During Initiation and Progression of Valve Disease

The normal aortic valve comprises three layers: the fibrosa, spongiosa, and ventricularis.[2] Importantly, each layer contains valvular interstitial cells, which play a critical role in the production, maintenance, and repair of each layer (Figure 3-1).[3] Both the aortic and ventricular sides of the valve are covered by an endothelial monolayer (Table 3-1).

Disruption of the aortic valve endothelium is thought to be one of the earliest histopathologic changes contributing to the initiation of fibrocalcific aortic valve disease in humans and experimental animals (see Figure 3-1).[4] This is typically accompanied by infiltration of T lymphocytes and macrophages.[4-7] The subsequent elaboration of profibrotic and inflammatory cytokines elicits increased extracellular matrix production and turnover, finally resulting in stiffening and fibrosis of the extracellular matrix in the early valve lesions.[8] Early valve lesions may also exhibit lipid accumulation of extracellular lipid, which is ultimately taken up by macrophages to become foam cells. Calcium deposition is commonly observed in early stages of fibrocalcific aortic valve disease and frequently co-localizes with areas showing inflammatory cell infiltration.[4,7]

During advanced stages of fibrocalcific valve disease there is massive accumulation of lipid and inflammatory cell infiltrate, as well as increased production of a disorganized, stiffened extracellular matrix and fragmented elastic lamina.[4,5,8] Extensive cusp calcification, however, is the hallmark histopathologic change associated with hemodynamically significant aortic valve stenosis.[4] As discussed in more detail later, accumulation of calcium can appear either amorphous (i.e., no clear organization/bone structure) or osteogenic (i.e., evidence of endochondral ossification, bone matrix, and hematopoietic marrow compartments).[1,4,5,9]

Risk Factors Converge on a Pathogenic Response to Chronic Injury

Risk factors for development of aortic valve disease are remarkably similar to those for atherosclerosis, and include increasing age, hypercholesterolemia, hypertension, smoking, and diabetes.[10,11] (See Figure 3-2 and Chapter 4.) The observation that the phenotypic penetrance of any one risk factor is highly variable suggests that there is a complex interplay between the environment and the genome (i.e., genetic propensity to mount an excessive response to injury) (Table 3-2). In the context of fibrocalcific aortic valve stenosis, this pathophysiologic response results in massive accumulation of calcium in the valve cusp.

The concept that osteogenic processes are a key pathogenic response to injury in fibrocalcific valve disease is supported by the following three key lines of evidence: (1) the observation that there can be bone matrix in aortic valves excised from humans with aortic stenosis, (2) reports that humans and experimental

TABLE 3-1   Classification of Aortic Valve Cell Origins and Phenotypes

CELL TYPE	ORIGIN	FUNCTION
Endothelium	Endothelial endocardial cushion	Paracrine regulation of VIC function Maintenance of VIC population through ECM
	Circulating endothelial progenitors	Repair in response to injury Maintenance of VIC population through ECM
Quiescent, resident interstitial cells	Endothelial endocardial cushion (via ECM) or neural crest	Maintenance of valve structure/connective tissue production Secretion of antiangiogenic factors Potential osteogenic precursor
Interstitial cells of extravalvular origin	Bone marrow/circulating progenitor cells	Repair in response to injury Potential osteogenic precursor
Activated interstitial cells (α-SMA⁺)	Resident or circulating ICs	Repair in response to injury (migration, proliferation) Angiogenic factor secretion with cusp thickening Robust ECM production/matrix remodeling enzyme expression Potential osteogenic precursor

ECM, Extracellular matrix; *IC,* immune complex; *SMA,* smooth muscle actin; *VIC,* valve interstitial cell.

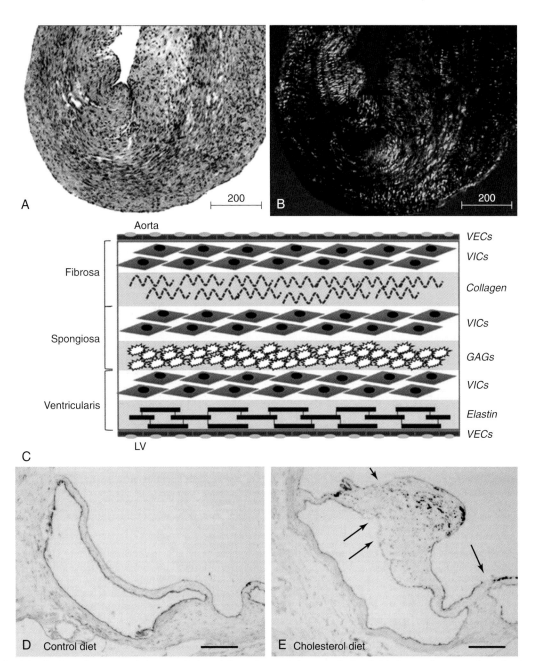

FIGURE 3-1   Key histologic and structural characteristics of the valve and changes during initiation and progression of valve disease. Movat's pentachrome staining **(A)** and polarized light **(B)** imaging of a normal porcine aortic valve cusp depicting the trilayered structure of the aortic valve. Note that the matricellular composition varies throughout the valve. In **A,** *black* indicates nuclei and elastic fibers, *yellow* collagen, *blue* mucin, *bright red* fibrin, and *dark red* muscle. **C,** Schematic depicting the different layers of the aortic valve cusp (layering/orientation is the same as in **A** and **B**). **D** and **E,** Micrographs depicting disruption of the aortic valve endothelium *(arrows)* in mice fed a western-type diet for 16 weeks (immunohistochemical staining using anti–endothelial nitric oxide synthase antibody). *Continued*

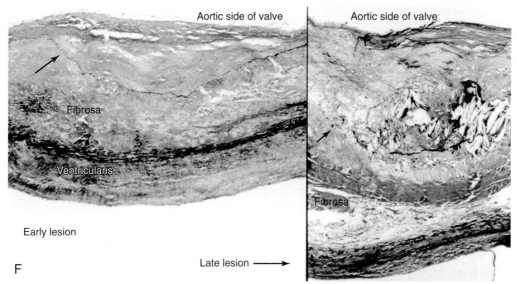

FIGURE 3-1, cont'd. **F,** Micrographs depicting cusp thickening in early stages of fibrocalcific aortic valve disease *(left)* and a massive calcific deposit in an aortic valve cusp during later stages of fibrocalcific aortic valve disease *(right)*. Note that calcification and matrix disruption predominantly affect the aortic side of the valve. *GAGs,* Glycosaminoglycans; *LV,* left ventricle; *VECs,* vascular endothelial cells; *VICs,* valve interstitial cells. (*A* and *B* from Simionescu DT, Chen J, Jaeggli M, et al. *Form follows function: advances in trilayered structure replication for aortic heart valve tissue engineering. J Healthc Eng 2012;3:179–202; **C** from Leopold JA. Cellular mechanisms of aortic valve calcification. Circ Cardiovasc Interv 2012;5:605–14; **D** and **E** from Matsumoto Y, Adams V, Jacob S, et al. Regular exercise training prevents aortic valve disease in low-density lipoprotein-receptor-deficient mice. Circulation 2010;121:759–67; **F** from Freeman RV, Otto CM. Spectrum of calcific aortic valve disease: pathogenesis, disease progression, and treatment strategies. Circulation 2005;111:3316–26.)*

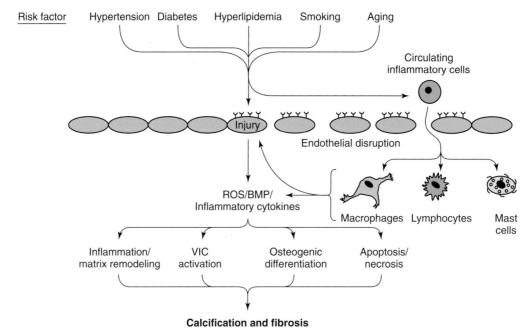

FIGURE 3-2 Schematic working model of the interplay between risk factors for fibrocalcific aortic valve disease and the dysfunctional "response to injury" that can increase propensity for development of valvular stenosis. Note that both valvular calcification and fibrosis are likely to play major roles in the development of hemodynamically significant aortic valve dysfunction. *BMP,* Bone morphogenic protein; *ROS,* reactive oxygen species; *VIC,* valvular interstitial cell. *(Modified from Miller JD, Weiss RM, Heistad DD. Calcific aortic valve stenosis: methods, models, and mechanisms. Circ Res 2011;108:1392–412.)*

animals with fibrocalcific aortic valve disease have robust induction of multiple osteogenic signaling cascades, and (3) reports that aortic valve interstitial cells have the capacity to redifferentiate into osteoblast-like cells in vitro.

Clinical Observations in Humans

In 2001, Mohler et al[1] reported that approximately 20% of aortic valves from humans with severe aortic stenosis had evidence of bone matrix at the time of valve surgery. Histologically, the bone matrix was associated with the presence of cells that

resembled osteoblasts and osteoclasts (Figure 3-3). These findings were particularly remarkable given the fact that aortic valve calcification was typically viewed as a passive, degenerative process by clinicians and scientists alike, and they represented a paradigm shift in the field of fibrocalcific aortic valve disease.

More recently, the role of fibrosis and matrix remodeling in the pathogenesis of aortic valve calcification and dysfunction has received a substantial amount of attention. Massive valvular calcification is nearly ubiquitously associated with increases in extracellular matrix accumulation and turnover.[12-14] While this was once thought to be an epiphenomenon, an emerging body of

TABLE 3-2	Risk Factors for Development of Fibrocalcific Aortic Valve Disease and Their Potential Molecular Mediators
RISK FACTOR	**POTENTIAL MOLECULAR MEDIATORS**
Hypertension	Angiotensin II
	Force/shear-initiated signaling pathways
	Reactive oxygen species
Diabetes	Hyperglycemia
	Receptor for advanced glycation end products (RAGE) activation
	Angiotensin II
	Reactive oxygen species
Hyperlipidemia	Low-density lipoprotein
	Lipoprotein-related receptor protein 5/6 activation
	Local angiotensin II generation
	Reactive oxygen species
Smoking	Reactive oxygen species
Aging	Epigenetics
	Reactive oxygen species

experimental data suggests that changes in the extracellular matrix of the valve may not only be a major modulator of valve interstitial cell function, but may also be sufficient to impair valvular dysfunction in advanced fibrocalcific aortic valve disease.

Experimental Models

Although description of cellular and molecular changes in human tissue is a critical component in research, empirical testing in animal models is an essential step in discerning whether a change is a pathophysiologic driver of fibrocalcific aortic valve disease or merely an epiphenomenon (Figure 3-4). When one is evaluating experimental data or deciding which model is useful for a particular study design, several important questions must be asked (Table 3-3):

- Does the model require genetically altered animals, and do the mutations relate to the specific question at hand?
- What is the underlying stimulus driving calcification (e.g., hyperlipidemia, hypertension)?
- Are the histopathologic changes relevant to human disease (e.g., fibrosis and calcification)?
- Do the animals develop hemodynamically significant aortic valve dysfunction and stenosis, or only aortic valve sclerosis?

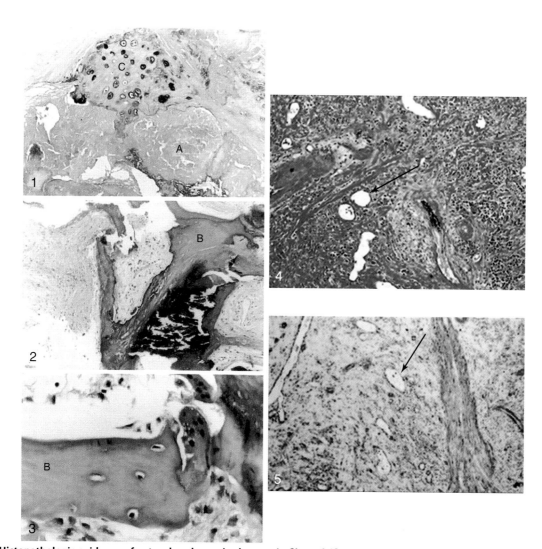

FIGURE 3-3 **Histopathologic evidence of osteochondrogenic changes in fibrocalcific aortic valve disease. Panel 1** shows atheromatous *(A)* and chondrocyte-like *(C)* changes. In contrast, **2** and **3** depict mature bone-like structures *(B)*. **4** and **5** depict massive valvular collagen accumulation/fibrosis (Masson's trichrome stain) and α-smooth muscle actin (immunohistochemistry) as well as areas of neovascularization *(arrows)*. *(Modified from Mohler 3rd ER, Gannon F, Reynolds C, et al. Bone formation and inflammation in cardiac valves. Circulation 2001;103:1522–8; and Rajamannan NM, Nealis TB, Subramaniam M, et al. Calcified rheumatic valve neoangiogenesis is associated with vascular endothelial growth factor expression and osteoblast-like bone formation. Circulation 2005;111:3296–301.)*

CH 3

CELLULAR AND MOLECULAR BASIS OF CALCIFIC AORTIC VALVE DISEASE

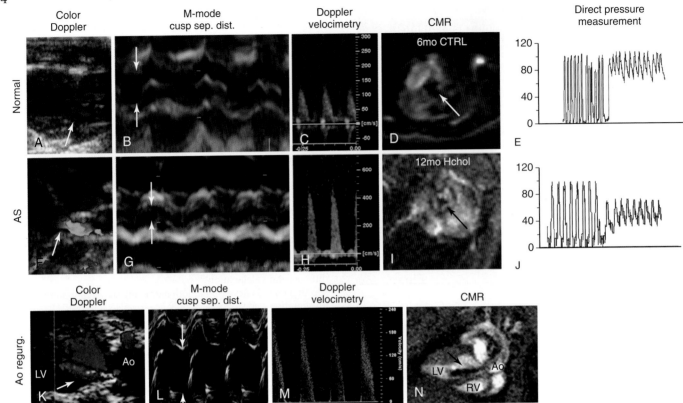

FIGURE 3-4 **Methods to evaluate aortic valve function in mice. A** through **C,** Measurements of aortic valve function using echocardiography in nonhypercholesterolemic mice (i.e., "normal" animals). Note that there is no evidence of aortic valve regurgitation on color-flow Doppler imaging, cusp separation distance is relatively large (>0.8 mm; *arrows*), and peak transvalvular velocities are relatively low (<2 m/sec). These data correspond to relatively large aortic valve orifice areas measured on cardiac magnetic resonance (CMR) **(D),** and low transvalvular pressure gradients measured directly with a Millar catheter **(E). F** through **H,** In mice with aortic stenosis (AS), note that there is again no evidence of aortic valve regurgitation (i.e., normal flow in *green* on the ventricular side of the valve during diastole in **F**), cusp separation distance is markedly reduced (<0.6 mm; *arrows*), and peak transvalvular velocity is markedly elevated (>4 m/sec). **I,** Subsequent measurement of aortic valve area using CMR showed clear reductions in aortic valve orifice area and **J,** dramatic increases in peak transvalvular pressures. **K** through **N,** The importance of using multiple measurements of valve function in mice; the presence of aortic valve regurgitation (Ao regurg) **(K, N)** dramatically elevates peak transvalvular velocity and gives the appearance of aortic valve dysfunction due to hyperdynamic cardiac function **(M).** In contrast, aortic valve regurgitation does not influence cusp separation distance *(arrows)* **(L).** *Ao,* Aorta; *CTRL,* control; *Hchol,* high cholesterol; *LV,* left ventricle; *RV,* right ventricle. *(From Miller JD, Weiss RM, Heistad DD. Calcific aortic valve stenosis: methods, models, and mechanisms. Circ Res 2011;108:1392–412.)*

Induction of Osteogenic Signaling Cascades

After the observation that osteoblast-like and osteoclast-like cells were present in stenotic human valves, a number of subsequent studies went on to perform molecular characterization of pathways contributing to osteogenic differentiation of cells in the stenotic valve. The ensuing sections focus on key pro-osteogenic and antiosteogenic mechanisms that have been identified in stenotic valves and provide a framework for osteogenic mechanisms that may ultimately be viable therapeutic targets for slowing progression of fibrocalcific aortic valve disease.

Bone Morphogenetic Protein Signaling

Numerous studies have reported increased expression of multiple bone morphogenetic protein (BMP) isoforms in diseased human valves, including BMP2, BMP4, and BMP6.[14-20] In general, BMP elaboration is thought to originate from the endothelium on the aortic face of the valve[21] (Figure 3-5), where shear forces are nonlaminar and inhibitors of BMP signaling are disproportionately low.[15] Binding of BMPs to their receptor complex on aortic valve interstitial cells results in Smad1/5/8 phosphorylation and subsequent translocation of the Smad complex to the nucleus, where it drives pro-osteogenic gene expression through its binding to Smad binding elements.[22,23] Although Smad6 appears to play a

major role in tonic suppression of BMP signaling (because Smad6-null mice have evidence of cardiovascular calcification at 2 weeks of age[24]), the role of other inhibitory molecules in the regulation of aortic valve calcification (e.g., Smurf1/2) remains poorly understood.

Bone morphogenetic protein signaling is also elevated in experimental animal models of fibrocalcific aortic valve disease. Importantly, increases in Smad1/5/8 phosphorylation precede aortic valve dysfunction in hypercholesterolemic mice,[6] suggesting that increases in BMP signaling are not simply an epiphenomenon associated with end-stage valve calcification and stenosis.

Wnt/β-Catenin Signaling

A second major osteogenic pathway activated in fibrocalcific aortic valve disease is Wnt/β-catenin signaling (Figure 3-6). In brief, activation of the canonical signaling pathway involves binding of Wnt ligands to a receptor complex that results in activation and nuclear translocation of β-catenin, which can subsequently drive pro-osteogenic gene expression.[25,26] Multiple components of this pathway have been implicated in calcified human and animal aortic valves, including Wnt ligands (Wnt3a, Wnt7a),[27-30] lipoprotein receptor–related protein (lrp) receptor complex components (LRP5/6, frizzled receptors),[29,31] and nuclear translocation of the β-catenin transcription factor complex.[28,30-32]

Wnt/β-catenin signaling can be negatively regulated at multiple levels, including through inhibition of Wnt binding, inhibition of

TABLE 3-3 Echocardiographic and Hemodynamic Changes in Animal Models of Aortic Valve Sclerosis and Stenosis

SPECIES/STRAIN	DIET (REFERENCE)	HISTOPATHOLOGIC CHANGES IN AORTIC VALVE	HEMODYNAMICALLY SIGNIFICANT STENOSIS?
Mice			
C57BL/6	HF[156]	Lipid deposition Modest calcification	No
ApoE[−/−]	Chow[157]	Lipid deposition Calcification Monocyte/Inflammatory cell infiltration	<2%
	HF/HC[118,158]	Lipid deposition Fibrosis[118,158] Calcification[118,158] Monocyte/Inflammatory cell infiltration[118,158]	<2%
Ldlr[−/−]	HF/HC[156,159]	Lipid deposition Calcification Monocyte/Inflammatory cell infiltration	No
Ldlr[−/−]/apoB[100/100]	Chow[160]	Lipid deposition Calcification Monocyte/Inflammatory cell infiltration Myofibroblast activation	Yes, ~30% of mice
	HF/HC[6,32]	Lipid deposition Calcification Fibrosis Monocyte/Inflammatory cell infiltration Myofibroblast activation	Yes, >50% of mice
EGFR[Wa2/Wa2]	Chow[161]	Fibrosis Calcification Inflammatory cell infiltration	Yes, but background strain dependent
eNOS[−/−]: Tricuspid offspring	Chow[162] HF/HC	Bicuspid aortic valves in ~40% of mice Calcification Fibrosis	No No
Bicuspid offspring	HF/HC	Calcification Fibrosis	Yes
Notch1[+/−]	HF/HC[108,163]	Calcification	No
Periostin[−/−]	Chow[164]	Calcification Fibrosis	Not known
	HF/HC[165]	Reduced valve thickening and fibrosis	No
MGP[−/−]	Chow[40]	Calcification	Not known
Klotho[−/−]	Chow	Calcification	No
Col1a2[Oim/Oim]	Chow	Fibrosis/extracellular matrix disruption	No
Twist1[Tg/0]	Chow	Hypercellular, thickened valves	No
Sox9[Fl/+]/Col2a1[Cre]	Chow	Calcification Fibrosis	No
Chm1[−/−]	Chow[166]	Neoangiogenesis Lipid deposition Calcification	Not known
Rabbits			
New Zealand White	HF/HC[31,85,96,167-178]	Lipid deposition Calcification Inflammatory cell infiltration	<10% Mostly moderate sclerosis
	Chow + hypertension[168]	Fibrosis Inflammation	<10%
Watanabe	HF/HC[31]	Lipid deposition Fibrosis Calcification Inflammatory cell infiltration	No
Pigs			
Yorkshire Landrace	HF/HC[21,179]	Lipid deposition	No

Apo, Apolipoprotein; *EGFR*, epidermal growth factor receptor; *eNOS*, endothelial nitric oxide synthetase; *HC*, high cholesterol; *HF*, high fat; *Ldlr*, low-density lipoprotein receptor; *MGP*, matrix Gla protein. Superscript numbers are reference citations.

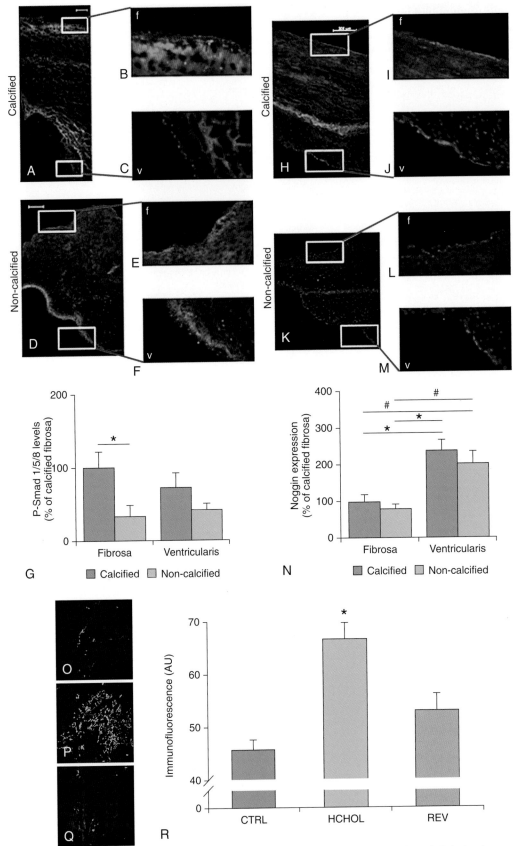

FIGURE 3-5 **Changes in bone morphogenetic protein signaling in fibrocalcific aortic valve disease. A** through **G** depict changes in levels of phospho-Smad1/5/8 (P-Smad), a key signal transduction molecule in bone morphogenic protein (BMP) signaling, in calcified and noncalcified regions of human aortic valves. **H** through **N** depict changes in levels of Noggin (an endogenous inhibitor of BMP signaling) in calcified and noncalcified regions of human aortic valves. Note that P-Smad1/5/8 levels are highest where Noggin levels are lowest, suggesting that reductions in endogenous inhibitors of BMP signaling are a key permissive step for increases in canonical pathway activation. **O** through **R** show P-Smad1/5/8 levels in aortic valves from hypercholesterolemic (HCHOL) mice with severe fibrocalcific aortic valve disease. Note that reduction of hyperlipidemia (REV) significantly reduces canonical BMP signaling, suggesting that this pathway is labile even in advanced stages of valve disease. (*A through N from Ankeny RF, Thourani VH, Weiss D, et al. Preferential activation of SMAD1/5/8 on the fibrosa endothelium in calcified human aortic valves—association with low BMP antagonists and SMAD6. PLoS One 2011;6:e20969; O through R from Miller JD, Weiss RM, Serrano KM, et al. Evidence for active regulation of pro-osteogenic signaling in advanced aortic valve disease. Arterioscler Thromb Vasc Biol 2010;30:2482-24862.*)

Continued

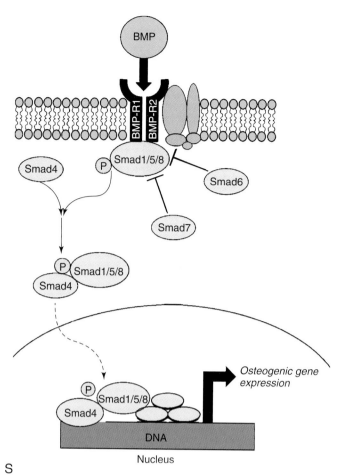

FIGURE 3-5, cont'd. S depicts canonical BMP signaling, in which binding of BMP ligand to its receptor complex results in phosphorylation (P) of Smad1/5/8, translocation of the activated Smad complex to the nucleus, and induction of osteogenic gene expression.

β-catenin activation, and proteasomal degradation of β-catenin.[25,26] The role of changes in endogenous inhibitors of the Wnt/β-catenin signaling pathway in the pathogenesis of fibrocalcific aortic valve disease remains poorly understood.

Transforming Growth Factor-β Signaling

Like BMP signaling, canonical tumor growth factor-β (TGF-β) signaling involves phosphorylation of Smad proteins (Smad2/3 in particular) and translocation of the activated Smad complex to the nucleus.[22,33] Increases in TGF-β expression, Smad2/3 phosphorylation, and multiple Smad2/3 target genes have been shown in humans and animals with fibrocalcific aortic valve disease[6,32,34-37] (Figure 3-7).

The role of canonical TGF-β signaling in the initiation and progression of calcification in aortic valve disease, however, is controversial. The key observation suggesting that TGF-β contributes to calcification in valve disease is that cultured aortic valve interstitial cells treated with exogenous TGF-β rapidly form calcified nodules via a caspase/apoptosis-dependent mechanism.[35,38] There are, however, several observations from in vivo model systems suggesting that TGF-β may not accelerate valve calcification in fibrocalcific aortic valve disease. First, lipid lowering in mice with advanced aortic valve disease reduces osteogenic gene expression and does not reduce Smad2/3 phosphorylation,[32] suggesting that TGF-β is not a primary driver of osteogenic gene expression in fibrocalcific aortic valve disease.

Second, mice that are deficient in one copy of Smad3 (i.e., Smad3[+/-] mice) have a higher bone mineral density than their wild-type littermates,[39] suggesting that TGF-β may suppress osteogenesis in bone. Finally, although canonical TGF-β signaling may not promote (or may even inhibit) valve calcification, emerging data suggest that TGF-β receptor activation may transactivate Wnt/β-catenin signaling,[30] which is likely to promote interstitial cell osteogenesis. Future studies with experimental manipulation of TGF-β signaling in robust, in vivo models of fibrocalcific aortic valve disease will be essential to define its role in valve calcification and stenosis.

Modulators of Osteogenic Differentiation

There is compelling evidence that the signaling pathways discussed in the preceding section can induce osteogenesis and accumulation of calcification (and perhaps even bone matrix) in stenotic valves, but we are only beginning to understand the primary events inciting these signaling cascades. Significant insights have been gained from genetically altered mouse models and in vitro experiments, however, in which deletion or overexpression of genes has allowed us to discern between molecular mechanisms that *initiate* and those that *modulate* osteogenic signaling.

Direct Inhibitors of Osteogenic Signaling

Reductions in expression of inhibitors of osteogenic signaling are likely to play a significant role in initiation and progression of fibrocalcific aortic valve disease. As mentioned previously, genetic deletion of Smad6 results in cardiovascular calcification in the absence of additional exogenous stressors,[24] suggesting that tonic suppression of BMP signaling is critical for prevention of valvular calcification. It would also appear that tonic BMP ligand sequestration/neutralization is important in preventing cardiovascular calcification because mice deficient in matrix Gla protein (which binds and inactivates BMP2) demonstrate spontaneous cardiovascular calcification early in life,[40] and mice overexpressing matrix Gla protein are protected against hypercholesterolemia-induced vascular calcification.[41] Although matrix Gla protein levels are under transcriptional and translational regulation, the posttranslational gamma-carboxylation of matrix Gla protein is required for binding to BMP2.[42-46] Clinically, several retrospective studies reported that drugs that inhibit gamma-carboxylase (e.g., warfarin) have been associated with increased risk of cardiovascular calcification and aortic valve stenosis.[47-50] Along these lines, administration of warfarin to juvenile rats results in significant vascular calcification.[51-55] Collectively, tonic suppression of BMP signaling, at both intracellular and extracellular levels, appears to be important in prevention of cardiovascular calcification.

Angiotensin II

Hypertension is a major risk factor for development of fibrocalcific aortic valve disease, and is frequently associated with systemic increases in activity of the renin-angiotensin system (RAS). It is often underappreciated, however, that the "local" RAS can be a major contributor to rises in tissue levels of angiotensin II. A large amount of work has shown that increases in tissue RAS activity are major contributors to inflammation, oxidative stress, fibrosis, and plaque expansion in atherosclerotic lesions.[56-58] In stenotic aortic valves, infiltrating macrophages are abundant and can be primary sources of greater local RAS activity and concomitant rises in tissue angiotensin II levels[6,7,59-61] (Figure 3-8). Interestingly, increases in chymase activity can also convert angiotensin I to angiotensin II, and macrophages express high levels of chymase.[58,59] Retrospective studies suggest that angiotensin-converting enzyme (ACE) inhibition may slow progression of aortic valve disease,[62] there are limited experimental data testing

CH
3

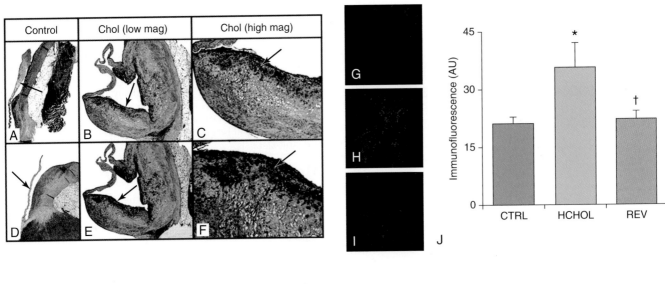

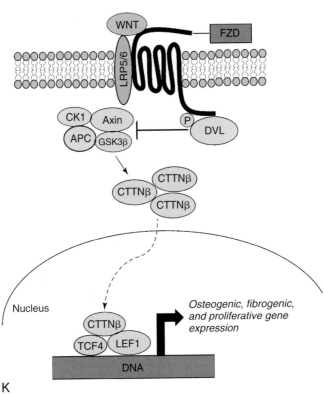

FIGURE 3-6 **Changes in Wnt/β-catenin signaling in experimental animal models of fibrocalcific aortic valve disease. A** through **F** are micrographs depicting changes in Wnt/β-catenin signaling in control rabbits (CTRL) and in rabbits with hypercholesterolemia-induced aortic valve disease (Chol). More specifically, **A** through **C** show changes in low-density lipoprotein receptor–related protein 5 (Lrp5), a receptor critical for Wnt ligand binding. **D** through **F** show changes in β-catenin levels. Note that levels of both Lrp5 and β-catenin are dramatically increased by hypercholesterolemia and that these increases occur preferentially on the aortic side of the valve. **G** through **J** depict changes in β-catenin immunofluorescence in aortic valves from hypercholesterolemic mice. **K,** Like BMP signaling (shown in Figure 3-5), β-catenin immunofluorescence can be markedly attenuated by a reduction in blood lipids in hypercholesterolemic mice with advanced fibrocalcific aortic valve disease. *APC,* Adenomatous Polyposis Coli tumor suppressor gene; *CK1,* Casein Kinase 1; *CTTNβ,* b-catenin protein; *DVL,* disheveled proteins; *FZD,* Frizzled proteins; *GSK3β,* glycogen synthetase kinase-3β; *HCHOL,* high-cholesterol diet; *LEF1,* lymphoid enhancer binding factor; *REV,* reversed; *TCF4,* Transcription Factor 4.

this hypothesis, and the fact that chymase activity is unaffected by ACE inhibitors makes it a less appealing target. Preclinical experiments in hypercholesterolemic rabbits, however, showed that angiotensin 1 receptor blockade attenuates aortic valve interstitial cell activation, endothelial disruption, and valvular inflammation in early stages of valve disease,[63] suggesting that angiotensin II and angiotensin 1 receptor activation may be important factors even in early stage fibrocalcific aortic valve disease.

Inflammatory Cell Infiltrate and Proinflammatory Cytokines

Inflammatory cells such as macrophages,[64] neutrophils,[65,66] and T cells[67] are ubiquitous findings in end-stage human aortic valve disease and in most animal models of fibrocalcific valve disease. Consistent with this finding, elaboration of proinflammatory cytokines—for example, tumor necrosis factor-α (TNFα) and interleukins IL-6 and IL-1—is also dramatically increased in

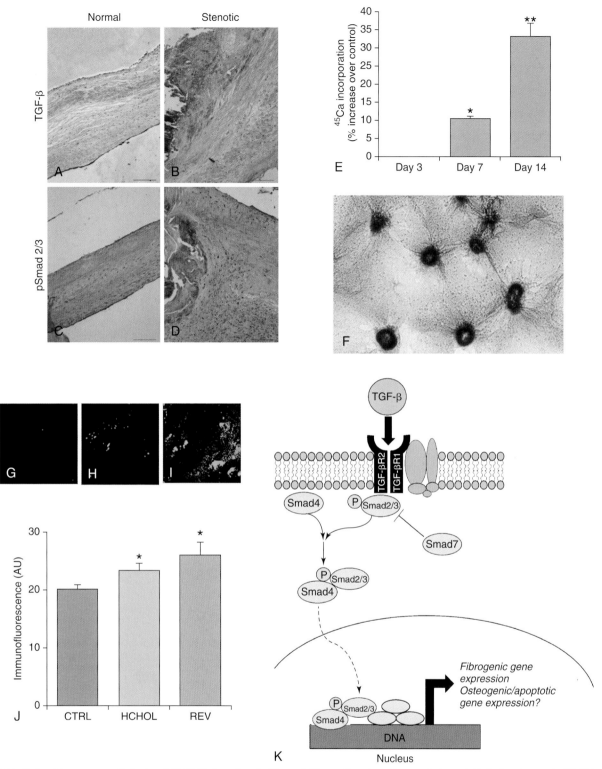

FIGURE 3-7   Role of tumor growth factor-β (TGF-β) signaling in fibrocalcific aortic valve disease. A through **D** depict changes in TGF-β levels and phospho-Smad2/3 levels in aortic valves from humans with severe fibrocalcific aortic valve disease. Note that phospho-Smad2/3 levels are increased most dramatically in pericalcific regions of the stenotic valve. **E** and **F** show changes in calcium (⁴⁵Ca) accumulation **(E)** and nodule formation **(F)** in aortic valve interstitial cells treated with exogenous TGF-β1. Note that prolonged exposure to TGF-β1 in cells plated directly on plastic culture plates results in robust calcium accumulation and Alizarin red–positive nodule formation. **G** through **J** depict changes in phospho-Smad2 levels in aortic valves from mice with severe fibrocalcific aortic valve disease. Note that canonical TGF-β signaling is increased in valves from mice with severe fibrocalcific aortic valve disease. In contrast to osteogenic signaling, however, reducing blood lipids does not effectively reduce TGF-β signaling in mice with advanced aortic valve dysfunction and stenosis. **K** depicts canonical TGF-β signaling, in which binding of TGF-β ligand to its receptor complex results in phosphorylation (P) of Smad2/3, translocation of the activated Smad complex to the nucleus, and induction of fibrogenic and osteogenic gene expression. *CTRL,* Control; *HCHOL,* high-cholesterol diet; *P,* phosphorylation; *REV,* reversed; *TGF-βR,* TGF-β receptor. *(**A** through **D** from Osman N, Grande-Allen KJ, Ballinger ML, et al. Smad2-dependent glycosaminoglycan elongation in aortic valve interstitial cells enhances binding of LDL to proteoglycans. Cardiovasc Pathol 2013;22:146–55; **E** and **F** from Jian B, Narula N, Li QY, et al. Progression of aortic valve stenosis: TGF-beta1 is present in calcified aortic valve cusps and promotes aortic valve interstitial cell calcification via apoptosis. Ann Thorac Surg 2003;75:457–65; **G** through **J** from from Miller JD, Weiss RM, Serrano KM, et al. Evidence for active regulation of pro-osteogenic signaling in advanced aortic valve disease. Arterioscler Thromb Vasc Biol 2010;30:2482–6.)*

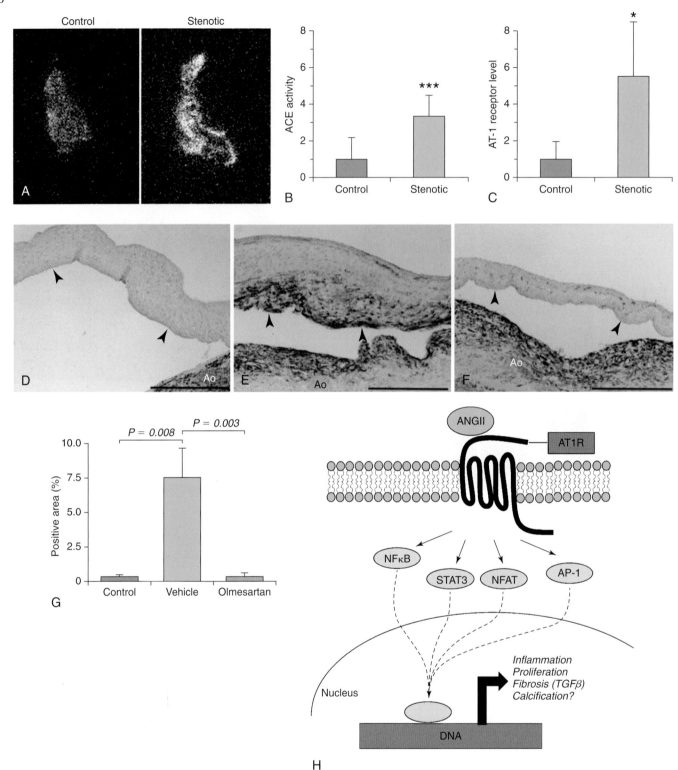

FIGURE 3-8 **Changes in angiotensin II (ANGII)–related molecules in fibrocalcific aortic valve disease. A** and **B,** Autoradiography imaging of angiotensin-converting enzyme (ACE) levels in control and stenotic valves, with quantitative measurement of image intensity in **B** and **C**. Note that local ACE levels are significantly increased in stenotic valves and are associated with dramatic increases in angiotensin type 1 receptor (AT1R) levels. **D** through **G** illustrate the effects of long-term AT1R inhibition (with olmesartan) on myofibroblast activation in a hypercholesterolemic rabbit model of fibrocalcific aortic valve disease. Note that long-term AT1R blockade significantly reduces the number of α-smooth muscle actin–positive myofibroblasts in this model. **H** depicts potential signaling cascades that may be activated following binding of ANGII to AT1R. Note that AT1R activation has the potential to elicit a broad range of responses, including induction of cellular inflammation, proliferation, fibrosis, and calcification. *AP-1,* activator protein-1; *NFAT,* nuclear factor of activated T-cells; *NFκB,* nuclear factor κB; *STAT,* signal transducer and activator of transcription. *(**A** through **C** from Helske S, Lindstedt KA, Laine M, et al. Induction of local angiotensin II-producing systems in stenotic aortic valves. JACC 2004;44:1859–66; **D** through **G** from Arishiro K, Hoshiga M, Negoro N, et al. Angiotensin receptor-1 blocker inhibits atherosclerotic changes and endothelial disruption of the aortic valve in hypercholesterolemic rabbits. JACC 2007;49:1482–9.)*

human and animals with fibrocalcific aortic valve disease.[68-72] Although few studies have examined the role of proinflammatory cytokines in the progression of fibrocalcific aortic valve disease, three lines of evidence suggest that TNFα may play a central role in the initiation and progression of disease.

First, aortic valves from interleukin-1 receptor antagonist (IL-1ra)–deficient mice are thickened, accumulate calcium, and develop mild aortic valve dysfunction (peak transvalvular velocity 2 m/sec)[68] (Figure 3-9). Importantly, this phenotype is abolished in IL-1ra/TNFα double-knockout mice, suggesting

that TNFα is the major downstream mediator of IL-1–induced inflammation.[68]

Second, a growing body of work suggests that activation of receptors for advanced glycosylation end products (RAGEs) is likely to accelerate cardiovascular calcification. Specifically, overexpression of S100A12 significantly accelerates vascular calcification in hypercholesterolemic mice by what appears to be a nicotinamide adenine dinucleotide phosphate (NAD[P]H) oxidase–dependent mechanism.[73-76] Furthermore, RAGE activation drives proinflammatory cytokine production and osteogenic

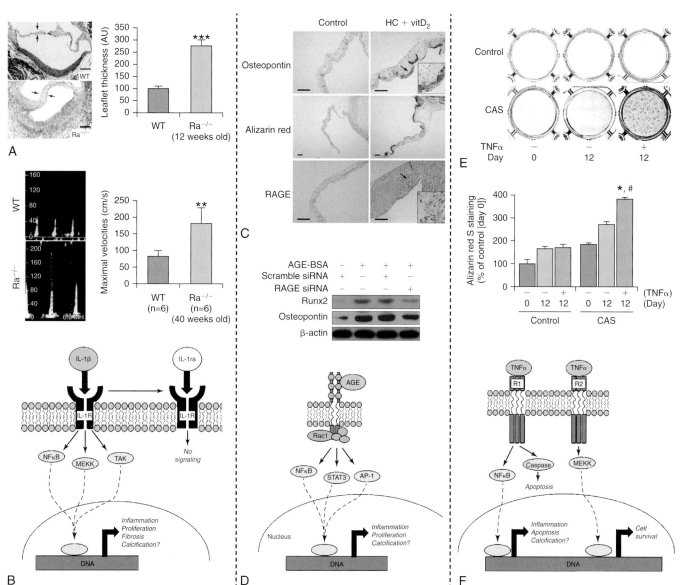

FIGURE 3-9 **Role of proinflammatory signaling in the pathogenesis of fibrocalcific aortic valve disease. A** and **B** illustrate histopathologic and functional changes in aortic valves from mice that are deficient (Ra$^{-/-}$) in an endogenous antagonist to interleukin 1 (IL-1ra); *WT,* wild type mice. Note that increasing IL-1β signaling dramatically increases leaflet thickness **(A)** and peak transvalvular velocity **(B)**. **C** and **D** depict changes in RAGE (receptor for advanced glycosylation end products) signaling in hypercholesterolemic rabbits (HC) receiving high-doses of vitamin D$_2$ (*vitD₂*) to induce fibrocalcific aortic valve disease. Note that both calcium accumulation and induction of osteopontin are associated with increases in RAGE levels in aortic valves from these animals. Furthermore, induction of osteogenic signaling by AGE–bovine serum albumin (AGE-BSA) can be markedly attenuated by knockdown of RAGE in aortic valve interstitial cells in vitro. **E** and **F** show changes in tumor necrosis factor α (TNFα)–induced calcification in valve interstitial cells from control/nonstenotic valves and from calcified stenotic valves (CAS). Note that TNFα-induced calcium accumulation is much more dramatic in cells from patients with aortic stenosis, suggesting that genetic and/or epigenetic changes are likely to increase the propensity for valve calcification and osteogenesis even after cells are taken out of the body/"fibrocalcific aortic valve disease milieu" and cultured. *AGE,* advanced glycosylation end products; *AP-1,* activator protein-1; *MEKK,* mitogen activated protein kinase kinase kinase; *Rac1,* ras-related C3 botulinum toxin substrate 1; *Runx2,* runt-related transcription factor 2; *siRNA,* small interfering RNA; *STAT,* signal transducer and activator of transcription; *TAK,* transforming growth factor-beta activated kinase. (*A* and *B* from Isoda K, Matsuki T, Kondo H, et al. Deficiency of interleukin-1 receptor antagonist induces aortic valve disease in balb/c mice. Arterioscler Thromb Vasc Biol 2010;30:708–15; *C* and *D* from Li F, Cai Z, Chen F, et al. Pioglitazone attenuates progression of aortic valve calcification via down-regulating receptor for advanced glycation end products. Basic Res Cardiol 2012;107:306; *E* and *F* from Yu Z, Seya K, Daitoku K, et al. Tumor necrosis factor-α accelerates the calcification of human aortic valve interstitial cells obtained from patients with calcific aortic valve stenosis via the BMP2-Dlx5 pathway. J Pharmacol Exp Ther 2011;337:16–23.)

gene expression in valve interstitial cells in vitro.[77] Although mechanisms contributing to increased oxidative stress differ dramatically between aorta and aortic valve (see later),[5,78] numerous studies have shown that RAGE activation is strongly associated with increases in TNFα,[79,80] which may be a point of convergence in inflammatory signals driving calcification in aortic valve and aorta.

Finally, addition of exogenous TNFα to cultured aortic valve interstitial cells amplifies BMP signaling and accelerates calcium accumulation in vitro.[20] Importantly, TNFα accelerated calcification only in cells from patients with fibrocalcific aortic valve disease (i.e., not in cells from nonstenotic control valves), suggesting that phenotypic and/or epigenetic changes that occur in vivo may persist in cultured interstitial cells in vitro.[20] The molecular mechanisms whereby TNFα promotes valve interstitial cell calcification are still under investigation, but work in aortic myofibroblasts suggests that reactive oxygen species (ROS) generated by TNF receptor 1 activation may be integral to the pro-osteogenic effects of TNFα.[81,82]

Oxidative Stress

Although NAD(P)H (nicotinamide adenine dinucleotide phosphate) oxidase–derived free radicals have been implicated in the pathogenesis of atherosclerosis for many years,[83,84] the role of oxidative stress in fibrocalcific aortic valve disease—and mechanisms contributing to increased ROS—is only beginning to be understood.

Superoxide and hydrogen peroxide levels are dramatically increased in stenotic aortic valves[5,6,32,78,85] (Figure 3-10). Interestingly, these increases occur almost exclusively in the calcified and pericalcific regions of the valve, and unlike atherosclerosis, are predominantly the result of uncoupled nitric oxide synthase (NOS) and reductions in antioxidant enzyme expression.[5,78] Although NAD(P)H oxidase–derived radicals appear to contribute to increased ROS levels in a subset of pericalcific regions,[85] global expression of most catalytic subunits of the oxidase are significantly reduced in human fibrocalcific aortic valve disease.[78]

Several observations suggest that ROS may play an important role in the pathogenesis of fibrocalcific aortic valve disease. First, increases in ROS occur prior to the onset of aortic valve dysfunction in hypercholesterolemic mice,[6] suggesting that elevations in ROS are not a consequence of aortic valve dysfunction per se. Second, there is a growing body of data demonstrating that ROS play a critical role in the transduction of multiple signaling cascades related to osteogenesis[86-90] (including TGF-β and BMP signaling). Third, increasing superoxide or hydrogen peroxide levels accelerates calcification of valve interstitial cells in vitro.[86] Finally, administration of α-lipoic acid (an antioxidant that reduces superoxide and hydrogen peroxide levels), but not tempol (which reduces only superoxide levels), reduces valvular calcification in a rabbit model of fibrocalcific aortic valve disease.[85]

However, other data suggest that ROS are not a primary driver of osteogenic signaling in fibrocalcific aortic valve disease. First, reduction of blood lipids in mice with severe valvular dysfunction and fibrocalcific aortic valve disease reduces BMP signaling, Wnt signaling, and valvular calcification, but does not lower ROS levels.[32] Second, although exogenous ROS do accelerate vascular smooth muscle cell calcification in vitro, increased ROS do not induce calcification in the absence of osteogenic stimuli.[91,92] Collectively, we are only beginning to understand the role of ROS in the pathogenesis of fibrocalcific aortic valve disease. Future studies examining the role of different ROS-generating systems and the role of ROS in different subcellular compartments will be critical for development of complementary treatments to slow progression of valve disease.

Nitric Oxide Signaling

As with oxidative stress, reductions in nitric oxide (NO) bioavailability and signaling are known to play a major role in vasomotor dysfunction and atherosclerosis,[93-95] and the role of NO is only beginning to be understood in fibrocalcific aortic valve disease.

Although endothelial NOS expression and protein levels are significantly reduced in fibrocalcific aortic valve disease,[96,97] the impact this reduction has on NO signaling is likely to be underestimated, given the observations that (1) ROS are increased in fibrocalcific aortic valve disease, resulting in formation of peroxynitrite (ONOO⁻),[98,99] (2) increases in ROS are known to result in oxidation of soluble guanylate cyclase, making it insensitive to increases in NO levels,[100] and (3) there is strong evidence for uncoupled NOS in fibrocalcific aortic valve disease, a condition in which ROS are produced instead of NO[78] (Figure 3-11). Although depletion of tetrahydrobiopterin is known to elicit increases in uncoupled NOS,[101] it remains unknown whether de novo synthesis or salvage pathways that maintain tetrahydrobiopterin levels are altered in fibrocalcific aortic valve disease.

Despite the strong association between fibrocalcific aortic valve disease and conditions that favor reduced NO signaling, few studies have experimentally examined the effects of NO bioavailability on osteogenic signaling and valve calcification. Early work suggested that treatment of hypercholesterolemic rabbits with statins was associated with increases in endothelial nitric oxide synthase (eNOS) levels and slower progression of fibrocalcific aortic valve disease.[96] Furthermore, subsequent studies demonstrated that addition of exogenous NO slowed progression of valvular interstitial cell calcification in vitro.[102] Interestingly, studies examining the role of NO in fibrocalcific aortic valve disease in vivo have reported that progression of aortic valve dysfunction was not accelerated in eNOS-deficient mice with tricuspid aortic valves but was in those with bicuspid aortic valves.[103] Collectively, there are two potential interpretations of these data: (1) reductions in NO levels do not play a major role in progression of tricuspid fibrocalcific aortic valve disease because reducing NO production does not accelerate valve disease, or (2) NO production already is dramatically reduced in fibrocalcific aortic valve disease, and further reducing NOS does not result in significant acceleration of valve dysfunction in an already compromised system. Regardless of the effects of reducing NO on valve function, the preponderance of the evidence suggests that increasing NO is likely to slow initiation and/or progression of fibrocalcific aortic valve disease.

Peroxisome Proliferator-Activated Receptor-γ Signaling

During the differentiation of multipotent cells (mesenchymal stem cells, aortic valve interstitial cells, etc.), there is a critical "decision point" at which cells enter either an osteoblast-like lineage or an adipocyte-like lineage.[104] This decision is typically governed by the balance between runt-related transcription factor 2 (Runx2), a master regulator of osteogenesis, and peroxisome proliferator-activated receptor-γ (PPARγ), a master regulator of adipogenesis.[104,105] Therefore, it is perhaps not surprising that administration of thiazolidinediones (TZDs), which activate PPARγ, significantly attenuated aortic valve calcification and dysfunction in hypercholesterolemic rabbits and mice.[77,106] Importantly, TZDs inhibit osteogenic differentiation in both cardiovascular tissues and in bone. Thus, administration of one of these agents at a dose that predominantly inhibits inflammation or preferentially affects cardiovascular calcification may allow administration of this drug class without negatively affecting skeletal ossification.

Notch1 Signaling

Several years ago, loss-of-function mutations in Notch1, a signaling protein involved in development, were shown to be strongly associated with bicuspid valve formation and severe valve cusp calcification in humans.[107] This observation formed the impetus for a series of studies in experimental animals and in vitro model systems examining the role of Notch1 in the initiation and progression of fibrocalcific aortic valve disease. The findings from these studies can be distilled down to two key points. First, the developmental consequences of loss-of-function mutations in Notch1 are highly context dependent because deletion of one copy of Notch1 in mice (i.e., Notch1[+/−]) does not result in bicuspid valve formation.[108] Second, reducing Notch1 levels accelerates aortic valve interstitial cell calcification both in vitro and in vivo.[108,109] Mechanistically, this finding appears to be attributed to permissive increases in Runx2 and β-catenin–dependent signaling[107] (Figure 3-12).

Matrix-Degrading Enzymes

Multiple matrix remodeling proteins (MMPs) are upregulated in human valves with fibrocalcific aortic valve disease, including matrix metalloproteinases MMP1,[110-112] MMP2,[113] MMP3,[14] and MMP9,[114] and cathepsins S,[115] K,[115] V,[115] and G[37] (Figure 3-13). There are two potential mechanisms whereby elevated matrix-remodeling proteins may affect valve calcification and stenosis. First, matrix remodeling may be an important permissive event

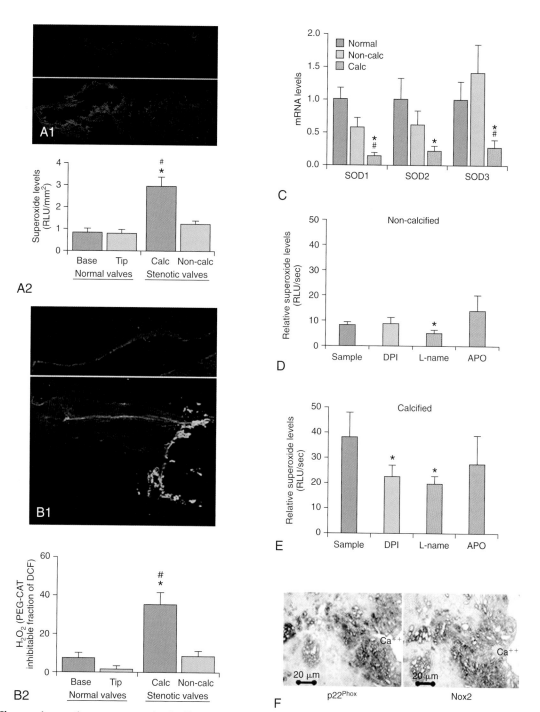

FIGURE 3-10   Changes in reactive oxygen species in fibrocalcific aortic valve disease. A1 and **A2,** Micrographs and quantitation of superoxide levels (dihydroethidium fluorescence) in normal and stenotic human aortic valves. **B1** and **B2,** Micrographs and quantitation of hydrogen peroxide levels (CM-H₂DCFDA fluorescence) in normal and stenotic human aortic valves. As shown in **C,** reductions in antioxidant enzyme expression are likely to contribute to increases in reactive oxygen species in stenotic valves, with these changes being most pronounced in the pericalcific regions of the valve. Furthermore, uncoupled nitric oxide synthase (L-NAME [L-NG-nitroarginine methyl ester]–inhibitable fraction of superoxide production in **D** and **E**) and NAD(P)H (nicotinamide adenine dinucleotide phosphate) oxidase (immunohistochemical evidence in **F**) are potential contributors to increased superoxide and hydrogen peroxide levels in calcifying microenvironments in stenotic valves.

Continued

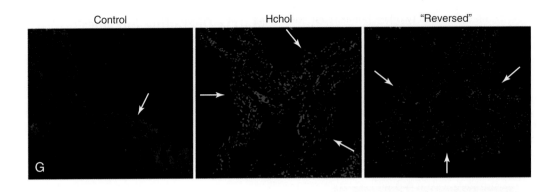

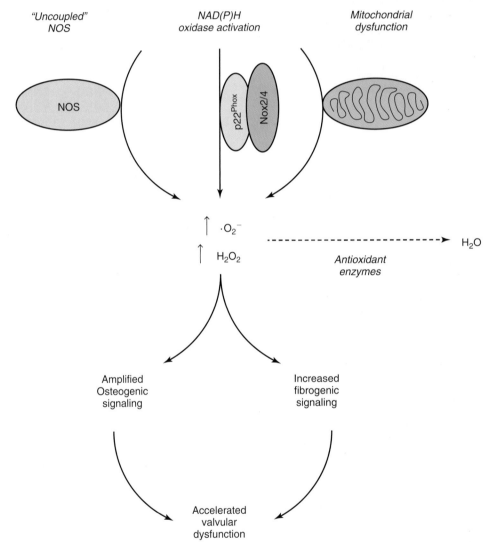

FIGURE 3-10, cont'd. **G,** Changes in superoxide levels (dihydroethidium fluorescence) in a hypercholesterolemic mouse model of fibrocalcific aortic valve disease. Note that prolonged hypercholesterolemia can dramatically increase valvular oxidative stress in the valve cusps *(arrows)*, which can be markedly reduced by lipid lowering in early stages of valve disease. *APO,* apocynin; *Calc,* calcified; *DCF,* dichlorofluorescein; *DPI,* diphenyliodonium; *Hchol,* high-cholesterol; *Non-calc,* noncalcified; *NOS,* nitric oxide synthase; *Nox2,* NAD(P)H oxidase catalytic subunit 2; *p22^{Phox},* cytochorome-b245 alpha polypeptide; *PEG-CAT,* polyethylene glycol conjugated catalase; *SOD,* superoxide dismutase. (***A** to **E** from Miller JD, Chu Y, Brooks RM, et al. Dysregulation of antioxidant mechanisms contributes to increased oxidative stress in calcific aortic valvular stenosis in humans. JACC 2008;52:843–50; **F** from Liberman M, Bassi E, Martinatti MK, et al. Oxidant generation predominates around calcifying foci and enhances progression of aortic valve calcification. Arterioscler Thromb Vasc Biol 2008;28:463–70; **G** from Miller JD, Weiss RM, Serrano KM, et al. Lowering plasma cholesterol levels halts progression of aortic valve disease in mice. Circulation 2009;119:2693–701.)*

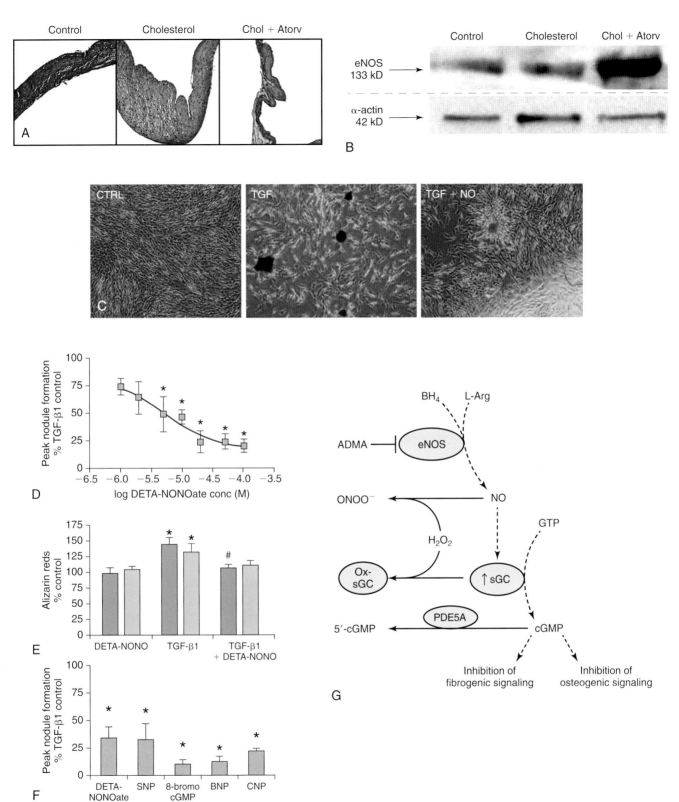

FIGURE 3-11 **Potential role of nitric oxide signaling in fibrocalcific aortic valve disease. A,** Changes in aortic valve cusp thickness in a hypercholesterolemic rabbit model of fibrocalcific aortic valve disease. Note that prolonged hypercholesterolemia elicits substantial cusp thickening *(middle panel)*, which can largely be prevented by lipid lowering with statins *(right panel)*. **B,** Note that the protective effect of statins is associated with dramatic increases in endothelial nitric oxide synthase (eNOS). **C** through **F** show evidence that nitric oxide signaling can play a major role in valve interstitial cell calcification. More specifically, tumor growth factor-β1 (TGF-β1)–induced nodule formation is dramatically attenuated by nitric oxide donors **(C** to **E)** and appears to be due in large part to increases in cyclic guanine monophosphate (cGMP) levels **(F).** *ADMA,* asymmetric dimethylarginine; *BNP,* brain natriuretic peptide; *CNP,* C-type natiuretic peptide; *DETA-NONOate,* Diethylenetriamine NONOate; *CTRL,* control; *GTP,* guanosine triphosphate; *L-Arg,* L-arginine; *PDE5A,* phosphodiesterase 5A; *sGC,* soluble guanylate cyclase; *SNP,* sodium nitroprusside. *(A* to *B from Rajamannan NM, Subramaniam M, Stock SR, et al. Atorvastatin inhibits calcification and enhances nitric oxide synthase production in the hypercholesterolaemic aortic valve. Heart 2005;91:806–10;* **C** *to* **F** *from Kennedy JA, Hua X, Mishra K, et al. Inhibition of calcifying nodule formation in cultured porcine aortic valve cells by nitric oxide donors. Eur J Pharmacol 2009;602:28–35.)*

CH
3

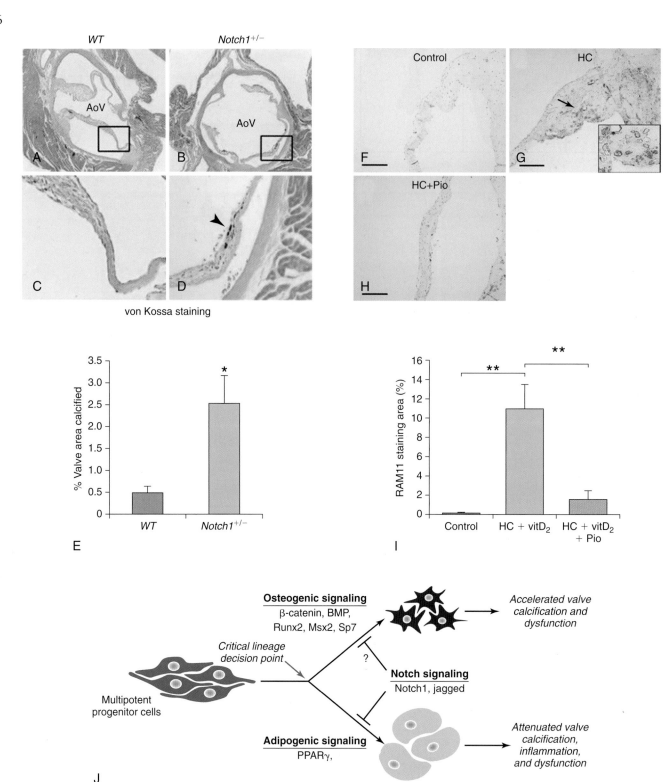

von Kossa staining

FIGURE 3-12 **Role of antiosteogenic pathways in the initiation and progression of fibrocalcific aortic valve disease.** Changes in valve calcification (micrographs **[A to D]** and quantitated data **[E]**) from wild-type (WT) and Notch1-haploinsufficient (Notch1⁺/⁻) mice. Boxes in panels **A** and **B** are shown under higher magnification in panels **C** and **D**, respectively. *Arrow in panel **D*** denotes positive Von Kossa staining in valves from Notch1⁺/⁻ mice. Note that deletion of one copy of Notch1 is sufficient to significantly increase calcium in the aortic valve (AoV), an effect that is likely due to de-repression of Wnt/β-catenin signaling. Changes in macrophage infiltration (micrographs **[F to H]** and quantitated data **[I]**) in control rabbits, hypercholesterolemic (HC) rabbits, and hypercholesterolemic rabbits treated with pioglitazone (Pio) *Arrow in panel **G*** denotes regions of high macrophage infiltration in valves from hypercholesterolemic rabbits. **J,** Note that increasing peroxisome proliferator–activated receptor gamma (PPARγ) signaling reduces valvular inflammation and is also likely to decrease osteogenesis by promoting entry of cells into an adipocyte-like lineage (i.e., instead of an osteoblast-like lineage). *BMP,* Bone morphogenetic protein; *Msx2,* msh homeobox 2; *Runx2,* runt-related transcription factor 2; *Sp7,* a transcription factor. (*A through **E** from Nigam V, Srivastava D. Notch1 represses osteogenic pathways in aortic valve cells. J Mol Cell Cardiol 2009;47:828–34; **F** through **I** from Li F, Cai Z, Chen F, Shi X, et al. Pioglitazone attenuates progression of aortic valve calcification via down-regulating receptor for advanced glycation end products. Basic Res Cardiol 2012;107:306.*)

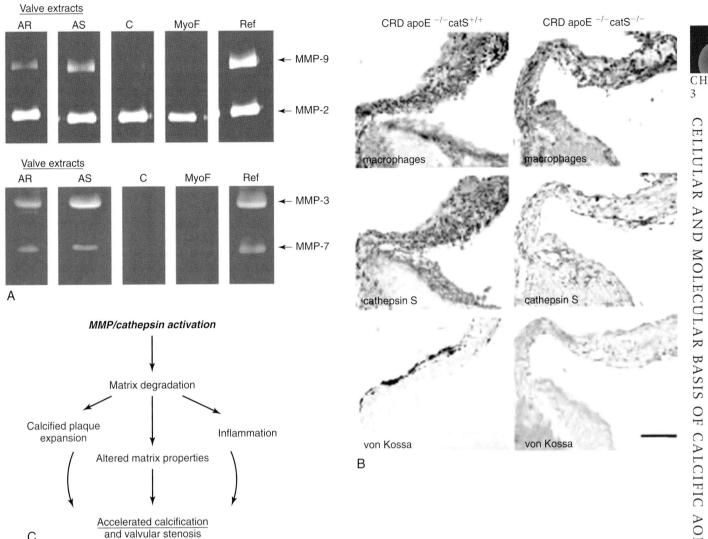

FIGURE 3-13 **Matrix-remodeling enzymes in fibrocalcific aortic valve disease. A** shows increases in matrix metalloproteinase (MMP) activity in valves from humans with aortic valve regurgitation (AR) and aortic valve stenosis (AS) in comparison with control/healthy valves. **B** shows the associations between inflammatory cell infiltrate, calcification, and cathepsin S (catS) levels in wild-type and cathepsin S–deficient mice. **C** shows potential mechanisms whereby alterations in matrix-remodeling protein activity may influence different aspects of fibrocalcific aortic valve disease. *ApoE*, Apolipoprotein E; *C*, control; *CRD*, chronic renal disease; *MyoF*, cultured myofibroblasts. (*A from Fondard O, Detaint D, Iung B, et al. Extracellular matrix remodelling in human aortic valve disease: the role of matrix metalloproteinases and their tissue inhibitors. Eur Heart J 2005;26:1333–41; **B** from Aikawa E, Aikawa M, Libby P, et al. Arterial and aortic valve calcification abolished by elastolytic cathepsin S deficiency in chronic renal disease. Circulation 2009;119:1785–94.*)

for expansion of amorphous, calcified plaques.[5] Second, generation of collagen fragments can induce inflammation in aortic valve interstitial cells, which may increase the propensity of these cells to undergo redifferentiation to an osteoblast-like phenotype.[116,117] The procalcific nature of matrix degradation is supported by the observation that genetic deletion of cathepsin S in hypercholesterolemic mice dramatically reduces valvular and vascular calcification in mice with chronic renal failure.[118] Future studies aimed at determining the therapeutic efficacy of MMP or cathepsin inhibitors will be a critical next step in this area of research.

Epigenetic Regulation of Osteogenic Signaling

Epigenetic modifications are emerging as major regulators of transcription factor binding and gene expression in numerous pathophysiologic conditions. Although little is known with regard to epigenetic regulation of gene expression in fibrocalcific aortic valve disease, data from literature on aging and other cardiovascular diseases suggest that alterations in both histone acetylation

and DNA methylation may play a significant role in the pathogenesis of valvular calcification and fibrosis.

Histone acetylation, which alters transcription factor binding and affinity, is regulated by class I to class IV histone deacetylases.[119] Class I deacetylases (such as histone deacetylase 3 [HDAC3]) and class III deacetylases (sirtuin proteins [Sirts]) have both been implicated in the regulation of proteins known to drive cardiovascular calcification. More specifically, HDAC3 has been shown to suppress activity of Runx2 and prevent osteoblastic differentiation[120] (i.e., exert a protective effect) and Sirt1 tonically suppresses vascular inflammation and endothelial cell activation.[121] Importantly, experimental reductions in Sirt1 and Sirt6 have been shown to increase histone acetylation, promote genomic instability, and increase NFκB binding in the nucleus.[122-124] Although age-related reductions in HDAC3 and/or Sirt1/ or 6 would be anticipated to increase cardiovascular calcification, changes in these deacetylase isoforms in the stenotic valve are not known.

Histone acetylation is thought to alter gene expression on a relatively large-scale basis, but changes in DNA methylation can alter expression of genes in a much more discrete manner.[125,126] Evidence that DNA methylation may play a role in regulation of aortic valve calcification can be drawn from the field of vascular calcification, in which induction of an osteogenic phenotype is associated with hypermethylation of the alpha-smooth muscle actin promoter and the addition of DNA demethylating agents (such as procaine) markedly reduces vascular smooth muscle cell calcification in vitro.[127] Whether DNA methylation silences expression of anticalcific genes in fibrocalcific aortic valve disease is unknown but remains an exciting area of future investigation.

Fibrosis and Matrix Modulation of Calcification

During the initiation and progression of fibrocalcific aortic valve disease, there are substantial changes in the composition, organization, and mechanical properties of the extracellular matrix in the aortic valve.[8] Although these changes were once thought to be simply contributors to increases in aortic valve stiffness and a direct mechanical impediment to valve function, a growing body of data now suggests that changes in the extracellular matrix can have profound effects on aortic valve interstitial cell signaling and differentiation (Figure 3-14). The interactions between valve interstitial cells and their environment can be functionally divided into four categories: matricellular signaling, matricrine signaling, mechanical signaling through changes in matrix elasticity, and mechanical signaling secondary to changes in external forces.

Matricellular signaling refers to induction of signals within the valve interstitial cell (VIC) by direct interactions with extracellular matrix components.[8] One example of this is the interaction between VICs and tenascin-C. Although tenascin-C levels are low in normal valves, expression of this molecule is markedly

upregulated in fibrocalcific aortic valve disease, its localization shifts from the subendothelium to the valve interstitium as severity of fibrocalcific aortic valve disease progresses, and it has been suggested that matricellular signals initiated by tenascin-C upregulate matrix metalloproteinase expression and alkaline phosphatase activity in VICs.[110,128]

Matricrine signaling refers to the ability of the matrix to modulate the bioavailability and binding of growth factors through their sequestration and localization.[8] Examples of this process are the regulation of latent TGF-β assembly and storage by fibronectin and the binding of TNFα by biglycan.[129] Upregulation of these extracellular matrix molecules may play a key role in the localization of profibrotic and proinflammatory molecules to sites of calcification and injury in the valve.[30]

The stiffness of the extracellular matrix can also have a profound effect on the differentiation of cells in response to various lineage-directing cues.[130] Recent reports clearly demonstrate that matrix stiffness not only can be an independent determinant of cellular differentiation but can also determine whether cells undergo apoptosis or osteogenesis following specific stimuli (e.g., TGF-β).[8,30,34] Collectively, increases in matrix stiffness with progression of fibrocalcific aortic valve disease are likely to perpetuate osteogenesis, apoptosis, and calcification in an independent manner.

Finally, changes in external mechanical forces are ultimately transmitted to aortic VICs via the extracellular matrix.[8] Hypertension, which is a major risk factor for development of fibrocalcific aortic valve disease, increases myofibroblast activation and appears to accelerate differentiate differentiation of cells to an osteoblast-like phenotype.[81,131-134] Detailed studies of changes in VIC biology in experimental models of hypertension (e.g., with or without genetic alterations in extracellular matrix proteins) will undoubtedly be critical to understanding the role of the extracellular matrix in the integration of physiologic and biochemical cues in vivo.

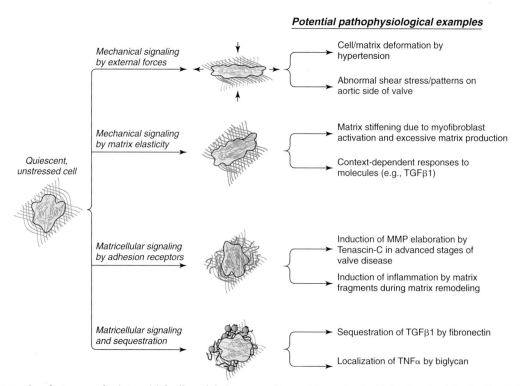

FIGURE 3-14 **Interactions between valve interstitial cells and their surrounding matrix, and potential pathophysiologic stimuli that may promote development of fibrocalcific aortic valve disease.** *MMP,* Matrix metalloproteinase; *TGF,* tumor growth factor; *TNF,* tumor necrosis factor. *(Modified from Chen JH, Simmons CA. Cell-matrix interactions in the pathobiology of calcific aortic valve disease: critical roles for matricellular, matricrine, and matrix mechanics cues. Circ Res 2011;108:1510–24.)*

Molecular Pathways Contributing to Nonosteogenic Calcification

Much of this chapter has focused on ectopic osteogenesis as a major contributor to calcification in fibrocalcific aortic valve disease, but it is clear from detailed histopathologic studies that nonosteogenic mechanisms may also contribute to accrual of calcium in the valve[5,9] (Figure 3-15). Two mechanisms whereby this may occur are accumulation of calcium secondary to cell death and reductions in molecules that prevent ectopic calcium accumulation.

Cell Death as a Contributor to Nonosteogenic Calcification

In general, cell death can occur via apoptosis (in which the internal and external cell membranes are preserved so that the cell and its contents can be cleared by phagocytosis), necrosis (in which membrane lysis releases cellular contents and results in inflammation), or apoptosis followed by secondary necrosis.[135-137]

The exact mechanisms whereby cellular death promotes valve calcification have yet to be determined experimentally. Several key observations, however, lend insight into how this process may occur. First, calcified nodules that form following induction of cell death typically have a crystalline ultrastructure and lack live cells within the core of the calcified mass itself.[1] Second,

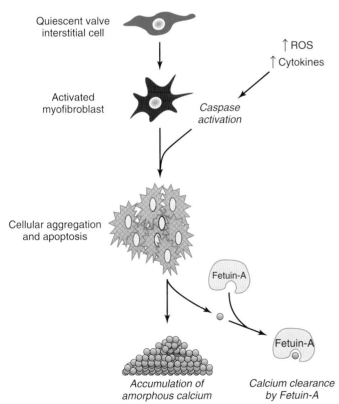

Quiescent valve interstitial cell

↑ROS
↑Cytokines

Activated myofibroblast

Caspase activation

Cellular aggregation and apoptosis

Fetuin-A

Fetuin-A

Accumulation of amorphous calcium

Calcium clearance by Fetuin-A

FIGURE 3-15 Potential mechanisms contributing to nonosteogenic valve calcification. Although mechanisms initiating nonosteogenic calcification have yet to be determined empirically, amorphous calcium accumulation is a common finding in humans with end-stage fibrocalcific aortic valve disease. Clearance of "excess" local calcium by fetuin-A is likely to be an important mechanism preventing accumulation of calcium in both early and late stages of fibrocalcific aortic valve disease, and it may be a reasonable therapeutic target in a subset of patients with nonosteogenic calcification. *ROS,* reactive oxygen species.

TGF-β1–induced calcification is strongly associated with caspase activation and programmed cell death/apoptosis in vitro, and co-treatment of cells with caspase inhibitors can markedly attenuate calcified nodule formation in vitro.[36] Although it is unclear whether cell death elicits VIC calcification through focal increases in the calcium/phosphorous product or via other mechanisms,[5] treatments such as caspase inhibitors and molecules that attenuate cell necrosis may prove to be efficacious treatments to slow progression of fibrocalcific aortic valve disease in many patients with nonosteogenic valve calcification.

Reduction of Fetuin-A Levels

Fetuin-A is a hepatic glycoprotein that is constitutively secreted into the circulation and serves to prevent accumulation of calcification at ectopic sites.[138-141] Evidence that fetuin-A is a major inhibitor of soft tissue calcification comes from the fetuin-A–deficient mouse, in which massive calcified deposits develop throughout the body,[142] and which shows dramatic increases in intimal plaque calcification when crossed with apolipoprotein E (ApoE)–deficient mice.[143] Furthermore, degradation of fetuin-A by matrix metalloproteinases significantly reduces its ability to attenuate calcium accumulation.[144] Clinically, reductions in serum fetuin-A levels are strongly associated with vascular and valvular calcification,[145] and may prove to be a useful biomarker for initiation of aggressive risk factor management in patients with early stages of valve disease.

Translation of Biological Findings to Therapeutic Interventions

In the development of novel therapeutic approaches to slow or potentially halt progression of valvular dysfunction in fibrocalcific aortic valve disease, it is likely that successful interventions will need to target both calcification and fibrosis in the stenotic aortic valve. This likelihood may require a multidrug approach, but several insights from preclinical and clinical studies are likely to help guide the field in the design of successful treatments for fibrocalcific aortic valve disease.

First, it would seem intuitive to most that targeting a specific risk factor, such as hypercholesterolemia, could slow progression of fibrocalcific aortic valve disease. When the risk factor is present, as is the case in animals or patients with severe fibrocalcific aortic valve disease, aggressive lipid lowering may slow or halt progression of valvular dysfunction.[6,32,146] It is important to note, however, that reducing blood lipids does not induce *regression* of valvular dysfunction under such conditions,[6,32] a lack that may be in part due to the absence of an effect of lipid lowering on valve fibrosis.[32] Furthermore, several large, randomized clinical trials have shown that statins do not effectively slow progression of fibrocalcific aortic valve disease in nonhypercholesterolemic patients,[147-149] suggesting that the off-target (or "pleiotropic") effects of statins are not sufficient to repress osteogenic or fibrogenic signaling in advanced fibrocalcific aortic valve disease in vivo. Collectively, these data would suggest that targeting a specific risk factor is most likely to be successful in well-defined subsets of patients (e.g., severely hypercholesterolemic patients) or when local activity of a signaling pathway associated with a risk factor is markedly upregulated (e.g., angiotensin II signaling/ACE activity in valve tissue).

Second, careful consideration of the by-products of treatments is critical for predicting success of most therapies. A common example can be found in treatments that attempt to reduce oxidative stress. Oxidative stress is a particularly attractive therapeutic target for slowing progression of fibrocalcific aortic valve disease in humans, because increases in oxidative stress are a nearly ubiquitous finding in valves from patients with fibrocalcific aortic valve disease,[78,85] and preclinical work suggested that reducing oxidative stress can slow progression of atherosclerosis.[150] When a superoxide dismutase mimetic was administered in a rabbit model of fibrocalcific aortic valve disease, however, progression of valve calcification and dysfunction was paradoxically *increased*.[85] This result is likely to be due to the fact that superoxide dismutase mimetics effectively reduce superoxide radicals but, in the process, increase hydrogen peroxide levels (which have been shown to accelerate vascular and valvular *calcification in vitro*).[85,151] Similarly, overexpression of NOS can effectively slow progression of atherosclerosis only when adequate cofactors (e.g., tetrahydrobiopterin [BH$_4$]) are available[152] because increases in epithelial NOS activity when the bioavailability of such cofactors is reduced result in increased free radical production as a result of uncoupled NOS activity. Prospectively, application of high-throughput "systems biology" approaches will probably be useful in the prediction of downstream/off-target side effects of novel therapeutics.

Finally, any treatment aimed at slowing the progression of valve calcification must not negatively affect skeletal/bone ossification. The vast majority of patients with fibrocalcific aortic valve disease are elderly, and emerging data suggest that many patients with this disease have lower bone mineral density than age-matched patients without valve disease.[153-155] Thus, treatments that may nondiscriminately reduce osteoblast activity in both cardiovascular and skeletal systems (e.g., many PPARγ agonists) may slow progression of fibrocalcific aortic valve disease but accelerate osteoporosis. Development of drugs that drive specific subcomponents of specific signaling cascades (e.g., the anti-inflammatory effects of PPARγ agonists) or preferentially activate signaling cascades in specific tissues may overcome such limitations.

REFERENCES

1. Mohler 3rd ER, Chawla MK, Chang AW, et al. Identification and characterization of calcifying valve cells from human and canine aortic valves. J Heart Valve Dis 1999;8:254–60.
2. Simionescu DT, Chen J, Jaeggli M, et al. Form follows function: advances in trilayered structure replication for aortic heart valve tissue engineering. J Healthc Eng 2012;3:179–202.
3. Leopold JA. Cellular mechanisms of aortic valve calcification. Circ Cardiovasc Interv 2012;5:605–14.
4. Freeman RV, Otto CM. Spectrum of calcific aortic valve disease: pathogenesis, disease progression, and treatment strategies. Circulation 2005;111:3316–26.
5. Miller JD, Weiss RM, Heistad DD. Calcific aortic valve stenosis: methods, models, and mechanisms. Circ Res 2011;108:1392–412.
6. Miller JD, Weiss RM, Serrano KM, et al. Lowering plasma cholesterol levels halts progression of aortic valve disease in mice. Circulation 2009;119:2693–701.
7. Otto CM, Kuusisto J, Reichenbach DD, et al. Characterization of the early lesion of 'degenerative' valvular aortic stenosis. histological and immunohistochemical studies. Circulation 1994;90:844–53.
8. Chen JH, Simmons CA. Cell-matrix interactions in the pathobiology of calcific aortic valve disease: critical roles for matricellular, matricrine, and matrix mechanics cues. Circ Res 2011;108:1510–24.
9. Mohler 3rd ER, Gannon F, Reynolds C, et al. Bone formation and inflammation in cardiac valves. Circulation 2001;103:1522–8.
10. Beckmann E, Grau JB, Sainger R, et al. Insights into the use of biomarkers in calcific aortic valve disease. J Heart Valve Dis 2010;19:441–52.
11. Messika-Zeitoun D, Bielak LF, Peyser PA, et al. Aortic valve calcification: determinants and progression in the population. Arterioscler Thromb Vasc Biol 2007;27:642–8.
12. Elmariah S, Mohler 3rd ER. The pathogenesis and treatment of the valvulopathy of aortic stenosis: beyond the seas. Curr Cardiol Rep 2010;12:125–32.
13. Cote C, Pibarot P, Despres JP, et al. Association between circulating oxidised low-throughput lipoprotein and fibrocalcific remodelling of the aortic valve in aortic stenosis. Heart 2008;94:1175–80.
14. Edep ME, Shirani J, Wolf P, et al. Matrix metalloproteinase expression in nonrheumatic aortic stenosis. Cardiovasc Pathol 2000;9:281–6.
15. Ankeny RF, Thourani VH, Weiss D, et al. Preferential activation of SMAD1/5/8 on the fibrosa endothelium in calcified human aortic valves—association with low bmp antagonists and SMAD6. PLoS One 2011;6:e20969.
16. Seya K, Yu Z, Kanemaru K, et al. Contribution of bone morphogenetic protein-2 to aortic valve calcification in aged rat. J Pharmacol Sci 2011;115:8–14.
17. Yanagawa B, Lovren F, Pan Y, et al. MiRNA-141 is a novel regulator of BMP-2-mediated calcification in aortic stenosis. J Thorac Cardiovasc Surg 2012;144:256–62.
18. Nagy JT, Foris G, Fulop Jr T, et al. Activation of the lipoxygenase pathway in the methionine enkephalin induced respiratory burst in human polymorphonuclear leukocytes. Life Sci 1988;42:2299–306.
19. Yang X, Meng X, Su X, et al. Bone morphogenic protein 2 induces Runx2 and osteopontin expression in human aortic valve interstitial cells: role of Smad1 and extracellular signal-regulated kinase 1/2. J Thorac Cardiovasc Surg 2009;138:1008–15.
20. Yu Z, Seya K, Daitoku K, et al. Tumor necrosis factor-alpha accelerates the calcification of human aortic valve interstitial cells obtained from patients with calcific aortic valve stenosis via the BMP2-DLX5 pathway. J Pharmacol Exp Ther 2011;337:16–23.
21. Simmons CA, Grant GR, Manduchi E, et al. Spatial heterogeneity of endothelial phenotypes correlates with side-specific vulnerability to calcification in normal porcine aortic valves. Circ Res 2005;96:792–9.
22. Massague J, Wotton D. Transcriptional control by the TGF-beta/Smad signaling system. EMBO J 2000;19:1745–54.
23. Heldin CH, Miyazono K, ten Dijke P. TGF-beta signalling from cell membrane to nucleus through Smad proteins. Nature 1997;390:465–71.
24. Galvin KM, Donovan MJ, Lynch CA, et al. A role for SMAD6 in development and homeostasis of the cardiovascular system. Nat Genet 2000;24:171–4.
25. Clevers H. Wnt/beta-catenin signaling in development and disease. Cell 2006;127:469–80.
26. Logan CY, Nusse R. The wnt signaling pathway in development and disease. Annu Rev Cell Dev Biol 2004;20:781–810.
27. Al-Aly Z, Shao JS, Lai CF, et al. Aortic msx2-wnt calcification cascade is regulated by TNF-alpha-dependent signals in diabetic ldlr-/- mice. Arterioscler Thromb Vasc Biol 2007;27:2589–96.
28. Alfieri CM, Cheek J, Chakraborty S, et al. Wnt signaling in heart valve development and osteogenic gene induction. Dev Biol 2010;338:127–35.
29. Caira FC, Stock SR, Gleason TG, et al. Human degenerative valve disease is associated with up-regulation of low-density lipoprotein receptor-related protein 5 receptor-mediated bone formation. J Am Coll Cardiol 2006;47:1707–12.
30. Chen JH, Chen WL, Sider KL, et al. β-Catenin mediates mechanically regulated, transforming growth factor-β1-induced myofibroblast differentiation of aortic valve interstitial cells. Arterioscler Thromb Vasc Biol 2011;31:590–7.
31. Rajamannan NM, Subramaniam M, Caira F, et al. Atorvastatin inhibits hypercholesterolemia-induced calcification in the aortic valves via the LRP5 receptor pathway. Circulation 2005;112:I229–34.
32. Miller JD, Weiss RM, Serrano KM, et al. Evidence for active regulation of pro-osteogenic signaling in advanced aortic valve disease. Arterioscler Thromb Vasc Biol 2010;30:2482–6.
33. Derynck R, Zhang YE. Smad-dependent and Smad-independent pathways in TGF-beta family signalling. Nature 2003;425:577–84.
34. Yip CY, Chen JH, Zhao R, et al. Calcification by valve interstitial cells is regulated by the stiffness of the extracellular matrix. Arterioscler Thromb Vasc Biol 2009;29:936–42.
35. Clark-Greuel JN, Connolly JM, Sorichillo E, et al. Transforming growth factor-beta1 mechanisms in aortic valve calcification: increased alkaline phosphatase and related events. Ann Thorac Surg 2007;83:946–53.
36. Jian B, Narula N, Li QY, et al. Progression of aortic valve stenosis: TGF-beta1 is present in calcified aortic valve cusps and promotes aortic valve interstitial cell calcification via apoptosis. Ann Thorac Surg 2003;75:457–65; discussion 465–456.
37. Helske S, Syvaranta S, Kupari M, et al. Possible role for mast cell-derived cathepsin g in the adverse remodelling of stenotic aortic valves. Eur Heart J 2006;27:1495–504.
38. Cushing MC, Liao JT, Anseth KS. Activation of valvular interstitial cells is mediated by transforming growth factor-beta1 interactions with matrix molecules. Matrix Biol 2005;24:428–37.
39. Balooch G, Balooch M, Nalla RK, et al. TGF-beta regulates the mechanical properties and composition of bone matrix. Proc Natl Acad Sci U S A 2005;102:18813–8.
40. Luo G, Ducy P, McKee MD, et al. Spontaneous calcification of arteries and cartilage in mice lacking matrix gla protein. Nature 1997;386:78–81.
41. Yao Y, Bennett BJ, Wang X, et al. Inhibition of bone morphogenetic proteins protects against atherosclerosis and vascular calcification. Circ Res 2010;107:485–94.
42. Wallin R, Cain D, Hutson SM, et al. Modulation of the binding of matrix Gla protein (MGP) to bone morphogenetic protein-2 (BMP-2). Thromb Haemost 2000;84:1039–44.
43. Wallin R, Cain D, Sane DC. Matrix Gla protein synthesis and gamma-carboxylation in the aortic vessel wall and proliferating vascular smooth muscle cells—a cell system which resembles the system in bone cells. Thromb Haemost 1999;82:1764–7.
44. Price PA, Fraser JD, Metz-Virca G. Molecular cloning of matrix gla protein: Implications for substrate recognition by the vitamin K-dependent gamma-carboxylase. Proc Natl Acad Sci U S A 1987;84:8335–9.
45. Price PA, Williamson MK. Primary structure of bovine matrix gla protein, a new vitamin K-dependent bone protein. J Biol Chem 1985;260:14971–5.
46. Price PA, Urist MR, Otawara Y. Matrix Gla protein, a new gamma-carboxyglutamic acid-containing protein which is associated with the organic matrix of bone. Biochem Biophys Res Commun 1983;117:765–71.
47. Yamamoto K, Yamamoto H, Yoshida K, et al. Prognostic factors for progression of early- and late-stage calcific aortic valve disease in Japanese: The Japanese Aortic Stenosis Study (JASS) retrospective analysis. Hypertens Res 2010;33:269–74.
48. Lerner RG, Aronow WS, Sekhri A, et al. Warfarin use and the risk of valvular calcification. J Thromb Haemost 2009;7:2023–7.
49. Danziger J. Vitamin K-dependent proteins, warfarin, and vascular calcification. Clin J Am Soc Nephrol 2008;3:1504–10.
50. Holden RM, Sanfilippo AS, Hopman WM, et al. Warfarin and aortic valve calcification in hemodialysis patients. J Nephrol 2007;20:417–22.
51. Liu C, Wan J, Yang Q, et al. Effects of atorvastatin on warfarin-induced aortic medial calcification and systolic blood pressure in rats. J Huazhong Univ Sci Technolog Med Sci 2008;28:535–8.
52. Schurgers LJ, Spronk HM, Soute BA, et al. Regression of warfarin-induced medial elastocalcinosis by high intake of vitamin K in rats. Blood 2007;109:2823–31.
53. Howe AM, Webster WS. Warfarin exposure and calcification of the arterial system in the rat. Int J Exp Pathol 2000;81:51–6.
54. Price PA, Faus SA, Williamson MK. Warfarin-induced artery calcification is accelerated by growth and vitamin d. Arterioscler Thromb Vasc Biol 2000;20:317–27.

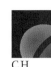

55. Price PA, Faus SA, Williamson MK. Warfarin causes rapid calcification of the elastic lamellae in rat arteries and heart valves. Arterioscler Thromb Vasc Biol 1998;18:1400–7.
56. Nguyen Dinh Cat A, Touyz RM. A new look at the renin-angiotensin system—focusing on the vascular system. Peptides 2011;32:2141–50.
57. Durante A, Peretto G, Laricchia A, et al. Role of the renin-angiotensin-aldosterone system in the pathogenesis of atherosclerosis. Curr Pharm Des 2012;18:981–1004.
58. Weir MR, Dzau VJ. The renin-angiotensin-aldosterone system: a specific target for hypertension management. Am J Hypertens 1999;12:205S-13S
59. Helske S, Lindstedt KA, Laine M, et al. Induction of local angiotensin II-producing systems in stenotic aortic valves. J Am Coll Cardiol 2004;44:1859–66.
60. Kitazono T, Padgett RC, Armstrong ML, et al. Evidence that angiotensin II is present in human monocytes. Circulation 1995;91:1129–34.
61. Potter DD, Sobey CG, Tompkins PK, et al. Evidence that macrophages in atherosclerotic lesions contain angiotensin II. Circulation 1998;98:800–7.
62. O'Brien KD, Probstfield JL, Caulfield MT, et al. Angiotensin-converting enzyme inhibitors and change in aortic valve calcium. Arch Intern Med 2005;165:858–62.
63. Arishiro K, Hoshiga M, Negoro N, et al. Angiotensin receptor-1 blocker inhibits atherosclerotic changes and endothelial disruption of the aortic valve in hypercholesterolemic rabbits. J Am Coll Cardiol 2007;49:1482–9.
64. Mehrabian M, Demer LL, Lusis AJ. Differential accumulation of intimal monocyte-macrophages relative to lipoproteins and lipofuscin corresponds to hemodynamic forces on cardiac valves in mice. Arterioscler Thromb 1991;11:947–57.
65. Kupreishvili K, Baidoshvili A, ter Weeme M, et al. Degeneration and atherosclerosis inducing increased deposition of type IIa secretory phospholipase A2, C-reactive protein and complement in aortic valves cause neutrophilic granulocyte influx. J Heart Valve Dis 2011;20:29–36.
66. ter Weeme M, Vonk AB, Kupreishvili K, et al. Activated complement is more extensively present in diseased aortic valves than naturally occurring complement inhibitors: a sign of ongoing inflammation. Eur J Clin Invest 2010;40:4–10.
67. Shuvy M, Ben Ya'acov A, Zolotarov L, et al. Beta glycosphingolipids suppress rank expression and inhibit natural killerT cell and CD8+ accumulation in alleviating aortic valve calcification. Int J Immunopathol Pharmacol 2009;22:911–8.
68. Isoda K, Matsuki T, Kondo H, et al. Deficiency of interleukin-1 receptor antagonist induces aortic valve disease in BALB/C mice. Arterioscler Thromb Vasc Biol 2010;30:708–15.
69. Cote N, Mahmut A, Bosse Y, et al. Inflammation is associated with the remodeling of calcific aortic valve disease. Inflammation 2013;36(3):573–81.
70. Lommi JI, Kovanen PT, Jauhiainen M, et al. High-density lipoproteins (HDL) are present in stenotic aortic valves and may interfere with the mechanisms of valvular calcification. Atherosclerosis 2011;219:538–44.
71. Mohty D, Pibarot P, Despres JP, et al. Association between plasma LDL particle size, valvular accumulation of oxidized ldl, and inflammation in patients with aortic stenosis. Arterioscler Thromb Vasc Biol 2008;28:187–93.
72. Kapadia SR, Yakoob K, Nader S, et al. Elevated circulating levels of serum tumor necrosis factor-alpha in patients with hemodynamically significant pressure and volume overload. J Am Coll Cardiol 2000;36:208–12.
73. Cecil DL, Terkeltaub RA. Arterial calcification is driven by rage in enpp1-/- mice. J Vasc Res 2010;48:227–35.
74. Gawdzik J, Mathew L, Kim G, et al. Vascular remodeling and arterial calcification are directly mediated by s100a12 (EN-RAGE) in chronic kidney disease. Am J Nephrol 2011;33:250–9.
75. Geroldi D, Falcone C, Emanuele E. Soluble receptor for advanced glycation end products: from disease marker to potential therapeutic target. Curr Med Chem 2006;13:1971–8.
76. Hofmann Bowman MA, Gawdzik J, Bukhari U, et al. S100a12 in vascular smooth muscle accelerates vascular calcification in apolipoprotein e-null mice by activating an osteogenic gene regulatory program. Arterioscler Thromb Vasc Biol 2011;31:337–44.
77. Li F, Cai Z, Chen F, et al. Pioglitazone attenuates progression of aortic valve calcification via down-regulating receptor for advanced glycation end products. Basic Res Cardiol 2012;107:306.
78. Miller JD, Chu Y, Brooks RM, et al. Dysregulation of antioxidant mechanisms contributes to increased oxidative stress in calcific aortic valvular stenosis in humans. J Am Coll Cardiol 2008;52:843–50.
79. Zhang H, Park Y, Wu J, et al. Role of TNF-alpha in vascular dysfunction. Clin Sci (Lond) 2009;116:219–30.
80. Csiszar A, Ungvari Z. Endothelial dysfunction and vascular inflammation in type 2 diabetes: interaction of AGE/RAGE and TNF-alpha signaling. Am J Physiol Heart Circ Physiol 2008;295:H475–6.
81. Warnock JN, Nanduri B, Pregonero Gamez CA, et al. Gene profiling of aortic valve interstitial cells under elevated pressure conditions: modulation of inflammatory gene networks. Int J Inflam 2011;2011:176412.
82. Lai CF, Shao JS, Behrmann A, et al. TNFR1-activated reactive oxidative species signals up-regulate osteogenic MSX2 programs in aortic myofibroblasts. Endocrinology 2012;153:3897–910.
83. Lassegue B, Griendling KK. Nadph oxidases: functions and pathologies in the vasculature. Arterioscler Thromb Vasc Biol 2010;30:653–61.
84. Rivera J, Sobey CG, Walduck AK, et al. NOX isoforms in vascular pathophysiology: insights from transgenic and knockout mouse models. Redox Rep 2010;15:50–63.
85. Liberman M, Bassi E, Martinatti MK, et al. Oxidant generation predominates around calcifying foci and enhances progression of aortic valve calcification. Arterioscler Thromb Vasc Biol 2008;28:463–70.
86. Branchetti E, Sainger R, Poggio P, et al. Antioxidant enzymes reduce DNA damage and early activation of valvular interstitial cells in aortic valve sclerosis. Arterioscler Thromb Vasc Biol 2013;33:e66–74.
87. Casalena G, Daehn I, Bottinger E. Transforming growth factor-beta, bioenergetics, and mitochondria in renal disease. Semin Nephrol 2012;32:295–303.
88. Csiszar A, Lehoux S, Ungvari Z. Hemodynamic forces, vascular oxidative stress, and regulation of Bmp-2/4 expression. Antioxid Redox Signal 2009;11:1683–97.
89. Jain M, Rivera S, Monclus EA, et al. Mitochondrial reactive oxygen species regulate transforming growth factor-beta signaling. J Biol Chem 2013;288:770–7.
90. Liberman M, Johnson RC, Handy DE, et al. Bone morphogenetic protein-2 activates nadph oxidase to increase endoplasmic reticulum stress and human coronary artery smooth muscle cell calcification. Biochem Biophys Res Commun 2011;413:436–41.
91. Byon CH, Javed A, Dai Q, et al. Oxidative stress induces vascular calcification through modulation of the osteogenic transcription factor Runx2by AKT signaling. J Biol Chem 2008;283:15319–27.
92. Byon CH, Sun Y, Chen J, et al. Runx2-upregulated receptor activator of nuclear factor κB ligand in calcifying smooth muscle cells promotes migration and osteoclastic differentiation of macrophages. Arterioscler Thromb Vasc Biol 2011;31:1387–396.
93. Anderson TJ. Nitric oxide, atherosclerosis and the clinical relevance of endothelial dysfunction. Heart Fail Rev 2003;8:71–86.
94. Shimokawa H. Primary endothelial dysfunction: atherosclerosis. J Mol Cell Cardiol 1999;31:23–37.
95. Channon KM, Qian H, George SE. Nitric oxide synthase in atherosclerosis and vascular injury: insights from experimental gene therapy. Arterioscler Thromb Vasc Biol 2000;20:1873–81.
96. Rajamannan NM, Subramaniam M, Stock SR, et al. Atorvastatin inhibits calcification and enhances nitric oxide synthase production in the hypercholesterolaemic aortic valve. Heart 2005;91:806–10.
97. Aicher D, Urbich C, Zeiher A, et al. Endothelial nitric oxide synthase in bicuspid aortic valve disease. Ann Thorac Surg 2007;83:1290–4.
98. Fukai T, Ushio-Fukai M. Superoxide dismutases: role in redox signaling, vascular function, and diseases. Antioxid Redox Signal 2011;15:1583–606.
99. Doughan AK, Harrison DG, Dikalov SI. Molecular mechanisms of angiotensin ii-mediated mitochondrial dysfunction: linking mitochondrial oxidative damage and vascular endothelial dysfunction. Circ Res 2008;102:488–96.
100. Stasch JP, Pacher P, Evgenov OV. Soluble guanylate cyclase as an emerging therapeutic target in cardiopulmonary disease. Circulation 2011;123:2263–73.
101. McNeill E, Channon KM. The role of tetrahydrobiopterin in inflammation and cardiovascular disease. Thromb Haemost 2012;108:832–9.
102. Kennedy JA, Hua X, Mishra K, et al. Inhibition of calcifying nodule formation in cultured porcine aortic valve cells by nitric oxide donors. Eur J Pharmacol 2009;602:28–35.
103. Rajamannan NM. Oxidative-mechanical stress signals stem cell niche mediated lrp5 osteogenesis in enos(-/-) null mice. J Cell Biochem 2012;113:1623–34.
104. Kawai M, Sousa KM, MacDougald OA, et al. The many facets of ppargamma: novel insights for the skeleton. Am J Physiol Endocrinol Metab 2010;299:E3–9.
105. Takada I, Kouzmenko AP, Kato S. Wnt and PPARgamma signaling in osteoblastogenesis and adipogenesis. Nat Rev Rheumatol 2009;5:442–7.
106. Chu Y, Lund DD, Weiss RM, et al. Pioglitazone attenuates valvular calcification induced by hypercholesterolemia. Arterioscler Thromb Vasc Biol 2013;33:523–32.
107. Garg V, Muth AN, Ransom JF, et al. Mutations in notch1 cause aortic valve disease. Nature 2005;437:270–4.
108. Nigam V, Srivastava D. Notch1 represses osteogenic pathways in aortic valve cells. J Mol Cell Cardiol 2009;47:828–34.
109. Hofmann JJ, Briot A, Enciso J, et al. Endothelial deletion of murine JAG1 leads to valve calcification and congenital heart defects associated with alagille syndrome. Development 2012;139:4449–60.
110. Jian B, Jones PL, Li Q, et al. Matrix metalloproteinase-2 is associated with tenascin-cC in calcific aortic stenosis. Am J Pathol 2001;159:321–7.
111. Kaden JJ, Dempfle CE, Grobholz R, et al. Inflammatory regulation of extracellular matrix remodeling in calcific aortic valve stenosis. Cardiovasc Pathol 2005;14:80–7.
112. Kaden JJ, Dempfle CE, Grobholz R, et al. Interleukin-1 beta promotes matrix metalloproteinase expression and cell proliferation in calcific aortic valve stenosis. Atherosclerosis 2003;170:205–11.
113. Kaden JJ, Vocke DC, Fischer CS, et al. Expression and activity of matrix metalloproteinase-2 in calcific aortic stenosis. Z Kardiol 2004;93:124–30.
114. Fondard O, Detaint D, Iung B, et al. Extracellular matrix remodelling in human aortic valve disease: the role of matrix metalloproteinases and their tissue inhibitors. Eur Heart J 2005;26:1333–41.
115. Helske S, Syvaranta S, Lindstedt KA, et al. Increased expression of elastolytic cathepsins S, K, and V and their inhibitor cystatin c in stenotic aortic valves. Arterioscler Thromb Vasc Biol 2006;26:1791–8.
116. Pacifici R, Carano A, Santoro SA, et al. Bone matrix constituents stimulate interleukin-1 release from human blood mononuclear cells. J Clin Invest 1991;87:221–8.
117. Qin X, Corriere MA, Matrisian LM, et al. Matrix metalloproteinase inhibition attenuates aortic calcification. Arterioscler Thromb Vasc Biol 2006;26:1510–6.
118. Aikawa E, Aikawa M, Libby P, et al. Arterial and aortic valve calcification abolished by elastolytic cathepsin s deficiency in chronic renal disease. Circulation 2009;119:1785–94.
119. de Ruijter AJ, van Gennip AH, Caron HN, et al. Histone deacetylases (HDACs): Characterization of the classical HDAC family. Biochem J 2003;370:737–49.
120. Schroeder TM, Kahler RA, Li X, et al. Histone deacetylase 3 interacts with Runx2 to repress the osteocalcin promoter and regulate osteoblast differentiation. J Biol Chem 2004;279:41998–2007.
121. Stein S, Schafer N, Breitenstein A, et al. Sirt1 reduces endothelial activation without affecting vascular function in apoE-/- mice. Aging (Albany NY) 2010;2:353–60.
122. Yang B, Zwaans BM, Eckersdorff M, et al. The sirtuin SIRT6 deacetylates H3 K56Ac in vivo to promote genomic stability. Cell Cycle 2009;8:2662–3.
123. Yuan J, Pu M, Zhang Z, et al. Histone H3-K56 acetylation is important for genomic stability in mammals. Cell Cycle 2009;8:1747–53.
124. Chua KF, Mostoslavsky R, Lombard DB, et al. Mammalian SIRT1 limits replicative life span in response to chronic genotoxic stress. Cell Metab 2005;2:67–76.

125. Baylin SB, Esteller M, Rountree MR, et al. Aberrant patterns of DNA methylation, chromatin formation and gene expression in cancer. Hum Mol Genet 2001;10:687–92.

126. Jaenisch R, Bird A. Epigenetic regulation of gene expression: how the genome integrates intrinsic and environmental signals. Nat Genet 2003;33(Suppl):245–54.

127. Montes de Oca A, Madueno JA, Martinez-Moreno JM, et al. High-phosphate-induced calcification is related to SM22alpha promoter methylation in vascular smooth muscle cells. J Bone Miner Res 2010;25:1996–2005.

128. Satta J, Melkko J, Pollanen R, et al. Progression of human aortic valve stenosis is associated with tenascin-C expression. J Am Coll Cardiol 2002;39:96–101.

129. Macri L, Silverstein D, Clark RA. Growth factor binding to the pericellular matrix and its importance in tissue engineering. Adv Drug Deliv Rev 2007;59:1366–81.

130. Engler AJ, Sen S, Sweeney HL, et al. Matrix elasticity directs stem cell lineage specification. Cell 2006;126:677–89.

131. Merryman WD, Lukoff HD, Long RA, et al. Synergistic effects of cyclic tension and transforming growth factor-beta1 on the aortic valve myofibroblast. Cardiovasc Pathol 2007;16:268–76.

132. Merryman WD, Youn I, Lukoff HD, et al. Correlation between heart valve interstitial cell stiffness and transvalvular pressure: implications for collagen biosynthesis. Am J Physiol Heart Circ Physiol 2006;290:H224–231.

133. Carruthers CA, Alfieri CM, Joyce EM, et al. Gene expression and collagen fiber micromechanical interactions of the semilunar heart valve interstitial cell. Cell Mol Bioeng 2012;5:254–65.

134. Thayer P, Balachandran K, Rathan S, et al. The effects of combined cyclic stretch and pressure on the aortic valve interstitial cell phenotype. Ann Biomed Eng 2011;39:1654–67.

135. Bonfoco E, Krainc D, Ankarcrona M, et al. Apoptosis and necrosis: two distinct events induced, respectively, by mild and intense insults with N-methyl-D-aspartate or nitric oxide/superoxide in cortical cell cultures. Proc Natl Acad Sci U S A 1995;92:7162–6.

136. Fiers W, Beyaert R, Declercq W, et al. More than one way to die: apoptosis, necrosis and reactive oxygen damage. Oncogene 1999;18:7719–30.

137. Kanduc D, Mittelman A, Serpico R, et al. Cell death: apoptosis versus necrosis (review). Int J Oncol 2002;21:165–70.

138. Mori K, Emoto M, Inaba M. Fetuin-a and the cardiovascular system. Adv Clin Chem 2012;56:175–95.

139. Mori K, Emoto M, Inaba M. Fetuin-a: a multifunctional protein. Recent Pat Endocr Metab Immune Drug Discov 2011;5:124–46.

140. Jahnen-Dechent W, Heiss A, Schafer C, et al. Fetuin-a regulation of calcified matrix metabolism. Circ Res 2011;108:1494–509.

141. Cozzolino M, Brenna I, Ciceri P, et al. Vascular calcification in chronic kidney disease: Aa changing scenario. J Nephrol 2011;24(Suppl 18):S3–10.

142. Schafer C, Heiss A, Schwarz A, et al. The serum protein alpha 2-Heremans-Schmid glycoprotein/fetuin-a is a systemically acting inhibitor of ectopic calcification. J Clin Invest 2003;112:357–66.

143. Westenfeld R, Schafer C, Kruger T, et al. Fetuin-a protects against atherosclerotic calcification in CKD. J Am Soc Nephrol 2009;20:1264–74.

144. Schure R, Costa KD, Rezaei R, et al. Impact of matrix metalloproteinases on inhibition of mineralization by fetuin. J Periodontal Res 2013;48:357–66.

145. Burke AP, Kolodgie FD, Virmani R. Fetuin-a, a valve calcification, and diabetes: what do we understand? Circulation 2007;115:2464–7.

146. Moura LM, Ramos SF, Zamorano JL, et al. Rosuvastatin affecting aortic valve endothelium to slow the progression of aortic stenosis. J Am Coll Cardiol 2007;49:554–61.

147. Chan KL, Teo K, Dumesnil JG, et al. Effect of lipid lowering with rosuvastatin on progression of aortic stenosis: results of the Aortic Stenosis Progression Observation: measuring effects of rosuvastatin (astronomer) trial. Circulation 2010;121:306–14.

148. Cowell SJ, Newby DE, Prescott RJ, et al. A randomized trial of intensive lipid-lowering therapy in calcific aortic stenosis. N Engl J Med 2005;352:2389–97.

149. Rossebo AB, Pedersen TR, Boman K, et al. Intensive lipid lowering with simvastatin and ezetimibe in aortic stenosis. N Engl J Med 2008;359:1343–56.

150. Barry-Lane PA, Patterson C, van der Merwe M, et al. P47phox is required for atherosclerotic lesion progression in apoe(-/-) mice. J Clin Invest 2001;108:1513–22.

151. Yang H, Roberts LJ, Shi MJ, et al. Retardation of atherosclerosis by overexpression of catalase or both Cu/Zn-superoxide dismutase and catalase in mice lacking apolipoprotein E. Circ Res 2004;95:1075–81.

152. Ozaki M, Kawashima S, Yamashita T, et al. Overexpression of endothelial nitric oxide synthase accelerates atherosclerotic lesion formation in apoe-deficient mice. J Clin Invest 2002;110:331–40.

153. Hjortnaes J, Butcher J, Figueiredo JL, et al. Arterial and aortic valve calcification inversely correlates with osteoporotic bone remodelling: a role for inflammation. Eur Heart J 2010;31:1975–84.

154. Skolnick AH, Osranek M, Formica P, et al. Osteoporosis treatment and progression of aortic stenosis. Am J Cardiol 2009;104:122–4.

155. Dweck MR, Newby DE. Osteoporosis is a major confounder in observational studies investigating bisphosphonate therapy in aortic stenosis. J Am Coll Cardiol 2012;60:1027; author reply 1027.

156. Drolet MC, Roussel E, Deshaies Y, et al. A high fat/high carbohydrate diet induces aortic valve disease in C57BL/6J mice. J Am Coll Cardiol 2006;47:850–5.

157. Tanaka K, Sata M, Fukuda D, et al. Age-associated aortic stenosis in apolipoprotein E-deficient mice. J Am Coll Cardiol 2005;46:134–41.

158. Aikawa E, Nahrendorf M, Sosnovik D, et al. Multimodality molecular imaging identifies proteolytic and osteogenic activities in early aortic valve disease. Circulation 2007;115:377–86.

159. Shao JS, Cheng SL, Charlton-Kachigian N, et al. Teriparatide (human parathyroid hormone (1–34)) inhibits osteogenic vascular calcification in diabetic low density lipoprotein receptor-deficient mice. J Biol Chem 2003;278:50195–202.

160. Weiss RM, Ohashi M, Miller JD, et al. Calcific aortic valve stenosis in old hypercholesterolemic mice. Circulation 2006;114:2065–9.

161. Barrick CJ, Roberts RB, Rojas M, et al. Reduced EGFR causes abnormal valvular differentiation leading to calcific aortic stenosis and left ventricular hypertrophy in C57BL/6J but not 129S1/SVIMJ mice. Am J Physiol Heart Circ Physiol 2009;297:H65–75.

162. Lee TC, Zhao YD, Courtman DW, et al. Abnormal aortic valve development in mice lacking endothelial nitric oxide synthase. Circulation 2000;101:2345–8.

163. Luna-Zurita L, Prados B, Grego-Bessa J, et al. Integration of a notch-dependent mesenchymal gene program and bmp2-driven cell invasiveness regulates murine cardiac valve formation. J Clin Invest 2010;120:3493–507.

164. Tkatchenko TV, Moreno-Rodriguez RA, Conway SJ, et al. Lack of periostin leads to suppression of Notch1 signaling and calcific aortic valve disease. Physiol Genomics 2009;39:160–8.

165. Hakuno D, Kimura N, Yoshioka M, et al. Periostin advances atherosclerotic and rheumatic cardiac valve degeneration by inducing angiogenesis and MMP production in humans and rodents. J Clin Invest 2010;120:2292–306.

166. Yoshioka M, Yuasa S, Matsumura K, et al. Chondromodulin-I maintains cardiac valvular function by preventing angiogenesis. Nat Med 2006;12:1151–9.

167. Cimini M, Boughner DR, Ronald JA, et al. Development of aortic valve sclerosis in a rabbit model of atherosclerosis: an immunohistochemical and histological study. J Heart Valve Dis 2005;14:365–75.

168. Cuniberti LA, Stutzbach PG, Guevara E, et al. Development of mild aortic valve stenosis in a rabbit model of hypertension. J Am Coll Cardiol 2006;47:2303–9.

169. Drolet MC, Couet J, Arsenault M. Development of aortic valve sclerosis or stenosis in rabbits: role of cholesterol and calcium. J Heart Valve Dis 2008;17:381–7.

170. Gkizas S, Koumoundourou D, Sirinian X, et al. Aldosterone receptor blockade inhibits degenerative processes in the early stage of calcific aortic stenosis. Eur J Pharmacol 2010;642:107–12.

171. Hekimian G, Passefort S, Louedec L, et al. High-cholesterol + vitamin D2 regimen: A questionable in-vivo experimental model of aortic valve stenosis. J Heart Valve Dis 2009;18:152–8.

172. Marechaux S, Corseaux D, Vincentelli A, et al. Identification of tissue factor in experimental aortic valve sclerosis. Cardiovasc Pathol 2009;18:67–76.

173. Ngo DT, Stafford I, Kelly DJ, et al. Vitamin D(2) supplementation induces the development of aortic stenosis in rabbits: interactions with endothelial function and thioredoxin-interacting protein. Eur J Pharmacol 2008;590:290–6.

174. Ngo DT, Stafford I, Sverdlov AL, et al. Ramipril retards development of aortic valve stenosis in a rabbit model: mechanistic considerations. Br J Pharmacol 2011;162:722–32.

175. Rajamannan NM, Sangiorgi G, Springett M, et al. Experimental hypercholesterolemia induces apoptosis in the aortic valve. J Heart Valve Dis 2001;10:371–4.

176. Rajamannan NM, Subramaniam M, Springett M, et al. Atorvastatin inhibits hypercholesterolemia-induced cellular proliferation and bone matrix production in the rabbit aortic valve. Circulation 2002;105:2660–5.

177. Speidl WS, Cimmino G, Ibanez B, et al. Recombinant apolipoprotein A-I Milano rapidly reverses aortic valve stenosis and decreases leaflet inflammation in an experimental rabbit model. Eur Heart J 2010;31:2049–57.

178. Zeng W, Chen W, Leng X, et al. Chronic angiotensin-(1-7) administration improves vascular remodeling after angioplasty through the regulation of the TGF-beta/Smad signaling pathway in rabbits. Biochem Biophys Res Commun 2009;389:138–44.

179. Guerraty MA, Grant GR, Karanian JW, et al. Hypercholesterolemia induces side-specific phenotypic changes and peroxisome proliferator-activated receptor-gamma pathway activation in swine aortic valve endothelium. Arterioscler Thromb Vasc Biol 2010;30:225–31.

CHAPTER 4

Clinical and Genetic Risk Factors for Calcific Valve Disease

David S. Owens and Kevin D. O'Brien

Key Points

- Calcific aortic valve disease (CAVD) is a common feature of aging that is regulated by active biologic processes.
- Early-stage CAVD shares important similarities with atherosclerosis and vascular calcification, including cardiovascular risk factors.
- Risk factors for CAVD initiation and progression may be age and stage specific.
- Atherosclerosis risk factors are associated weakly, if at all, with progression to late-stage CAVD.
- Randomized clinical trials of statin therapy in later-stage CAVD have not shown benefit in slowing progression of valve disease or delaying need for valve replacement.
- The presence of aortic valve calcium is a marker of increased cardiovascular risk across a wide range of age and ethnicities.

Calcific aortic valve disease, defined by aortic valve leaflet thickening and calcification, is a common feature of aging, being present in nearly 25% of individuals older than 65 years, and in more than 40% of individuals more than 75 years of age.[1] Because of its high prevalence among the elderly, CAVD was initially thought to be a degenerative process due to wear and tear of fragile leaflets. However, contemporary research has demonstrated CAVD to be an active biologic process marked by lipoprotein deposition, inflammatory cell infiltration, renin-angiotensin system activation, and calcium deposition (further discussed in Chapter 3).

To date, no lifestyle modifications or medical therapies have been shown to slow CAVD initiation or progression, and the mainstays of therapy remain careful observation and timely procedural intervention with surgical or transcutaneous aortic valve replacement (AVR) at the onset of valve-related symptoms.[2,3] CAVD is one of the most common indications for cardiac surgery, with approximately 75,000 AVR procedures performed annually in the United States.

CAVD is traditionally classified into two functional stages. Aortic sclerosis—early-stage disease—is marked by initial calcium deposition that is insufficient to impede blood flow across the valve. This stage may have an extremely long latent period, with slow progression over decades. Aortic stenosis—later-stage disease—is demarcated by the onset of measurable hemodynamic obstruction.

This chapter focuses on the clinical and genetic risk factors for valve calcification across the full disease spectrum, incorporating data from observational and epidemiologic studies and clinical trials. The relationship between valve calcification and nonvalvular clinical outcomes is also discussed.

Methods of Detection

On a clinical basis, CAVD is often first detected incidentally by means of noninvasive imaging techniques, such as echocardiography and computed tomography (CT). Aortic sclerosis appears on echocardiography as thickened leaflets with focal, echo-bright nodules but relatively preserved leaflet excursion. Because transvalvular flow remains at near-normal velocity, only semiquantitative assessment of aortic sclerosis severity can be performed. This problem has hampered research into the determinants of calcium and fibrosis progression in the earliest stages. In contrast, as valve calcification and fibrosis progress and begin to impair leaflet excursion, transvalvular velocity begins to increase, making transvalvular velocity a practical, noninvasive measure of disease progression. For this reason, clinical investigations into the determinants of CAVD progression have focused on this "echocardiographically amenable" but inherently late stage of the disease.

In contrast, CT is well validated as a modality for assessing CAVD presence and severity, particularly in the earlier disease stage.[4-6] Although its clinical role is limited because CT cannot assess the hemodynamic sequelae of valve calcification, it remains a powerful research tool. With use of the Agatston method, which estimates calcium volume and density from voxel intensity,[7] CT allows quantitative assessment of calcium burden in all stages of disease. Moreover, CT is relatively inexpensive and easily acquired and has been incorporated into many large epidemiologic studies. Modern, high-resolution CT technology may also permit assessment of valve morphology. Figure 4-1 shows the appearance of aortic stenosis (AS) on both echocardiography and CT.

Bicuspid Aortic Valves

Bicuspid aortic valve (BAV) disease—valve dysgenesis marked by the presence of two rather than three valve leaflets—is the most common congenital heart defect. It is present in 0.5% to 2% of the general population, with a 3:1 male predominance. BAV disease may result in perturbation in transvalvular flow in absence of secondary calcification. However, its association with other vascular structural abnormalities, including thoracic aortic aneurysm and aortic coarctation, suggests that largely unidentified genetic defects may underlie the pathogenesis of many cases of BAV.

Although valvular interventions are occasionally necessary in childhood, adults with BAV are at risk for early valve calcification, clinically significant AS, and surgical valve replacement. The importance of BAV in CAVD pathogenesis was demonstrated by rigorous, pathologic analyses of explanted aortic valves (Figure 4-2).[8,9] In a series of 932 patients undergoing AVR, Roberts et al[9] estimated that nearly 50% had a BAV disease and that patients with BAV underwent AVR approximately 2 decades earlier than those with normal trileaflet valves. BAV was present in about 62% of patients undergoing AVR who were aged 50 to 70 years, but in only 37% of those older than 70 years. An earlier, small case series of 43 patients found a 42% prevalence of BAV among surgically resected aortic valves.[10]

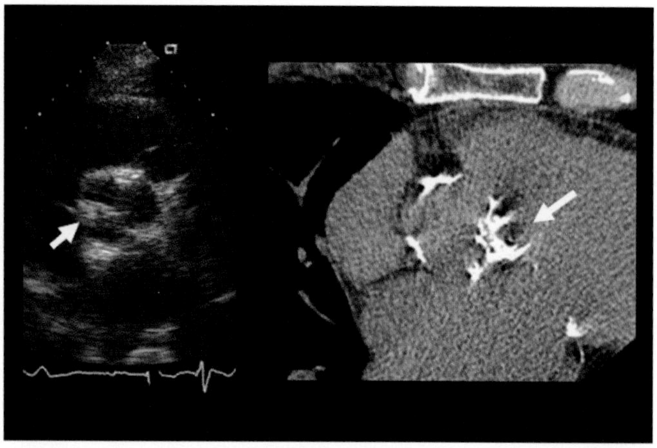

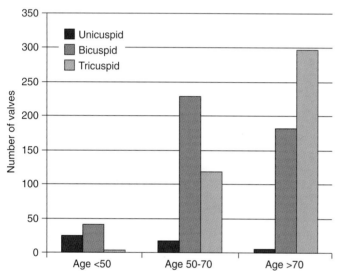

FIGURE 4-1 Aortic valve calcification. Depiction of a patient with severe aortic stenosis, showing the appearance of calcium on both echocardiography (*left*) and computed tomography (*right*). The regions of valvular calcium are shown by the *white arrows*. Mitral annular calcium is also present.

FIGURE 4-2 Valve morphology among subjects undergoing aortic valve replacement, classified by age. *(Data from Roberts WC, Ko JM. Frequency by decades of unicuspid, bicuspid, and tricuspid aortic valves in adults having isolated aortic valve replacement for aortic stenosis, with or without associated aortic regurgitation. Circulation 2005;111:920–5.)*

TABLE 4-1	General Summary of Strength of Associations Seen in Observational and Epidemiologic Studies of Clinical Risk Factors and Calcific Aortic Valve Disease		
	CAVD Analyses		
	CROSS-SECTIONAL	**INCIDENT**	**PROGRESSION**
Age	+++	+++	+++
Male gender	++/–	++	0
Height	++	++	0
BMI	++	++	0
Hypertension	++	++	0
Diabetes	+++	+++	0
Metabolic syndrome	++	++	+
Dyslipidemia	++	++	0
Smoking	++	++	+
Renal dysfunction	+	0	0
Inflammatory markers	+	0	0
Phosphorus	++	0	n/a
Calcium levels	0	0	n/a
Baseline calcium score	n/a	n/a	+++

+, Weak positive association; ++, modest positive association; +++, strong positive association; –, weak negative association; 0, no association seen; n/a, insufficient data available.

that genetic abnormalities may underlie the BAV phenotype and early valve calcification.

Clinical Risk Factors

Because of challenges associated with developing practical and representative animal models for CAVD, much of our knowledge about CAVD risk factors has arisen from observational studies using hospital registries and population investigations. Here a caveat is in order. Because valve calcium is often subclinical and often only incidentally detected, hospital or echocardiography laboratory databases may be prone to a selection bias, with over-representation of individuals with high cardiovascular risk. On the other hand, most population-based epidemiologic investigations were designed to focus on coronary artery disease risk and outcomes. Analyses of valve calcium risks have often been post hoc and dependent on previously collected coronary risk factor data. A shared limitation of both hospital- and population-based observational studies is the challenge of inferring causality from either cross-sectional or prospective associations.

This limitation aside, observational and epidemiologic studies have provided important insights into the risk factors for CAVD in varied stages. The earliest of these studies focused on cross-sectional risk associations in subjects with end-stage CAVD, whereas later studies have utilized CT to identify risk associations in earlier-stage disease. In general, traditional cardiovascular risk factors have shown strong associations with the presence of CAVD and incident CAVD but weak associations with CAVD progression (summarized in Table 4-1). The following discussion summarizes the major findings.

Older Age

CAVD primarily affects the elderly, and the prevalence of CAVD increases with advancing age. In the Cardiovascular Health Study,

Early family studies suggested that BAV disease may have a genetic basis. Initial reports of familial clustering prompted detailed family screening studies, which showed that approximately 9% of first-degree relatives of patients with BAV also had BAV morphology.[11,12] From these studies, it was estimated that the "heritability factor" for BAV disease was approximately 89%, suggesting a strong genetic basis with low phenotypic penetrance. Subsequent linkage analyses identified possible loci at 18q, 5q, and 13q, but exact genes were not identified.[13]

In a landmark study, Garg et al[14] studied a large family that had both highly penetrant BAV disease and other congenital heart abnormalities. Using linkage-guided gene sequencing, the researchers identified a stop mutation in the NOTCH1 gene. This result was further validated in an independent study of a BAV disease family, in whom a NOTCH1 frameshift mutation was then identified. NOTCH1 is highly expressed in aortic valve development and normally suppresses Runx2, a transcription factor that regulates osteoblastogenesis. Although mutations in NOTCH1 are extremely rare in the population, explaining only a small portion of BAV and CAVD, this proof-of-concept discovery demonstrates

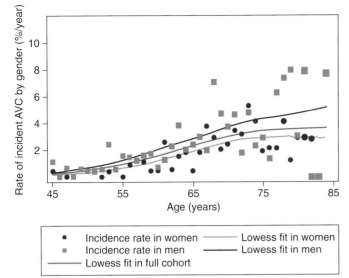

FIGURE 4-3 Incidence rate of new aortic valve calcium (AVC) by age. Data over a median follow-up of 2.7 years are shown for the 5142 participants in the Multi-Ethnic Study of Atherosclerosis who were free of baseline AVC. (The size of the scatter points is weighted for the number at risk in each age category.) A marked increase in the AVC incidence rate is seen with advancing age. (*From Owens DS, Katz R, Takasu J, et al. Incidence and progression of aortic valve calcium in the Multi-ethnic Study of Atherosclerosis [MESA]. Am J Cardiol 2010;105:701–8.*)

CAVD prevalence was 21% in subjects 65 to 74 years old, 38% in those 75 to 84 years old, and 52% in those 85 years or older.[1] Longitudinal analyses from the Multi-ethnic Study of Atherosclerosis (MESA) show not only that this increasing prevalence is due to accumulation of cases but also that the rate of new ("incident") CAVD also rises substantially with age. For example, the estimated CAVD incidence rate is 0.6% per year in subjects 50 to 54 years old and 3.5% per year in those 70 to 79 years old (Figure 4-3).[15]

Multiple studies have used multivariate regression to account for potential confounding factors. Nearly universally, age has been found to be an independent predictor of CAVD risk throughout all stages, including prevalent and incident disease as well as disease progression. The exact reasons for this strong association remain incompletely understood. On the one hand, age serves as a surrogate measure for duration of exposure to risk factors. On the other hand, longitudinal analyses (in which exposure to risk factors is age independent) suggest that age may be a marker of other, unmeasured factors. It is intriguing to consider whether biologic mechanisms implicated in the aging process, such as mitochondrial uncoupling and oxidative stress or epigenetic modification and DNA damage, may play a causal role in CAVD pathogenesis.

Age also has been shown to be an important modifier of the association between traditional cardiovascular risk factors and CAVD. Owens et al[16] demonstrated that age significantly modified the low-density lipoprotein cholesterol (LDL)–associated risk of CAVD, with LDL being a risk factor in younger but not older individuals within the MESA population. Similar findings were seen in a cohort of patients with AS undergoing AVR, in which elderly subjects had less atherogenic lipid profiles in general.[17] In a later study, a significant interaction between age and the metabolic syndrome was shown in patients with severe AS, such that the effect of metabolic syndrome was stronger in younger patients.[18] Overall, these findings suggest weaker influences of traditional cardiovascular risk factors in older subjects, which in turn has two implications. First, treatment of cardiovascular risk factors to prevent CAVD may be most beneficial in younger patients; and second, other mechanisms may be important in older individuals, in whom the rate of incident CAVD is the highest.

Male Gender

Gender influences many aspects of CAVD. Bicuspid aortic valves are nearly three times more common among men than women, and BAVs account for about 50% of aortic valve replacements. If all other factors were equal, these facts would translate into a nearly 3/2 male:female ratio among subjects undergoing AVR. Most studies examining the influence of gender on CAVD have not accounted for valve phenotype, but this problem is likely not as significant in analyses of earlier-stage CAVD, in which trileaflet valves account for the vast majority of cases.

On multivariate analyses, most studies have identified male gender to be associated with CAVD in both early-stage and late-stage disease. In the MESA, which utilized CT to identify early subclinical disease, male gender conferred a 1.87-fold (95% confidence interval (CI) 1.31-2.69) higher odds of valve calcium after adjustment for traditional cardiovascular risk factors.[19] One study, however, found a strong independent association between aortic sclerosis identified by echocardiography and female gender.[20]

Race/Ethnicity

Few studies have examined the relationship between CAVD and race/ethnicity, and the majority of clinical data surrounding CAVD is derived from Caucasian populations. One study examining interracial differences in BAVs demonstrated a significantly higher prevalence of BAVs among Caucasians than among African-Americans with a single-center cohort (1.1% versus 0.2%; *P* = 0.001).[21] The MESA used targeted oversampling of ethnic minority groups in its recruitment in order to enhance statistical power. In the MESA population, the baseline prevalence among the race/ethnic groups was 14% among white, 7% among Chinese, 11% among black, and 12% among Hispanic participants.[16] However, after baseline cardiovascular risk factors were accounted for, there was no significant difference among these race/ethnic groups in either cross-sectional or incident analyses.[16,19] However, on pathologic analysis of explanted stenotic aortic valves, African-Americans showed greater likelihood of heterotopic ossification (bone formation). Whether this is due to delayed surgical intervention from socioeconomic factors or an inherent tendency for bone formation is unclear.[22]

Anthropometry

Studies have accounted for body size in various manners, including assessment of height, weight, body mass index (BMI), and waist circumference. The relationship between height and CAVD appears complex. Within the Cardiovascular Health Study (CHS), greater height was associated with prevalent aortic sclerosis,[1] but short stature was associated with progression to AS.[23] Height may influence aortic pulse wave dynamics, thus altering shear forces across the aortic valve.

Body mass index has been more universally associated with CAVD in varied stages. Whether BMI is directly associated with CAVD, or whether it is mediated by dysglycemia and/or insulin resistance, is uncertain.

Hypertension

Multiple case-control, population, and prospective studies have shown an association between hypertension and CAVD. Linefsky et al[24] demonstrated that higher hypertension categories were more strongly associated with prevalent disease in the MESA population.

Additionally, Iwata et al[25] provide compelling data associating 24-hour ambulatory blood pressure with the cross-sectional prevalence of aortic sclerosis.[25] After adjustment for cardiovascular risk factors, 24-hour awake/asleep mean diastolic pressures—but not systolic pressures—were associated with aortic sclerosis. This finding is intriguing, because diastolic flow across the aortic side of the valve leaflets and into the coronary arteries creates shear forces that may contribute to disease initiation and progression. However, this finding has not been validated on a prospective basis, and data supporting a role for hypertension in disease progression are currently lacking.

Dysglycemia and the Metabolic Syndrome

Insulin resistance, diabetes, and the metabolic syndrome form a spectrum of metabolic abnormalities that have been shown to associate strongly with coronary atherosclerosis. The Homeostatic Model of Assessment—Insulin Resistance (HOMA-IR) has been associated with incident CAVD in prospective analysis of the MESA cohort, but this association was not independent of other cardiovascular risks.[26]

Similarly, overt diabetes has not been a consistent predictor of either cross-sectional CAVD or incident CAVD, nor a predictor of CAVD progression. Case-control studies have shown mixed results,[20,27,28] and diabetes was found to be associated with cross-sectional CAVD and incident CAVD in the MESA population.[29,30] However, this result was not found in either the Cardiovascular Heart Study or the Framingham Heart Study.[1,23,31] Interestingly, patients with diabetes had a lower rate of heterotopic ossification on histopathologic evaluation of explanted, severely calcified aortic valves of patients undergoing valve replacement.[22]

Metabolic syndrome is a constellation of clinical conditions that are often coexistent, including dysglycemia and insulin resistance, high blood pressure, dyslipidemia, central obesity, and microalbuminuria.[32-34] Patients with metabolic syndrome have a higher prevalence of CAVD[30] and are more likely to have incident CAVD (Figure 4-4).[29] Additionally, metabolic syndrome appears to influence the rate of hemodynamic progression of late-stage CAVD measured either by transvalvular velocity[18] or aortic valve area.[35] The metabolic syndrome has also been associated with faster deterioration of bioprosthetic aortic valves.[36,37] Although metabolic syndrome is one of the few clinical factors that have been shown to be associated with CAVD progression, the mechanisms underlying this association are unclear.

Dyslipidemia

Multiple observational studies have demonstrated significant associations between atherogenic dyslipidemia, including both total cholesterol and LDL concentrations, and both prevalent and incident CAVD.[1,19,20,23,31,38,39] However, the risk conferred by dyslipidemias appears to be clinically modest. Additionally, at least one study found an association between lipoprotein(a) [Lp(a)] concentrations and the presence of CAVD,[1] and Lp(a) has been shown to colocalize to regions of calcification.[40] These observational studies were bolstered by hyperlipidemic animal models,[41,42] in vitro studies,[43,44] and retrospective clinical analyses,[45-47] suggesting a beneficial effect of hydroxymethyl glutaryl–coenzyme A (HMG-CoA) reductase inhibition with statin therapy in slowing the progression of CAVD. Together, these findings, for a time, fostered a paradigm of CAVD as an atherosclerosis-like process.

Several randomized clinical trials were launched to test the hypothesis that statin therapy would slow progression of established CAVD (Table 4-2). The first of these, the Scottish Aortic Stenosis and Lipid Lowering Trial, Impact on Regression (SALTIRE),[48] tested whether 80 mg of atorvastatin daily would slow CAVD progression (as measured by aortic valve jet velocity and aortic valve calcium score) in 156 patients with established AS (mean jet velocity 3.4 m/s). Over a median follow-up of 25

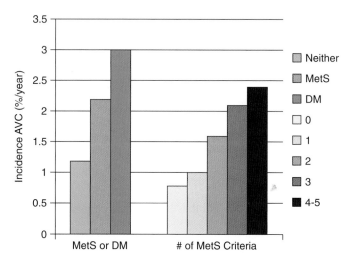

FIGURE 4-4   Rates of incident aortic valve calcification (AVC) in relationship to diabetes (DM) and metabolic syndrome (MetS). Data are shown for the 5723 participants in the Multi-ethnic Study of Atherosclerosis, according to (*left*) the presence of metabolic syndrome (by criteria of the Third Report of the Expert Panel on Detection, Evaluation, and Treatment of High Blood Cholesterol in Adults [ATP-III]) or diabetes and (*right*) the number of metabolic syndrome criteria present. (*Adapted from Katz R, Budoff MJ, Takasu J, et al. Relationship of metabolic syndrome with incident aortic valve calcium and aortic valve calcium progression: the Multi-Ethnic Study of Atherosclerosis (MESA). Diabetes 2009;58:813–9.*)

TABLE 4-2	Summary of Randomized Control Trials Testing Statin Therapy for Slowing the Progression of Calcific Aortic Valve Disease		
	SALTIRE[48]	**SEAS TRIAL[49]**	**ASTRONOMER TRIAL[50]**
AS severity			
Aortic velocity (m/s)	3.7	3.1	3.2
Aortic valve area (cm²)	1.0	1.3	1.5
Number of subjects	155	1873	269
Mean age (years)	68	67	58
BAV prevalence (%)	3	5	49
Baseline LDL (mg/dL)	135 ± 32	139 ± 35	122 ± 26
Statin tested	Atorvastatin 80 mg	Simvastatin 40 mg + ezetimibe 10 mg	Rosuvastatin 40 mg
Median follow-up (mo)	25	52	42
Valve outcomes assessed	1. Aortic velocity 2. Valve calcium score	1. Aortic valve events 2. Aortic velocity	1. Aortic valve peak gradient 2. Aortic valve area
Results	No benefit	Reduction in ischemic but not aortic valve events	No benefit

AS, aortic stenosis; ASTRONOMER, Aortic Stenosis Progression Observation: Measuring Effects of Rosuvastatin; BAV, bicuspid aortic valve; LDL, low-density lipoprotein cholesterol.

months, the rates of AS progression did not differ between the treated and untreated groups. A second, much larger trial, the Simvastatin and Ezetimibe in Aortic Stenosis (SEAS) study, tested whether simvastatin 40 mg plus ezetimibe 10 mg daily would slow CAVD progression[49] in 1873 patients with mild-to-moderate AS; after a median follow-up of 52 months, the between-group rate of aortic valve replacement did not differ (28.3% vs. 29.9%; $P = 0.97$). A third trial, the Aortic Stenosis Progression Observation: Measuring Effects of Rosuvastatin (ASTRONOMER),[50] randomly assigned 269 subjects with asymptomatic AS to receive either rosuvastatin 40 mg daily or placebo. Although this population was notable for being younger (mean age 58 years) and having a high prevalence of BAV morphology (49%), there was no significant difference between the groups in the transvalvular gradients or aortic valve areas at a mean follow-up of 3.5 years.

Taken together, these trials have been taken as a repudiation of the hypothesis that lipid lowering impacts CAVD progression, calling into question the paradigm that CAVD is regulated by an atherosclerosis-like process. Several observations are notable. First, these were trials of participants with AS, a relatively late stage in the spectrum of CAVD. In contrast, observational studies demonstrated the strongest statistical associations of dyslipidemia with early-stage disease initiation, and it remains uncertain whether lipid-lowering therapy, particularly in younger patients,[16] might affect disease progression. Second, statin therapy reduced the coronary revascularization rate in the SEAS study (hazard ratio [HR] 0.78; 95% CI 0.63-0.97).[49] Thus, although statin therapy may not impact valve-specific end points in those with late-stage CAVD, the overall clinical effect may be beneficial.

Smoking

Cigarette smoking is strongly linked to atherosclerosis, including coronary, carotid, and peripheral vascular disease, through varied mechanisms such as promotion of inflammation, alterations in lipids, vasomotor dysfunction, increased oxidative stress, and induction of a prothrombotic milieu.[51] Smoking has been linked with cross-sectional and incident CAVD in multiple studies.[1,19,31,52]

Markers of Inflammation

Studies in animal models and of human pathologic specimens have demonstrated a clear role for inflammatory cell infiltration and oxidative stress in CAVD pathogenesis with induction of osteogenic pathways.[53-57] However, to date no convincing associations have been found between systemic markers of inflammation and CAVD. C-reactive protein levels have failed to show associations with early- or late-stage disease or with disease initiation.[19,23,31,58] Moreover, several studies have examined the relationship between CAVD and soluble intercellular adhesion molecule-1 (sICAM-1), with mixed results.[58-60] Thus it seems that future clinical studies investigating the role of inflammation in CAVD will need more targeted strategies.[54]

Renal Dysfunction

Chronic kidney disease (CKD) reduces filtration of metabolites, minerals, and toxins, is often associated with albuminuria, and creates systemic perturbations in blood pressure, red blood cell production, and neurohormonal pathways.[61] In particular, end-stage renal disease is associated with hyperphosphatemia, hypocalcemia, and a secondary hyperparathyroidism that can cause osteopenia and progressive vascular calcifications[62,63] and is associated with cardiovascular events.[64] It has long been observed that patients with end-stage renal disease (ESRD) who are undergoing hemodialysis have premature vascular and valvular calcification,[65-68] and calcium-phosphorus metabolism is an important determinant in the rate of progression of CAVD in patients receiving hemodialysis.[69-71]

Whether less severe forms of CKD are associated with CAVD has been the study of several investigations. Mills et al[72] examined 118 patients with AS and normal renal function (serum creatinine <1.5 mg/dL) and found no association between the severity of AS and the calcium-phosphate product. Furthermore, Fox et al,[58] examining 3047 participants in the Framingham Offspring study, found a strong association between the presence of CKD (defined as estimated glomerular filtration rate (GFR) <60 mL/min per 1.73 m²) and mitral annular calcification (odds ratio [OR] 1.6; 95% CI 1.03-2.5), but found no association between CKD and CAVD (OR 1.1; 95% CI 0.7-1.7) after full adjustments.

An additional investigation of 6785 participants of the MESA utilized more robust measures of CKD, including estimated GFR and cystatin C concentrations and the presence of microalbuminuria.[73] The MESA population is generally healthy, and the prevalence of CKD (estimated GFR <60 mL/min per 1.73 m²) and CAVD were 10% and 13%, respectively. In this population, there were trends for associations between aortic valve calcium and both CKD (OR 1.23; 95% CI 0.99-1.14), and cystatin C (OR 1.06; 95% CI 0.99-1.14), but not with microalbuminuria (OR 1.11; 95% CI 0.89-1.40).

Taken together, these studies suggest that mild CKD is, at most, weakly associated with CAVD on a population basis, and thus renal dysfunction may only be a significant contributor to CAVD pathogenesis in ESRD. However, an intriguing study by Linefsky et al[74] found a significant relationship between phosphorus levels and the prevalence of CAVD among 1938 subjects in the Cardiovascular Heart Study. These subjects had normal renal function on average (estimated GFR 76.6 mL/min/1.73 m²) and 97% had phosphorus levels within the normal range. Each 0.5 mg/dL increase in serum phosphate concentrations was associated with greater adjusted odds of CAVD (OR 1.17; 95% CI 1.04-1.31), as shown in Figure 4-5. Significant associations were also seen between serum phosphate and aortic annular and mitral annular calcification, but no associations were seen with serum calcium, parathyroid hormone, or 25-OH vitamin D concentrations. This result is intriguing because phosphate uptake via the Pit-1

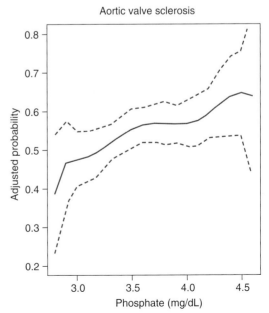

FIGURE 4-5 Probability of aortic sclerosis according to serum phosphate concentration among 1938 participants in the Cardiovascular Health Study. *Solid line* indicates fully adjusted cubic spline estimate; *dashed lines* indicate 95% confidence intervals. Higher phosphate concentrations—even within the normal range—are associated with a significant increase in probability of aortic sclerosis (P = 0.01). *(Taken from Linefsky et al, J Am Coll Cardiol. 2011 Jul 12;58(3):291-7.)*

receptor has been linked with pro-osteogenic gene expression patterns in calcified aortic valves.

Extent of Calcification

There is increasing evidence from preclinical and in vitro studies that CAVD is regulated by osteogenic pathways that induce biomineralization via distinct paracrine signaling mechanisms.[75,76] Resident fibroblasts have been shown to transdifferentiate down an osteoblastic phenotype,[77-79] and advanced CAVD may show regions of heterotopic ossification.[22,78] Several studies have implicated the osteoprotegerin and receptor activator of nuclear factor kappa β ligand (RANKL) axis in CAVD,[80] and this pathway has also been linked to osteoporosis, vascular calcification, and cardiovascular events.[81-84] Osteoprotegerin levels have been shown to predict mortality in patients with AS.[85] This pathway is intriguing because of the commercial availability of RANKL inhibitors, but to our knowledge, there have been no clinical studies investigating the role of these novel pathways on the progression of CAVD.

A consistent finding among studies that have examined risk factors for CAVD progression is that the baseline burden of disease—measured either by Agatston calcium scores or valvular hemodynamics—is a strong, independent predictor of progression[19,39,86] and outcomes.[87] There are two potential explanations for this finding. First, baseline disease severity may be a marker of the patient's previous rate of progression, and patients who previously experienced rapid progression will continue to do so in the future. Second, local, paracrine regulators of calcification may be influenced by disease severity ("calcium begets calcium"), and patients with high calcium burden have accelerated calcification. To date, there have been no efforts to determine which of these explanations is more suitable.

An intriguing new approach to studying the relative roles of inflammation and calcification in CAVD combines positron emission tomography (PET) imaging for metabolic imaging with CT for anatomic mapping. Both fluorodeoxyglucose F 18 (¹⁸F-FDG), which correlates with inflammatory activity, and ¹⁸F–sodium fluoride (¹⁸F-NaF), which correlates with active deposition of calcium, localize to the aortic valve in patients with AS, with higher signal intensities than seen in controls.[88,89] Preliminary data suggest a relatively higher rate of ¹⁸F-NaF activity than of ¹⁸F-FDG activity, suggesting a relatively greater role for metabolic processes regulating calcification, in comparison with that of inflammation, in the progression of established CAVD. Moreover, these methods appear to be reliable and reproducible[88,90] and may therefore provide novel means of studying the roles of valvular inflammation and calcification in disease progression.

Summary of Risk Associations

Thus far, the body of evidence suggests strong associations between many traditional cardiovascular risk factors and CAVD, especially in its early stages. These risk factors include age, male gender, hypertension, diabetes, metabolic syndrome, dyslipidemia, and smoking. Prospective analyses have suggested that these factors may play a causal role in disease development. This suggestion is supported by a study by Thanassoulis et al,[31] who examined the association between early adult risk factors and the presence of aortic valve calcium on later-life CT among 1323 participants of the Framingham Offspring study.[31] After a median 27-year follow-up, 39% had aortic valve calcium on CT. Risk factors for the subsequent development of valve calcification were age (P < 0.0001), male gender (P = 005), total cholesterol (P < 0.0001), and smoking P = 0.002), whereas higher levels of high-density cholesterol (HDL) were associated with a lower likelihood of valve calcification (P = 0.002). Framingham Risk Score in midlife was a strong predictor of the presence of aortic valve calcium, and the prevalences of aortic valve calcium were 33.0%, 52.8%, and 61.1% for low, intermediate and high

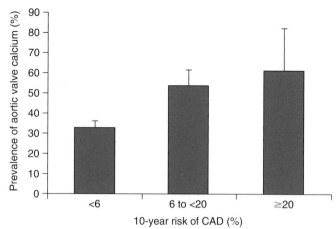

FIGURE 4-6 **Relationship between Framingham risk score in early adulthood and the presence of aortic valve calcium (AVC) after a median 27-year follow-up.** Categories are divided into low (<6%), intermediate (6% to <20%), and high (≥20%) 10-year risk for coronary artery disease (CAD). Higher aggregate risk scores were associated with a greater prevalence of AVC (P <0.001 for trend across groups). Error bars represent 95% confidence intervals. *(From Thanassoulis G, Massaro JM, Cury R, et al. Associations of long-term and early adult atherosclerosis risk factors with aortic and mitral valve calcium. J Am Coll Cardiol 2010;55:2491–8.)*

cardiovascular risk Framingham Risk Score categories, respectively (Figure 4-6). In contrast, renal dysfunction and systemic markers of inflammation have demonstrated weaker and variable correlations with CAVD, and their role in the pathogenesis of CAVD is uncertain.

Although atherosclerotic risk factors certainly contribute to the disease initiation and the presence of early-stage disease, there is currently little data to support their role in progression of established CAVD. This situation is highlighted by multiple randomized trials showing the failure of statin therapy to impact disease progression. Histopathologic analyses have demonstrated osteoblastic transformation within calcified valves, and it is intriguing to postulate that later-stage disease progression may be regulated by factors involved with systemic calcium and bone metabolism. However, currently there is scant clinical data to support a relationship between these factors and CAVD progression.

Genetic Associations with CAVD

Genetic factors may underlie the many, varied facets of CAVD, influencing valve morphology, plaque development, and progressive calcification. These factors may range from rare, single-gene mendelian mutations producing a large effect (e.g., *NOTCH1* mutations) or more common polymorphisms in multiple genes, each with a smaller effect.

The first investigations into the genetic basis of CAVD focused on identifying polymorphisms with candidate genes that were believed to be in the causal pathways for development of CAVD (Table 4-3). These smaller, case-control studies suggested a role for genetic variation in apolipoproteins AI and B,[91] vitamin D receptor,[92] estrogen receptor α,[93] interleukin-10 (IL-10),[94] chemokine receptor 5,[94] and paraoxonase 1 (PON1)[95] genes. Additionally, transforming growth factor-β (TGF-β) receptor polymorphisms were shown to significantly modify the effect of the estrogen receptor α polymorphisms.[93] In general, these early studies had marginal statistical power and lacked validation and replication cohorts. This problem is exemplified by several studies of the apolipoprotein E (*APOE*) gene,[91,96] with early studies showing associations between CAVD and the apo E ε2 allele and the apo E ε4 allele that were not validated in a larger (n = 1074) subject

TABLE 4-3   Summary of Candidate Gene Association Studies for Calcific Aortic Valve Disease

GENE	LOCATION	PHENOTYPE	CASES	RISK VARIANT	*P* VALUE
Vitamin D receptor[92]	12q12-q14	Severe AS	100	B allele	*P* = 0.001
ApoB[91]	2p24-p23	Severe AS	62	X+	*P* = 0.007
ApoE	19q13.2	AS	43	ApoE 2/4+3/4 genotypes	*P* = 0.03
Estrogen receptor α[93]	6q25.1	AVR	41	Pvull polymorphism	*P* = 0.03
TGF-β receptor1[93]	9q33-q34	AVR	41	Aocl polymorphism	*
Interleukin-10[94]	1q31-q32	Ex vivo atomic absorption	187	3 promoter polymorphisms	*P* = 0.03
Chemokine receptor 5[94]	3p21.31	Ex vivo atomic absorption	187	32–base pair deletion	*P* = 0.04[†]
Paraoxonase 1[95]	7q21-22	Moderate AS	67	Q192R polymorphisms	*P* = 0.03

Apo, apolipoprotein; *AS*, aortic stenosis; *AVR*, aortic valve replacement.
*Significantly modified the effect of the estrogen receptor Aocl polymorphisms (odds ratio 4.58; 95% confidence interval 1.68-12.51).
[†]*P* value represents significance for effect modification with the interleukin-10 polymorphisms.

cohort.[97] Thus, whether any of the alleles identified in these early studies is truly related to CAVD risk is somewhat suspect.

Advances in gene chip technology have facilitated gene association studies by using a compendium of reference single-nucleotide polymorphisms (SNPs). There have been several attempts to validate some of these initial candidate gene results using SNP-based analyses. A case-control analysis by Gaudreault et al[98] involving 457 patients with severe AS and 3294 control subjects. In this study, strong associations were found between SNPs in the *APOB* gene and in SNPs surrounding the IL-10 gene locus. The number of SNPs within the parathyroid hormone and vitamin D receptor genes failed to reach statistical significance. A separate study by Ellis et al[99] examined genetic associations with trileaflet aortic valves in an elderly (mean age 73 ± 7 years) cohort of 265 patients and 961 control subjects; they were able to identify significant associations between CAVD and SNPs within the myosin VIIA (*MYO7A*), angiotensin II receptor (*AGTR1*), and elastin (*ELN*) genes.[99] However, as with earlier studies, the lack of validation and replication cohorts calls into question the true strengths of associations, if any, of these candidate SNPs with CAVD.

In contrast, a genome-wide association study (GWAS), which utilizes gene chips with several hundred thousand SNPs throughout the genome, has both the advantage and disadvantage of being an unbiased method of assessing genetic associations. The first GWAS for the presence of aortic valve calcium, using CT-based phenotyping for discovery phase analyses, has been reported.[100] This study, which included 2245 patients with prevalent aortic valve calcium, discovered a strong association between genetic variation near the Lp(a) (*LPA*) gene locus and the presence of valvular calcium on CT scans among subjects of European descent. *LPA* is the gene that encodes apolipoprotein(a), an apolipoprotein that is covalently linked to an apolipoprotein B molecule in Lp(a) particles. Lp(a) levels have been associated with the presence of CAVD in population studies,[1] and apolipoprotein(a) colocalizes to regions of early calcification within explanted human aortic valves.[40]

Additional validation analyses demonstrated that the *LPA* SNP was associated with valve calcium in both Hispanic and black subjects, supporting its generalizability to non-Caucasian ethnic groups. Moreover, the *LPA* SNP also was associated with incident AS and the need for aortic valve replacement in two prospective European cohorts. Further, Mendelian randomization analyses suggested a causal role for *LPA* genotypes acting through Lp(a) levels. Thus the *LPA* genotype appears to strongly influence the development and progression of CAVD through its effect on circulating Lp(a) levels and may account for up to 10% of CAVD within the general population.

Although these genetic association studies are enticing, much of the genetic underpinnings of CAVD remain unexplained and are the subject of additional, ongoing investigations.

TABLE 4-4   Relative Risk of Cardiovascular Events According to the Presence or Absence of Aortic Sclerosis*

	Relative Risk (95% Confidence Intervals)	
	ADJUSTED FOR AGE & SEX	**ADJUSTED FOR AGE, SEX, & ASSOCIATED BASELINE FACTORS**
Death from any cause	1.42 (1.19-1.70)	1.35 (1.12-1.61)
Cardiovascular death	1.66 (1.23-2.23)	1.52 (1.12-2.05)
Myocardial infarction	1.46 (1.12-1.90)	1.40 (1.07-1.83)
Angina	1.23 (1.00-1.50)	1.17 (0.95-1.43)
Congestive heart failure	1.33 (1.05-1.68)	1.28 (1.01-1.63)
Stroke	1.31 (1.01-1.71)	1.25 (0.96-1.64)

Adapted from Otto CM, Lind BK, Kitzman DW, et al. Association of aortic-valve sclerosis with cardiovascular mortality and morbidity in the elderly. N Engl J Med 1999;341:142–7.
*Among 4271 subjects in the Cardiovascular Health Study without prevalent cardiovascular disease.

CAVD and Clinical Outcomes

Severe calcific AS is associated with a substantial increase in left ventricular afterload and subsequent changes to the left ventricular myocardium, including hypertrophy, fibrosis, and apoptosis. The onset of symptoms with severe AS is associated with an overall poor prognosis, with a collection of adverse events including angina, congestive heart failure, syncope, and sudden death. These events appear to be related—directly or indirectly—to the physiologic changes of increased afterload and higher filling pressures. What is more surprising is that early-stage CAVD, prior to hemodynamic perturbations, is also associated with an increased risk of cardiovascular events.

In a pivotal study, Otto et al[101] assessed the relationship between aortic sclerosis (defined by echocardiography) and clinical cardiovascular events among 5621 elderly (age ≥65 years) participants in the Cardiovascular Heart Study. After a mean 5-year follow-up, subjects with aortic sclerosis but no prior coronary heart disease had a 1.42-fold higher risk of death (95% CI 1.12-1.61), and a 1.66-fold higher risk of cardiovascular death (95% CI: 1.12-2.05) than those without aortic sclerosis, after adjustments were made for baseline cardiovascular risk factors (Table 4-4). Aortic sclerosis did not confer increased mortality among participants with established coronary disease but the study of this small subset (19%) of participants was probably insufficiently powered to examine this end point. In two other studies, aortic sclerosis was also associated with increased risk for development of myocardial infarction (relative risk [RR] 1.40; 95% CI 1.07-1.83) or congestive heart failure (RR 1.28; 95% CI 1.01-1.63), whereas no association was seen with angina (RR 1.17; 95% CI 0.95-1.43) or stroke (RR 1.25; 95% CI 0.96-1.64). Because of the observational nature of these analyses, it was not possible to determine whether valve calcification played a causal role or simply served as a risk marker.[102,103]

Several follow-up studies attempted to show that aortic sclerosis served as a marker of increased risk. Chandra et al[104] examined 425 patients who came to the emergency department complaining of chest pain and found that patients with aortic sclerosis had a higher rate of cardiovascular events (16.8% vs. 7.1%; $P = 0.002$) over the ensuing year. However, on multivariate analysis, aortic sclerosis was not independently associated with clinical events (cardiovascular death or myocardial infarction), whereas coronary artery disease, myocardial infarction at index admission, C-reactive protein levels, congestive heart failure, and age were independent predictors. The investigators concluded that aortic sclerosis served as a marker of increased risk because of its associations with coronary artery disease and inflammation.

In a later study, Owens et al[15] looked at the relationship between aortic valve calcium on CT and cardiovascular events in the MESA cohort, which excluded subjects with baseline coronary artery disease. In the relatively young and generally healthy MESA cohort, the presence of aortic valve calcium conferred increased risk for a combined end point of cardiovascular events (cardiovascular death, resuscitated arrest, myocardial infarction, fatal and nonfatal strokes) and coronary heart disease events (excluding strokes), with HRs of 1.50 (95% CI 1.10-2.04) and 1.72 (95% CI 1.19-2.49), respectively after adjustment for clinical risk factors. Coronary artery calcium scores, but not C-reactive protein levels, attenuated the risk associated with aortic valve calcium. Thus, subclinical atherosclerosis appears to mediate much of the association between aortic valve calcium and cardiovascular events, primarily because of the association of valve calcium with risk for myocardial infarction. In subset analysis, aortic valve calcium remained strongly and independently associated with cardiovascular mortality (HR 2.76; 95% CI 1.44-5.30).

The relationship between subclinical CAVD and stroke is intriguing. There is at least a theoretic possibility that calcific nodules could be a direct source of embolism, and there have been several reports of embolic strokes that were thought to be due to embolization from a calcified aortic valve.[105-108] However, no significant association between subclinical CAVD and clinical stroke has been seen on a population level. Rodriguez et al,[109] who examined the relationship between annular and valvular (aortic or mitral annular) calcium and subclinical brain infarcts on magnetic resonance imaging, showed that the presence and severity of calcification were associated with the presence of subclinical infarcts. When aortic sclerosis was examined as an individual marker, no association was seen. Moreover, in the Strong Heart Study, involving 2723 American Indians, mitral annular calcification but not aortic sclerosis was associated with incident stroke.[110] Thus, there is no conclusive evidence that embolization of calcific nodules from a sclerotic aortic valve is a significant cause of clinical stroke, and the relationship may more likely be mediated by coincident atherosclerotic disease of the thoracic aorta and/or carotid arteries.

Subclinical CAVD is clearly associated with increased cardiovascular morbidity and mortality, above and beyond traditional cardiovascular risk factors, probably in part because aortic sclerosis serves as a marker of subclinical atherosclerosis. There are two lingering issues. First, subclinical atherosclerosis does not appear to explain all of the excess risk captured by aortic sclerosis, and additional mechanisms are likely. Second, it is not known whether aortic sclerosis could be used to reclassify a patient's cardiovascular risk or whether more aggressive therapies (e.g., statin therapy) would reduce future cardiovascular event risk in those with aortic sclerosis.

Gaps in Knowledge and Future Studies

Our understanding of the biology of CAVD has been greatly enhanced over the past two decades. However, there are currently no therapeutic interventions to prevent or slow the progression of CAVD, highlighting the importance of ongoing research. Future treatment strategies may be stage specific, with different therapies targeting early- and late-stage CAVD. The following is a partial list of important topics that remain unanswered:

1. Does earlier treatment of cardiovascular risk factors favorably affect the progression of CAVD and/or reduce valve-specific outcomes?
2. What mechanisms underlie later-stage disease progression? What is the role of inflammation in this process?
3. What factors related to the biology of aging explain the exceedingly strong relationship between age and both incidence and progression of CAVD? Will treatment options be age specific?
4. What are the genetic bases of BAV?
5. Is aortic sclerosis/valve calcium a risk marker warranting more aggressive therapies to lower overall risk for cardiovascular events?

Conclusions

CAVD is a complex disease of dysregulated mineralization influenced by underlying valve morphology and sharing some features with atherosclerosis but also including local induction of osteogenic signaling pathways (See Chapter 3). Clinical epidemiologic and observational studies have shown a clear link between early-stage CAVD and traditional cardiovascular risk factors, an association that has not been seen with CAVD progression. The paradigm of CAVD progression as simply atherosclerosis of the valve is not supported by clinical data, and results of randomized trials of statin therapy have been uniformly negative about these agents' effectiveness. Therapeutic strategies aimed at preventing or slowing CAVD progression have proved elusive, and our current understanding of the disease process suggests that therapies may be stage and age specific. Cardiovascular risk factor reduction in younger subjects with early-stage CAVD (aortic sclerosis) may be beneficial, but these strategies do not appear to influence late-stage disease progression, particularly in older subjects, in whom the disease is most common. CAVD remains associated with excess cardiovascular morbidity and mortality beyond traditional risk factors, with excess cardiovascular mortality even beyond the severity of subclinical coronary artery disease. Insights into the genetics of CAVD and underlying osteogenic and biomineralization processes may offer novel strategies for treatment in the future.

REFERENCES

1. Stewart BF, Siscovick D, Lind BK, et al. Clinical factors associated with calcific aortic valve disease. Cardiovascular Health Study. J Am Coll Cardiol 1997;29:630–4.
2. Nishimura RA, Carabello BA, Faxon DP, et al. ACC/AHA 2008 guideline update on valvular heart disease: focused update on infective endocarditis: a report of the American College of Cardiology/American Heart Association Task Force on Practice Guidelines: endorsed by the Society of Cardiovascular Anesthesiologists, Society for Cardiovascular Angiography and Interventions, and Society of Thoracic Surgeons. Circulation 2008;118:887–96.
3. Bonow RO, Carabello BA, Kanu C, et al. ACC/AHA 2006 guidelines for the management of patients with valvular heart disease: a report of the American College of Cardiology/American Heart Association Task Force on Practice Guidelines (writing committee to revise the 1998 Guidelines for the Management of Patients With Valvular Heart Disease): developed in collaboration with the Society of Cardiovascular Anesthesiologists: endorsed by the Society for Cardiovascular Angiography and Interventions and the Society of Thoracic Surgeons. Circulation 2006;114:e84–231.
4. Koos R, Mahnken AH, Kuhl HP, et al. Quantification of aortic valve calcification using multislice spiral computed tomography: comparison with atomic absorption spectroscopy. Invest Radiol 2006;41:485–9.
5. Budoff MJ, Mao S, Takasu J, et al. Reproducibility of electron-beam CT measures of aortic valve calcification. Acad Radiol 2002;9:1122–7.
6. Pohle K, Dimmler A, Feyerer R, et al. Quantification of aortic valve calcification with electron beam tomography: a histomorphometric validation study. Invest Radiol 2004;39:230–4.

7. Agatston AS, Janowitz WR, Hildner FJ, et al. Quantification of coronary artery calcium using ultrafast computed tomography. J Am Coll Cardiol 1990;15:827–32.

8. Roberts WC, Ko JM, Hamilton C. Comparison of valve structure, valve weight, and severity of the valve obstruction in 1849 patients having isolated aortic valve replacement for aortic valve stenosis (with or without associated aortic regurgitation) studied at 3 different medical centers in 2 different time periods. Circulation 2005;112: 3919–29.

9. Roberts WC, Ko JM. Frequency by decades of unicuspid, bicuspid, and tricuspid aortic valves in adults having isolated aortic valve replacement for aortic stenosis, with or without associated aortic regurgitation. Circulation 2005;111:920–5.

10. Chui MC, Newby DE, Panarelli M, et al. Association between calcific aortic stenosis and hypercholesterolemia: is there a need for a randomized controlled trial of cholesterol-lowering therapy? Clin Cardiol 2001;24:52–5.

11. Cripe L, Andelfinger G, Martin LJ, et al. Bicuspid aortic valve is heritable. J Am Coll Cardiol 2004;44:138–43.

12. Huntington K, Hunter AG, Chan KL. A prospective study to assess the frequency of familial clustering of congenital bicuspid aortic valve. J Am Coll Cardiol 1997;30: 1809–12.

13. Martin LJ, Ramachandran V, Cripe LH, et al. Evidence in favor of linkage to human chromosomal regions 18q, 5q and 13q for bicuspid aortic valve and associated cardiovascular malformations. Hum Genet 2007;121:275–84.

14. Garg V, Muth AN, Ransom JF, et al. Mutations in NOTCH1 cause aortic valve disease. Nature 2005;437:270–4.

15. Owens DS, Budoff MJ, Katz R, et al. Aortic valve calcium independently predicts coronary and cardiovascular events in a primary prevention population. Cardiovasc Imaging 2012;5:619–25.

16. Owens DS, Katz R, Johnson E, et al. Interaction of age with lipoproteins as predictors of aortic valve calcification in the multi-ethnic study of atherosclerosis. Arch Intern Med 2008;168:1200–7.

17. Mohty D, Pibarot P, Despres JP, et al. Age-related differences in the pathogenesis of calcific aortic stenosis: the potential role of resistin. Int J Cardiol 2010;142: 126–32.

18. Capoulade R, Clavel MA, Dumesnil JG, et al. Impact of metabolic syndrome on progression of aortic stenosis: influence of age and statin therapy. J Am Coll Cardiol 2012;60:216–23.

19. Owens DS, Katz R, Takasu J, et al. Incidence and progression of aortic valve calcium in the Multi-ethnic Study of Atherosclerosis (MESA). Am J Cardiol 2010;105:701–8.

20. Boon A, Cheriex E, Lodder J, et al. Cardiac valve calcification: characteristics of patients with calcification of the mitral annulus or aortic valve. Heart 1997;78:472–4.

21. Chandra S, Lang RM, Nicolarsen J, et al. Bicuspid aortic valve: inter-racial difference in frequency and aortic dimensions. JACC Cardiovasc Imaging 2012;5:981–9.

22. Ing SW, Mohler Iii ER, Putt ME, et al. Correlates of valvular ossification in patients with aortic valve stenosis. Clinical and Translational Science 2009;2:431–5.

23. Novaro GM, Katz R, Aviles RJ, et al. Clinical factors, but not C-reactive protein, predict progression of calcific aortic-valve disease: the Cardiovascular Health Study. J Am Coll Cardiol 2007;50:1992–8.

24. Linefsky J, Katz R, Budoff M, et al. Stages of systemic hypertension and blood pressure as correlates of computed tomography-assessed aortic valve calcium (from the Multi-Ethnic Study of Atherosclerosis). Am J Cardiol 2011;107:47–51.

25. Iwata S, Russo C, Jin Z, et al. Higher ambulatory blood pressure is associated with aortic valve calcification in the elderly: a population-based study. Hypertension 2013;61(1): 55–60.

26. Tison GH, Blaha MJ, Budoff MJ, et al. The relationship of insulin resistance and extra-coronary calcification in the multi-ethnic study of atherosclerosis. Atherosclerosis 2011;218:507–10.

27. Ortlepp JR, Schmitz F, Bozoglu T, et al. Cardiovascular risk factors in patients with aortic stenosis predict prevalence of coronary artery disease but not of aortic stenosis: an angiographic pair matched case-control study. Heart 2003;89:1019–22.

28. Aronow WS, Schwartz KS, Koenigsberg M. Correlation of serum lipids, calcium, and phosphorus, diabetes mellitus and history of systemic hypertension with presence or absence of calcified or thickened aortic cusps or root in elderly patients. Am J Cardiol 1987;59:998–9.

29. Katz R, Budoff MJ, Takasu J, et al. Relationship of metabolic syndrome with incident aortic valve calcium and aortic valve calcium progression: the Multi-Ethnic Study of Atherosclerosis (MESA). Diabetes 2009;58:813–19.

30. Katz R, Wong ND, Kronmal R, et al. Features of the metabolic syndrome and diabetes mellitus as predictors of aortic valve calcification in the Multi-Ethnic Study of Atherosclerosis. Circulation 2006;113:2113–19.

31. Thanassoulis G, Massaro JM, Cury R, et al. Associations of long-term and early adult atherosclerosis risk factors with aortic and mitral valve calcium. J Am Coll Cardiol 2010;55:2491–8.

32. Alberti KG, Zimmet PZ. Definition, diagnosis and classification of diabetes mellitus and its complications. Part 1: diagnosis and classification of diabetes mellitus provisional report of a WHO consultation. Diabet Med 1998;15:539–53.

33. Balkau B, Charles MA. Comment on the provisional report from the WHO consultation. European Group for the Study of Insulin Resistance (EGIR). Diabet Med 1999;16: 442–3.

34. Grundy SM, Brewer Jr HB, Cleeman JI, et al. Definition of metabolic syndrome: Report of the National Heart, Lung, and Blood Institute/American Heart Association conference on scientific issues related to definition. Circulation 2004;109:433–8.

35. Briand M, Lemieux I, Dumesnil JG, et al. Metabolic syndrome negatively influences disease progression and prognosis in aortic stenosis. J Am Coll Cardiol 2006;47: 2229–36.

36. Briand M, Pibarot P, Despres JP, et al. Metabolic syndrome is associated with faster degeneration of bioprosthetic valves. Circulation 2006;114:I512–17.

37. O'Brien KD. Do bioprosthetic aortic valves deteriorate more rapidly in patients with the metabolic syndrome? Nat Clin Pract Cardiovasc Med 2007;4:192–3.

38. Aronow WS, Schwartz KS, Koenigsberg M. Correlation of serum lipids, calcium and phosphorus, diabetes mellitus, aortic valve stenosis and history of systemic hypertension with presence or absence of mitral anular calcium in persons older than 62 years in a long-term health care facility. Am J Cardiol 1987;59:381–2.

39. Messika-Zeitoun D, Bielak LF, Peyser PA, et al. Aortic valve calcification: determinants and progression in the population. Arterioscler Thromb Vasc Biol 2007;27:642–8.

40. O'Brien KD, Reichenbach DD, Marcovina SM, et al. Apolipoproteins B, (a), and E accumulate in the morphologically early lesion of "degenerative" valvular aortic stenosis. Arterioscler Thromb Vasc Biol 1996;16:523–32.

41. Rajamannan NM, Subramaniam M, Stock SR, et al. Atorvastatin inhibits calcification and enhances nitric oxide synthase production in the hypercholesterolaemic aortic valve. Heart 2005;91:806–10.

42. Rajamannan NM, Subramaniam M, Springett M, et al. Atorvastatin inhibits hypercholesterolemia-induced cellular proliferation and bone matrix production in the rabbit aortic valve. Circulation 2002;105:2660–5.

43. Monzack EL, Gu X, Masters KS. Efficacy of simvastatin treatment of valvular interstitial cells varies with the extracellular environment. Arterioscler Thromb Vasc Biol 2009;29:246–53.

44. Osman L, Yacoub MH, Latif N, et al. Role of human valve interstitial cells in valve calcification and their response to atorvastatin. Circulation 2006;114:I547–52.

45. Aronow WS, Ahn C, Kronzon I, et al. Association of coronary risk factors and use of statins with progression of mild valvular aortic stenosis in older persons. Am J Cardiol 2001;88:693–5.

46. Novaro GM, Tiong IY, Pearce GL, et al. Effect of hydroxymethylglutaryl coenzyme a reductase inhibitors on the progression of calcific aortic stenosis. Circulation 2001;104:2205–9.

47. Shavelle DM, Takasu J, Budoff MJ, et al. HMG CoA reductase inhibitor (statin) and aortic valve calcium. Lancet 2002;359:1125–6.

48. Cowell SJ, Newby DE, Prescott RJ, et al. A randomized trial of intensive lipid-lowering therapy in calcific aortic stenosis. N Engl J Med 2005;352:2389–97.

49. Rossebo AB, Pedersen TR, Boman K, et al. Intensive lipid lowering with simvastatin and ezetimibe in aortic stenosis. N Engl J Med 2008;359:1343–56.

50. Chan KL, Teo K, Dumesnil JG, et al. Effect of Lipid lowering with rosuvastatin on progression of aortic stenosis: results of the aortic stenosis progression observation: measuring effects of rosuvastatin (ASTRONOMER) trial. Circulation 2010;121:306–14.

51. Ambrose JA, Barua RS. The pathophysiology of cigarette smoking and cardiovascular disease: an update. J Am Coll Cardiol 2004;43:1731–7.

52. Mohler ER, Sheridan MJ, Nichols R, et al. Development and progression of aortic valve stenosis: atherosclerosis risk factors—a causal relationship? A clinical morphologic study. Clin Cardiol 1991;14:995–9.

53. Miller JD, Chu Y, Brooks RM, et al. Dysregulation of antioxidant mechanisms contributes to increased oxidative stress in calcific aortic valvular stenosis in humans. J Am Coll Cardiol 2008;52:843–50.

54. New SE, Aikawa E. Molecular imaging insights into early inflammatory stages of arterial and aortic valve calcification. Circulation Research 2011;108:1381–91.

55. O'Brien KD. Pathogenesis of calcific aortic valve disease: a disease process comes of age (and a good deal more). Arterioscler Thromb Vasc Biol 2006;26:1721–8.

56. Towler DA. Oxidation, inflammation, and aortic valve calcification peroxide paves an osteogenic path. J Am Coll Cardiol 2008;52:851–4.

57. Yang X, Fullerton DA, Su X, et al. Pro-osteogenic phenotype of human aortic valve interstitial cells is associated with higher levels of Toll-like receptors 2 and 4 and enhanced expression of bone morphogenetic protein 2. J Am Coll Cardiol 2009;53: 491–500.

58. Fox CS, Guo CY, Larson MG, et al. Relations of inflammation and novel risk factors to valvular calcification. Am J Cardiol 2006;97:1502–5.

59. Shavelle DM, Katz R, Takasu J, et al. Soluble intercellular adhesion molecule-1 (sICAM-1) and aortic valve calcification in the multi-ethnic study of atherosclerosis (MESA). The Journal of heart valve disease 2008;17:388–95.

60. Shahi CN, Ghaisas NK, Goggins M, et al. Elevated levels of circulating soluble adhesion molecules in patients with nonrheumatic aortic stenosis. Am J Cardiol 1997;79: 980–2.

61. Levey AS, Coresh J. Chronic kidney disease. Lancet 2012;379:165–80.

62. Giachelli CM. The emerging role of phosphate in vascular calcification. Kidney International 2009;75:890–7.

63. Tonelli M, Pannu N, Manns B. Oral phosphate binders in patients with kidney failure. N Engl J Med 2010;362:1312–24.

64. De Boer IH, Gorodetskaya I, Young B, et al. The severity of secondary hyperparathyroidism in chronic renal insufficiency is GFR-dependent, race-dependent, and associated with cardiovascular disease. Journal of the American Society of Nephrology 2002;13: 2762–9.

65. Michel PL. Aortic stenosis in chronic renal failure patients treated by dialysis. Nephrology, dialysis, transplantation: official publication of the European Dialysis and Transplant Association—European Renal Association 1998;13(Suppl 4):44–8.

66. Straumann E, Meyer B, Misteli M, et al. Aortic and mitral valve disease in patients with end stage renal failure on long-term haemodialysis. British heart journal 1992;67:236–9.

67. Maher ER, Young G, Smyth-Walsh B, et al. Aortic and mitral valve calcification in patients with end-stage renal disease. Lancet 1987;2:875–7.

68. Maher ER, Pazianas M, Curtis JR. Calcific aortic stenosis: a complication of chronic uraemia. Nephron 1987;47:119–22.

69. Hoshina M, Wada H, Sakakura K, et al. Determinants of progression of aortic valve stenosis and outcome of adverse events in hemodialysis patients. J Cardiol 2012;59: 78–83.

70. Perkovic V, Hunt D, Griffin SV, et al. Accelerated progression of calcific aortic stenosis in dialysis patients. Nephron Clinical Practice 2003;94:c40–5.

71. Urena P, Malergue MC, Goldfarb B, et al. Evolutive aortic stenosis in hemodialysis patients: analysis of risk factors. Nephrologie 1999;20:217–25.

72. Mills WR, Einstadter D, Finkelhor RS. Relation of calcium-phosphorus product to the severity of aortic stenosis in patients with normal renal function. Am J Cardiol 2004;94:1196–8.

73. Ix JH, Shlipak MG, Katz R, et al. Kidney function and aortic valve and mitral annular calcification in the Multi-Ethnic Study of Atherosclerosis (MESA). Am J Kidney Dis 2007;50:412–20.

74. Linefsky JP, O'Brien KD, Katz R, et al. Association of serum phosphate levels with aortic valve sclerosis and annular calcification: the cardiovascular health study. J Am Coll Cardiol 2011;58:291–7.

75. Bostrom KI, Rajamannan NM, Towler DA. The regulation of valvular and vascular sclerosis by osteogenic morphogens. Circulation Research 2011;109:564–77.

76. Mohler 3rd ER, Kaplan FS, Pignolo RJ. Boning-up on aortic valve calcification. J Am Coll Cardiol 2012;60:1954–5.

77. Rajamannan NM, Subramaniam M, Rickard D, et al. Human aortic valve calcification is associated with an osteoblast phenotype. Circulation 2003;107:2181–4.

78. Mohler 3rd ER, Gannon F, Reynolds C, et al. Bone formation and inflammation in cardiac valves. Circulation 2001;103:1522–8.

79. Miller JD, Weiss RM, Serrano KM, et al. Evidence for active regulation of pro-osteogenic signaling in advanced aortic valve disease. Arterioscler Thromb Vasc Biol 2010;30:2482–6.

80. Kaden JJ, Bickelhaupt S, Grobholz R, et al. Receptor activator of nuclear factor kappaB ligand and osteoprotegerin regulate aortic valve calcification. J Mol Cell Cardiol 2004;36:57–66.

81. Hofbauer LC, Schoppet M. Clinical implications of the osteoprotegerin/RANKL/RANK system for bone and vascular diseases. JAMA 2004;292:490–5.

82. Venuraju SM, Yerramasu A, Corder R, et al. Osteoprotegerin as a predictor of coronary artery disease and cardiovascular mortality and morbidity. J Am Coll Cardiol 2010;55:2049–61.

83. Kiechl S, Schett G, Wenning G, et al. Osteoprotegerin is a risk factor for progressive atherosclerosis and cardiovascular disease. Circulation 2004;109:2175–80.

84. Kiechl S, Werner P, Knoflach M, et al. The osteoprotegerin/RANK/RANKL system: a bone key to vascular disease. Expert review of cardiovascular therapy 2006;4:801–11.

85. Ueland T, Aukrust P, Dahl CP, et al. Osteoprotegerin levels predict mortality in patients with symptomatic aortic stenosis. J Intern Med 2011;270:452–60.

86. Sverdlov AL, Ngo DT, Chan WP, et al. Determinants of aortic sclerosis progression: implications regarding impairment of nitric oxide signalling and potential therapeutics. Eur Heart J 2012;33:2419–25.

87. Rosenhek R, Binder T, Porenta G, et al. Predictors of outcome in severe, asymptomatic aortic stenosis. N Engl J Med 2000;343:611–7.

88. Dweck MR, Jones C, Joshi NV, et al. Assessment of valvular calcification and inflammation by positron emission tomography in patients with aortic stenosis. Circulation 2012;125:76–86.

89. Marincheva-Savcheva G, Subramanian S, Qadir S, et al. Imaging of the aortic valve using fluorodeoxyglucose positron emission tomography increased valvular fluorodeoxyglucose uptake in aortic stenosis. J Am Coll Cardiol 2011;57:2507–15.

90. Dweck MR, Chow MW, Joshi NV, et al. Coronary arterial 18F-sodium fluoride uptake: a novel marker of plaque biology. J Am Coll Cardiol 2012;59:1539–48.

91. Avakian SD, Annicchino-Bizzacchi JM, Grinberg M, et al. Apolipoproteins AI, B, and E polymorphisms in severe aortic valve stenosis. Clinical Genetics 2001;60:381–4.

92. Ortlepp JR, Hoffmann R, Ohme F, et al. The vitamin D receptor genotype predisposes to the development of calcific aortic valve stenosis. Heart 2001;85:635–8.

93. Nordstrom P, Glader CA, Dahlen G, et al. Oestrogen receptor alpha gene polymorphism is related to aortic valve sclerosis in postmenopausal women. J Intern Med 2003;254:140–6.

94. Ortlepp JR, Schmitz F, Mevissen V, et al. The amount of calcium-deficient hexagonal hydroxyapatite in aortic valves is influenced by gender and associated with genetic polymorphisms in patients with severe calcific aortic stenosis. Eur Heart J 2004;25:514–22.

95. Moura LM, Faria S, Brito M, et al. Relationship of PON1 192 and 55 gene polymorphisms to calcific valvular aortic stenosis. Am J Cardiovasc Dis 2012;2:123–32.

96. Novaro GM, Sachar R, Pearce GL, et al. Association between apolipoprotein E alleles and calcific valvular heart disease. Circulation 2003;108:1804–8.

97. Ortlepp JR, Pillich M, Mevissen V, et al. APOE alleles are not associated with calcific aortic stenosis. Heart 2006;92:1463–6.

98. Gaudreault N, Ducharme V, Lamontagne M, et al. Replication of genetic association studies in aortic stenosis in adults. Am J Cardiol 2011;108:1305–10.

99. Ellis SG, Dushman-Ellis S, Luke MM, et al. Pilot candidate gene analysis of patients >/= 60 years old with aortic stenosis involving a tricuspid aortic valve. Am J Cardiol 2012;110:88–92.

100. Thanassoulis G, Campbell C, Owens DS, et al. Genetic Associations of Valve Calcification and Aortic Stenosis. N Engl J Med 2013;368(6):503–12.

101. Otto CM, Lind BK, Kitzman DW, et al. Association of aortic-valve sclerosis with cardiovascular mortality and morbidity in the elderly. N Engl J Med 1999;341:142–7.

102. Palmiero P, Maiello M, Passantino A, et al. Aortic valve sclerosis: is it a cardiovascular risk factor or a cardiac disease marker? Echocardiography 2007;24:217–21.

103. Otto CM. Why is aortic sclerosis associated with adverse clinical outcomes? J Am Coll Cardiol 2004;43:176–8.

104. Chandra HR, Goldstein JA, Choudhary N, et al. Adverse outcome in aortic sclerosis is associated with coronary artery disease and inflammation. J Am Coll Cardiol 2004;43:169–75.

105. Holley KE, Bahn RC, McGoon DC, et al. Spontaneous calcific embolization associated with calcific aortic stenosis. Circulation 1963;27:197–202.

106. Oliveira-Filho J, Massaro AR, Yamamoto F, et al. Stroke as the first manifestation of calcific aortic stenosis. Cerebrovasc Dis 2000;10:413–6.

107. Wilson JH, Cranley JJ. Recurrent calcium emboli in a patient with aortic stenosis. Chest 1989;96:1433–4.

108. Brockmeier LB, Adolph RJ, Gustin BW, et al. Calcium emboli to the retinal artery in calcific aortic stenosis. American heart journal 1981;101:32–7.

109. Rodriguez CJ, Bartz TM, Longstreth Jr WT, et al. Association of annular calcification and aortic valve sclerosis with brain findings on magnetic resonance imaging in community dwelling older adults: the cardiovascular health study. J Am Coll Cardiol 2011;57:2172–80.

110. Kizer JR, Wiebers DO, Whisnant JP, et al. Mitral annular calcification, aortic valve sclerosis, and incident stroke in adults free of clinical cardiovascular disease: the Strong Heart Study. Stroke 2005;36:2533–7.

CHAPTER 5

Left Ventricular Adaptation to Pressure and/or Volume Overload

Blase A. Carabello

Key Points

- Each valve lesion imparts a unique hemodynamic load on the left ventricle, wherein aortic stenosis creates a pure pressure overload, mitral regurgitation presents a pure volume overload, aortic regurgitation causes combined pressure and volume overload, and mitral stenosis leads to volume underload and potentially increased afterload. In turn, each lesion causes its own type of hypertrophy and remodeling.
- Individuals respond to similar load in very different ways, presumably on the basis of their genetic makeup.
- Hypertrophy can accrue not just from increased protein synthesis but also from reduced protein degradation.
- The terms *remodeling* and *hypertrophy* are not synonymous.
- In almost all cases hypertrophy is both adaptive and maladaptive.
- The transition from hypertrophy to heart failure is not a simplistic change in a single system but represents a complex biological cascade not yet completely defined.

Each form of valvular heart disease places a unique hemodynamic load on the left ventricle. The left ventricle is an amazingly complex sea of biological processes, but in fact, it can respond to these overloads using only three basic mechanisms. They are (1) activation of the Frank-Starling mechanism, (2) use of the adrenergic (and other) neurohumoral systems, and (3) chamber remodeling. This chapter attempts to summarize the response of the left ventricle to the load it faces in each of the four major left-sided valve lesions: aortic stenosis (AS), mitral regurgitation (MR), aortic regurgitation (AR), and mitral stenosis (MS).

Background

In 1973, Grossman et al[1] proposed the schema shown in Figure 5-1 as the foundation on which the left ventricle responds to valvular heart disease.[1] In this concept, the increased systolic stress (σ) caused by pressure overload induces sarcomere production in parallel, increasing myocyte width, and in turn increasing left ventricular (LV) wall thickness. Because $\sigma = p \times r/2h$, where $p =$ LV pressure, $r =$ LV radius, and $h =$ thickness, increased pressure in the numerator is offset by increased thickness in the denominator so that stress remains normal. Systolic wall stress is a reasonable surrogate for LV afterload. Because the ejection fraction varies inversely with afterload, the concentric hypertrophy and remodeling that occur through this process are thought of as initially compensatory because they help maintain LV function.

In the same hypothesis, volume overload increases diastolic stress that causes sarcomeres to be laid down in series, lengthening each myocyte and in turn increasing LV volume. Greater volume then allows total stroke volume to increase, helping to compensate for the wasted volume lost to regurgitation. Because this mechanism is a requisite to normalizing forward stroke volume, it too is considered compensatory, at least in part. Table 5-1 demonstrates the patterns of remodeling found in the left-sided overloading valve lesions.[2] AS, the classic pressure overload lesion, produces typical concentric LV hypertrophy (LVH) with the highest mass:volume (m/v) ratio and the lowest radius:thickness (r/h) ratio. MR is the prototypical volume overload lesion, leading to the lowest mass:volume ratio and the highest radius:thickness ratio. AR, a combined LV pressure and volume overload, causes the greatest amount of LVH with hybrid geometry between that of AS and MR.

Hypertrophy versus Remodeling

It has become fashionable to use the term *remodeling* when discussing changes in ventricular size and geometry, and most remodeling is associated with LVH. However, the two terms are not synonymous. *Hypertrophy* means an increase in mass, whereas *remodeling* indicates a change in geometry and/or volume. Thus, a situation in which increased wall thickness is accompanied by increased LV mass should be considered *concentric hypertrophy*, whereas one in which increased thickness is accompanied by a reduction in volume, leading to no change in LV mass,[3] should be termed *concentric remodeling*. Although the term remodeling is most often used in the context of LV dilation, a distinction should also be made between ventricles that enlarge with concomitant wall thinning, in which LV mass could remain the same (*pure remodeling*), and left ventricles that also increase their mass (*eccentric hypertrophy*) (Figure 5-2).

Aortic Stenosis

The normal aortic valve opens slightly, through not entirely understood mechanisms, before pressure in the left ventricle exceeds aortic pressure[4,5] and then offers almost no resistance to LV outflow. As the valve becomes diseased it stiffens and the orifice area diminishes. Even when aortic valve area is reduced by half, the LV pressure exceeds that of the aorta by only 5 to 10 mm Hg. However, further reductions in aortic valve area cause progressively greater pressure gradients across the valve. The transvalvular gradient represents the additional pressure that the left ventricle must generate to drive blood past the obstruction to outflow. It is generally agreed that this mechanical stress is transduced into a biological response, leading to hypertrophy and/or remodeling.

As noted previously, because the development of hypertrophy helps normalize afterload, thereby normalizing ejection performance, such hypertrophy has been viewed as compensatory. According to the paradigm proposed in Figure 5-1, just enough hypertrophy should develop to return wall stress to normal. Indeed, in some cases this expected course is borne out. However, such perfect compensation often fails to occur (Figures 5-3 and 5-4). Figure 5-3 demonstrates that frequently in patients with LV dysfunction, such dysfunction is due to afterload excess, indicating that not enough hypertrophy developed to normalize

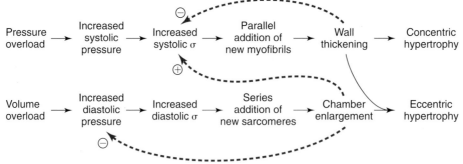

FIGURE 5-1 Effect of pressure and volume overload on development of left ventricular hypertrophy. The diagram shown is a framework for how mechanical stress (σ) is transduced into pressure versus volume overload hypertrophy. *(From Grossman W, Jones D, McLaurin LP. Wall stress and patterns of hypertrophy in the human left ventricle. J Clin Invest 1975;53:332–41.)*

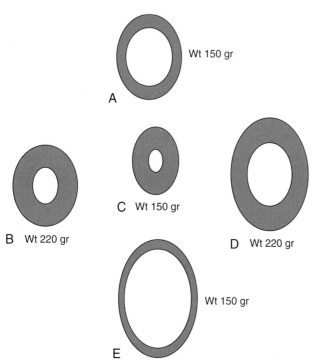

FIGURE 5-2 Schematic representation of the types of hypertrophy and remodeling that occur in valvular heart disease. A, Normal. **B,** Concentric left ventricular hypertrophy (LVH). **C,** Concentric remodeling. **D,** Eccentric LVH. **E,** Eccentric remodeling. *Wt,* weight.

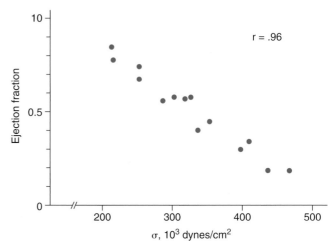

FIGURE 5-3 Wall stress and left ventricular systolic function in aortic stenosis. Ejection fraction is plotted against mean systolic wall stress (afterload; σ) for patients with aortic stenosis. As afterload increases from inadequate left ventricular hypertrophy, ejection fraction falls. *(From Gunther S, Grossman W. Determinants of ventricular function in pressure-overload hypertrophy in man. Circulation 1979;59:679–88.)*

TABLE 5-1	Hypertrophy in Human Left-Sided Overload Valve Lesions*		
	MASS INDEX (g/m²)	**r/h**	**m/v**
Normal	86 (259)	3.05 (88)	1.25 (225)
Mitral regurgitation	158 (146)	4.03 (64)	0.87 (117)
Aortic regurgitation	230 (148)	3.52 (31)	1.00 (141)
Aortic stenosis	178 (302)	2.35 (93)	1.55 (296)

m/v, ratio of left ventricular mass to volume; *r/h,* ratio of left ventricular radius to thickness. From Carabello BA. The relationship of left ventricular geometry and hypertrophy to left ventricular function in valvular heart disease. J heart Valve Dis 1995(Suppl 2):S132–8.
*Numbers in parentheses indicate numbers of subjects analyzed.

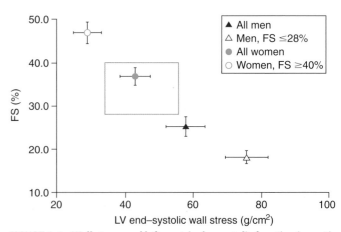

FIGURE 5-4 Wall stress and left ventricular systolic function in aortic stenosis. Fractional shortening (FS) is plotted against left ventricular (LV) systolic wall stress for patients with aortic stenosis. Some patients, especially women, have abnormally low stress and very high shortening fractions, suggesting that more left LV hypertrophy is present than that needed simply to normalize stress. *(From Carroll JD, Carroll EP, Feldman T, et al. Sex-associated differences in left ventricular function in aortic stenosis of the elderly. Circulation 1992;86:1099–107.)*

stress.[6] In fact, the majority of patients with AS have some element of afterload excess, indicating a lack of fully compensatory hypertrophy.[7]

The opposite end of the spectrum is shown in Figure 5-4.[8] In some patients, especially elderly women and children born with congenital AS,[9] there appears to be excessive hypertrophy. In such patients afterload is actually subnormal, leading to higher than expected ejection performance, at least at the endocardial level. It should be noted that assessment of LV function at the endocardial level often overestimates contractility. Ejection of blood from the LV cavity during systole is primarily a function of wall thickening. The more sarcomeres present in parallel, the more thickening occurs with shortening of the sarcomeres. Thus, in concentric remodeling and hypertrophy, subnormal shortening can still produce a normal ejection fraction.[10] Therefore, for accurate assessment of LV function in concentrically altered ventricles, midwall shortening should be evaluated; and when done, this evaluation may reveal diminished LV function, although not always.

In still other patients yet another response—concentric remodeling—develops to AS. In these patients there is no increase in LV mass.[3] Rather there is a reduction in LV volume together with an increase in LV wall thickness, acting to normalize stress without actual hypertrophy.

Variability in the Response to Pressure Overload

The question arises, why is there such inhomogeneity in the hypertrophic response to pressure overload? Is the differing LV geometry that occurs a response to different disease characteristics, such as valve area, rate of progression, or body habitus? Or is there an inherent difference in response to a similar pressure overload? Koide et al[11] addressed this question by creating a model of AS in which a gradually imposed gradient was identical in dogs of similar size and weight. The hypertrophy that subsequently developed recapitulated that seen in humans. Some animals had modest concentric hypertrophy, whereas others had severe hypertrophy. Of interest, the group with modest hypertrophy had persistently higher wall stress yet far less myocardial mass despite this greater stimulus for hypertrophy (Figure 5-5). These data suggest a different set point for response to the overload for which the stimulus was greater and the response less. It is likely that these inherent differences also explain the difference in the hypertrophic response noted in humans.

Concentric Hypertrophy and Left Ventricular Function

LV ejection is controlled by preload, afterload, and contractility. The reduction in the ejection fraction in AS stems from increased afterload, decreased contractility, or both.[7,12] Increased afterload occurs when remodeling fails to offset the greater systolic pressure required of the left ventricle. Whereas concentric LVH has long been considered a compensatory mechanism, this issue is not clear-cut. In studies of hypertrophy in general, LVH has led to increased cardiac mortality, especially in the presence of coronary artery disease.[13] Yet genetic maneuvers in mice that prevent or diminish the hypertrophic response have led to both increased mortality[14,15] and, conversely, beneficial effects,[16,17] leaving the question of the compensatory role of LVH in doubt. In the canine model already described, contractility was preserved at both sarcomere and LV chamber levels in the animals with extreme hypertrophy in which wall stress was normalized. In dogs with high afterload, contractility was depressed, at least in part owing to microtubular hyperpolymerization, which acted as an internal stent inhibiting sarcomere shortening.[18] Conversely, in a human study of AS, the best outcome was in patients without LVH who

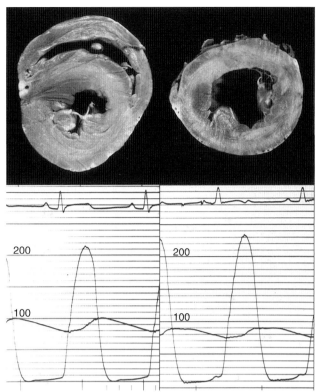

FIGURE 5-5   Heterogeneous response to pressure overload. Left ventricles from two dogs *(top)* with identical gradients *(bottom)* demonstrate different degrees of hypertrophy. *(From Koide M, Nagatsu M, Zile MR, et al. Premorbid determinants of left ventricular dysfunction in a novel mode of gradually induced pressure overload in the adult canine. Circulation 1997;95:1349–51.)*

underwent concentric remodeling.[3] LV mass was not greater, but increased relative wall thickness normalized afterload, allowing for compensated systolic function. This observation is not universal, however. In some patients the concentrically hypertrophied left ventricle is so reduced in volume that stroke volume is decreased. In turn, a small stroke volume reduces the transaortic gradient, potentially misleading the clinician into underestimating disease severity, thereby delaying therapy and leading to increased surgical risk.[19] In still another study, Duncan et al[20] propensity matched 964 pairs of patients with AS undergoing aortic valve replacement with and without concentric LVH and/or remodeling. Patients with concentric LVH had double the operative risk and double the postoperative morbidity in comparison with patients without this pattern.[20] It seems likely that intrinsic LV biological factors beyond the simple imaged geometry and mass of the LV account for these disparate results regarding the compensatory versus deleterious effects of LVH. Our future ability to understand and detect these factors should give us a better understanding of the role of LVH in AS.

When contractile dysfunction does occur, its mechanism is probably multifactorial. Concentric LVH clearly results in abnormal coronary blood flow and blood flow reserve.[21-23] Normally the subendocardium receives about 20% more blood flow than the epicardium, but this ratio is reversed in LVH.[24]

Thus, the myocardial layer with the highest oxygen demand receives the least oxygen supply. Further, coronary reserve is limited in concentric LVH. Whereas in normal individuals, coronary flow can increase by fivefold to eightfold in response to increased myocardial energy demands, flow reserve in AS is limited to an increase of twofold to threefold.[21] Abnormal flow reserve and flow distribution lead to subendocardial ischemia and contractile dysfunction during periods of stress.[24] It is also possible, but unproven, that this chronic imbalance could cause myocardial hibernation or stunning. The cytoskeletal abnormalities noted previously as well as disordered calcium handling and apoptosis also probably play a role.[25-27] Finally, there is the general belief that LVH transitions from a compensatory phase to a pathologic one.[28] Although certainly plausible, this concept, too, has been questioned. Animals destined to have contractile dysfunction demonstrated gene expression different from that in those who maintained normal function early in the course of pressure overload, suggesting that two separate patterns of hypertrophy exist rather than one that transitions into another,[29] consistent with the Koide dog model.

It is well recognized that diastolic function is abnormal in concentric LVH. Dysfunction accrues from delayed relaxation, increased wall thickness, and changes in myocardial structure with an increase in stiffness mediated by greater collagen content.[30,31]

In summary, the body of evidence supports the concept that concentric LVH is compensatory in the pressure overload of AS. However, concentric LVH is also associated with adverse outcomes, and the differences between compensatory LVH and pathologic LVH have yet to be clearly delineated but are not explained by magnitude alone.

Mitral Regurgitation

Whereas a variety of cardiac lesions are classified as volume overload lesions, most are actually combined pressure and volume overload lesions.[32,33] In conditions such as AR, anemia, and complete heart block, the additional volume pumped by the left ventricle is ejected into the aorta, where it increases stroke volume, widening pulse pressure and causing an element of systolic hypertension. Conversely, MR is a pure volume overload lesion. The extra volume pumped by the left ventricle in MR is ejected into the relatively low-pressure zone of the left atrium, and systemic systolic pressure tends to be reduced. Thus, MR is an ideal lesion in which to examine volume overload. As noted previously, the remodeling in MR is eccentric, with a large increase in LV radius and little, if any, increase in LV thickness. In fact, LV thickness in MR may even be less than normal.

This type of remodeling is beneficial for diastolic filling of the left ventricle but may impair systolic emptying. MR is one of the few cardiac diseases in which diastolic function is supernormal (Figure 5-6).[34,35] The thin-walled left ventricle in MR requires less filling pressure to fill it to any given filling volume. Thus, the ventricle is equipped to fill rapidly to accept the large blood volume

stored in the left atrium during systole that helps compensate for the volume wasted to regurgitation.

However, the large r/h ratio found in this type of remodeling (see Table 5-1) does not facilitate and may even impede LV ejection. The misconception that MR unloads the left ventricle by way of the low-impedance pathway for ejection into the left atrium is common. Although to some extent this concept must be valid, afterload is reduced only in acute MR. Thereafter, as the radius term in the Laplace equation increases, afterload returns to normal. As remodeling progresses, the enlarging r/h ratio actually causes afterload to become abnormally high, impeding rather than unloading the left ventricle during ejection.[36] If one reexamines Grossman's hypothesis, it appears that the pressure term in the Laplace equation is more effective than the radius term in causing LV thickening, because increased systolic stress from pressure overload but not from volume overload induces wall thickening. Alternatively it may be the lack of isovolumic pressure generation that causes this type of remodeling. In MR and ventricular septal defect, ejection from the left ventricle begins almost immediately, lacking the isovolumic period before the aortic valve opens, and in both cases the relative lack of LV muscle mass seems connected with reduced LV function.[2,33,36,37]

Left Ventricular Function in Mitral Regurgitation

Increased preload and normal afterload work in concert with initially normal contractility to maintain the LV ejection fraction at higher than normal levels. A "normal" ejection fraction in MR is about 70%. However, contractility eventually becomes impaired in severe prolonged MR, so that by the time ejection fraction falls to less than 60%, prognosis is impaired.[38,39]

Coronary blood flow is normal in MR and thus is not responsible for impaired contractile function.[40] Reduced contractility stems from loss of sarcomeric contractile elements (Figure 5-7) and impaired calcium handling.[41,42] The former can be reversed by correction of the volume overload or institution of beta-adrenergic blockade, implying sympathetic overdrive as a cause for the abnormal contractile function.[43,44] In a small randomized clinical trial, beta-blockade was compared with placebo in the treatment of patients with asymptomatic MR.[45] Beta-blockade prevented the reduction in LV ejection fraction seen in the placebo group after several months of therapy, adding further support to the concept that adrenergic overdrive is part of the pathophysiology of MR. It also raises the possibility that assessment of pathologic systems could add to the assessment of cardiac geometry and function in defining the proper timing for corrective surgery.

The force-frequency response in MR is impaired, with peak force occurring at relatively low heart rates, followed by an early descending limb of the force-frequency curve.[42] These data indicate impaired calcium handling. Forskolin also reverses contractile dysfunction, indicating that abnormal cyclic AMP (adenosine monophosphate) generation is also involved in abnormal contractility.[42]

Mechanisms of Hypertrophy in Aortic Stenosis versus Mitral Regurgitation

The contractile proteins of the myocardium are in constant flux, turning over every 10 days or so. For hypertrophy to occur, the rate of protein synthesis (K_s) must exceed the rate of protein degradation (K_d). Obviously, the only way for this to occur is for K_s to increase or for K_d to decrease. When an experimental animal is infused with a tritiated amino acid such as leucine, the rate of incorporation of new protein (K_s) can be determined. When a pressure overload is imposed on the canine left ventricle, K_s increases by 35% within 6 hours of the onset of the overload (Figure 5-8).[46] K_s then remains elevated for several days and

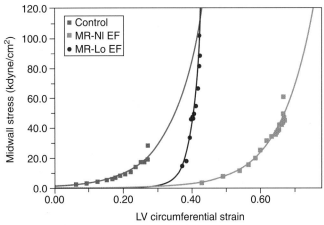

FIGURE 5-6 Stress-strain (stiffness) plots. Data are shown for normal (control) subjects, for patients with mitral regurgitation (MR) and normal left ventricular (LV) function (MR-NI EF), and for patients with MR and reduced LV function (MR-Lo EF) are demonstrated. Patients with MR and normal ejection fraction have reduced myocardial stiffness, their curve falling down and to the right of normal. *(From Corin WJ, Murakami T, Monrad ES, et al. Left ventricular passive diastolic properties in chronic mitral regurgitation. Circulation 1991;83: 797–807.)*

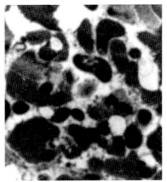
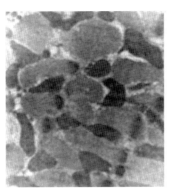
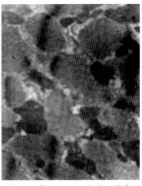

FIGURE 5-7 Effect of mitral regurgitation on myocardial ultrastructure. Photomicrographs are shown for a normal dog (*left*), a dog with severe mitral regurgitation (MR) (*center*), and a dog with severe MR that was corrected surgically (*right*). During severe MR there is a loss of contractile elements that is restored after surgery. *(From Spinale FG, Ishihara K, Zile M, et al. Structural basis for changes in left ventricular function and geometry because of chronic mitral regurgitation and after correction of volume overload. J Thorac Cardiovasc Surg 1993;106:1147–57.)*

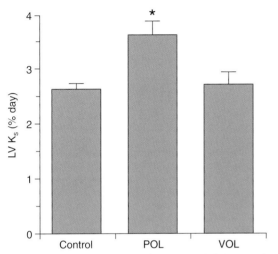

FIGURE 5-8 Myosin heavy chain synthesis rates (K_s). Data are shown for controls, for subjects with acute pressure overload (POL), and for subjects with acute volume overload (VOL). Whereas K_s increased substantially in POL, no increase could be detected in VOL. *LV,* left ventricular. *(From Imamura T, McDermott PJ, Kent RL, et al. Acute changes in myosin heavy chain synthesis rate in pressure versus volume overload. Circ Res 1994;75:418–25.)*

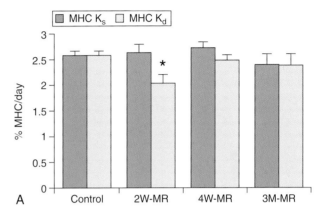
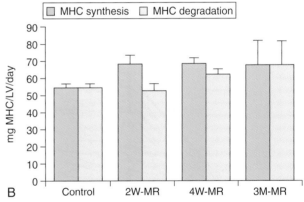

FIGURE 5-9 Myosin heavy chain (MHC) synthesis rate (K_s) and calculated degradation rate (K_d). A, Data are shown for controls and for dogs with mitral regurgitation (MR) at 2 weeks (2W-MR), 4 weeks (4W-MR), and 3 months (3M-MR) after creation of MR. An increase in K_s was not seen during the course of the lesion. Asterisk indicates significant difference ($p < 0.05$) compared to control. **B,** Calculated total myosin heavy chain weight per left ventricle per day. *(From Matsuo T, Carabello BA, Nagatomo Y, et al. Mechanisms of cardiac hypertrophy in canine volume overload. Am J Physiol 1998;275:H65–74, with permission.)*

returns to normal once afterload is normalized, strongly supporting Grossman's hypothesis.[47] Increased protein synthesis does not accrue from increased DNA transcription in this model but rather by enhanced message translation, because there is no increase in myosin message but there are increases in ribosomal number and polysome formation.

Conversely, even when severe MR was imposed on the canine left ventricle, no increase in K_s could be detected acutely nor at 2 weeks, 1 month, or 3 months after creation of MR (Figure 5-9).[46,48] Because eccentric LVH did occur, the lack of an increase in K_s implies that hypertrophy ensued by a decrease in K_d, an opposite mechanism for hypertrophy development from that of pressure overload. A rabbit model of MR produced similar findings.[49] In an isolated myocyte study in which load was imposed either during systole as it would be in pressure overload or in diastole as it would occur in volume overload, different signaling pathways were activated, again pointing to potentially differing mechanisms for generating pressure versus volume overload hypertrophy.[50]

Aortic Regurgitation: A Hybrid Disease

Although AR has long been lumped together with MR as a volume overload lesion, it is clear that AR is really a combined pressure

and volume overload.[32] Here the relatively high systolic pressure generated by the high total stroke volume ejected into the aorta combined with a large LV radius produces afterload that may be as high as that seen in AS, the traditional pressure overload. Not surprisingly then, both types of hypertrophy develop in AR. LV volume is increased and to a lesser extent so is LV wall thickness.[51] Thus, LV mass in AR is the highest of all valve lesions. Of interest, the mechanism of hypertrophy in AR also appears to be a hybrid of AS and MR, established by an increase in K_s but maintained by a decrease in K_d.[52]

Left Ventricular Function in Aortic Regurgitation

LV function in even severe AR may remain normal for years, and the rate of progression to LV dysfunction or symptom onset in asymptomatic patients is slow, probably less than 4% per year.[53] As with AS, when LV dysfunction does occur, it appears to be due both to excess afterload and to diminished contractility.[54] After aortic valve replacement, a depressed ejection fraction may improve dramatically, especially if the duration of dysfunction has been short (Figure 5-10).[55] Recovery is primarily due to a postoperative reduction in afterload.[56] If the ejection fraction is only mildly depressed preoperatively, it is likely to return to normal postoperatively. Even if the preoperative ejection fraction is severely reduced, significant improvement postoperatively is the rule because of the fall in afterload. The mechanisms of depressed contractility have been studied in a rabbit model,[57,58] in which there was an abundant growth of the noncollagen interstitial matrix, especially fibronectin. This abundant overgrowth appeared to "choke" existing contractile elements, often replacing them. To what extent this process is reversible after correction of the volume overload is unknown, as is the extent of its role in human AR.

Mitral Stenosis: The Underloaded Left Ventricle

Approximately one third of patients with MS have reduced LV ejection performance, a proportion that is perhaps surprising,

because this lesion "protects" the left ventricle from the consequences of MS.[59,60] Although the issue of whether the rheumatic process causes a contractile or "myocardial factor" leading to impaired myocardial function remains controversial, it does not appear to be operative in developed countries, where the consequences of rheumatic fever seem milder than in the developing world. Why then should LV ejection performance be reduced in MS? It appears that increased afterload is partly to blame. Although MS is not usually thought of as an afterload-excess lesion, systolic wall stress is increased in many patients with MS.[59] Increased afterload seems predicated on reduced wall thickness and reflexively increased systemic vascular resistance. At the same time, impaired LV filling prevents the use of the preload reserve to compensate for the afterload excess. These abnormalities are reversed after balloon mitral valvotomy.[61] It is plausible, although far from being proven, that reduced filling also impairs the ventricle from receiving the mechanical signals necessary for maintaining the mass and geometry needed for normalization of wall stress.

Conclusion

Each valve lesion creates its own, unique set of loading conditions that lead to LV remodeling and/or hypertrophy. These changes in many cases provide compensation for the load presented by the lesion, but remarkable differences exist among patients with similar types and severities of lesions, suggesting a great deal of modulation downstream from the initial mechanical signal. Although hypertrophy and remodeling may be compensatory, they often are not, instead leading to negative consequences such as heart failure and death. Future efforts to understand when and why these processes become pathologic are almost certain to augment our current armamentarium for deciding when to intervene in valvular heart disease.

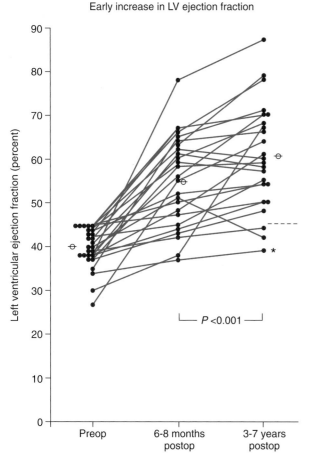

Early increase in LV ejection fraction

$P <0.001$

FIGURE 5-10 Left ventricular (LV) ejection fraction before (preop) and after (postop) aortic valve replacement in patients with aortic regurgitation. *(From Bonow RO, Dodd JT, Maron BJ, et al. Long-term serial changes in left ventricular function and reversal of ventricular dilation after valve replacement for chronic aortic regurgitation. Circulation 1988;78:1108–20.)*

REFERENCES

1. Grossman W, Jones D, McLaurin LP. Wall stress and patterns of hypertrophy in the human left ventricle. J Clin Invest 1975;53:332–41.
2. Carabello BA. The relationship of left ventricular geometry and hypertrophy to left ventricular function in valvular heart disease. J Heart Valve Dis 1995;4(Suppl 2):S132–8; discussion S138–S139.
3. Kupari M, Tutro H, Lommi J. Left ventricular hypertrophy in aortic valve stenosis—preventive or promotive of systolic dysfunction and heart failure? Eur Heart J 2005; 26:1790–6.
4. Rodriguez F, Green GR, Dagum P, et al. Left ventricular volume shifts and aortic root expansion during isovolumic contraction. J Heart Valve Dis 2006;15:465–73.
5. Pang DC, Choo SJ, Luo HH, et al. Significant increase of aortic root volume and commissural area occurs prior to aortic valve opening. J Heart Valve Dis 2000;9:9–15.
6. Gunther S, Grossman W. Determinants of ventricular function in pressure-overload hypertrophy in man. Circulation 1979;59:679–88.
7. Huber D, Grimm J, Koch R, et al. Determinants of ejection performance in aortic stenosis. Circulation 1981;64:126–34.
8. Carroll JD, Carroll EP, Feldman T, et al. Sex-associated differences in left ventricular function in aortic stenosis of the elderly. Circulation 1992;86:1099–107.
9. Donner R, Carabello BA, Black I, et al. Left ventricular wall stress in compensated aortic stenosis in children. Am J Cardiol 1983;51:946–51.
10. deSimone G, Devereux RB, Celentano A, et al. Left ventricular chamber and wall mechanics in the presence of concentric geometry. J Hypertens 1999;17:1001–6.
11. Koide M, Nagatsu M, Zile MR, et al. Premorbid determinants of left ventricular dysfunction in a novel mode of gradually induced pressure overload in the adult canine. Circulation 1997;95:1349–51.
12. Carabello BA, Green LH, Grossman W, et al. Hemodynamic determinants of prognosis of aortic valve replacement in critical aortic stenosis and advanced congestive heart failure. Circulation 1980;62:42–8.
13. Levy D, Garrison RJ, Savage DD, et al. Prognostic implications of echocardiographically determined left ventricular mass in the Framingham Heart Study. N Engl J Med 1990;322:1561–6.
14. Meguro T, Hong C, Asai K, et al. Cyclosporine attenuates pressure-overload hypertrophy in mice while enhancing susceptibility to decompensation and heart failure. Circ Res 1999;84:735–40.
15. Rogers JH, Tamirisa P, Kovacs A, et al. RGS4 causes increased mortality and reduced cardiac hypertrophy in response to overload. J Clin Invest 1999;104:567–76.
16. Esposito G, Rapacciuolo A, Naga Prasad SV, et al. Genetic alterations that inhibit in vivo pressure-overload hypertrophy prevent cardiac dysfunction despite increased wall stress. Circulation 2002;105:85–92.
17. Hill JA, Karimi M, Kutschke W, et al. Cardiac hypertrophy is not a required compensation response to short-term pressure overload. Circulation 2000;101:2863–9.

18. Koide M, Hamawaki M, Narishige T, et al. Microtubule depolymerization normalizes in vivo myocardial contractile function in dogs with pressure-overload left ventricular hypertrophy. Circulation 2000;102:1045–52.

19. Hachicha Z, Dumesnil JG, Bogaty P, et al. Paradoxical low-flow, low-gradient severe aortic stenosis despite preserved ejection fraction is associated with higher afterload and reduced survival. Circulation 2007;115(22):2856–64.

20. Duncan AI, Lowe BS, Garcia MJ, et al. Influence of concentric left ventricular remodeling on early mortality after aortic valve replacement. Ann Thorac Surg 2008;85(6):2030–9.

21. Marcus ML, Doty DB, Hiratzka LF, et al. Decreased coronary reserve: a mechanism for angina pectoris in patients with aortic stenosis and normal coronary arteries. N Engl J Med 1982;307:1362–6.

22. Julius BK, Spillman M, Vassali G, et al. Angina pectoris in patients with aortic stenosis and normal coronary arteries: mechanisms and pathophysiological concepts. Circulation 1997;95:892–8.

23. Rajappan K, Rimoldi OE, Dutka DP, et al. Mechanisms of coronary microcirculatory dysfunction in patients with aortic stenosis and angiographically normal coronary arteries. Circulation 2002;105:470–6.

24. Nakano K, Corin WJ, Spann Jr JF, et al. Abnormal subendocardial blood flow in pressure overload hypertrophy is associated with pacing-induced subendocardial dysfunction. Circ Res 1989;65:1555–64.

25. Tsutsui H, Oshihara K, Cooper GT. Cytoskeletal role in the contractile dysfunction of hypertrophied myocardium. Science 1993;260:682–7.

26. Ito K, Yan X, Feng X, et al. Transgenic expression of sarcoplasmic reticulum Ca²⁺ ATPase modifies the transition from hypertrophy to early heart failure. Circ Res 2001;89:422–9.

27. Olivetti G, Abbi R, Quaini F, et al. Apoptosis in the failing human heart. N Engl J Med 1997;336:1131–41.

28. Hein S, Arnon E, Kostin S, et al. Progression from compensated hypertrophy to failure in the pressure-overloaded human heart: structural deterioration and compensatory mechanisms. Circulation 2003;25(107):984–9.

29. Buermans HPJ, Redout EM, Schiel AE, et al. Micro-array analysis reveals pivotal divergent mRNA expression profiles early in the development of either compensated ventricular hypertrophy or heart failure. Physiol Genomics 2005;21:314–23.

30 Zile MR, Brutsaert DL. New concepts in diastolic dysfunction and diastolic heart failure: part II-causal mechanisms and treatment. Circulation 2002;105:1503–8.

31. Hess OM, Ritter M, Schneider J, et al. Diastolic stiffness and myocardial structure in aortic valve disease before and after valve replacement. Circulation 1984;69:855–65.

32. Wisenbaugh T, Spann JF, Carabello BA. Differences in myocardial performance and load between patients with similar amounts of chronic aortic versus chronic mitral regurgitation. J Am Coll Cardiol 1984;3:916–23.

33. Carabello BA. Mitral regurgitation. Part I: Basic pathophysiological principles. Mod Concepts Cardiovasc Dis 1988;57:53–8.

34. Zile MR, Tomita M, Nakano K, et al. Effects of left ventricular volume overload produced by mitral regurgitation on diastolic function. Am J Physiol 1991;261:H1471–80.

35. Corin WJ, Murakami T, Monrad ES, et al. Left ventricular passive diastolic properties in chronic mitral regurgitation. Circulation 1991;83:797–807.

36. Corin WJ, Monrad ES, Murakami T, et al. The relationship of afterload to ejection performance in chronic mitral regurgitation. Circulation 1987;76:59–67.

37. Corin WJ, Swindle MM, Spann Jr JF, et al. Mechanisms of decreased forward stroke volume in children and swine with ventricular septal defect and failure to thrive. J Clin Invest 1988;82:544–51.

38. Enriquez-Sarano M, Tajik AJ, Schaff HV, et al. Echocardiographic prediction of survival after surgical correction of organic mitral regurgitation. Circulation 1994;90:830–7.

39. Schuler G, Peterson KL, Johnson A, et al. Temporal response of left ventricular performance to mitral valve surgery. Circulation 1979;59:1218–31.

40. Carabello BA, Nakano K, Ishihara K, et al. Coronary blood flow in dogs with contractile dysfunction due to experimental volume overload. Circulation 1991;83:1063–75.

41. Spinale FG, Ishihara K, Zile M, et al. Structural basis for changes in left ventricular function and geometry because of chronic mitral regurgitation and after correction of volume overload. J Thorac Cardiovasc Surg 1993;106:1147–57.

42. Mulieri LA, Leavitt BJ, Martin BJ, et al. Myocardial force-frequency defect in mitral regurgitation heart failure is reversed by forskolin. Circulation 1993;88:2700–4.

43. Nakano K, Swindle MM, Spinale F, et al. Depressed contractile function due to canine mitral regurgitation improves after correction of the volume overload. J Clin Invest 1991;87:2077–86.

44. Tsutsui H, Spinale FG, Nagatsu M, et al. Effects of chronic β-adrenergic blockade on the left ventricular and cardiocyte abnormalities of chronic canine mitral regurgitation. J Clin Invest 1994;93:2639–48.

45. Ahmed MI, Aban I, Lloyd SG, et al. A randomized controlled phase IIb trial of beta(1)-receptor blockade for chronic degenerative mitral regurgitation. J Am Coll Cardiol 2012;60(9):833–8.

46. Imamura T, McDermott PJ, Kent RL, et al. Acute changes in myosin heavy chain synthesis rate in pressure versus volume overload. Circ Res 1994;75:418–25.

47. Nagatomo Y, Carabello BA, Hamawaki M, et al. Translational mechanisms accelerate the rate of protein synthesis during canine pressure-overload hypertrophy. Am J Physiol 1999;277:H2176–84.

48. Matsuo T, Carabello BA, Nagatomo Y, et al. Mechanisms of cardiac hypertrophy in canine volume overload. Am J Physiol 1998;275:H65–74.

49. Borer JS, Carter JN, Jacobson MH, et al. Myofibrillar protein synthesis rates in mitral regurgitation. Circulation 1997;96(Suppl 1):I-469.

50. Yamamoto K, Dang Q, Maeda Y, et al. Regulation of cardiomyocyte mechanotransduction by the cardiac cycle. Circulation 2001;103:1459–64.

51. Feiring AJ, Rumberger JA. Ultrafast computed tomography analysis of regional radius-to-wall thickness ratios in normal and volume-overloaded human left ventricle. Circulation 1992;85:1423–32.

52. Magid NM, Wallerson DC, Borer JS. Myofibrillar protein turnover in cardiac hypertrophy due to aortic regurgitation. Cardiology 1993;82:20–9.

53. Bonow RO, Lakatos E, Maron BJ, et al. Serial long-term assessment of the natural history of asymptomatic patients with chronic aortic regurgitation and normal left ventricular systolic function. Circulation 1991;84:1625–35.

54. Sutton M, Plappert T, Spegel A, et al. Early postoperative changes in left ventricular chamber size, architecture, and function in aortic stenosis and aortic regurgitation and their relation to intraoperative changes in afterload: a prospective two-dimensional echocardiographic study. Circulation 1987;76:77–89.

55. Bonow RO, Dodd JT, Maron BJ, et al. Long-term serial changes in left ventricular function and reversal of ventricular dilatation after valve replacement for chronic aortic regurgitation. Circulation 1988;78:1108–20.

56. Taniguchi K, Nakano S, Kawashima Y, et al. Left ventricular ejection performance, wall stress, and contractile state in aortic regurgitation before and after aortic valve replacement. Circulation 1990;82:798–807.

57. Borer JS, Truter S, Herrold EM, et al. Myocardial fibrosis in chronic aortic regurgitation: molecular and cellular responses to volume overload. Circulation 2002;105:1837–42.

58. Borer JS, Herrold EM, Carter JN, et al. Cellular and molecular basis of remodeling in valvular heart diseases. Heart Fail Clin 2006;2:415–24.

59. Gash AK, Carabello BA, Cepin D, et al. Left ventricular ejection performance and systolic muscle function in patients with mitral stenosis. Circulation 1983;67:148–54.

60. Horwitz LD, Mullins CB, Payne PM, et al. Left ventricular function in mitral stenosis. Chest 1973;64:609–14.

61. Fawzy ME, Choi WB, Mimish L, et al. Immediate and long-term effect of mitral balloon valvotomy on left ventricular volume and systolic function in severe mitral stenosis. Am Heart J 1996;132:356–60.

CHAPTER 6

Echocardiographic Evaluation of Valvular Heart Disease

Catherine M. Otto

Key Points

- Echocardiography provides an accurate diagnosis of the presence and cause of valve disease.
- Quantitative echocardiographic evaluation of left ventricular size and systolic function is a key factor in clinical decision making in adults with valvular heart disease.
- Aortic stenosis severity is defined by maximum aortic jet velocity, mean gradient, and continuity equation valve area.
- Mitral stenosis severity is defined by mean gradient and valve area, determined by three- or two-dimensional planimetry and by the pressure half-time method.
- Regurgitant severity is defined by vena contracta width, the continuous-wave Doppler velocity signal, and the presence of distal flow reversals. In selected cases, calculation of regurgitant volume and regurgitant orifice area is recommended.
- Other key echocardiographic data include left ventricular diastolic function, left atrial and thrombus formation, pulmonary pressure estimates, and evaluation of right heart function.
- Aortic dilation associated with aortic valve disease can be diagnosed by echocardiography, but other imaging modalities may be needed for complete evaluation.
- Primary indications for transesophageal imaging include detection of left atrial thrombus, evaluation of prosthetic mitral valves, mitral valve repair, aortic dilation, and nondiagnostic transthoracic data.
- Three-dimensional echocardiography now has a key role in evaluation of myxomatous mitral valve disease and for guidance of transcatheter valve procedures.
- Postoperative echocardiography is recommended in patients with prosthetic heart valves to serve as a baseline for long-term follow-up of prosthetic valve function.
- Transesophageal echocardiography has a higher sensitivity than transthoracic echocardiography for detection of vegetations and complications of endocarditis.

Echocardiography allows evaluation of valve anatomy, etiology of disease, severity of stenosis and regurgitation, and consequences of valve disease including left ventricular (LV) hypertrophy, dilation, systolic and diastolic function, effects on other cardiac chambers, and changes in pulmonary pressures or vascular resistance. In current clinical practice, echocardiography is the standard diagnostic approach to the patient with suspected or known valvular heart disease. This chapter provides a concise overview of echocardiographic evaluation of the patient with valvular heart disease; more detailed discussions are available in standard echocardiography texts.[1,2] The use of echocardiography for specific valve lesions is included in subsequent chapters in this book, including the role of echocardiography in evaluation of patients with endocarditis (see Chapter 25) and prosthetic valves (see Chapter 26).

Anatomic Imaging

The first step in evaluation of the patient with valvular heart disease is assessment of valve anatomy (Table 6-1). In many cases, the specific valve involved is known from the clinical history, physical examination, or previous diagnostic studies, but in other cases, the exact diagnosis may be unknown or may have been incorrectly inferred from clinical data. Thus, a careful examination of all four valves and screening for other lesions that might be mistaken for valvular disease are important aspects of the examination. For example, in a patient with a systolic murmur referred for suspected valvular aortic stenosis, other diagnostic possibilities include a subaortic membrane, mitral regurgitation, ventricular septal defect, and hypertrophic cardiomyopathy. An appropriate examination includes exclusion (or confirmation) of each differential diagnosis, as well as evaluation of the aortic valve itself.

Echocardiographic Valve Anatomy

Standard two-dimensional (2D) transthoracic echocardiography (TTE) in multiple image planes identifies involved valve and often allows precise definition of the etiology of valve disease, on the basis of the typical anatomic features of each disease process. When TTE image quality is suboptimal, transesophageal echocardiography (TEE) may be appropriate. Three-dimensional (3D) imaging is increasingly important in evaluation of valve disease, particularly for TEE evaluation of myxomatous mitral valve disease and for guidance of transcatheter valve interventions.[3-5]

Mitral stenosis most often is due to rheumatic disease with the pathognomonic features commissural fusion, thickening of the leaflet tips, and chordal thickening, fusion, and shortening, all of which are easily recognized on 2D and 3D imaging (Figures 6-1 and 6-2). In contrast, the occasional elderly patient with functional mitral stenosis due to extension of mitral annular calcification onto the valve leaflets has thin, mobile leaflet tips, with calcification and thickening at the leaflet bases. The specific anatomic features of the rheumatic mitral valve, including severity of leaflet calcification, extent of chordal fusion, and asymmetry in commisural calcification, are important factors in predicting prognosis and in decision making for percutaneous or surgical intervention, discussed in Chapter 17.

TABLE 6-1	Echocardiographic Evaluation of the Patient with Valvular Heart Disease

2D and 3D Imaging

Valve anatomy and etiology of disease
2D or 3D valve area
Quantitative LV dimensions, volumes, ejection fraction, and mass
Associated chamber enlargement (e.g., left atrium)
Right heart structure and function
Complications of valve disease (i.e., left atrial thrombus)
Aortic sinuses and ascending aortic anatomy and dimensions

Doppler Evaluation of Severity of Valve Disease

Valve Stenosis

Maximum velocity
Mean pressure gradient
Valve area (continuity equation and/or pressure half-time)
Other measures of stenosis severity, if needed

Valve Regurgitation

Vena contracta width
CW Doppler signal
Distal flow reversals
Regurgitant volume and orifice area

Speckle Tracking Strain Imaging

LV strain and strain rate

Other Doppler Data

LV diastolic function
Pulmonary pressures at rest and with exercise

2D, two-dimensional; *3D,* three-dimensional; *CW,* continuous wave; *LV,* left ventricular.

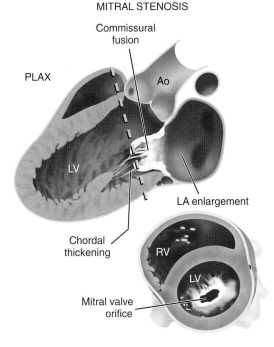

FIGURE 6-1 Anatomic findings in mitral stenosis. In the parasternal long-axis view (PLAX), commissural fusion with diastolic doming of the mitral leaflets is seen, as well as chordal thickening and fusion. In a parasternal short-axis view (PSAX), at the mitral valve orifice, the area of opening can be determined by planimetry at the white-black interface of the orifice. The plane of the short-axis view is indicated by a *dashed line* on the long-axis image. *Ao,* Aorta; *LV,* left ventricle; *RV,* right ventricle. *(From Otto CM. Textbook of clinical echocardiography. 5th ed. Philadelphia: Elsevier/Saunders; 2013.)*

Although aortic valve stenosis of any cause is characterized by thickened, stiff leaflets with reduced systolic opening, calcific aortic valve disease is typified by increased echogenicity and thickness in the body of the leaflets without evidence of commissural fusion, resulting in a stellate orifice in systole (Figure 6-3). It may be difficult to separate calcific changes superimposed on a bicuspid aortic valve from calcification of a trileaflet valve, although 3D TEE may help with this distinction. Rheumatic aortic valve disease is characterized by commissural fusion with increased thickening and echogenicity along the leaflet closure lines and is invariably associated with rheumatic mitral valve disease. Congenital aortic stenosis, seen in young adults, is characterized by a deformed (often unicuspid) valve that "domes" in systole with a restrictive orifice.

Evaluation of the etiology of a regurgitant lesion by echocardiography is more challenging, given the wide range of abnormalities that can lead to valvular incompetence. Mitral regurgitation may be due to abnormalities of the mitral annulus, leaflets, subvalvular apparatus, papillary muscle, or regional or global LV dysfunction (Figure 6-4). Echocardiographic imaging allows assessment of each of these valve components, so that the etiology of the regurgitant lesion can be discerned in many cases, as discussed in detail in Chapters 18 and 19. Selection of patients for surgical and percutaneous mitral valve interventions is discussed in Chapters 17, 21 and 22. In adults with secondary "functional" mitral regurgitation due to ischemic disease or dilated cardiomyopathy, imaging allows evaluation of both valve anatomy and the left ventricle. Quantitative evaluation of regurgitant severity also may be helpful in determining whether mitral regurgitation is the cause or consequence of ventricular dysfunction.

Aortic regurgitation may be due to abnormalities of the valve leaflets (such as a bicuspid valve and endocarditis), inadequate support of the valve structures (for example, a subaortic ventricular septal defect), or aortic root dilation (such as in Marfan syndrome or annuloaortic ectasia) (Figure 6-5). Echocardiographic imaging provides accurate measurements of aortic root dimensions and allows detailed evaluation of valve anatomy and

dynamics. A bicuspid valve is diagnosed on the basis of the typical appearance in *systole* of two open leaflets with two commissures; the closed valve in diastole may mimic a trileaflet valve if there is a raphe in one leaflet. Other recognized abnormalities of the valve leaflets that correspond to a specific etiology include valvular vegetations in endocarditis, redundant leaflets in myxomatous disease, and commissural thickening and associated mitral valve involvement in rheumatic disease, all of which can be recognized on echocardiographic imaging.

With aortic root disease, the specific pattern of root dilation and associated features may indicate a specific etiology, such as the "water balloon" appearance of the root in Marfan syndrome with loss of the normal tapering at the sinotubular junction and associated mitral valve abnormalities. In other cases, the pattern of root dilation is nonspecific, so incorporation of other clinical information is needed to determine the etiology of disease. For example, aortic root dilation in a patient with a systemic immune-mediated process (such as rheumatoid arthritis) is probably due to this systemic disease process. In contrast, dilation of the ascending aorta in a patient with a bicuspid aortic valve is likely related to bicuspid aortic valve disease.[6,7]

Right-sided valve abnormalities in adults most likely are due to residual congenital heart disease (e.g., congenital pulmonic stenosis, Ebstein anomaly of the tricuspid valve) or are secondary to left-sided heart disease (e.g., tricuspid annular dilation due to pulmonary hypertension in a patient with mitral stenosis). Again, 2D imaging usually allows determination of the valve anatomy and etiology of the valvular lesion, particularly when other aspects of the examination and clinical features are incorporated in the echocardiographic interpretation.

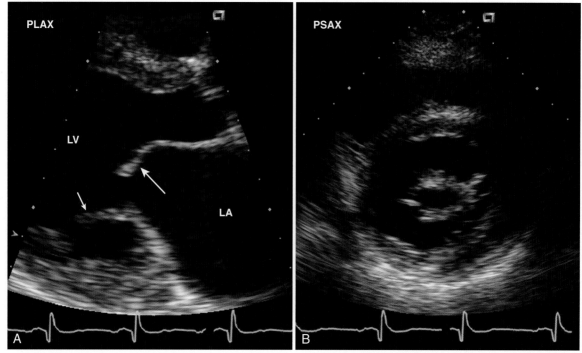

FIGURE 6-2 Mild rheumatic mitral stenosis. A, The parasternal long-axis view shows the typical doming *(long arrow)* of the anterior mitral leaflet due to commissural fusion as well as chordal shortening and fusion *(short arrow)*. Left atrial (LA) enlargement is present. **B,** The short-axis view allows accurate planimetry of the mitral orifice area if care is taken to identify the smallest opening by scanning slowly from apex toward the base. *LV,* left ventricle. *(From Otto CM. Textbook of clinical echocardiography. 5th ed. Philadelphia: Elsevier/Saunders; 2013.)*

Transthoracic versus Transesophageal Echocardiographic Imaging

TTE provides diagnostic images in the vast majority of patients with valvular heart disease and is the standard approach both for initial evaluation and for follow-up studies. However, TTE image quality may be suboptimal in patients in whom ultrasound access is poor because of body habitus, hyperexpanded lungs, or the postoperative state. Even when TTE images are adequate, TEE provides better image resolution for posterior structures, including the mitral valve, left atrium (LA), and atrial appendage. 3D TEE imaging provides a "surgical" view of the mitral valve from the perspective of the LA, demonstrating the presence, location, and severity of prolapse; identification of chordal rupture; and evaluation of the valve commissures (Figure 6-6).[8,9] TEE or intracardiac echocardiography is essential for excluding left atrial thrombus in candidates for balloon mitral valvotomy.

Other indications for TEE in patients with valvular disease include assessment of regurgitant severity when TTE images are nondiagnostic or when a prosthetic mitral valve is present, monitoring of surgical and transcatheter valve repair procedures (see Chapters 17 and 22), measurements for valve sizing with transcatheter valve procedures (Figures 6-7 and 6-8), and determining the exact level of obstruction in a patient with a differential diagnosis of valvular or subvalvular obstruction. Rarely, TEE is needed for evaluation of stenosis severity when TTE data are not diagnostic.

Evaluation of Stenosis Severity

Velocity Data and Pressure Gradients

The fluid dynamics of a stenotic valve are characterized by a high-velocity jet in the narrowed orifice; laminar, normal velocity flow proximal to the stenosis; and a flow disturbance distal to the obstruction.[10,11] The pressure gradient across the valve (ΔP) is related to the high-velocity jet (V_{max}) in the stenosis, the proximal velocity (V_{prox}), and the mass density of blood (ρ), as stated in the

Bernoulli equation, which includes terms for conversion of potential to kinetic energy (convective acceleration), the effects of local acceleration, and viscous (v) losses:

$$\Delta P = \tfrac{1}{2}\rho(V_{max}^2 - V_{prox}^2) + \rho(dv/dt)dx + R(v)$$
$$\text{Convective} \qquad \text{Local} \qquad \text{Viscous}$$
$$\text{acceleration} \qquad \text{acceleration} \qquad \text{losses}$$

where $(dv/dt)dx$ is the time varying velocity at each distance along the flow stream; and R is a constant describing the viscous losses for that fluid and orifice.

In clinical practice, the terms for acceleration and viscous losses are ignored, so that the following equation is used:

$$\Delta P = 4(V_{max}^2 - V_{prox}^2)$$

where the constant 4 accounts for the mass density of blood and conversion factors for measurement of pressure in mm Hg and velocity in m/s. When the proximal velocity is low (<1.5 m/s) and the jet velocity is high $(v_1^2 \ll v_2^2)$, this equation can be further simplified as follows:

$$\Delta P = 4V_{max}^2$$

Maximum instantaneous gradient is calculated from the maximum transvalvular velocity, whereas mean gradient is calculated by averaging the instantaneous gradients over the flow period.

The accuracy of the simplified Bernoulli equation in measuring transvalvular pressure gradients has been shown in in vitro studies, animal models, and clinical studies of patients with valvular disease (Table 6-2). However, accuracy depends on optimal data acquisition; specifically, care is needed to obtain a parallel intercept angle between the continuous-wave (CW) Doppler beam and the direction of blood flow in order to avoid underestimation of the velocity and, hence, pressure gradient across the valve. The high velocities encountered in aortic and pulmonic stenosis mandate the use of CW Doppler echocardiography to avoid signal aliasing. A dedicated small dual-crystal CW Doppler transducer is recommended. Pulsed or high pulse repetition frequency Doppler echocardiography can be used for evaluation of the lower velocities seen in mitral and tricuspid stenosis with

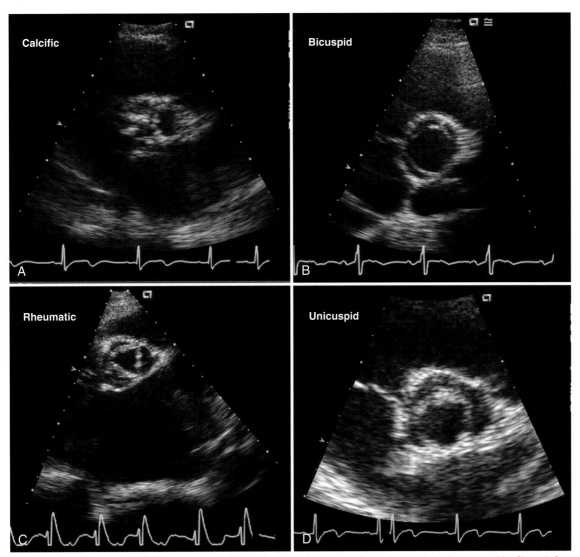

FIGURE 6-3   Causes of aortic stenosis. A, In a parasternal midsystolic short-axis view, calcific aortic stenosis is characterized by fibrocalcific masses on the aortic side of the leaflet that result in increased leaflet stiffness without commissural fusion. Calcific shadowing and reverberations limit image quality. **B,** With a congenital bicuspid valve, the two leaflets (with a raphe in the anterior leaflet) open widely in systole. **C,** The diagnostic features of rheumatic stenosis are commissural fusion and mitral valve involvement, with the characteristic triangular aortic valve opening in systole. **D,** The unicuspid valve has only one point of attachment (at the 6 o'clock position) with a funnel-shaped valve opening. *(From Otto CM. Textbook of clinical echocardiography. 5th ed. Philadelphia: Elsevier/Saunders; 2013.)*

TABLE 6-2	**Selected Studies Validating Doppler Pressure Gradients in Valvular Aortic Stenosis***				
FIRST AUTHOR (YEAR)	**N**	**STUDY GROUP/MODEL**	**R**	**RANGE (mm Hg)**	**SEE (mm Hg)**
Callahan (1985)	120	Supravalvular constriction (canines)	0.99 (ΔP_{max})	7-179	5.2
			0.98 (ΔP_{mean})	N/A	4.3
Smith (1985)	88	Supravalvular constriction (canines)	0.98 (ΔP_{max})	5-166	5.3
			0.98 (ΔP_{mean})	5-116	3.3
Currie (1985)	100	Adults with valvular aortic stenosis	0.92 (ΔP_{max})	2-180	15
			0.92 (ΔP_{mean})	0-112	10
Smith (1986)	33	Adults with valvular aortic stenosis	0.85 (ΔP_{max})	27-138	–
Simpson (1985)	24	Adults with valvular aortic stenosis	0.98 (ΔP_{max})	0-120	–
Burwash (1993)	98	Chronic valvular aortic stenosis (canines)	0.95 (ΔP_{max})	10-128	8.4
			0.91 (ΔP_{mean})	5-77	5.3

SEE, standard error of the estimate.

From Otto CM. Textbook of clinical echocardiography. 5th ed. Philadelphia: Elsevier/Saunders; 2013.

*Data from Callahan et al, Am J Cardiol 1985;56:989–993; Smith et al, J Am Coll Cardiol 1985;6:1306–1314; Currie et al, Circulation 1985;71:1162–1169; Smith et al, Am Heart J 1986;111:245–252; Simpson et al, Br Heart J 1985;53:636–639; Burwash et al, Am J Physiol 1993;265:H1734–H1743.

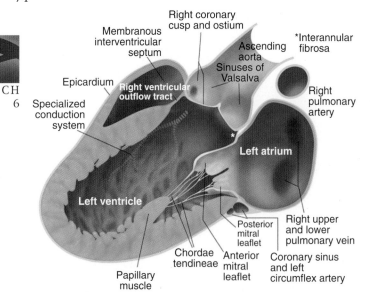

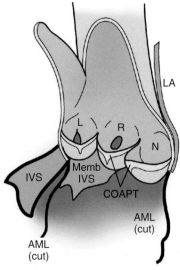

FIGURE 6-4 Cardiac valve anatomy in the long-axis view. The parasternal long-axis view in diastole shows: the closed right and noncoronary cusps of the aortic valve; the aortic sinuses, sinotubular junction, and proximal ascending aorta; the open anterior and posterior mitral valve leaflets; the basal and midventricular segments of the anterior septum and posterior LV wall; the RV outflow tract anteriorly; and the coronary sinus in the atrioventricular groove. The medial papillary muscle is shown for reference, although slight medial angulation is typically needed to visualize this structure in the long-axis view.

FIGURE 6-5 Aortic valve anatomy. Detailed view of the aortic valve with the aorta opened to show the valve leaflets and the interventricular septum (IVS) and anterior mitral leaflet (AML) bisected. The aortic valve consists of three leaflets and associated sinuses of Valsalva; the left (L) right (R), and noncoronary (N) leaflets and sinuses. Each leaflet-sinus pair forms a cup-shaped unit when the valve is closed. The load-bearing section of the leaflet appears linear when viewed in long axis but curved in cross-section, consistent with a hemicylindrical shape. The coaptation surfaces of the leaflets thicken toward the center of each leaflet with areas of prominent thickening termed the nodes of Arantius. Lambl excrescences, filamentous attachments on the ventricular side of the nodules of Arantius, are common in older subjects. *(From Otto CM. Textbook of clinical echocardiography. 5th ed. Philadelphia: Elsevier/Saunders; 2013.)*

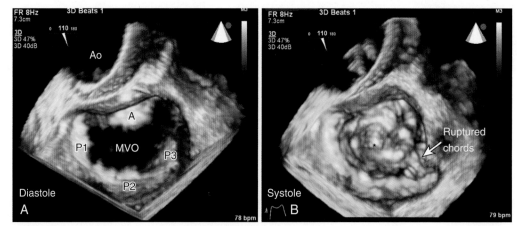

FIGURE 6-6 Three-dimensional images of the mitral valve. A, The surgeon's view from the left atrial side of the mitral valve with the aortic valve (Ao) at the top of the image, showing the anterior leaflet and posterior leaflet (with *P1, P2,* and *P3* scallops) are seen in diastole in the open position with a normal mitral valve orifice (MVO). **B,** In systole, severe prolapse of the anterior leaflet is seen. One bulging section *(asterisk)* and a flail segment with two small ruptured chords are particularly well visualized, which results in severe posteriorly directed mitral regurgitation. This patient also a bileaflet mechanical aortic prosthesis; the open leaflets can be seen in the systolic image. *(From Otto CM. Textbook of clinical echocardiography. 5th ed. Philadelphia: Elsevier/Saunders; 2013.)*

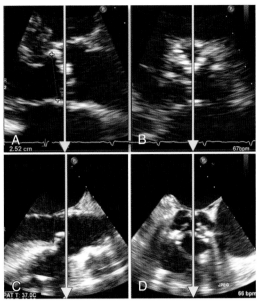

FIGURE 6-7 **Measurement of aortic annulus diameter for transcatheter aortic valve implantation. A** and **B,** Biplane echocardiographic imaging identifies the sagittal imaging plane that bisects the largest dimension of the aortic annulus. Biplane transthoracic imaging shows the sagittal **(A)** and corresponding transverse **(B)** planes. The *yellow arrows* define the imaging planes for the orthogonal view. The *red line* shows the appropriate annular measurement in the on-axis sagittal plane. **C** and **D,** Biplane transesophageal imaging shows the sagittal **(C)** and corresponding transverse **(D)** planes. *Red arrow* in **(C)** shows the appropriate annular measurement in the on-axis sagittal plane. *(From Bloomfield GS, Gillam LD, Hahn RT, et al. A practical guide to multimodality imaging of transcatheter aortic valve replacement. JACC Cardiovasc Imaging 2012;5:441–55.)*

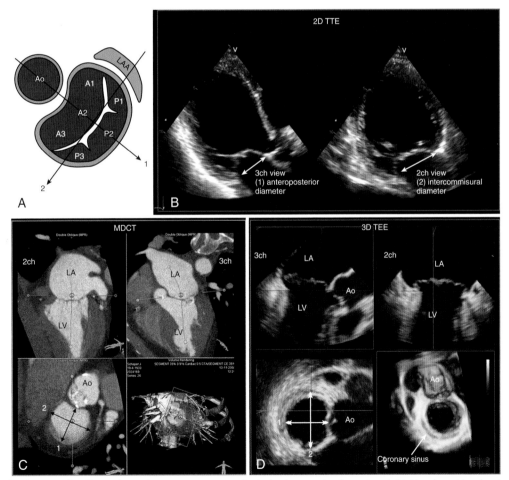

FIGURE 6-8 **Mitral valve annular dimensions.** Accurate assessment of mitral valve annular dimensions is highly relevant to planning of the therapeutic strategy. **A,** The anteroposterior (1) and intercommissural (2) diameters are commonly measured. **B,** With 2D TTE, the anteroposterior diameter *(arrow)* is measured at the apical three-chamber (3ch) view whereas the inter commissural diameter *(arrow)* can be measured in the apical two-chamber (2ch) view. Three-dimensional (3D) imaging techniques, such as multidetector computed tomography (MDCT) **(C)** and 3D transesophageal echocardiography (3D TEE) **(D),** permit correct alignment of the orthogonal multiplanar reformation planes to obtain the most accurate cross-sectional visualization of the mitral valve annulus. The maximum and minimum diameters can be assessed. These two orthogonal diameters commonly correspond to the intercommissural and anteroposterior diameters, respectively. *A1* to *A3,* Anterior mitral valve leaflet scallops; *Ao,* Aorta; *LA,* left atrium; *LV,* left ventricle; *P1* to *P3,* posterior mitral valve leaflet scallops . *(From Delgado V, Kapadia S, Marsan NA, et al. Multimodality imaging before, during, and after percutaneous mitral valve repair. Heart 2011;97:1704–14.)*

the advantage of a better signal-to-noise ratio and clearer definition of the diastolic deceleration slope than with CW Doppler echocardiography. Other potential technical sources of error in measuring transvalvular velocities include poor acoustic access with an inadequate flow signal, incorrect identification of the flow signal (e.g., mistaking the mitral regurgitation signal for aortic stenosis), respiratory motion, and measurement variability. In addition, physiologic sources of error include beat-to-beat variability with irregular rhythms and interim changes in volume flow rates leading to changes in velocity and pressure gradient.

For aortic stenosis, the maximum velocity across the stenotic valve provides the most important diagnostic and prognostic information. As indicated by the Bernoulli equation, there is a consistent relationship between maximum velocity and maximum pressure gradient. In addition, there is a consistent relationship between maximum velocity and *mean* gradient in native aortic valve stenosis, so that maximum velocity, maximum gradient, and mean gradient all convey the same information about the degree of valve narrowing. Increasingly, clinicians rely on velocity data alone in clinical decision making, without the intermediate step of converting velocities to pressure gradients.

Valve Area Concept and Measurement

Pressure gradients and velocities depend on the volume flow rate across the valve as well as the degree of valve narrowing. Valve area (or the size of the stenotic orifice) is a useful measure of stenosis severity that, at least in theory, more closely reflects valve anatomy independent of the flow rate across the valve. Valve area can be calculated from invasive data as discussed in Chapter 7 or noninvasively from 2D and Doppler echocardiographic data using the continuity equation.

IMAGING THE STENOTIC VALVE ORIFICE

The valve orifice in rheumatic mitral stenosis is a relatively planar structure with a constant shape and size throughout diastole (see Figure 6-2). From a parasternal short-axis view, the orifice can be imaged, with care taken to identify the minimum orifice area by scanning from the apex toward the base, using low gain settings, and tracing the inner border of the black-white interface.[12] Measurement of 2D mitral valve area has been well validated in comparison with direct measurement at surgery and with invasive valve area calculations (Table 6-3). Planimetry of the stenotic mitral valve orifice from a 3D volumetric data set or image ensures that the minimal orifice area at the leaflet tips is correctly measured; 3D measurements show improved reliability with less experienced sonographers (Figure 6-9).[13]

The anatomy of valvular aortic stenosis is variable and more complex than mitral stenosis. A congenitally unicuspid valve may have a relatively symmetric orifice that can be imaged in a single tomographic plane and is well seen on 3D imaging. Although the opening of a bicuspid valve often is clearly seen early in the disease course, superimposed calcific changes result in shadowing and reverberations, making planimetry of the stenotic valve orifice problematic, although 3D imaging may be helpful when calcification is not severe. The orifice of a calcified trileaflet valve may be quite complex with a nonplanar stellate shape. Although not routine clinical practice, 3D TEE imaging is helpful for planimetry of aortic valve area, in selected patients (Figure 6-10).[14,15]

CONTINUITY EQUATION

Valve area is calculated with use of the continuity equation (Figure 6-11), which is based on the principle of conservation of mass, specifically that the stroke volumes proximal to *(SV_Proximal)* and in *(SV_Stenotic orifice)* the stenotic orifice are equal:

$$SV_{Proximal} = SV_{Stenotic\ orifice}$$

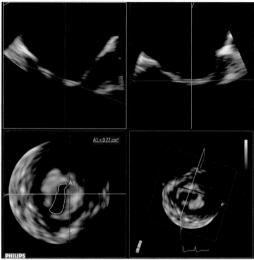

FIGURE 6-9   Three-dimensional measurement of mitral valve area. A full-volume image of the mitral valve was acquired in a patient with mitral stenosis and asymmetric fusion of the commissures. For measurement of the mitral valve area, offline analysis of the three-dimensional (3D) volume used three orthogonal planes (*x, y,* and *z,* shown in *red, green,* and *blue* to align an image plane at the tips of the stenotic valve. The resulting tomographic image at the minimal orifice area in diastole (*lower left*) was traced to determine mitral valve area (*A1*). (*From Otto CM. Textbook of clinical echocardiography. 5th ed. Philadelphia: Elsevier/Saunders; 2013.*)

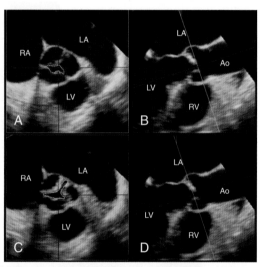

FIGURE 6-10   Measurement of aortic valve area by 3D transesophageal echocardiography. The tip of the aortic valve was obtained as the smallest possible area (*A1, A2*). The shape and area of the aortic valve changed (from *A1* to *B1*) as the green plane moved slightly from the tip to the base (from *A2* to *B2*). *Dotted lines* indicate aortic valve area at each level. *Ao,* Ascending aorta; *LA,* left atrium; *LV,* left ventricle; *RA,* right atrium. (*From Saitoh T, Shiota M, Izumo M, et al. Comparison of left ventricular outflow geometry and aortic valve area in patients with aortic stenosis by 2-dimensional versus 3-dimensional echocardiography. Am J Cardio 2012;109:1626–31.*)

Because stroke volume is the product of cross-sectional area *(CSA)* and the velocity-time integral of flow *(VTI)*:

$$CSA_{Proximal} \times VTI_{Proximal} = Area_{Stenotic\ orifice} \times VTI_{Stenotic\ orifice}$$

This equation then is solved for stenotic orifice area as follows:

$$Area_{Stenotic\ orifice} = (CSA_{Proximal} \times VTI_{Proximal})/VTI_{Stenotic\ orifice}$$

The continuity equation is used routinely for evaluation of aortic valve area,[16] with transaortic stroke volume measured in the LV outflow tract just proximal to the stenotic valve. The

TABLE 6-3   Selected Studies of Mitral Valve Area Determination*

FIRST AUTHOR (YEAR)	COMPARISON	N	STUDY GROUP	R	RANGE (cm²)	SEE (cm²)
Gorlin (1951)	MVA by Gorlin vs direct at autopsy or surgery	11	MS	0.89	0.5-1.5	0.15
Libanoff (1968)	T½ at rest vs exercise	20	Mitral valve disease	0.98	20-340 ms	21 ms
Henry (1975)	2D TTE vs direct measurement at surgery	20	Patients with MS undergoing surgery	0.92	0.5-3.5	—
Holen (1977)	MVA by Doppler vs Gorlin	10	MS	0.98	0.6-3.4	0.18
Hatle (1979)	T½ vs Gorlin MVA	32	MS	0.74	0.4-3.5	—
Smith (1986)	2D echo vs Gorlin	37	MS alone	0.83	0.4-2.3	0.26
		35	Prior commissurotomy	0.58		0.28
	T½ MVA vs Gorlin	(37)	MS alone	0.85		0.22
		(35)	Prior commissurotomy	0.90		0.14
Come (1988)	T½ MVA vs Gorlin	37	Pre-BMV	0.51	0.6-1.3	—
			Post-BMV	0.47	1.2-3.8	—
	Gorlin vs Gorlin		Repeat catheterization	0.74	0.4-1.4	—
Thomas (1988)	Predicted vs actual T½	18	Pre-BMV	0.93-0.96		
			Post-BMV	0.52-0.66		
Chen (1989)	T½ MVA vs Gorlin	18	Pre-BMV	0.81	0.4-1.2	0.11
			Immediately post-BMV	0.84	1.3-2.6	0.20
			24-48 hrs post-BMV	0.72	1.3-2.6	0.49
Faletra (1996)	2D TTE vs direct measurement	30	MS undergoing surgical MVR	0.95	0.6-2.0	0.06
	T½ vs direct measurement	30		0.80		0.09
	Continuity equation vs direct measurement	30		0.87		0.09
	Flow area vs direct measurement	30		0.54		0.10
						Bland Altman Mean Difference
Dreyfus (2011)		80	MS			
	MVA by 3D TEE vs. 2D TTE			0.79	0.45-2.20	0.0004 ± 0.21 cm²
Schlosshan (2011)		43	MS		0.5-2.5	Mean difference
	3D MVA on TEE vs. 2D MVA			0.87		−0.16 ± 0.22 cm²
	3D MVA on TEE vs. T½ MVA			0.73		−0.23 ± 0.28 cm²
	3D MVA on TEE vs continuity equation MVA			0.83		0.05 ± 0.22 cm²

2D, two-dimensional; *3D*, three-dimensional; *Gorlin*, Gorlin formula valve area; *BMV*, balloon mitral valvotomy; *MS*, mitral stenosis; *MVA*, mitral valve area; *SEE*, standard error of the estimate *T½*, pressure half-time; *TEE*, transesophageal echocardiography; *TTE*, transthoracic echocardiography.
From Otto CM. Textbook of clinical echocardiography. 5th ed. Philadelphia: Elsevier/Saunders; 2013.
*Data from Gorlin et al, Am Heart J 1951;41:1–29; Libanoff et al, Circulation 1968;38:144–150; Henry et al, Circulation 1975;51:827–831; Holen et al, Acta Med Scand 1977;201:83–88; Hatle et al, Circulation 1979;60:1096–1104; Smith et al, Circulation 1986;73:100–107; Come et al, Am J Cardiol 1988;61:817–825; Thomas et al, Circulation 1988;78:980–993; Chen et al, J Am Coll Cardiol 1989;13:1309–1313; Faletra et al, J Am Coll Cardiol 1996;28:1190–1197; Dreyfus et al, Eur J Echocardiogr 2011;12:750–755; Schlosshan et al, JACC Cardiovasc Imaging 2011;4:580–588.

high-velocity aortic jet signal is recorded with CW Doppler from the window yielding the highest velocity signal.

Continuity equation valve area calculations have been validated in comparison with invasive measures of valve area in both animal models and clinical studies, and the utility of this measurement in patient management is clear (Table 6-4). In an experienced laboratory, with meticulous attention to technical details, the reproducibility of continuity equation valve area measurements is 5% to 8%, so an interim change of more than 0.15 cm² is clinically significant.[1] Although detailed imaging of aortic valve anatomy suggests that the outflow tract is not strictly circular, and thus, measuring its area may not be the ideal approach for selecting the size of a transcatheter prosthetic valve, this simple measurement still provides a reasonable approximation for valve area calculations.

PRESSURE HALF-TIME

In contrast to stenosis of a semilunar valve, where ventricular ejection drives blood across the narrowed orifice, resulting in a characteristic ejection-type velocity curve, the time course of the decline in velocity (or pressure gradient) across a narrowed atrioventricular valve is a passive process, largely dependent on the area of the stenotic valve. This rate of pressure decline across the stenotic valve is independent of heart rate and volume flow rate

and is inversely related to valve area. The rate of pressure decline typically is measured as the pressure half-time *(T½)* defined as the time interval between the maximum initial gradient and the point at which this gradient has declined to half the initial value (Figure 6-12). Although this method was initially described as using invasive pressure measurement, it now is used noninvasively, with the pressure half-time measured from the Doppler velocity curve as the time from the maximum velocity to the maximum velocity divided by the square root of 2 (given the quadratic relationship between velocity and pressure) (see Table 6-3). A normal pressure half-time is 40 to 60 msec, with progressively longer half-times indicating more severe stenosis. For the stenotic native mitral valve, an empiric constant of 220 is used to convert the half-time (in milliseconds) to mitral valve area *(MVA* in cm²):

$$MVA = 220/T\tfrac{1}{2}$$

The pressure half-time concept also can be applied to the stenotic tricuspid valve and to prosthetic valves, although it is preferable to report only the half-time itself because the empiric constant has not been as well validated in these situations.

A major assumption of the pressure half-time method is that valve area is the predominant factor affecting ventricular diastolic filling. Although this assumption is appropriate in clinically stable patients with severe mitral stenosis, caution is needed in other

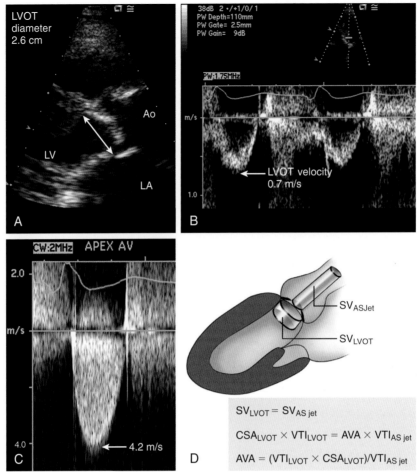

FIGURE 6-11 Continuity equation for aortic valve area (AVA). Calculation requires measurement of left ventricular outflow tract (LVOT) diameter from a parasternal long-axis view *(upper left)* for circular cross-sectional area (CSA) calculation, pulsed Doppler recording of the LVOT velocity-time integral (VTI) from an apical approach *(upper right)* and CW Doppler recording of the aortic stenosis (AS) velocity-time integral (VTI$_{AS jet}$) from whichever window gives the highest-velocity signal *(lower left)*. *Ao,* Aorta; *LA,* left atrium; *SV,* stroke volume. *(From Otto CM. Textbook of clinical echocardiography. 5th ed. Philadelphia: Elsevier/Saunders; 2013.)*

clinical situations. For example, when mitral stenosis is not severe, the time course of the pressure decline between the LA and LV in diastole is determined by the diastolic compliance of the two chambers, the initial (or opening) gradient across the valve, and atrial contractile function in addition to the effect of the restrictive mitral orifice. Similarly, in the patient undergoing balloon mitral valvotomy, changing ventricular and atrial compliances in the immediate postprocedure period can lead to inaccuracies. Another potential concern is coexisting aortic regurgitation, because LV diastolic filling is due to both antegrade transmitral and retrograde transaortic flows, although this theoretic concern does not appear to significantly affect the accuracy of the pressure half-time in the clinical setting.

Other Measures of Stenosis Severity

Several other echocardiographic measures of stenosis severity have been proposed for aortic stenosis, including valve resistance, stroke work loss, and valve impedance. These proposed measures have not gained wide acceptance, although studies are ongoing to determine whether any might provide better prediction of symptom onset and long-term clinical outcome than standard measures of maximum velocity, mean gradient, and valve area.[11,16]

A simplified version of the continuity equation is the velocity ratio—the dimensionless ratio of the maximum velocity proximal to a stenosis (LV outflow velocity; *LVOT*) to the maximum velocity in the stenotic aortic orifice *(AS-V$_{max}$)*:

$$\text{Velocity ratio} = \frac{V_{LVOT}}{AS - V_{max}}$$

A normal velocity ratio is slightly less than 1, with smaller ratios indicating more severe stenosis. For example, a velocity ratio of 0.25 implies that the valve opening is reduced to one-fourth its normal size. In one sense, the velocity ratio is a simplification of the continuity equation, with elimination of the term for cross-sectional area of the proximal flow stream. In another sense, the velocity ratio is a more robust descriptor of stenosis severity. Normal valve area is a function of body size, so stenotic valve areas need to be interpreted in the context of patient size, specifically by indexing valve area to body surface area. The velocity ratio has the advantage that is already "indexed" to body size. Normal intracardiac velocities are similar in people of all ages and sizes; differences in stroke volume relate to differences in the cross-sectional area of flow rather than to flow velocities. Being concerned with velocities alone, the velocity ratio assumes that the proximal cross-sectional area is "normal" for that patient and thus the resulting descriptor of stenosis severity is already indexed for body size.

Stenosis Severity with Changes in Flow Rate

The velocity and pressure gradients across a stenotic valve increase and decrease in parallel with changes in transvalvular volume flow rate as predicted by the mathematical relationship between velocity and flow rate. When anatomic valve area is

TABLE 6-4 Selected Studies of Aortic Valve Area Determination*

FIRST AUTHOR (YEAR)	COMPARISON	N	STUDY GROUP	$R^{\dagger}$	RANGE (cm²)	SEE (cm²)†
Hakki (1981)	Simplified vs original Gorlin	60	Aortic stenosis	0.96	0.2-2.0	0.10
Zoghbi (1986)	Cont eq vs Gorlin	39	Aortic stenosis	0.95	0.4-2.0	0.15
Otto (1988)	Cont eq vs Gorlin	103	Aortic stenosis	0.87	0.2-3.7	0.34
Oh (1988)	Cont eq vs Gorlin	100	Aortic stenosis	0.83	0.2-1.8	0.19
Danielson (1989)	Cont eq vs Gorlin	100	Aortic stenosis	0.96	0.4-2.0	—
Cannon (1985)	Gorlin vs videotape of valve opening	42	Porcine valves in pulsatile flow model	0.87	0.6-2.5	0.28
	New formula vs actual orifice area	42	Porcine valves in pulsatile flow model	0.98	0.6-2.5	0.11
Segal (1987)	Cont eq vs actual valve area		In vitro pulsatile flow with orifice plates	0.99	0.05-0.5	0.016
	Gorlin vs actual valve area			0.87		0.047
Cannon (1988)	Gorlin vs known valve area	135	Prosthetic aortic valves	0.39	0.6-2.3	—
Nishimura (1988)	Cont eq vs Gorlin	55	Pre-BAV	0.72	0.2-0.9	0.10
			Post-BAV	0.61	0.5-1.3	0.17
Desnoyers (1988)	Cont eq vs Gorlin	42	Pre-BAV	0.74	0.3-1.3	—
Tribouilloy (1994)	TEE vs cont eq	54	Aortic stenosis	0.96	0.3-2.0	0.11
	TEE vs Gorlin			0.90		0.12
Kim (1997)	TEE vs Gorlin	81	Aortic stenosis	0.89	0.4-2.0	0.04
						Bland-Altman Mean Difference
Goland (2007)	3D TEE vs 2D TTE AVA	33	Aortic stenosis	0.99	0.45-1.98	0.00(−0.15 to 0.15) cm²
	3D TEE vs Gorlin AVA	15		0.86	0..4-1.4	0.01 (−0.20 to 0.22) cm²
de la Morena (2010)	3D TEE AVA vs 2D TTE AVA	59	Aortic stenosis	0.72†	0.30-1.3	0.04 (−0.37 to 0.45) cm²
Furukawa (2012)	3D TEE AVA vs 2D TEE AVA	25	Aortic stenosis	0.95	0.40-1.10	−0.14 (range −0.41 to 0.12) cm²

2D, Two-dimensional; *3D*, three-dimensional; *AVA*, aortic valve area; *BAV*, balloon aortic valvuloplasty; *cont eq*, continuity equation; *Gorlin*, Gorlin formula for AVA; *TEE*, transesophageal echocardiography; *TTE*, transthoracic echocardiography.

From Otto CM. Textbook of clinical echocardiography. 5th ed. Philadelphia: Elsevier/Saunders; 2013.

*Data from Hakki et al, Circulation 1981;63:1050–1055; Zoghbi et al, Circulation 1986;73:452–459; Otto et al, Arch Intern Med 1988;148:2553–2560; Oh et al, J Am Coll Cardiol 1988;11:1227–1234; Danielson et al, Am J Cardiol 1989;63:1107–1111; Cannon et al, Circulation 1985;71:1170–1178; Segal et al, J Am Coll Cardiol 1987;9:1294–1305; Cannon et al, Am J Cardiol 1988;62:113–116; Nishimura et al, Circulation 1988;78:791–799; Desnoyers et al, Am J Cardiol 1988;62:1078–1084; Tribouilloy et al, Am Heart J 1994;128:526–532; Kim et al, Am J Cardiol 1997;79:436–441. Goland et al, Heart 2007;93:801–807; de la Morena et al, Eur J Echocardiogr 2010;11:9–13. Furukawa et al, J Cardiol. 2012;59:337–343.

†If not stated in the publication, statistics were calculated from the raw data provided in tables. A blank indicates that data for this calculation were not available.

fixed, for example, with rheumatic mitral stenosis, increases in flow rate result in expected increases in pressure gradient, with little change in calculated effective valve area because opening of the fused commissures is constant at all flow rates. In contrast, a calcified aortic valve is "stiff" and the degree of leaflet opening depends on the applied force, or volume flow rate in the clinical setting. In fact, the degree of change in stenosis severity relative to a change in volume flow rate can provide a useful index of disease severity. For example in adults with concurrent aortic stenosis and reduced LV ejection fraction, the change in valve area with changes in flow rate helps distinguish patients with only moderate valve obstruction from those with severe aortic stenosis resulting in LV dysfunction. This evaluation typically is performed with a low-dose dobutamine stress test, measuring the maximum velocity, mean gradient, stroke volume, and valve area at each stage of the protocol (Figure 6-13).[17-19]

Evaluation of Valvular Regurgitation

Echocardiographic assessment of valvular regurgitation includes integration of data from imaging of the valve and ventricle, as well as Doppler measures of regurgitant severity. No single Doppler method provides a definitive measure of regurgitant severity, nor can findings with this modality be interpreted in the absence of evaluation of LV size and function. The standard examination in a patient with valvular disease includes vena contracta measurement on color-flow imaging, CW Doppler velocity curves, evaluation for distal flow reversals, and transvalvular volume flow velocity data. Quantitative measures of regurgitant severity, including regurgitant orifice area and regurgitant volume, are increasingly utilized, particularly when regurgitation is moderate on qualitative evaluation or when the cause of LV dilation is not clear.[20-22]

Qualitative Measures of Regurgitation Severity

Color-flow imaging provides a 2D display of blood flow direction and velocity superimposed on the 2D image. Doppler color-flow imaging can also be displayed on 3D images, although the frame rate is quite low, limiting clinical utility of this modality. The physics of color-flow Doppler imaging are complex and numerous factors affect the final display, but the color-flow image provides an intuitive and appealing real-time display of blood flow patterns in the heart. Color-flow Doppler imaging has high sensitivity (nearly 100%) and specificity (nearly 100%) for identification of valvular regurgitation based on identification of the flow disturbance in the receiving chamber, exceeding the detection rates for auscultation and angiography. With a meticulous examination, a small degree of valvular regurgitation is seen in many normal individuals; tricuspid regurgitation is detectable in 80% to 90% of

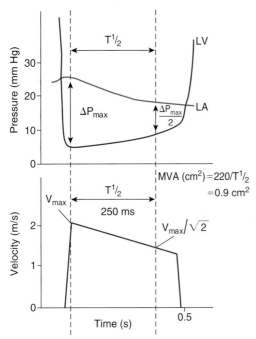

FIGURE 6-12   Mitral pressure half-time valve area measurement. *Top,* Schematic diagram showing the relationship between left ventricular (LV) and left atrial (LA) pressures. *Bottom,* The transmitral velocity curve recorded with Doppler ultrasound. The shape of the pressure gradient is reflected in the Doppler velocity curve. The pressure half-time (T½) is the same whether measured from the pressure data or from the velocity data. Mitral valve area (MVA) is calculated using an empiric constant as 220/T½, where valve area is in cm² and T½ is in milliseconds (ms). ΔP_{max}, maximum pressure difference; V_{max}, maximum velocity. *(From Otto CM. Textbook of clinical echocardiography. 5th ed. Philadelphia: Elsevier/Saunders; 2013.)*

normal individuals, pulmonic regurgitation in 70% to 80%, mitral regurgitation in 70% to 80%, and aortic regurgitation in 5% to 10%, with an increasing frequency of detectable regurgitation with age. Physiologic or "normal" regurgitation is characterized by a small volume of backflow with only a small area of flow disturbance seen on color-flow imaging and a weak CW Doppler signal.

Pathologic regurgitation is associated with a larger area of flow disturbance on color-flow imaging. Although it is tempting to interpret the size of the flow disturbance as synonymous with the severity of regurgitation, the color-flow display is affected by numerous factors other than regurgitant severity and is not recommended as a measure of regurgitant severity. However, the origin and direction of the regurgitant jet may be helpful in determining the anatomic mechanism of regurgitation, particularly with mitral valve disease (Figure 6-14).

VENA CONTRACTA

Color-flow Doppler evaluation of regurgitation severity focuses on the geometry of the regurgitant signal as is passes through the narrowed orifice (Figure 6-15). The narrowest segment of the flow stream, the vena contracta, typically occurs just beyond the regurgitant orifice. The size of the vena contracta does not depend on flow rate or pressure and is less sensitive to instrument setting than the downstream size of the jet.

For aortic regurgitation, vena contracta width is measured as the smallest flow diameter, immediately beyond the flow convergence region, in the parasternal long-axis view. An aortic regurgitant vena contracta width greater than 6 mm indicates severe aortic regurgitation, and a width smaller than 3 mm indicates mild regurgitation.[22,23] For mitral regurgitation, the vena contracta also is best imaged in the parasternal long-axis view, taking

advantage of the axial resolution at this depth. However, identification of the vena contracta is most reliable when both the proximal convergence zone and the distal expansion of the jet can be seen, with the vena contracta as the narrow segment joining these two regions. Thus, a mitral regurgitant vena contracta often is better visualized in an apical four-chamber or long-axis view. Vena contracta width should not be measured in a two-chamber view because this is a tangential plane through the flow signal. A mitral regurgitant vena contracta jet width greater than 7 mm indicates severe regurgitation, and a width less than 3 mm indicates mild regurgitation.[22]

CONTINUOUS-WAVE DOPPLER DATA

Two types of data are inherent in the CW Doppler spectral recording of a regurgitant jet velocity curve. First, the signal strength, especially relative to antegrade flow, is directly related to the volume of regurgitation. Although acoustic attenuation and instrumentation variability make quantitation of signal strength problematic, qualitative assessment is a simple and useful clinical measure.

Second, the time-velocity curve reflects the time course of the instantaneous pressure difference across the regurgitant valve. For each instantaneous velocity, the pressure difference across the valve is $4v^2$ (as stated in the Bernoulli equation), so inferences about intracardiac pressures and the time course of pressure changes can be derived from the Doppler data.

For aortic regurgitation, the rate of pressure decline between the aorta and LV in diastole relates to chronicity of disease and LV compensation, as illustrated in Figure 6-16. In addition, the end-diastolic velocity across the regurgitant aortic valve corresponds to the end-diastolic pressure gradient, which, when subtracted from the cuff diastolic blood pressure, provides an approximation of LV end-diastolic pressure, although wide measurement variability limits the clinical utility of this estimate.

The mitral regurgitant signal is characterized by a high maximum velocity, reflecting the high LV systolic pressure and low left atrial pressure in compensated disease. Typically, this high velocity persists through most of systole. However, when left atrial pressure rises in late systole (e.g., a v wave) because of severe and/or acute mitral regurgitation, the velocity curve shows a steep decline in velocity in late systole, the Doppler "v wave." On the right side of the heart, the tricuspid regurgitant jet velocity corresponds to the difference between right ventricular and right atrial pressures in systole, so that right ventricular (and pulmonary systolic) pressure can be calculated from the maximum tricuspid regurgitant jet, on the basis of the Bernoulli equation. As for mitral regurgitation, severe or acute tricuspid regurgitation may result in a right atrial v wave, seen as a late systolic rapid decline in the velocity curve.

The pulmonic regurgitant jet velocity is related to the diastolic pressure difference between the pulmonary artery and right ventricle and, given that the normal pressure difference is low, is typically low. When pulmonary hypertension is present, pulmonic regurgitant velocities are increased with the early-diastolic velocity in combination with an estimate of right atrial pressure, allowing calculation of diastolic pulmonary pressure.

DISTAL FLOW REVERSALS

When atrioventricular valve regurgitation is severe, the backflow across the valve not only fills the atrium but extends into the veins, resulting in reversal of the normal flow pattern in systole. Severe tricuspid regurgitation results in retrograde systolic flow in the venae cavae and hepatic veins, which can be demonstrated from the subcostal view using pulsed Doppler recordings. Severe mitral regurgitation results in systolic flow reversal in the pulmonary veins. Examination of all four pulmonary veins on TEE is especially helpful with an eccentric regurgitant jet because the pattern of systolic flow reversal may not be uniform. However,

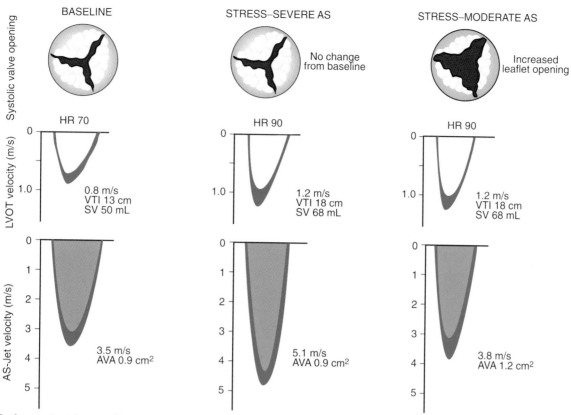

FIGURE 6-13   Low-output, low-gradient aortic stenosis. Changes in aortic valve opening and Doppler flows with dobutamine stress echocardiography for low-output, low-gradient aortic stenosis (AS). *Left,* The baseline data show a hypothetical patient with an ejection fraction (EF) of 35% and limited aortic valve systolic opening, an aortic jet (AS-jet) velocity of 3.5 m/s, and an aortic valve area (AVA) of 0.9 cm². *Middle,* If true severe AS is present, as EF increases from 35% to 45% with stress, transaortic flow rate increases but aortic opening is fixed, resulting in a marked increase in aortic velocity (and pressure gradient) with no change in valve area. *Right,* in a patient with the same baseline data but "pseudo–severe AS," the increase in EF and transaortic stroke volume with stress "push" the aortic leaflets to open more, so there is a smaller increase in aortic velocity in association with an increase in AVA. Current diagnostic testing relies on Doppler data with dobutamine stress testing because direct imaging of valve anatomy is not adequate for visualization of the exact systolic orifice. *HR,* heart rate in beats/min; *SV,* stroke volume; *VTI,* velocity-time integral. *(From Otto CM, Owens DS. Stress testing for structural heart disease. In: Gillam LD, Otto CM, editors. Advanced approaches in echocardiography. Philadelphia: Elsevier/Saunders; 2012.)*

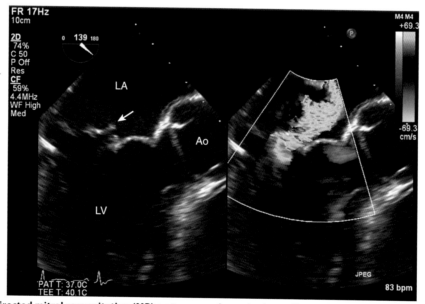

FIGURE 6-14   Anteriorly directed mitral regurgitation (MR) on transesophageal echocardiography (TEE). *Left,* The long-axis TEE view shows a partial flail posterior mitral leaflet *(arrow).* *Right,* The anteriorly directed jet seen on color Doppler imaging *(right)* confirms that MR is due to isolated posterior leaflet dysfunction, and the width of the jet as it crosses the mitral valve, the vena contracta, is consistent with severe regurgitation. The proximal isovelocity surface area (PISA) on the ventricular side of the valve is shown. *Ao,* Aorta; *LA,* left atrium; *LV,* left ventricle. *(From Otto CM. Textbook of clinical echocardiography. 5th ed. Philadelphia: Elsevier/Saunders; 2013.)*

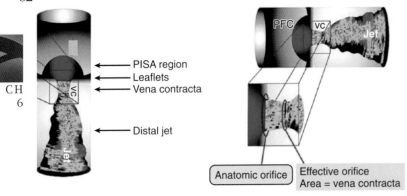

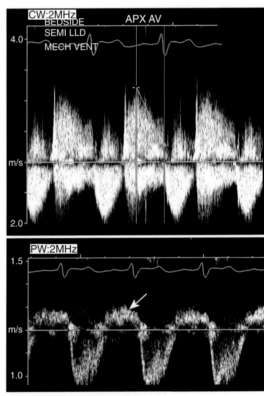

FIGURE 6-15 **Fluid dynamics of a regurgitant jet.** *Left,* The proximal isovelocity surface area (PISA) region—also referred to as proximal flow convergence (PFC) region at *right*—vena contracta (VC), and distal jet. *Right,* The effective regurgitant orifice area is the orifice area defined by the narrowest regurgitant flow stream and typically occurs distal to the anatomic orifice defined by the valve leaflets. *(From Otto CM. Textbook of clinical echocardiography. 5th ed. Philadelphia: Elsevier/Saunders; 2013; adapted from Roberts BJ, Grayburn P. Color flow imaging of the vena contracta in mitral regurgitation: technical considerations. J Am Soc Echocardiogr 2003;16:1002–6.)*

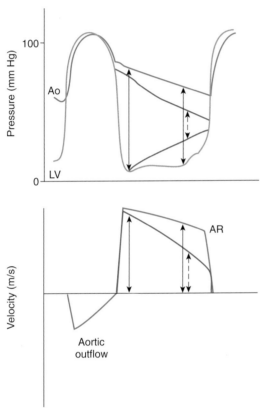

FIGURE 6-16 **Transvalvular pressure-velocity relationships.** Left ventricular (LV) and central aortic (Ao) pressures and the corresponding Doppler velocity curve are shown for chronic *(green lines)* and acute *(blue lines)* aortic regurgitation (AR). The shape of the velocity curve is related to the instantaneous pressure differences across the valve, as stated in the Bernoulli equation. With acute aortic regurgitation, aortic pressure falls more rapidly and ventricular diastolic pressure rises more rapidly, resulting in a steeper deceleration slope on the Doppler curve. *(From Otto CM. Textbook of clinical echocardiography. 5th ed. Philadelphia: Saunders/Elsevier; 2013.)*

FIGURE 6-17 **Doppler findings with acute severe aortic regurgitation.** CW Doppler recording shows a dense signal with a steep deceleration slope *(top).* Holodiastolic flow reversal is seen in the descending thoracic aorta recorded from a suprasternal notch window with pulsed wave (PW) Doppler imaging *(bottom).* *(From Otto CM. Textbook of clinical echocardiography. 5th ed. Philadelphia: Saunders/Elsevier; 2013.)*

other physiologic factors affect atrial inflow patterns, including respiratory phase, cardiac rhythm, atrial and venous compliances, ventricular diastolic filling, and patient age. The presence and severity of venous systolic flow reversal is a useful adjunct in the evaluation of atrioventricular valve regurgitant severity, but its presence is not a pathognomonic finding and should not be relied on when the patient is not in normal sinus rhythm.

For the semilunar valves (aortic and pulmonic), severe regurgitation results in diastolic flow reversal in the associated great vessels as blood flows back into the ventricular chamber across the incompetent valve. The distance that holodiastolic flow reversal extends down the aorta correlates with regurgitant severity; this finding in the proximal abdominal aorta indicates severe aortic regurgitation, whereas holodiastolic flow reversal in the descending thoracic aorta is seen with both moderate and severe regurgitation (Figure 6-17). When signal-to-noise ratio is adequate and wall filters are set at a low velocity, this approach is a simple and reliable method for qualitative evaluation of regurgitant severity. False-negative results are due to poor examination technique or limited acoustic access. False-positive results are due to other sources of diastolic runoff in the aorta, such as a patent ductus

TABLE 6-5 Validation of Quantitative Evaluation of Regurgitant Severity Using Doppler Echocardiography*

FIRST AUTHOR (YEAR)	METHOD	STANDARD OF REFERENCE	N	R	SEE
Color Jet Area					
Spain (1989)	Color jet area	Angio LV, TD-CO	15 pts with MR	0.62 (RF)	—
Tribouilloy (1992)	Regurgitant jet width at origin	Angio LV, TD-CO	31 pts with MR	0.85 (RSV)	—
Enriquez-Sarano (1993)	Color jet area	Doppler SV at two sites	80 pts with MR	0.69 (RF)	4.4 cm²
Vena Contracta					
Tribouilloy (2000)	Vena contracta width	Doppler ROA and RSV	79 pts with AR	0.89 (ROA) 0.90 (RSV)	0.08 cm² 18 mL
Hall (1997)	Vena contracta width	Doppler ROA and RSV	80 pts with MR	0.86 (RSV) 0.85 (ROA)	0.15 cm² 20 mL
PISA					
Recusani (1991)	PISA (hemispherical)	Rotometer	In vitro, constant flow	0.94-0.99 (flow rate)	1-1.6 L/min
Utsunomiya (1991)	PISA (hemispherical)	Actual flow rate stopwatch and cylinder	In vitro, pulsatile flow	0.99 (flow rate)	0.53 L/min
Vandervoort (1993)	PISA	Actual flow rate	In vitro, steady flow	0.98-0.99 (flow rate)	—
Giesler (1993)	PISA	Angio LV, Fick CO	16 pts with MR	0.88 (RSV)	17 mL
Chen (1993)	PISA	Doppler SV at two sites	46 pts with MR	0.94 (RSV)	18 mL
CW Doppler					
Teague (1986)	AR half-time	Angio LV, Fick CO	32 pts with AR	−0.88 (RF)	11%
Masuyama (1986)	AR half-time	Angio LV, ID-CO	20 pts with AR	−0.89 (RF)	—
Volume Flow at Two Sites					
Ascah (1985)	Transmitral vs transaortic SV	EM-flow	30 flow rates in canine model	0.83 (RF)	—
Kitabatake (1985)	Transaortic vs transpulmonic SV	Angio LV, TD-CO	20 pts with AR	0.94 (RF)	—
Rokey (1986)	Transmitral vs transaortic SV	Angio LV, TD-CO	19 pts with MR and 6 with AR	0.91 (RF)	7%
Distal Flow Reversals					
Boughner (1975)	Diastolic flow reversal in descending Ao	Angio LV, Fick CO	15 pts with AR	0.91 (RF)	—
Touche (1985)	Diastolic flow reversal in descending Ao	Angio LV, TD-CO	30 pts with AR	0.92 (RF)	8.8%
					Bland Altman Mean Difference
Marsan 2009	3DE vena contracta	CMR	64 pts with functional MR	0.94	−0.08 (−7.7 to 7.6) mL/beat
Zeng 2011	3DE vena contracta	Quantitative Doppler	49 pts with MR	r²=0.86	SEE = 0.02 cm²
Perez de Isla 2012	3DE vena contracta	CMR	32 pts with AR	0.88	—

3DE, Three-dimensional echocardiography; *angio*, angiography; *Ao*, aorta; *AR*, aortic regurgitation; *CMR*, cardiac magnetic resonance imaging; *CO*, cardiac output; *EM-flow*, volume flow rate measured by electromagnetic flowmeter; *ROA*, regurgitant orifice area; *Fick CO*, Fick cardiac output; *ID*, indicator dilation; *LV*, left ventricle; *MR*, mitral regurgitation; *PISA*, proximal isovelocity surface area method; *pts*, patients; *RF*, regurgitant fraction; *RSV*, regurgitant stroke volume; *SEE*, standard error of the estimate; *SV*, stroke volume; *TD*, thermodilution.
From Otto CM. Textbook of clinical echocardiography. 5th ed. Philadelphia: Elsevier/Saunders; 2013.
* Data from Boughner et al, Circulation 1975;52:874–879; Touche et al, Circulation 1985;72:819–824; Ascah et al, Circulation 1985;72:377–383; Kitabatake et al, Circulation 1985;72:523–529; Rokey et al, J Am Coll Cardiol 1986;7:1273–1278; Teague et al, J Am Coll Cardiol 1986;8:592–599; Masuyama et al, Circulation 1986;73:460–466; Spain et al, J Am Coll Cardiol 1989;13:585–590; Tribouilloy et al, Circulation 1992;85:1248–1253; Enriquez-Sarano et al, J Am Coll Cardiol 1993;21:1211–1219; Rescusani et al, Circulation 1991;83:594–604; Utsunomiya et al, J Am Soc Echocardiogr 1991;4:338–348; Vandervoort et al, J Am Coll Cardiol 1993;22:535–541; Giesler et al, Am J Cardiol 1993;71:217–224; Chen et al, J Am Coll Cardiol 1993;21:374–383; Tribouilloy CM et al. Circulation 2000;102:558–564; Hall SA et al. Circulation 1997;95: 636–642. Marsan et al, JACC Cardiovasc Imaging 2009;2:1245–1252; Zeng et al, Circ Cardiovasc Imaging 2011;4:506–513; Perez de Isla et al, Int J Cardiol 2011 Dec 20 [epub ahead of print].

arteriosus, or misinterpretation of the normal early diastolic flow reversal.

Regurgitant Volume and Orifice Area

Regurgitant stroke volume (RSV) and regurgitant fraction (RF)—the absolute and relative amount of backflow across the valve—and regurgitant orifice area (ROA)—the cross-sectional area of the flow stream—all can be calculated from imaging and Doppler data (Table 6-5). Methods for these calculations include: (1) the proximal isovelocity surface area (PISA) approach, (2) measurement of volume flow rate across the regurgitant valve compared with that for a normal valve, and (3) 2D or 3D imaging for measurement of total LV stroke volume with Doppler measurement of forward stroke volume.

PROXIMAL FLOW CONVERGENCE

Blood flow accelerates on the upstream side of a regurgitant valve, resulting in successively higher velocities as flow approaches the regurgitant orifice, which can be seen on color-flow Doppler imaging (Figure 6-18). Color-flow imaging utilizes pulsed Doppler technology, so signal aliasing occurs when velocity exceeds a value determined by instrument settings and depth. Aliasing is displayed as a change in color from blue to red (or vice versa), with the color change occurring at a specific velocity. Thus, visualization of the hemisphere of flow acceleration proximal to a regurgitant orifice represents an isovelocity surface area where flow is equal to the aliasing velocity (*v*) on the color-flow image. By definition, the instantaneous flow rate (*Q*) at this site (e.g., regurgitant flow rate) is the cross-sectional area of flow times

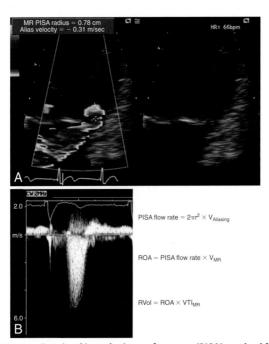

FIGURE 6-18 Proximal isovelocity surface area (PISA) method for calculation of regurgitant volume (RVol) and regurgitant orifice area (ROA). In the apical view that best demonstrated a PISA on color-flow Doppler imaging, the baseline was shifted in the direction of MR to obtain an aliasing velocity between 30 and 40 cm/s. A narrow sector width and a shallow depth were used to optimize scan line density and frame rate. PISA radius (r) was measured from the aliasing velocity ($V_{aliasing}$) to the level of the valve orifice. The regurgitant jet was recorded with CW Doppler for measurement of maximum velocity (V_{MR}) and the velocity-time integral (VTI_{MR}). For mitral regurgitant *(MR)* jets, which are not pansystolic, only the Doppler signal that represents mitral regurgitation is traced. *HR,* Heart rate. *(From Cawley PJ, Hamilton-Craig C, Owens DS, et al. Prospective comparison of valve regurgitation quantitation by cardiac magnetic resonance imaging and transthoracic echocardiography. Circ Cardiovasc Imaging 2013;6:48–57.)*

velocity. The area of flow can be calculated as the area of a hemisphere (with radius *r*), so that:

$$Q = 2\pi r^2 v$$

Based on the continuity equation principle, this flow rate then can be used to calculate an instantaneous regurgitant orifice area, in conjunction with the maximal CW Doppler velocity *(V)* through the regurgitant orifice[20]:

$$ROA = Q/V$$

In the clinical setting this approach is most useful for evaluation of mitral regurgitation because imaging of proximal acceleration is more difficult for aortic regurgitation.[20] The PISA method also can be used to estimate regurgitant stroke volume by multiplying orifice area by the velocity time integral of the mitral regurgitant jet *(VTI_{MR})*:

$$RSV = ROA \times VTI_{MR}$$

The PISA approach is most accurate for holosystolic flow with a constant regurgitant orifice area. However, many causes of mitral regurgitation are associated with a dynamic orifice area, as seen with late systolic mitral regurgitation due to mitral valve prolapse. In this situation, PISA-based calculations may overestimate regurgitant severity. Even so, clinical outcome studies have shown the prognostic value of these measurements both in adults with functional mitral regurgitation and in those with mitral valve prolapse. A mitral regurgitant orifice area greater than 0.4 cm^2 corresponds to severe regurgitation, and an area smaller than 0.2 cm^2 indicates mild regurgitation.[22]

Another approach to calculation of regurgitant volume is measurement of transvalvular flow at two intracardiac sites using 2D and pulsed Doppler echocardiography (Figure 6-19). Regurgitant stroke volume is equal to the total stroke volume *(TSV)* antegrade across the regurgitant valve minus the forward stroke volume (the amount of blood delivered to the body) across a normal valve. For aortic regurgitation *(AR)*, total stroke volume is measured in the LV outflow tract *(LVOT)* and forward stroke volume across the mitral or pulmonic *(PA)* annulus:

$$RSV_{AR} = (CSA_{LVOT} \times VTI_{LVOT}) - (CSA_{PA} \times VTI_{PA})$$

For mitral regurgitation *(MR)*, total stroke volume is measured across the mitral annulus *(MA)*, and forward stroke volume across the LVOT or pulmonic valve:

$$RSV_{MR} = (CSA_{MA} \times VTI_{MA}) - (CSA_{LVOT} \times VTI_{LVOT})$$

Regurgitant fraction then is the ratio of regurgitant stroke volume to total stroke volume:

$$RF = RSV/TSV$$

The validity of this method has been demonstrated in animal and clinical studies of valvular but is challenging in the clinical setting with considerable physiologic and measurement variability. Echocardiographic quantitation of aortic regurgitant severity shows more interobserver variability than cardiac magnetic resonance (CMR) imaging (Figure 6-20). Reproducibility for quantitation of mitral regurgitation is similar for echocardiography compared to CMR imaging.[24] Given the potential error of this approach, and the complexity of data acquisition and measurement, most laboratories perform these calculations only in selected cases.

A third approach to quantitation of mitral regurgitation is to use the 2D biplane or 3D volumetric LV stroke volume, instead of transmitral flow, for total stroke volume. Then, regurgitant volume and orifice area are calculated with use of the forward stroke volume measured by pulsed Doppler velocity recording in the LV outflow tract. This approach utilizes measurements performed as part of a routine examination and avoids the measurement variability inherent in determination of mitral annulus diameter. However, LV volumes often are underestimated on 2D imaging, so this approach may underestimate regurgitant severity.

Integration of Regurgitant Parameters

A stepwise approach to the use of Doppler measures of regurgitant severity is recommended by the American Society of Echocardiography.[22] For both mitral regurgitation and aortic regurgitation, the initial step is measurement of vena contracta diameter. With mitral regurgitation and a small (<0.3 cm) or very large (>0.7 cm) vena contracta diameter, further evaluation is not typically needed, particularly if the CW Doppler signal confirms mild or severe regurgitation (Figure 6-21). For a vena contracta diameter of 0.3 to 0.7 cm, regurgitant severity may be further quantitated by the PISA or volume flow method. With aortic regurgitation, the combination of vena contracta diameter, CW Doppler signal strength, and holodiastolic flow reversal in the aorta is usually adequate, with further quantitation only if regurgitant severity remains uncertain (Figure 6-22).

Evaluation of Left Ventricular Geometry and Function

Evaluation of the LV response to pressure and/or volume overload is a critical step in echocardiographic examination of the patient with left-sided valvular heart disease.

Volumes and Ejection Fraction

Quantitative evaluation of LV volumes and ejection fraction is recommended in all patients with valvular heart disease.[25,26] The

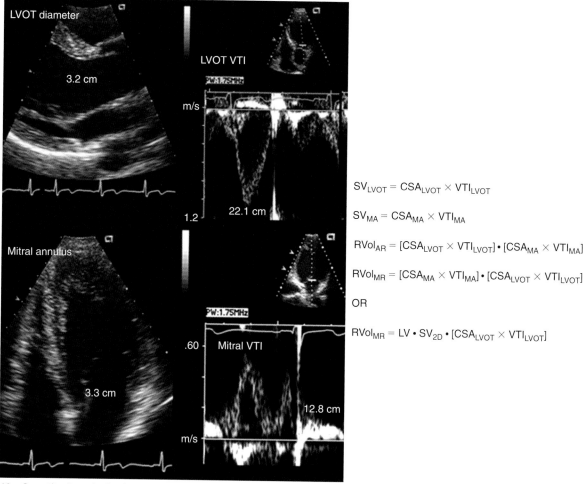

$$SV_{LVOT} = CSA_{LVOT} \times VTI_{LVOT}$$

$$SV_{MA} = CSA_{MA} \times VTI_{MA}$$

$$RVol_{AR} = [CSA_{LVOT} \times VTI_{LVOT}] \cdot [CSA_{MA} \times VTI_{MA}]$$

$$RVol_{MR} = [CSA_{MA} \times VTI_{MA}] \cdot [CSA_{LVOT} \times VTI_{LVOT}]$$

OR

$$RVol_{MR} = LV \cdot SV_{2D} \cdot [CSA_{LVOT} \times VTI_{LVOT}]$$

FIGURE 6-19   Quantitation of mitral regurgitation (MR) severity based on volume flow across two valves. Left ventricular (LV) outflow tract (LVOT) diameter was measured at the aortic valve leaflet insertion points in midsystole to calculate a circular cross-sectional area (CSA). LVOT velocity-time integral (VTI) was recorded from the apical window, with the sample volume just on the LV side of the aortic valve. Mitral annulus (MA) diameter (D) was measured from the apical four-chamber view during early diastole (E wave). From an apical window, the Doppler sample volume was positioned at the mitral annulus, and modal velocity was traced for the VTI. Stroke volume (SV) at each site was used to calculate regurgitant volume (RVol) for aortic regurgitation (AR) and MR as shown. Total stroke volume also was calculated from two-dimensional LV volumes (LV-SV2D). *(From Cawley PJ, Hamilton-Craig C, Owens DS, et al. Prospective comparison of valve regurgitation quantitation by cardiac magnetic resonance imaging and transthoracic echocardiography. Circ Cardiovasc Imaging 2013;6:48–57.)*

simplest quantitative measures of LV size are 2D-guided M-mode recordings at the midventricular level (see Table 6-2) for end-diastolic dimension (EDD) and end-systolic dimension (ESD). The American College of Cardiology/American Heart Association and European Society of Cardiology guidelines for the management of valvular heart disease recommend ventricular dimension values for clinical decision making because our evidence base currently depends on studies using these measurements.[25,26] Using both long- and short-axis views from a parasternal window, the 2D image is used to ensure that the M-mode beam is centered in the LV chamber and is perpendicular to the long axis of the LV. The advantages of M-mode measurements, compared with measurements from 2D images, are dependence on the axial resolution of the ultrasound system (rather than the less accurate lateral resolution) and a much higher temporal resolution, allowing better identification of endocardial borders. The disadvantages of M-mode data are that an oblique orientation of the M-mode beam or incorrect identification of endocardial borders leads to measurement errors; in this situation, 2D measurements should be used instead.[27]

2D imaging–guided LV diameter measurements are reasonably reproducible when performed by experienced laboratories using careful recording and measurement techniques, and are frequently substituted for M-mode measurements in clinical practice. On serial studies, side-by-side comparisons of image planes and measurement sites are needed to ensure consistency in recording and measurement techniques on serial examinations. With any measurement approach, end-diastolic dimensions may change if there are differences in preload due to volume status or medications. End-systolic dimensions are less dependent on preload but may be affected by afterload.

Quantitative 2D measurements also include LV end-diastolic volume *(EDV)* and end-systolic volume *(ESV)* with calculation of the ejection fraction *(EF)*:

$$EF = (EDV - ESV)/EDV$$

LV volumes are calculated using the apical biplane method from 2D images acquired in apical four-chamber and two-chamber views with tracing of endocardial borders at end-diastole and end-systole, as follows:

$$V = (\pi/4) \sum_{i=1}^{20} a_i b_i \times (L/20)$$

where *a* and *b* represent the minor axis dimensions in two image planes at each of 20 intervals *(i)* perpendicular to the long axis of the ventricle, from apex to the base, with a length *(L)*. Accurate

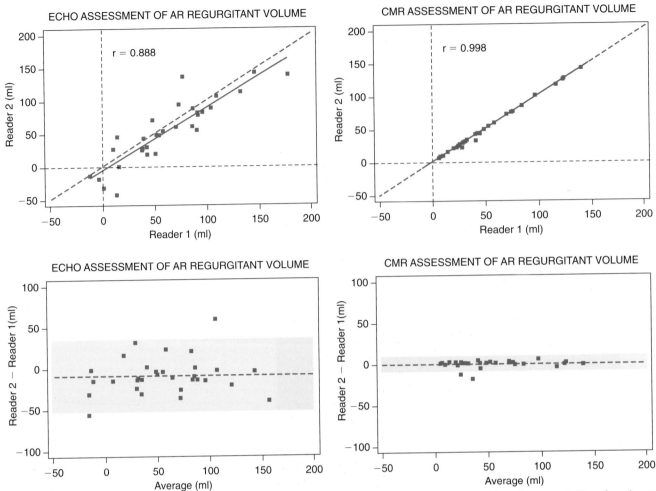

FIGURE 6-20 **Measurement variability for echocardiographic** *ECHO* **and cardiac magnetic resonance (CMR) imaging quantitation of aortic regurgitation (AR) severity.** Linear regression *(top)* and Bland-Altman plots *(bottom)* for aortic regurgitation (AR) volume measurement variability with echocardiography *(left)* and cardiac magnetic resonance imaging *(right)*. In the *top* panels, *dashed line* indicates line of identity, and *solid line,* linear regression line. In the *bottom* panels, *dashed line* is mean difference. *(From Cawley PJ, Hamilton-Craig C, Owens DS, et al. Prospective comparison of valve regurgitation quantitation by cardiac magnetic resonance imaging and transthoracic echocardiography. Circ Cardiovasc Imaging 2013;6:48–57.)*

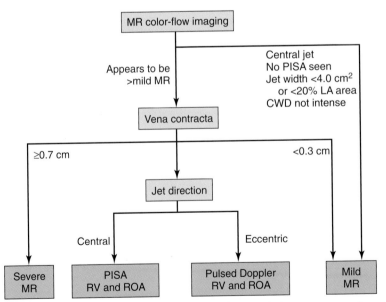

FIGURE 6-21 **Approach to quantitation of mitral regurgitation (MR) severity.** Other quantitative measures may be needed in some patients with a vena contracta width ≥0.7 cm². Evaluation of systolic flow reversal in the pulmonary veins provides useful additional information in patients with sinus rhythm. Transesophageal echocardiography (TEE) is often needed for complete evaluation of MR severity in patients with moderate to severe disease. *CWD,* continuous-wave Doppler; *PISA,* proximal isovelocity surface area; *ROA,* regurgitant orifice area; *RV,* regurgitant volume. *(From Otto CM. Textbook of clinical echocardiography. 5th ed. Philadelphia: Elsevier/Saunders; 2013.)*

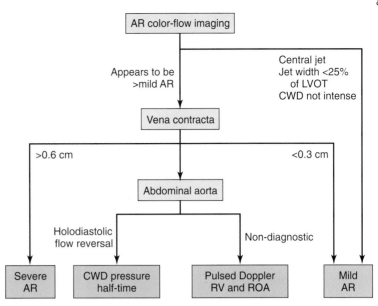

FIGURE 6-22 **Approach to echocardiographic quantitation of aortic regurgitation (AR) severity.** In some cases, quantitation using pulsed and CW Doppler (CWD) techniques may be helpful when vena contracta width is >0.6 cm. *LVOT*, left ventricular outflow tract; *ROA*, regurgitant orifice area; *RV*, regurgitant volume. *(From Otto CM. Textbook of clinical echocardiography. 5th ed. Philadelphia: Elsevier/ Saunders; 2013.)*

LV volume measurements on 2D imaging depend on correct image plane orientation and inclusion of the true long axis of the ventricle in the image (see Table 6-2). Use of a cutout in the bed to allow positioning of the transducer on the apex with the patient in a steep left lateral decubitus position helps avoid inadvertent foreshortening of the apex. Accuracy also depends on correct identification of endocardial borders. Manual tracing of borders by an experienced observer is currently used for calculation of volumes from 2D images, but automated border detection or newer approaches such as speckle tracking may become standard in the future. During image acquisition, care is taken to optimize endocardial definition based on patient positioning, transducer frequency and focusing, subtle adjustments in transducer position and orientation, preprocessing and postprocessing curves, and gray-scale and gain settings. Harmonic imaging markedly improves endocardial definition in most patients and should be used whenever possible for assessment of ventricular function. Contrast echocardiography to opacify the LV chamber is recommended for quantitation of LV function whenever endocardial definition is suboptimal.

3D image acquisition is now possible at many centers and allows more reproducible automated calculation of LV volumes, based on 3D endocardial borders, rather than the use of geometric assumptions as with the apical biplane 2D method (Figure 6-23). Unfortunately, there is little data on the utility of either 2D or 3D volume measurements for optimizing timing of intervention in patients with valvular heart disease. Despite this knowledge gap, 3D echocardiographic measurement of LV volumes should be acquired when possible.[8] It is hoped that future clinical studies on disease progression and clinical outcome in adults with chronic valve regurgitation will incorporate the more robust measures of LV volumes instead of linear chamber dimensions, in studies.

Mechanics

LV mechanics can be evaluated by echocardiography using Doppler tissue imaging or speckle tracking strain imaging (Figure 6-24). Speckle tracking strain imaging measurements allow evaluation of global longitudinal strain, which reflects myocardial contractile function.[28-30] In addition, regional differences in the degree and timing of myocardial function can be quantitated and graphically displayed. Changes in LV mechanics may precede overt evidence of LV dilation or systolic dysfunction and might provide more sensitive markers for optimizing the timing of intervention in patients with chronic valve disease.

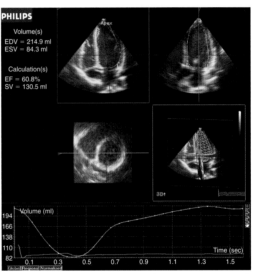

FIGURE 6-23 **Three-dimensional (3D) left ventricular (LV) volumes.** LV volumes are derived from a 3D volume acquisition with three orthogonal planes corresponding to four-chamber, two-chamber, and short-axis views shown along with the 3D volume rendered from semiautomated border tracing. *Bottom,* The LV volume curve is shown at the bottom starting with the largest volume at end-diastole (EDV) and the smallest (end-systolic) volume (ESV) at the nadir of the curve. *EF,* ejection fraction; *SV,* stroke volume. *(From Otto CM. Textbook of clinical echocardiography. 5th ed. Philadelphia: Elsevier/ Saunders; 2013.)*

Diastolic Function

LV diastolic function is reflected in the Doppler velocity patterns of ventricular inflow, myocardial tissue velocities, and left atrial filling curves (see Figure 6-24).[31,32] LV diastolic inflow is recorded from the transthoracic approach in the apical four-chamber view with the sample volume positioned at the mitral leaflet tips in diastole. The normal pattern of LV diastolic filling in young, healthy individuals consists of a short isovolumic relaxation time, a high early diastolic filling velocity (E-velocity), a steep early diastolic deceleration slope, and a smaller late diastolic filling velocity following atrial contraction (A-velocity) with a high ratio of early to late diastolic filling velocities (E/A ratio).

LV tissue-Doppler imaging (TDI) velocities are recorded with the sample volume positioned in the basal septum, adjacent to

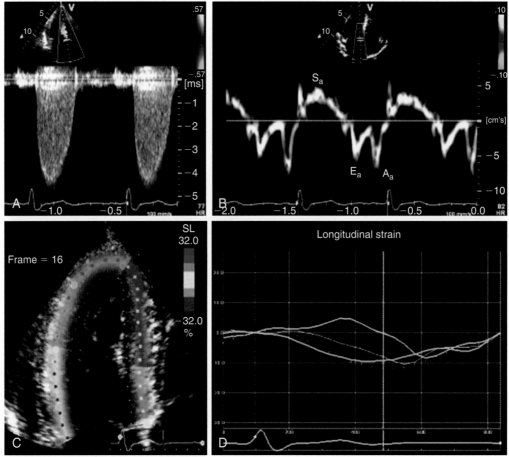

FIGURE 6-24 Longitudinal left ventricular mechanics in asymptomatic severe aortic stenosis. A, Continuous-wave Doppler signal across the stenotic aortic valve shows a peak and a mean gradient of 80 and 44 mm Hg, respectively. **B,** Pulsed-wave tissue Doppler imaging from the septal corner of the mitral valve annulus shows a reduced peak early diastolic longitudinal relaxation velocity (5 cm/s). **C** and **D,** Longitudinal strain obtained by speckle tracking (2D Strain, GE Healthcare, Milwaukee, Wisconsin) shows attenuated peak longitudinal strain from apical *(green curve)*, mid *(yellow curve)*, and basal *(blue curve)* positions of the lateral wall of the left ventricle (peak strain values <10%). *Dotted white line* in **D** also shows a reduced global longitudinal strain, averaged from the septum and lateral wall of the left ventricle (global strain = 12%). A_a, Peak late diastolic annular velocity; E_a, peak early diastolic annular velocity; S_a, peak systolic velocity during ejection. *(From Dal-Bianco JP, Khandheria BK, Mookadam F, et al. Management of asymptomatic severe aortic stenosis. J Am Coll Cardiol 2008;52:1279–92.)*

the mitral annulus, in the apical four-chamber view. The normal tissue Doppler imaging velocity curves shows an early (E′) and late diastolic (A′) velocity toward the transducer, similar to the mitral inflow velocity curve but with lower peak velocities.

Pulmonary vein flow is recorded from the apical four-chamber view on TTE with the sample volume positioned in the right inferior pulmonary vein. Higher-quality pulmonary vein flow signals can be obtained from the TEE approach with the sample volume positioned in the left superior pulmonary vein. Normal pulmonary vein flow patterns show systolic and diastolic flow into the atrium with diastolic flow (D) exceeding systolic flow (S) in young normal individuals. A small flow reversal following atrial contraction (a-reversal) is also seen.

With diastolic dysfunction due to impaired LV relaxation, the E-velocity is reduced and the A-velocity is increased, resulting in a low E/A ratio. In addition, the isovolumic relaxation time is prolonged and the deceleration slope is reduced. Tissue Doppler imaging also shows an E′ velocity less than the A′ velocity. Pulmonary vein flow shows a reduced diastolic filling velocity, prominent systolic filling velocity, and increased atrial reversal.

With diastolic dysfunction due to decreased compliance of the left ventricle, the pattern of LV diastolic filling is characterized by an increased E-velocity and a reduced A-velocity, resulting in a high E/A ratio, in conjunction with a reduced isovolumic relaxation time and an increased early diastolic deceleration slope. Tissue Doppler imaging shows a low E′ velocity (<0.10 m/s) and

a high A′ velocity. An elevated ratio of the mitral E-velocity to tissue Doppler imaging E′ velocity indicates elevated filling pressures. The pulmonary venous inflow curve shows a reduced systolic filling and increased diastolic filling curve, with increases in the velocity and duration of the atrial reversal velocity curve.

Between these two extremes, diastolic dysfunction may cause a "pseudonormal" pattern in which the LV filling curve appears normal yet the pulmonary vein flow pattern shows reduced diastolic filling and an increased atrial reversal velocity. A pseudonormal pattern can be identified from the presence of a reduced E′/A′ ratio on tissue Doppler imaging.

Unfortunately, although the Doppler velocity curves accurately portray LV diastolic filling, evaluation of LV diastolic *function* by echocardiography is limited by the numerous technical and physiologic factors other than the diastolic properties of the ventricle that affect diastolic *filling*. First, these parameters of LV diastolic filling reflect abnormal transmitral flow dynamics in patients with mitral stenosis or mitral regurgitation, not LV diastolic function. In adults with aortic valve disease, LV diastolic filling is affected by technical factors such as sample volume position and intercept angle; normal physiologic variations, including respiration, heart rate, age, and PR interval; and other physiologic variables such as preload, coexisting mitral regurgitation, LV systolic function, and atrial contractile function.[32] Pulmonary vein flow is affected by age, left atrial size, left atrial pressure, atrial contractile function, and cardiac rhythm in addition to LV and left atrial compliance, LV diastolic relaxation, and the gradient from the pulmonary veins to the left ventricle. Thus, evaluation of diastolic function in an individual patient must take into consideration whether technical or physiologic factors may affect the findings. With knowledge of these potential limitations, clinically useful information about LV diastolic function can be derived from the Doppler patterns of LV inflow and pulmonary vein flow in patients with valvular heart disease.

Other Echocardiographic Data

Echocardiographic evaluation of the patient with valvular heart disease also includes assessment of other parameters, depending on the specific valve involved and the severity of valve disease. For example, in a patient with mitral stenosis, measurement of left atrial size and estimation of pulmonary pressures are important components of the examination. In a patient with severe aortic stenosis and heart failure symptoms despite normal LV systolic function, evaluation of diastolic ventricular function may be needed.

Left Atrial Enlargement and Thrombus Formation

Left atrial size can be assessed on 2D transthoracic imaging from parasternal, apical, and subcostal views. Methods for calculation of left atrial volume based on planimetry of atrial area in two views have been validated and provide quantitative measures of atrial size, but in most clinical situations, a single anterior-posterior diameter, in conjunction with 2D visual estimates of atrial size, provides adequate information for patient management.

The specificity of identification of a left atrial thrombus on transthoracic imaging is high (95%-99%), but sensitivity is low (about 60%) owing to poor image quality at the depth of the left atrium and difficulty in visualizing the atrial appendage. TEE provides high-quality images of the left atrium and atrial appendage, resulting in very high sensitivity (nearly 100%) and specificity (nearly 100%) for detection of atrial thrombus. Thus, when atrial thrombus is suspected clinically, TEE is necessary for reliable exclusion of this potential diagnosis.

Determination of Pulmonary Pressures

Pulmonary pressure is estimated on the basis of measurement of tricuspid regurgitant jet velocity in combination with an estimate of right atrial pressure.[33] A small degree of tricuspid regurgitation is present in most normal individuals, with an even higher prevalence in patients with valvular disease. Because the velocity of the regurgitant jet relates to the pressure difference across the valve, and not to the volume of regurgitation, this degree of tricuspid regurgitation, although not hemodynamically significant, allows recording of jet velocity and calculation of pulmonary pressures.

The velocity in the tricuspid regurgitant jet *(TR_{jet})* reflects the difference between right ventricular and right atrial systolic pressures, as stated in the Bernoulli equation. Addition of right atrial pressure *(RAP)* to this pressure difference yields right ventricular systolic pressure, which in the absence of pulmonic stenosis, equals pulmonary artery systolic pressure *(PA_{systolic})*:

$$PA_{systolic} = 4(TR_{jet})^2 + RAP$$

Right atrial pressure is estimated from the appearance of the inferior vena cava at its entrance into the right atrium as imaged from a subcostal view during normal respiration. Because this method depends on normal intrathoracic pressure changes with respiration, it is not applicable in the mechanically ventilated patient. Examination of the tricuspid regurgitant jet from parasternal and apical windows with careful transducer angulation to record the highest-velocity signal is essential to avoid underestimation of jet velocity (and hence pulmonary artery pressures). When a clear maximum regurgitant jet velocity cannot be identified, or only an incomplete waveform is obtained, pulmonary pressures cannot be reliable determined with this method. Instead, indirect evidence for pulmonary hypertension (e.g., midsystolic notching and short time to peak velocity in the pulmonary artery velocity wave, abnormal septal motion) or another method must be used. In patients with mitral stenosis, assessment of the rise in pulmonary pressures with exercise provides insight into the relationship between hemodynamic severity and clinical symptoms. Exercise Doppler echocardiographic data also may be useful in determining the optimal timing of intervention in patients with mitral stenosis in order to prevent the development of irreversible pulmonary hypertension (see Chapter 17).

Right Heart Structure and Function

Qualitative evaluation of right ventricular size and systolic function on 2D echocardiography is an important component of the examination in patients with valvular heart disease.[34] The right ventricle is imaged in the parasternal short-axis and right ventricular inflow views, and in apical and subcostal four-chamber views. Right ventricular size is described as normal or mildly, moderately, or severely enlarged on the basis of integration of data from these views. Similarly, right ventricular systolic function is graded on a scale from normal to severely reduced. The pattern of ventricular septal motion also is helpful in diagnosis of right ventricular pressure or volume overload. In addition to qualitative evaluation of the right ventricle, at least one quantitative measurement is recommended both for size and systolic function. A normal basal diastolic chamber dimension in the four-chamber view is 4.2 cm or less, and the normal tissue Doppler imaging systolic velocity is at least 10 cm/s. Right ventricular longitudinal shortening or the tricuspid annular plane systolic excursion (TAPSE) is another simple measure of systolic function. The tricuspid annular plane systolic excursion is measured from an apical M-mode recording as the difference between the diastolic and systolic positions of the annulus, with normal being at least 1.6 cm. When right heart valve disease is present and quantitative evaluation of right ventricular function is needed, CMR imaging may be considered.

Aortic Anatomy and Dilation

Aortic dilation often accompanies aortic valve disease. On echocardiography, the aortic annulus, sinuses, and proximal ascending aorta are well visualized in parasternal views. Additional views of the ascending aorta can often be obtained from a higher intercostal space, the aortic arch can be imaged from a suprasternal notch approach, and portions of the descending thoracic and proximal abdominal aorta are seen on apical and subcostal views, respectively.

Basic measurements on echocardiography include the maximum end-diastolic diameter of the aortic root, typically at the sinus level, measured from a 2D long-axis image. If this measurement is abnormal, or if there is effacement of the sinotubular junction, measurements are taken at multiple sites in the aortic root. The American Society of Echocardiography recommends calculation of an expected aortic root size on the basis of age and body size.[35,36] Additional imaging with chest computed tomography or CMR imaging may be helpful when aortic involvement is suspected or known.

REFERENCES

1. Otto CM. Textbook of Clinical Echocardiography. 5th ed. Philadelphia: Elsevier Saunders; 2013.
2. Otto CM. The Practice of Clinical Echocardiography. 4th ed. Philadelphia: Elsevier-Saunders; 2012.
3. Lang RM, Tsang W, Weinert L, et al. Valvular heart disease. The value of 3-dimensional echocardiography. J Am Coll Cardiol 2011;58(19):1933–44.

4. Bloomfield GS, Gillam LD, Hahn RT, et al. A practical guide to multimodality imaging of transcatheter aortic valve replacement. JACC Cardiovasc Imaging 2012;5(4):441–55.

5. Delgado V, Kapadia S, Marsan NA, et al. Multimodality imaging before, during, and after percutaneous mitral valve repair. Heart 2011;97(20):1704–14.

6. Schaefer BM, Lewin MB, Stout KK, et al. Usefulness of bicuspid aortic valve phenotype to predict elastic properties of the ascending aorta. Am J Cardiol 2007;99(5):686–90.

7. Fedak PW, Verma S, David TE, et al. Clinical and pathophysiological implications of a bicuspid aortic valve. Circulation 2002;106(8):900–4.

8. Lang RM, Badano LP, Tsang W, et al. EAE/ASE recommendations for image acquisition and display using three-dimensional echocardiography. J Am Soc Echocardiogr 2012;25(1):3–46.

9. Levine RA. Dynamic mitral regurgitation–more than meets the eye. N Engl J Med 2004;351(16):1681–4.

10. Garcia D, Kadem L, Savery D, et al. Analytical modeling of the instantaneous maximal transvalvular pressure gradient in aortic stenosis. J Biomech 2006;39(16):3036–44.

11. Baumgartner H, Hung J, Bermejo J, et al. Echocardiographic assessment of valve stenosis: EAE/ASE recommendations for clinical practice. Eur J Echocardiogr 2009; 10(1):1–25.

12. Iung B, Vahanian A. Echocardiography in the patient undergoing catheter balloon mitral valvotomy: patient selection, hemodynamic results, complications and long term outcome. In: Otto CM, editor. The Practice of Clinical Echocardiography. 3rd ed. Philadelphia: Elsevier-Saunders; 2012. p. 389–407.

13. Xie MX, Wang XF, Cheng TO, et al. Comparison of accuracy of mitral valve area in mitral stenosis by real-time, three-dimensional echocardiography versus two-dimensional echocardiography versus Doppler pressure half-time. Am J Cardiol 2005;95(12): 1496–9.

14. Goland S, Trento A, Iida K, et al. Assessment of aortic stenosis by three-dimensional echocardiography: an accurate and novel approach. Heart 2007;93(7):801–7.

15. Saitoh T, Shiota M, Izumo M, et al. Comparison of left ventricular outflow geometry and aortic valve area in patients with aortic stenosis by 2-dimensional versus 3-dimensional echocardiography. Am J Cardiol 2012;109(11):1626–31.

16. Rosenhek R. Aortic stenosis: disease severity, progression, timing of intervention and role in monitoring transcatheter valve implanation. In: Otto CM, editor. The Practice of Clinical Echocardiography. 4th ed. Philadelphia: Elsevier/Saunders; 2012. p. 425–49.

17. Awtry E, Davidoff R. Low-flow/low-gradient aortic stenosis. Circulation 2011;124(23): e739–41.

18. Pibarot P, Dumesnil JG. Low-flow, low-gradient aortic stenosis with normal and depressed left ventricular ejection fraction. J Am Coll Cardiol 2012;60(19):1845–53.

19. Owens DS, Otto CM. Stress testing for structural heart disease. In: Gillam LD, Otto CM, editors. Advanced Appoaches in Echocardiography. Philadelphia: Elsevier-Saunders; 2012. p. 171–98.

20. Hung J. Mitral valve anatomy, quantification of mitral regurgitation and timing of surgical intervention for mitral regurgitation. In: Otto CM, editor. The Practice of Clinical Echocardiography. 4th ed. Philadelphia: Elsevier-Saunders; 2012. p. 330–50.

21. Evangelista A, Tornos P. Aortic valve regurgitation: quantitation of disease severity and timing of surgical intervention. In: Otto CM, editor. The Practice of Clinical Echocardiography. 4th ed. Philadelphia: Elsevier-Saunders; 2012. p. 367–88.

22. Zoghbi WA, Enriquez-Sarano M, Foster E, et al. Recommendations for evaluation of the severity of native valvular regurgitation with two-dimensional and Doppler echocardiography. J Am Soc Echocardiogr 2003;16(7):777–802.

23. Tribouilloy CM, Enriquez-Sarano M, Bailey KR, et al. Quantification of tricuspid regurgitation by measuring the width of the vena contracta with Doppler color flow imaging: a clinical study. J Am Coll Cardiol 2000;36(2):472–8.

24. Cawley PJ, Hamilton-Craig C, Owens DS, et al. Prospective comparison of valve regurgitation quantitation by cardiac magnetic resonance imaging and transthoracic echocardiography. Circ Cardiovasc Imaging 2013;6(1):48–57.

25. Bonow RO, Carabello BA, Kanu C, et al. ACC/AHA 2006 guidelines for the management of patients with valvular heart disease: a report of the American College of Cardiology/ American Heart Association Task Force on Practice Guidelines (writing committee to revise the 1998 Guidelines for the Management of Patients With Valvular Heart Disease): developed in collaboration with the Society of Cardiovascular Anesthesiologists: endorsed by the Society for Cardiovascular Angiography and Interventions and the Society of Thoracic Surgeons. Circulation 2006;114(5):e84–231.

26. Vahanian A, Alfieri O, Andreotti F, et al. Guidelines on the management of valvular heart disease (version 2012). Eur Heart J 2012;33(19):2451–96.

27. Lang RM, Bierig M, Devereux RB, et al. Recommendations for chamber quantification: a report from the American Society of Echocardiography's Guidelines and Standards Committee and the Chamber Quantification Writing Group, developed in conjunction with the European Association of Echocardiography, a branch of the European Society of Cardiology. J Am Soc Echocardiogr 2005;18(12):1440–63.

28. Marwick TH. Strain and strain rate imaging. In: Gillam LD, Otto CM, editors. Advanced Approaches in Echocardiography. Philadelphia: Elsevier-Saunders; 2012. p. 84–102.

29. Smiseth OA, Edvardsen T. Myocardial mechanics: velocity, strain, strain rate, cardiac synchrony and twist. In: Otto CM, editor. The Practice of Clinical Echocardiography. 4th ed. Philadephia: Elsevier-Saunders; 2012. p. 177–96.

30. Dal-Bianco JP, Khandheria BK, Mookadam F, et al. Management of asymptomatic severe aortic stenosis. J Am Coll Cardiol 2008;52(16):1279–92.

31. Redfield MM, Jacobsen SJ, Burnett Jr JC, et al. Burden of systolic and diastolic ventricular dysfunction in the community: appreciating the scope of the heart failure epidemic. JAMA 2003;289(2):194–202.

32. Plana JC, Desai MY, Klein AL. Assessment of diastolic function by echocardiography. In: Otto CM, editor. The Practice of Clinical Echocardiography. 4th ed. Philadephia: Elsevier-Saunders; 2012. p. 197–217.

33. Milan A, Magnino C, Veglio F. Echocardiographic indexes for the non-invasive evaluation of pulmonary hemodynamics. J Am Soc Echocardiogr 2010;23(3):225–39.

34. Rudski LG, Lai WW, Afilalo J, et al. Guidelines for the echocardiographic assessment of the right heart in adults: a report from the American Society of Echocardiography endorsed by the European Association of Echocardiography, a registered branch of the European Society of Cardiology, and the Canadian Society of Echocardiography. J Am Soc Echocardiogr 2010;23(7):685–713.

35. Lang RM, Bierig M, Devereux RB, et al. Recommendations for chamber quantification: a report from the American Society of Echocardiography's Guidelines and Standards Committee and the Chamber Quantification Writing Group, developed in conjunction with the European Association of Echocardiography, a branch of the European Society of Cardiology. J Am Soc Echocardiogr 2005;18(12):1440–63.

36. Roman MJ, Devereux RB, Kramer-Fox R, et al. Two-dimensional echocardiographic aortic root dimensions in normal children and adults. Am J Cardiol 1989;64:507–12.

CHAPTER 7

Evaluation of Valvular Heart Disease by Cardiac Catheterization and Angiocardiography

David M. Shavelle

Key Points

- Cardiac catheterization and angiocardiography is useful in patients:
  - Who require coronary angiography prior to surgical intervention
  - With complex multivalve disease when data from echocardiography and cardiac catheterization must be integrated
  - With suboptimal echocardiographic imaging (large body habitus, obesity, chronic lung disease)
  - In whom discrepancies exist between the clinical information and findings from echocardiography
  - In whom the diagnosis remains uncertain despite echocardiography and additional noninvasive imaging studies
  - With low-gradient aortic stenosis when the administration of dobutamine can differentiate between true and "pseudo"–aortic stenosis
  - Being considered for transcutaneous aortic valve implantation
- Accurate and detailed measurements are essential in patients with valvular heart disease so that the subsequently derived data (valve area, valve area index) remain accurate.
- Evaluation of left ventricular systolic function includes ventriculography, measurement of cardiac output, and measurement of left ventricular pressures throughout the cardiac cycle.
- The principles of evaluating the severity of stenosis of each of the cardiac valves are similar and involve:
  - Measurement of the pressure gradient
  - Analysis of the pressure waveforms
  - Measurement of cardiac output
  - Calculation of the valve area
  - Occasionally, angiocardiography of the chamber upstream to the site of stenosis
- The pressure gradient between the left ventricle and the aorta in aortic stenosis is described by three invasive measurements: the mean gradient, the peak-to-peak gradient, and the maximum gradient. The mean and maximum gradients are used to evaluate stenosis severity.
- True severe aortic stenosis and a low gradient can be differentiated from pseudo-aortic stenosis on the basis of the hemodynamic response during a dobutamine infusion. True severe aortic stenosis is present when dobutamine increases cardiac output >50% above baseline, the mean aortic valve gradient is >30 mm Hg and the aortic valve area remains ≤1.0 cm^2.
- Angiographic evaluation of regurgitant severity is based on injection of contrast agent into the chamber downstream of the affected valve with imaging of contrast agent reflux into the chamber receiving the regurgitant volume.

Basic Principles

Cardiac catheterization and angiocardiography continue to play an important role in the management of patients with valvular heart disease.[1] Although in the majority of patients, information obtained from the history, physical examination, and noninvasive imaging studies (electrocardiogram, chest radiograph, and echocardiogram) is sufficient to establish the correct diagnosis and allow appropriate clinical decision making, including referral for percutaneous or surgical intervention, cardiac catheterization and angiocardiography are often required in select patients with valvular heart disease. They include patients (1) who require coronary angiography prior to surgical intervention, (2) who have complex multivalve disease for which data from echocardiography and cardiac catheterization must be integrated, (3) who have suboptimal echocardiographic imaging results (large body habitus, obesity, chronic lung disease), (4) in whom discrepancies exist between the clinical information and findings from echocardiography, (5) in whom the diagnosis remains uncertain despite echocardiography and additional no-invasive imaging studies, (6) with low-gradient aortic stenosis (AS) when the administration of dobutamine can differentiate between true and "pseudo"–aortic stenosis, and (7) being evaluated for transcutaneous aortic valve implantation.

Various protocols can be used in the cardiac catheterization laboratory to evaluate patients with valvular heart disease (Table 7-1). The fundamental basis of each approach relies on the premise that obtaining accurate and detailed measurements during the procedure is essential so that the subsequently derived data remain accurate. Pressure and cardiac output measurements should be performed prior to angiocardiography. A number of potential sources of error can be present during the cardiac catheterization laboratory procedure (Table 7-2). The specific methods and techniques used during a cardiac catheterization procedure are selected to provide answers to specific clinical questions. The significance of the hemodynamic findings must be integrated with the complete set of clinical data, including information from the history, physical examination, electrocardiogram, chest radiograph, and echocardiogram.

Pressures

Direct measurement of left ventricular (LV) pressures throughout the entire cardiac cycle provide valuable data on LV systolic

TABLE 7-1   Protocol for Evaluation of Valvular Heart Disease at Cardiac Catheterization

PRESSURE MEASUREMENTS	CARDIAC OUTPUT	ANGIOCARDIOGRAPHY	CALCULATED VALUES
Right heart (including pulmonary capillary wedge pressure) Left ventricle Left atrium (for mitral stenosis evaluation) Aorta Transvalvular gradients—simultaneous pressure recordings on both sides of stenotic valve	Thermodilution and Fick methods (simultaneous with transvalvular gradient)	Left ventricle—end-diastolic volume, end-systolic volume, stroke volume, ejection fraction Aortic root—for evaluation of ascending aorta and aortic regurgitation Coronary—for assessment of coexisting coronary artery disease	Valve areas—Gorlin and Gorlin formula, Hakki formula Use transvalvular volume flow rate Pulmonary vascular resistance—baseline and following vasodilator challenge Systemic vascular resistance Regurgitant volume and fraction

TABLE 7-2   Potential Sources of Error in Evaluation of Valvular Heart Disease at Catheterization

PRESSURE DATA	Cardiac Output		ANGIOGRAPHY	VALVE AREA CALCULATIONS
	FICK METHOD	THERMODILUTION METHOD		
Frequency response Side-hole vs. end-hole catheters Catheter whip and impact artifacts Signal damping Calibration and zero Recorder sweep speed and scale Peripheral amplification	Measurement of O_2 consumption Timing of arterial and venous O_2 samples Site of arterial and venous sampling	Uneven mixing of injectate within right atrium (tricuspid regurgitation) Poor accuracy at low outputs (extrapolation of curve)	Geometric assumptions Endocardial border identification Catheter positioning Cardiac rhythm	Transvalvular volume flow rate Pressure measurements Empirical constant

function, although the effect of concurrent valvular disease must also be taken into account. The rate of rise of LV pressure (*dP/dt*) during isovolumic contraction provides a relatively load-independent measure of LV systolic function, which is particularly useful in patients with altered loading conditions due to valvular disease.

Pressure-Volume Loops

The relationship between LV pressure and volume throughout the cardiac cycle can be examined in detail by graphing instantaneous pressure (on the vertical axis) against volume (on the horizontal axis). LV stroke volume is the distance on the horizontal axis between end-diastole and end-systole, whereas LV stroke work (the integral of pressure times volume over the cardiac cycle) is the area enclosed by the pressure-volume loop. When pressure-volume loops are recorded under different loading conditions, the slope of the end-systolic pressure-volume relationship, termed elastance or E_{max}, provides a load-independent measure of LV systolic function.[2,3]

Valvular heart disease characterized by pressure overload of the left ventricle results in a taller pressure-volume loop that is shifted upwards, reflecting the higher ventricular systolic pressures and greater LV stroke work. Volume overload of the left ventricle also increases stroke work, resulting in a larger loop that is shifted upwards and to the right. However, despite these shifts in the pressure-volume loop, the slope of the end-systolic pressure-volume relationship remains normal in patients with valvular disease and compensated ventricular systolic function. A reduced slope indicates impaired contractility superimposed on the pressure and/or volume overload state.

In practice, measurement of pressure-volume loops is technically demanding and often not required for clinical decision making. Ventricular pressures must be recorded with high-fidelity catheters, and volumes must be determined at multiple points in the cardiac cycle using either contrast or radionuclide angiography or experimental approaches such as a conductance catheter.[4] Thus, although this approach provides insight into the pathophysiology of disease and provides essential information in research studies, it is rarely used in the routine clinical management of patients with valvular heart disease.[5]

Evaluation of Left Ventricular Systolic Function

Evaluation of LV systolic function includes ventriculography, measurement of cardiac output, and measurement of LV pressures throughout the cardiac cycle. *Contractility* is defined as the intrinsic ability of the myocardium to shorten, independent of loading conditions. However, measurement of LV contractility in the clinical setting is problematic. The reason is that most conventional measures of LV systolic function depend on both ventricular preload and afterload, as well as myocardial contractility. Increased *preload*, defined as LV end-diastolic volume or pressure, increases myocardial shortening as described by the Frank-Starling relationship. In contrast, *afterload*, defined as the resistance or impedance to LV ejection, is inversely related to myocardial shortening. Loading conditions are frequently altered in patients with valvular heart disease. For example, with AS, afterload is increased and with aortic regurgitation, both afterload and preload are increased. These alterations complicate the assessment of LV systolic function.

Angiocardiography

LV end-diastolic volume (EDV) and end-systolic volume (ESV) can be calculated by tracing the respective endocardial boundaries on angiographic images and applying a validated geometric formula for volume calculation. Stroke volume (SV) is calculated as follows:

$$SV = EDV - ESV$$

and ejection fraction (EF) as:

$$EF = \frac{SV}{EDV}$$

The stroke volume (cardiac output divided by heart rate) calculated by angiocardiography represents the total amount of blood ejected by the ventricle, whether that blood is ejected forward into the aorta or backward into the left atrium across an incompetent mitral valve. Thus, angiographic stroke volume is termed "total" stroke volume.

The geometric formulas for angiographic calculation of volume (V) typically assume a prolate ellipsoid shape of the left ventricle. Endocardial border tracings from two orthogonal views of the ventricle (right and left anterior oblique projections) are used to measure the area (A) and length (L) of the ventricle with the minor axis diameter (D) calculated for each view as:

$$D = (4A)/\pi L$$

$$V_c = (\pi/6)(L \times D_a \times D_b)$$

where D_a and D_b are the minor axis dimensions in the two orthogonal views.

In the clinical setting, a single-plane right anterior oblique angiogram using the modified for mula of Dodge and Sandler[6] also provides acceptable results:

$$V_c = (8A^2)/(3\pi L) \text{ OR } V_c = (\pi/6)(LD^2)$$

Although both angiography and echocardiography depend on manual border tracing, a slight, but consistent, overestimation of LV volumes by angiography is due to filling of the ventricular trabeculations by contrast agent so that the traced endocardial border represents the outer edge of the myocardial trabeculations, in contrast to echocardiography, in which ultrasound is reflected from the inner edge of the myocardial trabeculations so that the volume tends to be underestimated slightly.[7-9] In addition, the volume occupied by the papillary muscles (which are excluded from the endocardial border tracing) needs to be taken into account. Regression equations have been derived in an attempt to correct for the overestimation of volume on angiography resulting from these two factors, such as the following:[10-12]

$$V = 0.81 V_c + 1.9$$

where V_c is the calculated volume and V is the corrected volume.

With careful angiographic technique, tracing of endocardial borders by an experienced observer, and use of appropriate correction factors, ventricular volumes derived from angiography correlate well with directly measured volumes and with echocardiographic volumes.[13-16] A biplane imaging approach, using borders traced from both the right and left anterior oblique radiographic projections,[17,18] provides accurate results with a mean difference for measurement variability of 6 to 10 mL for end-systolic and 7 to 20 mL for end-diastolic volumes.[19]

Technical factors important in the performance of ventricular angiography include the need for complete opacification of the ventricle with clear definition of the endocardial borders at both end-diastole and end-systole. This goal can be achieved with a 6 French side-hole pigtail catheter, a power contrast injector, and use of an injection rate and volume appropriate to the type of catheter, ventricular chamber size, and hemodynamics. A nonionic contrast agent is optimal in patients with valvular disease to avoid myocardial depression and/or hemodynamic changes. Correct positioning of the catheter in the midventricle is needed to completely opacify the chamber, to prevent movement of the catheter during the contract injection, and to minimize the risk of arrhythmias. Optimal catheter positioning also avoids artifactual mitral regurgitation due to entrapment of the catheter in the mitral valve apparatus. In addition, a correction factor for the effect of magnification must be determined by filming a calibrated grid at the estimated level of the ventricle. Other factors that affect the accuracy and reproducibility of angiographic volumes are image quality, the experience of the individual tracing the endocardial borders, heart rate and rhythm, and the potential cardiodepressant effect of the contrast agent.

Methods for determining LV mass by angiographic techniques have been described, with LV mass calculated on the basis of the thickness (h) of the anterior wall (assuming a symmetric thickness around the ventricle), ventricular diameter in anterior-posterior (D_{AP}) and lateral (D_{lat}) views, long-axis length (L), and ventricular volume (V), as follows:

$$\text{LV mass (g)} = \left(\frac{4}{3}\pi \left[\frac{D_{AP}}{2} + h \right]\left[\frac{D_{lat}}{2} + h \right]\left[\frac{L}{2} + h \right] - V \right) \times 1.05$$

However, ventricular mass calculations are limited by the inaccuracy in measuring LV wall thickness from the angiographic image and thus are not widely used clinically.[20,21]

LV angiography also allows qualitative and quantitative assessment of wall motion in patients with valvular heart disease and concurrent coronary artery disease.[22,23]

Cardiac Output

Cardiac output can be calculated during cardiac catheterization by the dilution of a known concentration of an indicator (e.g., dye, oxygen, or cold saline) as it passes through the vascular bed. This concept is illustrated by the injection of a known volume and concentration of dye (typically indocyanine green) into the venous circulation. From the rate at which this dye appears in the arterial circulation, the volume of blood the dye was diluted in (i.e., the cardiac output) can be calculated. Although indicator dilution dye curves provide accurate measurement of cardiac output, the procedure is time consuming and depends on meticulous technique, and other methods are now more commonly used.

FICK TECHNIQUE

Oxygen serves as the "indicator" for cardiac output calculations in the Fick method. The Fick principle states that the uptake or release of oxygen by a tissue is the product of the amount of oxygen delivered to the tissue times the difference in oxygen content between the blood entering and the blood leaving the tissue.[24] Thus, for the uptake of oxygen by the lungs:

$$\text{Oxygen uptake} = \frac{\text{Pulmonary blood flow}}{(O_2 \text{ content}_{PV} - O_2 \text{ content}_{PA})}$$

If the amount of oxygen consumed by the patient (oxygen uptake), and the oxygen content of pulmonary arterial (PA) and pulmonary venous (PV) blood are measured, this equation can be solved for pulmonary blood flow, as follows:

$$\text{Pulmonary blood flow} = \frac{O_2 \text{ consumption}}{(O_2 \text{ content}_{PV} - O_2 \text{ content}_{PA})}$$

In the absence of an intracardiac shunt, pulmonary and systemic blood flows are equal, so this method provides a measure of systemic (or forward) cardiac output, which can be calculated as follows:

$$\text{Cardiac output} = \frac{O_2 \text{ consumption}}{[(O_2 \text{ content})_{arterial} - (O_2 \text{ content})_{venous}]}$$

where O_2 consumption is measured in mL O_2/min and O_2 content as mL O_2/100 mL blood (often referred to as "volume percent").

To ensure that the sample of venous blood represents total venous return with adequate mixing of the sample, a pulmonary artery blood sample is used for mixed systemic venous oxygen content in this equation (in the absence of an intracardiac shunt). Although pulmonary venous blood provides the most accurate sample of oxygenated blood, the arterial sample is obtained from a systemic artery or the left ventricle. When an intracardiac shunt is present, separate calculations for systemic and pulmonary blood flows (using the appropriate arterial and venous oxygen contents) allow determination of the shunt ratio.

In clinical practice, oxygen consumption is usually measured by the polarographic O_2 method or by the paramagnetic method. Collection of expired air using the Douglas bag method is rarely used. The polarographic method uses a hood or face mask with the rate of air flow through the servo unit controlled by an oxygen sensor cell to maintain a constant fractional content of oxygen. Oxygen consumption (VO_2) then is calculated from the fractional content of oxygen and flow rates of air entering and exiting the patient mask, assuming a respiratory quotient of 1.0. The paramagnetic method measures both oxygen and carbon dioxide in expired air, allowing calculation of the respiratory quotient for each patient. In recent years, there has been a trend to estimate oxygen consumption with the use of derived equations.[25] However, use of these derived equations is inaccurate, especially in patients with increased body mass index.[26]

The arteriovenous oxygen difference is calculated from measurement of oxygen content in simultaneously drawn samples of arterial and mixed venous blood collected midway during the oxygen consumption measurement. Oxygen content is typically calculated as oxygen saturation multiplied by the theoretic oxygen capacity, which is estimated from the patient's hemoglobin (Hgb) level as follows:

$$O_2 \text{ content} = \text{Hgb (g/dL)} \times 1.36 \text{ (mL } O_2/g \text{ of Hgb)} \times 10 \times \% \text{ saturation}$$

For accurate cardiac output calculations, it is important that the arterial and venous oxygen samples are collected from the correct sites with prompt processing of the samples and that oxygen consumption and content measurements are simultaneous. Even with careful technique, the average error in measuring oxygen consumption is approximately 6%[27] and the error in measurement of the arteriovenous oxygen difference is approximately 5%,[28] resulting in an error in cardiac output measurement of about 10% by the Fick method.[29] Measurements are more inaccurate if physiologic changes that affect cardiac output, such as heart rate and loading conditions, occur during the analysis period. Use of an assumed, rather than measured, oxygen consumption also leads to significant error because there is wide variation in the normal rate of oxygen consumption in adults.[30,31] Fick cardiac outputs tend to be more accurate for low outputs, and thermodilution outputs are more accurate at high flow rates.

THERMODILUTION METHOD

Measurement of cardiac output by the thermodilution method is widely used in the evaluation of patients with valvular heart disease. With the thermodilution method, a known volume of cold saline is injected into the right atrium while a thermistor in the pulmonary artery continuously records temperature (Figure 7-4). Cardiac output is then calculated from the known temperature (T) and volume (V) of the injectate, and the integral of temperature over time ($\Delta T/dt$) in the pulmonary artery.[32,33]

$$\text{Cardiac output} = \frac{\text{Constant } [V_{injectate} \times (T_{blood} - T_{injectate})]}{(\Delta T/dt)}$$

where the constant incorporates factors for the specific gravity and specific heat of blood and the injectate (1.08 if the injectate is 5% dextrose). In addition, an empirical correction factor (multiplication by 0.825) is needed for the effect of warming of the injectate as it passes through the catheter.[34,35]

As with the Fick method, the thermodilution method measures the "forward" cardiac output, specifically the output of the right heart. Advantages of the thermodilution method include ease and repeatability of use, thus allowing multiple measurements over short time intervals with a reasonable accuracy (a reproducibility of about 5%-10% with proper technique).[36] Disadvantages include relatively poor accuracy at low cardiac outputs[37] and dependence on careful attention to technique, in particular the avoidance of warming of the injectate. Because this method depends on even mixing of the injectate with the right atrial (RA) blood, thermodilution output measurements are inaccurate when significant tricuspid regurgitation is present. Significant tricuspid regurgitation results in a prolonged decay in the temperature-over-time curve.

Evaluation of Stenosis Severity

Measurement of Pressure Gradients

Normal cardiac valves offer little to no resistance to blood flow when the valve is open in either systole (semilunar valves—aortic

and pulmonic) or diastole (atrioventricular valves—tricuspid and mitral). In the setting of disease, restriction to leaflet opening (stenosis) occurs and blood flow across the valve is hindered. Resistance to blood flow results in a pressure drop or gradient across the valve. The principles of evaluating the severity of stenosis of each of the cardiac valves are similar and involve: (1) measurement of the pressure gradient, (2) analysis of the pressure waveforms, (3) measurement of cardiac output, (4) calculation of the valve area and, occasionally, (5) angiocardiography of the chamber upstream of the site of stenosis.

BASIC PRINCIPLES

Pressure gradients are most accurately measured with use of two transducers that allow for simultaneous measurement of the upstream and downstream pressures. A systematic approach to the review of pressure waveforms includes assessment of: (1) cardiac rhythm, (2) pressure scale and pressure per division, (3) recording speed (i.e., paper speed), (4) pressure values across the valve, (5) pressures in all adjacent cardiac chambers (Table 7-3), (6) the rate and shape of the upslope and downslope of pressure waveforms, and (6) recording artifacts. Both technical and physiologic factors can affect the measured pressure gradients (see Table 7-2).

TABLE 7-3	Normal Values at Cardiac Catheterization (Supine, Resting Adults)	
ANGIOGRAPHIC LEFT VENTRICULAR VOLUMES		**MEAN ± 1 SD**
End-diastolic volume		70 ± 20 mL/m^2
End-systolic volume		24 ± 0 mL/m^2
Ejection fraction		0.67 ± 0.08
LV mass		92 ± 16 g/m^2
CARDIAC OUTPUT		**MEAN ± 1 SD**
Rest		3.0 L/min/m^2
Exercise		18.0 L/min/m^2
O_2 consumption (resting)		126 ± 26 mL/min/m^2
Arterial O_2 saturation		95%
Venous O_2 saturation		75%
Arteriovenous oxygen difference		40 mL/L (volume %)
PRESSURES (mm Hg)	**SYSTOLIC/ DIASTOLIC**	**MEAN**
Right atrium	a3-6, v1-4	1-5
Right ventricle	20-30/2-7	
Pulmonary artery	16-30/4-13	9-18
Pulmonary wedge	4-14/v 6-16	5-12
Left atrial	a4-14, v6-16	6-11
Left ventricular	90-140/6-12	
Aorta	90-140/70-90	70-110
VASCULAR RESISTANCE	**MEAN ± 1 SD**	**INDEXED TO BSA**
Pulmonary resistance Wood units (mm Hg-L^{-1}-min)	67 ± 30 0.8-1.1 ± 0.3-0.5	123 ± 54
Systemic resistance (dynes-s-cm^{-5})	1170 ± 270	2130 ± 450
VALVE AREAS (cm^2)[90]	**OVERALL**	**MALE**	**FEMALE**
Aortic	4.6 ± 1.1	4.8 ± 1.3	3.7 ± 1.0
Mitral	7.8 ± 1.9	8.3 ± 2.0	6.7 ± 1.3
Tricuspid	10.6 ± 2.6	11.5 ± 2.5	8.8 ± 1.7
Pulmonic	4.7 ± 1.2	4.9 ± 1.3	4.3 ± 1.0

TECHNICAL FACTORS

Technical factors can significantly affect the accuracy of the reported transvalvular gradients. The frequency response of the pressure measurement system significantly affects the recorded pressure waveform. Although micromanometer-tipped catheters have an optimal frequency response (at least 20 cycles/second) for intracardiac pressure recording, these catheters are expensive and require meticulous technique. In the clinical setting, the fluid-filled catheters and strain-gauge external transducers that are commonly used have a frequency response of only 10 to 20 cycles/second. The frequency response can be optimized by use of stiff wide-bore catheters, a short length of connecting tubing, and a low-density liquid.

External pressure transducers are subject to a phenomenon called "ring-down," which results from the conversion of pressure energy to an electrical signal, similar to the sound resulting from striking a bell. The use of a fluid-filled catheter between the chamber of interest and the transducer amplifies this phenomenon, leading to apparent fluctuations in the recorded pressure signal. This phenomenon, called "underdamping," is characterized by a waveform consisting of diminishing harmonic oscillations of the underlying pressure signal. To counter this effect, the recording system is damped just enough to avoid excessive oscillations while maintaining the frequency response of the system. "Overdamping" must also be avoided as it can lead to underestimation of pressure gradients. Damping can typically be optimized by using short, stiff tubing to connect the catheter to the pressure transducer, minimizing the number of connections in the system, and using a contrast agent (instead of saline) to fill the catheter.

Pressure recording systems must be zeroed and calibrated both before and after data collection. Calibration is optimally performed with the use of a known input pressure, such as with a mercury manometer, but many systems now include an electronic calibration that is usually adequate. The zero and the reference standard need to be rechecked periodically during and at completion of the study to avoid erroneous data interpretations. When two catheters are used to measure pressures simultaneously on both sides of a stenotic valve, the calibrations are checked together, and if possible, data are re-recorded after the transducers are switched to the other catheters to avoid any systematic bias.

Pressures are recorded at a fast sweep speed to allow accurate time measurements and to display the waveform in enough detail to allow analysis of the degree of damping and the subtleties of the pressure waveform. The vertical axis is adjusted, depending on the pressures being recorded, to utilize the full height of the recording while including the pressure waveforms of interest on the scale. For example, left atrial (LA) and LV pressures across a stenotic mitral valve might be recorded on a 0 to 25 mm Hg scale, whereas severe AS might require a 0 to 200 mm Hg scale.

PHYSIOLOGIC FACTORS

The exact locations of the pressures recorded upstream and downstream of a stenotic valve can significantly affect the measured transvalvular gradient, and occurs for several reasons. First, the timing of the pressure waveform is different closer to the valve from that at a greater distance from the valve, so that realignment of the waveforms may be needed for accurate gradient calculations. For example, the femoral artery pressure upstroke is delayed in comparison with the central aortic pressure as predicted by the velocity of pressure propagation between these two sites. If a femoral artery waveform is used in place of central aortic pressure to calculate the aortic transvalvular gradient, this timing difference needs to be taken into account. Similarly, if the diastolic pressure curve uses the the pulmonary capillary wedge pressure in place of directly measured LA pressure in a patient with mitral stenosis, failure to consider timing differences may lead to erroneous mitral gradient calculations.

Second, the shape of the waveform adjacent to the valve and that of a more distal waveform may affect the apparent transvalvular gradient. This is most evident in comparison of central aortic and peripheral arterial (e.g., femoral artery) pressures. Because of summation of the transmitted and reflected pressure waveforms, the femoral artery pressure curve is narrower with a higher peak than the central aortic pressure curve, a phenomenon known as "peripheral amplification." Simultaneously measured central aortic and LV pressures are used whenever possible for calculation of transaortic pressure gradients, but if only a femoral pressure is available, realignment of timing and correction of the peripheral amplification are needed.

The third physiologic issue that may affect the measured transvalvular gradient is the phenomenon of pressure recovery that occurs distal to a site of stenosis. Pressure recovery is especially important with AS.[38-40] As the high-velocity jet flows through the stenotic orifice, it decelerates and expands distal to the valve. The associated turbulence results in an increase in aortic pressure ("pressure recovery") such that the pressure difference between the left ventricle and the distal ascending aorta is less than the pressure difference between the left ventricle and the stenotic orifice itself. Although pressure recovery may account for some of the observed discrepancies between Doppler and catheter-based data and conceivably could lead to underestimation of stenosis severity, the magnitude of this effect in the clinical setting appears to be small (approximately 5-10 mm Hg) and is unlikely to affect clinical decision making. Pressure recovery is greatest when stenosis severity is mild and aortic root dimension is small, and is least with severe stenosis and poststenotic dilation. Potential underestimation of stenosis severity due to pressure recovery can be avoided by recording pressures immediately adjacent to the valve on the downstream side of the stenosis.

Several other factors may also affect recorded pressure gradients. Transaortic pressure gradient may be affected by the presence of the catheter itself in the stenotic orifice. The catheter may increase the transvalvular pressure gradient either by further decreasing the cross-sectional flow area or by inducing aortic regurgitation.[41] Other physiologic variables that may affect the pressure gradient are the effect of atrial contraction, cardiac arrhythmias, and the compliance of the receiving chamber when regurgitation is present. Irregular heart rhythms affect measured pressure gradients in valvular stenosis because of the varying volume flow rates across the valve, necessitating averaging of several beats for clinical interpretation.

Aortic Valve

The most commonly encountered valvular heart disease condition in the cardiac catheterization laboratory in recent years is AS. With the widespread use of echocardiography, the diagnosis and severity of AS are frequently known prior to referral of the patient to the cardiac catheterization laboratory. With more elderly patients being offered treatment for AS with minimally invasive options (e.g., transcatheter aortic valve implantation), the number of patients with AS referred for invasive hemodynamics will continue to rise. The cardiac catheterization procedure therefore usually involves confirming the findings of echocardiography. Occasionally, however, the diagnosis and/or severity of stenosis remains in question, and cardiac catheterization is requested to further clarify the situation. In this setting, it is essential to obtain complete, accurate, and reliable data during the procedure. Patients with low-output and/or low-gradient AS represent a unique and challenging subset and are discussed separately.

PRESSURE GRADIENTS

All pressures should be measured prior to contrast ventriculography and angiography. A variety of catheters and techniques can be used to the cross the aortic valve in a retrograde manner to measure the pressure gradient. A 0.038-inch standard straight wire in combination with a pigtail catheter, Judkins right, or Amplatz left coronary catheter is commonly used.[42] Occasionally, a catheter specifically designed to cross the aortic valve, called a Feldman catheter, may be required.[43] When the straight wire cannot be passed across the valve, supravalvular angiography may be useful to localize the position and orientation of the valve orifice. The position and movement of calcium within the valve leaflets may also suggest the location of the valve orifice. Although hydrophilic straight wires can also be used to cross the aortic valve, the hydrophilic wire coating may increase the risk for valve leaflet perforation. Probing the aortic valve orifice with the wire should be done in less than 2-minute increments, with the wire removed and the catheter carefully flushed prior to reinsertion and another attempt to cross the valve. Although the risk of retrograde passage of a catheter across a narrowed and diseased aortic valve is small, one study has found that 3% of patients undergoing cardiac catheterization experienced a clinically significant neurologic event and 22% had magnetic resonance imaging evidence of an acute cerebral embolic event.[44] In the setting of severe aortic valve calcification or critical AS, or when coexisting mitral stenosis is present, transseptal puncture should be considered.

The pressure gradient between the left ventricle and the aorta can be described by three invasive measurements: (1) the mean gradient, (2) the peak-to-peak gradient, and (3) the maximum gradient (Figure 7-1). The mean gradient represents the area under the LV-aortic pressure curve and corresponds to the mean gradient measured by echocardiography. The peak-to-peak gradient has no true physiologic meaning and represents the difference between maximum aortic and the maximum LV pressures. Note that these maximum pressures do not occur at the same time and that the peak-to-peak gradient is not the same as the maximum gradient. Although the peak-to-peak gradient is easily measured with computer-assisted software, it is not useful in classifying the severity of AS. The maximum gradient represents the maximum difference that can be measured between the left ventricle and aorta during systole and corresponds to the maximum instantaneous gradient measured by echocardiography. The

maximum gradient occurs early during ventricular ejection, before the peak LV pressure.

In the absence of AS, there occasionally may be a small, early gradient between the left ventricle and aorta that is referred to as an "impulse" gradient (Figure 7-2).[45] This gradient can be detected only with high-fidelity micromanometer-tipped catheters and may be present during high-flow states such as exercise.[46]

Five invasive methods can be used to measure pressure gradients between the left ventricle and the aorta. The single-catheter "pullback technique" is not recommended because spontaneous changes in cardiac cycle length, especially in the setting of atrial and/or ventricular arrhythmias, result in significant variations in the measured gradient.[47] Simultaneous measurement of the proximal aortic and the LV pressures using two transducers yields the most accurate data. The first method is the most commonly used and involves a single arterial puncture with placement of a 6 French sheath within the femoral artery and advancement of a 6 French double-lumen catheter (Langston dual-lumen catheter, Vascular Solutions, Minneapolis, MN) into the left ventricle. This catheter provides simultaneous measurement of the aortic and LV pressures through ports within these locations.[48] Following measurement of the gradient, contrast agent can be injected through the LV port of the catheter to perform a left ventriculogram.

The second method requires two arterial punctures with one catheter positioned within the left ventricle and a second catheter (from the second arterial puncture site) located within the ascending aorta. The third method uses femoral venous access to allow transseptal puncture with subsequent positioning of a catheter that is advanced from the left atrium into the left ventricle and a second catheter (from an arterial puncture) positioned into the ascending aorta. The fourth method uses a single arterial puncture with placement of a standard, short 6 French sheath within the femoral artery and advancement of a 4 or 5 French pigtail catheter (through the 6 French sheath) into the left ventricle. The femoral artery pressure is measured via the side-arm of the sheath and is used as a surrogate to the central aortic pressure. By nature of its peripheral location, the femoral artery pressure is delayed and higher than the central aortic pressure. When this delay is accounted for by realignment of the pressures, the mean LV-to-aortic gradient is underestimated by approximately 10 mm Hg. Without realignment, the mean gradient is overestimated by approximately 9 mm Hg (Figures 7-3 and 7-4).[49] Therefore, to obtain accurate data, the central aortic pressure should

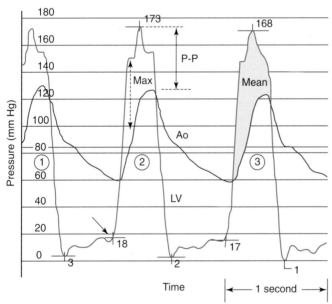

FIGURE 7-1 Transaortic pressure gradient. The gradient between the left ventricle (LV) and the aorta (Ao) in aortic stenosis can be described by three invasive measures. The mean gradient (beat #3) represents the area under the left ventricular–aortic pressure curve. The peak-to-peak (P-P) gradient (beat #2) is the difference between the maximum aortic pressure and the maximum left ventricular systolic pressure. The maximum (Max) gradient (beat #2) is the maximum difference that can be measured between the left ventricle and aorta during systole.

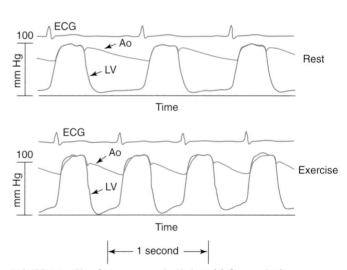

FIGURE 7-2 Simultaneous aortic (Ao) and left ventricular pressure (LV) measured at rest (top) and at exercise (bottom). A small early systolic gradient between the left ventricle and aorta is present during exercise; it is referred to as an impulse gradient. *(From Pasipoularides A. Clinical assessment of ventricular ejection dynamics with and without outflow obstruction. J Am Coll Cardiol 1990;15:859–82.)*

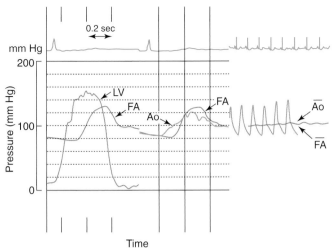

FIGURE 7-3 Comparison of central aortic and femoral artery pressure waveforms in aortic stenosis. Sequential recording of the left ventricular (LV) pressure and simultaneous ascending aortic (Ao) (*left panel*) and femoral artery (FA) pressures (*middle panel*). The femoral artery pressure is delayed and higher than the aortic pressure (*middle panel*). The mean aortic and mean femoral artery pressures are similar (*right panel*). (*From Folland ED, Parisi AF, Carbone C. Is peripheral arterial pressure a satisfactory substitute for ascending aortic pressure when measuring aortic valve gradients? J Am Coll Cardiol 1984;4:1207–12.*)

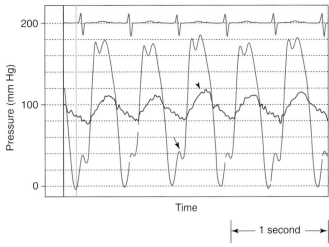

FIGURE 7-5 Hemodynamics in critical aortic stenosis. Simultaneous left ventricular (*blue*) and aortic (*red*) pressures measured with two catheters in a patient with critical aortic stenosis. The mean and maximum gradients are 68 and 90 mm Hg, respectively. The aortic valve area is 0.48 cm². The aortic upstroke (*arrowhead*) is delayed. The left ventricular end-diastolic pressure (*arrow*) is elevated at 38 mm Hg.

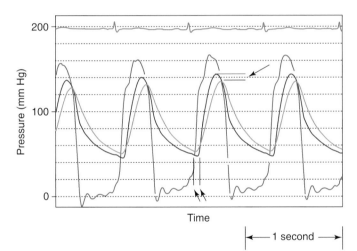

FIGURE 7-4 Left ventricular, aortic, and femoral pressures. Simultaneous measurement of the left ventricular (*blue*), aortic (*yellow*) and femoral artery (*red*) pressures in a patients with moderate aortic stenosis. Measurements were made with three transducers and catheters placed within the left ventricle (*yellow*) and aorta (*red*). The femoral arterial pressure was measured using the side arm of a the arterial sheath. The femoral arterial pressure (*red*) is higher (*single arrow*) than the aortic pressure (*yellow*) and is delayed in comparison with the aortic pressure (*double arrows*).

be measured, and the use of the femoral artery pressure as a "surrogate" to the central aortic pressure should be avoided. The fifth method uses a single arterial puncture with placement of a long (55 or 90 cm) 6 French sheath into the ascending aorta with a smaller 4 or 5 French sheath advanced through the long sheath into the left ventricle.[50] The side-arm of the long sheath is used to measure the central aortic pressure.

An additional, novel method has been introduced to simultaneously measure both aortic and LV pressures. Bertog et al[51] described performing a single arterial puncture with placement of a 4 French catheter into the ascending aorta. LV pressure is measured using a 0.014-inch pressure wire (placed through the 4

French catheter), which is the same wire used to measure fractional flow reserve. In this small series of 4 patients, correlation with traditional methods to measure the aortic valve gradient was excellent. Using this method in a larger series of 18 patients with AS, Bae et al[52] also found high correlation with traditional methods to measure the aortic valve gradient with an average procedure time of 36 minutes.

In the setting of critical AS, the presence of a catheter positioned across the aortic valve can influence the pressure gradient, as initially described by Carabello[53] in 1987. In the setting of an aortic valve area less than 0.6 cm², Carabello observed an increase of 10 mm Hg in the peripheral arterial pressure when the catheter was withdrawn from the left ventricle across the aortic valve. This rise was believed to be related to the catheter's further narrowing the orifice of the severely narrowed valve.

ANALYSIS OF PRESSURE WAVEFORMS

In the absence of AS, the slope and magnitude of the aortic and LV systolic pressures are similar and rise together to a midsystolic peak. With AS, the pressure in the aorta rises slowly and achieves a late systolic peak (Figure 7-5). In an attempt to reduce wall stress, the left ventricle responds to the pressure overload of AS by developing hypertrophy. LV hypertrophy limits the ability of the left ventricle to fill at a normal pressure, resulting in a higher end-diastolic pressure.

VALVE AREA

GENERAL CONCEPTS. In their classic 1951 article, Gorlin and Gorlin[54] described data derived from hydraulic systems that were used to determine the orifice of various cardiac valves. The calculated valve area from the formula was validated by directly measuring the valve orifice from autopsy or surgical specimens in 11 patients. The formula states that the area of a valve (cm²) is equal to the flow across the valve (mL/sec) divided by the product of two constants and the square root of the pressure difference (mm Hg) across the valve. The first constant (C) is an empirical constant that accounts for energy loss and issues related to orifice contraction. For the aortic, pulmonic, and tricuspid valve, C is assumed to be 1.0. For the mitral valve, the researchers initially assumed C to be 0.7; this value was revised in 1972 to 0.85.[55] The second constant is equal to the square root of twice the gravity

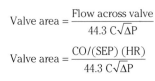

acceleration factor (980 cm/sec^{-1}) and is 44.3. The formula is as follows:

$$\text{Valve area} = \frac{\text{Flow across valve}}{44.3\ C\sqrt{\Delta P}}$$

$$\text{Valve area} = \frac{\text{CO/(SEP) (HR)}}{44.3\ C\sqrt{\Delta P}}$$

where ΔP is the mean pressure gradient, *CO* is cardiac output, *SEP* is the systolic ejection period, and *HR* is heart rate.

A simplified formula for calculating valve areas was proposed in 1981 by Hakki et al.[56] The Hakki equation for valve area uses cardiac output (liters/min) divided by the square root of the pressure difference across the valve, as follows:

$$\text{Valve area} = \frac{\text{CO}}{\sqrt{\Delta P_{mean}}}$$

For the aortic valve, either the mean or the peak-to-peak pressure gradient can be used; for the mitral valve, the mean pressure gradient should be used. In a series of 100 patients with mitral stenosis or AS, the correlation coefficient for the simplified Hakki equation in comparison with the Gorlin formula was 0.94 or 0.96, respectively.[56]

MEASUREMENT OF AORTIC VALVE AREA. Worksheets can be useful to organize the measured and derived data when one is determining the aortic valve area (Table 7-4). Simultaneous aortic and LV pressures are measured using one of the techniques already discussed. Traditionally, gradients were measured from the printout using handheld planimeter devices. Currently, however, computer-based monitoring systems can accurately determine the mean, maximum, and peak-to-peak gradients. Manual confirmation of the computer-measured gradients can be performed with a grid-based system (Figure 7-6). If sinus rhythm is present, 5 cardiac beats should be used to determine the gradients. If atrial fibrillation or other arrhythmias are present, 10 cardiac beats should be used for accurate results. The cardiac output is measured by both thermodilution and Fick methods. The systolic ejection period (SEP) is measured from the opening of the aortic valve (LV pressure exceeds aortic pressure) to the closing of the aortic valve (LV pressures falls below aortic pressure) in units of seconds per beat. The SEP should also be measured for 5 beats, and an average taken. Aortic valve area is reported using the cardiac output as measured by both the Fick and thermodilution methods. The aortic valve area index is calculated as the aortic valve area divided by the body surface area. Both the aortic valve area and the aortic valve index should be used as indicators of AS severity (see Chapter 11).

LIMITATIONS. There are often discrepancies among the aortic valve area, aortic valve index, and transvalvular gradients measured by cardiac catheterization and Doppler-echocardiography. When these discrepancies are systematically evaluated, the aortic valve area tends to be higher when measured with cardiac catheterization than with Doppler-echocardiography.[57-59] These discrepancies are due to the

pressure recovery phenomenon,[60,61] changes in hemodynamics (transaortic flow rate and heart rate) between the time of the studies,[62] and suboptimal echocardiographic recording of the aortic jet velocity. In the setting of coexisting aortic regurgitation, the valve area calculated by the Gorlin equation can provide only a minimum value for the aortic valve area.

LOW-GRADIENT AORTIC STENOSIS

Up to 30% of patients with a calculated aortic valve area in the severe range have low-gradient AS.[63] These patients can be further characterized as having: (1) normal-flow, low-gradient AS or (2) low-flow, low-gradient AS (Figure 7-7). Although the majority of patients with low-flow, low-gradient AS have decreased systolic function, as many as 35% have an ejection fraction higher than 50%.[64] The reasons for a low stroke volume in the setting of normal LV function include high aortic impedance and a small LV cavity; low stroke volume itself may be an early marker for intrinsic myocardial dysfunction.[65]

The Gorlin equation is flow dependent, particularly when the cardiac output is less than 4 liters/min. Differentiating true, severe AS from mild AS with a coexisting cardiomyopathy (so-called

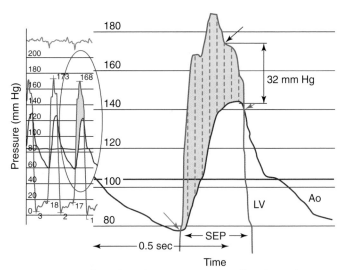

FIGURE 7-6 **Confirmation of mean pressure gradient in aortic stenosis.** Simultaneous left ventricular (LV; *blue*) and aortic (Ao; *red*) pressure tracings in a patient with severe aortic stenosis. The systolic ejection period (SEP) begins with the opening of the aortic valve (*orange arrow*) and ends with closure of the aortic valve (*orange arrowhead*). The *shaded area* represents the mean gradient throughout systole. To confirm the computer-measured pressure gradients, a grid-based system can be used. Eight vertical lines are drawn at equal spaces throughout systole. Each line is measured to determine the gradient at that time period. For example, the sixth line from the left (*black arrow*) shows a gradient of 32 mm Hg. Summing all of the values together and dividing by 8 (8 lines were drawn) yields manual confirmation of the mean gradient.

TABLE 7-4	Valve Area Calculation Worksheet for Aortic and Mitral Valves
Aortic valve area (valve constant = 1)	1. Determine the average gradient for 5 cardiac beats if in sinus rhythm and 10 cardiac beats if in atrial fibrillation 2. Determine the mean systolic ejection period (SEP) for 5 cardiac beats 3. Heart rate = beats/min 4. Cardiac output = mL/min 5. Valve area $= \dfrac{\text{cardiac output (heart rate} \times \text{systolic ejection period)}}{44.3 \times \sqrt{\text{mean gradient}}}$
Mitral valve area (valve constant = 37.7)	1. Determine the average gradient for 5 cardiac beats if in sinus rhythm and 10 cardiac beats if in atrial fibrillation 2. Determine the mean diastolic filling period (DFP) for 5 cardiac beats 3. Heart rate = beats/min 4. Cardiac output = mL/min 5. Valve area $= \dfrac{\text{cardiac output (heart rate} \times \text{diastolic filling period)}}{37.7\sqrt{\text{mean gradient}}}$

pseudo–aortic stenosis) is clinically important because the former group of patients derive benefit from aortic valve replacement.[66]

The widely accepted definition of low-gradient AS is a mean aortic valve gradient lower than 40 mm Hg in the setting of an ejection fraction less than 40%.[67] For patients with pseudo–aortic stenosis, medications that increase cardiac output usually increase the calculated aortic valve area. In contrast, for patients with true, severe AS, an increase in cardiac output does not result in a significant increase in the calculated aortic valve area. Intravenous dobutamine can be used in the cardiac catheterization laboratory to differentiate true AS from pseudo–aortic stenosis. A standard protocol involves obtaining baseline measurements of cardiac output, heart rate, and simultaneous LV and aortic pressures and initiating dobutamine by continuous infusion at 5 µg/kg/min.[68] The dose is then increased by 3 to 10 µg/kg/min every 5 minutes until a maximum dose of 40 µg/kg/min is achieved, the mean gradient increases to more than 40 mm Hg, cardiac output increases by 50%, heart rate increases to more than 140 beats per minute (bpm), or intolerable symptoms or side effects (arrhythmias) occur. Patients with true, severe AS can be identified

following dobutamine infusion as those with: (1) mean aortic valve gradient greater than 30 mm Hg and (2) an aortic valve area that remains 1.0 cm² or less (Figure 7-8).[69] In patients with pseudo–aortic stenosis (1) cardiac output increases and (2) mean aortic valve gradient remains less than 30 mm Hg; these findings indicate a component of a primary cardiomyopathy and mild to moderate AS. Occasionally, dobutamine does not increase the stroke volume or cardiac output, signifying poor contractile reserve.

AORTIC VALVE RESISTANCE

Aortic valve resistance has been proposed as another measure to assess the severity of AS.[70,71] Aortic valve resistance is calculated as the mean pressure gradient divided by the flow rate ratio and is expressed in units of dyne-seconds-cm⁻⁵, as follows:

$$\text{Aortic valve resistance} = \frac{1.33\sqrt{\Delta P_{mean}}}{(CO/HR) \times SEP}$$

A cutoff value of 300 dyne-seconds-cm⁻⁵ is commonly used to identify patients with severe AS.[72] It was previously believed that calculated aortic valve resistance was less flow dependent than the Gorlin formula-derived aortic valve area. However, in vitro and clinical studies now suggest that aortic valve resistance is flow dependent and is not superior to aortic valve area for the assessment of AS.[73,74]

ANGIOCARDIOGRAPHY

Left ventriculography should be routinely performed in patients with AS because it provides assessment of LV systolic function, the anatomy of the aortic valve, and coexisting mitral regurgitation. The aortic valve should be assessed for calcification, leaflet morphology (bicuspid), and leaflet mobility. A bicuspid aortic valve may show systolic doming of the leaflets.

Pulmonic Valve

Most cases of valvular pulmonic stenosis are congenital in origin. Adults commonly present with dyspnea and exertional fatigue secondary to the inability to increase cardiac output sufficiently

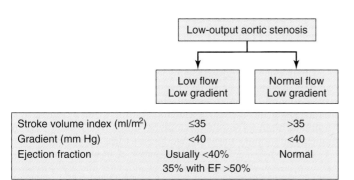

FIGURE 7-7 Classification of low-output aortic stenosis. Low-output aortic stenosis can be further classified as either (1) normal flow, low gradient or (2) low flow, low gradient. The stroke volume index is ≤35 mL/m² in patients with low-flow, low-gradient aortic stenosis. The ejection fraction is normal in those with normal-flow, low-gradient aortic stenosis. In those with low-flow, low-gradient aortic stenosis, the ejection fraction is usually <40%, but it can be >50% in up to 35% of patients.

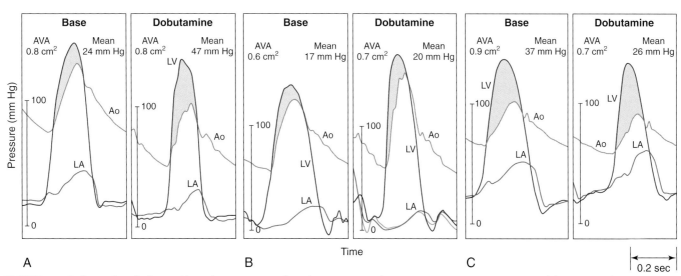

FIGURE 7-8 Dobutamine challenge. Hemodynamic tracings from three patients with aortic stenosis receiving intravenous dobutamine: with measurement of left ventricular (LV), aortic (Ao) and left atrial (LA) pressures, showing changes in the systolic transaortic gradient (*blue shaded area*). **A,** Cardiac output and aortic valve gradient increased in response to dobutamine, and the aortic valve area (AVA) remained 0.8 cm². This patient was found at the time of valve surgery to have severe aortic stenosis. **B,** Dobutamine infusion resulted in increases in cardiac output and aortic valve gradient. Final aortic valve area was 0.7 cm². The patient was found at the time of valve surgery to only have mild aortic stenosis. **C,** Dobutamine infusion did not change cardiac output, and the mean aortic valve gradient decreased from 37 to 26 mm Hg. Dobutamine was stopped because of hypotension. This patient was found at the time of valve surgery to have severe aortic stenosis. *(From Nishimura RA, Grantham JA, Connolly HM, et al. Low-output, low-gradient aortic stenosis in patients with depressed left ventricular systolic function: the clinical utility of the dobutamine challenge in the catheterization laboratory. Circulation 2002;106:809–13.)*

during exercise. Patients are frequently diagnosed by Doppler ultrasound and echocardiography, and cardiac catheterization is usually performed only prior to balloon valvotomy.

PRESSURE GRADIENT

The severity of valvular pulmonic stenosis is evaluated on the basis of the peak-to-peak gradient between the right ventricle and pulmonary artery. A peak-to-peak gradient larger than 30 mm Hg is considered hemodynamically significant and warrants consideration for balloon valvotomy. Unlike in the assessment of AS, the gradient between the right ventricle and pulmonary artery can be measured by pullback technique using an end-hole catheter. Using the peak-to-peak gradient, the severity of pulmonic stenosis is classified as mild (25-49 mm Hg), moderate (50-79 mm Hg), or severe (≥80 mm Hg).[75]

PRESSURE WAVEFORM ANALYSIS

Pressure waveform analysis in valvular pulmonic stenosis is notable for showing an elevated right ventricular (RV) systolic pressure, the gradient across the pulmonic valve, and a pulmonary artery pressure that rises slowly to achieve a late systolic peak (Figure 7-9).

VALVE AREA

The normal pulmonary valve orifice is greater than 2.0 cm²/m², and in the absence of disease, there is no gradient across the valve.[76] However, the concept of valve area is not used in the evaluation of pulmonic stenosis, and decisions regarding therapy are based on the peak-to-peak gradient.

ANGIOCARDIOGRAPHY

Right ventriculography in a left lateral projection displays the pulmonic valve, the right ventricle, and the proximal portion of the main pulmonary artery in a relatively straight line. With valvular pulmonic stenosis, the valve appears thickened and "domes" during systole. RV function and the presence and severity of tricuspid regurgitation should also be assessed. A right anterior oblique projection with 25 to 30 degrees of cranial angulation allows visualization of the right ventricle and also profiles the pulmonic valve.

Mitral Valve

Patients with mitral stenosis are usually referred to the cardiac catheterization laboratory for evaluation of disease severity prior to percutaneous mitral balloon valvotomy or mitral valve replacement. Complete assessment consists of right and left heart catheterization, simultaneous measurement of LA (or pulmonary capillary wedge) and LV pressures, and measurement of cardiac output.

PRESSURE GRADIENT

Transseptal puncture is required for accurate assessment of LA pressure. A transseptal sheath is placed into the left atrium, and simultaneous measurements of LA and LV pressure are performed. This can be done using the side-arm of the transseptal sheath to measure LA pressure; LV pressure can be measured by insertion of an undersized pigtail catheter through the transseptal sheath into the left ventricle. The mean and maximum pressure gradients should be recorded at various paper speeds and scales. The optimal paper speed and pressure scale are usually 100 mm/s and 0-40 mm Hg, respectively. Mean gradients are measured by averaging the instantaneous gradients over the flow period using carefully recorded and correctly aligned tracings of the LA and LV pressure curves.

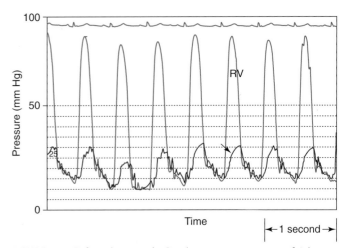

FIGURE 7-9 Pulmonic stenosis. Simultaneous measurement of right ventricular (RV; *blue*) and pulmonary artery (PA; *red*) pressures in a patient with severe pulmonic stenosis. The upstroke of the pulmonary artery tracing is delayed (*arrow*), consistent with severe pulmonic stenosis. The maximum gradient is 65 mm Hg.

In clinical practice, the pulmonary capillary wedge pressure is often used as a surrogate of the LA pressure to assess the severity of mitral stenosis (Figure 7-10). If an accurate pulmonary capillary wedge pressure has been obtained, the mean pulmonary capillary wedge pressure should be less than the mean pulmonary artery pressure and the saturation of blood should be greater than 95%. After systematic study, Lange et al[77] found that the pulmonary capillary wedge pressure overestimates the LA pressure by 1.7 ± 0.6 mm Hg. Conditions in which the pulmonary capillary wedge pressure overestimates the LA pressure include acute respiratory failure, chronic obstructive pulmonary disease, pulmonary hypertension, pulmonary venoocclusive disease, and impaired LA compliance (prior mitral valve replacement).[78]

PRESSURE WAVEFORM ANALYSIS

Atrial fibrillation may be present in patients with long-standing mitral stenosis and results in loss of the a wave in the LA (and pulmonary capillary wedge) pressure tracing. Left atrial v waves, which are frequently prominent, are thought to be the result of reduced compliance of the LA (Figure 7-11). The presence of v waves may also indicate coexisting mitral regurgitation.

VALVE AREA

The normal mitral valve area is more than 4.0 to 6.0 cm². When the mitral valve area is reduced to 1.0 cm², a significant diastolic gradient at rest is present. At this severity of mitral stenosis, increases in cardiac output result in a significant elevation in LA pressure and pulmonary edema. Increases in heart rate preferentially shorten diastole more than systole and therefore limit the time available for flow across the mitral valve.

The Gorlin equation for the mitral valve is as follows:

$$\text{Valve area} = \frac{\text{CO}/(\text{DFP})\,(\text{HR})}{44.3\,\text{C}\sqrt{\Delta P_{mean}}}$$

where ΔP_{mean} is the mean pressure gradient, *DFP* is the diastolic filling period, and *C* is an empirical constant that is 0.85.

A worksheet to determine the mitral valve area is shown in Table 7-4. LA (or pulmonary capillary wedge) and LV pressures are measured simultaneously. Manual confirmation of the computer-measured gradients can be performed using the grid-based system as discussed in the assessment of AS. If sinus rhythm is present, 5 cardiac beats should be used to determine the mean gradient. If atrial fibrillation is present, 10 cardiac beats

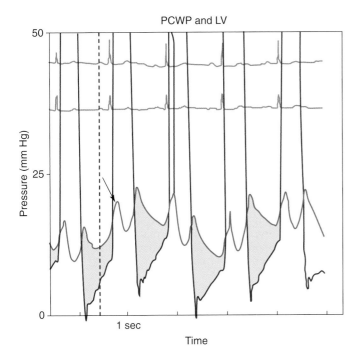

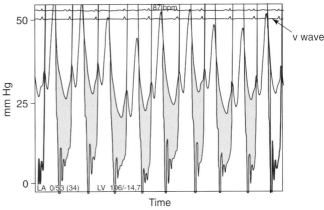

FIGURE 7-11 Left atrial pressure in mitral stenosis. Simultaneous left atrial (LA, obtained from transeptal puncture) and left ventricular (LV) pressures in a patient with critical mitral stenosis. The mean and maximum gradients are 23 and 54 mm Hg, respectively. The v waves (*arrow*) are prominent and approach 52 mm Hg.

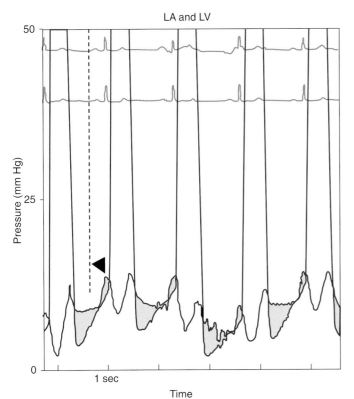

FIGURE 7-10 Severe mitral stenosis. Example of a good-quality pulmonary capillary wedge pressure tracing that mirrors the left atrial pressure tracing in a patient with severe mitral stenosis. *Upper panel,* Simultaneous pulmonary capillary wedge pressure (*blue*) and left ventricular pressure (*purple*) tracings. The *vertical dotted line* marks the beginning of the P wave in the electrocardiogram. The a wave in the pulmonary capillary wedge pressure tracing (*arrow*) occurs approximately 120 msec after the P wave. *Lower panel,* Simultaneous left atrial (*blue*) and left ventricular pressure (*purple*) tracings in the same patient with severe mitral stenosis. Note that the gradient (*blue shaded area*) is higher when the pulmonary capillary wedge pressure tracing is used instead of the left atrial pressure. The a wave in the left atrial pressure tracing occurs 80 msec after the P wave.

is required for accurate results. The cardiac output is measured by both the thermodilution and Fick methods. The diastolic filling period (DFP) is measured from the opening of the mitral valve (LA pressure exceeds LV pressure) to the closing of the mitral valve (LA pressure falls below LV pressure) in units of seconds per beat. The DFP should also be measured for 5 beats, and an average taken. Mitral valve area using cardiac output as measured by both the Fick and thermodilution methods is reported.

Tricuspid Valve

Prior to technologic advances in echocardiography, cardiac catheterization was used to confirm the presence and severity of tricuspid stenosis. Simultaneous recordings of the RA and RV diastolic pressures were needed for accurate assessment because the pressure gradients are small and there is considerable respiratory variation in the pressure waveforms.

PRESSURE GRADIENT

The gradient between the right atrium and right ventricle should be measured simultaneously with two catheters. This can be accomplished with a long 6 French sheath advanced into the right atrium and an end-hole (multipurpose) catheter placed through the sheath and into the right ventricle. Alternatively, a double-lumen catheter (Langston dual-lumen catheter) can also be used. A mean gradient of 2 mm Hg or greater throughout diastole indicates tricuspid stenosis.[79]

PRESSURE WAVEFORM ANALYSIS

Characteristic findings in tricuspid stenosis include a prominent a wave and blunting or or absence of the y descent in the RA pressure waveform.

VALVE AREA

The Gorlin formula can be employed to determine the tricuspid valve area using a constant of 1.0. Significant tricuspid stenosis is present when the valve area is less than 1.3 cm[2].

ANGIOCARDIOGRAPHY

Right ventriculography performed in a right anterior oblique projection may be useful in the evaluation of tricuspid stenosis. The tricuspid valve may be calcified with decreased mobility, and associated tricuspid regurgitation is frequently present.[80]

Evaluation of Valvular Regurgitation

Valvular regurgitation is evaluated by cardiac catheterization with direct measurement of intracardiac pressures and analyais of pressure waveforms, semiquantitative evaluation of regurgitant severity by angiocardiography, and calculation of regurgitant fraction. Inspection of the pressure waveforms on both sides of the regurgitant valve allows determination of the severity and chronicity of the regurgitant lesion. Angiographic evaluation of regurgitant severity is based on injection of contrast agent into the chamber downstream of the affected valve with imaging of contrast reflux into the chamber receiving the regurgitant volume. The regurgitant fraction is calculated as the difference between the angiographic (total) and forward (Fick or thermodilution method) stroke volume.

Aortic Regurgitation

PRESSURE WAVEFORM ANALYSIS

Aortic regurgitation results in a systolic pressure gradient across the aortic valve (even in the absence of coexisting stenosis) because of the high volume flow rate. This pressure gradient occurs predominantly in early systole. Although the magnitude of the systolic pressure gradient is related to volume flow rate, pressure gradients in isolated severe aortic regurgitation are usually small, with mean gradients ranging from 5 to 20 mm Hg. Higher pressure gradients indicate associated AS or another cause of LV outflow obstruction.

In diastole, central aortic pressure falls more rapidly than normal, owing to the diastolic runoff into the left ventricle, so that aortic end-diastolic pressure is lower than normal (Figure 7-12). Conversely, LV diastolic pressure rises more rapidly than normal because of rapid ventricular filling retrograde across the incompetent aortic valve as well as antegrade across the mitral valve. With acute severe aortic regurgitation, the fall in aortic and rise in ventricular diastolic pressures result in equalization of aortic

and ventricular pressures at end-diastole. Thus, the rate of equalization of aortic and LV diastolic pressures relates to regurgitant severity. This concept serves as the basis for using the diastolic slope of the Doppler velocity curve as a measure of regurgitant severity (see Chapter 6). This approach is limited because chronic aortic regurgitation results in compensatory changes in LV diastolic compliance such that the LV end-diastolic pressure may remain low even with severe regurgitation. Thus, interpretation of the pressure waveforms must take disease chronicity, as well as severity, into account.

This combination of systolic and diastolic pressure abnormalities leads to the most characteristic hemodynamic feature of chronic aortic regurgitation, that is, an increased pulse pressure. Because systolic pressure is increased and end-diastolic pressure is decreased, the pulse pressure is increased. However, the magnitude of the increase in pulse pressure only modestly correlates with regurgitation severity.[81] Even so, this simple measure of regurgitant severity should be integrated with other imaging and hemodynamic data in patient evaluation.

ANGIOCARDIOGRAPHY

For angiocrdiographic evaluation of aortic regurgitation, a contrast agent is injected into the aortic root and regurgitation is graded on a semiquantitative 1+ to 4+ scale as shown in Table 7-5.[82,83] Angiographic grading of regurgitation severity has several limitations.[84] First, interobserver variability in grading of regurgitant severity can be considerable unless there is strict adherence to the definitions outlined in Table 7-5. Although mild regurgitation is distinct from severe regurgitation, intermediate grades are often difficult to estimate and differentiate. Second, technical factors may lead to an erroneous interpretation. The volume and rate of contrast injection must provide complete opacification of the upstream chamber. The catheter should be positioned close to the valve but should not interfere with valve closing. The angiocardiogram should be recorded from an angle and with an image size that include both the upstream and downstream chambers without overlapping the structures. For aortic regurgitation, a 45-degree left anterior oblique view with 10% to 15% cranial angulation results in an image perpendicular to the valve plane and allows accurate assessment of the degree of reflux from the aortic root into the left ventricle. Third, physiologic factors, including heart rate, cardiac rhythm, preload, and afterload, affect the severity of regurgitation so that images recorded under conditions

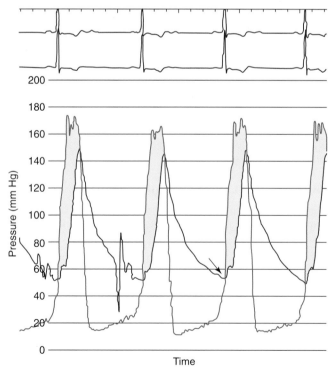

FIGURE 7-12 Hemodynamics in severe aortic regurgitation. Simultaneous aortic and left ventricular pressures in a patient with mild aortic stenosis and severe aortic regurgitation. Note that the pulse pressure is wide (approximately 100 mm Hg) and the aortic diastolic pressure (*arrow*) is low.

TABLE 7-5	Angiographic Grading of Regurgitation Severity	
AORTIC REGURGITATION		**MITRAL REGURGITATION**
1+	Contrast refluxes from the aorta into the left ventricle (LV) but clears on each beat	Contrast refluxes into the left atrium but clears on each beat
2+	Contrast refluxes into the LV with a gradually increasing density of contrast in the LV that never equals contrast intensity in the aorta	Left atrial contrast density gradually increases but never equals LV density
3+	Contrast refluxes into the LV with a gradually increasing density such that LV and aortic densities are equal after several beats	The densities of contrast in the atrium and ventricle equalize after several beats
4+	Contrast fills the LV rapidly, resulting in equivalent radiographic densities in the LV and aorta on the first beat	The left atrium becomes as dense as the LV on the first beat, and contrast is seen refluxing into the pulmonary veins

Modified from Sellers RD, Levy MJ, Aplatz K, Lillehei CW. Left retrograde cardioangiography in acquired cardiac disease: technic, indications and interpretations in 700 cases. Am J Cardiol 1964;14:437–447.

disparate from the patient's baseline hemodynamic state may not accurately reflect disease severity.

REGURGITANT FRACTION

Regurgitant volume and fraction can be calculated at cardiac catheterization on the basis of measurement of the amount of blood ejected by the left ventricle (total stroke volume) and the amount of blood delivered to the body (forward stroke volume). Total SV is calculated from the left ventriculogram as the difference between the end-diastolic and end-systolic LV volumes. The forward SV is calculated by dividing the measured cardiac output (by either Fick or thermodilution method) by the heart rate. The regurgitant SV is calculated as follows:

Regurgitant SV = Total SV − Forward SV

The regurgitation fraction is the regurgitant SV divided by the total SV. A regurgitation fraction less than 20% indicates mild, of 20% to 40% moderate, of 40% to 60% moderately severe, and more than 60% severe regurgitation. Although this method has the potential to provide a quantitative measure of regurgitant severity, it is rarely used in clinical practice now that reliable noninvasive measures of regurgitation severity are available.

Regurgitation volume index is calculated by dividing the regurgitant volume by the body surface area and is another measure of regurgitation severity. A regurgitation volume index lower than 700 mL/min/m^2 indicates mild, of 700 to 1700 mL/min/m^2 moderate, of 1700 to 3000 mL/min/m^2 severe, and more than 3000 mL/min/m^2 very severe regurgitation.

Mitral Regurgitation

PRESSURE WAVEFORM ANALYSIS

Mitral regurgitation results in an increase in LA pressure, which peaks in late systole and is represented by the v wave. The height of the v wave relates to regurgitation severity, although other factors, such as LA size and compliance, also play a role. The LA pressure curve is variably transmitted to the pulmonary capillary wedge pressure tracing, again in relation to the modulating effects of the size and compliance of the pulmonary vascular bed. For example, a patient with a prosthetic mitral valve and mild mitral regurgitation may show a prominent v wave owing to a noncompliant pulmonary vascular bed. In contrast, a patient with chronic severe mitral regurgitation may have no v wave because of compensatory changes in the left atrium and pulmonary vasculature. Thus, although a v wave is often considered the hallmark of mitral regurgitation, its presence is not sensitive for the diagnosis, nor is the absolute value a reliable predictor of regurgitation severity.[85]

LA pressure is not routinely measured in patients with mitral regurgitation, and information from the pulmonary artery and pulmonary capillary wedge pressure tracings is therefore used. A large v wave may result in a bifid appearance to the pulmonary artery pressure tracing. A large v wave in the pulmonary capillary wedge pressure tracing may occasionally give the appearance of a pulmonary artery pressure tracing (Figure 7-13).[86]

The rate of rise of LV pressure during "isovolumic" contraction (dP/dt) provides a measure of LV systolic function in patients with mitral regurgitation. Normally dP/dt is higher than 1000 mm Hg/sec, and lower values reflect progressively more severe impairment of LV contractility. Peak LV systolic pressure is typically normal in patients with mitral regurgitation, although severe regurgitation associated with decreased forward cardiac output may lead to decreased LV systolic pressure and subsequent hypotension.

ANGIOCARDIOGRAPHY

A 30-degree right anterior oblique view separates the LV and the LA in a plane perpendicular to the mitral valve annulus. The

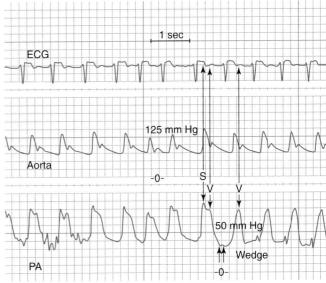

FIGURE 7-13 Acute severe mitral regurgitation. Electrocardiogram (ECG), aortic (Aorta), pulmonary artery (PA) pressure (*left*), and pulmonary capillary wedge (wedge) pressure (*right*) tracings in a patient with acute severe mitral regurgitation. A prominent v wave is present in both the pulmonary artery and wedge pressure tracings. The pulmonary artery pressure is bifid because of the presence of both the pulmonary artery systolic wave (S) and the v wave. The large v wave can cause the wedge tracing to be confused with a pulmonary artery tracing. *(From Sharkey SW. Beyond the wedge: clinical physiology and the Swan-Ganz catheter. Am J Med 1987;83:111–22.)*

descending aortic shadow is superimposed on the LA in this view, so contrast agent in the descending aorta may be mistaken for mitral regurgitation. A left ventriculogram should be performed with a sufficient amount of contrast agent to completely opacify the LV. Mitral regurgitation is graded on the same semiquantitative scale (1+ to 4+) as used for aortic regurgitation (see Table 7-5).

REGURGITANT FRACTION

Regurgitant fraction for mitral regurgitation is calculated in the same manner as for aortic regurgitation.

Tricuspid Regurgitation

PRESSURE WAVEFORM ANALYSIS

Severe tricuspid regurgitation results in elevation in the RA pressure, a prominent RA v wave (or *c*–v wave) and a prominent and sharp y descent (Figure 7-14). The prominent v or c-v wave causes "ventricularization" of the RA pressure waveform. The RV end-diastolic pressure is elevated. Kussmaul's sign, which is the lack of a decrease or even a small rise in mean RA pressure with inspiration, may be present.[87] Elevated pulmonary artery pressures (>60 mm Hg) suggest that the cause of tricuspid regurgitation is secondary (i.e., RV dilation resulting from pulmonary hypertension).

ANGIOCARDIOGRAPHY

As with mitral regurgitation, a 30-degree right anterior oblique view on angiocardiography separates the right ventricle and the right atrium in a plane perpendicular to the tricuspid valve annulus. The presence of a catheter across the tricuspid valve may cause a small amount (usually negligible) of tricuspid regurgitation. The presence of ventricular tachycardia during right ventriculography precludes assessment of tricuspid regurgitation. An angled pigtail catheter placed into the body of the right ventricle usually provides adequate imaging. Tricuspid regurgitation is

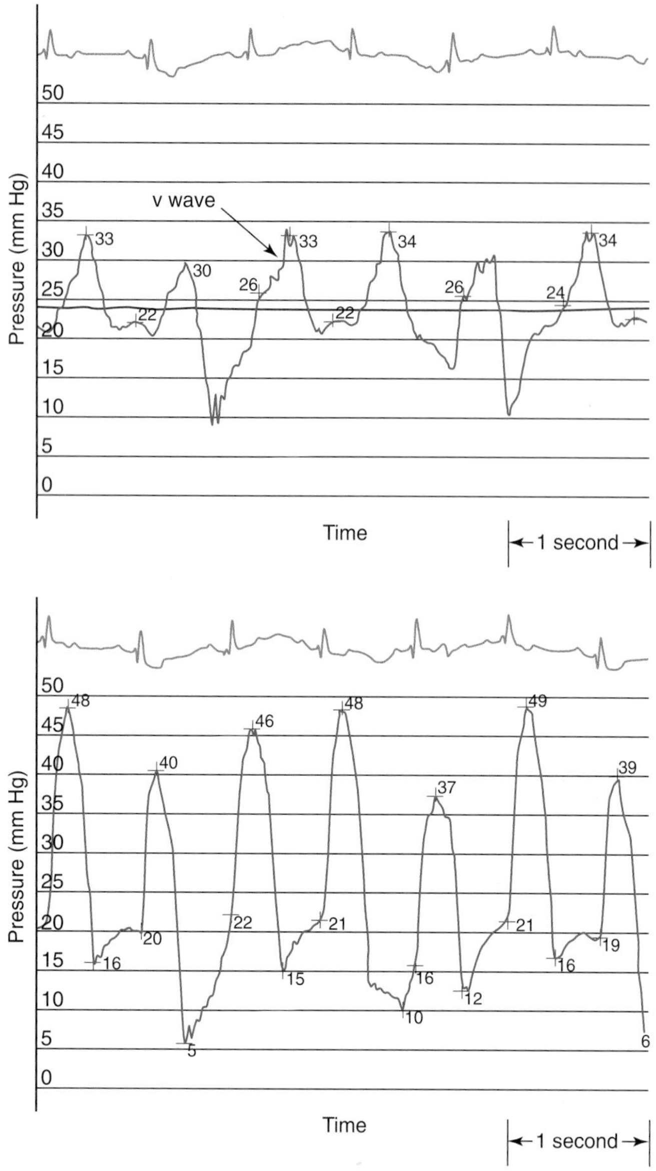

FIGURE 7-14 **Severe tricuspid regurgitation.** Right atrial (*top*) and right ventricular (*bottom*) pressure tracings in a patient with severe tricuspid regurgitation. The right atrial pressure is elevated, and there is a prominent v wave that reaches 34 mm Hg. The right ventricular end-diastolic pressure is also elevated, at 21 mm Hg.

graded on the same semiquantitative scale (1+ to 4+) as discussed previously (see Table 7-5).

REGURGITANT FRACTION

Calculation of the regurgitant fraction for right heart valves is problematic owing to the difficulties in calculating RV volumes from angiographic data.

Pulmonic Regurgitation

Pulmonic regurgitation is infrequently evaluated in the cardiac catheterization laboratory and is usually the result of repaired tetralogy of Fallot or severe pulmonary hypertension. Pulmonic regurgitation results in a diminished diastolic pulmonary artery pressure and an increased diastolic RV pressure, with the rate of pressure equalization related to the severity and chronicity of disease. Angiocardiography is rarely performed because the catheter used to perform it crosses the pulmonic valve and may cause artifactual regurgitation.

Other Catheterization Data

In addition to evaluation of valvular and ventricular function, cardiac catheterization provides data that allows calculation of pulmonary and systemic vascular resistance. Cardiac catheterization also allows direct measurement of LV end-diastolic pressure, which may be essential for management of the decompensated patient.

Pulmonary Artery Pressures and Resistance

Direct measurement of pulmonary artery pressures at catheterization is needed when noninvasive data are nondiagnostic or are discordant with other clinical data. In AS, pulmonary artery pressures should be measured before the catheter crosses the aortic valve because an average increase in mean pulmonary pressure of 4 mm Hg (range up to 19 mm Hg) has been reported when a catheter is lying across the valve.[88] There is a slight increase in normal pulmonary artery pressures with maximal exercise in young adults, from a resting pulmonary artery systolic pressure of 15 to 20 mm Hg to a maximum of 25 to 35 mm Hg.

Pulmonary artery pressure depends not only on the resistance to flow imposed by the pulmonary vascular bed but also on the volume flow rate and the pulmonary venous (or LA) pressure. The rise in pulmonary pressure that occurs "passively" secondary to an elevated LA pressure (e.g., in mitral stenosis) reverses when LA pressure is lowered. Similarly, high pulmonary pressures due to a high volume flow rate revert toward normal with a reduction in the flow rate. Thus, it is important to calculate pulmonary vascular resistance (PVR), which takes volume flow rate and the pressure drop across the circuit into account, as follows:

$$PVR = \frac{(PA_{mean} - LA_{mean})}{\text{pulmonary blood flow}}$$

where PA_{mean} is mean pressure in pulmonary artery and LA_{mean} is mean pressure in left atrium. When pressures are measured in mm Hg and blood flow in L/min, this equation results in Wood units of resistance, which can be converted to dynes-sec-cm^{-5} by multiplying by 80.

Although pulmonary vascular resistance describes the component of pulmonary hypertension that is due to the pulmonary vasculature, some of the increase in vascular resistance may be reversible after relief of the initiating cause and some may represent an irreversible increase. The degree of reversibility of an elevated pulmonary vascular resistance often is difficult to predict in patients with valvular heart disease.

Systemic Vascular Resistance

Systemic vascular resistance, in dyne-sec-cm^{-5}, can be calculated as follows:

Systemic vascular resistance $= [(Ao_{mean} - RA_{mean})/\text{cardiac output}] \times 80$

where Ao_{mean} is mean pressure in the aorta. In patients with valvular regurgitation, an elevated systemic vascular resistance may contribute to the total load imposed on the left ventricle and thus can lead to increased LV wall stress and clinical symptoms.

Left Ventricular Diastolic Function

The most widely used clinical measure of LV diastolic function is the LV end-diastolic pressure, which is measured directly at cardiac catheterization. In situations in which second measurements are needed, an indwelling pulmonary artery catheter is used, with the assumption that the pulmonary artery wedge pressure reflects the pressure in the left atrium, which in turn reflects LV end-diastolic pressure.

Although LV end-diastolic pressure is typically normal at rest in patients with chronic valvular disease, significant elevations can occur with acute regurgitation or in the decompensated patient with chronic regurgitation. For example, in the patient with acute aortic regurgitation, severe elevation in LV end-diastolic pressure is seen because of the acute volume overload imposed on the LV, which has not had time to dilate. Similarly, a superimposed systemic disease (e.g., fever, anemia, sepsis) in a patient with LV diastolic dysfunction (e.g., in the patient with compensatory hypertrophy secondary to AS) may result in acute decompensation with significant elevation in LV diastolic pressure. Other measures of diastolic function, such as the time constant of relaxation, can also be measured at catheterization but require special recording and analysis of data and are rarely performed in the clinical setting.

Coronary Angiography

Coronary angiography is often needed in patients with valvular heart disease either as part of the preoperative evaluation or to evaluate for other potential causes of clinical symptoms.[89] Current guidelines suggest that coronary angiography should be performed prior to valve surgery in patients with chest pain, objective evidence of ischemia, or a prior history of coronary artery disease, in men 35 years or older, in premenopausal woman aged 35 years and older with coronary risk factors, and in postmenopausal woman.[89]

REFERENCES

1. Cheitlin MD. Valvular heart disease: management and intervention. Clinical overview and discussion. Circulation 1991;84(3 Suppl):I259–64.
2. Grossman W, Braunwald E, Mann T, et al. Contractile state of the left ventricle in man as evaluated from end-systolic pressure-volume relations. Circulation 1977;56(5): 845–52.
3. Mirsky I, Tajimi T, Peterson KL. The development of the entire end-systolic pressure-volume and ejection fraction-afterload relations: a new concept of systolic myocardial stiffness. Circulation 1987;76(2):343–56.
4. Kass DA, Midei M, Graves W, et al. Use of a conductance (volume) catheter and transient inferior vena caval occlusion for rapid determination of pressure-volume relationships in man. Cathet Cardiovasc Diagn 1988;15(3):192–202.
5. Starling MR, Kirsh MM, Montgomery DG, et al. Impaired left ventricular contractile function in patients with long-term mitral regurgitation and normal ejection fraction. J Am Coll Cardiol 1993;22(1):239–50.
6. Sandler H, Dodge HT. The use of single plane angiocardiograms for the calculation of left ventricular volume in man. Am Heart J 1968;75(3):325–34.
7. Dodge HT, Sandler H, Ballew DW, et al. The use of biplane angiocardiography for the measurement of left ventricular volume in man. Am Heart J 1960;60:762–76.
8. Greene DG, Carlisle R, Grant C, et al. Estimation of left ventricular volume by one-plane cineangiography. Circulation 1967;35(1):61–9.
9. Wynne J, Green LH, Mann T, et al. Estimation of left ventricular volumes in man from biplane cineangiograms filmed in oblique projections. Am J Cardiol 1978;41(4): 726–32.
10. Sandler H, Dodge HT. The use of single plane angiocardiograms for the calculation of left ventricular volume in man. Am Heart J 1968;75(3):325–34.
11. Kennedy JW, Trenholme SE, Kasser IS. Left ventricular volume and mass from single-plane cineangiocardiogram. A comparison of anteroposterior and right anterior oblique methods. Am Heart J 1970;80(3):343–52.
12. Graham Jr TP, Jarmakani JM, Canent Jr RV, et al. Left heart volume estimation in infancy and childhood. Reevaluation of methodology and normal values. Circulation 1971;43(6): 895–904.
13. Greene DG, Carlisle R, Grant C, et al. Estimation of left ventricular volume by one-plane cineangiography. Circulation 1967;35(1):61–9.
14. Kennedy JW, Trenholme SE, Kasser IS. Left ventricular volume and mass from single-plane cineangiocardiogram. A comparison of anteroposterior and right anterior oblique methods. Am Heart J 1970;80(3):343–52.
15. Kasser IS, Kennedy JW. Measurement of left ventricular volumes in man by single-plane cineangiocardiography. Invest Radiol 1969;4(2):83–90.
16. Sheehan FH, Mitten-Lewis S. Factors influencing accuracy in left ventricular volume determination. Am J Cardiol 1989;64(10):661–4.
17. Dodge HT, Sandler H, Ballew DW, et al. The use of biplane angiocardiography for the measurement of left ventricular volume in man. Am Heart J 1960;60:762–76.
18. Wynne J, Green LH, Mann T, et al. Estimation of left ventricular volumes in man from biplane cineangiograms filmed in oblique projections. Am J Cardiol 1978;41(4): 726–32.
19. Chaitman BR, DeMots H, Bristow JD, et al. Objective and subjective analysis of left ventricular angiograms. Circulation 1975;52(3):420–5.
20. Rackley CE, Dodge HT, Coble Jr YD, et al. A method for determining left ventricular mass in man. Circulation 1964;29:666–71.
21. Kennedy JW, Reichenbach DD, Baxley WA, et al. Left ventricular mass. A comparison of angiocardiographic measurements with autopsy weight. Am J Cardiol 1967;19(2): 221–3.
22. Sheehan FH, Bolson EL, Dodge HT, et al. Advantages and applications of the centerline method for characterizing regional ventricular function. Circulation 1986;74(2): 293–305.
23. Sheehan FH, Schofer J, Mathey DG, et al. Measurement of regional wall motion from biplane contrast ventriculograms: a comparison of the 30 degree right anterior oblique and 60 degree left anterior oblique projections in patients with acute myocardial infarction. Circulation 1986;74(4):796–804.
24. Fick A. Uber die Messung des Blutquantums in de Herzventrikeln. Verh Physik Med Ges Wurzburg 2:16–28, 1870.
25. LaFarge CG, Miettinen OS. The estimation of oxygen consumption. Cardiovasc Res 1970;4(1):23–30.
26. Narang N, Gore MO, Snell PG, et al. Accuracy of estimating resting oxygen uptake and implications for hemodynamic assessment. Am J Cardiol 2012;109(4):594–8.
27. Barratt-Boyes BG, Wood EH. The oxygen saturation of blood in the venae cavae, right-heart chambers, and pulmonary vessels of healthy subjects. J Lab Clin Med 1957;50(1):93–106.
28. Selzer A, Sudrann RB. Reliability of the determination of cardiac output in man by means of the Fick principle. Circ Res 1958;6(4):485–90.
29. Visscher MB, Johnson JA. The Fick principle: analysis of potential errors in its conventional application. J Appl Physiol 1953;5(10):635–8.
30. Kendrick AH, West J, Papouchado M, et al. Direct Fick cardiac output: are assumed values of oxygen consumption acceptable? Eur Heart J 1988;9(3):337–42.
31. Dehmer GJ, Firth BG, Hillis LD. Oxygen consumption in adult patients during cardiac catheterization. Clin Cardiol 1982;5(8):436–40.
32. Branthwaite MA, Bradley RD. Measurement of cardiac output by thermal dilution in man. J Appl Physiol 1968;24(3):434–8.
33. Ganz W, Donoso R, Marcus HS, et al. A new technique for measurement of cardiac output by thermodilution in man. Am J Cardiol 1971;27(4):392–6.
34. Forrester JS, Ganz W, Diamond G, et al. Thermodilution cardiac output determination with a single flow-directed catheter. Am Heart J 1972;83(3):306–11.
35. Weisel RD, Berger RL, Hechtman HB. Current concepts measurement of cardiac output by thermodilution. N Engl J Med 1975;292(13):682–4.
36. Weisel RD, Berger RL, Hechtman HB. Current concepts measurement of cardiac output by thermodilution. N Engl J Med 1975;292(13):682–4.
37. van Grondelle A, Ditchey RV, Groves BM, et al. Thermodilution method overestimates low cardiac output in humans. Am J Physiol 1983;245(4):H690–2.
38. Levine RA, Cape EG, Yoganathan AP. Pressure recovery distal to stenoses: expanding clinical applications of engineering principles. J Am Coll Cardiol 1993;21(4):1026–8.
39. Voelker W, Reul H, Stelzer T, et al. Pressure recovery in aortic stenosis: an in vitro study in a pulsatile flow model. J Am Coll Cardiol 1992;20(7):1585–93.
40. Laskey WK, Kussmaul WG. Pressure recovery in aortic valve stenosis. Circulation 1994;89(1):116–21.
41. Cujec B, Welsh R, Aboguddah A, et al. Comparison of Doppler echocardiography and cardiac catheterization in patients requiring valve surgery: search for a 'gold standard'. Can J Cardiol 1992;8(8):829–38.
42. Kern MJ. Catheter selection for the stenotic aortic valve. Cathet Cardiovasc Diagn 1989;17(3):190–1.
43. Feldman T, Carroll JD, Chiu YC. An improved catheter design for crossing stenosed aortic valves. Cathet Cardiovasc Diagn 1989;16(4):279–83.
44. Meine TJ, Harrison JK. Should we cross the valve: the risk of retrograde catheterization of the left ventricle in patients with aortic stenosis. Am Heart J 2004;148(1):41–2.
45. Pasipoularides A. Clinical assessment of ventricular ejection dynamics with and without outflow obstruction. J Am Coll Cardiol 1990;15(4):859–82.
46. Criley JM, Siegel RJ. Has 'obstruction' hindered our understanding of hypertrophic cardiomyopathy? Circulation 1985;72(6):1148–54.
47. Kern MJ, Deligonul U. Interpretation of cardiac pathophysiology from pressure waveform analysis: I. The stenotic aortic valve. Cathet Cardiovasc Diagn 1990;21(2): 112–20.
48. Jayne JE, Catherwood E, Niles NW, et al. Double-lumen catheter assessment of aortic stenosis: comparison with separate catheter technique. Cathet Cardiovasc Diagn 1993;29(2):157–60.
49. Folland ED, Parisi AF, Carbone C. Is peripheral arterial pressure a satisfactory substitute for ascending aortic pressure when measuring aortic valve gradients? J Am Coll Cardiol 1984;4(6):1207–12.
50. Hays J, Lujan M, Chilton R. Aortic stenosis catheterization revisited: a long sheath single-puncture technique. J Invasive Cardiol 2006;18(6):262–7.
51. Bertog SC, Smith A, Panetta CJ. Feasibility assessment of aortic valve area in patients with aortic stenosis using a pressure wire through a 4 French system and single femoral arterial access. J Invasive Cardiol 2005;17(11):E24–6.
52. Bae JH, Lerman A, Yang E, et al. Feasibility of a pressure wire and single arterial puncture for assessing aortic valve area in patients with aortic stenosis. J Invasive Cardiol 2006;18(8):359–62.
53. Carabello BA. Advances in the hemodynamic assessment of stenotic cardiac valves. J Am Coll Cardiol 1987;10(4):912–19.
54. Gorlin R, Gorlin SG. Hydraulic formula for calculation of the area of the stenotic mitral valve, other cardiac valves, and central circulatory shunts. I. Am Heart J 1951;41(1): 1–29.
55. Cohen MV, Gorlin R. Modified orifice equation for the calculation of mitral valve area. Am Heart J 1972;84(6):839–40.
56. Hakki AH, Iskandrian AS, Bemis CE, et al. A simplified valve formula for the calculation of stenotic cardiac valve areas. Circulation 1981;63(5):1050–5.
57. Chambers JB, Sprigings DC, Cochrane T, et al. Continuity equation and Gorlin formula compared with directly observed orifice area in native and prosthetic aortic valves. Br Heart J 1992;67(2):193–9.

58. Oh JK, Taliercio CP, Holmes Jr DR, et al. Prediction of the severity of aortic stenosis by Doppler aortic valve area determination: prospective Doppler-catheterization correlation in 100 patients. J Am Coll Cardiol 1988;11(6):1227–34.

59. Danielsen R, Nordrehaug JE, Vik-Mo H. Factors affecting Doppler echocardiographic valve area assessment in aortic stenosis. Am J Cardiol 1989;63(15):1107–11.

60. Garcia D, Dumesnil JG, Durand LG, et al. Discrepancies between catheter and Doppler estimates of valve effective orifice area can be predicted from the pressure recovery phenomenon: practical implications with regard to quantification of aortic stenosis severity. J Am Coll Cardiol 2003;41(3):435–42.

61. Razzolini R, Manica A, Tarantini G, et al. Discrepancies between catheter and Doppler estimates of aortic stenosis: the role of pressure recovery evaluated 'in vivo'. J Heart Valve Dis 2007;16(3):225–9.

62. Aghassi P, Aurigemma GP, Folland ED, et al. Catheterization-Doppler discrepancies in nonsimultaneous evaluations of aortic stenosis. Echocardiography 2005;22(5):367–73.

63. Jander N, Minners J, Holme I, et al. Outcome of patients with low-gradient "severe" aortic stenosis and preserved ejection fraction. Circulation 2011;123(8):887–95.

64. Hachicha Z, Dumesnil JG, Bogaty P, et al. Paradoxical low-flow, low-gradient severe aortic stenosis despite preserved ejection fraction is associated with higher afterload and reduced survival. Circulation 2007;115(22):2856–64.

65. Awtry E, Davidoff R. Low-flow/low-gradient aortic stenosis. Circulation 2011;124(23): e739–41.

66. Connolly HM, Oh JK, Schaff HV, et al. Severe aortic stenosis with low transvalvular gradient and severe left ventricular dysfunction: result of aortic valve replacement in 52 patients. Circulation 2000;101(16):1940–6.

67. Monin JL, Monchi M, Gest V, et al. Aortic stenosis with severe left ventricular dysfunction and low transvalvular pressure gradients: risk stratification by low-dose dobutamine echocardiography. J Am Coll Cardiol 2001;37(8):2101–7.

68. Nishimura RA, Grantham JA, Connolly HM, et al. Low-output, low-gradient aortic stenosis in patients with depressed left ventricular systolic function: the clinical utility of the dobutamine challenge in the catheterization laboratory. Circulation 2002;106(7): 809–13.

69. Pibarot P, Dumesnil JG. Low-flow, low-gradient aortic stenosis with normal and depressed left ventricular ejection fraction. J Am Coll Cardiol 2012;60(19):1845–53.

70. Cannon Jr JD, Zile MR, Crawford Jr FA, et al. Aortic valve resistance as an adjunct to the Gorlin formula in assessing the severity of aortic stenosis in symptomatic patients. J Am Coll Cardiol 1992;20(7):1517–23.

71. Ford LE, Feldman T, Chiu YC, et al. Hemodynamic resistance as a measure of functional impairment in aortic valvular stenosis. Circ Res 1990;66(1):1–7.

72. Nishimura RA, Carabello BA. Hemodynamics in the cardiac catheterization laboratory of the 21st century. Circulation 2012;125(17):2138–50.

73. Mascherbauer J, Schima H, Rosenhek R, et al. Value and limitations of aortic valve resistance with particular consideration of low flow-low gradient aortic stenosis: an in vitro study. Eur Heart J 2004;25(9):787–93.

74. Burwash IG, Hay KM, Chan KL. Hemodynamic stability of valve area, valve resistance, and stroke work loss in aortic stenosis: a comparative analysis. J Am Soc Echocardiogr 2002;15(8):814–22.

75. Nadas AS. Report from the Joint Study on the Natural History of Congenital Heart Defects. I. General introduction. Circulation 1977;56(1 Suppl):I3–4.

76. Almeda FQ, Kavinsky CJ, Pophal SG, et al. Pulmonic valvular stenosis in adults: diagnosis and treatment. Catheter Cardiovasc Interv 2003;60(4):546–57.

77. Lange RA, Moore Jr DM, Cigarroa RG, et al. Use of pulmonary capillary wedge pressure to assess severity of mitral stenosis: is true left atrial pressure needed in this condition? J Am Coll Cardiol 1989;13(4):825–31.

78. Kern MJ. When should you question your wedge and use a long iron (transseptal needle) instead? Catheter Cardiovasc Interv 2011;78(7):1029–31.

79. Yousof AM, Shafei MZ, Endrys G, et al. Tricuspid stenosis and regurgitation in rheumatic heart disease: a prospective cardiac catheterization study in 525 patients. Am Heart J 1985;110(1 Pt 1):60–4.

80. Yousof AM, Shafei MZ, Endrys G, et al. Tricuspid stenosis and regurgitation in rheumatic heart disease: a prospective cardiac catheterization study in 525 patients. Am Heart J 1985;110(1 Pt 1):60–4.

81. Judge TP, Kennedy JW. Estimation of aortic regurgitation by diastolic pulse wave analysis. Circulation 1970;41(4):659–65.

82. Lehman JS, Boyle Jr JJ, Debbas JN. Quantitation of aortic valvular insufficiency by catheter thoracic aortography. Radiology 1962;79:361–70.

83. Sellers RD, Levy MJ, Mplatz K, et al. Left retrograde cardioangiography in acquired cardiac disease: technic, indications and interpretations in 700 cases. Am J Cardiol 1964;14:437–47.

84. Croft CH, Lipscomb K, Mathis K, et al. Limitations of qualitative angiographic grading in aortic or mitral regurgitation. Am J Cardiol 1984;53(11):1593–8.

85. Snyder RW, Glamann DB, Lange RA, et al. Predictive value of prominent pulmonary arterial wedge V waves in assessing the presence and severity of mitral regurgitation. Am J Cardiol 1994;73(8):568–70.

86. Sharkey SW. Beyond the wedge: clinical physiology and the Swan-Ganz catheter. Am J Med 1987;83(1):111–22.

87. Lingamneni R, Cha SD, Maranhao V, et al. Tricuspid regurgitation: clinical and angiographic assessment. Cathet Cardiovasc Diagn 1979;5(1):7–17.

88. Tamari I, Borer JS, Goldberg HL, et al. Hemodynamic changes during retrograde left-heart catheterization in patients with aortic stenosis. Cardiology 1991;78(3): 171–8.

89. American College of Cardiology/American Heart Association Task Force on Practice Guidelines; Society of Cardiovascular Anesthesiologists; Society for Cardiovascular Angiography and Interventions; Society of Thoracic Surgeons, Bonow RO, Carabello BA, Kanu C, et al. ACC/AHA 2006 guidelines for the management of patients with valvular heart disease: a report of the American College of Cardiology/American Heart Association Task Force on Practice Guidelines (writing committee to revise the 1998 Guidelines for the Management of Patients With Valvular Heart Disease): developed in collaboration with the Society of Cardiovascular Anesthesiologists: endorsed by the Society for Cardiovascular Angiography and Interventions and the Society of Thoracic Surgeons. Circulation 2006;114(5):e84–231.

90. Westaby S, Karp RB, Blackstone EH, et al. Adult human valve dimensions and their surgical significance. Am J Cardiol 1984;53(4):552–6.

CHAPTER 8

Evaluation of Valvular Heart Disease by Cardiac Magnetic Resonance and Computed Tomography

Mario J. Garcia

Key Points

- Echocardiography is the modality of choice for the evaluation of the heart valves, providing both anatomic and functional information with high temporal and spatial resolution. Cardiac computed tomography (CT) and cardiac magnetic resonance (CMR) may be useful, however, in patients with suboptimal acoustic windows and in those in whom more detailed information of the cardiac and vascular anatomy is needed.
- CMR may be useful in patients with valvular heart disease when symptoms are out of proportion to the echocardiographic findings, particularly patients with regurgitant valve lesions.
- CMR may be useful for the assessment of ventricular function and viability, such as in patients with functional mitral or tricuspid regurgitation.
- CT should be considered to evaluate the extent of aortic valve calcification in patients with left ventricular dysfunction and suspected low-gradient severe aortic stenosis (AS), and is critical for the evaluation of the aortic root anatomy and the femoral arteries in patients being considered for transcatheter aortic valve implantation (TAVI).
- CT is useful to visualize the motion of mechanical disk valves and the presence of thrombus, pannus, or infection in patients with suspected prosthetic dysfunction.
- CT may be used as an alternative to invasive coronary angiography in patients undergoing valve surgery who are at low to intermediate risk for coronary artery disease (CAD), such as those with mitral valve myxomatous degeneration or congenital valve anomalies, but has low specificity and should be avoided in groups with high prevalence of CAD, such as elderly patients with degenerative AS.
- CT may also be useful in patients at high risk for complications from invasive angiography, such as those with aortic valve endocarditis and large vegetations, and in patients with mechanical valves.

Cardiac magnetic resonance (CMR) and computed tomography (CT) imaging provide complementary information about valve anatomy and hemodynamic function that could be relevant for management decisions in selected patients. In addition, patients undergoing CMR and CT for a variety of indications are often incidentally found to have unsuspected valve disease. This chapter reviews the principles and use of these imaging techniques as applied to the evaluation of the cardiac valves.

Indications for, relative utility of, and appropriate use criteria of CT and CMR for the evaluation of patients with valvular heart disease are listed in Tables 8-1 to 8-3.

Principles and Instrumentation

Cardiac Magnetic Resonance

Magnetic resonance imaging is without doubt one of the most sophisticated and versatile noninvasive diagnostic tools. With the use of electrocardiogram (ECG)–gated acquisition coupled to dedicated surface coils, high-resolution static and moving images of the heart and cardiovascular system may be obtained. A powerful helium-cooled superconductor generates a high-strength magnetic field in which nuclei with unpaired numbers of protons and electrons are forced to behave like small magnets, aligning their poles in the direction of the magnetic field (T1 or longitudinal relaxation) and precess at a frequency proportional to the magnetic field strength (T2 or transverse relaxation). The most common magnetic field strength used for cardiac applications is 1.5 Tesla (1500 times the earth's magnetic field strength).

To generate images, surface coils emit sequences of radio signal pulses that excite the nuclei to briefly flip out of alignment, while receiving coils measure the magnetic signals produced by the nuclei as they return to their baseline state of relaxation. The magnitude of the signals received depends on the magnetic field strength, the concentration of odd nuclei (primarily the hydrogen ion [H⁺]), and the T1 and the T2 relaxation times, which are tissue-specific. Paramagnetic contrast agents, such as gadolinium compounds, specifically alter the T1 and T2 times and are used to highlight the blood pool and areas of fibrosis or edema, where they gradually accumulate. Field magnetic gradients permit identification of the spatial location of each signal being received, allowing acquisition of images in any location and plane within the center of the magnet. Different pulse sequences are designed to acquire images that are preferentially based on the distribution of tissue. Cardiac images may be acquired from a single heartbeat and displayed in near-real time or derived from a series of consecutive heartbeats acquired during a 20- to 40-second breath-hold or respiratory gating. The spatial and temporal resolution of CMR images depends on the magnitude of the magnetic field and the acquisition time. Therefore, real-time imaging is done at low resolution and is limited to specific applications or to patients

TABLE 8-1 Comparison of Echocardiography, CT, and CMR for Characterizing Cardiovascular Structural and Functional Parameters in Valvular Disease*			
PARAMETER	ECHO	CT	CMR
Leaflet mobility	++++	++	+++
Valvular calcification	++	++++	+
Annular geometry	++	++++	+++
Annular calcification	++	++++	+
Stenotic orifice area	++++	+++	++
Transvalvular pressure gradients	++++	−	+++
Regurgitant jet morphology	++++	−	+++
Regurgitant volume	+++	+	++++
Aortic root morphology	+++	++++	++++
LV dimensions	+++	++++	++++
LV function	+++	+++	++++
RV dimensions	++	+++	++++
RV function	++	+++	++++
LV contractile reserve	++++	−	+++
Myocardial viability	+++	+	++++
Coronary anatomy	+	++++	++

*Ratings: −, unable; +, very limited; ++, marginal; +++, adequate; ++++, excellent.
CT, computed tomography; *CMR*, cardiac magnetic resonance; *Echo*, echocardiography; *LV*, left ventricular; *RV*, right ventricular.

TABLE 8-2 CT and CMR Methods for Evaluating Stenotic and Regurgitant Lesions		
VALVULAR LESION	MODALITY	METHOD
Stenosis	CT	Calcium scoring
	CT	Stenotic orifice planimetry
	CMR	Stenotic orifice planimetry
	CMR	PC-VENC pressure gradients
	CMR	PC-VENC continuity valve area
	CMR	PC-VENC pressure half-time (mitral)
Regurgitation	CT	Regurgitant orifice planimetry
	CT	Regurgitant volume (LV-RV stroke volume difference)
	CMR	PC-VENC aortic regurgitant volume
	CMR	Regurgitant volume (LV-RV stroke volume difference)
	CMR	Regurgitant volume (Ao-PA stroke volume difference)
	CMR	Regurgitant volume (Ao–mitral valve inflow stroke volume difference)
	CMR	Vena contracta
	CMR	Flow acceleration radius
	CMR	Signal void area

Ao, aortic; *CT*, computed tomography; *CMR*, cardiac magnetic resonance; *LV*, left ventricular; *PA*, pulmonary artery; *PC-VENC*, phase-contrast velocity–encoding; *RV*, right ventricular.

who have severe heart rate variability and/or are unable to comply with breath-holding.

A particularly useful CMR application called phase-contrast velocity–encoded mapping may be applied to interrogate flow across the cardiac valves. After excitation, moving targets produce a signal that is proportional to the velocity at which they travel through an imaging plane. Flow may be calculated as the product of area times velocity within a conduit, and pressure gradients across valves may be estimated, as in echocardiography, with use of the Bernoulli equation.

TABLE 8-3 Criteria for Appropriate Use of CMR in Patients with Valvular Heart Disease	
INDICATION	APPROPRIATENESS CRITERIA (MEDIAN SCORE)
Assessment of complex congenital heart disease, including anomalies of coronary circulation, great vessels, and cardiac chambers and valves Procedures may include LV/RV mass and volumes, CMR angiography, quantification of valvular disease, and contrast enhancement	A (9)
Quantification of LV function Discordant information that is clinically significant from prior tests	A (8)
Characterization of native and prosthetic cardiac valves, including planimetry of stenotic disease and quantification of regurgitant disease Patients with technically limited images from echocardiogram or transesophageal echocardiography	A (8)

A, appropriate; *CMR*, cardiac magnetic resonance; *LV*, left ventricular; *RV*, right ventricular.
From Hendel RC, Patel MR, Kramer CM, et al. ACCF/ACR/SCCT/SCMR/ASNC/NASCI/SCAI/SIR 2006 appropriateness criteria for cardiac computed tomography and cardiac magnetic resonance imaging. J Am Coll Cardiol 2006;48:1475–97.

A typical CMR study performed for the evaluation of valvular disease may include 30 to 60 acquisitions obtained from different imaging planes and using varying pulse sequences. Thus, a complete study may take 30 to 90 minutes, making the examination of clinically unstable patients difficult.

Cardiac Computed Tomography

Electron-beam computed tomography (EBCT) and multidetector computed tomography (MDCT) allow ECG-gated images to be obtained with sufficient temporal and spatial resolution to visualize the beating heart. The most common applications of cardiac CT are evaluation of coronary calcification and detection of coronary stenosis. Both EBCT and MDCT systems basically contain an X-ray source and a detector array of crystals that receive the X-rays after traveling through the body and convert photons into electrical impulses. Unlike plain fluoroscopy, in CT imaging the x-ray data need to be collected for a minimum of 180 degrees. From the precise spatial and temporal location of each x-ray photon detected, a three-dimensional (3D) data set is reconstructed using filtered back-projection. In addition, CT imaging requires ECG-gated temporal registration to match data collected at the same time during the cardiac cycle, given the continuous motion of the heart.

With EBCT, a rapidly rotating electron beam generates x-rays, which are electronically steered to sweep over tungsten targets arranged in a stationary semicircular array under the patient table. Even though this system has the advantage of high temporal resolution (33 to 50 ms) for each slice acquisition because of the lack of rotating parts, it has limited speed to cover the *z*-axis (moving from one slice to the next) and has limited x-ray power, producing poor-quality images in large patients. MDCT imaging involves a rotating x-ray source that emits a fan-shaped beam of x-rays that passes through the body and is detected by a moving detector array panel set at the opposite end of a doughnut-shaped gantry. Coverage in the *z*-axis is obtained by moving the table through the gantry during image acquisition in a "spiral" or "helical" movement. The superior spatial resolution and x-ray power have established MDCT as the preferred CT technology for cardiac imaging. Nevertheless, temporal resolution is limited because of the weight of the moving components (100 to 250 ms for single-source and 50 to 100 ms for the newer dual-source scanners). Moreover, radiation exposure may be considerable (8 to 25 mSv), and the use of intravenous iodine contrast material is required, limiting the utility of this method for routine cardiac valve evaluation. In selected patients, however, CT may provide very useful information, such as the extent of valvular calcification and dimensions of stenotic orifices.

A typical CT study has one to three data sets (noncontrast, contrast-enhanced, and postcontrast) acquired over a 5- to 15-second period each. Each set contains data acquired over multiple sequential cardiac cycles. Each cardiac cycle corresponds to a different series of craniocaudal axial images. Thus, significant changes in heart rate may produce misregistration artifacts that may be relevant to accurate visualization of the cardiac valve anatomy.

Ventricular Volumes, Mass, and Function

The Left Ventricle

In patients with chronic valvular disease, changes in left ventricular (LV) size, mass, and function are critical for establishing the timing of surgical intervention. CMR is a superior method for quantifying LV volumes, ejection fraction, and mass. Cine (bright-blood) ECG-gated two-dimensional images may be obtained in any of the conventional two-chamber, three-chamber, or four-chamber long-axis or cross-sectional short-axis planes. For the purpose of quantification, a stack of 10 to 20 contiguous 5- to 10-mm-thick short-axis images are acquired from the base to the apex of the left ventricle, during breath-holding.[1] These images may be then traced offline in a dedicated computer workstation. Volumetric quantification is based on the Simpson rule, for which the volume of the left ventricle equals the sum of the 10 to 20 cross-sectional discs. LV mass is calculated by subtracting the endocardially from the epicardially traced volumes and multiplying by a muscle weight–specific constant. CMR yields more accurate values than angiographic or echocardiographic planar imaging methods, especially when the ventricular shape deviates from the normal geometric model, because in the latter methods, fewer images are used and most of the data are interpolated.[2,3] In addition, CMR is superior for visualization of the true LV apex, which is often outside the acoustic echocardiographic windows. Several studies have validated CMR measurements of LV volumes, mass, and function using quantitative reference techniques, such as indicator dilution, radionuclide angiography, and studies of postmortem examination.[4-6]

CMR is the best method for longitudinal follow-up of LV mass and volumes to determine the effect of therapeutic interventions owing to its excellent interstudy reproducibility with an intertest variability less than 5%.[7-10] CMR has been used to evaluate sequential changes in LV and right ventricular (RV) geometry in response to chronic mitral regurgitation.[11] CMR is been used increasingly in clinical trials, allowing reduction in the sample size required to detect a difference between treatment arms.[12-14]

CMR is also useful for calculating LV wall stress using measurements of wall thickness and chamber dimensions in conjunction with cuff blood pressures and a carotid pulse tracing. Increased wall stress in patients with chronic valvular regurgitation has been shown to predict adverse events and deterioration of LV function.[15]

CT also allows accurate quantification of LV volumes, ejection fraction, and mass.[16,17] In fact, early studies suggested that EBCT was a reference standard for evaluation of other methods of calculating LV volumes in patients with valvular heart disease.[18] The main advantage of CT is its isotropic, submillimeter spatial resolution, which allows easy, direct 3D volumetric assessment, in many cases with the use of automated border detection algorithms. However, the limited temporal resolution of CT may result in overestimation of the true end-systolic volume, particularly in patients with elevated heart rate. Moreover, the rapid infusion of contrast material and use of beta-blockers may result in slightly larger LV volumes and reduced ejection fractions.

In many patients with valvular disease, in particular those with AS, diastolic dysfunction is an important contributor to symptoms and prognosis. CMR has been used to evaluate diastolic filling on the basis of regional myocardial diastolic velocities and strain.[19] In addition, the 3D pattern of LV filling and pulmonary venous flow has been evaluated with phase-contrast velocity–encoded data.[20,21] In patients with LV hypertrophy due to AS, CMR-determined early filling and atrial contraction velocities have been shown to correlate with Doppler echocardiographic measurements and have shown a higher atrial contribution to ventricular filling in the patients than in control subjects.[22]

The Right Ventricle

CMR is the most reliable way to assess regional and global RV function quantitatively.[23,24] Furthermore, CMR may give an unrestricted view of the RV outflow tract. The end-diastolic and end-systolic velocities are calculated by the manual drawing of endocardial contours at end-diastole and end-systole, respectively, on cine loops, oriented in the axial plane or along the short axis of the left ventricle. Ejection fraction and RV mass are determined in a fashion similar to that used in the left ventricle. Several studies have validated CMR volume measurements of dimensions and function of the right ventricle using quantitative catheterization, postmortem, and radionuclide techniques.[25-28] Thus, this approach offers the potential for more reliable evaluation of RV size and function in patients with valvular disease than with echocardiography. Assessment of RV volumes and function is important in patients with severe tricuspid or pulmonary regurgitation, including assessment after repair of tetralogy of Fallot.[29] In these patients, RV function is an important determinant of long-term prognosis after surgical correction.[30]

CT may also be used to evaluate RV volumes and ejection fraction. In order to visualize the RV endocardium, the contrast injection protocol is modified, with use of a biphasic or triphasic contrast injection, depending on what additional information is sought in the study. CT may be useful to evaluate RV size and function in patients with poor acoustic transthoracic echocardiography (TTE) windows and in those with contraindications to CMR, such as implanted left-ventricular assist devices.[31]

Valvular Stenosis

The use of CMR is well established for detecting the presence of and quantifying the severity of valve stenosis (Table 8-4). Cine gradient-echo CMR can identify valvular stenosis or regurgitation because areas of turbulent flow create a signal void in the high-intensity blood pool (Video 8-1).[32] This signal void may allow identification of the site of obstruction, for example, differentiating subvalvular from valvular stenosis.[33]

The quantitative assessment of stenotic valves with CMR primarily involves (1) evaluating the valve area using direct planimetry and (2) determining peak and average velocities across the valve to estimate pressure gradients with the modified Bernoulli equation, as follows:

$$\Delta P = 4V_{max}^2$$

where ΔP is pressure and V is velocity. To obtain the maximal velocity, the plane of interrogation must be set perpendicular to the direction of flow, and then several phase-contrast sections are obtained near the vena contracta of the jet to identify the maximum velocity. The velocity-encoding gradient needs to be adjusted often to encompass the predicted velocity range. As in Doppler echocardiography, aliasing occurs if the measured velocity exceeds the interrogation range. There is good agreement between CMR-determined aortic valve pressure gradients and other reference techniques, with reported accuracy rates of 85% and interobserver reproducibility of 93%. Calculation of continuity equation aortic valve orifice area, using phase-contrast velocity mapping, have also been found to be reliable, with a reported

110

TABLE 8-4	Criteria for Appropriate Use of CT in Patients with Valvular Heart Disease
INDICATION	**APPROPRIATENESS CRITERIA (MEDIAN SCORE, 1-9)**
Assessment of complex adult congenital heart disease	A (8)
Characterization of native cardiac valves Suspicion of clinically significant valvular dysfunction Inadequate images from other noninvasive methods	U (6)
Characterization of prosthetic cardiac valves Suspicion of clinically significant valvular dysfunction Inadequate images from other noninvasive methods	A (8)
Coronary evaluation before noncoronary cardiac surgery: Low probability of CAD Intermediate probability of CAD High probability of CAD	A (8) A (7) I (3)

A, appropriate; *CAD*, coronary artery disease; *I*, inappropriate; *U*, uncertain.
Modified from Taylor AJ, Cerqueira M, Hodgson JM, et al. ACCF/SCCT/ACR/AHA/ASE/ASNC/NASCI/SCAI/SCMR 2010 Appropriate Use Criteria for Cardiac Computed Tomography. Circulation 2010;122:e525–55.

accuracy of 81% in comparison with that for the Doppler-derived continuity equation and the Gorlin formula.[34]

Stenotic lesions of the semilunar valves lead to concentric hypertrophy and/or ventricular dilation. Poststenotic dilation of the pulmonary trunk or the ascending aorta may be present as well. These hemodynamic sequelae can be detected by both CMR and CT. CT may also detect pulmonary vein dilation and interstitial and alveolar lung edema, which are all signs of increased left atrial pressure and left-sided heart failure. Similarly, dilation of the right heart chambers and superior and inferior vena cava, pleuropericardial effusions, and ascites are suggestive of pulmonary hypertension and/or RV heart failure.

Aortic Stenosis

Echocardiography remains the most useful modality for the evaluation of AS. However, in many patients, the transvalvular gradient determined by continuous-wave Doppler echocardiography may underestimate stenosis severity because of an inadequate Doppler angle of interrogation or reduced cardiac output. The continuity-equation aortic valve area (AVA) may also be inaccurate owing to inadequate measurements of LV outflow tract dimensions or incorrect sampling of pulsed Doppler velocities.[35] Direct planimetry (Figure 8-1) of the aortic orifice is another method for determination of stenosis severity, but the accuracy is limited by TTE and even by transesophageal echocardiography (TEE) because of the acoustic shadowing produced by heavy leaflet calcification.

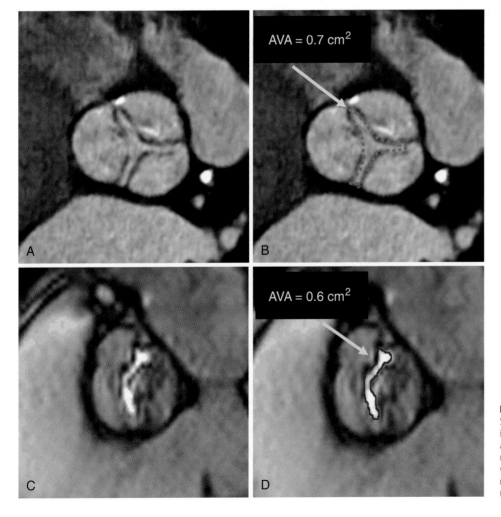

FIGURE 8-1 Calcific aortic stenosis. Short-axis cardiac computed tomography images obtained in a patient with stenosis of a trileaflet aortic valve **(A, B)** and cardiac magnetic resonance image obtained in a patient with bicuspid aortic valve **(C, D),** showing the method for determination of aortic valve area (AVA) by planimetry.

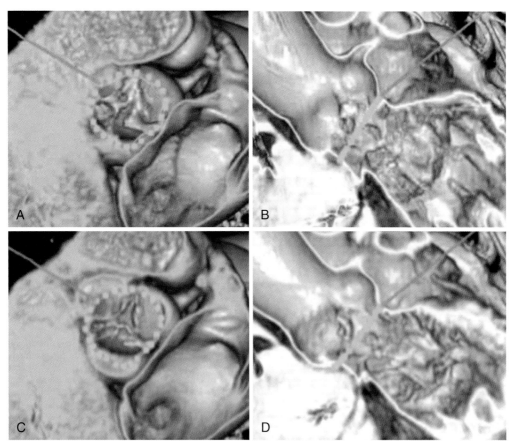

FIGURE 8-2 **Aortic annulus size and shape.** Short-axis **(A, C)** and long-axis **(B, D)** zoomed, volume-rendered cardiac computed tomography images of a stenotic aortic valve displayed at end-diastole **(A, B)** and end-systole **(C, D)** obtained from a patient evaluated for transcatheter aortic valve implantation (TAVI). Measurement of the annular diameter and area are obtained to determine the new valve size.

In a study in which 40 consecutive patients underwent cardiac catheterization, TEE, and CMR,[36] AVA was determined by direct planimetry on CMR and TEE, and calculated pressure gradients from cardiac catheterization and Doppler echocardiography were also compared. By CMR mean AVA was 0.91 ± 0.25 cm^2, by TEE AVA was 0.89 ± 0.28 cm^2, and by catheterization, AVA was 0.64 ± 0.26 cm^2. The correlation between CMR-derived and TEE-derived AVA values was $r = 0.96$, significantly higher than the correlations between TEE and catheterization and between CMR and catheterization.

Calcific AS of a trileaflet valve or congenitally bicuspid valve is invariably accompanied by calcification. Severe calcification is associated with a faster rate of stenosis progression and higher rates of cardiac events. Echocardiography may detect the presence of calcification but has limited ability to quantify its severity. Aortic valve calcification can be accurately quantified with CT. Studies have shown excellent interscan reproducibility (>90%).[37-39] The amount of calcification is directly correlated with stenosis severity, although the relationship is nonlinear. The incremental value of the information derived from the aortic valve calcium score may be particularly useful to evaluate stenosis severity in patients with low cardiac output and reduced transvalvular gradients.

Contrast-enhanced CT can precisely evaluate valve morphology and accurately differentiate trileaflet from bicuspid valves. Planimetric determinations of the AVA have shown excellent correlation with echocardiographic measurements.[40,41]

Transcatheter Aortic Valve Implantation

Surgical valve replacement is the procedure of choice for treating severe AS. However, as many as 30% of patients with AS are not referred for surgery or are turned down because of comorbidities and expected high perioperative mortality.[42] Transcatheter aortic valve implantation (TAVI) constitutes a new alternative for high-risk surgical candidates.[43] Before valve implantation, patients require an extensive workup to assess the anatomy of the aortic root and of the coronary and peripheral arteries, which is relevant for valve sizing and for positioning and access planning (Figure 8-2). CT can noninvasively provide relevant information about the anatomy of the aortic root.[44] The aortic annulus diameters and location of coronary ostia can be assessed reliably with ECG gating. In a 2010 study,[45] TTE was unable to identify the anatomy of the aortic valve in 20% of patients with severe AS because of extensive calcification. In contrast, CT was able to provide direct visualization of the aortic valve and thus could correctly identify the valve anatomy in 98%. This information is important before the procedure because TAVI is currently not recommended for bicuspid valves owing to the potential risk of an unfavorable deployment. CT allows detailed analysis of the quantification and localization of aortic valve calcification. Studies have shown a strong linear correlation between the degree of aortic regurgitation (AR) immediately after TAVI and the severity of existing calcification in the aortic root[46] and at the valve commissures.[47] Bulky calcification at the edge of native valvular leaflets has also been related to increased risk of coronary occlusion when the new prosthetic valve is displaced over the coronary ostium.[48]

Severe calcification, tortuosity, and small diameter (<6 mm) of the iliac arteries constitute contraindications to the transfemoral approach. CT provides an accurate diagnostic technique for evaluating these parameters (Figure 8-3).

Mitral Stenosis

CMR can easily demonstrate the thickened leaflets and reduced diastolic opening of the valve in patients with mitral stenosis. The

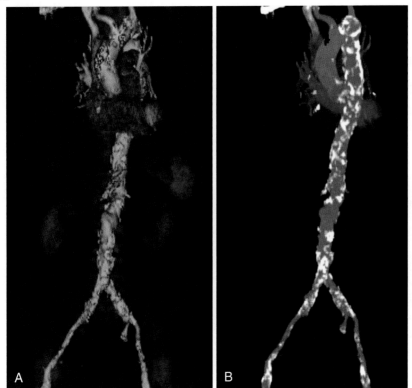

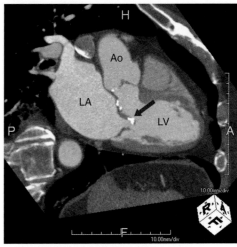

FIGURE 8-3 CT aortography in a candidate for trans-catheter aortic valve implantation (TAVI). Volume-rendered **(A)** images show the aortic luminal anatomy. Maximum intensity projection (MIP) computed tomography images **(B)** show extensive aortic and iliac calcifications.

maximal extent of leaflet opening determined by CMR correlates with stenosis severity.[49]

In-plane as well as through-plane velocity mapping by CMR has been used to measure the transmitral peak velocity in mitral stenosis. Compared with Doppler echocardiography, an accuracy rate of 87% has been reported, with an interobserver reproducibility rate of 96%.[50,51] CMR-determined peak early filling (r = 0.99) and atrial contraction (r = 0.99) velocities and estimated mitral valve area by the pressure half-time method (r = 0.94) have been validated against those obtained with Doppler echocardiography.[52]

The presence of calcium in the mitral annulus is associated with systemic atherosclerosis and has negative prognostic implications. The amount of mitral annular calcium can also be quantified with CT, although reproducibility appears to be somewhat lower than that for the aortic valve. In rheumatic mitral stenosis, calcification can extend to the leaflets, commissures, subvalvular apparatus, or even the left atrial wall (Figure 8-4). CT has been reported to be useful in evaluating mitral valve morphology in patients undergoing balloon mitral commissurotomy.[53]

Mitral stenosis is often accompanied by marked atrial enlargement involving the appendage. The presence or absence of thrombus can be determined after contrast agent administration with very high sensitivity although lower specificity, because slow flow may often impair contrast agent opacification in the left atrial appendage. Planimetry of the mitral opening by CT provides accurate assessment of stenosis severity.[54]

Pulmonic and Tricuspid Valve Stenosis

Thickened tricuspid valve leaflets in patients with rheumatic or carcinoid heart disease can be recognized on both CMR and CT imaging.[55] CMR can assess 3D morphology in patients with pulmonary stenosis and congenital heart disease without exposure to x-rays. The morphology of the RV outflow tract may vary significantly in these patients.[56] CMR has been proposed as a method to determine which patients may be candidates for percutaneous pulmonary valve replacement. Moreover, pulmonic valvuloplasty

FIGURE 8-4 Rheumatic mitral stenosis. Long-axis cardiac computed tomography image from a patient with rheumatic mitral stenosis showing thickened and mildly calcified leaflets (*arrow*). *A*, anterior; *Ao*, aorta, *F*, foot; *H*, head; *LA*, left atrium; *LV*, left ventricle; *P*, posterior.

and valve replacement may be performed under CMR guidance, reducing the need for radiation exposure.

Valvular Regurgitation

CMR evaluation of patients with regurgitant valve disease includes (1) anatomic assessment of valves, great vessels, and the cardiac chamber, (2) estimation of ventricular volumes and function, and (3) quantification of valvular regurgitant volume and fraction. Numerous studies have documented the accuracy and reliability of these methods.[57-61]

Regurgitant jets may be visualized in cine images as a region of signal void. This is achieved by dephasing of the spins caused by turbulence. The presence of a signal void provides accurate identification of the presence of aortic or mitral regurgitation with sensitivity greater than 93% and specificity greater than 89% in comparison with Doppler flow imaging or angiography.[62] Further, as with color Doppler flow imaging, the 3D spatial distribution of the signal void is related to regurgitant severity, allowing separation of mild from severe degrees of regurgitation.[63] However, the magnitude of signal void depends on multiple imaging parameters, such as echo time and flip angle used on the acquisition sequence. Moreover, turbulence may actually decrease in the presence of severe regurgitation, when the flow becomes laminar. Thus, direct semiquantitative assessment of regurgitant lesion severity on the basis of jet visualization alone is limited.

In many patients, the acceleration of flow proximal to the regurgitant orifice may be visualized by CMR as an area of signal loss (Figure 8-5). As with the Doppler echocardiography proximal isovelocity surface area method, the diameter and persistence of the detected proximal convergence zone is a marker of regurgitant flow severity.[64,65]

CMR ventricular volumes may be used for quantification of valvular regurgitation. In the absence of valvular regurgitation, the difference between LV and RV stroke volumes is less than 5%.[66,67] In the presence of single valvular regurgitation, regurgitant volume may be calculated as the difference between LV and RV stroke volumes, and regurgitant fraction as the ratio of LV to RV stroke volumes. The use of CMR for calculation of regurgitant volume using the latter approach has been demonstrated for isolated mitral and aortic regurgitation.[68]

Most commonly, mitral regurgitant volume is measured as the difference between total LV stroke volume and phase-contrast velocity–determined forward stroke volume across the aortic valve. CMR has been shown to measure regurgitant fractions with 90% accuracy in comparison with radionuclide ventriculography[69] and echocardiography.[70] Alternatively, the difference between aortic and pulmonic phase-contrast velocity-encoded flow can be used to quantify the severity of either aortic or pulmonic regurgitation.[71]

The evaluation of regurgitant lesions by CT is limited by the fact that its acquisition is not dynamic, so regurgitant flow cannot be visualized or quantified. However, in isolated regurgitant lesions, the regurgitant volume (and fraction) can be derived from the difference between the left and right stroke volumes.[72] Significant regurgitation of any valve eventually causes ipsilateral ventricular dilation, often accompanied by eccentric hypertrophy.

Aortic Regurgitation

Aortic regurgitant volume is usually determined from the phase-contrast velocity–encoded diastolic regurgitant flow velocities at the aortic root (Figure 8-6). Phase-contrast velocity–encoded CMR of the ascending and descending aorta has been used to identify patients with severe AR. Like the Doppler method, CMR identifies severe AR as the presence of holodiastolic flow reversal.[73] However, this method has several limitations. Normally, 3% to 15% of the forward aortic flow is reversed during diastole into the coronary arteries.[74] In addition, the normal movement of the imaging plane from a position between the aortic valve and the coronary ostia to a position 2 cm distal to the sinotubular junction may lead to a 30% to 70% underestimation of regurgitant volume.[75] Nevertheless this method has been validated in several studies, revealing accuracy of 90%, an interstudy reproducibility rate of 95%, and an interobserver reproducibility rate of 94%.[76] This technique has been used to demonstrate the beneficial effects of vasodilator therapy in chronic AR.[77]

CT may be useful in evaluating the mechanism leading to AR. In degenerative valve disease there is increased leaflet thickness and calcification, and the area of lack of coaptation may be visualized in diastolic phase reconstructions centrally or at the commissures, often providing accurate visualization of the anatomic regurgitant orifice (Figure 8-7). Direct planimetry of the AR orifice by CT has been shown to correlate with the degree of AR severity measured by echocardiography.[78] Planimetric assessment is

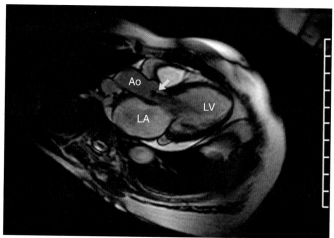

FIGURE 8-5   Aortic regurgitation. Cine cardiac magnetic resonance mid-diastolic image obtained in a patient with moderate to severe aortic regurgitation. Notice the proximal acceleration zone and the vena contracta at the regurgitant orifice (*arrow*). *Ao,* aorta, *LA,* left atrium; *LV,* left ventricle.

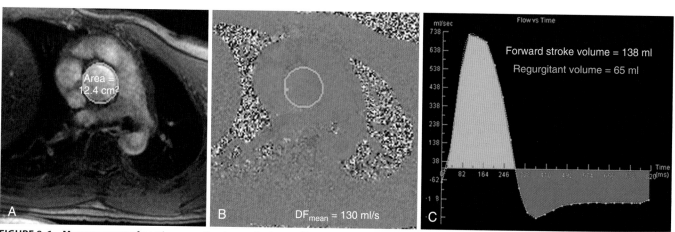

FIGURE 8-6   Measurement of aortic regurgitant severity by cardiac magnetic resonance (CMR). Magnitude **(A)** and phase-contrast velocity–encoded flow **(B)** CMR images obtained at the aortic root in a patient with severe aortic regurgitation. The areas under the curves shown in **C** represent the forward (*yellow*) and regurgitant (*blue*) flows. *DF$_{mean}$* diastolic mean flow velocity.

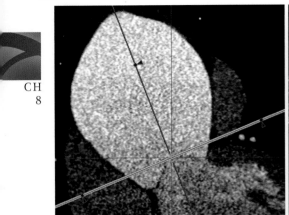

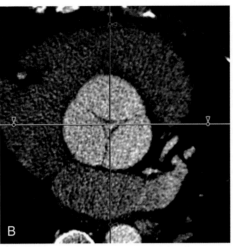

FIGURE 8-7 Aortic valve images. End-diastolic Long-axis **(A)** cardiac computed tomography imaging shows a dilated proximal ascending aorta with the regurgitant valve orifice seen at the junction of the long axis (*red line*) and a short axis plane (*yellow line*) placed at the valve leaflet tips. In the short axis view **(B),** the central gap indicates the area of incomplete leaflet coaptation exactly centered in the valve in boht the vertical long axis (*red line*) and horizonal long axis (*green line*) image planes.

feasible in patients with degenerative AR and in those with AR secondary to aortic root dilation but is difficult to perform in patients with eccentric regurgitant jets, such as those with bicuspid valves. The aortic regurgitant volume cannot be accurately established by CT, because this modality cannot visualize flow. However, in cases of severe regurgitation, CT may demonstrate LV dilation and/or a significant difference between the LV and RV stroke volumes.

Evaluation of the Aorta

In AR due to enlargement of the aortic root, the regurgitant orifice is typically located centrally. Other causes of AR that can be detected include interposition of an intimal flap in dissection, valve distortion or perforation in endocarditis, and leaflet prolapse, often observed in dissection and Marfan syndrome. CMR also allows evaluation of the thickness and compliance of the aortic root. It is increasingly being recognized that many patients with AR may have an aortopathy because CMR shows edema of the aortic wall.

The thoracic aorta and main branches may be imaged by CMR using either ECG-gated static spin-echo (black-blood), gradient-echo (cine bright-blood), or contrast-enhanced magnetic resonance angiography (MRA). Each technique has several potential advantages and disadvantages. Spin-echo and gradient-echo images are acquired in multiple two-dimensional planes, whereas contrast-enhanced MRA involves a 3D reconstruction, which allows reorientation and measurements in any direction and plane. MRA may, however, result in overestimation of the aortic root size because of cardiac motion artifacts. This technique provides the measurement of the lumen, whereas the others provide the external diameter, including the aortic wall.

CT is accepted as the most accurate method for obtaining measurements of the aorta, owing to its high isotropic spatial resolution. With the use of ECG gating, motion artifacts are virtually eliminated. One important disadvantage, however, is the required radiation exposure, a consideration for younger patients undergoing serial follow-up examinations.

Measurements of the thoracic aorta are typically performed at multiple levels, including the annulus, sinus of Valsalva, sinotubular junction, mid-ascending (pulmonary artery bifurcation) arch, and midthoracic levels. Measurements are typically done from outside to outside edge, at end-diastole, and in oblique planes perpendicular to the long axial orientation of each segment. Off-line digital measurements performed in computer workstations with 3D reconstruction capability have helped eliminate the overestimation that often occurred when measurements were performed from plain films in a straight axial orientation.

Mitral Regurgitation

Mitral regurgitant volume may be determined by CMR as the difference between (1) forward stroke volumes across the mitral annulus and the aortic annulus, (2) LV and RV stroke volumes, or (3) LV stroke volume and forward aortic stroke volume. The estimation of forward volume flow through the mitral annulus has shown accuracy of 90% but may be unreliable in patients with eccentric jets and atrial fibrillation problems. Accordingly, the quantitative assessment of mitral regurgitant volume is most commonly calculated as the difference between the LV stroke volume, as determined by planimetry, and the forward flow in the ascending aorta. The accuracy for this technique has been reported as 91%, and the interobserver reproducibility as 90%.

CMR is particularly useful for the evaluation of patients with ischemic mitral regurgitation. CMR studies have shown a strong relationship among LV end-systolic volume, interpapillary muscle distance, distance between anterior mitral annulus to medial and lateral papillary muscle, and functional ischemic mitral regurgitation.[79,80] Mitral systolic tenting area and scarring of the anterolateral region (Figure 8-8) have been shown to be independent predictors of mitral regurgitation severity.[81]

In patients with mitral valve prolapse, CT can demonstrate the presence of leaflet thickening or the degree and location of prolapse (Figure 8-9). In patients with mitral regurgitation due to annular enlargement, dimensions of the annulus can be accurately quantified, and a central area of insufficient leaflet coaptation may be observed. Although quantifying severity of mitral regurgitation may be difficult, one study suggested that planimetry of the regurgitant orifice by CT correlates well with echocardiographic grading of mitral regurgitation severity.[82]

Pulmonic and Tricuspid Valve Regurgitation

Management decisions in patients with right-side regurgitant lesions are usually more difficult than in patients with mitral and/or AR. Although previously the right-side lesions were always considered benign, we now know that many patients with tricuspid and pulmonic valve disease experience severe RV dysfunction and irreversible heart failure. Evaluation of RV function is notoriously difficult. RV volume and ejection fraction measurements are less reproducible than LV measurements. Geometric assumptions are usually erroneous because the geometry of the RV is distorted with chronic pressure and/or volume overload. CMR provides accurate determination of RV volumes and ejection fraction because volume determinations do not require any specific geometric assumptions. The accuracy rates for velocity mapping of pulmonary regurgitant volume and regurgitant fraction by CMR have been reported to be 78% and 76%,

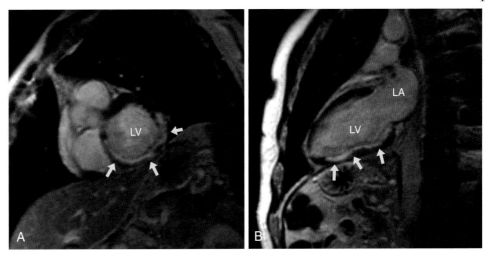

FIGURE 8-8 Ischemic mitral regurgitation. Left ventricular short-axis **(A)** and two-chamber **(B)** cardiac magnetic resonance images show near-transmural delayed enhancement in the inferolateral segments (*arrows*) in a patient with mitral regurgitation and previous myocardial infarction. *LA*, left atrium; *LV*, left ventricle.

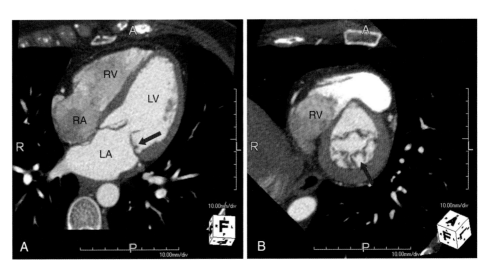

FIGURE 8-9 Mitral valve prolapse. Four-chamber **(A)** and short-axis **(B)** cardiac computed tomography images demonstrating thickened leaflets (*arrows*) in a patient with myxomatous mitral valve disease. *LA*, left atrium; *LV*, left ventricle; *R*, right; *RA*, right atrium; *RV*, right ventricle.

respectively.[83] CT is unreliable for evaluation of tricuspid regurgitation. Nevertheless, dilation and contrast opacification of the inferior vena cava and hepatic veins may be seen in patients with severe tricuspid regurgitation.[84]

Prosthetic Valves

At a magnetic field strength of 1.5 Tesla, all valvular prostheses, except some ball-and-cage models, can be safely imaged.[85] Most prosthetic valves are visible on bright-blood CMR as areas of signal loss (see Figure 8-8). The extent of the artifact depends on the type of prosthesis, magnetic field strength, and type of sequence used. The assessment of mechanical valve prosthesis dysfunction may be limited, and intravalvular or perivalvular prosthetic valve regurgitation may be easily hidden by the signal loss around the prosthesis. CMR has shown good agreement with TEE in separating pathologic from physiologic paravalvular and intravalvular prosthetic valve regurgitation.[86] Measurement of prosthetic valve gradients and evaluation of flow profiles with phase-contrast velocity–encoded CMR also have been reported.[87]

Many of the aforementioned features of native valvular heart disease apply also to the evaluation of cardiac prostheses. Several studies suggest that CT can help assess mechanism of dysfunction in mechanical prosthetic heart valve disorders, including pannus and thrombus formation as well as opening and closing angles (Figure 8-10).[88,89] CT also allows visualization of bioprosthetic aortic valve leaflets and provides morphologic and functional information regarding the mechanism underlying dysfunction of bioprosthetic valves. One study demonstrated that direct planimetric assessment of prosthetic valve orifice

correlates well with TTE–continuity equation valve area determinations.[90] Finally, heterografts and homografts can be evaluated completely by CT, including the distal anastomosis and the patency of the coronary arteries if these were reimplanted.

Infective Endocarditis

The diagnosis of infective endocarditis relies on the visualization of vegetations, for which TTE and TEE are usually superior to CT because vegetations are often mobile and thus require imaging at high temporal resolution. However, CT can be particularly useful in the demonstration of paravalvular abscesses as fluid-filled collections (Figure 8-11).[91] In a study of 19 consecutive patients who underwent aortic valve replacement for endocarditis, the sensitivity, specificity, positive predictive value, and negative predictive value of CT for detecting aortic valve vegetations is suboptimal at 71.4%, 100%, 100%, and 55.5%, respectively. On the other hand, the sensitivity, specificity, positive predictive value, and negative predictive value of CT for depicting aortic valve pseudoaneurysms is excellent at 100%, 87.5%, 91.7%, and 100%, respectively.[92] Aortic valve vegetations and complications of endocarditis may be recognized on CMR in some patients.[93,94]

Coronary Artery Disease in Patients with Valvular Heart Disease

The most common primary indication for CT is the assessment of the coronary arteries. CT coronary angiography is accurate for excluding the diagnosis of coronary artery disease, with slightly

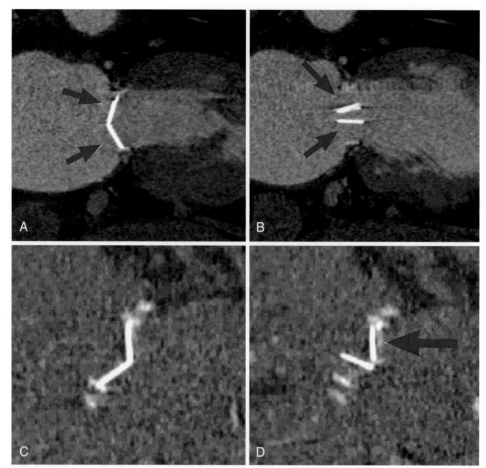

FIGURE 8-10 Mitral mechanical prosthetic valve. Cine cardiac computed tomography images show a normal bileaflet mechanical mitral prosthesis in the closed position at end-systole **(A)** and open **(B)** position with the leaflet positions showing full motion of the leaflet occluders. In a patient with a malfunctioning mechanical aortic prosthesis valve closure is normal at end-diastole **(C)** but the systolic image **(D)** shows a "frozen" disk (*arrow*).

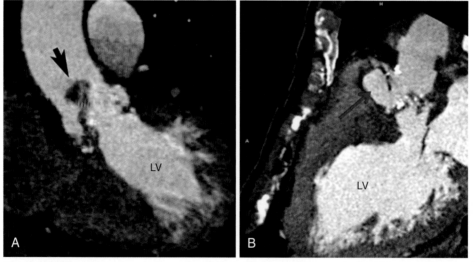

FIGURE 8-11 Prosthetic valve endocarditis. Long-axis cine cardiac computed tomography images obtained from two different patients with bioprosthetic valves with a large vegetation (*arrow*, **A**) and an abscess cavity (*arrow*, **B**). *LV*, left ventricle.

lower diagnostic yield in patients with AS because of the frequent coexistence of both aortic and coronary calcifications.[95,96] These studies have demonstrated high negative predictive value but low positive predictive value for the CT detection of significant coronary stenosis. Thus, patients who have been referred for surgical repair of valvular lesions and in whom absence of significant coronary stenosis is demonstrated by CT may safely avoid invasive coronary angiography. On the other hand, patients who seem to have more than a mild degree of luminal stenosis or extensive calcifications need to undergo confirmatory catheterization. In a study that enrolled 133 consecutive patients undergoing noncoronary cardiovascular surgery, CT was diagnostic in 108 (81%). In this study, patients in whom CT was nondiagnostic had significantly higher Agatston calcium scores

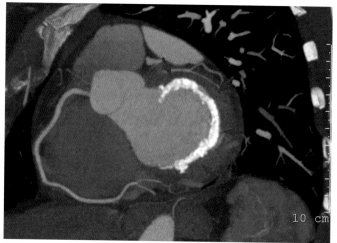

FIGURE 8-12 Mitral annular calcification. Mitral annular calcification. Sagittal cardiac computed tomography image demonstrating a normal right coronary artery and extensive annular calcification (*arrows*) in a patient with mitral valve prolapse obtained before repair surgery.

(1089, range 505-2305) than those with diagnostic CT (Agatston calcium score 10, range 0-218; P <0.001). Among patients with diagnostic evaluations, 93 of 108 had no significant CAD.[97] For this reason, it is prudent to consider CT for this application only in selected patients with low or intermediate pretest probability of having obstructive coronary artery disease. (Figure 8-12; Table 8-3), such as younger patients with mitral valve disease. In patients with aortic valve endocarditis and highly mobile vegetations, CT offers an alternative to invasive coronary angiography.

Summary

CMR and CT imaging are useful and complementary methods for the evaluation of valvular disease. However, the limitations of these techniques need to be considered in selection of patients who may derive a benefit. In CMR, choosing the correct value for the velocity-encoding gradient is important because the range must be appropriate to encompass the expected peak velocities. If the value is set too low, the peak gradient may be underestimated. Conversely, when the value is set too high, sensitivity for slow flow is reduced. Selecting the correct plane of interrogation is important, because the maximal velocity is detected at a specific spatial location and in a plane perpendicular to the direction of flow. High spatial and temporal resolutions are important to localize the peak velocity. Improved spatial resolution can be achieved by decreasing the field of view or increasing the acquisition matrix. Temporal resolution is much lower than in Doppler echocardiography; thus, peak velocities may occasionally be underestimated by CMR. CMR, however, has the advantage of not being limited to specific acoustic windows for interrogation, which is the main limitation of Doppler echocardiography. CMR and CT are superior to echocardiography for the assessment of ventricular function and aortic dimensions. CT is also emerging as an important tool for the evaluation and guidance of transcatheter valve procedures, given its ability to provide detailed information about the cardiac and vascular anatomy.

REFERENCES

1. Barkhausen J, Ruehm SG, Goyen M, et al. MR evaluation of ventricular function: true fast imaging with steady-state free precession versus fast low-angle shot cine MR imaging: feasibility study. Radiology 2001;219:264–9.
2. Bellenger NG, Burgess MI, Ray SG, et al. Comparison of left ventricular ejection fraction and volumes in heart failure by echocardiography, radionuclide ventriculography and cardiovascular magnetic resonance. Are they interchangeable? Eur Heart J 2000;21:1387–96.
3. Grothues F, Smith GC, Moon JC, et al. Comparison of interstudy reproducibility of cardiovascular magnetic resonance with two-dimensional echocardiography in normal subjects and in patients with heart failure or left ventricular hypertrophy. Am J Cardiol 2002;90:29–34.
4. Møgelvang J, Stockholm KH, Saunamäki K, et al. Assessment of left ventricular volumes by magnetic resonance in comparison with radionuclide angiography, contrast angiography and echocardiography. Eur Heart J 1992;13:1677–83.
5. Markiewicz W, Sechtem U, Kirby R, et al. Measurement of ventricular volumes in the dog by nuclear magnetic resonance imaging. J Am Coll Cardiol 1987;10:170–7.
6. Katz J, Milliken MC, Stray-Gundersen J, et al. Estimation of human myocardial mass with MR imaging. Radiology 1988;169:495–8.
7. Ostrzega E, Maddahi J, Honma H, et al. Quantification of left ventricular myocardial mass in humans by nuclear magnetic resonance imaging. Am Heart J 1989;117:444–52.
8. Keller AM, Peshock RM, Malloy CR, et al. In vivo measurement of myocardial mass using nuclear magnetic resonance imaging. J Am Coll Cardiol 1986;8:113–7.
9. Shapiro EP, Rogers WJ, Beyar R, et al. Determination of left ventricular mass by magnetic resonance imaging in hearts deformed by acute infarction. Circulation 1989;79:706–11.
10. Semelka RC, Tomei E, Wagner S, et al. Normal left ventricular dimensions and function: interstudy reproducibility of measurements with cine MR imaging. Ann Thorac Surg 1990;174:763–8.
11. Young AA, Orr R, Smaill BH, et al. Three-dimensional changes in left and right ventricular geometry in chronic mitral regurgitation. Am J Physiol 1996;271:H2689–700.
12. Doherty III NE, Seelos KC, Suzuki J, et al. Application of cine nuclear magnetic resonance imaging for sequential evaluation of response to angiotensin-converting enzyme inhibitor therapy in dilated cardiomyopathy. J Am Coll Cardiol 1992;19:1294–302.
13. Bellenger NG, Davies LC, Francis JM, et al. Reduction in sample size for studies of remodeling in heart failure by the use of cardiovascular magnetic resonance. J Cardiovasc Magn Reson 2000;2:271–8.
14. Bellenger NG, Rajappan K, Rahman SL, et al. Effects of carvedilol on left ventricular remodeling in chronic stable heart failure: a cardiovascular magnetic resonance study. Heart 2004;90:760–4.
15. Auffermann W, Wagner S, Holt WW, et al. Noninvasive determination of left ventricular output and wall stress in volume overload and in myocardial disease by cine magnetic resonance imaging. Am Heart J 1991;121:1750–8.
16. Rumberger JA, Reiring AJ, Rees MR, et al. Quantitation of left ventricular mass and volume in normal patients using cine computed tomography. J Am Coll Cardiol 1986;7:173.
17. Orazkai SH, Orazkai RH, Nasir K, et al. Assessment of cardiac function using multidetector row computed tomography. J Comput Assist Tomogr 2006;30:555–63.
18. Rihal CS, Nishimura RA, Rumberger JA, et al. Quantitative echocardiography: a comparison with ultrafast computed tomography in patients with chronic aortic regurgitation. J Heart Valve Dis 1994;3:417–24.
19. Karwatowski SP, Brecker SJ, Yang GZ, et al. A comparison of left ventricular myocardial velocity in diastole measured by magnetic resonance and left ventricular filling measured by Doppler echocardiography. Eur Heart J 1996;17:795–802.
20. Kim WY, Walker PG, Pedersen EM, et al. Left ventricular blood flow patterns in normal subjects: a quantitative analysis by three-dimensional magnetic resonance velocity mapping. J Am Coll Cardiol 1995;26:224–38.
21. Hartiala JJ, Mostbeck GH, Foster E, et al. Velocity-encoded cine MRI in the evaluation of left ventricular diastolic function: measurement of mitral valve and pulmonary vein flow velocities and flow volume across the mitral valve. Am Heart J 1993;125:1054–66.
22. Hartiala JJ, Foster E, Fujita N, et al. Evaluation of left atrial contribution to left ventricular filling in aortic stenosis by velocity-encoded cine MRI. Am Heart J 1994;127:593–600.
23. Grothues F, Moon JC, Bellenger NG, et al. Interstudy reproducibility of right ventricular volumes, function, and mass with cardiovascular magnetic resonance. Am Heart J 2004;147:218–23.
24. Pattynama PM, Lamb HJ, Van der Velde EA, et al. Reproducibility of MRI-derived measurements of right ventricular volumes and myocardial mass. Magn Reson Imaging 1995;13:53–63.
25. Markiewicz W, Sechtem U, Higgins CB. Evaluation of the right ventricle by magnetic resonance imaging. Am Heart J 1987;113:8–15.
26. Møgelvang J, Stubgaard M, Thomsen C, et al. Evaluation of right ventricular volumes measured by magnetic resonance imaging. Eur Heart J 1988;9:529–33.
27. Doherty NE, Fujita N, Caputo GR, et al. Measurement of right ventricular mass in normal and dilated cardiomyopathic ventricles using cine magnetic resonance imaging. Am J Cardiol 1992;69:1223–8.
28. Mackey ES, Sandler MP, Campbell RM, et al. Right ventricular myocardial mass quantification with magnetic resonance imaging. Am J Cardiol 1990;65:529–32.
29. Helbing WA, de Roos A. Clinical applications of cardiac magnetic resonance imaging after repair of tetralogy of Fallot. Pediatr Cardiol 2000;21:70–9.
30. Helbing WA, de Roos A. Optimal imaging in assessment of right ventricular function in tetralogy of Fallot with pulmonary regurgitation. Am J Cardiol 1998;82:1561–2.
31. Garcia-Alvarez A, Fernandez-Friera L, Lau JF, et al. Evaluation of right ventricular function and post-operative findings using cardiac computed tomography in patients with left ventricular assist devices. J Heart Lung Transplant 2011;30(8):896–903.
32. Evans AJ, Blinder RA, Herfkens RJ, et al. Effects of turbulence on signal intensity in gradient echo images. Invest Radiol 1988;23:512–8.
33. Globits S, Higgins CB. Assessment of valvular heart disease by magnetic resonance imaging. Am Heart J 1995;129:369–81.
34. Søndergaard L, Stahlberg F, Thomsen C, et al. Accuracy and precision of MR velocity mapping in measurement of stenotic cross-sectional area, flow rate, and pressure gradient. J Magn Reson Imaging 1993;3:433–7.
35. Danielsen R, Nordrehaug JE, Vik-Mo H. Factors affecting Doppler echocardiographic valve area assessment in aortic stenosis. Am J Cardiol 1989;63:1107–11.
36. John AS, Dill T, Brandt RR, et al. Magnetic resonance to assess the aortic valve area in aortic stenosis: how does it compare to current diagnostic standards? J Am Coll Cardiol 2003;42:519–26.

37. Koos R, Mahnken AH, Kuhl HP, et al. Quantification of aortic valve calcification using multislice spiral computed tomography: comparison with atomic absorption spectroscopy. Invest Radiol 2006;41:485–9.

38. Messika-Zeitoun D, Aubry M-C, Detaint D, et al. Evaluation and clinical implications of aortic valve calcification measured by electron-beam computed tomography. Circulation 2004;110:356–62.

39. Budoff MJ, Takasu J, Katz R, et al. Reproducibility of CT measurements of aortic valve calcification, mitral annulus calcification, and aortic wall calcification in the multiethnic study of atherosclerosis. Acad Radiol 2006;13:166–72.

40. Alkadhi H, Wildermuth S, Plass A, et al. Aortic stenosis: comparative evaluation of 16-detector row CT and echocardiography. Radiology 2006;240:47–55.

41. Feuchtner GM, Dichtl W, Friedrich GJ, et al. Multislice computed tomography for detection of patients with aortic valve stenosis and quantification of severity. J Am Coll Cardiol 2006;47:1410–7.

42. Iung B, Cachier A, Baron G, et al. Decision-making in elderly patients with severe aortic stenosis: why are so many denied surgery? Eur Heart J 2005;26:2714–20.

43. Vahanian A, Alfieri O, Al-Attar N, et al. European Association of Cardio-Thoracic Surgery; European Society of Cardiology; European Association of Percutaneous Cardiovascular Interventions. Transcatheter valve implantation for patients with aortic stenosis: a position statement from the European Association of Cardio-Thoracic Surgery (EACTS) and the European Society of Cardiology (ESC), in collaboration with the European Association of Percutaneous Cardiovascular Interventions (EAPCI). Eur Heart J 2008;29:1463–70.

44. Tops LF, Wood DA, Delgado V, et al. Noninvasive evaluation of the aortic root with multislice computed tomography: implications for transcatheter aortic valve replacement. JACC Cardiovasc Imaging 2008;1:321–30.

45. Tanaka R, Yoshioka K, Niinuma H, et al. Diagnostic value of cardiac CT in the evaluation of bicuspid aortic stenosis: comparison with echocardiography and operative findings. Am J Roentgenol 2010;195:895–9.

46. John D, Buellesfeld L, Yuecel S, et al. Correlation of device landing zone calcification and acute procedural success in patients undergoing transcatheter aortic valve implantations with the self-expanding CoreValve prosthesis. JACC Cardiovasc Interv 2010;3:233–43.

47. Delgado V, Ng ACT, Van de Veire NR, et al. Transcatheter aortic valve implantation: role of multidetector row computed tomography to evaluate prosthesis positioning and deployment in relation to valve function. Eur Heart J 2010;31:1114–23.

48. Webb JG, Chandavimol M, Thompson CR, et al. Percutaneous aortic valve implantation retrograde from the femoral artery. Circulation 2006;113:842–50.

49. Casolo GC, Zampa V, Rega L, et al. Evaluation of mitral stenosis by cine magnetic resonance imaging. Am Heart J 1992;123:1252–60.

50. Kilner PJ, Manzara CC, Mohiaddin RH, et al. Magnetic resonance jet velocity mapping in mitral and aortic valve stenosis. Circulation 1993;87:1239–48.

51. Heidenreich PA, Steffens J, Fujita N, et al. Evaluation of mitral stenosis with velocity encoded cine-magnetic resonance imaging. Am J Cardiol 1995;75:365–9.

52. Lin SJ, Brown PA, Watkins MP, et al. Quantification of stenotic mitral valve area with magnetic resonance imaging and comparison with Doppler ultrasound. J Am Coll Cardiol 2004;44:133–7.

53. White ML, Grover MM, Weiss RM, et al. Prediction of change in mitral valve area after mitral balloon commissurotomy using cine computed tomography. Invest Radiol 1994;29:827–33.

54. Messika-Zeitoun D, Serfaty JM, Laissy JP, et al. Assessment of the mitral valve area in patients with mitral stenosis by multislice computed tomography. J Am Coll Cardiol 2006;48:411–3.

55. Mirowitz SA, Gutierrez FR. MR and CT diagnosis of carcinoid heart disease. Chest 1993;103:630–1.

56. Schievano S, Coats L, Migliavacca F, et al. Variations in right ventricular outflow tract morphology following repair of congenital heart disease: implications for percutaneous pulmonary valve implantation. J Cardiovasc Magn Reson 2007;9:687–95.

57. Sondergaard L, Lindvig K, Hildebrandt P, et al. Quantification of aortic regurgitation by magnetic resonance velocity mapping. Am Heart J 1993;125:1081–90.

58. Ambrosi P, Faugere G, Desfossez L, et al. Assessment of aortic regurgitation severity by magnetic resonance imaging of the thoracic aorta. Eur Heart J 1995;16:406–9.

59. Honda N, Machida K, Hashimoto M, et al. Aortic regurgitation: quantitation with MR imaging velocity mapping. Radiology 1993;186:189–94.

60. Kizilbash AM, Hundley WG, Willett DL, et al. Comparison of quantitative Doppler with magnetic resonance imaging for assessment of the severity of mitral regurgitation. Am J Cardiol 1998;81:792–5.

61. Hundley WG, Hong FL, Willard JE, et al. Magnetic resonance imaging assessment of the severity of mitral regurgitation: comparison with invasive techniques. Circulation 1995;92:1151–8.

62. Wagner S, Auffermann W, Buser P, et al. Diagnostic accuracy and estimation of the severity of valvular regurgitation from the signal void on cine magnetic resonance images. Am Heart J 1989;118:760–7.

63. Aurigemma G, Reichek N, Schiebler M, et al. Evaluation of aortic regurgitation by cardiac cine magnetic resonance imaging: planar analysis and comparison to Doppler echocardiography. Cardiology 1991;78:340–7.

64. Yoshida K, Yoshikawa J, Hozumi T, et al. Assessment of aortic regurgitation by the acceleration flow signal void proximal to the leaking orifice in cinemagnetic resonance imaging. Circulation 1991;83:1951–5.

65. Cranney GB, Benjelloun H, Perry GJ, et al. Rapid assessment of aortic regurgitation and left ventricular function using cine nuclear magnetic resonance imaging and the proximal convergence zone. Am J Cardiol 1993;71:1074–81.

66. Sechtem U, Pflugfelder PW, Gould RG, et al. Measurement of right and left ventricular volumes in healthy individuals with cine MR imaging. Radiology 1987;163:697–702.

67. Lorenz CH, Walker ES, Morgan VL, et al. Normal human right and left ventricular mass, systolic function, and gender differences by cine magnetic resonance imaging. J Cardiovasc Magn Reson 1999;1:7–21.

68. Sechtem U, Pflugfelder PW, Cassidy MM, et al. Mitral or aortic regurgitation: quantification of regurgitant volumes with cine MR imaging. Ann Thorac Surg 1988;167:425–30.

69. Underwood SR, Klipstein RH, Firmin DN, et al. Magnetic resonance assessment of aortic and mitral regurgitation. Br Heart J 1986;56:455–62.

70. Sechtem U, Pflugfelder PW, Cassidy MM, et al. Mitral or aortic regurgitation: quantification of regurgitant volumes with cine MR imaging. Radiology 1988;167:425–30.

71. Fujita N, Chazouilleres AF, Hartiala JJ, et al. Quantification of mitral regurgitation by velocity-encoded cine nuclear magnetic resonance imaging. J Am Coll Cardiol 1994;23:951–8.

72. Reiter SJ, Rumberger JA, Stanford W, et al. Quantitative determination of aortic regurgitant volumes in dogs by ultrafast computed tomography. Circulation 1987;76:728–35.

73. Ambrosi P, Faugere G, Desfossez L, et al. Assessment of aortic regurgitation severity by magnetic resonance imaging of the thoracic aorta. Eur Heart J 1995;16:406–9.

74. Bogren HG, Klipstein RH, Firmin DN, et al. Quantitation of antegrade and retrograde blood flow in the human aorta by magnetic resonance velocity mapping. Am Heart J 1989;117:1214–22.

75. Chatzimavroudis GP, Oshinski JN, Franch RH, et al. Quantification of the aortic regurgitant volume with magnetic resonance phase velocity mapping: a clinical investigation of the importance of imaging slice location. J Heart Valve Dis 1998;7:94–101.

76. Dulce MC, Mostbeck GH, O'Sullivan M, et al. Severity of aortic regurgitation: interstudy reproducibility of measurements with velocity-encoded cine MR imaging. Radiology 1992;185:235–40.

77. Globits S, Blake L, Bourne M, et al. Assessment of hemodynamic effects of angiotensin-converting enzyme inhibitor therapy in chronic aortic regurgitation by using velocity-encoded cine magnetic resonance imaging. Am Heart J 1996;131:289–93.

78. Jeon MH, Choe YH, Cho SJ, et al. Multidetector CT for aortic regurgitation: a comparison with the use of echocardiography. Korean J Radiol 2010;11:169–77.

79. Yu HY, Su MY, Liao TY, et al. Functional mitral regurgitation in chronic ischemic coronary artery disease: analysis of geometric alterations of mitral apparatus with magnetic resonance imaging. J Thorac Cardiovasc Surg 2004;128:543–51.

80. Kaji S, Nasu M, Yamamuro A, et al. Annular geometry in patients with chronic ischemic mitral regurgitation: three-dimensional magnetic resonance imaging study. Circulation 2005;112:409–14.

81. Srichai MB, Grimm RA, Stillman AE, et al. Ischemic mitral regurgitation: impact of the left ventricle and mitral valve in patients with left ventricular systolic dysfunction. Ann Thorac Surg 2005;80:170–8.

82. Alkadhi H, Wildermuth S, Bettex DA, et al. Mitral regurgitation: quantification with 16-detector row CT—initial experience. Radiology 2005;238:454–63.

83. Rebergen SA, Chin JGJ, Ottenkamp J, et al. Pulmonary regurgitation in the late postoperative follow-up of tetralogy of Fallot: volumetric quantitation by nuclear magnetic resonance velocity mapping. Circulation 1993;88:2257–66.

84. Collins MA, Pidgeon JW, Fitzgerald R. Computed tomography manifestations of tricuspid regurgitation. Br J Radiol 1995;68:1058–60.

85. Shellock FG, Crues JV. MR procedures: biologic effects, safety, and patient care. Radiology 2004;232:635–52.

86. Deutsch HJ, Bachmann R, Sechtem U, et al. Regurgitant flow in cardiac valve prostheses: diagnostic value of gradient echo nuclear magnetic resonance imaging in reference to transesophageal two-dimensional color Doppler echocardiography. J Am Coll Cardiol 1992;19:1500–7.

87. Di Cesare E, Enrici RM, Paparoni S, et al. Low-field magnetic resonance imaging in the evaluation of mechanical and biological heart valve function. Eur J Radiol 1995;20:224–8.

88. Teshima H, Hayashida N, Fukunaga S, et al. Usefulness of a multidetector-row computed tomography scanner for detecting pannus formation. Ann Thorac Surg 2004;77:523–6.

89. Konen E, Goitein O, Feinberg MS, et al. The role of ECG-gated MDCT in the evaluation of aortic and mitral mechanical valves: initial experience. AJR Am J Roentgenol 2008;191:26–31.

90. Chenot F, Montant P, Goffinet C, et al. Evaluation of anatomic valve opening and leaflet morphology in aortic valve bioprosthesis by using multidetector CT: comparison with transthoracic echocardiography. Radiology 2010;255:377–85.

91. Gilkeson RC, Markowitz AH, Balgude A, et al. MDCT evaluation of aortic valvular disease. AJR Am J Roentgenol 2006;186:350–60.

92. Gahide G, Bommart S, Demaria R, et al. Preoperative evaluation in aortic endocarditis: findings on cardiac CT. Am J Roentgen 2010;194:574–8.

93. Caduff JH, Hernandez RJ, Ludomirsky A. MR visualization of aortic valve vegetations. J Comput Assist Tomogr 1996;20:613–5.

94. Winkler ML, Higgins CB. MRI of perivalvular infectious pseudoaneurysms. AJR Am J Roentgenol 1986;147:253–6.

95. Meijboom WB, Mollet NR, Van Mieghem CA, et al. Pre-operative computed tomography coronary angiography to detect significant coronary artery disease in patients referred for cardiac valve surgery. J Am Coll Cardiol 2006;48:1658–65.

96. Gilard M, Cornily J-C, Pennec P-Y, et al. Accuracy of multislice computed tomography in the preoperative assessment of coronary disease in patients with aortic valve stenosis. J Am Coll Cardiol 2006;47:2020–4.

97. Catalán P, Leta R, Hidalgo A, et al. Ruling Out Coronary Artery Disease with Noninvasive Coronary Multidetector CT Angiography before Noncoronary Cardiovascular Surgery. Radiology 2011;258:426–34.

CHAPTER 9

Basic Principles of Medical Therapy in the Patient with Valvular Heart Disease

Catherine M. Otto

> ### Key Points
>
> - Patients with valvular heart disease are best cared for in the context of a multidisciplinary Heart Valve Clinic.
> - Many adverse outcomes in adults with valvular heart disease are due to sequelae of the disease process, including atrial fibrillation, embolic events, left ventricular (LV) dysfunction, pulmonary hypertension, and endocarditis.
> - Medical therapy in adults with valvular heart disease focuses on prevention and treatment of complications because there are no specific therapies to prevent progression of the valve disease itself.
> - Endocarditis prophylaxis guidelines recommend antibiotics therapy before dental procedures, or other procedures associated with bacteremia, in adults with prosthetic valves but not in patients with native valve disease.
> - Periodic evaluation of disease severity and the LV response to chronic volume and/or pressure overload allows optimal timing of surgical and percutaneous interventions.
> - General health maintenance is important, including evaluation and treatment of coronary disease risk factors, regular exercise, standard immunizations, and optimal dental care.
> - Management of concurrent cardiovascular disease follows standard approaches with modification, as needed, based on the potential confounding effects of valve hemodynamics.
> - In patients with valvular disease undergoing noncardiac surgery, management focuses on an accurate assessment of disease severity and symptom status, with appropriate hemodynamic monitoring and optimization of loading conditions in the perioperative period.
> - Evaluation of coronary anatomy usually is needed before valve surgery because of the high prevalence of coronary disease and improved surgical outcomes with concurrent coronary revascularization.

The Heart Valve Clinic

In patients with valvular heart disease, the basic principles of management are to:
- Obtain an accurate diagnosis of the specific valvular lesion and quantitative disease severity using Doppler echocardiography and other advanced imaging modalities
- Prevent complications of the disease process, such as endocarditis, atrial fibrillation (AF), and embolic events
- Periodically reevaluate ventricular size and function to identify early ventricular dysfunction and optimize the timing of surgical or percutaneous intervention
- Provide optimal management of associated conditions

- Provide patient education regarding the disease process, expected outcomes, and potential medical or surgical therapies

These goals are best met with an interdisciplinary health-care team structured as a Heart Valve Clinic. Valvular heart disease is relatively uncommon in comparison with other cardiac conditions, such as coronary disease, heart failure, and AF, so general cardiologists often have little experience in managing the complex care that patients with valvular heart disease need. Data from the Euro Heart Surveys shows that many patients are not treated according to current guidelines—some patients are inappropriately denied interventions that would improve survival and quality of life; others undergo intervention earlier in the disease course than necessary.[1] In addition, optimal decision making requires input from cardiologists with expertise in valve disease, interventional cardiologists, imaging specialists, and cardiovascular surgeons. The European Society of Cardiology has published a position paper on the need for Heart Valve Clinics with specific recommendations for goals (Table 9-1), patient population, clinic structure (Figure 9-1), and the tasks for each member of the Heart Valve Clinic team.[2]

Diagnosis of Valve Disease

Valvular heart disease may first be diagnosed in the setting of an acute medical event, such as heart failure, pulmonary edema, AF, or infective endocarditis. More often, the diagnosis of valvular heart disease is initially suspected prior to the onset of overt symptoms on the basis of the physical examination finding of a cardiac murmur, during screening of relatives in a family with a history of a genetic disorder, or because of abnormal findings on an electrocardiograph, chest radiograph, or echocardiogram requested for unrelated reasons. Worldwide, many patients are first diagnosed with valvular heart disease when a cardiac murmur is heard during an episode of acute rheumatic fever.

In patients with a cardiac murmur, the first step is clinical assessment based on the history and physical examination.[3,4] If clinical evaluation indicates a high likelihood of significant valvular disease, the next step is echocardiography to confirm the diagnosis and evaluate valve anatomy and function.[5,6] A condensed version of indications for echocardiography in patients with suspected or known valve disease is shown in Table 9-2.[7]

In a patient with cardiac or respiratory symptoms and a cardiac murmur on auscultation, it is prudent to obtain an echocardiogram to evaluate for possible valvular disease. When symptoms are present, it is difficult to reliably exclude significant valvular disease with physical examination because findings may be subtle.[8] For example, some patients with severe aortic stenosis (AS) have only a grade 2 or 3 murmur on examination and the carotid upstroke may appear normal because of coexisting atherosclerosis.[9-11] Diagnosis may be even more difficult in other situations. For example, only 50% of patients with acute mitral regurgitation (MR) have an audible murmur.[12]

In *asymptomatic* patients with a murmur on physical examination, those with a benign flow murmur should be distinguished from those with a pathologic murmur.[13] Although there are no absolutely reliable criteria for making this distinction, a reasonable estimate of the pretest likelihood of disease can be derived from the history and physical examination findings. Flow

murmurs, defined as audible systolic murmurs in the absence of structural heart disease, are most common in younger patients and those with high-output states. Thus, a flow murmur is a normal finding in pregnancy, being appreciated in more than 80% of pregnant women.[5,6] Flow murmurs also are likely in patients who are anemic or febrile. Typically a flow murmur is systolic, of low intensity (grade 1 to 2) and loudest at the base with little radiation, ends before the second heart sound, and has a crescendo-decrescendo or "ejection" shape with an early systolic peak. Flow murmurs are related to rapid ejection into the aorta or pulmonary artery in patients with normal valve function, high flow rates, and good transmission of sound to the chest wall.[4,14] The yield of echocardiography is very low in asymptomatic patients with a typical flow murmur on examination, no history of cardiac problems, and no cardiac symptoms on careful questioning.

In contrast, echocardiographic examination usually is appropriate in asymptomatic patients with a diastolic or continuous murmur, a systolic murmur of grade 3 or higher, an ejection click or midsystolic click, a holosystolic (rather than ejection) murmur, or an atypical pattern of radiation, even if the patient is asymptomatic. To some extent, the loudness of the murmur correlates with disease severity but is not reliable for decision making in an individual patient.[15,16] Echocardiography allows differentiation of valve disease from a flow murmur, identification of the specific valve involved, definition of the etiology of valve disease, and quantitation of the hemodynamic severity of the lesion along with LV size and function. On the basis of these data, the expected prognosis, need for preventive measures, and timing of subsequent examinations (if any) can be determined.

In older adults, distinguishing a benign from a pathologic murmur is more difficult than in younger patients, because many older patients have some degree of aortic valve sclerosis or mild MR that can be appreciated on auscultation, and many also have mild symptoms that may or may not be related to heart disease.[10,17-19] In this setting, a baseline echocardiogram may be prudent. The finding of aortic sclerosis is associated with an increased risk of adverse cardiovascular events, and some patients have progressive valve obstruction. A soft mitral regurgitant murmur is most likely associated with mild to moderate regurgitation due to mitral annular calcification, but establishing the diagnosis with a baseline echocardiogram and excluding

TABLE 9-1 Specific Aims of the Heart Valve Clinic

- To improve the outcome of patients with valvular heart disease (VHD)
- To ensure optimal communication and coordination among all health-care professionals involved in the management of the patient with VHD
- To perform or coordinate relevant diagnostic tests to obtain a complete evaluation of the severity of VHD and its implications for symptomatic status, cardiac function, and risk of future adverse events
- To ensure rational utilization of diagnostic tests according to the recommendations of international guidelines
- To standardize and centralize the collection and interpretation of the results of these tests and provide all health-care professionals involved in management of the patient with complete and accurate information concerning the diagnosis and prognosis of VHD
- To optimize patient education concerning compliance with medical therapy and prompt reporting of symptoms relating to VHD
- To assist the general cardiologist with regard to prescription of appropriate pharmacologic treatment and determination of the most appropriate timing for clinical evaluation, imaging, exercise testing, and follow-up before and after valve procedures
- To assist the general cardiologist in the determination of the optimal timing and mode of intervention
- To enhance adherence to international guidelines for the evaluation and management of patients with VHD

From Lancellotti P, Rosenhek R, Pibarot P, et al; ESC Working Group on Valvular Heart Disease Position Paper—heart valve clinics: organization, structure, and experiences. Eur Heart J 2013;Jan 4.

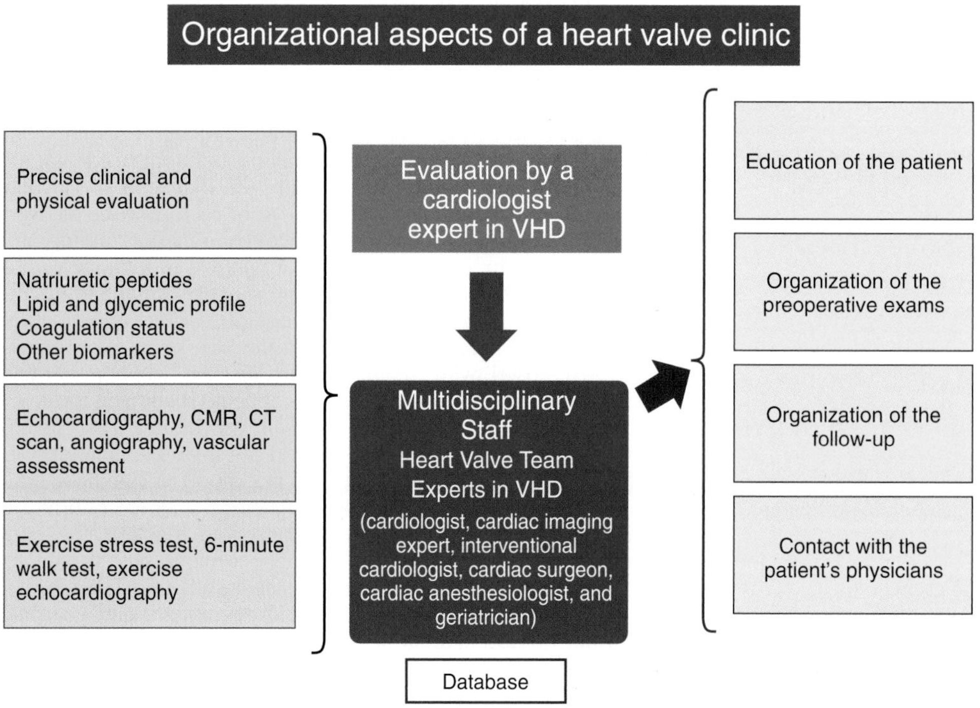

FIGURE 9-1 Functioning of the advanced heart valve clinic. CMR, cardiac magnetic resonance; CT, computed tomography; Echo, echocardiography; VHD, valvular heart disease. (From Lancellotti P, Rosenhek R, Pibarot P, et al. ESC Working Group on Valvular Heart Disease Position Paper—heart valve clinics: organization, structure, and experiences. Eur Heart J 2013;Jan 4. [Epub ahead of print])

TABLE 9-2	Indications for Echocardiography in Adults with Suspected or Known Valvular Heart Disease

Suspected Valvular Disease

- Cardiac murmur in a patient with cardiorespiratory symptoms
- Murmur suggestive of structural heart disease, even if asymptomatic:
  - Diastolic murmur
  - Continuous murmur
  - Holosystolic or late systolic murmur
  - Murmur associated with an ejection click or radiation to neck or back
  - Grade 3 or louder midpeaking systolic murmur

Native Valve Disease

- Stenosis:
  - Initial diagnosis and assessment of hemodynamic severity
  - Assessment of left and right ventricular size, function, and hemodynamics
  - Reevaluation for changing signs or symptoms
  - Assessment of changes in valve or ventricular function during pregnancy
  - Periodic reevaluation as shown in Table 9-10
  - Assessment of pulmonary pressures with exercise in patients with mitral stenosis when there is a discrepancy between symptoms and resting hemodynamics
  - TEE before balloon mitral valvotomy in patients with mitral stenosis
- Regurgitation:
  - Initial diagnosis and assessment of hemodynamic severity
  - Initial evaluation of left and right ventricular size, function, and hemodynamics
  - Assessment of aortic regurgitation when aortic root enlargement is present
  - Reevaluation with a change in symptoms
  - Periodic reevaluation even in asymptomatic patients, as in Table 9-10
  - Reassessment of valve and ventricular function during pregnancy
- Mitral valve prolapse:
  - Assessment of leaflet morphology, hemodynamic severity, and ventricular compensation
- Infective endocarditis*:
  - Detection of valvular vegetations with or without positive blood culture results
  - Characterization of hemodynamic severity with known endocarditis
  - Detection of complications, such as abscesses, fistulas, and shunts
  - Reevaluation in high-risk patients (virulent organism, clinical deterioration, persistent or recurrent fever, new murmur, persistent bacteremia)

Interventions for Valvular Disease

- Selection of alternate therapies for mitral valve disease (balloon mitral valvotomy, surgical valve repair vs. replacement)*
- Monitoring interventional techniques in the catheterization laboratory (3D TEE, ICE, or TTE)
- Intraoperative TEE for valve repair surgery
- Intraoperative TEE for stentless bioprosthetic, homograft, or autograft valve replacement surgery
- Intraoperative TEE for valve surgery of infective endocarditis

Prosthetic Valves

- Baseline postoperative study (at hospital discharge or 6-8 weeks)
- Annual evaluation of bioprosthetic valves after 5 years of implantation
- Changing clinical signs and symptoms or suspected prosthetic valve dysfunction*
- Prosthetic valve endocarditis:
  - Detection of endocarditis and characterization of valve and ventricular function
  - Detection of endocarditis complications and reevaluation in complex endocarditis*
  - Persistent fever without bacteremia or a new murmur*
  - Bacteremia without known source*

ICE, intracardiac echocardiography; *TEE,* transesophageal echocardiography; *TTE,* transthoracic echocardiography; *3D,* three dimensional.
* Transesophageal echocardiography usually required.
Summarized and updated from Bonow RO, Carabello BA, Chatterjee K, et al. ACC/AHA 2006 guidelines for the management of patients with valvular heart disease: a report of the American College of Cardiology/American Heart Association Task Force on Practice Guidelines (writing Committee to Revise the 1998 guidelines for the management of patients with valvular heart disease) developed in collaboration with the Society of Cardiovascular Anesthesiologists endorsed by the Society for Cardiovascular Angiography and Interventions and the Society of Thoracic Surgeons. J Am Coll Cardiol 2006;48:e1–148.

TABLE 9-3	Updated Jones Criteria for the Diagnosis of Initial Attacks of Rheumatic Fever

Major Criteria

- Carditis (may involve endocardium, myocardium, and pericardium)
- Polyarthritis (most frequent manifestation, usually migratory)
- Chorea (documentation of recent Group A streptococcal infection may be difficult)
- Erythema marginatum (distinctive, evanescent rash on trunk and proximal extremities)
- Subcutaneous nodules (firm, painless nodules on extensor surfaces of elbows, knees, and wrists)

Minor Criteria

- Clinical findings (arthralgia, fever)
- Laboratory findings (elevation of erythrocyte sedimentation rate or C-reactive protein)
- Electrocardiography (prolonged PR interval)

Evidence of Antecedent Group A Streptococcal Infection

- Positive throat culture or rapid streptococci antigen test result
- Elevated or rising streptococcal antibody titer

High Probability of Rheumatic Fever

Evidence of preceding Group A Streptococcal infection
PLUS
2 major criteria OR 1 major and 2 minor criteria

Modified from Guidelines for the diagnosis of rheumatic fever: Jones Criteria, 1992 update (in Circulation 1993;87:302–7) as updated in Ferrieri P. Jones Criteria Working Group. Proceedings of the Jones Criteria workshop. Circulation 2002;106:2521–153.

other causes of MR, such as ischemic disease and mitral valve prolapse, is appropriate.

Although echocardiography is the primary diagnostic modality used for evaluation of valve disease, cardiac magnetic resonance (CMR) imaging and computed tomography (CT) are useful in some cases, as discussed in Chapter 8. Diagnostic cardiac catheterization continues to be useful in selected patients, particularly when echocardiographic data are nondiagnostic or discrepant with other clinical data, as discussed in Chapter 7.

Preventive Measures

Diagnosis and Prevention of Rheumatic Fever

Rheumatic fever is a multiorgan inflammatory disease that occurs 10 days to 3 weeks after group A streptococcal pharyngitis. The clinical diagnosis is based on the conjunction of an antecedent streptococcal throat infection and classic manifestations of the disease, including carditis, polyarthritis, chorea, erythema marginatum, and subcutaneous nodules.[20-22] Clinical guidelines for the diagnosis of rheumatic fever allow greater specificity because many of the manifestations of rheumatic fever are seen in other conditions as well (Table 9-3). Some studies show that strict adherence to these guidelines may result in underdiagnoses,[23] and additional echocardiographic criteria have been suggested. Although these guidelines are helpful in the initial diagnosis of rheumatic fever, exceptions do occur, so consideration of the diagnosis is of central importance in the recognition of this disease. Poststreptococcal reactive arthritis has some overlap in symptoms and signs with acute rheumatic fever but has no cardiac involvement.[24,25]

The carditis associated with rheumatic fever is a pancarditis; there may be involvement of the pericardium, myocardium, and valvular tissue. Rheumatic disease preferentially affects the mitral valve, with MR being characteristic of the acute episode and mitral stenosis (MS) characteristic of the long-term effect of the disease process.[26] It has been suggested that echocardiography can improve the early diagnosis of rheumatic fever by detection of valvular regurgitation.[27] However, a slight degree of MR is common in normal individuals so it is not a specific finding.

TABLE 9-4   Recommendations for Prevention of Rheumatic Fever

Primary Prevention (Treatment of Group A Streptococcal Tonsillopharyngitis)		
	ADULTS	**CHILDREN (≤27 KG)**
PENICILLINS		
Oral penicillin V* (phenoxymethyl penicillin)	500 mg two to three times daily for 10 days or	250 mg two to three times daily for 10 days
IM penicillin, single dose	Benzathine penicillin G 1.2 million units IM once or	Benzathine penicillin G 600,000 U IM once
Amoxicillin	50 mg/kg orally once daily (maximum 1000 mg/day) or	50 mg/kg per day orally (maximum 1000 mg/day) for 10 days
FOR INDIVIDUALS ALLERGIC TO PENICILLIN		
Narrow-spectrum cephalosporin*	Variable oral dose for 10 days	Variable oral dose for 10 days
Azithromycin	12 mg/kg once daily (maximum 500 mg/day) orally for 5 days or	12 mg/kg orally once daily for 5 days
Clarithromycin	15 mg/kg per day divided bid (maximum 250 bid) orally for 10 days or	15 mg/kg per day divided bid (maximum 250 bid) orally for 10 days
Clindamycin	20 mg/kg/day (maximum 1.8 gm/day) orally in three equally divided doses for 10 days	20 mg/kg per day orally in three equally divided doses for 10 days
Secondary Prevention (of Recurrent Rheumatic Fever)		
	ADULTS	**CHILDREN (≤27 KG)**
Penicillin G benzathine	1.2 million U intramuscularly every 4 weeks (every 3 weeks in high-risk situations)	600,000 units every 4 weeks (every 3 weeks in high-risk situations)
Penicillin V	250 mg orally twice daily	250 mg orally twice daily
Sulfadiazine	1000 mg orally daily	500 mg orally once daily
For Patients Allergic to Penicillin and Sulfadiazine		
Macrolide or azalide	Variable	Variaible
DURATION OF SECONDARY PROPHYLAXIS		
Rheumatic fever with carditis and residual valve disease (including after valve surgery)	10 years or until age 40 years (whichever is longer); sometimes lifelong	
Rheumatic fever with carditis but no residual valve disease	10 years or until age 21 years (whichever is longer)	
Rheumatic fever without carditis	5 years or until age 21 years (whichever is longer)	

*To be avoided in those with immediate (Type I) hypersensitivity to a penicillin.
From Gerber MA, Baltimore RS, Eaton CB, et al. Prevention of rheumatic fever and diagnosis and treatment of acute streptococcal pharyngitis: a scientific statement from the American Heart Association Rheumatic Fever, Endocarditis, and Kawasaki Disease Committee of the Council on Cardiovascular Disease in the Young, the Interdisciplinary Council on Functional Genomics and Translational Biology, and the Interdisciplinary Council on Quality of Care and Outcomes Research. Circulation 2009;119:1541–51. Copyright © 2009 Lippincott Williams & Wilkins.

Primary prevention of rheumatic fever is based on treatment of streptococcal pharyngitis with appropriate antibiotics for a sufficient time.[21] Patients with a history of rheumatic fever are at high risk for recurrent disease, leading to repeated episodes of valvulitis and increased damage to the valvular apparatus. Because recurrent streptococcal infections may be asymptomatic, secondary prevention is based on the use of continuous antibiotic therapy (Table 9-4). The risk of recurrent disease is related to the number of previous episodes, time interval since the last episode, the risk of exposure to streptococcal infections (contact with children or crowded situations), and patient age. A longer duration of secondary prevention is recommended in patients with evidence of carditis or persistent valvular disease than in those with no evidence of valvular damage.

Prevention of Infective Endocarditis

Infective endocarditis occurs when bacteremia results in bacterial adherence and proliferation at sites of platelet and fibrin deposition on disrupted endothelial surfaces. Patients with native and prosthetic heart valve disease are at increased risk for infective endocarditis because of endothelial disruption on the valve leaflets secondary to high-velocity and turbulent blood flow patterns (see Chapter 25). About 50% of patients with endocarditis have underlying native valve disease, and endocarditis may precipitate the diagnosis of valve disease in a previously asymptomatic patient.

Prevention of bacterial endocarditis is based on short-term antibiotic therapy at times of anticipated bacteremia in patients at the highest risk of endocarditis. The American Heart Association has published revised guidelines for groups of patients at highest risk (Table 9-5), procedures likely to cause significant bacteremia (Table 9-6), and appropriate antibiotic regimens for dental procedures (Table 9-7).[28] Prophylaxis for other procedures should include antibiotics active against the organisms most likely to be present, as detailed in these guidelines. Antibiotics also are recommended at the time of surgical implantation of prosthetic cardiac valves or other intracardiac material.

On the basis of a careful review of the published literature and expert opinion, current guidelines no longer recommend endocarditis prophylaxis for patients with native valvular heart disease.[28] The key elements underlying the current recommendations are: (1) the recognition that bacteremia due to normal daily activities, like tooth brushing, flossing, and chewing, is much

TABLE 9-5 Cardiac Conditions for which Endocarditis Prophylaxis for Dental Procedures Is Reasonable

- Prosthetic cardiac valve or prosthetic material used for cardiac valve repair*
- Previous infective endocarditis
- Congenital heart disease (CHD)[†]:
  - Unrepaired cyanotic CHD, including palliative shunts and conduits
  - Completely repaired CHD with prosthetic material or device, whether placed by surgery or catheter intervention, during the first 6 months after the procedure[‡]
  - Repaired CHD with residual defects at the site or adjacent to the site of a prosthetic patch or prosthetic device (which inhibits endothelialization)
- Cardiac transplant recipients in whom valve disease develops

* Prophylaxis is not needed for patients with only coronary artery stents.
† Except for the conditions listed here, antibiotic prophylaxis is no longer recommended for any form of CHD.
‡ Prophylaxis is reasonable because endothelialization of prosthetic material occurs within 6 months after the procedure.
Modified from Wilson W, Taubert KA, Gewitz M, et al. Prevention of infective endocarditis: guidelines from the American Heart Association. Circulation 2007;116:1736–54.

TABLE 9-6 Dental or Surgical Procedures for which Endocarditis Prophylaxis Is Recommended*

Prophylaxis Recommended for Patients Meeting Criteria in Table 9-5

- All dental procedures that involve manipulation of gingival tissue or the periapical region of teeth or perforation of the oral mucosa (Class IIa, LOE C)
- Invasive procedures of the respiratory tract that involve incision or biopsy, including tonsillectomy and adenoidectomy (Class IIa, LOE C)
- Infections of the GI or GU tract, including an antibiotic active against enterococci (Class IIb, LOE B)
- Elective cystoscopy or other urinary tract manipulation only in patients with an enterococcal urinary tract infection or colonization, using an agent active against enterococci (Class IIb, LOE B)
- Procedures on infected skin or musculoskeletal tissue including agents active against staphylococci and b-hemolytic streptococci (Class IIb, LOE C)

Prophylaxis Recommended for ALL Patients

- Surgical placement of prosthetic heart valves or prosthetic intravascular or intracardiac material, (Class I, LOE B) using a first-generation cephalosporin (Class I, LOE A) or vancomycin at centers with high prevalence of methicillin-resistant *Staphylococcus epidermidis* (Class IIb, LOE C). Prophylaxis should begin immediately before surgery and should be continued for less than 48 hours (Class IIa, LOE B).

Prophylaxis Solely to Prevent Endocarditis NOT Needed
Minor Dental Procedures

- Routine anesthetic injections through noninfected tissue
- Dental radiographs
- Placement, removal, or adjustment of prosthodontic or orthodontic appliances
- Placement of orthodontic brackets
- Shedding of deciduous teeth
- Bleeding from trauma to the lips and/or oral mucosa

Respiratory Procedure

- Bronchoscopy without incision of the respiratory tract mucosa

GU and GI Procedures

- All GI and GU procedures, including diagnostic esophagogastroduodenoscopy and colonoscopy
- Vaginal delivery and hysterectomy

Skin and Musculoskeletal Procedures

- Tattooing
- Body piercing

GI, gastrointestinal; *GU*, genitourinary; *LOE*, level of evidence.
* ACC/AHA classification of recommendations (I, IIa, IIb) and level of evidence (A, B, C) are used (see Appendix A).
Summarized from Wilson W, Taubert KA, Gewitz M, et al. Prevention of infective endocarditis: guidelines from the American Heart Association. Circulation 2007;116:1736–54.

more frequent than bacteremia related to dental procedures, (2) there are no controlled studies showing that short-term antibiotic therapy at the time of anticipated bacteremia prevents endocarditis, and estimates of total benefit are exceedingly small, (3) the risk of an adverse reaction to the antibiotic outweighs any potential benefit, and (4) the most important factor in reducing daily bacteremia is maintaining optimal oral health and hygiene, including regular dental care.[29,30] Analysis of large data sets from the United Kingdom and United States showed that the current recommendations have resulted in an approximately 80% decrease in the use of antibiotic prophylaxis with no evidence of an increase in endocarditis cases.[31,32]

Prevention of Embolic Events

Prevention of embolic events in patients with valvular heart disease, particularly those with prosthetic valves, MS, or AF, is a key component of optimal medical therapy[7,33-38] (Table 9-8). While anticoagulation in patients with prosthetic valves is discussed in Chapter 26, this section discusses anticoagulation in adults with native valve disease. A systemic embolic event can have devastating consequences and may occur even in previously asymptomatic patients. Systemic embolism is usually due to left atrial (LA) thrombus formation in patients with low blood flow in a dilated LA chamber, with or without concurrent AF (Figure 9-2).[39-44] Embolic events due to calcific debris from the aortic or mitral valves are much less common but may occur when a catheter is passed across the aortic valve.[45-47]

CHOICE OF ANTITHROMBOTIC THERAPY

Therapy for prevention of embolic events in patients with valvular heart disease typically includes antiplatelet agents or long-term warfarin anticoagulation. There is little data on the use of newer anticoagulants, such as direct thrombin inhibitors and anti-Xa agents, for prevention of embolic events in patients with valve disease. In patients with mechanical prosthetic valves, these newer agents should not be used because of (1) a higher incidence of thromboembolic events in several case reports involving such patients and (2) early termination of RE-ALIGN (Randomized, phase II study to evaluate the safety and pharmacokinetics of oral dabigatran etexilate in patients after heart valve replacement) owing to a higher rate of valve thrombosis, stroke, and myocardial infarction in subjects randomly assigned to dabigatran compared to those receiving warfarin.[48-50] These findings prompted a U.S. Food and Drug Administration (FDA) "black box" warning on the package insert for dabigatran against its use

in patients with mechanical heart valves.[51] In addition, patients with AF associated with rheumatic mitral valve disease are at much higher risk for embolic events than those without valve disease, so the current expert clinical consensus is to use warfarin in patients with rheumatic mitral valve disease and indications for anticoagulation. However, the choice of warfarin or newer agents in patients with AF and aortic valve disease or nonrheumatic mitral valve disease is less clear, and most experts believe that these patients should be treated by following the same guidelines as in patients without valve disease, particularly if valve disease is only mild or moderate in severity.[52,53]

ANTICOAGULATION CLINICS

Warfarin therapy is monitored by means of the international normalized ratio (INR), because it provides a consistent measure of the degree of anticoagulation. Management by hospital-based anticoagulation clinics results in lower complication rates than standard care (Figure 9-3).[54,55] Anticoagulation clinics also are cost effective because they are associated with lower rates of

TABLE 9-7 American Heart Association Recommendations for Endocarditis Prophylaxis for Dental Procedures

SITUATION	AGENT	Regimen: Single Dose 30 to 60 Min Before Procedure	
		ADULTS	CHILDREN
Oral	Amoxicillin	2 g	50 mg/kg
Unable to take oral medications	Ampicillin OR	2 g IM or IV	50 mg/kg IM or IV
	Cefazolin or ceftriaxone	1 g IM or IV	50 mg/kg IM or IV
Allergic to penicillins or ampicillin—oral	Cephalexin*† **OR**	2 g	50 mg/kg
	Clindamycin **OR**	600 mg	20 mg/kg
	Azithromycin or clarithromycin	500 mg	15 mg/kg
Allergic to penicillins or ampicillin and unable to take oral medications	Cefazolin or ceftriaxone† **OR**	1 g IM or IV	50 mg/kg IM or IV
	Clindamycin	600 mg IM or IV	20 mg/kg IM or IV

IM, intramuscularly; IV, intravenously.
*Or other first- or second-generation oral cephalosporin in equivalent adult or pediatric dosage.
†Cephalosporins should not be used in individuals with anaphylaxis, angioedema, or urticaria penicillin or ampicillin.
From Wilson W, Taubert KA, Gewitz M, et al. Prevention of infective endocarditis: guidelines from the American Heart Association. Circulation 2007;116:1736–54.

TABLE 9-8 Recommendations for Anticoagulation in Patients with Native Valvular Heart Disease

VALVE LESION	RECOMMENDATION
Mitral valve disease with AF	Warfarin, INR 2.0-3.0
Rheumatic mitral valve stenosis:	
Paroxysmal, persistent or permanent AF	Warfarin, INR 2.0-3.0
Previous embolic event or LA thrombus (even with NSR)	Warfarin, INR 2.0-3.0
Recurrent systemic emboli despite adequate anticoagulation	Add aspirin 80-100 mg qd OR dipyridamole 400 mg qd OR ticlopidine 250 mg bid
Mitral valve prolapse:	
TIAs	Long-term (75-325 mg qd) aspirin
AF and age <65 years with no other risk factors	Long-term (75-325 mg qd) aspirin
AF plus at least 1 other risk factor (age > 65 years, hypertension, MR murmur, or history of HF)	Warfarin, INR 2.0-3.0
CVA with AF, MR, or LA thrombus	Warfarin, INR 2.0-3.0
Infective endocarditis:	
Native valve or tissue prosthesis	Anticoagulation therapy contraindicated
Mechanical valve	Continue or restart anticoagulation (heparin or warfarin) when neurologic condition allows
Nonbacterial thrombotic endocarditis:*	
With systemic emboli	Heparin anticoagulation
Debilitating disease with aseptic vegetations on echocardiography	Heparin anticoagulation

AF, atrial fibrillation; HF, Heart failure; CVA, cerebrovascular accident; INR, international normalized ratio; LA, left atrial; MR, mitral regurgitation; NSR, normal sinus rhythm; TIA, transient ischemic attack.
*This recommendation is not based on guidelines but is based on review of references 7, 33-37, and 115.

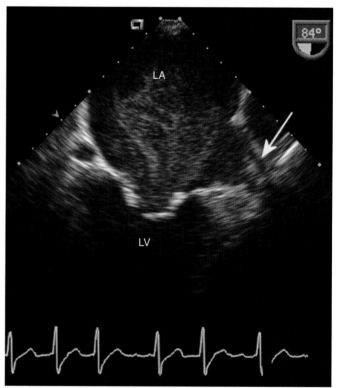

FIGURE 9-2 Left atrial spontaneous contrast. Transesophageal imaging in a patient with rheumatic mitral stenosis shows diffuse mobile echodensities in the left atrium consistent with blood flow stasis. *Arrow* indicates the left atrial appendage with a possible thrombus. *LA*, left atrium; *LV*, left ventricle. *(From Otto CM. Textbook of clinical echocardiography. 5th ed. Philadelphia: Elsevier, 2013.)*

bleeding and hemorrhagic complications.[56-76] Long-term management is equally effective with periodic direct patient contact and with telephone encounters.[57,77,78] The typical anticoagulation clinic is staffed by pharmacists with special expertise in anticoagulation management, who use written policies and procedures developed in collaboration with the responsible physicians.

Another option is self-management of anticoagulation by the patient using a small home monitoring device that uses a finger-stick blood sample. In randomized trials, conventional therapy and home management showed similar rates of anticoagulation control, with an INR in the therapeutic range about two thirds of the time in both groups, although the rate of major complications was lower in the home management group.[79,80] A meta-analysis of 14 randomized studies of home monitoring of warfarin therapy demonstrated lower rates of thromboembolic events, all-cause mortality, and major hemorrhage.[81] Investigators in all of these studies emphasize that home monitoring is appropriate only in selected patients and requires careful education and supervision.[82]

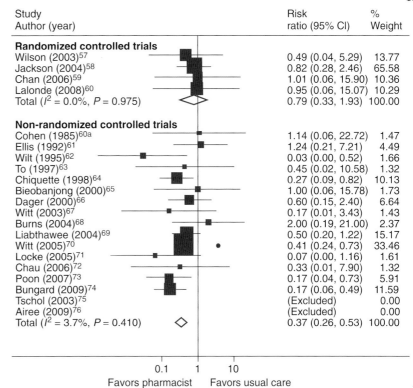

Study Author (year)	Risk ratio (95% CI)	% Weight
Randomized controlled trials		
Wilson (2003)[57]	0.49 (0.04, 5.29)	13.77
Jackson (2004)[58]	0.82 (0.28, 2.46)	65.58
Chan (2006)[59]	1.01 (0.06, 15.90)	10.36
Lalonde (2008)[60]	0.95 (0.06, 15.07)	10.29
Total (I^2 = 0.0%, P = 0.975)	0.79 (0.33, 1.93)	100.00
Non-randomized controlled trials		
Cohen (1985)[60a]	1.14 (0.06, 22.72)	1.47
Ellis (1992)[61]	1.24 (0.21, 7.21)	4.49
Wilt (1995)[62]	0.03 (0.00, 0.52)	1.66
To (1997)[63]	0.45 (0.02, 10.58)	1.32
Chiquette (1998)[64]	0.27 (0.09, 0.82)	10.13
Bieobanjong (2000)[65]	1.00 (0.06, 15.78)	1.73
Dager (2000)[66]	0.60 (0.15, 2.40)	6.64
Witt (2003)[67]	0.17 (0.01, 3.43)	1.43
Burns (2004)[68]	2.00 (0.19, 21.00)	2.37
Liabthawee (2004)[69]	0.50 (0.20, 1.22)	15.17
Witt (2005)[70]	0.41 (0.24, 0.73)	33.46
Locke (2005)[71]	0.07 (0.00, 1.16)	1.61
Chau (2006)[72]	0.33 (0.01, 7.90)	1.32
Poon (2007)[73]	0.17 (0.04, 0.73)	5.91
Bungard (2009)[74]	0.17 (0.06, 0.49)	11.59
Tschol (2003)[75]	(Excluded)	0.00
Airee (2009)[76]	(Excluded)	0.00
Total (I^2 = 3.7%, P = 0.410)	0.37 (0.26, 0.53)	100.00

0.1   1   10

Favors pharmacist   Favors usual care

FIGURE 9-3 Effect of pharmacist-led clinical care versus usual care on thromboembolic events. Data from a metaanalysis of 24 studies with 728,377 patients show the relative benefit of a pharmacist-led anticoagulation clinic versus standard care in terms of the incidence of thromboembolic events. Patients in these studies were receiving warfarin anticoagulation for a variety of indications, including atrial fibrillation and a mechanical heart valve. *Diamonds* indicate the summary risk ratios and 95% confidence intervals (CIs). The sizes of the *squares* are proportional to the reciprocals of the variance of the studies. *(From Saokaew S, Permsuwan U, Chaiyakunapruk N, et al. Effectiveness of pharmacist-participated warfarin therapy management: a systematic review and meta-analysis. J Thromb Haemost 2010;8:2418–27.)*

At the initiation of therapy, a target INR and acceptable range are defined by the referring physician for each patient on the basis of published guidelines and clinical factors unique to that patient. The pharmacist interviews each patient with specific attention to current medications, diet, lifestyle, and any other factors that may affect long-term anticoagulation therapy. In addition, patient education about anticoagulation, possible dietary and drug interactions, recognition of complications of therapy, and the need for careful monitoring of the INR is provided verbally and through the use of a variety of media (such as pamphlets, recorded presentations, and computer-based material).

Typically, the INR is measured weekly (or more frequently) at the initiation of therapy with a typical interval of 4 weeks for patients on a stable therapeutic regimen. At each visit, the timing of the next INR measurement is determined on the basis of the current INR and any trends over the past several visits. In addition, further patient education and counseling are provided as needed. The pharmacist monitors concurrent medical therapy for any potential drug interaction, and the patient or physician can contact the pharmacist before starting new prescription or nonprescription medications either to avoid possible interactions by choosing an alternate agent or to alert the pharmacist of the need for more frequent INR determinations if an effect is likely (Figures 9-4 and 9-5).

Minor bleeding complications may be managed by the anticoagulation clinic in consultation with the physician, depending on the specific protocol at each institution. If major bleeding episodes or thromboembolic events occur, the patient is triaged promptly for acute medical care. The anticoagulation clinic also manages changes in therapy necessitated by surgical or invasive procedures, according to policies developed in conjunction with the referring physician.

ANTICOAGULATION WITH NATIVE VALVE DISEASE

Paroxysmal, persistent, or permanent AF should be treated with anticoagulation, as stated in current guidelines, when aortic valve or nonrheumatic mitral valve disease is present.[52] The risk of atrial thrombus and embolism is particularly high for AF in adults with

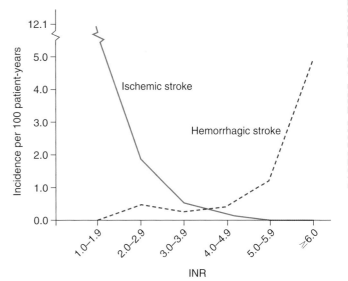

FIGURE 9-4 Stroke risk with mechanical valves. Incidence of ischemic and hemorrhagic stroke in patients with mechanical heart valves according to international normalized ratio (INR) category. *(From Cannegieter SC, Rosendaal FR, Wintzen AR, et al. optimal oral anticoagulant therapy in patients with mechanical heart valves. N Engl J Med 1995;333:11–7.)*

MS; in these patients warfarin anticoagulation to maintain an INR of 2.0 to 3.0 is recommended. Warfarin anticoagulation also is recommended in patients with a previous embolic event or a LA thrombus, even with normal sinus rhythm (Figure 9-6).[7,83-85] Some data support the use of warfarin anticoagulation in patients with MS and normal sinus rhythm with a LA dimension greater than 55 mm as well as in those with prominent spontaneous contrast on echocardiography, because of the high risk of atrial thrombus formation even in the absence of AF,[86-89] but this clinical decision is also influenced by the severity of stenosis and the presence of comorbid conditions.

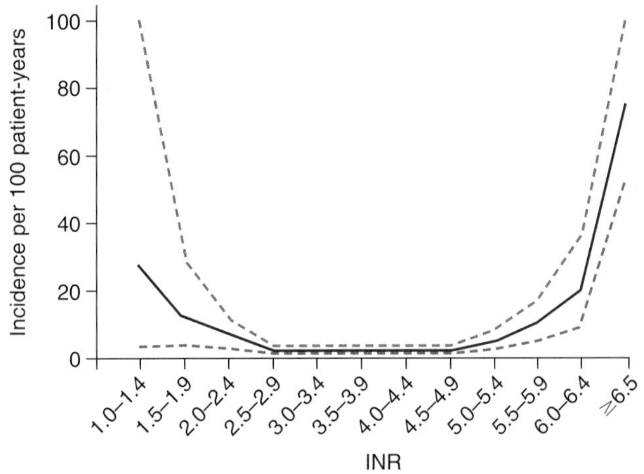

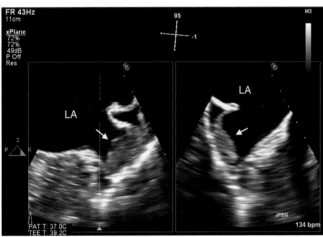

FIGURE 9-5   Risk of adverse events in patients with a mechanical valve. International normalized ratio (INR)–specific incidence of all adverse events (all episodes of thromboembolism, all major bleeding episodes, and unclassified stroke). The *dotted lines* indicate the 95% confidence interval. *(From Cannegieter SC, Rosendaal FR, Wintzen AR, et al. Optimal oral anticoagulant therapy in patients with mechanical heart valves. N Engl J Med 1995;333:11–17.)*

FIGURE 9-6   Left atrial thrombus. In this 45-year-old woman with severe mitral stenosis referred for balloon valvotomy, transesophageal biplane orthogonal images of the left atrial (LA) appendage show an irregular mass (arrow) consistent with atrial thrombus. *(From Otto CM Textbook of Clinical Echocardiography. 5th ed. Philadelphia: Elsevier, 2013.)*

In the absence of AF, anticoagulation is not indicated for patients with aortic valve disease or asymptomatic mitral valve prolapse because of the low risk of embolic events with these lesions. Although elderly patients with mitral annular calcification appear to be at higher risk for embolic events, there is no evidence that anticoagulation is beneficial unless they have concurrent AF.[90-93] If patients with mitral prolapse have unexplained transient ischemic attacks, treatment with aspirin is recommended. Long-term warfarin anticoagulation is indicated in the patient with mitral valve prolapse, with or without a documented systemic embolic event, who is in AF and has at least one other risk factor (age >65 years, MR, or LA thrombus).

In younger patients (<65 years) with mitral prolapse and AF, aspirin therapy is recommended unless there is a history of stroke, hypertension, MR, or LA thrombus—situations in which warfarin is appropriate. However, some clinicians would also consider warfarin therapy in the patient with mitral prolapse who has had a stroke and show excessive leaflet thickening (>5 mm) or redundancy (even without AF or other risk factors) and in the patient with persistent transient ischemic attacks despite aspirin therapy.[7]

In patients with infective endocarditis, anticoagulation should be avoided in general, given an increased risk of hemorrhagic transformation of embolic stroke in such patients and the lack of evidence of benefit.[94-97] The major exception to the avoidance of anticoagulation in endocarditis is the presence of a mechanical valve. In this situation, most studies suggest, long-term anticoagulation should be continued, unless the patient experiences a stroke.[98-100] The choice of intravenous (IV) heparin rather than warfarin therapy, so that anticoagulation can be promptly stopped in the event of a stroke, is controversial and depends on the specific clinical circumstances of each case. If warfarin is used, close monitoring is needed because many antibiotics affect its metabolism.

General Health Maintenance

Adults with mild to moderate asymptomatic valve disease should be encouraged to maintain normal body weight and to remain physically fit with regular dynamic physical activity. There are no restrictions on participation in competitive sports for asymptomatic patients with valve disease who are in normal sinus rhythm, have normal LV size and systolic function, and have normal pulmonary pressures at rest and with exercise. Even those with severe asymptomatic valve disease should also be encouraged to participate in regular low-level aerobic activity, although they should avoid participation in competitive sports and strenuous activity, as summarized in Table 9-9.[101] Recommendations regarding competitive sports are more problematic in patients with moderate disease and should be individualized according to the presence of LV dilation or dysfunction and the patient's hemodynamic response to exercise. Patients undergoing long-term anticoagulation for AF or a prosthetic valve should avoid sports with the potential for bodily contact or falls.

Both pneumococcal and annual influenza vaccinations are recommended for all adults older than 65 years and are especially important in patients with valvular disease, in whom the increased hemodynamic demands of an acute infection may lead to cardiac decompensation. In younger patients with valve disease, routine immunization is indicated only if conditions associated with immunocompromise are also present.

Patients with heart valve disease should undergo assessment of risk factors for coronary artery disease and aggressive risk factor modification as appropriate. Because aortic valve sclerosis is associated with an increased risk of myocardial infarction and cardiac death, the finding of aortic sclerosis on echocardiography should prompt a careful evaluation and initiation of treatment for known cardiac risk factors (see Chapter 4).[102,103] In addition, many patients with valvular disease need eventual surgical intervention, and both surgical mortality and morbidity rates are markedly increased when coronary disease complicates valvular heart disease. The negative impact of coexisting coronary disease is particularly striking for patients with MR, with coronary disease conferring an fourfold increase in surgical mortality[104] and a 5-year survival half that of patients without coronary disease.[105] In AS, concurrent coronary disease is associated with an approximate doubling of surgical mortality.[104,106-109]

Monitoring Disease Progression

Periodic noninvasive monitoring is essential for optimal timing of interventions in patients with valve dysfunction. Disease progression may be evident as changes in valve anatomy or motion; an increase in the severity of valve stenosis or regurgitation; LV dilation, hypertrophy, or dysfunction in response to pressure and/or volume overload; or secondary effects of the valvular lesion, such as pulmonary hypertension or AF. The frequency of periodic evaluations is tailored to each case, depending on the severity of the lesion at the initial evaluation, the known natural history of the disease, indications for surgical intervention, and other clinical factors in each patient. Clearly, there is no simple set of rules

TABLE 9-9	Recommendations for Participation in Competitive Sports for Adults with Asymptomatic Valvular Heart Disease*

Patients with Following Conditions Should Not Participate in Any Competitive Sports

- Severe MS
- MS of any degree with an exercise PA pressure >50 mm Hg
- Severe MR with pulmonary hypertension, LV dilation (EDD 60 mm or greater) or LV systolic dysfunction
- Severe AS
- Severe AR and LV dilation (EDD >65 mm)

Avoid Sports with Risk of Bodily Contact

- All patients with valvular heart disease on long-term anticoagulation

Can Participate in All Competitive Sports

- Mild MS in NSR and an exercise PA pressure <50 mm Hg
- Mild to moderate MR in NSR with normal LV size and function
- Mild AS (with annual evaluation of AS severity)
- Mild to moderate AR with normal LV size

AS, aortic stenosis; AR, aortic regurgitation; EDD, end-diastolic dimension; LV, left ventricular; MR, mitral regurgitation; MS, mitral stenosis; NSR, normal sinus rhythm; PA, pulmonary artery.
* Recommendations in patients with moderate asymptomatic valve disease are individualized according to the type and level of activity and objective measures of the patient's exercise response.
Summarized from Bonow RO, Cheitlin MD, Crawford JH, et al. Task Force 3: valvular heart disease. J Am Coll Cardiol 2005;45:1334–40.

TABLE 9-10	Framework for Periodic Echocardiography in Patients with Valvular Heart Disease

Step 1: Initial Diagnostic Study
A comprehensive baseline echocardiographic and Doppler examination. Transesophageal imaging should be considered if transthoracic images are nondiagnostic.

Step 2: Basic Frequency of Examination
The basic frequency of echocardiographic examination, given in the following table, provides a starting point for each patient that will be modified as appropriate in Steps 3 and 4.

VALVE LESION	SEVERITY	BASIC FREQUENCY
Aortic stenosis	Mild (V_{max} <3.0 m/s)	3-5 years
	Moderate (V_{max} 3-4 m/s)	1-2 years
	Severe (V_{max} >4.0 m/s)	Annually
Aortic regurgitation	Mild	2-3 years
	Moderate, normal LV size	1-2 years
	Severe, normal LV size	Annually
	Severe, LV dilation	6-12 months
Mitral stenosis	Mild (MVA >2.0 cm^2)	2-3 years
	Moderate (MVA 1-2 cm^2)	Annually
	Severe (MVA <1.0 cm^2)	6-12 months
Mitral regurgitation	Mild	2-3 years
	Moderate	1-2 years
	Severe, normal LV size	Annually
	Severe, change in LV size or function	6 months

Step 3: Modifiers of Examination Frequency
Modifiers that Increase Frequency

Interim change in symptoms or physical examination findings
New-onset atrial fibrillation
Evidence for progressive LV dilation and/or early contractile dysfunction
Evidence for increasing pulmonary pressures

Modifiers that Decrease Frequency

Stable findings over 2-3 examination intervals

Step 4: Special Situations
Preoperative evaluation before noncardiac surgery
Pregnancy
Monitoring interventional procedures
Assessment of complications and hemodynamic results after an intervention
Intraoperative transesophageal monitoring

LV, left ventricular; MVA, mitral valve area; V_{max}, maximal velocity across the valve.

that defines the optimal or most cost-effective frequency of evaluation. However, on the basis of our current understanding of the natural history of valve disease, a framework for periodic evaluation can be devised (Table 9-10). First, an initial complete diagnostic echocardiographic study is performed to define disease severity, LV size and systolic function, pulmonary pressures, and any associated abnormalities. Next, a basic frequency of repeat examinations is suggested for each valve lesion, depending on the severity of valve disease and, for valve regurgitation, the LV response to chronic volume overload.

However, the specific timing of repeat studies may need to be modified according to interim changes in symptoms or physical examination findings, new-onset AF, evidence of progressive LV dilation or early contractile dysfunction, or evidence of increasing pulmonary pressures. For example, an apparent increase in ventricular dimensions in a patient with chronic regurgitation prompts a repeat evaluation at a shorter interval to distinguish a pathologic change from normal physiologic or measurement variation. Similarly, a change in symptom status in a patient with myxomatous mitral valve disease warrants reevaluation because a sudden change in regurgitant severity due to chordal rupture may have occurred. In addition, more frequent examinations are warranted when quantitative parameters are approaching the values defined as optimal for timing of surgical intervention.

In other clinical situations, reevaluation may be indicated to assess hemodynamics under changing physiologic conditions (such as during pregnancy), to guide a surgical or interventional procedure, or to assess results and complications after an intervention. In patients with comorbid diseases, such as those undergoing noncardiac surgery, a repeat echocardiographic examination may be needed to assist in medical and/or surgical management.

Medical Therapy of Valvular Heart Disease

Primary Treatment

Ideally, the treatment of patients with primary disease of the valve leaflets should be directed toward the underlying disease process

affecting valve anatomy and function. Worldwide, primary prevention of rheumatic heart disease would have a dramatic impact on the incidence of valve dysfunction. In patients with rheumatic heart disease, prevention of recurrent episodes of rheumatic fever is critical for preventing further valve damage and progressive disease. However, currently no specific therapies are available to prevent or reverse the primary disease processes in other types of valve disease.

The recognition that calcific valve disease is an active disease process with similarities to atherosclerosis led to the hypothesis that disease progression might be prevented by lipid-lowering therapy (see Chapters 3 and 4). However, well-designed randomized prospective trials of lipid-lowering therapy in adults with mild to moderate calcific aortic valve disease have shown no effect on disease progression or the need for valve replacement (see Chapter 11).[110-112] It is to be hoped that further research will lead to targeted therapy to prevent disease progression in adults with calcific valve disease.

Prevention of Left Ventricular Contractile Dysfunction

As discussed in Chapter 5, the basic response of the left ventricle to the chronic volume overload imposed by aortic or mitral regurgitation is an increase in chamber size. Initially, LV systolic function is normal; however, with long-standing disease, contractile dysfunction may supervene and may not improve after intervention to correct the regurgitant lesion. Most patients demonstrate symptoms that prompt consideration of valve surgery, but in a subset of patients, LV dysfunction occurs prior to symptom onset.[113,114] Thus, a major focus of the medical management of patients with chronic valvular regurgitation is periodic noninvasive evaluation to monitor LV size and systolic function. The rationale for sequential monitoring is that surgical intervention can be performed just before (or soon after) the onset of contractile dysfunction.

A more elusive goal in the medical therapy of patients with chronic regurgitation is to prevent or delay progressive LV dilation and contractile dysfunction, thus delaying the need for surgical intervention. Afterload reduction therapy improves acute hemodynamics, but clinical studies have yielded variable results on the potential benefit of afterload reduction to prevent progressive LV dilation in response to chronic aortic or mitral regurgitation (see Chapters 12 and 18). There currently are no Class I indications for afterload reduction therapy in nonhypertensive adults with chronic asymptomatic aortic or mitral regurgitation.[7,38,115,116] However, adults with chronic regurgitation and elevated blood pressure, which is common in this patient group, should receive appropriate antihypertensive therapy. Instead of altering systemic vascular resistance, another approach to therapy is to prevent adverse effects on the LV myocardium. A pilot study of beta-blocker therapy in patients with MR showed a favorable trend in prevention of LV systolic dysfunction by this therapy in comparison with the placebo.[117] These data may stimulate larger prospective trials of therapy directed toward preserving LV function in adults with valve dysfunction.[118]

In patients with asymptomatic valvular AS, the development of LV contractile dysfunction is uncommon, occurring in less than 1%,[119] so the timing of surgical intervention is based on symptom onset rather than on changes in LV geometry or function.[120] There are no known medical therapies to prevent or modify the development of LV hypertrophy in adults with AS, and it is not clear that preventing this adaptive response would improve outcome. However, speckle tracking echocardiographic strain imaging has shown that subclinical changes in LV longitudinal shortening occur early in the disease process.[121] There also has been considerable interest in the changes in diastolic ventricular dysfunction that occur in patients with AS.[122-124] It has been hypothesized that surgical intervention prior to the development of irreversible changes in the myocardium might improve long-term clinical outcome.[125-128] Again, however, no medical therapy is known to prevent early systolic or diastolic dysfunction in patients with pressure overload hypertrophy.

Prevention of Left Atrial Enlargement and Atrial Fibrillation

Progressive LA enlargement and AF typically complicate the clinical course of mitral valve disease. Both MR and MS are associated with LA dilation due to the pressure and/or volume overload of the left atrium.[129-131] AF occurs frequently, particularly in older patients and in patients with severe and long-standing disease. Atrial enlargement and fibrillation occasionally complicate aortic valve disease, typically late in the disease course, and may worsen hemodynamics substantially as a result of the loss of the atrial contribution to ventricular filling.[132]

Medically, there is no specific therapy to prevent these complications of the disease process, although it has been proposed that earlier surgical or percutaneous intervention might prevent atrial enlargement and eventual AF. Surgical intervention for MR soon after the onset of AF (within 3 months) is more likely to restore sinus rhythm than surgical intervention in patients with AF of longer duration but is not uniformly successful.[133,134] In patients with MS, AF usually recurs or persists after intervention.

Prevention of Pulmonary Hypertension

The chronic elevation in LA pressure associated with mitral valve disease results in a passive increase in pulmonary pressures that resolves when LA pressure decreases after surgical or percutaneous intervention. However, reactive changes in the pulmonary vasculature may become superimposed on this passive rise in pressure with secondary histologic changes, leading to irreversible pulmonary hypertension. Intervention prior to the onset of irreversible changes is desirable to avoid long-term complications of right heart failure. In some patients, an excessive rise in pulmonary pressures with exercise may be the first clue that intervention is needed to prevent further irreversible changes in the pulmonary vasculature.[135]

In adults with aortic valve disease, pulmonary hypertension is a risk factor for operative mortality and long-term survival.[136] Preliminary studies suggest that phosphodiesterase type 5 inhibitors might be beneficial in reducing systemic and pulmonary vascular resistance in patients with AS.[137]

Medical Treatment of Symptomatic Disease

Although the goal in management of patients with valvular disease is to avoid symptoms and the need for medical therapy by optimizing the timing of surgical intervention, some patients have persistent symptoms after surgery, have symptoms only in response to a superimposed hemodynamic stress (such as pregnancy), or are not candidates for surgical intervention. In these situations, medical therapy is based primarily on adjustment of loading conditions and control of heart rate and rhythm.

Patients with pulmonary congestion are treated with diuretics to decrease LA and pulmonary venous pressures whether elevated LA pressures are due to LV dysfunction, MR, or MS. However, when MS is present, care is needed to ensure that LA pressures allow adequate LV diastolic filling across the narrowed valve. In patients with AS, diuretics should be used cautiously because pulmonary congestion often is due to diastolic dysfunction rather than volume overload. The further decrease in ventricular diastolic volume induced by diuretics may worsen symptoms as mid-cavity ventricular obstruction develops in the small, hypertrophied, hyperdynamic left ventricle.

Afterload reduction is most beneficial for treatment of heart failure symptoms in patients with acute aortic or mitral regurgitation. With acute regurgitation, a continuous intravenous infusion of nitroprusside may be used. Intraaortic balloon counterpulsation provides effective afterload reduction while maintaining coronary diastolic perfusion pressures in patients with acute MR. However, an intraaortic balloon is contraindicated in patients with aortic regurgitation (AR), because the increase in aortic diastolic pressure results in more severe valve regurgitation. In symptomatic patients with chronic regurgitation, standard therapy for heart failure is reasonable, including afterload reduction, only if surgery is not an option or if heart failure occurs in the setting of a reversible hemodynamic stress. In patients with MS, afterload reduction is not helpful because the ventricle typically is small with normal systolic function.

In the past, there was concern that afterload reduction in adults with severe AS might result in a precipitous fall in blood pressure due to peripheral vasodilation, because only a fixed stroke volume can be pumped though the rigid orifice.[138,139] However, other studies suggest that cautious use of afterload reduction is well tolerated and may be beneficial.[140,141] Most likely the benefit of afterload reduction is a greater degree of leaflet motion and increase in functional valve area, when cardiac output is increased.[142,143] Particularly when there is coexisting LV dysfunction, the decrease in systemic vascular resistance may lead to improved LV contractility and an increase in LV output as a result of greater opening of the valve leaflets.[144]

Management of Concurrent Cardiovascular Conditions

Hypertension

Concurrent hypertension is common in adults, with prevalence close to 50% after age 65 years. Thus, many patients with valve disease also have hypertension, which should be treated according to established guidelines. Treatment of hypertension is well tolerated in patients with mitral valve disease so modification in therapy is rarely needed because of the valve lesions.

Treatment of hypertension in patients with aortic valve disease is especially important to reduce total ventricular afterload, which includes both the load imposed by the valve lesions and the systemic vascular resistance. With AR, two factors are important in treatment of hypertension. First, severe AR is characterized by a wide pulse pressure; overtreatment of systolic pressure that is high due to large total stroke volume may result in excessively low diastolic pressure. In theory, the low pressure could compromise diastolic coronary blood flow. Second, therapy that lowers heart rate may result in a higher systolic blood pressure as a result of an even larger stroke volume with a longer diastolic filling period. Thus, if a beta-blocker is used, additional therapy with an afterload-reducing agent may be needed.

In patients with AS, treatment of hypertension should follow standard approaches, except that therapy should be initiated at low doses and slowly titrated to the therapeutic dose to avoid hypotension. Diuretics should be avoided, particularly in elderly women with AS, who typically have a small hypertrophied ventricle, because any decrease in preload would reduce forward cardiac output. Despite concerns in the past that systemic vasodilation might result in hypotension because of lack of a compensatory increase in stroke volume across the narrowed valve as systemic resistance decreases, angiotensin-converting enzyme inhibitor therapy is well tolerated in adults with moderate AS.[145] Afterload reduction therapy has been proposed as having potential, but unproven, benefit for preservation of ventricular systolic and diastolic function in AS.[146,147] The presence of hypertension may affect the accuracy of measures of AS severity, so blood pressure should be controlled before assessment of valve disease severity.[148-151]

Coronary Artery Disease

Coronary artery disease also is common in adults with heart valve disease as expected on the basis of age, sex, and clinical risk factors in this patient group.[152] In most patients undergoing valve surgery, coronary angiography is needed because concurrent coronary artery bypass grafting is recommended when significant disease is present. Similarly, the timing of valve intervention may be affected by the presence and severity of coronary disease, particularly when a patient with asymptomatic AS is referred for valve surgery (Table 9-11).

In adults with asymptomatic valve disease, prevention of coronary disease based on risk factor evaluation and modification is essential. When symptoms occur, particularly angina, it may be difficult to distinguish whether symptoms are due to coronary or valve disease.[153] The resting electrocardiogram (ECG) often shows LV hypertrophy and ST changes due to valve disease. Both exercise and pharmacologic stress testing are less accurate for detection of coronary stenoses when valve disease is present because exercise duration may be limited by valve, not coronary,

TABLE 9-11 Indications for Evaluation of Coronary Anatomy in Adults with Valvular Heart Disease

Prior to Surgical or Percutaneous Valve Procedures in Patients with:
- Chest pain
- Objective evidence of ischemia
- Decreased left ventricular (LV) systolic function
- History of coronary disease
- Coronary risk factors (including age):*
  - Men ≥35 years
  - Postmenopausal women
  - Women ≥35 years with coronary risk factors

Mild to Moderate Valve Disease in Patients with:
- Progressive angina
- Objective evidence of ischemia
- Decreased LV systolic function
- Heart failure

*Patients undergoing balloon mitral valvotomy do not need coronary angiography solely on the basis of coronary disease risk factors.
Summarized from Class I indications in Bonow RO, Carabello BA, Chatterjee K, et al. ACC/AHA 2006 guidelines for the management of patients with valvular heart disease: a report of the American College of Cardiology/American Heart Association Task Force on Practice Guidelines (writing Committee to Revise the 1998 guidelines for the management of patients with valvular heart disease) developed in collaboration with the Society of Cardiovascular Anesthesiologists endorsed by the Society for Cardiovascular Angiography and Interventions and the Society of Thoracic Surgeons. J Am Coll Cardiol 2006;48:e1–148.

disease, and coronary flow patterns are affected by valve hemodynamics.[154-156] Thus, direct imaging of coronary anatomy, usually by coronary angiography but alternatively with high-resolution CT, may be needed. If the cause of symptoms remains unclear after consideration of the severity of valve and coronary disease, it may be appropriate to consider a percutaneous coronary intervention. If symptoms resolve, continued treatment of coronary disease is reasonable; persistence of symptoms suggests that the cause is the valve disease. Standard approaches to percutaneous and medical therapy of coronary disease are appropriate in adults with valvular heart disease.

Aortic Disease

Aortic valve dysfunction may be due to or associated with abnormalities of the aortic root. In adults with a bicuspid valve, dilation of the aortic sinuses or ascending aorta is common, and patients with a bicuspid aortic valve have an increased risk of aortic dissection (see Chapter 13). In adults with a primary abnormality of the aorta, such as Marfan syndrome, AR may be the result of aortic dilation with relatively normal valve anatomy. Tomographic imaging using a wide field of view, either cardiac CT or CMR, is typically needed in addition to echocardiography for evaluation and monitoring of the location and degree of aortic dilation, because echocardiography cannot reliably evaluate the entire length of the aorta. When aortic dilation is present, the severity of aortic involvement may be the primary driver for repeat imaging and for the timing of surgical intervention.[157]

Arrhythmias

In patients with mitral valve disease and AF, restoration and maintenance of sinus rhythm is of high priority both to prevent atrial thrombus formation (as discussed previously) and to preserve the atrial contribution to LV diastolic filling. Approaches to restoring and maintaining sinus rhythm are no different in these patients from those in patients without valve disease, other than the increased awareness of embolic risk and need for appropriate anticoagulation (see Table 9-3).[52] There is growing interest in concurrent procedures, such as the maze procedure, to restore sinus rhythm at the time of surgical intervention for mitral valve disease.[158,159] AF ablation is unlikely to be successful when significant valve disease is present unless the hemodynamic abnormality also is corrected. Often the onset of AF is the first sign of hemodynamic decompensation in patients with chronic slowly progressive valve diseases.

When sinus rhythm cannot be maintained, ventricular rate is controlled with standard approaches. Rate control is especially important in patients with MS because a shortened diastolic filling time may result in a symptomatic decrease in forward cardiac output.[160,161]

Even when sinus rhythm is present, heart rate control may be needed in patients with valve disease. For example, the increased heart rate (and shortened diastolic filling time) associated with pregnancy in a patient with MS leads to inadequate ventricular filling and a reduced cardiac output. Slowing the heart rate with a beta-blocker improves diastolic filling and restores a normal cardiac output.[162,163] Another example is the elderly patient with AS. Bradycardia may develop in such a patient, as a result of either calcification of the conduction system with heart block or sick sinus syndrome, which further reduces the total cardiac output across the stenotic valve, leading to cardiac symptoms. Symptoms due to bradycardia resolve after placement of a pacemaker, possibly allowing deferral of aortic valve surgery.

There is an increased risk of sudden death in patients with significant LV dilation or dysfunction due to chronic AR,[164] which is prevented by aortic valve replacement. Mitral valve prolapse also is associated with an increased risk of sudden death, but use of antiarrhythmic therapy or placement of an automated implanted defibrillator is based on standard indications for these procedures, not on the presence of valve disease alone.[165]

Heart Failure

Heart failure due to valve stenosis or regurgitation is an indication for surgical or transcatheter intervention with either aortic or mitral valve disease. When severe valve disease is present, it is likely that heart failure is due to the valve lesion. For example, severe AR results in LV dilation and systolic dysfunction. With prompt valve replacement, ventricular size and function return to normal.

However, when only mild to moderate valve disease is present and there is evidence of heart failure, evaluation for other causes is appropriate. The combination of moderate to severe AS and moderate to severe LV dysfunction is a particular clinical challenge because it can be difficult to distinguish whether AS resulted in ventricular dysfunction or whether the poor ventricular function contributes to reduced aortic valve opening (see Chapter 11).

When heart failure is not due to valve dysfunction, standard approaches to medical therapy and continued sequential monitoring of valve disease are reasonable. In the patient with AS, therapy may need to be started at low doses and titrated upwards slowly to avoid hypotension due to an abrupt change in systemic vascular resistance. Evaluation of volume status should include consideration of the effects of valve dysfunction on ventricular filling as well as standard parameters. For example, in the patient with MS, the left ventricle may still be underfilled when central venous and pulmonary venous pressures are elevated.

Heart failure also may be the cause of valve dysfunction. For example, primary ventricular dilation and dysfunction result in secondary (or functional) MR due to distortion of the normal mitral annular-ventricular geometry, even when the mitral valve is structurally normal. Primary MR and secondary MR are distinguished by the relative time courses of ventricular and valvular dysfunction, valve anatomy, and the absence of other causes for myocardial dysfunction. In patients with secondary MR, treatment of ventricular dysfunction may result in a decrease in regurgitant severity (see Chapter 19).

Noncardiac Surgery in Patients with Valve Disease

Most adults with valvular heart disease can safely undergo noncardiac surgery, particularly when they have only mild or moderate disease.[166] The key principles in management of patients with valvular heart disease undergoing noncardiac surgery are as follows:
- Accurate assessment of the severity of valve disease
- Determination of symptom status
- Hemodynamic monitoring in the perioperative period
- Optimization of loading conditions

Most adverse outcomes of noncardiac surgery in adults with valve disease are due to failure to recognize the presence of valve disease preoperatively.[167] When valve disease is suspected from history or physical examination findings, echocardiography is appropriate to identify and define the severity of any valve lesions.

In asymptomatic patients, valve regurgitation, even if severe, is generally well tolerated during noncardiac surgery. However, patients with moderate to severe left-sided valve obstruction are at higher risk because an elevated preload results in pulmonary edema and a low preload results in hypotension due to a low cardiac output. Such patients also tolerate peripheral vasodilation poorly because of the inability to increase stroke volume when systemic vascular resistance falls. In asymptomatic patients with stenotic lesions, invasive hemodynamic monitoring is often helpful, beginning in the preoperative setting, to allow optimization of loading conditions, and continuing for 48 to 72 hours postoperatively, during the period of major changes in volume status. Intraoperative echocardiography and participation of an experienced cardiac anesthesiologist also are recommended. When left-sided valve obstruction is very severe, relief of stenosis prior to noncardiac surgery may be considered, depending on the urgency of the noncardiac surgery and whether a percutaneous approach to relief of valve obstruction is possible.[168]

Symptoms due to valve disease are an indication for a corrective valve procedure. Thus, elective noncardiac surgery should be deferred until after treatment of the valve lesion whenever possible. With urgent surgery, symptomatic valve regurgitation is managed with the use standard heart failure regimens based on hemodynamic parameters. Symptomatic severe left-sided valve obstruction can sometimes be managed with the combination of invasive hemodynamic monitoring, intraoperative echocardiography, and an experienced cardiac anesthesiologist. However, in the patient with MS, balloon mitral valvotomy should be considered if valve anatomy is suitable and there is no LA thrombus. In the patient with severe symptomatic AS who needs an urgent noncardiac surgical procedure, balloon mitral valvotomy or percutaneous valve implantation may be considered. Management of women with valve disease during pregnancy is discussed in Chapter 27.

Patient Education

Patient education is the key to compliance with periodic noninvasive monitoring, prevention of complications, and the early recognition of symptoms in patients with valvular heart disease. Each patient should understand the expected long-term prognosis, potential complications, typical symptoms, the rationale for sequential monitoring, and the indications for surgical intervention. Appropriate education avoids needless concern and prompts early reporting of symptoms, allowing optimal timing of surgical intervention. Increasingly, patients are actively involved in decisions about timing of surgery and choice of intervention.

Patients also should be knowledgeable about the risk of infective endocarditis and the importance of maintaining optimal oral hygiene, including regular dental care. Education about the clinical presentation of endocarditis and the importance of obtaining blood cultures before antibiotics are started allows the patient to make sure primary care physicians consider the possibility of endocarditis with a febrile illness. The patient with a prosthetic valve should be aware of situations in which endocarditis prophylaxis is needed and the specific antibiotic regimen to be used.

Patients undergoing long-term anticoagulation need both education and a reliable and available source for consultation regarding warfarin dose, interactions with other medications, and prompt evaluation of any complications.

All patients with valvular heart disease should be evaluated for risk factors for coronary artery disease and should receive education and appropriate therapy for coronary risk factor reduction.

Because the risk of pregnancy in patients with valve dysfunction ranges from normal to very high, this risk should be estimated and discussed with the patient (see Chapter 27). In patients with very high-risk valve lesions, surgical correction prior to a planned pregnancy should be considered. In women undergoing long-term anticoagulation, the issue of warfarin versus heparin anticoagulation during pregnancy should be addressed. In addition, contraception options should be reviewed with all women with valvular disease.

In patients with inherited forms of valve disease, such as Marfan syndrome, the physician should make every effort to ensure that other family members are screened for the disease. With the greater understanding of the genetic basis of myxomatous mitral valve disease and bicuspid aortic valve, screening of family members also may be appropriate for patients with these conditions, particularly if there is a family history of sudden death or aortic dissection.

REFERENCES

1. Iung B, Cachier A, Baron G, et al. Decision-making in elderly patients with severe aortic stenosis: why are so many denied surgery? Eur Heart J 2005;26(24):2714–20.
2. Lancellotti P, Rosenhek R, Pibarot P, et al. ESC Working Group on Valvular Heart Disease Position Paper–heart valve clinics: organization, structure, and experiences. Eur Heart J 2013. [Epub before print].
3. Giuliani ER, Brandenburg RO, Fuster V. Evaluation of cardiac murmurs. Cardiovasc Clin 1980;10(3):1–18.
4. Perloff JK. Physical examination of the heart and circulation. Philadelphia: W. B. Saunders; 1982.
5. Mishra M, Chambers JB, Jackson G. Murmurs in pregnancy: an audit of echocardiography. BMJ 1992;304:1413–4.
6. Northcote RJ, Knight PV, Ballantyne D. Systolic murmurs in pregnancy: value of echocardiographic assessment. Clin Cardiol 1985;8(6):327–8.
7. Bonow RO, Carabello BA, Chatterjee K, et al. ACC/AHA 2006 guidelines for the management of patients with valvular heart disease: a report of the American College of Cardiology/American Heart Association Task Force on Practice Guidelines (writing Committee to Revise the 1998 guidelines for the management of patients with valvular heart disease) developed in collaboration with the Society of Cardiovascular Anesthesiologists endorsed by the Society for Cardiovascular Angiography and Interventions and the Society of Thoracic Surgeons. J Am Coll Cardiol 2006;48(3):e1–148.
8. Jaffe WM, Roche AHG, Coverdale HA, et al. Clinical evaluation versus Doppler echocardiography in the quantitative assessment of valvular heart disease. Circulation 1988;78:267–75.
9. Lombard JT, Selzer A. Valvular aortic stenosis. A clinical and hemodynamic profile of patients. Ann Intern Med 1987;106(2):292–8.
10. Aronow WS, Kronzon I. Correlation of prevalence and severity of valvular aortic stenosis determined by continuous-wave Doppler echocardiography with physical signs of aortic stenosis in patients aged 62 to 100 years with aortic systolic ejection murmurs. Am J Cardiol 1987;60(4):399–401.
11. Forssell G, Jonasson R, Orinius E. Identifying severe aortic valvular stenosis by bedside examination. Acta Med Scand 1985;218(4):397–400.
12. Sutton GC, Craige E. Clinical signs of severe acute mitral regurgitation. Am J Cardiol 1967;20(1):141–4.
13. Etchells E, Glenns V, Shadowitz S, et al. A bedside clinical prediction rule for detecting moderate or severe aortic stenosis. J Gen Intern Med 1998;13(10):699–704.
14. Spooner PH, Perry MP, Brandenburg RO, Pennock GD. Increased intraventricular velocities: an unrecognized cause of systolic murmur in adults. J Am Coll Cardiol 1998;32(6):1589–95.
15. Desjardins VA, Enriquez Sarano M, Tajik AJ, et al. Intensity of murmurs correlates with severity of valvular regurgitation. Am J Med 1996;100(2):149–56.
16. Munt B, Legget ME, Kraft CD, et al. Physical examination in valvular aortic stenosis: correlation with stenosis severity and prediction of clinical outcome. Am Heart J 1999;137(2):298–306.
17. Sainsbury R, White T, Wray R. Echocardiography in elderly patients with systolic murmurs. Age Ageing 1981;10(4):225–30.
18. Vigna C, Impagliatelli M, Russo A, et al. Systolic ejection murmurs in the elderly: aortic valve and carotid arteries echo-Doppler findings. Angiology 1991;42(6):455–61.
19. Wong M, Tei C, Shah PM. Degenerative calcific valvular disease and systolic murmurs in the elderly. J Am Geriatr Soc 1983;31(3):156–63.
20. Guidelines for the diagnosis of rheumatic fever. Jones Criteria, 1992 update. Special Writing Group of the Committee on Rheumatic Fever, Endocarditis, and Kawasaki Disease of the Council on Cardiovascular Disease in the Young of the American Heart Association. JAMA 1992;268(15):2069–73.
21. Gerber MA, Baltimore RS, Eaton CB, et al. Prevention of rheumatic fever and diagnosis and treatment of acute Streptococcal pharyngitis: a scientific statement from the American Heart Association Rheumatic Fever, Endocarditis, and Kawasaki Disease Committee of the Council on Cardiovascular Disease in the Young, the Interdisciplinary Council on Functional Genomics and Translational Biology, and the Interdisciplinary Council on Quality of Care and Outcomes Research: endorsed by the American Academy of Pediatrics. Circulation 2009;119(11):1541–51.
22. Ferrieri P. Proceedings of the Jones Criteria workshop. Circulation 2002;106(19):2521–3.
23. Carapetis JR, Currie BJ. Rheumatic fever in a high incidence population: the importance of monoarthritis and low grade fever. Arch Dis Child 2001;85(3):223–7.
24. Barash J, Mashiach E, Navon-Elkan P, et al. Differentiation of post-streptococcal reactive arthritis from acute rheumatic fever. J Pediatr 2008;153(5):696–9.
25. van Bemmel JM, Delgado V, Holman ER, et al. No increased risk of valvular heart disease in adult poststreptococcal reactive arthritis. Arthritis Rheum 2009;60(4):987–93.
26. Marcus RH, Sareli P, Pocock WA, Barlow JB. The spectrum of severe rheumatic mitral valve disease in a developing country. Correlations among clinical presentation, surgical pathologic findings, and hemodynamic sequelae. Ann Intern Med 1994;120(3):177–83.
27. Abernethy M, Bass N, Sharpe N, et al. Doppler echocardiography and the early diagnosis of carditis in acute rheumatic fever. Aust N Z J Med 1994;24(5):530–5.
28. Wilson W, Taubert KA, Gewitz M, et al. Prevention of Infective Endocarditis. Guidelines From the American Heart Association. A Guideline From the American Heart Association Rheumatic Fever, Endocarditis, and Kawasaki Disease Committee, Council on Cardiovascular Disease in the Young, and the Council on Clinical Cardiology, Council on Cardiovascular Surgery and Anesthesia, and the Quality of Care and Outcomes Research Interdisciplinary Working Group. Circulation 2007;116:1736–54.
29. Seto TB. The case for infectious endocarditis prophylaxis: time to move forward. Arch Intern Med 2007;167(4):327–30.
30. Morris AM. Coming clean with antibiotic prophylaxis for infective endocarditis. Arch Intern Med 2007;167(4):330–2.
31. Thornhill MH, Dayer MJ, Forde JM, et al. Impact of the NICE guideline recommending cessation of antibiotic prophylaxis for prevention of infective endocarditis: before and after study. BMJ 2011;342:d2392.
32. Desimone DC, Tleyjeh IM, Correa de Sa DD, et al. Incidence of infective endocarditis caused by viridans group streptococci before and after publication of the 2007 American Heart Association's endocarditis prevention guidelines. Circulation 2012;126(1):60–4.
33. Whitlock RP, Sun JC, Fremes SE, et al; American College of Chest Physicians. Antithrombotic and thrombolytic therapy for valvular disease: antithrombotic therapy and prevention of thrombosis, 9th ed: American College of Chest Physicians Evidence-Based Clinical Practice Guidelines. Chest 2012;141(2 Suppl):e576S–600S.
34. Vongpatanasin W, Hillis LD, Lange RA. Prosthetic heart valves. New Eng J Med 1996;335:407–16.
35. Cannegieter SC, Rosendaal FR, Wintzen AR, et al. Optimal oral anticoagulant therapy in patients with mechanical heart valves. N Engl J Med 1995;333(1):11–7.
36. Altman R, Rouvier J, Gurfinkel E, et al. Comparison of high-dose with low-dose aspirin in patients with mechanical heart valve replacement treated with oral anticoagulant. Circulation 1996;94(9):2113–6.
37. Acar J, Iung B, Boissel JP, et al. AREVA: multicenter randomized comparison of low-dose versus standard-dose anticoagulation in patients with mechanical prosthetic heart valves. Circulation 1996;94(9):2107–12.
38. Vahanian A, Alfieri O, Andreotti F, et al. Guidelines on the management of valvular heart disease (version 2012). Eur Heart J 2012;33(19):2451–96.
39. Aberg H. Atrial fibrillation. I. A study of atrial thrombosis and systemic embolism in a necropsy material. Acta Med Scand 1969;185(5):373–9.
40. Hwang JJ, Li YH, Lin JM, et al. Left atrial appendage function determined by transesophageal echocardiography in patients with rheumatic mitral valve disease. Cardiology 1994;85(2):121–8.
41. Coulshed N, Epstein EJ, McKendrick CS, et al. Systemic embolism in mitral valve disease. Br Heart J 1970;32(1):26–34.
42. Hinton RC, Kistler JP, Fallon JT, et al. Influence of etiology of atrial fibrillation on incidence of systemic embolism. Am J Cardiol 1977;40(4):509–13.
43. Wolf PA, Dawber TR, Thomas HE Jr, et al. Epidemiologic assessment of chronic atrial fibrillation and risk of stroke: the Framingham study. Neurology 1978;28(10):973–7.
44. Chiang CW, Lo SK, Kuo CT, et al. Noninvasive predictors of systemic embolism in mitral stenosis. An echocardiographic and clinical study of 500 patients. Chest 1994;106(2):396–9.
45. Brockmeier LB, Adolph RJ, Gustin BW, et al. Calcium emboli to the retinal artery in calcific aortic stenosis. Am Heart J 1981;101(1):32–7.
46. Pleet AB, Massey EW, Vengrow ME. TIA, stroke, and the bicuspid aortic valve. Neurology 1981;31(12):1540–2.
47. Chambers J, Bach D, Dumesnil J, et al. Crossing the aortic valve in severe aortic stenosis: no longer acceptable? J Heart Valve Dis 2004;13(3):344–6.
48. Chu JW, Chen VH, Bunton R. Thrombosis of a mechanical heart valve despite dabigatran. Ann Intern Med 2012;157(4):304.
49. Price J, Hynes M, Labinaz M, et al. Mechanical valve thrombosis with dabigatran. J Am Coll Cardiol 2012;60(17):1710–11.
50. Stewart RA, Astell H, Young L, et al. Thrombosis on a mechanical aortic valve whilst anti-coagulated with dabigatran. Heart Lung Circ 2012;21(1):53–5.

51. FDA drug safety communication: Pradaxa (dabigatran etexilate mesylate) should not be used in patients with mechanical prosthetic heart valves. *http://www fda gov/Drugs/DrugSafety/ucm332912 htm* dated 12/19/2012. Accessed 04/18/2013.
52. Fuster V, Ryden LE, Cannom DS, et al. 2011 ACCF/AHA/HRS focused updates incorporated into the ACC/AHA/ESC 2006 guidelines for the management of patients with atrial fibrillation: a report of the American College of Cardiology Foundation/American Heart Association Task Force on practice guidelines. Circulation 2011;123(10):e269–e367.
53. Wann LS, Curtis AB, Ellenbogen KA, et al. 2011 ACCF/AHA/HRS focused update on the management of patients with atrial fibrillation (update on dabigatran): a report of the American College of Cardiology Foundation/American Heart Association Task Force on practice guidelines. Circulation 2011;123(10):1144–50.
54. Saokaew S, Permsuwan U, Chaiyakunapruk N, et al. Effectiveness of pharmacist-participated warfarin therapy management: a systematic review and meta-analysis. J Thromb Haemost 2010;8(11):2418–27.
55. Oake N, Jennings A, Forster AJ, et al. Anticoagulation intensity and outcomes among patients prescribed oral anticoagulant therapy: a systematic review and meta-analysis. CMAJ 2008;179(3):235–44.
56. Aziz F, Corder M, Wolffe J, et al. Anticoagulation monitoring by an anticoagulation service is more cost-effective than routine physician care. J Vasc Surg 2011;54(5):1404–7.
57. Wilson SJ, Wells PS, Kovacs MJ, et al. Comparing the quality of oral anticoagulant management by anticoagulation clinics and by family physicians: a randomized controlled trial. CMAJ 2003;169(4):293–8.
58. Jackson SL, Peterson GM, House M, et al. Point-of-care monitoring of anticoagulant therapy by rural community pharmacists: description of successful outcomes. Aust J Rural Health 2004;12(5):197–200.
59. Chan FW, Wong RS, Lau WH, et al. Management of Chinese patients on warfarin therapy in two models of anticoagulation service - a prospective randomized trial. Br J Clin Pharmacol 2006;62(5):601–9.
60. Lalonde L, Martineau J, Blais N, et al. Is long-term pharmacist-managed anticoagulation service efficient? A pragmatic randomized controlled trial. Am Heart J 2008;156(1):148–54.
60a. Cohen IA, Hutchison TA, Kirking DM, et al. Evaluation of a pharmacist-managed anticoagulation clinic. J Clin Hosp Pharm 1985;10:167–75.
61. Ellis RF, Stephens MA, Sharp GB. Evaluation of a pharmacy-managed warfarin-monitoring service to coordinate inpatient and outpatient therapy. Am J Hosp Pharm 1992;49(2):387–94.
62. Wilt VM, Gums JG, Ahmed OI, et al. Outcome analysis of a pharmacist-managed anticoagulation service. Pharmacotherapy 1995;15(6):732–9.
63. To EK, Pearson GJ. Implementation and evaluation of a pharmacist assisted warfarin dosing program. Can J Hosp Pharm]50, 169–75. 1997.
64. Chiquette E, Amato MG, Bussey HI. Comparison of an anticoagulation clinic with usual medical care: anticoagulation control, patient outcomes, and health care costs. Arch Intern Med 1998;158(15):1641–7.
65. Bieobanjong S. The Clinical Outcomes of Pharmaceutical Care onWarfarin in Out-Patients at Chiangrai Regional Hospital Chiang Mai University, China; 2000.
66. Dager WE, Branch JM, King JH, et al. Optimization of inpatient warfarin therapy: impact of daily consultation by a pharmacist-managed anticoagulation service. Ann Pharmacother 2000;34(5):567–72.
67. Witt DM, Humphries TL. A retrospective evaluation of the management of excessive anticoagulation in an established clinical pharmacy anticoagulation service compared to traditional care. J Thromb Thrombolysis 2003;15(2):113–8.
68. Burns N. Evaluation of warfarin dosing by pharmacists for elderly medical in-patients. Pharm World Sci 26, 232–7. 2004.
69. Liabthawee W. Impact of Education and Conseling by Clinical Pharmacists on Anticoagulation Therapy in Patients With Mechanical Heart Valves [thesis]. Bangkok, Thailand; Mahidol University, 2004.
70. Witt DM, Sadler MA, Shanahan RL, et al. Effect of a centralized clinical pharmacy anticoagulation service on the outcomes of anticoagulation therapy. Chest 2005;127(5):1515–22.
71. Locke C, Ravnan SL, Patel R, et al. Reduction in warfarin adverse events requiring patient hospitalization after implementation of a pharmacist-managed anticoagulation service. Pharmacotherapy 2005;25(5):685–9.
72. Chau T, Rotbard M, King S, et al. Implementation and evaluation of a warfarin dosing service for rehabilitation medicine:report from a pilot project. Can J Hosp Pharm 59, 136–47. 2006.
73. Poon IO, Lal L, Brown EN, Braun UK. The impact of pharmacist-managed oral anticoagulation therapy in older veterans. J Clin Pharm Ther 2007;32(1):21–9.
74. Bungard TJ, Gardner L, Archer SL, et al. Evaluation of a pharmacist-managed anticoagulation clinic: Improving patient care. Open Med 2009;3(1):e16–e21.
75. Tschol N, Lai DK, Tilley JA, et al. Comparison of physician- and pharmacist-managed warfarin sodium treatment in open heart surgery patients. Can J Cardiol 2003;19(12):1413–7.
76. Airee A, Guirguis AB, Mohammad RA. Clinical outcomes and pharmacists' acceptance of a community hospital's anticoagulation management service utilizing decentralized clinical staff pharmacists. Ann Pharmacother 2009;43(4):621–8.
77. Anderson RJ. Cost analysis of a managed care decentralized outpatient pharmacy anticoagulation service. J Manag Care Pharm 2004;10(2):159–65.
78. Wittkowsky AK, Nutescu EA, Blackburn J, et al. Outcomes of oral anticoagulant therapy managed by telephone vs in-office visits in an anticoagulation clinic setting. Chest 2006;130(5):1385–9.
79. Beyth RJ, Quinn L, Landefeld CS. A multicomponent intervention to prevent major bleeding complications in older patients receiving warfarin. A randomized, controlled trial. Ann Intern Med 2000;133(9):687–95.
80. Menendez-Jandula B, Souto JC, Oliver A, et al. Comparing self-management of oral anticoagulant therapy with clinic management: a randomized trial. Ann Intern Med 2005;142(1):1–10.
81. Heneghan C, Alonso-Coello P, Garcia-Alamino JM, et al. Self-monitoring of oral anticoagulation: a systematic review and meta-analysis. Lancet 2006;367(9508):404–11.
82. Ansell J, Jacobson A, Levy J, et al. Guidelines for implementation of patient self-testing and patient self-management of oral anticoagulation. International consensus guidelines prepared by International Self-Monitoring Association for Oral Anticoagulation. Int J Cardiol 2005;99(1):37–45.
83. Fleming HA. Anticoagulants in rheumatic heart-disease. Lancet 1971;2(722):486.
84. Petersen P, Boysen G, Godtfredsen J, et al. Placebo-controlled, randomised trial of warfarin and aspirin for prevention of thromboembolic complications in chronic atrial fibrillation. The Copenhagen AFASAK study. Lancet 1989;1(8631):175–9.
85. Stroke Prevention in Atrial Fibrillation Investigators. Warfarin versus aspirin for prevention of thromboembolism in atrial fibrillation: Stroke Prevention in Atrial Fibrillation II Study. Lancet 1994;343(8899):687–91.
86. Fatkin D, Herbert E, Feneley MP. Hematologic correlates of spontaneous echo contrast in patients with atrial fibrillation and implications for thromboembolic risk. Am J Cardiol 1994;73(9):672–6.
87. Black IW, Hopkins AP, Lee LC, Walsh WF. Left atrial spontaneous echo contrast: a clinical and echocardiographic analysis. J Am Coll Cardiol 1991;18(2):398–404.
88. Bernhardt P, Schmidt H, Hammerstingl C, et al. Patients with atrial fibrillation and dense spontaneous echo contrast at high risk a prospective and serial follow-up over 12 months with transesophageal echocardiography and cerebral magnetic resonance imaging. J Am Coll Cardiol 2005;45(11):1807–12.
89. Stroke prevention in atrial fibrillation investigators. Stroke Prevention in Atrial Fibrillation Study. Final results. Circulation 1991;84(2):527–39.
90. de Bono DP, Warlow CP. Mitral-annulus calcification and cerebral or retinal ischaemia. Lancet 1979;2(8139):383–5.
91. Fulkerson PK, Beaver BM, Auseon JC, Graber HL. Calcification of the mitral annulus: etiology, clinical associations, complications and therapy. Am J Med 1979;66(6):967–77.
92. Benjamin EJ, Plehn JF, D'Agostino RB, et al. Mitral annular calcification and the risk of stroke in an elderly cohort. New Eng J Med 1992;327:374–9.
93. Hart RG, Easton JD. Mitral valve prolapse and cerebral infarction. Stroke 1982;13(4):429–30.
94. Pruitt AA, Rubin RH, Karchmer AW, Duncan GW. Neurologic complications of bacterial endocarditis. Medicine Baltimore 1978;57(4):329–43.
95. Salem DN, Stein PD, Al Ahmad A, et al. Antithrombotic therapy in valvular heart disease—native and prosthetic: the Seventh ACCP Conference on Antithrombotic and Thrombolytic Therapy. Chest 2004;126(3 Suppl):457S–82S.
96. Tornos P, Almirante B, Mirabet S, et al. Infective endocarditis due to Staphylococcus aureus: deleterious effect of anticoagulant therapy. Arch Intern Med 1999;159(5):473–5.
97. Chan KL, Tam J, Dumesnil JG, et al. Effect of long-term aspirin use on embolic events in infective endocarditis. Clin Infect Dis 2008;46(1):37–41.
98. Wilson WR, Geraci JE, Danielson GK, et al. Anticoagulant therapy and central nervous system complications in patients with prosthetic valve endocarditis. Circulation 1978;57(5):1004–7.
99. Leport C, Vilde JL, Bricaire F, et al. Fifty cases of late prosthetic valve endocarditis: improvement in prognosis over a 15 year period. Br Heart J 1987;58(1):66–71.
100. Delahaye JP, Poncet P, Malquarti V, et al. Cerebrovascular accidents in infective endocarditis: role of anticoagulation. Eur Heart J 1990;11(12):1074–8.
101. Bonow RO, Cheitlin MD, Crawford MH, Douglas PS. Task Force 3: valvular heart disease. J Am Coll Cardiol 2005;45(8):1334–40.
102. Otto CM, Lind BK, Kitzman DW, et al. Association of aortic-valve sclerosis with cardiovascular mortality and morbidity in the elderly. N Engl J Med 1999;341(3):142–7.
103. Owens DS, Budoff MJ, Katz R, et al. Aortic valve calcium independently predicts coronary and cardiovascular events in a primary prevention population. JACC Cardiovasc Imaging 2012;5(6):619–25.
104. Fremes SE, Goldman BS, Ivanov J, et al. Valvular surgery in the elderly. Circulation 1989;80(Supp I):I77–I90.
105. Hendren WG, Nemec JJ, Lytle BW, et al. Mitral valve repair for ischemic mitral insufficiency. Ann Thorac Surg 1991;52(6):1246–51.
106. Craver JM, Weintraub WS, Jones EL, et al. Predictors of mortality, complications, and length of stay in aortic valve replacement for aortic stenosis. Circulation 1988;78(3):2185–90.
107. Freeman WK, Schaff HV, O'Brien PC, et al. Cardiac surgery in the octogenarian: perioperative outcome and clinical follow-up. J Am Coll Cardiol 1991;18(1):29–35.
108. Culliford AT, Galloway AC, Colvin SB, et al. Aortic valve replacement for aortic stenosis in persons aged 80 years and over. Am J Cardiol 1991;67(15):1256–60.
109. Elayda MA, Hall RJ, Reul RM, et al. Aortic valve replacement in patients 80 years and older. Operative risks and long-term results. Circulation 1993;88:II11–6.
110. Cowell SJ, Newby DE, Prescott RJ, et al. A randomized trial of intensive lipid-lowering therapy in calcific aortic stenosis. N Engl J Med 2005;352(23):2389–97.
111. Rossebo AB, Pedersen TR, Boman K, et al. Intensive lipid lowering with simvastatin and ezetimibe in aortic stenosis. N Engl J Med 2008;359(13):1343–56.
112. Chan KL, Teo K, Dumesnil JG, et al. Effect of Lipid lowering with rosuvastatin on progression of aortic stenosis: results of the aortic stenosis progression observation: measuring effects of rosuvastatin (ASTRONOMER) trial. Circulation 2010;121(2):306–14.
113. Carabello BA. The current therapy for mitral regurgitation. J Am Coll Cardiol 2008;52(5):319–26.
114. Carabello BA. Left ventricular adaptation to pressure or volume overload. In: Otto CM, Bonow RO, editors. Valvular Heart Disease: A Companion to Braunwald's Heart Disease. 3rd ed. Philadelphia: Saunders/Elsevier; 2009.
115. Levine HJ, Gaasch WH. Vasoactive drugs in chronic regurgitant lesions of the mitral and aortic valves. J Am Coll Cardiol 1996;28:1083–91.
116. Evangelista A, Tornos P, Sambola A, et al. Long-term vasodilator therapy in patients with severe aortic regurgitation. N Engl J Med 2005;353(13):1342–9.
117. Ahmed MI, Aban I, Lloyd SG, et al. A randomized controlled phase IIb trial of beta(1)-receptor blockade for chronic degenerative mitral regurgitation. J Am Coll Cardiol 2012;60(9):833–8.

118. Carabello BA. Beta-blockade for mitral regurgitation: could the management of valvular heart disease actually be moving into the 21st century? J Am Coll Cardiol 2012;60(9):839–40.

119. Henkel DM, Malouf JF, Connolly HM, et al. Asymptomatic left ventricular systolic dysfunction in patients with severe aortic stenosis: characteristics and outcomes. J Am Coll Cardiol 2012;60(22):2325–9.

120. Otto CM, Burwash IG, Legget ME, et al. A prospective study of asymptomatic valvular aortic stenosis: clinical, echocardiographic, and exercise predictors of outcome. Circulation 1997;95:2262–70.

121. Kearney LG, Lu K, Ord M, et al. Global longitudinal strain is a strong independent predictor of all-cause mortality in patients with aortic stenosis. Eur Heart J Cardiovasc Imaging 2012;13(10):827–33.

122. Douglas PS, Otto CM, Mickel MC, et al. Gender differences in left ventricular geometry and function in patients undergoing balloon dilation of the aortic valve for isolated aortic stenosis. Br Heart J 1995;73:548–54.

123. Villari B, Campbell SE, Hess OM, et al. Influence of collagen network on left ventricular systolic and diastolic function in aortic valve disease. J Am Coll Cardiol 1993;22(5):1477–84.

124. Villari B, Campbell SE, Schneider J, et al. Sex-dependent differences in left ventricular function and structure in chronic pressure overload. Eur Heart J 1995;16(10):1410–9.

125. Carabello BA. Timing of valve replacement in aortic stenosis. Moving closer to perfection [editorial; comment]. Circulation 1997;95(9):2241–3.

126. Lund O. Valve replacement for aortic stenosis: the curative potential of early operation. Scand J Thorac Cardiovasc Surg Suppl 1993;40:1–137.

127. Kang DH, Park SJ, Rim JH, et al. Early surgery versus conventional treatment in asymptomatic very severe aortic stenosis. Circulation 2010;121(13):1502–9.

128. Gada H, Scuffham PA, Griffin B, Marwick TH. Quality-of-life implications of immediate surgery and watchful waiting in asymptomatic aortic stenosis: a decision-analytic model. Circ Cardiovasc Qual Outcomes 2011;4(5):541–8.

129. Pape LA, Price JM, Alpert JS, et al. Relation of left atrial size to pulmonary capillary wedge pressure in severe mitral regurgitation. Cardiology 1991;78(4):297–303.

130. Burwash IG, Blackmore GL, Koilpillai CJ. Usefulness of left atrial and left ventricular chamber sizes as predictors of the severity of mitral regurgitation. Am J Cardiol 1992;70(7):774–9.

131. Sanfilippo AJ, Abascal VM, Sheehan M, et al. Atrial enlargement as a consequence of atrial fibrillation. A prospective echocardiographic study. Circulation 1990;82(3):792–7.

132. Braunwald E, Frahm CJ. Studies on Starling's law of the heart. IV. Observations on the hemodynamic functions of the left atrium in man. Circulation 1961;24:633.

133. Chua YL, Schaff HV, Orszulak TA, Morris JJ. Outcome of mitral valve repair in patients with preoperative atrial fibrillation. Should the maze procedure be combined with mitral valvuloplasty? J Thorac Cardiovasc Surg 1994;107(2):408–15.

134. Bum KJ, Suk MJ, Yun SC, et al. Long-term outcomes of mechanical valve replacement in patients with atrial fibrillation: impact of the maze procedure. Circulation 2012;125(17):2071–80.

135. Leavitt JI, Coats MH, Falk RH. Effects of exercise on transmitral gradient and pulmonary artery pressure in patients with mitral stenosis or a prosthetic mitral valve: a Doppler echocardiographic study. J Am Coll Cardiol 1991;17(7):1520–6.

136. Melby SJ, Moon MR, Lindman BR, et al. Impact of pulmonary hypertension on outcomes after aortic valve replacement for aortic valve stenosis. J Thorac Cardiovasc Surg 2011;141(6):1424–30.

137. Lindman BR, Bonow RO, Otto CM. Current management of calcific aortic stenosis circulation research. IN PRESS. 2012.

138. Richards AM, Nicholls MG, Ikram H, et al. Syncope in aortic valvular stenosis. Lancet 1984;2(8412):1113–6.

139. Johnson AM. Aortic stenosis, sudden death, and the left ventricular baroceptors. Br Heart J 1971;33(1):1–5.

140. Khot UN, Novaro GM, Popovic ZB, et al. Nitroprusside in critically ill patients with left ventricular dysfunction and aortic stenosis. N Engl J Med 2003;348(18):1756–63.

141. Chockalingam A, Venkatesan S, Subramaniam T, et al. Safety and efficacy of angiotensin-converting enzyme inhibitors in symptomatic severe aortic stenosis: Symptomatic Cardiac Obstruction-Pilot Study of Enalapril in Aortic Stenosis (SCOPE-AS). Am Heart J 2004;147(4):E19.

142. Bermejo J, Antoranz JC, Burwash IG, et al. In-vivo analysis of the instantaneous transvalvular pressure difference-flow relationship in aortic valve stenosis: implications of unsteady fluid-dynamics for the clinical assessment of disease severity. J Heart Valve Dis 2002;11(4):557–66.

143. Burwash IG, Thomas DD, Sadahiro M, et al. Dependence of Gorlin formula and continuity equation valve areas on transvalvular volume flow rate in valvular aortic stenosis. Circulation 1994;89:827–35.

144. Zile MR, Gaasch WH. Heart failure in aortic stenosis—improving diagnosis and treatment. N Engl J Med 2003;348(18):1735–6.

145. O'Brien KD, Zhao XQ, Shavelle DM, et al. Hemodynamic effects of the angiotensin-converting enzyme inhibitor, ramipril, in patients with mild to moderate aortic stenosis and preserved left ventricular function. J Investig Med 2004;52(3):185–91.

146. Routledge HC, Townend JN. ACE inhibition in aortic stenosis: dangerous medicine or golden opportunity? J Hum Hypertens 2001;15(10):659–67.

147. Nadir MA, Wei L, Elder DH, et al. Impact of renin-angiotensin system blockade therapy on outcome in aortic stenosis. J Am Coll Cardiol 2011;58(6):570–6.

148. Kadem L, Dumesnil JG, Rieu R, et al. Impact of systemic hypertension on the assessment of aortic stenosis. Heart 2005;91(3):354–61.

149. Otto CM. Valvular aortic stenosis: disease severity and timing of intervention. J Am Coll Cardiol 2006;47(11):2141–51.

150. Bermejo J. The effects of hypertension on aortic valve stenosis. Heart 2005;91(3):280–2.

151. Little SH, Chan KL, Burwash IG. Impact of blood pressure on the Doppler echocardiographic assessment of severity of aortic stenosis. Heart 2007;93(7):848–55.

152. Grundy SM, Pasternak R, Greenland P, et al. AHA/ACC scientific statement: Assessment of cardiovascular risk by use of multiple-risk-factor assessment equations: a statement for healthcare professionals from the American Heart Association and the American College of Cardiology. J Am Coll Cardiol 1999;34(4):1348–59.

153. Julius BK, Spillmann M, Vassalli G, et al. Angina pectoris in patients with aortic stenosis and normal coronary arteries. Mechanisms and pathophysiological concepts. Circulation 1997;95(4):892–8.

154. Kupari M, Virtanen KS, Turto H, et al. Exclusion of coronary artery disease by exercise thallium-201 tomography in patients with aortic stenosis. Am J Cardiol 1992;70:635–40.

155. Rask P, Karp KL, Eriksson MP, Moore T. Dipyridamole thallium-201 single photon emission tomography in aortic stenosis: gender differences. Eur J Nuclear Med 1995;22:1155–62.

156. Samuels B, Kiat H, Friedman JD, Berman DS. Adenosine pharmacologic stress myocardial perfusion tomographic imaging in patients with significant aortic stenosis: diagnostic efficacy and comparison of clinical, hemodynamic and electrocardiographic variable with 100 age-matched control subjects. J Am Coll Cardiol 1995;25:99–106.

157. Hiratzka LF, Bakris GL, Beckman JA, et al. 2010 ACCF/AHA/AATS/ACR/ASA/SCA/SCAI/SIR/STS/SVM guidelines for the diagnosis and management of patients with Thoracic Aortic Disease: a report of the American College of Cardiology Foundation/American Heart Association Task Force on Practice Guidelines, American Association for Thoracic Surgery, American College of Radiology, American Stroke Association, Society of Cardiovascular Anesthesiologists, Society for Cardiovascular Angiography and Interventions, Society of Interventional Radiology, Society of Thoracic Surgeons, and Society for Vascular Medicine. Circulation 2010;121(13):e266–e369.

158. Gillinov AM, Bhavani S, Blackstone EH, et al. Surgery for permanent atrial fibrillation: impact of patient factors and lesion set. Ann Thorac Surg 2006;82(2):502–13.

159. Doty JR, Doty DB, Jones KW, et al. Comparison of standard Maze III and radiofrequency Maze operations for treatment of atrial fibrillation. J Thorac Cardiovasc Surg 2007;133(4):1037–44.

160. Patel JJ, Dyer RB, Mitha AS. Beta adrenergic blockade does not improve effort tolerance in patients with mitral stenosis in sinus rhythm. Eur Heart J 1995;16(9):1264–8.

161. Ashcom TL, Johns JP, Bailey SR, Rubal BJ. Effects of chronic beta-blockade on rest and exercise hemodynamics in mitral stenosis. Cathet Cardiovasc Diagn 1995;35(2):110–5.

162. Stoll BC, Ashcom TL, Johns JP, et al. Effects of atenolol on rest and exercise hemodynamics in patients with mitral stenosis. Am J Cardiol 1995;75(7):482–4.

163. al Kasab SM, Sabag T, al Zaibag M, et al. Beta-adrenergic receptor blockade in the management of pregnant women with mitral stenosis. Am J Obstet Gynecol 1990;163(1):137–40.

164. Bonow RO, Rosing DR, McIntosh CL, et al. The natural history of asymptomatic patients with aortic regurgitation and normal left ventricular function. Circulation 1983;68(3):509–17.

165. Grigioni F, Enriquez-Sarano M, Ling LH, et al. Sudden death in mitral regurgitation due to flail leaflet. J Am Coll Cardiol 1999;34(7):2078–85.

166. Fleisher LA, Beckman JA, Brown KA, et al. ACC/AHA 2006 guideline update on perioperative cardiovascular evaluation for noncardiac surgery: focused update on perioperative beta-blocker therapy: a report of the American College of Cardiology/American Heart Association Task Force on Practice Guidelines (Writing Committee to Update the 2002 Guidelines on Perioperative Cardiovascular Evaluation for Noncardiac Surgery): developed in collaboration with the American Society of Echocardiography, American Society of Nuclear Cardiology, Heart Rhythm Society, Society of Cardiovascular Anesthesiologists, Society for Cardiovascular Angiography and Interventions, and Society for Vascular Medicine and Biology. Circulation 2006;113(22):2662–74.

167. Rohde LE, Polanczyk CA, Goldman L, et al. Usefulness of transthoracic echocardiography as a tool for risk stratification of patients undergoing major noncardiac surgery. Am J Cardiol 2001;87(5):505–9.

168. Torsher LC, Shub C, Rettke SR, Brown DL. Risk of patients with severe aortic stenosis undergoing noncardiac surgery. Am J Cardiol 1998;81(4):448–52.

CHAPTER 10

Risk Assessment for Valvular Heart Disease

Michael J. Mack

Key Points

- Risk scores are predicted probabilities calculated from a multivariable logistic regression model calibrated on data from within a fixed time.
- Risk algorithms are accurate only for the population and in the time frame in which they are developed and validated. Risk algorithms cannot reliably be applied to populations and treatments other than those in which they were developed.
- Risk adjustment loses accuracy at the extremes of the population studied when there are too few patients upon which to build a statistically valid model. This accounts for some of the overestimation of risk seen with many models.
- Risk algorithms cannot account for variables not collected or analyzed.
- Unless the factors upon which the risk algorithm is formulated are based on complete and accurate data, it is likely that an inaccurate predictor will result.
- Risk adjustment allows for a more meaningful analysis of hospitals or therapies for comparative safety and/or effectiveness of treatment. Public reporting of surgical outcomes in the United States is by risk-adjusted results, in which the observed outcome divided by the expected outcome is based on known patient risk factors.
- Current risk predictive models developed for surgical aortic valve replacement are inaccurate, are not applicable, and yield misinformation if applied to evaluation of candidates for transcatheter aortic valve implantation (TAVI). Patients being assessed for TAVI are at the extremes of risk, where the current risk models fail because there are too few patients at the higher extremes of risk to yield robust discrimination of risk. The risk models were neither developed nor validated for TAVI and are therefore highly likely to be invalid for it. They do not take into account variables that may play a significant role in risk, including porcelain aorta, previous radiation therapy, liver disease, and frailty.

Background

Outcomes data from medical procedures are commonly used to compare treatments or providers. Early databases were originally used to assess outcomes from cardiac surgical procedures, most commonly coronary artery bypass grafting (CABG). These registries were first constructed in the United States from administrative data from the U.S. Health Care Financing Administration (HCFA), the precursor to the current Center for Medicare and Medicaid Services (CMS). Although the purpose of publishing these database registries was to assess outcomes in various clinical programs, providers correctly argued that such data did not account for various patient-specific factors that may impact outcomes.[1,2] This objection led directly to the development of a number of high-quality clinical databases and risk models to account for these patient-specific factors, especially in cardiac surgery.[3,4]

Because patient outcomes may be influenced by severity of illness, treatment effectiveness, and chance, such comparisons must account for differences in the prevalence of patient risk factors, a concept termed "case mix."[5-9] It is possible to reduce or eliminate outcome variability due to case mix through a number of methods, including randomization, which should balance both known and unknown risk factors. However, this is possible only in randomized controlled trials, which have their own shortcomings, such as the "generalizability" of the outcomes. Therefore, we have come to rely on registries when comparing outcomes among various treatments or providers. The use of covariate matching or propensity score matching techniques, which balance known risk factors, can be used to balance patient variables. However, in the majority of observational studies, risk adjustment has been used to account for case mix.[10,11] With the use of statistical modeling techniques, most commonly multivariable regression analysis, the association between individual risk factors, known as *predictor variables* or *covariates*, and outcomes can be determined.[12] Once the impact of each risk factor is determined from a given population sample, it becomes possible to estimate the probability of the outcome for patients having particular combinations of these risk factors.

Although risk models have been utilized for many years, their broader applicability and critical importance became more fully appreciated after the aforementioned 1986 release of unadjusted hospital outcome data by HCFA. Soon after this release, The Society of Thoracic Surgeons (STS) established an Ad Hoc Committee on Risk Factors for Coronary Artery Bypass Surgery.[13] Subsequently, a committee began work on the development of The STS National Cardiac Database, which was formally established in 1989.[14] Subsequently, risk models have been utilized to adjust cardiac surgery outcomes for preoperative patient characteristics and disease severity.[15] Many other clinical databases have been established to assess outcomes not only in cardiac surgery but also in cardiology and other fields. Many of them have developed risk models based on those registries. There is significant variability among these models, which are accounted for by the population studied, the period of the data collection, and the statistical techniques used to develop the model. This chapter examines the intricacies of how these factors bear on the assessment of risk in patients with valvular heart disease.

How Risk Algorithms Are Constructed

Risk scores are predicted probabilities calculated from a multivariable logistic regression model calibrated on data from within a fixed time. It is, of course, a given that no risk adjustment model is better than the data on which it is based. Administrative databases, such as the CMS Medicare Provider Analysis and Review (MEDPAR) file, provide a readily available source of data on millions of patients. However, the file is based on claims data used for administrative billing purposes and does not capture key clinical data fields, such as ejection fraction, that may play a significant role in clinical outcomes. Hence, the first key component in constructing a robust risk model is the use of a clinical database with as complete and accurate data as possible. The second key factor is to use statisticians with sufficient experience in risk modeling because different multivariable equations can be developed from the same data.[15]

Three techniques have been used for construction of cardiac surgery risk models. Bayesian models were initially used for the STS database to account for the significant amount of missing data. As data completeness improved, logistic regression models were used; The most common statistical technique used currently, logistic regression is employed not only by the STS but also by the models constructed by New York State,[16] the Veterans Administration,[17] and the Northern New England Cardiovascular Disease Study Group.[18] Other models, such as the Parsonnet score[19] and the European System for Cardiac Operative Risk Evaluation (EuroSCORE),[20] use simple additive scores with weights derived from logistic regression models. There is some evidence that logistic regression models perform better.[21]

For development of a risk model, the study population is usually divided into a development or training sample and a validation or test sample. For the STS Isolated Valve Risk model, the study population was randomly divided into a 60% development sample and a 40% validation sample. The development sample was then used to identify predictor variables and estimate model coefficients. Data from the validation sample were used to assess model fit, discrimination, and calibration.[22] *Discrimination* refers to the model's ability to separate two groups studied, for example, survivors and nonsurvivors. An area under the receiver operating characteristic curve (AUROC) is calculated using the c-index, with ranges between 0.5 and 1.0. The higher the value of the c-index, the better the discrimination, whereas values closer to 0.5 indicate that the model's ability to discriminate is no better than random chance or the "flip of a coin."[23] In most risk prediction models used for cardiac surgery, the AUROC ranges between 0.75 and 0.80.

Limitations of Risk Algorithms

In the employment of risk adjustment, important limitations have to be taken into account in order that valid information and not "misinformation" is obtained from the "correction."[24] First, risk algorithms are accurate only for the population and in the time frame in which they are developed and validated. Second, risk adjustment loses accuracy at the extremes of the population studied, where there are too few patients upon which to build a statistically valid model. This "tail of the bell-shaped curve" is where high-risk patients with aortic stenosis "reside," accounting for some of the overestimation of risk seen with many models.[25,26] Third, risk algorithms cannot reliably be applied directly to populations and treatments other than those in which they were developed. The implication is that although both surgical aortic valve replacement (AVR) and transcatheter aortic valve implantation (TAVI) are used in treating patients with aortic stenosis, AVR risk algorithms are based on "surgical" AVR outcomes and therefore may not to be directly applicable to TAVI.

Fourth, risk algorithms cannot account for variables not collected or analyzed. This lack of accounting has one of two causes: (1) the occurrence of the factor or condition is so infrequent that its impact cannot be measured (e.g., porcelain aorta) or (2) the factor either may have not been previously known to be a factor that was causal or cannot be accurately measured or quantified. The role of frailty and its impact on outcomes of treatment is a case in point. Fifth, all risk predictors fall prey to the phenomenon "garbage in equals garbage out." Unless the factors upon which the algorithm is formulated are based on complete and accurate data, an inaccurate predictor will result. A corollary is that the risk predictor must be "user friendly." The greater number of variables collected in formulation of the risk algorithm, the more accurate the prediction of risk; however, the more burdensome the collection of data required, the less complete and accurate will be the information. So there must be a balance between including all information that is likely to be a factor in causing risk and

"user-friendliness" in order to facilitate complete and accurate collection and ensure that the tool is routinely employed in decision making. Indeed, one risk algorithm for aortic stenosis, the Age, Creatinine, Ejection Fraction (ACEF) score, provides reasonable prediction using only the three factors in its name: age, serum creatinine level, and ejection fraction.[27]

Uses of Risk Algorithms

Profiling risk in patients undergoing medical procedures serves many purposes.[28] First, it allows outcomes prediction for individual patients so that both patient and caregiver can be better informed in making decisions regarding the advisability and risks of a specific medical procedure. Second, patients undergoing medical procedures frequently have comorbidities that cause varying levels of risk and therefore may adversely affect the outcomes of a procedure. When different modalities of treatment or different caregivers are compared, risk adjustment allows for a balanced analysis of outcomes by accounting for the risk factor variation among different patient cohorts. This correction allows for a "more level playing field" of outcomes assessment; also, this achievement of an "apples-to-apples" comparison is one of the advantages of clinical outcomes databases over administrative databases, which have limited ability to adjust risk.

Risk adjustment, therefore, allows for a more meaningful analysis of hospitals or therapies for comparative safety and/or effectiveness of treatment. One could, for example, compare two standard procedures (e.g., CABG surgery and percutaneous coronary intervention) or a new procedure with an existing standard (e.g., TAVI and surgical AVR) for outcomes comparisons in different centers. Public reporting of surgical outcomes in the United States is by risk adjusted results, in which the observed outcome divided by the expected outcome is based on known patient risk factors. This approach creates an observed-to-expected ratio (O/E) that is a multiplier of the observed mortality. An O/E ratio of less than 1 is indicative of a better-than-expected outcome, whereas a ratio greater than 1 means the outcome is worse than expected on the basis of the patient's existing comorbidities or risk factors. Without the risk adjustment that takes into account these patient specific factors that may adversely affect outcomes, meaningful comparison is not possible.

What Can Be Predicted?

The earliest and most common use of risk prediction was for evaluating early mortality after isolated CABG. Because the procedure was performed commonly and outcomes were publicly reported, risk prediction for an "apples-to-apples" comparison among surgical centers performing CABG became common. "Early mortality," as defined by the STS, includes all deaths occurring before 30 days whether in or out of the hospital and any death occurring in the hospital at any time. Other risk prediction models for early mortality include only in-hospital mortality, which misses approximately 10% of the early deaths. The advantage of reporting in-hospital mortality is that the data are more easily collected and probably more accurate. The disadvantage, however, is that very ill postoperative patients who are quite likely to die are frequently discharged to long-term acute care or skilled nursing facilities less than 30 days after surgery and are therefore not counted. In a 2012 analysis of EuroSCORE II outcome data, for example, in which hospital mortality is around 4%, adding 30-day mortality increases the reported mortality by about 0.6%, and adding 90-day mortality increases it further by about 0.9%.[29] When one is comparing various risk predictors, it is important to be sure that the same data definitions are being used by each model.

Risk prediction models for early mortality after cardiac surgery have been expanded to use for other procedures. In addition isolated CABG (c-index 0.78), risk prediction is available for isolated surgical AVR, isolated mitral valve repair or replacement,

CABG combined with AVR, and CABG with mitral valve repair or replacement. The weighting of the various risk factors is recalibrated with each new version of the STS Adult Cardiac Database according to the most recent data uploaded by the 1,005 cardiac surgery programs in the United States that participate in the database. Rankin et al[30] have published a risk prediction for multiple valve operations, including aortic and mitral valve operation, mitral and tricuspid and aortic valve operation, and mitral and tricuspid operation, that has acceptable discrimination (c-index 0.711 to 0.727).[30] In addition to early mortality, the STS risk prediction algorithm has been demonstrated to be predictive of long-term survival for isolated CABG, with survival at 1,3,5 and 10 years having similar AUROC values to the value of 30-day survival (0.794).[31] A composite score of mortality and major morbidity after surgical AVR has also been published.[32] The STS AVR composite score is based solely on outcomes, including risk-standardized mortality and any-or-none risk-standardized morbidity (occurrence of sternal infection, reoperation, stroke, renal failure, or prolonged ventilation). The STS online risk calculator is capable of calculating major morbidity in addition to mortality after surgical AVR.[33]

Available Risk Algorithms for Aortic Stenosis

At least 12 risk algorithms have been constructed in various populations and differing periods to predict outcomes after surgical AVR (Table 10-1). The two most widely used are the Logistic EuroSCORE and the STS Predicted Risk of Mortality.[28,34,35] The Logistic EuroSCORE was developed in 1995 as an additive score (Additive EuroSCORE) and later converted to a logistic regression model. It was derived from a data set from eight European countries and was based on a population sample of almost 15,000 patients undergoing all types of cardiac operations. There were 12 covariates identified that were predictive of early mortality. The benefit of the Logistic EuroSCORE is its user-friendliness, in that it requires only 18 data fields for the calculation. The shortcoming for use in the United States is that the algorithm is calculated on a relatively small sample size from nearly 20 years ago in a population outside the country. These factors make the applicability of the risk model to the current patients undergoing surgical AVR, especially in the United States, quite questionable. The Logistic EuroSCORE has been repeatedly demonstrated to over-predict actual risk in the assessment of patients for whom surgery poses a high risk.[25,26] This problem is due to factors mentioned previously, including too few patients at high risk to be accurately analyzed and the fact that they underwent surgery in an earlier time. In order to address some of these shortcomings, the Logistic EuroSCORE has been updated as the EuroSCORE II.[36]

This updated risk predictor was derived from more than 22,000 patients operated on in 2010 in 43 countries worldwide. It includes all cardiac procedures and now has 18 covariates predictive of surgical aortic valve mortality. Whether the accuracy of the EuroSCORE II model has been improved is a subject of debate. Pooling contemporaneous multi-institutional data, Grant et al[37] found that EuroSCORE II performed well overall in the United Kingdom and was an acceptable contemporary generic cardiac surgery risk model. However, they also found that the model was poorly calibrated for isolated CABG surgery and in both the highest-risk and lowest-risk patients. These investigators recommended that regular revalidation of EuroSCORE II will be needed to identify calibration drift or clinical inconsistencies, which commonly emerge in clinical prediction models. Chalmers et al[38] applied the model to a 5500-patient cohort and concluded that EuroSCORE II is globally better calibrated than the EuroSCORE and found better overall discrimination, with a c-index of 0.79 (old model 0.77) and its best performance in mitral (0.87) and coronary (0.79) surgery; Euro SCORE II was weakest in isolated AVR (c-index 0.69), only marginally better than the old model (0.67).[38] A third study also found better performance of the EuroSCORE II model[39] (Table 10-2).

The STS Predicted Risk of Mortality (PROM) has generally correlated better with clinical outcomes. The model was developed in a later era (2002-2006) in the United States with use of data from 67,000 patients undergoing only isolated AVR.[22] Twenty-four covariates for mortality have been identified. At least two series have found the STS Predicted Risk of Mortality to be a better predictor of early mortality than the Logistic EuroSCORE, especially in the higher-risk patients undergoing AVR.[40,41] However, there still is the tendency for the STS instrument to under predict risk. The STS Predicted Risk of Mortality has now been updated from version 2.61 to version 2.73. The updated version includes multiple potential risk factors not previously collected, such as previous radiation exposure, liver disease, and frailty as measured by gait speed. As with all risk algorithms, calibration drift occurs as the original data set becomes dated, and the algorithm will need to be updated once sufficient numbers of patients are available for the new version that has in addition captured the new possible predictors.

Many other risk prediction models have been constructed but are not widely used. The Ambler Score was developed from a national database from the Society of Cardiothoracic Surgeons of Great Britain and Ireland on 32,839 patients who underwent heart valve surgery between April 1995 and March 2003.[42] This risk predictor has largely been supplanted by the Logistic EuroSCORE and STS Predicted Risk of Mortality.

The Northern New England risk model was derived from eight Northern New England Medical Centers in the period

TABLE 10-1	Risk Algorithms in Various Populations and Differing Time Periods to Predict Outcomes after Surgical Aortic Valve Replacement

Society of Thoracic Surgeons Predicted Risk of Mortality v2.73
Logistic EuroSCORE
EuroSCORE (Additive)
Ambler (United Kingdom)
Northern New England
New York State
Providence Health System
Veterans Affairs Risk Score
Age, Creatinine, Ejection Fraction (ACEF) Score
Australian AVR Score
EuroSCORE II
German Aortic Valve Score

AVR, aortic valve replacement.

TABLE 10-2	Comparison of Logistic EuroSCORE, STS PROM, and EuroSCORE II		
	LOGISTIC EUROSCORE	SOCIETY OF THORACIC SURGEONS PREDICTED RISK OF MORTALITY (STS PROM)	EUROSCORE II
Year of population analysis	1995	2002-2006	May-July 2010
Place	Europe (8 countries)	United States	43 countries worldwide
Number of operations	14,799	67,292	22,381
Type of operations	All cardiac	Aortic valve only	All cardiac
Covariates for aortic valve mortality	12	24	18

January 1991 through December 2001. In this model, 8943 patients undergoing heart valve surgery were analyzed, and 11 variables in the aortic model were found to be predictive of adverse outcomes.[43] They included older age, lower body surface area, prior cardiac operation; elevated serum creatinine level, prior stroke, New York Heart Association (NYHA) functional class IV, heart failure, atrial fibrillation, acuity, year of surgery, and concomitant CABG.

In efforts to simplify risk prediction, two additional algorithms have been developed. The Age, Creatinine, Ejection Fraction score, previously mentioned, analyzed 29,659 consecutive patients who underwent elective cardiac operations in 14 Italian institutions from 2004 to 2009.[44,45] Using only three variables, age serum creatinine and ejection fraction, Ranucci et al[44,45] found that for all deciles of risk distribution, the Logistic EuroSCORE significantly overestimated mortality risk and that the Age, Creatinine, Ejection Fraction score slightly overestimated the mortality risk in very-low-risk patients and significantly underestimated the mortality risk in very-high-risk patients, correctly estimating the risk in 7 of 10 deciles. The accuracy of the Age, Creatinine, Ejection Fraction score was acceptable (AUROC 0.702) and at least comparable to the Logistic EuroSCORE calculation.

Another algorithm specific for patients undergoing surgical AVR has been developed in Australia.[46] The Australian AVR score is based on 3544 AVR procedures performed between 2001 and 2008. It contains the following predictors: age, NYHA functional class, left main disease, infective endocarditis, cerebrovascular disease, renal dysfunction, previous cardiac surgery, and estimated ejection fraction. The final model (AVR-Score) obtained an average AUROC of 0.78 for early mortality

Risk Algorithms in Transcatheter Aortic Valve Implantation

An intense interest has developed in predictive modeling for the management of patients with aortic stenosis because of the introduction of TAVI. This has unfortunately led to the overuse and, indeed, frank abuse of the risk algorithms for applications for which they were not developed nor originally intended.[47] Overenthusiastic supporters of TAVI have touted the benefits of the catheter-based procedure because of the observed early mortality, which is better than the expected mortality based on the predictive model. In point of fact, these better outcomes are illusory because of misuse of risk prediction algorithms. This abuse has been particularly prevalent with use of the Logistic EuroSCORE to estimate risk and report outcomes in patients undergoing TAVI. The reasons that current risk predictive models developed for surgical AVR are inaccurate, are not applicable, and in fact yield misinformation in the evaluation of candidates for TAVI have already been detailed. Among the factors leading to inaccuracy include the fact that the patients being assessed for TAVI are at the extremes of risk, where the current risk models fail because there are too few patients at the higher extremes of risk to be able to have robust discrimination of risk. Furthermore, the risk predictors are being used for procedures in which the risk models were neither developed nor validated and therefore are highly likely to be invalid. They also do not take into account variables that may play significant roles in risk, including porcelain aorta, previous radiation therapy, liver disease, and frailty. These factors were not considered either because the data were not collected or there were too few occurrences of the factor to accurately incorporate it into the risk modeling. There are many studies attesting to the inaccuracies of the Logistic EuroSCORE in both CABG and AVR populations,[36,48-55] and its use in TAVI further compounds the inaccuracy.

In order to help address some of the inadequacies of the current risk prediction models in adults undergoing aortic valve procedures, the German Aortic Valve Registry (GARY) has developed the German Aortic Valve Score.[56] It is based on 11,794 patients

undergoing surgical AVR or TAVI in Germany in 2008. Using multiple logistic regression, Kötting et al[55] identified 15 risk factors influencing in-hospital mortality. Among the most important factors determined to predict risk were age, body mass index, renal disease, urgent status, and left ventricular function. The risk model had a high degree of discrimination, with an AUROC of 0.808.

This is the first attempt to develop a risk algorithm that can be applied with some degree of accuracy in patients who are currently undergoing all types of aortic valve procedures. It is the first step in a long journey of risk prediction in TAVI. The model does, however, have many limitations, including the fact that it was developed on the basis of patients treated in 2008 and may already be not applicable to current treatment because the field of TAVI is evolving so rapidly with new devices and techniques continuously introduced (see Chapter 15). Second, patients undergoing TAVI constituted only 5.1% (573/11,147) of the study population, limiting the specific application to transcatheter valve risk prediction. Also, TAVI was performed in only 25 of the 81 participating institutions, again limiting the "generalizability" of the score. It should also be noted that the model was developed for interhospital comparisons only and therefore can predict only overall outcomes in German hospitals. Comparisons can be made of overall program outcomes between various centers, but the German Aortic Valve Score cannot be used to discriminate among different procedures, approaches, or devices. With this risk score, one cannot as yet determine whether an individual patient should undergo surgical AVR or TAVI or whether a specific device or approach is preferable.

Another limitation of the German Aortic Valve Score is the methodology by which the risk model was constructed. As detailed previously, most risk models are developed with use of a portion of the overall analyzed population, usually 50% to 60% of the study population to construct a weighted risk model and then the remaining sample to validate it. Because of the small sample size of TAVI procedures in the study, this validation was not done, so the model needs to be validated externally in other populations.

Because the German Aortic Valve score model includes overall outcomes of surgical AVR and TAVI, its value lies in comparing the overall outcomes of a program and not necessarily surgical AVR or TAVI outcomes per se. Indeed, it is also likely that different factors constitute different risk profiles for different procedures. For example, frailty may be weighted more when when considering surgical AVR compared to TAVI. The risks may not be the same for the different approaches for TAVI, because severe lung disease may be a significant factor impacting outcomes with the transapical approach but not the transfemoral approach.

It should also be noted that this model is based on in-hospital mortality, which is lower than the 30-day definition of mortality used by the STS algorithm. It is likely that TAVI-specific risk algorithms will soon be developed that predict both short- and long-term results and outcomes other than mortality. The linkage of clinical databases, which capture early outcomes, with administrative databases, which capture long-term outcomes, will allow the development of models predictive of long-term survival. The current TAVI trials in intermediate-risk patients have a primary endpoint of death and stroke at 2 years. One can envision the eventual construction of risk models that will predict composite outcomes including mortality, stroke, and functional quality of life. The current STS model predicts not only 30-day mortality but also, individually and as a composite, six components of major morbidity including stroke.

A true TAVI-specific risk model needs to be developed, and at least two efforts are under way. The European registries of the SAPIEN Valve (Edwards Lifesciences, Irvine, California), the U.S. Placement of AoRTic TraNscathetER Valve (PARTNER) Trial, and data obtained in Continued Access patients are being collated and analyzed to develop a TAVI-specific algorithm, and the STS/ American College of Cardiology Transcatheter Valve Therapy

(STS/ACC TVT) Registry in the United States now has sufficient patients enrolled for a risk algorithm to be developed. Validation of a TAVI-specific risk algorithm between these two populations is planned.

Summary

Analysis of adult patients with aortic stenosis undergoing procedures is a rich area of outcomes and comparative effectiveness research. Although a single universal risk prediction model based on the minimal number of important risk factors and widely applicable to all patients undergoing treatment of valvular heart disease is desirable, the realities are that multiple algorithms will exist and will have to be continuously updated as calibration drift occurs and as treatment strategies, patient selection, procedures, and procedure performance evolve.

REFERENCES

1. Chassin MR, Hannan EL, DeBuono BA. Benefits and hazards of reporting medical outcomes publicly. N Engl J Med 1996;334:394–8.
2. Grover FL, Hammermeister KE, Shroyer ALW. Quality initiatives and the power of the database: what they are and how they run. Ann Thorac Surg 1995;60:1514–21.
3. Clark RE. The development of The Society of Thoracic Surgeons voluntary national database system: genesis, issues, growth, and status. Best Pract Benchmarking Healthc 1996;1:62–9.
4. Hammermeister KE, Johnson R, Marshall G, et al. Continuous assessment and improvement in quality ofcare: a model from the Department of Veterans Affairs cardiac surgery. Ann Surg 1994;219:281–90.
5. Daley J. Criteria by which to evaluate risk-adjusted outcomes programs in cardiac surgery. Ann Thorac Surg 1994;58:1827–35.
6. Iezzoni LI. The risks of risk adjustment. JAMA 1997;278:1600–7.
7. Iezzoni LI. Risk adjustment for measuring healthcare outcomes. Chicago: Health Administration Press; 1997.
8. Tu JV, Sykora K, Naylor CD. Assessing the outcomes of coronary artery bypass graft surgery: how many risk factors are enough? Steering Committee of the Cardiac Care Network of Ontario. J Am Coll Cardiol 1997;30:1317–23.
9. Luft HS, Romano PS. Chance, continuity, and change in hospital mortality rates. Coronary artery bypass graft patients in California hospitals, 1983 to 1989. JAMA 1993;270:331–7.
10. Grunkemeier GL, Payne N, Jin R, et al. Propensity score analysis of stroke after off-pump coronary artery bypass grafting. Ann Thorac Surg 2002;74:301–5.
11. Blackstone EH. Comparing apples and oranges. J Thorac Cardiovasc Surg 2002;123:8–15.
12. Harrell FE Jr. Regression modeling strategies with applications to linear models, logistic regression, and survival analysis. New York: Springer-Verlag; 2001.
13. Kouchoukos NT, Ebert PA, Grover FL, et al. Report of the Ad Hoc Committee on Risk Factors for Coronary Artery Bypass Surgery. Ann Thorac Surg 1988;45:348–9.
14. Edwards FH. Evolution of The Society of Thoracic Surgeons National Cardiac Surgery Database. J Invasive Cardiol 1998;10:485–8.
15. Shahian DM, Blackstone EH, Edwards FH, et al. Cardiac surgery risk models: a position article. Ann Thorac Surg 2004;78:1868–77.
16. Hannan EL, Kilburn H Jr, O'Donnell JF, et al. Adult open heart surgery in New York State: an analysis of risk factors and hospital mortality rates. JAMA 1990;264:2768–74.
17. Grover FL, Shroyer AL, Hammermeister KE. Calculating risk and outcome: the Veterans Affairs database. Ann Thorac Surg 1996;62:S6–11.
18. O'Connor GT, Plume SK, Olmstead EM, et al. Multivariate prediction of in-hospital mortality associated with coronary artery bypass graft surgery. Northern New England Cardiovascular Disease Study Group. Circulation 1992;85:2110–18.
19. Parsonnet V, Dean D, Bernstein AD. A method of uniform stratification of risk for evaluating the results of surgery in acquired adult heart disease. Circulation 1989;79: I3–I12.
20. Nashef SA, Roques F, Michel P, et al. European system for cardiac operative risk evaluation (EuroSCORE). Eur J Cardiothorac Surg 1999;16:9–13.
21. Marshall G, Grover FL, Henderson WG, et al. Assessment of predictive models for binary outcomes: an empirical approach using operative death from cardiac surgery. Stat Med 1994;13:1501–11.
22. O'Brien SM, Shahian DM, Filardo G. The Society of Thoracic Surgeons 2008 Cardiac Surgery Risk Models: Part 2—Isolated Valve Surgery. Ann Thorac Surg 2009;88: S23–42.
23. Zou KH, O'Malley AJ, Mauri L. Receiver-operating characteristic analysis for evaluating diagnostic tests and predictive models Circulation 2007;115:654–7.
24. Nashef SA, Sharples LD, Roques F, et al. EuroSCORE II and the art and science of risk modeling. Eur J Cardiothorac Surg 2013;43:695–6.
25. Osswald BR, Gegouskov V, Badowski-Zyla D, et al. Overestimation of aortic valve replacement risk by EuroSCORE: implications for percutaneous valve replacement. Eur Heart J 2009;30:74–80.
26. Leontyev S, Walther T, Borger MA, et al. Aortic valve replacement in octogenarians: utility of risk stratification with EuroSCORE. Ann Thorac Surg 2009;87:1440–5.
27. Ranucci M, Castelvecchio S, Conte M, et al. The easier, the better: age, creatinine, ejection fraction score for operative mortality risk stratification in a series of 29,659 patients undergoing elective cardiac surgery. J Thorac Cardiovasc Surg 2011;142:581–6.
28. Kappetein AP, Head SJ. Predicting prognosis in cardiac surgery: a prophecy? Eur J Cardiothorac Surg 2012;41:732–3.
29. Nashef SA, Roques F, Sharples LD, et al. EuroSCORE II. Eur J Cardiothorac Surg 2012;41:734–44.
30. Rankin SJ, He X, O'Brien SM. The Society of Thoracic Surgeons Risk Model for Operative Mortality After Multiple Valve Surgery. Ann Thorac Surg 2013;95:1484–90.
31. Puskas JD, Kilgo PD,Thourani VH, et al. The Society of Thoracic Surgeons 30-Day Predicted Risk of Mortality Score also predicts long-term survival. Ann Thorac Surg 2012;93:26–35.
32. Shahian DM, He X, Jacobs JP. The Society of Thoracic Surgeons Isolated Aortic Valve Replacement (AVR) Composite Score: a report of the STS Quality Measurement Task Force. Ann Thorac Surg 2012;94:2166–71.
33. Online STS Risk Calculator. Available at <http://riskcalc.sts.org>.
34. Roques F, Nashef SAM, Michel P, et al. Risk factors and outcome in European cardiac surgery: analysis of the EuroSCORE multinational database of 19,030 patients. Eur J Cardiothorac Surg 1999;15:816–23.
35. Roques F, Michel P, Goldstone AR, et al. The logistic EuroSCORE. Eur Heart J 2003;24: 881–2.
36. EuroSCORE Interactive Calculator. available at <http://www.euroscore.org/calc>.
37. Grant SW, Hickey GL, Dimarakis I, et al. How does EuroSCORE II perform in UK cardiac surgery; an analysis of 23,740 patients from the Society for Cardiothoracic Surgery in Great Britain and Ireland National Database. Heart 2012;98:1566–72.
38. Chalmers J, Pullan M, Fabri B, et al. Validation of EuroSCORE II in a modern cohort of patients undergoing cardiac surgery. Eur J Cardiothorac Surg 2013;43:688–94.
39. Di Dedda U, Pelissero G, Agnelli B, et al. Accuracy, calibration and clinical performance of the new EuroSCORE II risk stratification system. Eur J Cardiothorac Surg 2013;43:27–32.
40. Dewey T, Brown D, Ryan WH, et al. Reliability of risk algorithms in predicting early and late operative outcomes in high risk patients undergoing aortic valve replacement. J Thorac Cardiovasc Surg 2008;135:180–7.
41. Conradi L, Seiffert M, Treede H, et al. Transcatheter aortic valve implantation versus surgical aortic valve replacement: a propensity score analysis in patients at high surgical risk. J Thorac Cardiovasc Surg 2012;143:64–71.
42. Ambler G, Omar RZ, Royston P, et al. Generic, simple risk stratification model for heart valve surgery. Circulation 2005;112:224–31.
43. Nowicki ER, Birkmeyer NJ, Weintraub RW, et al. Multivariable prediction of in-hospital mortality associated with aortic and mitral valve surgery in Northern New England. Ann Thorac Surg 2004;77:1966–77.
44. Ranucci M, Castelvecchio S, Menicanti L, et al. Risk of Assessing mortality risk in elective cardiac operations: age, creatinine, ejection fraction, and the Law of Parsimony. Circulation 2009;119:3041–3.
45. Ranucci M, Castelvecchio S, Conte M. The easier, the better: age, creatinine, ejection fraction score for operative mortality risk stratification in a series of 29,659 patients undergoing elective cardiac surgery. J Thorac Cardiovasc Surg 2011;142:581–6.
46. Ariyaratne TV, Billah B, Yap CH, et al. An Australian risk prediction model for determining early mortality following aortic valve replacement. Eur J Cardiothorac Surg 2011;39: 815–21.
47. Sergeant P, Meuris B, Pettinari M. EuroSCORE II, illum qui est gravitates magni observe. Eur J Cardiothorac Surg 2012;41:729–31.
48. Gummert JF, Funkat A, Osswald B, et al. EuroSCORE overestimates the risk of cardiac surgery: results from the national registry of the German Society of Thoracic and Cardiovascular Surgery. Clin Res Cardiol 2009;98:363–9.
49. Biancari F, Kangasniemi OP, Aliasim Mahar M, et al. Changing risk of patients undergoing coronary artery bypass surgery. Interact Cardiovasc Thorac Surg 2009;8:40–4.
50. Nilsson J, Algotsson L, Höglund P, et al. Comparison of 19 pre-operative risk stratification models in open-heart surgery. Eur Heart J 2006;27:867–74.
51. Bridgewater B, Neve H, Moat N, et al. Predicting operative risk for coronary artery surgery in the United Kingdom: a comparison of various risk prediction algorithms. Heart 1998;79:350–5.
52. Bhatti F, Grayson AD, Grotte G, et al. The logistic EuroSCORE in cardiac surgery: how well does it predict operative risk? Heart 2006;92:1817–20.
53. Bode C, Kelm M. EUROSCORE: still gold standard or less? Clin Res Cardiol 2009;98: 353–4.
54. Zheng Z, Li Y, Zhang S, et al, Chinese CABG Registry Study. The Chinese coronary artery bypass grafting registry study: how well does the EuroSCORE predict operative risk for Chinese population? Eur J Cardiothorac Surg 2009;35:54–8.
55. Grossi EA, Schwartz CF, Yu PJ, et al. High-risk aortic valve replacement: are the outcomes as bad as predicted? Ann Thorac Surg 2008;85:102–6.
56. Kötting J, Schiller W, Beckmann A, et al. German Aortic Valve Score: a new scoring system for prediction of mortality related to aortic valve procedures in adults. Eur J Cardiothorac Surg 2013;43:971–7.

CHAPTER 11

Aortic Stenosis

Raphael Rosenhek and Helmut Baumgartner

Key Points

- Aortic stenosis is the most frequent reason for valve interventions in North America and Europe.
- Echocardiography is the key diagnostic tool for diagnosis, quantification of stenosis severity, and assessment of secondary changes.
- Aortic stenosis is a progressive disease and the possibility of rapid hemodynamic progression needs to be considered.
- Patients with symptoms (dyspnea, angina, dizziness/syncope with exertion) require urgent surgery.
- A watchful waiting approach is generally safe in asymptomatic patients under the condition of regular echocardiographic and clinical examinations.
- Risk stratification is useful in asymptomatic patients, in that it allows identification of patients who may benefit from early elective surgery.
- Key elements in risk stratification include leaflet calcification, rate of hemodynamic progression, the absolute degree of stenosis severity, and exercise testing in physically active patients.
- There is no established medical therapy for aortic stenosis.

Pathophysiology

The primary determinant of disease severity in patients with valvular aortic stenosis (AS) is the degree of obstruction to left ventricular (LV) outflow. In addition, valve obstruction leads to secondary effects on the left ventricle, peripheral vasculature, and coronary artery blood flow that impact both the clinical presentation of disease and subsequent outcome. The pathophysiologic mechanisms involved in the initiation and progression of the disease process are described in Chapters 3 and 4.

Valvular Hemodynamics

PRESSURE GRADIENTS

Obstruction at the aortic valve level results in an increased antegrade velocity across the narrowed valve corresponding to the systolic pressure gradient between the left ventricle and aorta. For any given transvalvular volume flow rate, both antegrade velocity and transaortic pressure gradient rise with increasing degrees of valvular narrowing. However, for any given valve area, the magnitude of increase in jet velocity and pressure gradient varies with the volume flow rate across the valve. Thus, patients with severe stenosis and a low stroke volume have only a moderate increase in antegrade velocity and systolic pressure gradient, whereas those with moderate stenosis and a high transaortic flow rate have a high jet velocity and systolic pressure gradient.

The rate of rise and fall of the antegrade velocity and the timing of the pressure gradient across the valve are also related to disease severity. With mild stenosis, the maximum velocity and maximum pressure difference across the valve occur in early systole, prior to the peak volume flow rate across the valve, at a time point corresponding to the maximum rate of flow acceleration.[1,2] As stenosis becomes more severe, the maximum velocity and pressure difference occur later in systole, eventually coinciding with the maximum volume flow rate across the valve. In addition to stenosis severity, the shape of the velocity curve and timing of the pressure gradient may be affected by other factors that alter LV or aortic pressure, such as coexisting aortic regurgitation (AR) and increased systemic vascular resistance.

The antegrade (or jet) velocity across the aortic valve is usually described in terms of the maximum instantaneous velocity. The maximum instantaneous velocity relates to the maximum instantaneous pressure gradient across the valve as stated in the Bernoulli equation. Although theoretically more complicated, the relationship can be simplified for most clinical applications so that the pressure gradient is equal to the velocity squared multiplied by 4 (i.e., "simplified Bernoulli equation").[3-6] At cardiac catheterization, the difference between peak LV and peak aortic pressures (the peak-to-peak gradient) is often reported. Because the peak LV and aortic pressures usually are not simultaneous, the difference between these two pressures is not a physiologic measurement and does not correspond to the maximum or any other instantaneous velocity obtained with Doppler echocardiography.

Mean transaortic pressure gradients can be derived from Doppler echocardiographic data or invasive pressure recordings by averaging the instantaneous pressure gradients over the systolic ejection period. In adults with valvular AS, maximum and mean pressure gradients are linearly related, with a close correlation.[7,8] The predictive value of mean gradient is also well established for both invasive and noninvasive assessment and this measurement should be included in diagnostic reports.

The phenomenon of pressure recovery distal to the stenotic valve contributes to some of the confusion surrounding comparisons of invasive and noninvasive transaortic gradients, because Doppler velocities reflect the pressure drop in the orifice itself, whereas catheter pressure data may include pressure recovery distal to the orifice, depending on the exact location of the catheter relative to the stenotic orifice.[9-11] The geometry of the flow obstruction in AS with its abrupt widening from the stenotic orifice to a comparatively large ascending aorta causes extensive turbulence with dissipation of kinetic energy into heat. This pattern precludes the occurrence of pressure recovery with clinically relevant magnitude in the majority of patients. Only in the case of a small aorta with a favorable ratio of orifice to cross-sectional aortic area—in this setting the occurrence of turbulences is reduced—will pressure recovery reach a magnitude that causes clinically relevant differences between Doppler gradient (pressure drop from ventricle to vena contracta) and net pressure gradient (drop from ventricular to distal, recovered pressure).[9,11] In the clinical setting, this becomes likely when the aortic root diameter is smaller than 3 cm.[11,12] In case of significant pressure recovery, the Doppler gradient overestimates the pathophysiologic consequence of a stenosis. In this case less proximal pressure and, consequently, workload are required to maintain an adequate peripheral pressure than in a clinical setting with the same Doppler gradient but no pressure recovery.

VALVE AREA

Aortic valve area, defined as the extent of aortic valve opening in systole, provides a clinically useful measure of stenosis severity that is less dependent on volume flow rate than pressure gradients. Valve area can be calculated from Doppler data using the continuity equation based on the principle that the volume flow rates are equal just proximal to and in the stenotic orifice[13-16] (see Chapter 6). Valve area also can be calculated at cardiac catheterization, using the Gorlin equation, on the basis of measurement of transaortic volume flow rate and mean systolic pressure gradient across the valve[17-21] (see Chapter 7).

Although less flow dependent than pressure gradients, aortic valve area also varies with transaortic volume flow rate, especially in patients with calcific stenosis.[22-25] The unfused commissures allow variation in the degree of valve opening, depending on the interaction between the stiffness of the cusps and the force directed against the valve in systole.[21,26-31] The variable opening of stiff aortic valve leaflets is not surprising, given the common echocardiographic observation in patients with dilated cardiomyopathy that changes in flow rate are associated with changes in the extent of aortic cusp opening, even in the absence of leaflet thickening. With aortic valve stenosis, the increase in LV outflow velocity with exercise may result in an increase in the extent of valve opening if the leaflets still have some flexibility. Initial concerns, that the observed increase was related to the mathematical assumptions of the calculations or to changes in the fluid dynamics across the valve, have been resolved by direct observation of valve opening,[32] so that most investigators now concur that leaflet opening varies with flow rate. With disease progression, the gradual increase in the degree of leaflet thickening and calcification eventually reaches a point at which valve area is fixed over the physiologic range of force that can be generated by the left ventricle.

The time course of valve opening, or the rate of change in valve area during a single cardiac cycle, reflects valve stiffness, inertia, and elasticity.[33] Stenotic aortic valves open and close more slowly than normal valves[34] and the rate of change in valve area during systole is a predictor of clinical outcome.[35]

Flow dependence of valve area becomes particularly important in the presence of low cardiac output most frequently due to LV dysfunction. Reduced opening forces may then cause a mildly or moderately stenotic valve to open to a valve area of only less than 1 cm^2. The term "pseudosevere stenosis" has been proposed for this condition.[36,37] Transvalvular gradient is typically low (mean gradient < 30-40 mm Hg) in this situation (low-flow, low-gradient AS). Although many patients with reduced LV function in a late stage of severe AS (afterload mismatch, see section titled Left Ventricular Pressure Overload) maintain a surprisingly high gradient (>40 mm Hg mean gradient),[38] some of them may also present with low gradients just because of severe flow reduction. Low-dose dobutamine can be used during echocardiography to stimulate myocardial contraction and increase flow rate. With increasing flow, one would assume that valve area increases with little change in gradient in the presence of pseudosevere stenosis and that primarily velocity and gradient should increase with less

change in valve area when there is fixed severe stenosis.[37] The test, of course, requires that there is indeed contractile reserve.

In addition to flow-related changes in geometric orifice area, it has been suggested that effective orifice area may increase with flow even without changes in anatomic area.[39] At normal flow rates, the kinetic energy of the fluid crossing the obstruction is sufficient to break down the vortex structures generated downstream from the stenosis and thus enables the formation of a large and well-established flow jet. However, at low flow rates, the reduction in kinetic energy may predispose to the formation of vortices, which tend then to squeeze the flow jet and thus the vena contracta, resulting in a smaller effective orifice.[39] The phenomenon is certainly less important in the presence of very small orifices but may become clinically relevant in moderately severe "low-flow AS." These findings once more emphasize that clinical judgment should not rely only on the absolute number of calculated valve area but should take into account all available hemodynamic and morphologic information.[40]

OTHER INDICES OF STENOSIS SEVERITY

Some investigators have explored the concept of valve resistance as a measure of AS severity.[31,41,42] Because valve resistance is calculated as the simple ratio of pressure gradient to flow across the valve, the underlying assumption of this approach is that there is a linear relationship between pressure gradient and transvalvular flow rate. This assumption is inconsistent with the Bernoulli equation, which assumes a quadratic relationship between pressure gradient and flow rate. Some disagreement persists as to the exact relationship between pressure and flow across a stenotic valve, but in fact, careful fluid dynamic studies support the concept of a quadratic relationship.[43] Although experimental studies suggest that valve resistance provides better discrimination of the extent of valve stiffness for valves 100 to 200 times stiffer than normal, disease progression and symptoms occur in the clinical setting in the range of valve stiffness from 20 to 100 times normal, a range where valve area provides better quantitation of disease severity.[44] Valve resistance has also been proposed for the evaluation of low-flow, low-gradient AS, with the argument that it is less flow dependent.[41] However, this concept cannot be supported by fluid dynamics theory, nor can it be supported experimentally or by clinical observation.[11,29,43,45] The studies examining the issue demonstrated that valve resistance certainly has no advantages over valve area with regard to flow dependence. The fact that valve resistance may indeed obscure actual changes in valve area, because the resistance may change only slightly when valve area increases with increasing flow rate, makes it even less useful for the evaluation of AS. As a matter of fact, an increase in flow must necessarily result in an increase in resistance unless it is compensated by a concomitant increase in effective valve area.[11,45] In addition, the calculation of valve "resistance" has no clear advantages over jet velocities, pressure gradients, and valve areas in predicting clinical outcome.[46,47]

The fluid dynamics of AS are more complex than those of mitral stenosis, in that the pressure gradient and volume flow rate across the valve depend on the force of LV contraction as well as the characteristics of the valve itself. Thus, another approach to describing AS severity is to estimate the total work performed by the ventricle in opening the aortic valve. In concept, total LV stroke work is calculated as the integral of flow times pressure. Effective stroke work (aortic pressure times flow) then is subtracted to yield the stroke work "lost" across the valve.[48,49] Although LV stroke work loss does correlate with other measures of stenosis severity, it also varies with flow rate (even when normalized for stroke volume), is an unfamiliar concept for most physicians, and offers no obvious clinical advantages. In addition, the calculation of stroke work loss accounts mainly for the potential energy components of total work, whereas kinetic energy losses, which are more difficult to estimate, may be even more important in valvular AS.[29]

Because aortic valve hemodynamics depend on aortic valve anatomy, LV mechanics, and the characteristics of the vascular system downstream from the valve, a complete description of AS severity would include all three of these components. Obviously, this type of descriptor is conceptually complex and may be difficult to derive in the clinical setting. A step toward an integrated descriptor of AS severity is the concept of ventricular-vascular coupling with the inclusion of components to describe the effect of the abnormal valve in the system.[50] Results of preliminary studies in this area are of interest but are not yet clinically applicable.

Left Ventricular Pressure Overload

The basic response of the left ventricle to the chronic and gradually progressive pressure overload of valvular AS is concentric hypertrophy. However, not all patients demonstrate hypertrophy, even with severe stenosis, and there are significant gender differences in the degree and pattern of hypertrophy.[51-54] In pathophysiologic terms, LV hypertrophy occurs as a mechanism to maintain normal wall stress as LV pressure rises through an increase in wall thickness (see Chapter 5). Typically, contractility is normal and ejection fraction (EF) is preserved until late in the disease course. However, even when contractility is normal, LV systolic performance may appear to be impaired in patients with severe outflow obstruction for at least three reasons. First, EF may decline owing to the excessive increase in afterload, often termed "afterload mismatch." Second, ventricular preload may be shifted to the left on the Starling curve because of a small, hypertrophied, noncompliant ventricle. Third, the temporal sequence of myocardial contraction is often asynchronous in pressure overload hypertrophy, with an "uncoordinated" ventricular contraction. The resultant fall in the peak rate of circumferential shortening correlates with an increase in systolic wall stress.[55] This pattern of discordant contraction, and the apparent decrease in ventricular function, resolves after relief of AS.

When LV mass measurements are normalized for body size and gender, hypertrophy is seen in 54% of men and 81% of women with AS.[52] The pattern of hypertrophy in women with AS is characterized by a small ventricular chamber with increased wall thickness, normal or hypercontractile systolic function, and early diastolic dysfunction.[51-54,56] In men with AS, the more common pattern is a normal or only mildly increased wall thickness and impaired systolic function.

Diastolic dysfunction occurs early in the disease course of AS[57] in association with an increase in the total collagen volume of the myocardium and an increase in the orthogonal collagen fiber network.[58] As for ventricular hypertrophy, significant gender differences in diastolic function are seen. Specifically, men have a higher constant of myocardial stiffness in association with a greater degree of endocardial fibrosis and an abnormal myocardial collagen pattern.[56] Age also affects the severity of diastolic dysfunction, with more severe LV hypertrophy and diastolic dysfunction seen in elderly patients (>65 years).[59]

The Peripheral and Pulmonary Vasculature

In patients with AS, the need to correct for peripheral amplification if femoral artery, rather than central aortic, pressures are used for invasive calculation of valve area has long been appreciated.[60] However, there is little data on the influence of systemic factors on valve or ventricular function in these patients. Although LV afterload is predominantly affected by the severity of obstruction at the valvular level, both factors internal to the left ventricle and characteristics of the systemic vascular circuit also contribute to total afterload.[50] To date, few studies have evaluated the impact of systemic vascular resistance (or impedance), wave reflections, or aortic elastance on the hemodynamics of valvular AS.

Prospective follow-up shows that pulmonary hypertension is common in patients with isolated AS.[47] In a series of 388 symptomatic patients with isolated AS, mild pulmonary hypertension was present in 35%, moderate in 50%, and severe (systolic pressure >50 mm Hg) in 15%.[61] In addition, a higher prevalence of moderate to severe pulmonary hypertension (seen in as high as 71% of patients) has been noted in some surgical series.[62] The degree of pulmonary hypertension correlates with LV end-diastolic pressure but not with the severity of AS or the LV EF.[61] The presence of pulmonary hypertension is a risk factor for cardiac surgery,[63] but pulmonary pressure usually returns to normal after valve replacement for AS, even when it was severely elevated.[62,64]

Coronary Blood Flow

Abnormalities in coronary blood flow, even in the absence of significant coronary atherosclerosis, contribute to the clinical presentation and long-term outcome of patients with valvular AS. Although coronary artery size, and thus blood flow, is increased in patients with AS, the increase in coronary artery size often is inadequate for the increase in muscle mass and, in addition, coronary flow reserve is limited.[65-68] Coronary flow reserve is most impaired in the subendocardium, with the severity of impairment related to AS severity.[69] After aortic valve replacement, coronary flow reserve improves in conjunction with regression of LV hypertrophy.[70] LV hypertrophy also is associated with decreased capillary density and increased diffusion distances.[71] Other factors that may impact coronary blood flow in patients with AS are a decreased diastolic perfusion time, impaired early diastolic relaxation, and increased diastolic wall stresses, all leading to a reduction in subendocardial blood flow.[72]

Transthoracic echocardiographic evaluation of phasic coronary blood flow in adults with AS shows reversal of early systolic flow and delayed forward flow in diastole, both of which resolve after aortic valve replacement.[73] These findings were further elucidated in both transthoracic and transesophageal echocardiographic studies showing that systolic coronary flow decreases in inverse relationship to the increase in LV wall stress, whereas diastolic flow increases in direct relationship to the transaortic pressure gradient, with these changes being particularly marked in symptomatic patients.[74,75] Coronary flow, measured by an intracoronary Doppler flow catheter, also shows retrograde systolic flow at rest, which correlates with the peak transaortic pressure gradient.[76] With stress induced by pacing and/or dobutamine, retrograde systolic flow increases, total systolic flow decreases, and forward diastolic flow increases in patients with AS; in normal control subjects, both systolic and diastolic flow increase proportionately.[76] These data suggest that an inadequate increase in total coronary blood flow in response to stress may contribute to the clinical presentation of AS, specifically the symptom of angina in patients with normal coronary arteries.

Further imbalance in myocardial oxygen demand and supply occurs late in the disease course as LV wall stress (and oxygen demands) increase out of proportion to the increase in coronary blood flow.[77] Angina, in the absence of coexisting coronary artery disease (CAD), is associated with an increased LV wall stress as a result of inadequate hypertrophy in conjunction with increased ventricular systolic pressures.[71] This increase in wall stress leads to an increase in myocardial oxygen consumption. The combination of increased myocardial oxygen demand and limited coronary blood flow leads to myocardial ischemia and symptoms of coronary regurgitation.

Exercise Physiology

Even asymptomatic patients with AS have a slight decrease in exercise tolerance in comparison with normative age standards. The hemodynamic response to exercise is characterized by a normal increase in heart rate to age-predicted maximums, but only a 50% increase in cardiac output. The increase in cardiac output is mediated by an increase in heart rate as stroke volume is unchanged or decreases slightly with upright exercise.[23,24,29,30,48,78] Although total stoke volume does not increase, there is a rise in the maximum instantaneous and mean systolic flow rates across the aortic valve because the systolic ejection period shortens as a result of the increase in heart rate. Transaortic velocity, maximum gradient, and mean gradient increase as the flow rate rises, although the extent of increase often is less than predicted by the resting valve area.[23,24,30,31,79]

Measures of LV diastolic function are also abnormal with exercise in adults with AS. Micromanometer pressure recordings demonstrate that resting diastolic pressures are higher, diastolic pressures increase further with exercise, and both the rate of diastolic pressure decay and the isovolumic contraction interval fail to decrease with exercise, in comparison with observations in normal control subjects.[80]

With exercise, valve area enlarges, on average, by 0.2 cm^2, accounting for the smaller increase in jet velocity and gradient than expected for resting valve area.[23,24,30] The increase in valve area with exercise allows ejection of a relatively normal stroke volume across the valve and an appropriate increase in cardiac output. As the disease becomes more severe and the leaflets become more rigid and stiff, the degree of valve opening is progressively limited, resulting in a drop in transaortic stroke volume and a failure of cardiac output to increase adequately with exercise.[24,29]

The increase in valve stiffness at adequate cardiac output results in a higher increase in gradient with exercise, which has been shown to be a predictor of outcome.[81]

Clinical Presentation

Clinical History

Valvular AS is a gradually progressive disease in which patients remain asymptomatic for many years.[82-86] Typically AS is first diagnosed from the finding of a systolic murmur on auscultation. Because the increase in hemodynamic severity occurs slowly, many patients do not recognize early symptoms, emphasizing the importance of patient education in medical management, including a discussion of the classic symptoms of AS (e.g., heart failure, angina, and syncope). In addition, the clinician must carefully question the patient to elicit symptoms, specifically asking the patient to compare current activity levels with activities at a set point in the past. In particular, older patients often unconsciously tend to avoid activities that may cause symptoms and then still describe themselves as asymptomatic.

The most common initial symptom of valvular AS is decreased exercise tolerance due to exertional dyspnea or fatigue.[47,87] The mechanism of this symptom most often is an elevated LV end-diastolic pressure due to a noncompliant, hypertrophied ventricle.[88] Exercise intolerance may also be due to LV systolic dysfunction or coexisting CAD in some patients. Over time, exertional dyspnea may progress to frank heart failure, with symptoms seen at rest in patients with long-standing severe valvular obstruction. Some patients present with the sudden onset of heart failure or pulmonary edema, often in relation to an acute infectious process, anemia, or other hemodynamic stress or to new-onset atrial fibrillation.

Exertional angina also is a common initial symptom in adults with valvular AS; it is due to an increase in oxygen demand by the hypertrophied myocardium, even in the absence of coexisting epicardial CAD.[47,87] As mentioned, angina may be precipitated by other hemodynamic stresses, such as pregnancy, anemia, and febrile disease.

The third classic symptom of AS is exertional lightheadedness or syncope. Several potential mechanisms of syncope in AS have been proposed, including ventricular arrhythmias and LV systolic dysfunction, but there is most support for an acute drop in blood pressure due to an inappropriate LV baroreceptor response.[89-91] The elevated ventricular pressure activates baroreceptors, which

mediate peripheral vasodilation. In the setting of a restricted aortic orifice, cardiac output fails to rise, so blood pressure falls and the patient losses consciousness.

Physical Examination

The key features in the physical examination of patients with suspected AS are palpation of the carotid pulse contour and amplitude; auscultation of the location, loudness, timing, and radiation of the systolic murmur; assessment of the splitting of the second heart sound; and examination for signs of heart failure.[92,93]

The timing and amplitude of the carotid pulse contour reflect central aortic pressure. As AS becomes more severe, the peak aortic pressure occurs later in systole (pulsus tardus) and the pulse amplitude is decreased (pulsus parvus). Both the timing and amplitude of the carotid pulse correlate with AS severity.[94,95] However, the pulse contour is affected by factors other than stenosis severity, particularly in adult patients.[96] The pulse amplitude may be diminished with a reduced cardiac output and only mild to moderate stenosis, as a result of the low volume flow rate into the aorta, although the timing of the impulse is typically normal in this situation. Conversely, the pulse amplitude and timing may appear to be normal with coexisting atherosclerosis because the stiff vessels lead to a rapid and excessive rise in aortic pressure even when severe stenosis is present. Thus, a slow-rising, low-amplitude carotid pulse has a relatively high specificity for the diagnosis of severe valvular obstruction. However, the sensitivity of this finding is poor, and severe stenosis cannot be excluded in adults with an apparently normal carotid upstroke.

The systolic murmur of AS is most often loudest at the base, over the right second intercostal space. In general, the loudness of the murmur correlates with jet velocity or pressure gradient.[95,97,98] The presence of systolic thrill in the aortic region (i.e., a grade IV murmur) is highly specific for severe valvular obstruction. Conversely, severe stenosis is unlikely with a grade I murmur. Unfortunately, there is considerable overlap in disease severity with the intermediate grades of murmur (II-III), so further evaluation is needed, depending on the clinical setting.[87,95] Besides the systolic pressure gradient across the valve, the loudness of the murmur is modulated by the volume flow rate across the valve, transmission of the murmur to the chest wall, and the direction of the turbulent jet. Thus, even with severe stenosis, the murmur may be soft if cardiac output is low or if obesity or lung disease diminishes its transmission to the chest wall.

The murmur of AS radiates to the carotid arteries in the majority of patients as the turbulent jet is directed superiorly into the ascending aorta, allowing transmission of sound through the aorta to the carotids. In a minority of patients, the murmur radiates to the apex, a pattern referred to as the Gallavardin phenomenon.[99]

The murmur of AS has a crescendo-decrescendo pattern of amplitude, corresponding the shape of the pressure difference between the left ventricle and aorta during the ejection period. As stenosis becomes more severe, the maximum instantaneous gradient occurs later in systole, so a late-peaking murmur is appreciated on auscultation. Conditions that are associated with a high transaortic volume flow rate, such as AR, may lead to early peaking of the murmur. Thus, although a late-peaking murmur is quite specific for the presence of severe stenosis, its sensitivity is low.

The second heart sound in severe AS typically is single; the aortic component is inaudible owing to the impaired motion of the thickened valve leaflets. Earlier in the disease course, the second heart sound may show reversed splitting with respiration as a result of a prolonged LV ejection time.

An S4 gallop may be appreciated in many patients with AS, reflecting a greater atrial contribution to ventricular filling.[100] Other physical examination findings in AS patients depend on whether hemodynamic decompensation has occurred, leading to typical signs of heart failure.

Chest Radiography and Electrocardiography

The chest radiograph may be entirely normal in patients with valvular AS, although dilation of the ascending aorta may be appreciated in some cases, even early in the disease course. Such aortic dilation has previously been called "poststenotic." However, it is not related to hemodynamic severity and appears to be caused by intrinsic abnormalities of the aortic wall rather than by the stenosis itself, particularly in patients with bicuspid valves.[101] The cardiac silhouette typically is normal because LV hypertrophy due to an increased wall thickness with a normal chamber dimension is not evident on a standard chest film. Calcification of the aortic valve rarely is evident on chest radiography but may be seen with fluoroscopy in a high percentage of patients with severe valvular obstruction.[102] Mitral annular calcification, which often accompanies degenerative aortic valve disease, may also be seen. With long-standing disease, LV dilation and signs of heart failure are present. Radiographic evidence of pulmonary hypertension may also be evident late in the disease course.

The classic electrocardiographic finding in AS is LV hypertrophy. However, many adults and children with severe AS do not have electrocardiographic criteria for LV hypertrophy.[103,104] Other nonspecific electrocardiographic changes in adults with AS are left atrial enlargement, left axis deviation, and left bundle branch block. Although early studies suggested that T wave changes correlate with the degree of AS, this finding has not been reliable in clinical practice.[105,106]

Electrocardiographic changes with exercise, specifically ST depression, are common in adults with AS. Significant (>1 mm) flat or downsloping ST depression is observed in about two thirds of patients, even with only mild to moderate valve obstruction. Even when their resting electrocardiography findings are normal, half of patients with AS have ST depression with exercise. The presence or severity of ST changes with exercise in adults with AS does not correlate with the presence or absence of epicardial CAD.[47]

Echocardiography

The standard echocardiographic evaluation of a patient with known or suspected AS includes assessment of stenosis severity, degree of coexisting AR and LV size and function, estimation of pulmonary pressures, and identification of any other cardiac abnormalities.[47] With an experienced examiner, diagnostic data are obtained on transthoracic examination in nearly all patients. The most clinically useful measures of stenosis severity are maximum aortic jet velocity, mean pressure gradient (highly flow dependent), and continuity equation valve area (less flow dependent) (Table 11-1). For details see also Chapter 6. Despite several potential limitations, the validity and accuracy of Doppler measures of AS severity for clinical purposes are well established both in comparison with catheterization data[5,6,107-111] and in terms of clinical outcome.[8,47] Nevertheless, it has to be emphasized that in clinical practice, careful consideration of all three measurements in conjunction with other findings, such as valve morphology and LV function, should be the basis for the final judgment of stenosis severity that will guide clinical management.

Current guidelines define severe AS as a peak velocity higher than 4 m/s, a mean gradient greater than 40 mm Hg, and AVA less than 1.0 cm^2,[112,113] but it has to be noted that discrepant findings regarding these criteria are common in patients with the disease (Table 11-2). Most frequently, a patient has a small AVA (<1.0 cm^2) but nevertheless lower values for peak velocity (<4.0 m/s) and gradient (<30-40 mm Hg). Low-flow, low-gradient AS in the presence of LV dysfunction as one reason for this finding has already been discussed. The most challenging group, however, remains patients with small valve area and low gradients in the presence of preserved EF.

The entity of severe paradoxical low-flow, low-gradient AS with preserved EF has been described,[114] with a stroke volume index of 35 mL/m^2 or less being defined as a "low flow." This situation may be observed in the presence of severe LV hypertrophy with a small LV cavity. Prior to diagnosis of severe paradoxical low-flow AS, it is essential to rule out potential underestimation of flow and, consequently, of valve area by the continuity equation (see previous discussion). Furthermore, it must be noted that currently used cutoff values for valve area and gradient are not entirely consistent. A mean gradient of 40 mm Hg requires, at normal flow rates, a valve area closer to 0.8 cm^2 than 1.0 cm^2. Finally, the patient with small stature may also have a small valve area but low gradient without having severe AS. In the initial retrospective study of this entity, a worse outcome was described in patients with paradoxical low-flow AS who were managed conservatively than in those undergoing aortic valve replacement.[114] In contrast, an analysis of data from the prospective Simvastatin and Ezetimibe in Aortic Stenosis (SEAS) cohort described an outcome that was comparable to that for patients with moderate AS.[115] The populations of these studies differed markedly, however, perhaps explaining the differences in the results. Although it is premature to draw final conclusions with regard to the management of patients with low-flow, low-gradient AS with preserved EF, decisions need to be individualized and explanations other than the presence of severe AS must be carefully excluded when a small valve area and low gradients are found despite normal LV EF.[116]

Coexisting AR is present in 70% to 80% of adults with predominant AS.[7,47]

LV chamber dimensions and volumes, wall thickness, mass, EF, and diastolic dysfunction are calculated by means of standard techniques. LV meridional and circumferential wall stress can be calculated from echocardiographic data in conjunction with a cuff blood pressure measurement, as described in Chapter 6. Although useful in clinical research studies, wall stress calculations are rarely performed routinely because these measurements are tedious to perform, and their clinical utility has not yet been convincingly demonstrated.

Other important information derived from the echocardiographic examination includes left atrial size, pulmonary artery systolic pressure, right ventricular size and systolic function, and mitral valve anatomy and function. Mitral annular calcification is seen about 50% of adults with AS,[47] and about 90% of patients have mild coexisting mitral regurgitation, with a smaller number having moderate mitral regurgitation. In patients with rheumatic disease, evaluation of the severity of mitral stenosis and/or regurgitation is also needed for clinical decision making.

Stress Testing

Exercise testing can be safely performed in patients with minimal or no symptoms.[29,47,117] The study should be promptly stopped if there is any decline in blood pressure, symptom onset, or the occurrence of significant arrhythmias.

Exercise testing may be used to clarify symptom status in patients with equivocal symptoms, denial of apparent symptoms, or a decrease in exercise tolerance as perceived by other family members. A normal exercise test result indicates a very low likelihood of symptom development or other complications within the following 6 to 12 months.[118-120] Symptoms on exercise indicate a high likelihood of symptom development or complications within 12 months in physically active patients, particularly those younger than 70 years.[120] Shortness of breath during exercise in patients with little physical activity in daily life, however, particularly the elderly, may be a nonspecific finding. Abnormal blood pressure response and/or ST segment depression has a low positive predictive value.[120]

Stress testing is also indicated to objectively measure the exercise capacity and to define the parameters of a safe exercise program in the asymptomatic patient. Although patients with AS should not participate in competitive sports or extremely vigorous activities, they usually tolerate moderate levels of recreational activity well.[121,122]

CH
11

TABLE 11-1 Measures of Aortic Stenosis Severity Obtained by Doppler Echocardiography

MEASURE	UNIT	FORMULA/METHOD	CUTOFF VALUE FOR SEVERE AS	CONCEPT	ADVANTAGES	LIMITATIONS
AS jet velocity[8-12]	m/s	Direct measurement	4.0	Velocity increases as stenosis severity increase	Direct measurement of velocity; Strongest predictor of clinical outcome	Correct measurement requires parallel alignment of ultrasound beam; Flow dependent
Mean gradient[8-10]	mm Hg	$\Sigma 4v^2 / N$	40	Pressure gradient calculated from velocity using the Bernoulli equation	Mean gradient is averaged from the velocity curve; Units comparable to invasive measurements	Accurate pressure gradients depend on accurate velocity data; Flow dependent
Continuity equation valve area[16,17,23]	cm^2	$AVA = \dfrac{(CSA_{LVOT} \times VTI_{LVOT})}{VTI_{AS}}$	1.0	Volume flow proximal to and in the stenotic orifice is equal	Measures effective orifice area; Feasible in nearly all patients; Relatively flow independent	Requires LVOT diameter and flow velocity data, along with aortic velocity; Measurement error more likely
Simplified continuity equation[18,23]	cm^2	$AVA = \dfrac{(CSA_{LVOT} \times V_{LVOT})}{V_{AS}}$	1.0	The ratio of LVOT to aortic velocity is similar to the ratio of VTIs with native aortic valve stenosis	Uses more easily measured velocities instead of VTIs	Less accurate if shape of velocity curves is atypical
Velocity ratio[15,18]	None	$VR = \dfrac{V_{LVOT}}{V_{AS}}$	0.25	Effective aortic valve area expressed as a proportion of the LVOT area	Doppler-only method; No need to measure LVOT size, less variability than continuity equation	Limited longitudinal data; Ignores LVOT size variability beyond patient size dependence
Planimetry of anatomic valve area[26,34]	cm^2	TTE, TEE, 3D-echo	1.0	Anatomic (geometric) cross-sectional area of the aortic valve orifice as measured by 2D or 3D-echo	Useful if Doppler measurements are unavailable	Contraction coefficient (anatomic/effective valve area) may be variable; Difficult with severe valve calcification
LV stroke work loss[27]	%	$\%SWL = \dfrac{\overline{\Delta P}}{\overline{\Delta P} + SBP} \cdot 100$	25	Work of the LV wasted each systole for flow to cross the aortic valve, expressed as a % of total systolic work	Very easy to measure. Related to outcome in one longitudinal study	Flow-dependent; Limited longitudinal data
Recovered pressure gradient[13,32]	mm Hg	$P_{distal} - P_{vc} = 4 \cdot v^2 \cdot 2 \cdot \dfrac{AVA}{AA}\left(1 - \dfrac{AVA}{AA}\right)$	—	Pressure difference between the LV and the aorta, slightly distal to the *vena contracta*, where distal pressure has increased	Closer to the global hemodynamic burden caused by AS in terms of adaptation of the cardiovascular system; Relevant at high-flow states and in patients with small ascending aorta	Introduces complexity and variability related to the measurement of the ascending aorta; No prospective studies showing real advantages over established methods
Energy loss index[35]	cm^2/m^2	$ELI = \dfrac{AVA \cdot AA}{AA - AVA} \Big/ BSA$	0.5	Equivalent to the concept of AVA, but correcting for distal recovered pressure in the ascending aorta	(As above) Most exact measurement of AS in terms of flow-dynamics; Increased prognostic value in one longitudinal study	Introduces complexity and variability related to the measurement of the ascending aorta
Valvuloarterial impedance[31]	mm Hg/ml/m^2	$Z_{VA} = \dfrac{\overline{\Delta P_{net}} + SBP}{SVI}$	5	Global systolic load imposed on the LV, where the numerator represents an accurate estimation of total LV pressure	Integrates information on arterial bed to the hemodynamic burden of AS, and systemic hypertension is a frequent finding in calcific-degenerative disease	Although named "impedance," only the steady-flow component (i.e., mean resistance) is considered; No longitudinal prospective study available
Aortic valve resistance[28,29]	dynes-sec-cm^{-5}	$AVR = \dfrac{\overline{\Delta P}}{Q} = \dfrac{4 \cdot v^2}{\pi \cdot r_{LVOT}^2 \cdot v_{LVOT}} \cdot 1333$	280	Resistance to flow caused by AS, assuming the hydrodynamics of a tubular (nonflat) stenosis	Initially suggested to be less flow-dependent in low-flow AS, but subsequently shown to not be true	Flow dependence; Limited prognostic value; Unrealistic mathematic modeling of flow dynamics of AS
Projected valve area at normal flow rate[30]	cm^2	$AVA_{proj} = AVA_{rest} + VC \cdot (250 - Q_{rest})$	1.0	Estimation of AVA at normal flow rate by plotting AVA vs. flow and calculating the slope of regression (DSE)	Accounts for the variable changes in flow during DSE in low-flow, low-gradient AS; provides improved interpretation of AVA changes	Clinical impact still to be shown; Outcome of low-flow AS appears closer related to the presence/absence of LV contractility reserve

Recommendation for clinical application: (1) appropriate in all patients with AS (*yellow*); (2) reasonable when additional information is needed in selected patients (*green*); and (3) not recommended for clinical use (*blue*). *3D-echo*, three-dimensional echocardiography; *A*, size of the ascending aorta; *AS*, aortic stenosis velocity; *AVA*, continuity-equation derived aortic valve area; *AVA$_{proj}$*, projected aortic valve area; *AVA$_{rest}$*, aortic valve area at rest; *AVR*, aortic valve resistance; *BSA*, body-surface area; $\overline{\Delta P}$, mean transvalvular systolic pressure gradient; *ELI*, energy-loss coefficient; *LVOT*, left ventricular outflow tract; *P$_{vc}$*, pressure at the *vena contracta*; *Q$_{rest}$*, mean systolic transvalvular flow-rate; *Q$_{rest}$*, mean systolic flow at rest; *DSE*, dobutamine stress echocardiography; *r*, radius; *SBP*, systolic blood pressure; *P$_{distal}$*, pressure at the ascending aorta; *SWL*, stroke work loss; *TTE*, transthoracic echocardiography; *TEE*, transesophageal echocardiography; *VTI*, velocity-time integral; *v*, velocity; *VC*, valve compliance derived as the slope of regression line fitted to the AVA versus Q plot; *VR*, velocity ratio; *Z$_{VA}$*, valvuloaortic impedance.

TABLE 11-2 Classification of Aortic Stenosis Severity

	LEFT VENTRICULAR FUNCTION (EJECTION FRACTION)	PEAK AORTIC JET VELOCITY (m/s)	MEAN GRADIENT (mm HG)	AORTIC VALVE AREA (cm²)
"Classic" aortic stenosis:				
Mild	Normal	2.5-3.0	<25	>1.5
Moderate	Normal	3.0-4.0	25-50	1.0-1.5
Severe	Normal	≥4.0	≥40	≤1.0
Very severe	Normal	≥5.0 (≥5.5)	≥60	<0.9
Severe aortic stenosis despite reduced LV EF	Reduced	≥4.0	≥40	≤1.0
Low-flow, low-gradient aortic stenosis	Reduced	≤4.0	≤40	≤1.0
"Paradoxical" low-flow, low-gradient aortic stenosis	Normal*	≤4.0	≤40	≤1.0

*In the presence of reduced stroke volume: An indexed stroke volume (SVi) ≤ 35 ml/m² has been proposed as a cutoff value.

Exercise electrocardiography is not helpful for the detection of coexisting CAD in patients with valvular AS. Although the increase in mean pressure gradient as assessed by exercise echocardiography has been reported to predict outcome and provide information beyond a regular exercise test,[81,123] more data are required to validate this finding and support its use in clinical practice.

Echocardiographic evaluation of the change in valve area with changes in flow rate in response to intravenous infusion of dobutamine may be helpful in the subgroup of patients with AS and significant LV systolic dysfunction who present with low gradient but small valve area.[37,124-130] For a description of the hemodynamic principles, see the earlier discussion Valvular Hemodynamics. More data are required to confirm that the distinction between truly severe and pseudosevere AS by dobutamine stress echocardiography is clinically useful and should guide clinical management, but contractile reserve—defined as a stroke volume increase of 20% or more—has been shown to be a potent predictor of outcome.[126] However, contractile reserve, surprisingly, has not been found to be an independent predictor of postoperative LV function.[131] In several studies, patients without contractile reserve prior to surgery had a higher perioperative mortality, but those who survived aortic valve replacement were found to have an increase in EF similar to that in those with contractile reserve[131] and to have a significantly better 5-year survival than patients managed conservatively.[132] Measuring the degree of aortic valve calcification by multislice computed tomography (CT) may be useful for the evaluation of AS severity, especially in difficult cases, such as patients with reduced EF and those without contractile reserve.[133]

Cardiac Catheterization

Aortic stenosis severity is routinely quantified using Doppler echocardiography. Invasive measurement of the transaortic gradient and calculation of valve area using the Gorlin formula is needed only in cases in which echocardiographic data are nondiagnostic or inconclusive (see Chapter 7).

Coronary angiography may be indicated to ascertain whether anginal symptoms are due to coexisting coronary disease in patients with mild or moderate AS. This procedure is routinely performed before aortic valve surgery unless the pretest likelihood of disease is extremely low, as, for example, in a young woman with congenital AS. Coronary CT angiography may be useful for the preoperative evaluation of patients at low risk of coronary disease when all major coronary branches can be properly visualized.

Disease Course

Clinical Outcome

ASYMPTOMATIC PATIENTS

In adults with valvular AS, obstruction to LV outflow develops gradually over many years.[83,85,86] In many patients, AS is coincidentally diagnosed when echocardiography is performed for other reasons or after the finding of a systolic murmur on examination, while they are still asymptomatic. Asymptomatic patients are found across the whole spectrum of AS severity, including a significant number with severe AS. In some patients a substantial decrease in valve area and an increase in transaortic velocity occur prior to symptom onset. The occurrence of symptoms clearly presents a turning point in the natural history of the disease (Table 11-3).

Patients with congenital AS may become symptomatic in early childhood or adolescence; in particular, patients with unicuspid valves tend to present with early symptoms. Later, at young adult age—typically between 20 and 30 years—these patients may also present with symptoms due to restenosis after a surgical valvotomy in childhood.[134,135] In the patient with congenital bicuspid stenotic aortic valve, surgery is typically performed between ages 50 and 70 years.[136-138] In the adult patient with degenerative calcific valve disease, symptom onset may already have occurred at age 50 but typically occurs in the elderly, between 70 and 90 years.[138] Rheumatic AS becomes symptomatic over a wider age range, with patients most often presenting between age 20 and 50 years.

In the absence of overt symptoms, clinical outcome with AS is excellent (Figure 11-1). However, some investigators suggest that irreversible changes of the ventricular myocardium occur even prior to symptom onset.[139]

With conservative follow-up of asymptomatic patients with AS, the risk of sudden death is one of the major concerns. In three studies that included significant numbers of patients with nonsevere stenosis, no sudden death was reported. Otto et al[47] followed up 123 patients with an average peak velocity of 3.6 ± 0.6 m/s for 30 months. The two other series, with 51[140] and 37 patients,[141] had follow-up periods of 1.5 and 2.0 years, respectively. Only two studies reported the outcome of larger cohorts of patients with exclusively severe stenosis, as defined by a peak aortic jet velocity 4.0 m/s or higher. Pellikka et al[142] observed 2 sudden deaths among 113 patients during a mean follow-up of 20 months. Both patients, however, had experienced symptoms at least 3 months before death. In a later published study, which is the largest to date, 11 sudden deaths were observed among 622 patients who had been followed up for a mean of 5.4 years.[143] However, as the investigators state, medical follow-up was limited in about half of the patients. It thus remained unclear in this study whether these patients had eventually experienced symptoms in the months prior to death. Rosenhek et al[144] reported 1 sudden death that was not preceded by any symptoms among 104 patients followed for 27 months on average. Even in a later report on 116 patients with very severe AS (peak velocity ≥ 5.0 m/s), only 1 sudden death was observed during a median follow-up of 3.4 years.[145] Thus, sudden death may indeed occur even in the absence of preceding symptoms in patients with AS but appears to be a very uncommon event, with a rate of probably less than 1% per year during the asymptomatic phase of the disease. Finally, it has to be considered that sudden death has been reported even after successful valve replacement in patients with AS, at an incidence of about

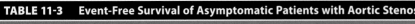

TABLE 11-3   Event-Free Survival of Asymptomatic Patients with Aortic Stenosis

FIRST AUTHOR	YR	ENTRY CRITERIA	N	AGE (YEARS)	FOLLOW-UP (MONTHS)	AS SEVERITY	EVENT-FREE SURVIVAL
Kelly[140]	1988	$V_{max} \geq 3.5$ m/s	51	63 ± 19	15 ± 10	ΔP 68 ± 19 mm Hg	60% at 2 yrs
Pellikka[142]	1990	$V_{max} \geq 4.0$ m/s	143	72 (40-94)	20	V_{max} 4.4 (4-6.4) m/s	62% at 2 yrs
Kennedy[243]	1991	Moderate AS at catheterization	66	67 ± 10	35	AVA 0.9 2 ± 0.13 cm²	59% at 4 yrs
Otto[47]	1997	Abnormal valve with V_{max} >2.6 m/s	123	63 ± 16	30	V_{max} <3.0 m/s V_{max} 3-4 m/s V_{max} >4 m/s	84% at 2 yrs 66% at 2 yrs 21% at 2 yrs
Rosenhek[144]	2000	$V_{max} \geq 4.0$ m/s	128	60 ± 18	22 ± 18	V_{max} 5.0 ± 0.7 m/s	67% at 1 yr 56% at 2 yrs 33% at 4 yrs
Rosenhek[148]	2004	Abnormal valve with V_{max} 2.5-3.9 m/s	176	58 ± 19	48 ± 19	V_{max} 3.1 ± 0.4 m/s	95% at 1 yr 75% at 2 yrs 60% at 5 yrs
Pellikka[143]	2005	$V_{max} \geq 4.0$ m/s	622	72 ± 11	65 ± 48	V_{max} 4.4 ± 0.4 m/s	82% at 1 yr 67% at 2 yrs 33% at 5 yrs
Rossebø[180]	2008	V_{max} 2.5 to 4.0 m/s	1873	68 ± 9	52 (median)	V_{max} 3.1 ± 0.55 m/s	Approx. 65% at 5 yrs
Lancellotti[155]	2010	AVAi ≤0.6 cm²/m²	163	70 ± 10	20 ± 19	≤0.6 cm²/m²	50% at 2 yrs 44% at 4 yrs
Kang[189]	2010	$V_{max} \geq 4.5$ m/s	95	63 ± 12	58 (median)	4.9 ± 0 4 m/s	71±5% at 2 yrs 47±5% at 4 yrs 28±6% at 6 yrs
Rosenhek[145]	2010	$V_{max} \geq 5.0$ m/s	116	67 ± 15	41 (median)	V_{max} 5.0-5.5 m/s $V_{max} \geq 5.5$ m/s	43% at 2 yrs 25% at 2 yrs

AS, aortic stenosis; *AVA*, aortic valve area; *AVAi*, indexed aortic valve area; *ΔP*, pressure gradient; *V_{max}*, maximum aortic jet velocity.

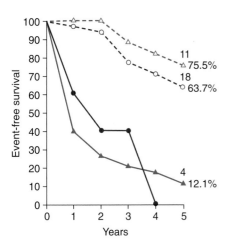

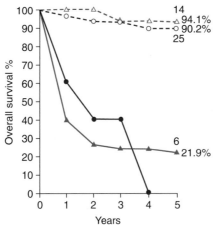

FIGURE 11-1 Event-free survival with aortic valve disease. Survival curves are shown for hemodynamically severe aortic stenosis and combined lesions (*triangles and blue lines*) as well as aortic regurgitation (*circles and red lines*) in severely symptomatic (*solid lines*) and asymptomatic or mildly symptomatic (*dashed lines*) patients. Event free survival at 5 years, and the number of remaining subjects, are shown at the end of each line. (*From Turina J, Hess O, Sepulcri F, Krayenbuehl HP. Spontaneous course of aortic valve disease. Eur Heart J 1987;8:471–83.*)

0.3%, so the risk cannot be entirely eliminated by surgical treatment.[146,147]

Overall, a watchful waiting strategy, which consists of regularly following up patients as long as they are asymptomatic and referring them for surgery once they become symptomatic, results in a good survival that is not statistically different from that of an age- and gender-matched control population (Figure 11-2).[144]

RISK STRATIFICATION IN ASYMPTOMATIC PATIENTS

In initially asymptomatic patients, the rate of symptom onset ranges from less than 1% to 15% per year. Predictors of symptom onset include older age, male gender, AS severity, and functional status. One of the most important predictors of outcome in patients with AS is the degree of stenosis severity. The necessity for subsequent aortic valve surgery is directly related to peak aortic jet velocity over the whole spectrum of disease, with event rates being lowest in patients with mild stenosis, followed by those with moderate and then severe stenosis.[47,144,148] The rate of symptom onset is about 8% per year in those with a jet velocity less than 3.0 m/s, 17% per year in those with a jet velocity of 3.0 to 4.0 m/s, and 40% per year in those with a jet velocity more than 4.0 m/s (Figure 11-3).

Significant calcification, age, and the presence of CAD indicated higher event rates in patients with mild to moderate AS.[148]

In addition, the rate of increase in aortic jet velocity over time is a strong predictor of clinical outcome.[47,144,148-150] In severe asymptomatic AS, the rate of symptom onset is higher in patients older than 50 years and in those with significant valve calcification, suggesting that calcific disease progresses more rapidly than rheumatic aortic valve stenosis.[144,151] Among 126 patients with asymptomatic severe AS, it was shown that the presence of a

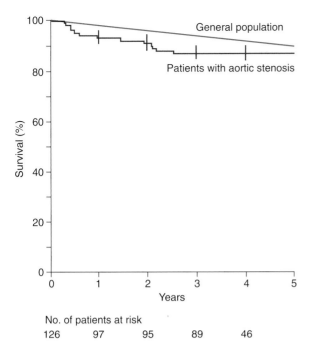

FIGURE 11-2 Asymptomatic severe aortic stenosis. Kaplan-Meier estimates of overall survival among 126 patients with asymptomatic but severe aortic stenosis, as compared with age- and sex-matched persons in the general population. This analysis included perioperative and postoperative deaths among patients who required valve replacement during follow-up. *The vertical bars indicate standard errors. (From Rosenhek R, Binder T, Porenta G, Lang I, Christ G, Schemper M, et al. Predictors of outcome in severe, asymptomatic aortic stenosis. N Engl J Med 2000;343:611–7.)*

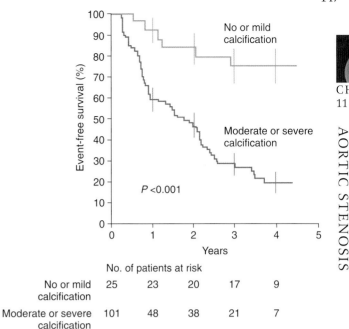

FIGURE 11-4 Effect of leaflet calcification on outcome in asymptomatic severe aortic stenosis. Kaplan-Meier estimates of event-free survival among 25 patients with no or mild aortic valve calcification compared with that among 101 patients with moderate or severe calcification. All patients had an aortic jet velocity of at least 4 m/s at study entry. The vertical bars indicate standard errors. *(From Rosenhek R, Binder T, Porenta G, Lang I, Christ G, Schemper M, et al. Predictors of outcome in severe, asymptomatic aortic stenosis. N Engl J Med 2000;343:611–7.)*

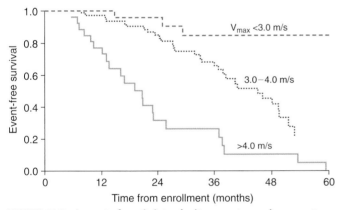

FIGURE 11-3 Impact of aortic jet velocity on outcome in asymptomatic aortic stenosis. Cox regression analysis showing event-free survival in 123 initially asymptomatic adults with valvular aortic stenosis, defined by maximum aortic jet velocity (V_{max}) at entry (P <0.001 by log-rank test). *(From Otto CM, Burwash IG, Legget ME, Munt BI, Fujioka M, Healy NL, et al. Prospective study of asymptomatic valvular aortic stenosis: clinical, echocardiographic, and exercise predictors of outcome. Circulation 1997;95:2262–70.)*

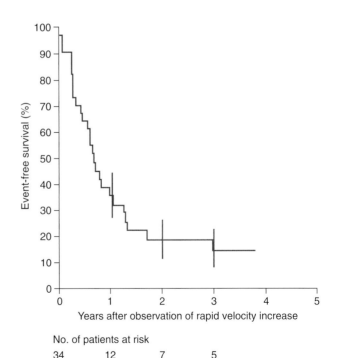

FIGURE 11-5 Effect of change in aortic velocity on clinical outcome. Kaplan-Meier estimates of event-free survival among 34 patients with moderate or severe calcification of the aortic valve and a rapid increase in aortic jet velocity (at least 0.3 m/s within 1 year). In this analysis, follow-up started with the visit at which the rapid increase was identified. *The vertical bars indicate standard errors. (From Rosenhek R, Binder T, Porenta G, et al. Predictors of outcome in severe, asymptomatic aortic stenosis. N Engl J Med 2000; 343: 611–7.)*

moderately to severely calcified aortic valve was associated with a significantly increased event rate, and 80% of these 126 patients experienced symptoms warranting aortic valve replacement or died within 4 years (Figure 11-4).[144] The combination of a calcified aortic valve with a rapid hemodynamic progression, defined as an increase in peak aortic jet velocity of more than 0.3 m/s within 1 year, identified a patient group at particularly high risk, with an event rate of 79% within 2 years (Figure 11-5).[144] The echocardiographic determination of aortic valve calcification has the advantage of being fast and easily obtainable at the moment of the echocardiographic exam. Although it is a semiquantitative

CH
11

AORTIC STENOSIS

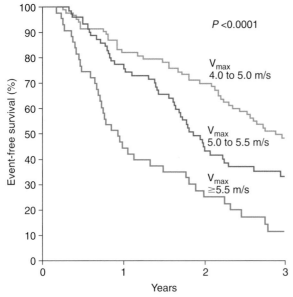

P <0.0001

V_{max}... V_{max} 4.0 to 5.0 m/s

V_{max} 5.0 to 5.5 m/s

V_{max} ≥5.5 m/s

Patients with V_{max} from 4.0 to 5.0 m/s
Pts. at risk: 82   69   59   38
Patients with V_{max} from 5.0 to 5.5 m/s
Pts. at risk: 72   53   29   18
Patients with V_{max} from ≥5.5 m/s
Pts. at risk: 44   20   11   5

FIGURE 11-6   **Outcomes with very severe aortic stenosis.** Kaplan-Meier event-free survival estimates for patients with a maximum aortic valve jet velocity (V_{max}) between 4.0 and 5.0 m/s (*yellow line*; n = 82), between 5. 0 and 5.5 m/s (*blue line*; n = 72), and ≥5.5 m/s (*green line*; n = 44). *(From Rosenhek R, Zilberszac R, Schemper M, Czerny M, Mundigler G, Graf S, et al. Natural history of very severe aortic stenosis. Circulation 2010;121:151–6.)*

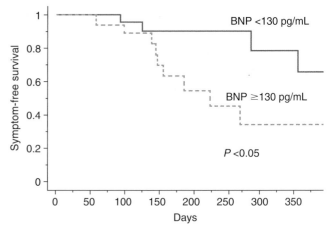

FIGURE 11-7   **Relationship between brain natriuretic peptide (BNP) levels and outcome in aortic stenosis.** Kaplan-Meier estimates of symptom-free survival for patients with severe aortic stenosis and a a baseline BNP <130 pg/mL (n = 25) versus ≥130 pg/mL (n = 18). *(From Bergler-Klein J, Klaar U, Heger M, Rosenhek R, Mundigler G, Gabriel H, Binder T, et al. Natriuretic peptides predict symptom-free survival and postoperative outcome in severe aortic stenosis. Circulation 2004;109:2302–8.)*

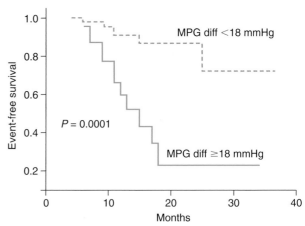

FIGURE 11-8   **Exercise change in pressure gradient and clinical outcome.** Event-free survival curves according to exercise-induced changes in mean transaortic pressure gradient (MPG diff) in 69 consecutive patients with severe aortic stenosis. *(From Lancellotti P, Lebois F, Simon M, Tombeux C, Chauvel C, Pierard LA. Prognostic importance of quantitative exercise Doppler echocardiography in asymptomatic valvular aortic stenosis. Circulation 2005;112:I377–82).*

method, the differentiation between no or mild and moderate to severe calcification can be easily made. The finding that aortic valve calcification is associated with a poor outcome was also confirmed by a study that assessed the degree of aortic valve calcification by electron-beam tomography.[152] Patients with very severe AS are also at an increased risk of experiencing a rapid symptom onset. Event-free survival rates at 3 years were found to 49%, 33%, and 11% for patients with peak aortic jet velocities between 4.0 and 5.0 m/s, between 5.0 and 5.5 m/s, and more than 5.5 m/s, respectively (Figure 11-6).[145] Most patients with an aortic jet velocity higher than 5.0 m/s are already symptomatic at presentation, and those who are still asymptomatic have a high likelihood of a rapid symptom onset, in particular when their peak aortic jet velocity exceeds 5.5 m/s. These findings strongly support the need to define the entity of "very severe" AS.

Monin et al[153] have proposed a risk score for the identification of patients with AS at high risk of adverse events that includes both information on stenosis severity and brain natriuretic peptide (BNP) levels as follows:

$$Score = [peak\ velocity\ (m/s) \times 2] + (\ln\ of\ BNP \times 1.5) + 1.5\ (if\ female\ sex)$$

BNP was previously demonstrated to predict symptom onset and operative outcome in several other studies[154-156] (Figure 11-7).

Lancellotti et al[81] assessed the value of exercise Doppler echocardiographic measurements in 69 patients with severe asymptomatic AS. In this study, an exercise-induced increase in mean transaortic gradient of 18 mm Hg or more (Figure 11-8), an abnormal exercise test result, and an aortic valve area less than 0.75 cm² were significant predictors of subsequent events in multivariate analysis, and all had an incremental value when they occurred together. In 135 asymptomatic AS patients with a normal

exercise response, an exercise-induced increase in mean transvalvular gradient of more than 20 mm Hg was described as an independent risk predictor, suggesting that exercise stress echocardiography may provide prognostic information additional to that obtained from standard exercise testing and resting echocardiography.[123] Using receiver operating characteristic curve analysis in 163 patients with moderate to severe AS, Lancellotti et al[155] identified a peak aortic jet velocity of 4.4 m/s or higher, an LV longitudinal myocardial deformation of 15.9% or less, a valvular-arterial impedance of 4.9 mm Hg/mL/m² or greater, and an indexed left atrial area of 12.2 cm²/m² or more as associated in an integrative way with events. In patients with severe AS, impaired multidirectional LV strain and strain rate are present even with preserved LV EF, but a significant improvement occurs after aortic valve replacement.[157] Significantly higher event-free survival rates were described for patients with appropriate and inappropriate LV mass, respectively, being 78% and 56% at 1 year, 68% and 29% at 3 years, and 56% and 10% at 5 years (all *P* < 0.01) (Figure 11-9).[158] However, in patients with calcific AS who have a

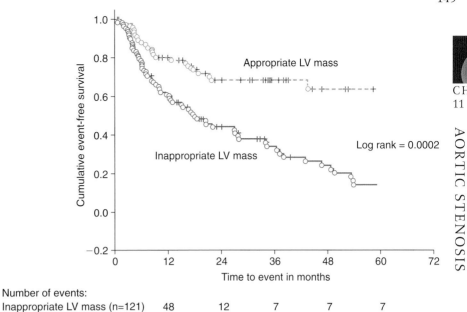

FIGURE 11-9 LV Mass and clinical outcome in aortic stenosis. Event-free survival curves in patients with appropriate (*yellow line*; n = 88) or inappropriately high (*blue line*; n = 121) left ventricular (LV) mass. *(From Cioffi G, Faggiano P, Vizzardi E, Tarantini L, Cramariuc D, Gerdts E, de Simone G. Prognostic effect of inappropriately high left ventricular mass in asymptomatic severe aortic stenosis. Heart 2011;97:301–7.)*

Number of events:					
Inappropriate LV mass (n=121)	48	12	7	7	7
Appropriate LV mass (n=88)	17	7	0	2	0

normal LV EF, the severity of stenosis is the most important correlate of symptomatic deterioration, and tissue Doppler imaging measurements of LV systolic and diastolic function and LV mass provide limited predictive information after for the severity of stenosis is accounted for.[159]

Interestingly, there is a wide range of hemodynamic severity at symptom onset in adults with valvular AS.[47,134,160,161] In the Balloon Valvuloplasty Registry study, symptomatic patients had aortic jet velocities ranging from 2.3 to 6.6 (mean 4.4 ± 0.8) m/s, mean transaortic pressure gradients ranging from 13 to 120 (mean 48 ± 18) mm Hg, and aortic valve areas ranging from 0.1 to 1.4 (mean 0.6 ± 0.2) cm^2.[7] In this study, there may have been bias toward overestimation of disease severity at symptom onset because some patients may have been symptomatic for several months or years prior to study entry. However, a prospective study of initially asymptomatic adults with valvular AS also found a wide range of hemodynamic severity at symptom onset, with an average jet velocity of 4.6 ± 0.8 m/s, a mean transaortic gradient of 49 ± 18 mm Hg, and a mean valve area of 0.93 ± 0.31 cm^2.[47] The range of hemodynamic severity at symptom onset is similar if indexed to body surface area, indicating that these differences between patients are not due simply to differences in body size. Other clinical series also show a substantial overlap in hemodynamic severity between symptomatic and asymptomatic patients.[134,161]

These clinical observations support the hypothesis that symptom onset is due to the interaction of valve stiffness, LV ejection force, and the metabolic requirements in each individual. Symptoms typically occur initially with conditions that increase total tissue oxygen demands, such as exertion, pregnancy, febrile illness, and anemia, as a result of the inability of the heart to increase cardiac output across the narrowed valve. Thus, the specific degree of valve narrowing associated with clinical symptoms shows considerable individual variability. In addition, concurrent conditions such as AR and CAD also modify the specific extent of hemodynamic perturbation associated with symptoms.

SYMPTOMATIC PATIENTS

Once definite symptoms of AS are present, outcome is very poor without surgical intervention. Using data from earlier autopsy series, one study projected that the average time from symptom onset to death is 2 years for patients with exertional syncope, 3 years for those with heart failure symptoms, and 5 years for those with angina.[85] Later series of adults who refused surgical intervention indicate survival rates with severe symptomatic AS of only 15% to 50% at 5 years.[82,134,161,162] Recently the poor outcome of inoperable patients with symptomatic severe AS has been confirmed in cohort B of the U.S. Placement of AoRTic TraNscathetER Valve (PARTNER) trial, with a mortality of 50% at 1 year.[163] More intense symptoms are associated with worse outcome.

This finding emphasizes the importance of patient education, the need for periodic clinical evaluation, and the importance of intervention for any symptom due to AS.

In adults with symptomatic AS, predictors of survival are transaortic velocity or gradient, functional status, LV systolic function, comorbid disease, and gender.[162] In a patient with symptoms due to severe AS, prognosis is better in the presence of a high gradient (or jet velocity), because a low gradient and low transaortic velocity in the setting of severe valve narrowing is the reflection of a reduced cardiac output.

Not surprisingly, BNP levels predict survival in this group of patients.[164] Often these patients have symptoms with minimal exertion or at rest and many have recurrent hospital admissions for decompensated heart failure. Medical therapy may enable alleviation of episodes of acute decompensation, for example, the use of diuretics for acute pulmonary edema, but does not prevent recurrent episodes of decompensation or prolong life.

Patients with paradoxical low-flow, low-gradient AS and preserved EF may present with severe symptoms, although the interpretation of symptoms may be difficult because of the common coexistence of hypertension. It has been shown that such patients have a reduced longitudinal LV function, a higher degree of interstitial fibrosis in biopsy samples, and more late enhancement on magnetic resonance imaging.[165]

AORTIC SCLEROSIS AND MILD TO MODERATE AORTIC STENOSIS

The presence of aortic valve sclerosis is associated with a significantly increased cardiovascular and all-cause mortality in the absence of hemodynamic obstruction to blood flow.[166] Also, mild to moderate AS is not a benign disease, being associated with increased cardiovascular and noncardiac deaths.[47,148] Thus aortic sclerosis and mild to moderate AS are markers of a poor overall prognosis.

In addition the prognosis of patients with the disease is influenced by hemodynamic progression of the disease. The Cardiovascular Health Study showed that aortic sclerosis progresses to significant AS within five years in about 9% of patients.[167] The interval between observation of aortic valve "sclerosis" on echocardiography and clinical evidence of severe stenosis may be as short as five years.[168] In addition, the progression to severe, hemodynamically significant stenosis is common and may be more rapid than previously assumed.[148]

Hemodynamic Progression

Understanding the progressive nature of AS and awareness of progression rates are fundamental to appropriate patient management and individualization of follow-up intervals in patients who have mild or moderate AS. Studies have aimed to define hemodynamic progression of AS during the phase prior to symptom onset, to predict prognosis, to identify predictors of rapid disease progression, and to improve our understanding of the relationship between hemodynamic severity and symptom onset.[35,141,144,148,150,169-173] Intervention studies, designed to assess the effects of statin therapy in halting or delaying the progression of AS, provide additional information on hemodynamic progression[174-178] (Table 11-4). Overall, these studies showed an average rate of increase in aortic jet maximum velocity between 0.2 and 0.4 m/s/year, and mean pressure gradient of about 8 mm Hg per year, with a decrease in valve area of 0.15 cm² per year. However, there is marked individual variability in the rate of hemodynamic progression. Factors predicting rapid hemodynamic progression are the presence of a calcified aortic valve, CAD, and age (Figure 11-10).[148] Although Doppler echocardiographic studies have the advantage of larger patient numbers and potentially less

selection bias (a repeat echocardiographic study is likely to be requested more often than a repeat cardiac catheterization), many of these studies are retrospective, the data having been extracted from ongoing clinical databases. Thus, patients with rapid progression, those demonstrating symptoms, or those requiring surgical intervention may be overrepresented. Conversely, repeat studies may not have been performed in clinically stable patients. The results of more recently published studies may avoid some of these biases.[47,144,176,179-181]

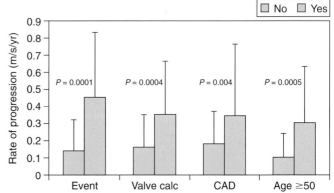

FIGURE 11-10 **Hemodynamic progression rates.** Rates of hemodynamic progression expressed as increases in peak aortic jet velocity among patients with mild to moderate aortic stenosis. *Valve calc,* calcified aortic valve leaflets; *CAD,* coronary artery disease. (*From Rosenhek R, Klaar U, Schemper M, Scholten C, Heger M, Gabriel H, Binder T, et al. Mild and moderate aortic stenosis: natural history and risk stratification by echocardiography. Eur Heart J 2004;25:199–205.*)

TABLE 11-4 Hemodynamic Progression of Valvular Aortic Stenosis

FIRST AUTHOR	YEAR	TYPE OF STUDY	CLINICAL STATUS AT ENTRY	N	MEAN FOLLOW-UP (yrs)	INCREASE IN MEAN ΔP (mm Hg/yr)	INCREASE IN V_{MAX} (m/s/yr)	DECREASE IN AVA (cm²/yr)
Echocardiographic Studies								
Otto[170]	1989	Prospective	Asymptomatic	42	1.7	8 (−7 to 23)	0.36 ± 0.31	0.1
Roger[173]	1990	Retrospective	AS on echo	112	2.1		0.23 ± 0.37	
Faggiano[141]	1992	Prospective	AS on echo	45	1.5		0.4 ± 0.3	0.1 ± 0.13
Peter[172]	1993	Retrospective	AS on echo	49	2.7	7.2		
Brener[169]	1995	Retrospective	AS on echo	394	6.3			0.14
Otto[47]	1997	Prospective	Asymptomatic	123	2.5	7 ± 7	0.32 ± 0.34	0.12 ± 0.19
Bahler[150]	1999	Retrospective	AS on echo	91	1.8	2.8	0.2	0.04
Palta[171]	2000	Retrospective	AS on echo	170	1.9			0.10 ± 0.27
Rosenhek[144]	2000	Prospective	V_{max} >4.0m/s	128	1.8	Slow	0.14 ± 0.18	
						Rapid	0.45 ± 0.38	
Rosenhek[148]	2004	Retrospective	V_{max} 2.5 to 3.9 m/s	176	3.8		0.24 ± 0.30	
Echocardiographic Intervention Studies								
Novaro[177]	2001	Retrospective	AVA 1.0 to 1.8 cm²	174	1.7	Statin therapy		0.06 ± 0.16
						No statin		0.11 ± 0.18
Bellamy[175]	2002	Retrospective	AVA <2.0 cm²	156	3.7	Statin therapy		0.04 ± 0.15
						No statin		0.09 ± 0.17
Rosenhek[178]	2004	Retrospective	V_{max} >2.5 m/s	211	2.0	Statin therapy	0.1 ± 041	
						No statin	0.39 ± 0.42	
Cowell[176]	2005	Prospective	V_{max} >2.5 m/s	134	2.1	Statin therapy	0.2 ± 0.21	0.08 ± 0.11
						No statin	0.2 ± 0.21	0.08 ± 0.11
Moura[179]	2007	Prospective	AVA 1.0 to 1.5 cm²	121	1.4	Statin therapy	0.4 ± 0.38	0.05 ± 0.12
						No statin	0.24 ± 0.30	0.1 ± 0.09
Chan[181]	2010	Prospective	V_{max} 2.5 to 4.0 m/s	269	3.5	Statin therapy		0.08 ± 0.21
						No statin		0.07 ± 0.15

AS, aortic stenosis; *AVA,* aortic valve area; *ΔP,* pressure gradient; *echo,* echocardiography; *V_{max},* maximum aortic jet velocity.

As the disease progresses, growing obstruction to LV outflow is most often reflected by a decrease in valve area and increases in jet velocity and pressure gradient. However, if there is a concurrent decrease in transaortic volume flow rate, a decrease in valve area alone may be seen, with no change in jet velocity or transaortic gradient. This situation may occur secondary to comorbid disease, such as increasing mitral regurgitation or myocardial infarction, but may also be due to a decrease in LV function late in the disease course. On the other hand, increases in jet velocity and pressure gradient with no change in valve area may be observed if transaortic stroke volume is increased as a result of hyperdynamic states (e.g., anemia, fever, pregnancy) or increasing AR.

In general, the rate of hemodynamic progression is fairly linear. However, episodes of more abrupt progression preceding the appearance of symptoms have been observed. Such abrupt progression might appear at the point at which leaflet stiffness exceeds the capacity of ventricular ejection force to adequately open the valve.

Coexisting Coronary Artery Disease

About 50% of adults undergoing valve replacement for AS have significant CAD. The concurrence of valvular AS and CAD complicates both the diagnosis and management in individual patients and the interpretation of outcome studies.

Only between 20% and 60% of patients with AS and symptoms of angina have coronary disease, whereas 0 to 54% (mean 16%) of those without angina also have significant CAD.[182] In the patient with previously asymptomatic AS, it is difficult to ascertain whether the onset of angina is due to the severe valvular stenosis or whether angina is due to coexisting CAD. Alcalai et al[183] described a series of 38 consecutive symptomatic patients with significant AS and CAD who underwent percutaneous coronary intervention (surgery was not performed because of patient preference, high surgical risk, and cardiologist recommendation). After the intervention, 35 of these patients reported relief of their symptoms.

On a general basis, even though the symptoms might not always be unequivocally attributable to AS, aortic valve replacement should not be deferred in symptomatic patients because of the unfavorable natural history of severe symptomatic AS. When stenosis severity is intermediate, decision making is more difficult, especially given that symptoms can occur with a relatively wide range of stenosis severity. Often, coronary angiography is needed to clarify the contribution of coronary disease to symptoms in these patients. The decision should incorporate coronary morphology, severity of AS, and expected progression rates.

In clinical studies of the natural history of AS, it rarely is possible to separate outcomes due to coexisting coronary disease from those due to valvular obstruction, given the high rate of concordance of these diseases. Of the four cardiac deaths in a prospective study of 123 adults with asymptomatic AS, two were due to coexisting CAD and the other two patients had severe AS but refused aortic valve replacement.[47]

Coronary angiography is routinely performed prior to planned surgical intervention. The operative mortality for patients with AS and coexisting CAD ranges from 1.1% to 4.8% if coronary artery bypass grafting is performed at the time of valve replacement but may be as high as 4% to 13.2% if no revascularization is performed in the setting of significant coronary disease, most likely because of inadequate myocardial perfusion immediately after cardiopulmonary bypass and in the early postoperative period.[139,184] Noninvasive tests are generally of limited use in the preoperative assessment. Especially older patients with calcific AS, who often have a significant risk profile and a high rate of associated CAD, should systematically undergo preoperative coronary angiography. Ruling out the presence of CAD with CT angiography might be an option in younger patients at low risk for the presence of CAD.

Surgical Intervention and Postoperative Outcome

Timing of Surgical Intervention

SYMPTOM ONSET

Surgical intervention for AS is indicated at symptom onset in adults because of the dramatic improvement in survival with surgical in comparison with medical therapy and the high likelihood of symptom relief after valve replacement. Surgery can be deferred in asymptomatic adults, in whom survival and clinical outcome are excellent without surgical intervention.[144] The only clinical difficulty with this approach is defining at what point the patient can be considered symptomatic.

Symptom onset in adults is so gradual that many patients fail to recognize early symptoms and first appear for medical attention with a syncopal episode, frank heart failure, or unstable angina. Surgical intervention clearly is needed in these patients. In contrast, patients followed up prospectively who are educated about the possible symptoms tend to present with a history of gradually decreasing exercise tolerance and increasing exertional dyspnea that is elicited only by focused and detailed questions. Physical examination typically shows severe AS but fails to reveal evidence of hemodynamic decompensation. Thus, it often is unclear whether these patients are truly symptomatic or whether these nonspecific symptoms are due to age, intercurrent illness, or comorbid conditions.

In general, if severe AS is present even mild symptoms should be considered to be due to AS, and the patient referred promptly for surgical intervention. Support for this approach includes natural history studies showing the high rate of symptom onset and death with Doppler echocardiographic evidence of severe stenosis, so that even if surgery is deferred initially, the patient is likely to experience more severe symptoms requiring surgical intervention within a relatively short time.[47,185,186] Additional support for surgical intervention for mild symptoms is the growing evidence that systolic dysfunction may be irreversible in some patients with AS and that nearly all patients have significant diastolic dysfunction that persists for several years after valve replacement. Some investigators suggest that even earlier intervention is needed (e.g., in the asymptomatic patient) to prevent the secondary LV changes of this disease process.[139]

Another clinical difficulty in the timing of surgical intervention in AS is determining whether symptoms are caused by AS when obstruction is not severe. In the patient with symptoms, such as angina, but only mild valve obstruction, it is clear that AS is not the cause of the symptoms. However, when symptoms are present and stenosis appears "moderate," the relationship between the valve obstruction and symptoms is less clear, especially in light of the observation that there is substantial overlap in hemodynamic severity between symptomatic and asymptomatic patients. There is no simple method to establish a cause-and-effect relationship between valve obstruction and symptoms in these cases. A careful history and search for alternate causes of symptoms may resolve the issue. If not, exercise testing for objective evaluation of exercise tolerance, hemodynamic response, and symptoms may be helpful.

SURGERY IN ASYMPTOMATIC PATIENTS

Although there is consensus now that surgery is indicated in symptomatic AS even if symptoms are mild,[112,113] the management of asymptomatic AS remains a matter of controversy.[187,188] Kang et al[189] recently reported a better outcome for 102 patients with asymptomatic AS with a peak aortic jet velocity of more than 4.5 m/s who underwent elective aortic valve replacement than for patients who were initially followed up conservatively. However, this study was nonrandomized and the mortality in the group of patients initially managed conservatively was unexpectedly high; it was 24% at 6 years and the majority of deaths indeed occurred in patients who had eventually demonstrated symptoms but nevertheless did not undergo surgery. Another study that proposed elective surgery in asymptomatic AS actually demonstrated that patients who underwent surgery while still asymptomatic had identical operative and long-term outcomes as those for patients who underwent surgery when they became symptomatic.[190] However, these data have not confirmed a better outcome with an early elective surgery strategy.

There is consensus that the very rare asymptomatic patient with AS and impaired LV systolic function that cannot be explained by other causes should be referred for surgery. Despite the data showing overall good outcome for all other truly asymptomatic patients and the low risk of sudden death during the asymptomatic phase of the disease, many physicians are reluctant to follow up these patients for several reasons. There is the previously discussed difficulty to clearly distinguish between asymptomatic and mildly symptomatic status and the fact that patients frequently do not present immediately when symptoms develop. Furthermore, operative risk significantly increases with symptoms and their severity. A large surgical registry reports an operative mortality of less than 2% for patients in New York Heart Association (NYHA) functional class I or II heart failure, compared with 3.7% and 7% for patients in NYHA classes III and IV, respectively.[191] In addition, there remains concern that severe myocardial hypertrophy and fibrosis may develop during the asymptomatic phase and preclude a later optimal surgical outcome.[192] Because it appears nevertheless unlikely from current data that the potential benefit of valve replacement in asymptomatic patients can outweigh the risk of surgery and the long-term risk of prosthesis-related complications in all patients, surgery for severe AS can certainly not be recommended in general before symptom onset. However, risk stratification should be considered to identify patients who are likely to benefit from elective surgery.[188]

Risk stratification has been discussed previously (see Clinical Outcome). It has to be noted that in all the studies that identified predictors of outcome in asymptomatic AS, the vast majority of events was symptom development that required valve replacement. Thus, these variables have primarily been shown to predict a shorter time to symptom onset but not mortality. No study could so far demonstrate that elective surgery in asymptomatic patients based on such risk factors has significant impact on survival. For this reason, current guidelines are rather cautious with recommendations.[112,113] Because patients with peak aortic jet velocity above 5.5 m/s[145] and those with moderate to severe calcification of the valve and rapid increase in transvalvular velocity (≥0.3m/s within 1 year)[144] are in particular likely to experience symptoms and rapid deterioration very soon, the revised European Guidelines recommend that surgery should be considered (class IIaC; see Table 11-5).

Stress testing as a predictor of outcome has also been discussed previously. Patients with normal exercise capacity can be

TABLE 11-5 Indications for Aortic Valve Replacement in Aortic Stenosis as Recommended by Current Practice Guidelines

INDICATION CLASS	EVIDENCE LEVEL	ACC/AHA GUIDELINES[244]	ESC GUIDELINES[113]
I	B	Symptomatic patient with severe AS	Symptomatic patient with severe AS
	C	Patient with severe AS and EF <0.50	Patient with severe AS and EF <0.50
	C	Patient with severe AS undergoing CABG or surgery on the aorta or other heart valves	Patient with severe AS undergoing CABG or surgery on the aorta or other heart valves
	C		Asymptomatic patient developing symptoms during exercise test
IIa	C	Patient with moderate AS undergoing CABG or surgery on the aorta or other heart valves	Patient with moderate AS undergoing CABG or surgery on the aorta or other heart valves
	C		Asymptomatic patient with severe AS and fall of blood pressure below baseline during exercise test
	C		Asymptomatic patients, with normal EF and none of the above-mentioned exercise test abnormalities, if the surgical risk is low and one or more of the following findings is present: • Very severe AS defined by a peak transvalvular velocity >5.5 m/s or • Severe valve calcification and a rate of peak transvalvular velocity progression ≥0.3 m/s per year
	C		AS with low gradient (<40 mm Hg) with LV dysfunction and contractile reserve
	C		Symptomatic patients with low-flow, low-gradient (<40 mm Hg) AS with normal EF only after careful confirmation of severe AS
IIb	C	Asymptomatic patient with severe AS and abnormal response to exercise (e.g., development of symptoms or asymptomatic hypotension)	Asymptomatic patients with severe AS, normal EF and none of the above-mentioned exercise test abnormalities, if surgical risk is low and one or more of the following findings is present:
	C	Asymptomatic patient with severe AS and high likelihood of rapid progression (age, calcification, and CAD) or if surgery might be delayed at the time of symptom onset	Markedly elevated natriuretic peptide levels confirmed by repeated measurements without other explanations
	C	Patient with mild AS undergoing CABG when there is evidence, such as moderate to severe calcification, that progression may be rapid	Increase of mean pressure gradient with exercise by >20 mm Hg
	C	Asymptomatic patient with extremely severe AS (valve area <0.6 cm², mean gradient >60 mm Hg, jet velocity >5.0 m/s) when expected operative mortality ≤1%	Excessive LV hypertrophy in the absence of hypertension AS with low gradient (<40 mm Hg) and LV dysfunction without contractile reserve

ACC, American College of Cardiology; AHA, American Heart Association; AS, aortic stenosis; CABG, coronary artery bypass graft surgery; CAD, coronary artery disease; EF, ejection fraction; ESC, European Society of Cardiology; LV, left ventricle.

considered at low risk and safely followed up. Symptom development during exercise test indicates surgery, particularly in physically active patients (class I in Europe, IIb in United States). However, it has to be kept in mind that breathlessness on exercise may be difficult to interpret in patients normally engaging in only low physical activity, particularly the elderly, making decisions more difficult. Asymptomatic patients with drops in blood pressure below baseline during exercise testing should also be considered for surgery by consensus.

Arrhythmias upon exercise, excessive LV hypertrophy, marked increase in mean gradient during exercise, and elevated neurohormones are more controversial and/or clear cutoffs for clinical decision making are poorly defined. Therefore, these risk factors are ranked rather low (IIbC).[112,113]

BNP levels are particularly helpful when they are normal or only slightly elevated, indicating a good short-term outcome. However, the positive predictive value of this measurement needs to be viewed cautiously because of its nonspecificity and the fact that several cutoff values were proposed in different studies to indicate a poor outcome.[154,193,194] Nevertheless, markedly elevated BNP without any other explanation must prompt further evaluation. Furthermore, high plasma levels of neurohormones have been reported to be associated with high operative mortality and worse postoperative outcome with regard to LV function and symptomatic status.[154] Finally, neurohormone measurements may help to better distinguish between asymptomatic and early symptomatic state or to relate shortness of breath to AS in a patient with an additional pulmonary cause of this symptom.

Recommendations for surgery according to current U.S.[112] and European[113] guidelines are summarized in Table 11-5 as well as in Figures 11-11 and 11-12.

INTERVENTION IN THE ELDERLY

The assessment of the interventional risk is particularly important in elderly patients. Objective parameters to assess interventional risk and thus to predict the risk of surgery and to identify high-risk patients who would benefit from percutaneous procedures are needed.[195] In that regard, reliable risk scores that predict surgical mortality would be helpful. The EuroSCORE, still widely used in Europe, was not developed for this specific patient group, has major limitations, and frequently overestimates the 30-day mortality.[196] Although surgical mortality is higher in elderly patients, they also experience significantly prolonged life expectancy after valve replacement. When intervention is being considered in elderly patients, it is helpful to consult age-adjusted life tables so that expected survival after surgery (as for age-matched adults without AS) can be compared with the expected survival without surgical intervention.[195] Also, in octogenarians, survival after aortic valve replacement is favorable even with concomitant bypass surgery, and more than half of patients survive more than 6 years after surgery, with a median survival between 6 and 7 years—similar to the life expectancy in the general population.[197] Patients with severe AS who are no longer considered suitable for conventional surgery have a significantly improved outcome with transfemoral transcatheter aortic valve implantation (TAVI) than with standard therapy (2-year all-cause mortality 43.3% vs. 68.0%, respectively) (Figure 11-13).[198] TAVI has also become an accepted therapy for patients with severe AS for whom surgery poses a high risk. In a randomized controlled trial comparing TAVI and conventional valve replacement, noninferiority was proven for TAVI (2-year all-cause mortality 33.9% and 35.0%, respectively) (Figure 11-14),[199] although there were important differences in

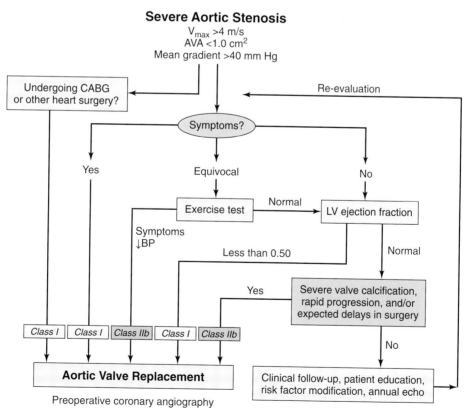

FIGURE 11-11 **Algorithm representing the management strategy for patients with severe aortic stenosis from the American College of Cardiology/ American Heart Association Guidelines.** Preoperative coronary angiography should be performed routinely as determined by age, symptoms, and coronary risk factors. Cardiac catheterization and angiography may also be helpful when there is discordance between clinical and echocardiographic findings. *AVA*, aortic valve area; *BP*, blood pressure; *CABG*, coronary artery bypass graft surgery; *echo*, echocardiography; *LV*, left ventricular; *V~max~*, maximal velocity across aortic valve as determined by Doppler echocardiography.

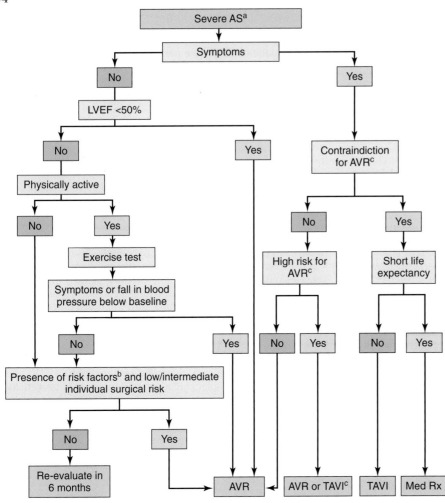

FIGURE 11-12 Algorithm representing the management strategy for patients with severe aortic stenosis (AS) from the European Society of Cardiology (ESC) Guidelines. *AVR*, aortic valve replacement; *LVEF*, left ventricular ejection fraction; *Med Rx*, medical therapy; *TAVI*, transcatheter aortic valve implantation. *(From Vahanian A, Alfieri O, Andreotti F, Antunes MJ, Barón-Esquivias G, Baumgartner H, et al. Guidelines on the management of valvular heart disease [version 2012]: the Joint Task Force on the Management of Valvular Heart Disease of the European Society of Cardiology (ESC) and the European Association for Cardio-Thoracic Surgery [EACTS]. Eur Heart J 2012;424:S1–44.)*
[a]Severity definition
[b]Risk factors
[c]Heart team decision

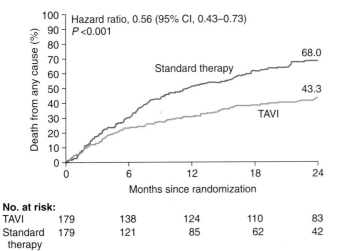

No. at risk:

	0	6	12	18	24
TAVI	179	138	124	110	83
Standard therapy	179	121	85	62	42

FIGURE 11-13 Transcatheter aortic valve replacement in inoperable patients with severe symptomatic aortic stenosis. Kaplan-Meier survival estimates for symptomatic patients with severe aortic stenosis who were not suitable candidates for surgery and who received standard therapy (n = 179) or transcatheter aortic valve implantation (TAVI) (n = 179). *CI*, confidence interval *(From Makkar RR, Fontana GP, Jilaihawi H, Kapadia S, Pichard AD, Douglas PS, et al. Transcatheter aortic-valve replacement for inoperable severe aortic stenosis. N Engl J Med 2012;366:1696–704.)*

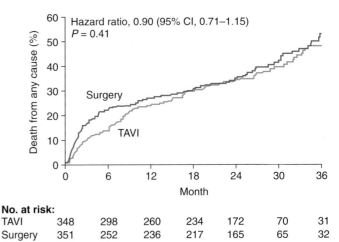

No. at risk:

	0	6	12	18	24	30	36
TAVI	348	298	260	234	172	70	31
Surgery	351	252	236	217	165	65	32

FIGURE 11-14 Transcatheter aortic valve implantation versus surgical aortic valve replacement in high-risk patients. Kaplan-Meier survival estimates for high-risk patients with severe aortic stenosis receiving surgical aortic valve replacement therapy (*Surgery*) (n = 351) or transcatheter aortic valve implantation (TAVI) (n = 348). *CI*, confidence interval. *(From Kodali SK, Williams MR, Smith CR, Svensson LG, Webb JG, Makkar RR, et al. Two-year outcomes after transcatheter or surgical aortic-valve replacement. N Engl J Med 2012;366:1686–95.)*

periprocedural risks, with more frequent vascular complications in the TAVI group (11.0% vs. 3.2%; *P* <0.001) and more frequent major bleeding and new-onset atrial fibrillation in those undergoing surgery.[200] AR is more frequent after TAVI,[200] and long-term outcome data are still missing. Therefore, TAVI must still be restricted to use in patients with high surgical risk. The choice between TAVI and surgical valve replacement in this group remains challenging and should be made by a cardiac team including cardiologists and surgeons.

Despite convincing data on the benefits of aortic valve intervention in the elderly, the rate of referral of elderly patients for aortic valve intervention is low, with studies estimating that only about 33% appropriate candidates are referred for surgical intervention.[201] Inappropriate reasons are often used to justify deferring valve surgery in such patients, such as older age, poor LV function, and response to medical therapy, indicating that improved education of primary care physicians about the benefits of intervention in this age group is needed.[201] Another reason for not referring elderly patients for surgery is frequent comorbidities.

AORTIC VALVE REPLACEMENT AT THE TIME OF CORONARY ARTERY BYPASS SURGERY

Given that many patients with AS also have significant CAD, it is not surprising that in some cases surgical intervention is required for coronary disease prior to the development of severe valvular obstruction. Subsequent progression of stenosis severity then leads to the need for aortic valve surgery at a later date in many of these patients. Unfortunately, the operative mortality for aortic valve replacement in patients with previous cardiac surgery is very high, ranging from 14% to 30%, although long-term outcome is more promising, with an approximate 5-year survival rate of 75%.[202,203]

One study with a long interval (9 years) between the two surgical procedures reported that there was no evidence of AS at the time of the initial procedure.[202] However, in a study with a shorter interval (6 years) between procedures, it was noted that evidence of mild to moderate AS was present at the first procedure in many patients.[204] These observations have generated controversy about the role of aortic valve replacement for mild to moderate AS in patients undergoing coronary bypass procedures. The rationale for not replacing the aortic valve is based on the hypothesis that disease progression is slow and does not occur in all patients, so valve surgery may never be needed or can be deferred to a much later date. The rationale for "prophylactic" replacement of the aortic valve is that disease progression is inevitable so a second surgical intervention will be needed at a predictable point, depending on baseline stenosis severity. Later studies on the natural history of mild to moderate AS support the latter of these two rationales and suggest that "prophylactic" valve replacement be considered when the aortic valve is anatomically abnormal and the antegrade velocity is increased. The rate of hemodynamic progression in specific subgroups appears to be quite predictable, even though there is some variability in the individual rate of progression.[47,141]

Of asymptomatic patients with an anatomically abnormal aortic valve and an aortic jet velocity higher than 4.0 m/s, almost 80% need aortic valve replacement within 2 years, suggesting that valve surgery at the time of coronary artery surgery is appropriate to prevent early reoperation. Of asymptomatic patients with a jet velocity between 3 and 4 m/s, the rate of valve replacement still is high, with about 40% requiring valve surgery by 2 years and nearly 80% needing surgery within 5 years. In this latter group, the decision about "prophylactic" valve replacement should be individualized, depending on the jet velocity within this range, the extent of valve calcification on two-dimensional echocardiography and on fluoroscopy, and other clinical factors, such as age, comorbid disease, and patient preference. When aortic sclerosis is present but the jet velocity is less than 3.0 m/s, it is appropriate to defer valvular intervention because the rate of

symptom development is considerably slower, being only 16% at 2 years.

This approach will be refined as additional data on the natural history of mild-moderate AS become available and also will be modified as improved surgical procedures for AS are developed. The major reasons to postpone valve replacement in a patient already undergoing cardiac surgery include the increased operative risk, the complications and inconvenience of long-term anticoagulation, suboptimal prosthetic valve hemodynamics, and the risk of prosthetic valve dysfunction or infection, so improvements in any of these factors might tip the balance toward earlier intervention. Conversely, the use of minimally invasive surgical approaches might argue against performing valve surgery until it is absolutely necessary, because the coronary and valve procedures are performed from different approaches. In any case, a history of aortic valve disease or a pathologic murmur on auscultation mandates a careful evaluation of valve anatomy and function in the patient undergoing coronary artery surgery. When Doppler echocardiography shows moderate or severe disease, concurrent aortic valve surgery should be considered.

AORTIC STENOSIS WITH LEFT VENTRICULAR DYSFUNCTION

LV systolic dysfunction is a risk factor for operative mortality; valve replacement for AS carries a threefold higher mortality in elderly patients with an EF less than 20% than for those with an EF higher than 60% (15% versus 6%, respectively).[205] However, clinical outcome is even worse without surgical intervention with a 12-month survival of only 20% to 50% in adults with AS and severely reduced LV function.[162] When LV systolic dysfunction is due to increased afterload with normal myocardial contractility, systolic function is expected to improve after relief of outflow obstruction. Even with superimposed myocardial dysfunction, ventricular ejection performance should improve because of the afterload-reducing effect of valve replacement.[206] In a series of 154 patients with severe AS and an EF of 35% or less, operative mortality was only 9%. Even though more than 50% of these patients underwent concurrent coronary artery bypass grafting, most had a better EF and decreased symptoms after surgical intervention.[38]

In patients with severe AS, a low gradient, and LV dysfunction, dobutamine stress echocardiography has been suggested as an approach to distinguish those with contractile reserve from those unlikely to benefit from surgical intervention.[125] Although this approach may be useful in some cases, caution is warranted because there are not sufficient outcome studies addressing whether this approach should be used to deny surgical intervention to any of these patients. In one study, patients with a small aortic valve area and a low transvalvular mean gradient (<30 mm Hg) had poor outcomes, with an operative mortality of 21% and a 3-year survival of only 62%, compared with 68% for patients with AS, LV dysfunction, and a mean gradient of 30 mm Hg or higher.[207] However, those who survived surgery had improved functional status, and EF improved by about 10 EF units. In a nonrandomized comparison of medical and surgical therapy for low-gradient AS, survival was 78% at 4 years in the surgical group compared with 15% in the medical group.[208] A multicenter registry of patients with low-flow, low-gradient AS reported that patients without contractile reserve had a markedly worse outcome than those with contractile reserve. However, survival was better with valve replacement even in the absence of contractile reserve (Figure 11-15).[126] More importantly, survivors showed similar improvement in LV function regardless of the presence of contractile reserve.[131] Thus, although the surgical risk is high, the dismal outcome with medical therapy gives weight to the consideration of surgical intervention for patients with low-flow, low-gradient severe AS even without contractile reserve. In particular, 5-year survival in patients with low-flow, low-gradient AS without contractile reserve was higher in AVR patients undergoing aortic valve replacement than in medically managed patients (54 ± 7%

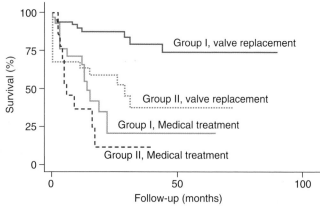

FIGURE 11-15 Outcomes for patients with low-flow low-gradient aortic stenosis. Kaplan-Meier survival estimates for 136 consecutive patients with low-flow low-gradient aortic stenosis. Group I (n = 92) represents patients with contractile reserve determined by low-dose dobutamine echocardiography, Group II represents the group of patients with absence of contractile reserve (n = 44). Survival estimates are represented according to contractile reserve and treatment strategy (aortic valve replacement versus medical treatment). *(From Monin JL, Quere JP, Monchi M, Petit H, Baleynaud S, Chauvel C, et al. Low-gradient aortic stenosis: operative risk stratification and predictors for long-term outcome: a multicenter study using dobutamine stress hemodynamics. Circulation 2003;22;108:319–24.)*

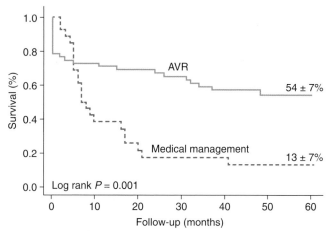

FIGURE 11-16 Effect of aortic valve replacement on outcome in low-flow low-gradient aortic stenosis. Prognostic impact of aortic valve replacement in patients with low-flow, low-gradient aortic stenosis in whom dobutamine stress echocardiography demonstrated absence of contractile reserve (n = 81). Kaplan-Meier survival estimates according to whether aortic valve replacement (AVR) was performed or patients received medical management. *(From Tribouilloy C, Levy F, Rusinaru D, Petit-Eisenmann H, Baleynaud S, Jobic Y, et al. Outcome after aortic valve replacement for low-flow/low-gradient aortic stenosis without contractile reserve on dobutamine stress echocardiography. J Am Coll Cardiol 2009;53:1865–73.)*

vs. 13 ± 7%, respectively; $P = 0.001$) despite an operative mortality of 22% (Figure 11-16).[132]

The controversial issue of paradoxical low-flow, low-gradient AS with preserved EF was already discussed (see Echocardiography). Before severe AS is considered in this subset, other reasons for the findings, such as underestimation of transaortic flow by Doppler echocardiography, inconsistency of grading criteria, and small body size, must be carefully excluded. Because such patients are typically elderly with hypertension and other comorbidities, the evaluation remains difficult even after confirmation of hemodynamic data. LV hypertrophy and fibrosis as well as symptoms or elevation of neurohormones may rather (or partially) be due to hypertensive heart disease and so may not help confirm

a diagnosis of severe AS. Furthermore, it remains unclear how to exclude pseudo–severe AS, and the severity of valve calcification may currently be the only clue in this context.[133] How to identify those patients who definitely have severe AS and who are most likely to benefit from surgery still needs to be better defined.[116]

Operative Mortality and Long-Term Survival

Currently, the operative mortality for aortic valve replacement for AS is low, and long-term outcomes after aortic valve surgery are excellent. Nevertheless an increased operative mortality can be expected in elderly patients and in the presence of comorbidity.[191] The topic is discussed in further detail in Chapter 14.

Changes in Left Ventricular Hypertrophy Geometry and Function

POSTOPERATIVE INTRACAVITARY OBSTRUCTION

In a subset of patients with AS, dynamic midventricular outflow obstruction occurs in the early postoperative period. Intracavitary obstruction is most likely in the presence of a small hypertrophied left ventricle with preserved systolic function. After valve replacement, the acute decrease in LV afterload results in hyperdynamic ventricular function with midcavity obstruction. These patients do not have asymmetric septal hypertrophy, and systolic anterior motion of the mitral valve is only rarely seen. The late-peaking systolic velocity curve may have maximum velocities ranging from 1.8 to 6.8 m/s, corresponding to maximum gradients of 13 to 185 mm Hg.[209-211] The mean gradients corresponding to these maximum velocities are lower than those seen with valvular obstruction, given the late-peaking shape of the velocity curve with low velocities in early and mid systole.

Dynamic outflow obstruction is more likely in the early postoperative period, being recognized in as many as 50% of patients immediately postoperatively and in about 14% of patients when echocardiography is performed within 10 days of surgery, averaging about 25% of patients overall.[209-211] In patients without evidence for obstruction at rest, an intracavitary gradient can be induced in an additional 13% with use of a nitroprusside and/or dobutamine infusion to decrease afterload and increase contractility.[210]

Dynamic intracavitary obstruction should be recognized because patients with such obstruction often have significant hypotension and dyspnea due to an impaired outflow from the small, hyperdynamic left ventricle. Prevention and treatment depend on maintaining an adequate preload and increasing (rather than further decreasing) afterload. Some studies show no differences in 1-year survival rates,[210] whereas other studies suggest that excessive ventricular hypertrophy, specifically in women, is associated with a higher postoperative mortality.[212]

LEFT VENTRICULAR SYSTOLIC FUNCTION

LV ejection performance improves after aortic valve replacement as a result of the favorable effects of valve surgery on afterload. A small increase in EF is observed even in patients with a normal preoperative EF, and dramatic increases in EF may be seen in patients with impaired systolic function at baseline.[213,214]

Of patients in whom preoperative ventricular function was normal, about 90% have preserved systolic function postoperatively.[215] Ventricular ejection performance predictably improves after relief of AS if the cause of impaired ventricular function was increased afterload due to valvular obstruction. Intraoperative transesophageal echocardiographic studies suggest that end-systolic wall stress decreases within 30 minutes of aortic valve replacement.[216] Even when preoperative LV function is severely impaired, with an EF less than 35%, an improvement of LV function can even be expected in the majority of patients.[207] However, the extent of improvement is minimal if irreversible changes in

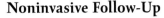

the myocardium are present, for example, in patients with previous myocardial infarction or cardiomyopathy.

Nevertheless, despite pathophysiologic arguments that ventricular function should improve after surgery for AS, it is preferable to operate before the onset of ventricular dysfunction.[139] Although most patients with AS who are followed up prospectively have definite symptoms before there is any evidence of ventricular dysfunction, the onset of LV systolic dysfunction rarely coincides with symptom onset.

REGRESSION OF LEFT VENTRICULAR HYPERTROPHY

LV hypertrophy gradually resolves after surgery for AS.[56,217] However, in most patients, some degree of LV hypertrophy persists indefinitely after aortic valve replacement and might be a marker of irreversible myocardial damage.[218] The pathophysiology of persistent hypertrophy is probably multifactorial, with both permanent structural changes in the myocardium and the persistent, although less severe, outflow obstruction imposed by the prosthetic valve. Myocardial fibrosis has been found to be associated with an unfavorable postoperative outcome and in one study was found to be irreversible in a postoperative follow-up of 9 months.[192]

PERSISTENT POSTOPERATIVE DIASTOLIC DYSFUNCTION

The muscular component of LV hypertrophy resolves more rapidly than the fibrous component, so early on and up to 2 years after valve replacement, the proportion of fibrous tissue in the myocardium increases in comparison with the amount of myocardium. This relative increase in fibrous tissue is associated with an increase in myocardial stiffness early after valve replacement and a decrease in early diastolic relaxation rate, concurrent with a reduction in the degree of LV hypertrophy.[56,219]

The interstitial fibrosis component of ventricular hypertrophy regresses slowly, so the balance between muscular and nonmuscular tissue does not normalize for several years after surgery. The prolonged persistence of diastolic dysfunction after surgery for AS has significant clinical implications in terms of exercise capacity and functional status.[220] As surgical approaches to AS improve in the future, the question whether surgery should be performed earlier in the disease course to prevent diastolic dysfunction will have to be addressed.

Exercise Capacity and Functional Status

After aortic valve replacement, in the absence of coexisting LV dysfunction or uncorrected CAD, nearly all patients have resolution of symptoms of angina, syncope, dizziness, or overt heart failure. Most patients also report an improvement in functional class, with all 6-month survivors assigned to NYHA functional class I or II in a series of patients older than 80 years.[221] Improvement in symptomatic status can also generally be expected to occur in the majority of patients with depressed preoperative LV function.[207,208]

In a prospective study of 34 patients undergoing valve replacement for AS, although LV systolic function improved and LV mass decreased, there was no objective improvement in treadmill exercise performance at 8 and 20 months after surgery, a finding that might be attributable to persistent diastolic dysfunction.[214] Preoperative peak systolic strain rate has been suggested to predict reverse remodeling, with a cutoff value of greater than 2/s predicting favorable symptomatic recovery after aortic valve replacement.[222]

Medical Therapy

In the asymptomatic patient with valvular AS, medical therapy is directed toward prevention of complications, patient education, and prompt recognition of symptom onset. Once symptoms supervene, surgical intervention is needed to improve outcome and relieve symptoms. Pharmacologic therapy alone is appropriate only in those symptomatic patients who are not surgical candidates because of comorbid conditions or who refuse surgical intervention.

Noninvasive Follow-Up

Echocardiographic evaluation is indicated at the time of diagnosis to ensure that valvular stenosis is present, to quantitate disease severity, and to evaluate any coexisting lesions. Many patients with an aortic outflow murmur have either no obstruction or only minimal sclerotic changes of the valve leaflets with only a minor increase in antegrade velocity. Because some of these patients may progress to having AS, routine repeat examinations at extended intervals are recommendable.

Once the initial diagnosis of AS has been confirmed, the frequency of noninvasive follow-up is tailored to disease severity and other clinical factors for the individual patient. Because the timing of surgical intervention is based on symptom onset, it is essential to follow up the patient's functional status. Patient education aimed at recognizing and promptly reporting the typical symptoms of AS is fundamental in severe but also in mild to moderate AS, because rapid progression and symptomatic deterioration are not infrequent. Further risk stratification should consider the extent of aortic valve calcification and hemodynamic progression.

Repeat echocardiographic examination is indicated for any change in clinical status and prior to any major noncardiac surgical procedures or events (such as pregnancy). In the absence of new symptoms, routine evaluation every 6 to 12 months is appropriate for patients with moderate or severe stenosis (aortic jet velocity > 3.0 m/s). With mild AS (jet velocity 2.0 to 3.0 m/s), evaluation every 2 to 3 years is reasonable, in the absence of any change in clinical status or physical examination findings. The objective of the follow-up visit is best summarized as, "Listen to the Patient, Look at the Valve."[223]

Management of Arterial Hypertension

Approximately 40% of patients with AS have concomitant hypertension.[47,148] Patients with AS are a population at high risk for cardiovascular events,[148,166] so hypertension is a risk factor that needs to be adjusted. Additionally, the presence of arterial hypertension results in an increased LV wall stress.

Hypertension must be treated cautiously in patients with AS, and negative inotropic drugs such as beta-blockers should be avoided. There is also a concern that use of vasodilators may lead to a reduction of the coronary perfusion pressure. Classically, the use of angiotensin-converting enzyme (ACE) inhibitors in AS was considered to be contraindicated.[224]

Although it was not designed to assess the safety of ACE inhibitor use in patients with AS, the findings of a retrospective study indicate that a significant number of patients with AS seen in daily clinical practice receive treatment with ACE inhibitors because of concomitant arterial hypertension (102 of 211 patients).[178] The observation, that about 30% of patients with documented AS receive ACE inhibitors, is also shared by O'Brien et al.[225] The initiation of ACE inhibitor therapy was shown to be safe and well tolerated in a group of 13 patients with mild to moderate AS and preserved LV function.[225]

In the Symptomatic Cardiac Obstruction–Pilot Study of Enalapril in Aortic Stenosis (SCOPE-AS), symptomatic patients with severe AS and normal LV function who were not candidates for surgery were randomly allocated to treatment with enalapril or placebo.[226] ACE inhibitors were well tolerated in these patients, although those with reduced LV function were prone to development of hypotension.

Finally, Jimenez-Candil et al[227] designed an elegant drug withdrawal study involving 20 patients with moderate to severe AS already receiving ACE inhibitor therapy.[227] Both the withdrawal and the careful reintroduction of the drug were well tolerated. While taking the ACE inhibitor, patients had a lower blood pressure and higher transvalvular gradients but exercise capacity and symptom status were unchanged.

These data suggest that ACE inhibitor therapy may be used cautiously in patients with AS. It has to be considered that with an increasing severity of the stenosis, reducing the dosage of antihypertensive might be necessary, because hypertension may become less accentuated and even hypotension may develop as a result of further narrowing of the aortic valve.

Management during Periods of Hemodynamic Stress

Asymptomatic patients with severe valvular AS undergoing noncardiac surgery are at risk of decompensation, with development of symptoms and potential hemodynamic instability. These concerns also apply to patients with AS and an intercurrent illness, particularly if accompanied by fever or anemia, and to the increased hemodynamic demands of pregnancy in a woman with AS. Several factors contribute to clinical decompensation in these situations, including changes in blood volume, fluid balance shifts, increased metabolic demands, decreased myocardial oxygen delivery, pain, and greater sympathetic system activity. During pregnancy, hemodynamic changes include increases in cardiac output, heart rate, and blood volume and a decrease in systemic vascular resistance.[228] Additional physiologic changes occur during labor (further increases in cardiac output, heart rate, and blood pressure as well as an increase in systemic vascular resistance) and after the delivery of the placenta (increase in afterload and preload).[228] Whenever possible, AS severity should be evaluated prior to pregnancy or a surgical procedure.

Symptomatic patients with severe AS and asymptomatic patients with impaired LV function or a pathologic exercise test result should be counseled against pregnancy, and valvuloplasty or surgery should be performed prior to pregnancy.[229] Pregnancy in patients with severe AS is associated with significant maternal morbidity and a high necessity of cardiac surgery after pregnancy.[230-232] However, in the asymptomatic patient with severe AS, pregnancy is associated with a relatively low mortality and may be well sustained if she remains asymptomatic.[229] According to the recent European Society of Cardiology guidelines on the management of cardiovascular diseases during pregnancy, pregnancy need not be discouraged in asymptomatic patients, even those with severe AS, when LV size and function as well as the exercise test results are normal, severe LV hypertrophy (<15 mm) has been excluded, and there is no evidence of recent progression of AS.[229]

Two studies describe an acceptable operative risk for noncardiac surgery performed in patients with severe AS in whom valve replacement was refused or judged to be too high a risk.[233,234] In another study, severe AS has been reported to significantly increase the risks for perioperative mortality and nonfatal myocardial infarction.[235] In this study, the risk of perioperative mortality was associated with a high risk score for CAD, suggesting that a screening for CAD is helpful in the assessment of the operative risk. In any case, meticulous planning and monitoring in the perioperative period are required.

Patients with asymptomatic mild or moderate AS can successfully undergo noncardiac surgery or pregnancy, although they need close care.[146,231,232,236]

Echocardiographic evaluation of stenosis severity and LV function is needed. Procedures must be planned (e.g., induction of labor rather than spontaneous labor) to allow invasive hemodynamic monitoring and to enable prevention or alleviation of pain (e g., using an epidural anesthetic for vaginal delivery). Invasive hemodynamic monitoring is required to optimize loading conditions both during the procedure and in the postoperative period. It is especially important to continue postoperative monitoring until fluid shifts have stabilized.

With the use of this approach, adults with AS have undergone noncardiac surgery with an acceptable mortality and morbidity,[236] and women with AS have undergone successful pregnancy with delivery of a normal infant at a low maternal mortality and morbidity.[146,231,232] The development of a second, superimposed hemodynamic stress, such as a febrile illness, during pregnancy in a woman with AS may tip the balance toward hemodynamic instability. In our experience these patients can be managed with monitoring in the intensive care unit, but surgical intervention during pregnancy may be needed in extreme cases.[135,237]

Prevention of Disease Progression

The similarities between AS and atherosclerosis in terms of associated clinical factors, histopathologic changes, and clinical outcomes indicate that calcific AS is an active disease process that may be amenable to medical therapy. It has been hypothesized that therapies directed at associated factors such as hyperlipidemia, inflammation, and calcification might slow or prevent disease progression. Although experimental and several retrospective studies appeared to support the concept that statins might slow AS progression,[174,175,177,178] this concept was not confirmed in randomized controlled trials.[176,180,181] The major difference between the retrospective and prospective studies was that patients who actually had hyperlipidemia were excluded because it was judged to be unethical to deprive them of statin therapy.[238] The currently available data therefore support an aggressive control of hyperlipidemia (using statins as a first-line therapy) in all patients with aortic sclerosis and stenosis. However, no data are available to support lipid-lowering therapies in patients with AS who have normal cholesterol levels. Because patients with AS and even patients with aortic sclerosis are known to have increased cardiovascular morbidity and mortality,[166] statin therapy might ultimately be beneficial. Shah et al[239] demonstrated that patients with known CAD and a sclerotic aortic valve who were not receiving statin therapy had a 2.4-fold higher risk for the occurrence of myocardial infarction than patients with a normal aortic valve. These investigators also showed that this risk might be attenuated by statin therapy.

An association of ACE with low-density lipoprotein was shown in sclerotic and stenotic but not in normal human aortic valves in one study.[240] Furthermore, in a retrospective study, O'Brien et al[241] found an association between the use of ACE inhibitors and a lower rate of aortic valve calcium accumulation, as determined by electron-beam CT scans. However, another retrospective study found no effect of ACE inhibitors on echocardiographically determined hemodynamic progression.[178] A large retrospective study has suggested that ACE and angiotensin-receptor blocker therapy may improve the survival in patients with AS.[242] Although experimental work proposes a positive modulation of the LV response to AS by renin angiotensin system blockade as a possible mechanism, a randomized prospective trial would be required to confirm this hypothesis.

REFERENCES

1. Clark C. Relation between pressure difference across the aortic valve and left ventricular outflow. Cardiovasc Res 1978;12:276–87.
2. Pasipoularides A. Clinical assessment of ventricular ejection dynamics with and without outflow obstruction. J Am Coll Cardiol 1990;15:859–82.
3. Bermejo J, Antoranz JC, Burwash IG, et al. In-vivo analysis of the instantaneous transvalvular pressure difference-flow relationship in aortic valve stenosis: implications of unsteady fluid-dynamics for the clinical assessment of disease severity. J Heart Valve Dis 2002;11:557–66.
4. Otto CM, Pearlman AS, Gardner CL, et al. Experimental validation of Doppler echocardiographic measurement of volume flow through the stenotic aortic valve. Circulation 1988;78:435–41.
5. Hatle L, Angelsen BA, Tromsdal A. Non-invasive assessment of aortic stenosis by Doppler ultrasound. Br Heart J 1980;43:284–92.

6. Currie PJ, Seward JB, Reeder GS, et al. Continuous-wave Doppler echocardiographic assessment of severity of calcific aortic stenosis: a simultaneous Doppler-catheter correlative study in 100 adult patients. Circulation 1985;71:1162–9.
7. Otto CM, Nishimura RA, Davis KB, et al. Doppler echocardiographic findings in adults with severe symptomatic valvular aortic stenosis. Balloon Valvuloplasty Registry Echocardiographers. Am J Cardiol 1991;68:1477–84.
8. Otto CM, Pearlman AS. Doppler echocardiography in adults with symptomatic aortic stenosis. Diagnostic utility and cost-effectiveness. Arch Intern Med 1988;148:2553–60.
9. Laskey WK, Kussmaul WG. Pressure recovery in aortic valve stenosis. Circulation 1994;89:116–21.
10. Levine RA, Jimoh A, Cape EG, et al. Pressure recovery distal to a stenosis: potential cause of gradient "overestimation" by Doppler echocardiography. J Am Coll Cardiol 1989;13:706–15.
11. Niederberger J, Schima H, Maurer G, et al. Importance of pressure recovery for the assessment of aortic stenosis by Doppler ultrasound. Role of aortic size, aortic valve area, and direction of the stenotic jet in vitro. Circulation 1996;94:1934–40.
12. Baumgartner H, Stefenelli T, Niederberger J, et al. "Overestimation" of catheter gradients by Doppler ultrasound in patients with aortic stenosis: a predictable manifestation of pressure recovery. J Am Coll Cardiol 1999;33:1655–61.
13. Otto CM, Pearlman AS, Comess KA, et al. Determination of the stenotic aortic valve area in adults using Doppler echocardiography. J Am Coll Cardiol 1986;7:509–17.
14. Zoghbi WA, Farmer KL, Soto JG, et al. Accurate noninvasive quantification of stenotic aortic valve area by Doppler echocardiography. Circulation 1986;73:452–9.
15. Teirstein P, Yeager M, Yock PG, et al. Doppler echocardiographic measurement of aortic valve area in aortic stenosis: a noninvasive application of the Gorlin formula. J Am Coll Cardiol 1986;8:1059–65.
16. Ohlsson J, Wranne B. Noninvasive assessment of valve area in patients with aortic stenosis. J Am Coll Cardiol 1986;7:501–8.
17. Gorlin R, Gorlin SG. Hydraulic formula for calculation of the area of the stenotic mitral valve, other cardiac valves, and central circulatory shunts. I. Am Heart J 1951;41:1–29.
18. Cannon SR, Richards KL, Crawford MH, et al. Inadequacy of the Gorlin formula for predicting prosthetic valve area. Am J Cardiol 1988;62:113–6.
19. Cannon SR, Richards KL, Crawford M. Hydraulic estimation of stenotic orifice area: a correction of the Gorlin formula. Circulation 1985;71:1170–8.
20. Richards KL, Cannon SR, Miller JF, et al. Calculation of aortic valve area by Doppler echocardiography: a direct application of the continuity equation. Circulation 1986;73:964–9.
21. Segal J, Lerner DJ, Miller DC, et al. When should Doppler-determined valve area be better than the Gorlin formula?: Variation in hydraulic constants in low flow states. J Am Coll Cardiol 1987;9:1294–305.
22. Montarello JK, Perakis AC, Rosenthal E, et al. Normal and stenotic human aortic valve opening: in vitro assessment of orifice area changes with flow. Eur Heart J 1990;11:484–91.
23. Bache RJ, Wang Y, Jorgensen CR. Hemodynamic effects of exercise in isolated valvular aortic stenosis. Circulation 1971;44:1003–13.
24. Otto CM, Pearlman AS, Kraft CD, et al. Physiologic changes with maximal exercise in asymptomatic valvular aortic stenosis assessed by Doppler echocardiography. J Am Coll Cardiol 1992;20:1160–7.
25. Shively BK, Charlton GA, Crawford MH, et al. Flow dependence of valve area in aortic stenosis: relation to valve morphology. J Am Coll Cardiol 1998;31:654–60.
26. Tardif JC, Rodrigues AG, Hardy JF, et al. Simultaneous determination of aortic valve area by the Gorlin formula and by transesophageal echocardiography under different transvalvular flow conditions. Evidence that anatomic aortic valve area does not change with variations in flow in aortic stenosis. J Am Coll Cardiol 1997;29:1296–302.
27. Badano L, Cassottano P, Bertoli D, et al. Changes in effective aortic valve area during ejection in adults with aortic stenosis. Am J Cardiol 1996;78:1023–8.
28. Bermejo J, Garcia-Fernandez MA, Torrecilla EG, et al. Effects of dobutamine on Doppler echocardiographic indexes of aortic stenosis. J Am Coll Cardiol 1996;28:1206–13.
29. Burwash IG, Pearlman AS, Kraft CD, et al. Flow dependence of measures of aortic stenosis severity during exercise. J Am Coll Cardiol 1994;24:1342–50.
30. Burwash IG, Thomas DD, Sadahiro M, et al. Dependence of Gorlin formula and continuity equation valve areas on transvalvular volume flow rate in valvular aortic stenosis. Circulation 1994;89:827–35.
31. Casale PN, Palacios IF, Abascal VM, et al. Effects of dobutamine on Gorlin and continuity equation valve areas and valve resistance in valvular aortic stenosis. Am J Cardiol 1992;70:1175–9.
32. Chambers JB, Sprigings DC, Cochrane T, et al. Continuity equation and Gorlin formula compared with directly observed orifice area in native and prosthetic aortic valves. Br Heart J 1992;67:193–9.
33. Bermejo J, Antoranz JC, Garcia-Fernandez MA, et al. Flow dynamics of stenotic aortic valves assessed by signal processing of Doppler spectrograms. Am J Cardiol 2000;85:611–7.
34. Arsenault M, Masani N, Magni G, et al. Variation of anatomic valve area during ejection in patients with valvular aortic stenosis evaluated by two-dimensional echocardiographic planimetry: comparison with traditional Doppler data. J Am Coll Cardiol 1998;32:1931–7.
35. Lester SJ, McElhinney DB, Miller JP, et al. Rate of change in aortic valve area during a cardiac cycle can predict the rate of hemodynamic progression of aortic stenosis. Circulation 2000;101:1947–52.
36. Carabello BA, Green LH, Grossman W, et al. Hemodynamic determinants of prognosis of aortic valve replacement in critical aortic stenosis and advanced congestive heart failure. Circulation 1980;62:42–8.
37. deFilippi CR, Willett DL, Brickner ME, et al. Usefulness of dobutamine echocardiography in distinguishing severe from nonsevere valvular aortic stenosis in patients with depressed left ventricular function and low transvalvular gradients. Am J Cardiol 1995;75:191–4.
38. Connolly HM, Oh JK, Orszulak TA, et al. Aortic valve replacement for aortic stenosis with severe left ventricular dysfunction. Prognostic indicators. Circulation 1997;95:2395–400.
39. Kadem L, Rieu R, Dumesnil JG, et al. Flow-dependent changes in Doppler-derived aortic valve effective orifice area are real and not due to artifact. J Am Coll Cardiol 2006;47:131–7.
40. Baumgartner H. Hemodynamic assessment of aortic stenosis: are there still lessons to learn? J Am Coll Cardiol 2006;47:138–40.
41. Cannon JD Jr, Zile MR, Crawford FA Jr, et al. Aortic valve resistance as an adjunct to the Gorlin formula in assessing the severity of aortic stenosis in symptomatic patients. J Am Coll Cardiol 1992;20:1517–23.
42. Ford LE, Feldman T, Chiu YC, et al. Hemodynamic resistance as a measure of functional impairment in aortic valvular stenosis. Circ Res 1990;66:1–7.
43. Voelker W, Reul H, Nienhaus G, et al. Comparison of valvular resistance, stroke work loss, and Gorlin valve area for quantification of aortic stenosis. An in vitro study in a pulsatile aortic flow model. Circulation 1995;91:1196–204.
44. Frank A, Chung C. The aortic valve hemodysnamics under degenerative leaflet calcification: a computer modeling approach. Bioengineering Conference 2001;50:655–75.
45. Blais C, Pibarot P, Dumesnil JG, et al. Comparison of valve resistance with effective orifice area regarding flow dependence. Am J Cardiol 2001;88:45–52.
46. Burwash IG, Hay KM, Chan KL. Hemodynamic stability of valve area, valve resistance, and stroke work loss in aortic stenosis: a comparative analysis. J Am Soc Echocardiogr 2002;15:814–22.
47. Otto CM, Burwash IG, Legget ME, et al. Prospective study of asymptomatic valvular aortic stenosis. Clinical, echocardiographic, and exercise predictors of outcome. Circulation 1997;95:2262–70.
48. Sprigings DC, Chambers JB, Cochrane T, et al. Ventricular stroke work loss: validation of a method of quantifying the severity of aortic stenosis and derivation of an orifice formula. J Am Coll Cardiol 1990;16:1608–14.
49. Tobin JR Jr, Rahimtoola SH, Blundell PE, et al. Percentage of left ventricular stroke work loss. A simple hemodynamic concept for estimation of severity in valvular aortic stenosis. Circulation 1967;35:868–79.
50. Laskey WK, Kussmaul WG, Noordergraaf A. Valvular and systemic arterial hemodynamics in aortic valve stenosis. A model-based approach. Circulation 1995;92:1473–8.
51. Carroll JD, Carroll EP, Feldman T, et al. Sex-associated differences in left ventricular function in aortic stenosis of the elderly. Circulation 1992;86:1099–107.
52. Douglas PS, Otto CM, Mickel MC, et al. Gender differences in left ventricle geometry and function in patients undergoing balloon dilatation of the aortic valve for isolated aortic stenosis. NHLBI Balloon Valvuloplasty Registry. Br Heart J 1995;73:548–54.
53. Aurigemma GP, Silver KH, McLaughlin M, et al. Impact of chamber geometry and gender on left ventricular systolic function in patients > 60 years of age with aortic stenosis. Am J Cardiol 1994;74:794–8.
54. Legget ME, Kuusisto J, Healy NL, et al. Gender differences in left ventricular function at rest and with exercise in asymptomatic aortic stenosis. Am Heart J 1996;131:94–100.
55. Jin XY, Pepper JR, Gibson DG. Effects of incoordination on left ventricular force-velocity relation in aortic stenosis. Heart 1996;76:495–501.
56. Villari B, Campbell SE, Schneider J, et al. Sex-dependent differences in left ventricular function and structure in chronic pressure overload. Eur Heart J 1995;16:1410–9.
57. Douglas PS, Berko B, Lesh M, et al. Alterations in diastolic function in response to progressive left ventricular hypertrophy. J Am Coll Cardiol 1989;13:461–7.
58. Villari B, Campbell SE, Hess OM, et al. Influence of collagen network on left ventricular systolic and diastolic function in aortic valve disease. J Am Coll Cardiol 1993;22:1477–84.
59. Villari B, Vassalli G, Schneider J, et al. Age dependency of left ventricular diastolic function in pressure overload hypertrophy. J Am Coll Cardiol 1997;29:181–6.
60. Folland ED, Parisi AF, Carbone C. Is peripheral arterial pressure a satisfactory substitute for ascending aortic pressure when measuring aortic valve gradients? J Am Coll Cardiol 1984;4:1207–12.
61. Faggiano P, Antonini-Canterin F, Ribichini F, et al. Pulmonary artery hypertension in adult patients with symptomatic valvular aortic stenosis. Am J Cardiol 2000;85:204–8.
62. Tracy GP, Proctor MS, Hizny CS. Reversibility of pulmonary artery hypertension in aortic stenosis after aortic valve replacement. Ann Thorac Surg 1990;50:89–93.
63. Aragam JR, Folland ED, Lapsley D, et al. Cause and impact of pulmonary hypertension in isolated aortic stenosis on operative mortality for aortic valve replacement in men. Am J Cardiol 1992;69:1365–7.
64. Snopek G, Pogorzelska H, Zielinski T, et al. Valve replacement for aortic stenosis with severe congestive heart failure and pulmonary hypertension. J Heart Valve Dis 1996;5:268–72.
65. Kaufmann P, Vassalli G, Lupi-Wagner S, et al. Coronary artery dimensions in primary and secondary left ventricular hypertrophy. J Am Coll Cardiol 1996;28:745–50.
66. Marcus ML, Doty DB, Hiratzka LF, et al. Decreased coronary reserve: a mechanism for angina pectoris in patients with aortic stenosis and normal coronary arteries. N Engl J Med 1982;307:1362–6.
67. Nadell R, DePace NL, Ren JF, et al. Myocardial oxygen supply/demand ratio in aortic stenosis: hemodynamic and echocardiographic evaluation of patients with and without angina pectoris. J Am Coll Cardiol 1983;2:258–62.
68. Villari B, Hess OM, Kaufmann P, et al. Effect of aortic valve stenosis (pressure overload) and regurgitation (volume overload) on left ventricular systolic and diastolic function. Am J Cardiol 1992;69:927–34.
69. Rajappan K, Rimoldi OE, Dutka DP, et al. Mechanisms of coronary microcirculatory dysfunction in patients with aortic stenosis and angiographically normal coronary arteries. Circulation 2002;105:470–6.
70. Hildick-Smith DJ, Shapiro LM. Coronary flow reserve improves after aortic valve replacement for aortic stenosis: an adenosine transthoracic echocardiography study. J Am Coll Cardiol 2000;36:1889–96.

71. Julius BK, Spillmann M, Vassalli G, et al. Angina pectoris in patients with aortic stenosis and normal coronary arteries. Mechanisms and pathophysiological concepts. Circulation 1997;95:892–8.
72. Gould KL. Why angina pectoris in aortic stenosis. Circulation 1997;95:790–2.
73. Kenny A, Wisbey CR, Shapiro LM. Profiles of coronary blood flow velocity in patients with aortic stenosis and the effect of valve replacement: a transthoracic echocardiographic study. Br Heart J 1994;71:57–62.
74. Omran H, Fehske W, Rabahieh R, et al. Relation between symptoms and profiles of coronary artery blood flow velocities in patients with aortic valve stenosis: a study using transoesophageal Doppler echocardiography. Heart 1996;75:377–83.
75. Isaaz K, Bruntz JF, Paris D, et al. Abnormal coronary flow velocity pattern in patients with left ventricular hypertrophy, angina pectoris, and normal coronary arteries: a transesophageal Doppler echocardiographic study. Am Heart J 1994;128:500–10.
76. Petropoulakis PN, Kyriakidis MK, Tentolouris CA, et al. Changes in phasic coronary blood flow velocity profile in relation to changes in hemodynamic parameters during stress in patients with aortic valve stenosis. Circulation 1995;92:1437–47.
77. Smucker ML, Tedesco CL, Manning SB, et al. Demonstration of an imbalance between coronary perfusion and excessive load as a mechanism of ischemia during stress in patients with aortic stenosis. Circulation 1988;78:573–82.
78. Anderson FL, Tsagaris TJ, Tikoff G, et al. Hemodynamic effects of exercise in patients with aortic stenosis. Am J Med 1969;46:872–85.
79. Ettinger PO, Frank MJ, Levinson GE. Hemodynamics at rest and during exercise in combined aortic stenosis and insufficiency. Circulation 1972;45:267–76.
80. Movsowitz C, Kussmaul WG, Laskey WK. Left ventricular diastolic response to exercise in valvular aortic stenosis. Am J Cardiol 1996;77:275–80.
81. Lancellotti P, Lebois F, Simon M, et al. Prognostic importance of quantitative exercise Doppler echocardiography in asymptomatic valvular aortic stenosis. Circulation 2005;112:I377–382.
82. Chizner MA, Pearle DL, deLeon AC Jr. The natural history of aortic stenosis in adults. Am Heart J 1980;99:419–24.
83. Frank S, Johnson A, Ross J Jr. Natural history of valvular aortic stenosis. Br Heart J 1973;35:41–6.
84. Rapaport E. Natural history of aortic and mitral valve disease. Am J Cardiol 1975;35:221–7.
85. Ross J Jr, Braunwald E. Aortic stenosis. Circulation. 1968;38:61–7.
86. Selzer A. Changing aspects of the natural history of valvular aortic stenosis. N Engl J Med 1987;317:91–8.
87. Lombard JT, Selzer A. Valvular aortic stenosis. A clinical and hemodynamic profile of patients. Ann Intern Med 1987;106:292–8.
88. Faggiano P, Sabatini T, Rusconi C, et al. Abnormalities of left ventricular filling in valvular aortic stenosis. Usefulness of combined evaluation of pulmonary veins and mitral flow by means of transthoracic Doppler echocardiography. Int J Cardiol 1995;49:77–85.
89. Johnson AM. Aortic stenosis, sudden death, and the left ventricular baroceptors. Br Heart J 1971;33:1–5.
90. Richards AM, Nicholls MG, Ikram H, et al. Syncope in aortic valvular stenosis. Lancet 1984;2:1113–16.
91. Schwartz LS, Goldfischer J, Sprague GJ, et al. Syncope and sudden death in aortic stenosis. Am J Cardiol 1969;23:647–58.
92. Eddleman EE Jr, Frommeyer WB Jr, Lyle DP, et al. Critical analysis of clinical factors in estimating severity of aortic valve disease. Am J Cardiol 1973;31:687–95.
93. Jaffe WM, Roche AH, Coverdale HA, et al. Clinical evaluation versus Doppler echocardiography in the quantitative assessment of valvular heart disease. Circulation 1988;78:267–75.
94. Bonner AJ Jr, Sacks HN, Tavel ME. Assessing the severity of aortic stenosis by phonocardiography and external carotid pulse recordings. Circulation 1973;48:247–52.
95. Munt B, Legget ME, Kraft CD, et al. Physical examination in valvular aortic stenosis: correlation with stenosis severity and prediction of clinical outcome. Am Heart J 1999;137:298–306.
96. Judge TP, Kennedy JW. Estimation of aortic regurgitation by diastolic pulse wave analysis. Circulation 1970;41:659–65.
97. Aronow WS, Kronzon I. Prevalence and severity of valvular aortic stenosis determined by Doppler echocardiography and its association with echocardiographic and electrocardiographic left ventricular hypertrophy and physical signs of aortic stenosis in elderly patients. Am J Cardiol 1991;67:776–7.
98. Aronow WS, Schwartz KS, Koenigsberg M. Correlation of serum lipids, calcium and phosphorus, diabetes mellitus, aortic valve stenosis and history of systemic hypertension with presence or absence of mitral anular calcium in persons older than 62 years in a long-term health care facility. Am J Cardiol 1987;59:381–2.
99. Perloff J. Physical examination of the heart and circulation. Philadelphia: WB Saunders, 1982.
100. Caulfield WH, de Leon AC Jr, Perloff JK, et al. The clinical significance of the fourth heart sound in aortic stenosis. Am J Cardiol 1971;28:179–82.
101. Bonderman D, Gharehbaghi-Schnell E, Wollenek G, et al. Mechanisms underlying aortic dilatation in congenital aortic valve malformation. Circulation 1999;99:2138–43.
102. Szamosi A, Wassberg B. Radiologic detection of aortic stenosis. Acta Radiol Diagn (Stockh) 1983;24:201–7.
103. Braunwald E, Goldblatt A, Aygen MM, et al. Congenital aortic stenosis. I. Clinical and hemodynamic findings in 100 patients. II. Surgical treatment and the results of operation. Circulation 1963;27:426–62.
104. Hugenholtz PG, Lees MM, Nadas AS. The scalar electrocardiogram, vectorcardiogram, and exercise electrocardiogram in the assessment of congenital aortic stenosis. Circulation 1962;26:79–91.
105. Abdin ZH. The electrocardiogram in aortic stenosis. Br Heart J 1958;20:31–40.
106. Fowler RS. Ventricular repolarization in congenital aortic stenosis. Am Heart J 1965;70:603–11.
107. Callahan MJ, Tajik AJ, Su-Fan Q, et al. Validation of instantaneous pressure gradients measured by continuous-wave Doppler in experimentally induced aortic stenosis. Am J Cardiol 1985;56:989–93.
108. Simpson IA, Houston AB, Sheldon CD, et al. Clinical value of Doppler echocardiography in the assessment of adults with aortic stenosis. Br Heart J 1985;53:636–9.
109. Burwash IG, Forbes AD, Sadahiro M, et al. Echocardiographic volume flow and stenosis severity measures with changing flow rate in aortic stenosis. Am J Physiol 1993;265:H1734–1743.
110. Smith MD, Dawson PL, Elion JL, et al. Correlation of continuous wave Doppler velocities with cardiac catheterization gradients: an experimental model of aortic stenosis. J Am Coll Cardiol 1985;6:1306–14.
111. Smith MD, Kwan OL, DeMaria AN. Value and limitations of continuous-wave Doppler echocardiography in estimating severity of valvular stenosis. Jama 1986;255:3145–51.
112. Bonow RO, Carabello BA, Chatterjee K, et al. ACC/AHA 2006 guidelines for the management of patients with valvular heart disease: a report of the American College of Cardiology/American Heart Association Task Force on Practice Guidelines (writing Committee to Revise the 1998 guidelines for the management of patients with valvular heart disease) developed in collaboration with the Society of Cardiovascular Anesthesiologists endorsed by the Society for Cardiovascular Angiography and Interventions and the Society of Thoracic Surgeons. J Am Coll Cardiol 2006;48:e1–148.
113. Vahanian A, Alfieri O, Andreotti F, et al. Guidelines on the management of valvular heart disease (Version 2012): The Joint Task Force on the Management of Valvular Heart Disease of the European Society of Cardiology (ESC) and the European Association for Cardio-Thoracic Surgery (EACTS). Eur Heart J 2012.
114. Hachicha Z, Dumesnil JG, Bogaty P, et al. Paradoxical low-flow, low-gradient severe aortic stenosis despite preserved ejection fraction is associated with higher afterload and reduced survival. Circulation 2007;115:2856–64.
115. Jander N, Minners J, Holme I, et al. Outcome of patients with low-gradient "severe" aortic stenosis and preserved ejection fraction. Circulation 2011;123:887–95.
116. Baumgartner H. Low-flow, low-gradient aortic stenosis with preserved ejection fraction - still a challenging condition. J Am Coll Cardiol 2012;59.
117. Clyne CA, Arrighi JA, Maron BJ, et al. Systemic and left ventricular responses to exercise stress in asymptomatic patients with valvular aortic stenosis. Am J Cardiol 1991;68:1469–76.
118. Alborino D, Hoffmann JL, Fournet PC, et al. Value of exercise testing to evaluate the indication for surgery in asymptomatic patients with valvular aortic stenosis. J Heart Valve Dis 2002;11:204–9.
119. Amato MC, Moffa PJ, Werner KE, et al. Treatment decision in asymptomatic aortic valve stenosis: role of exercise testing. Heart 2001;86:381–6.
120. Das P, Rimington H, Chambers J. Exercise testing to stratify risk in aortic stenosis. Eur Heart J 2005;26:1309–13.
121. Bonow RO, Cheitlin MD, Crawford MH, et al. Task Force 3: valvular heart disease. J Am Coll Cardiol 2005;45:1334–40.
122. Maron BJ, Thompson PD, Puffer JC, et al. Cardiovascular preparticipation screening of competitive athletes. A statement for health professionals from the Sudden Death Committee (clinical cardiology) and Congenital Cardiac Defects Committee (cardiovascular disease in the young), American Heart Association. Circulation 1996;94:850–6.
123. Marechaux S, Hachicha Z, Bellouin A, et al. Usefulness of exercise-stress echocardiography for risk stratification of true asymptomatic patients with aortic valve stenosis. European heart journal 2010;31:1390–7.
124. Lin SS, Roger VL, Pascoe R, et al. Dobutamine stress Doppler hemodynamics in patients with aortic stenosis: feasibility, safety, and surgical correlations. Am Heart J 1998;136:1010–16.
125. Monin JL, Monchi M, Gest V, et al. Aortic stenosis with severe left ventricular dysfunction and low transvalvular pressure gradients: risk stratification by low-dose dobutamine echocardiography. J Am Coll Cardiol 2001;37:2101–7.
126. Monin JL, Quere JP, Monchi M, et al. Low-gradient aortic stenosis: operative risk stratification and predictors for long-term outcome: a multicenter study using dobutamine stress hemodynamics. Circulation 2003;108:319–24.
127. Nishimura RA, Grantham JA, Connolly HM, et al. Low-output, low-gradient aortic stenosis in patients with depressed left ventricular systolic function: the clinical utility of the dobutamine challenge in the catheterization laboratory. Circulation 2002;106:809–13.
128. Otto CM. Clinical practice. Evaluation and management of chronic mitral regurgitation. N Engl J Med 2001;345:740–6.
129. Schwammenthal E, Vered Z, Moshkowitz Y, et al. Dobutamine echocardiography in patients with aortic stenosis and left ventricular dysfunction: predicting outcome as a function of management strategy. Chest 2001;119:1766–77.
130. Takeda S, Rimington H, Chambers J. The relation between transaortic pressure difference and flow during dobutamine stress echocardiography in patients with aortic stenosis. Heart 1999;82:11–4.
131. Quere JP, Monin JL, Levy F, et al. Influence of preoperative left ventricular contractile reserve on postoperative ejection fraction in low-gradient aortic stenosis. Circulation 2006;113:1738–44.
132. Tribouilloy C, Levy F, Rusinaru D, et al. Outcome after aortic valve replacement for low-flow/low-gradient aortic stenosis without contractile reserve on dobutamine stress echocardiography. J Am Coll Cardiol 2009;53:1865–73.
133. Cueff C, Serfaty JM, Cimadevilla C, et al. Measurement of aortic valve calcification using multislice computed tomography: correlation with haemodynamic severity of aortic stenosis and clinical implication for patients with low ejection fraction. Heart 2011;97:721–6.
134. Horstkotte D, Loogen F. The natural history of aortic valve stenosis. Eur Heart J 1988;9(Suppl E):57–64.
135. Lao TT, Adelman AG, Sermer M, et al. Balloon valvuloplasty for congenital aortic stenosis in pregnancy. Br J Obstet Gynaecol 1993;100:1141–2.

136. Beppu S, Suzuki S, Matsuda H, et al. Rapidity of progression of aortic stenosis in patients with congenital bicuspid aortic valves. Am J Cardiol 1993;71:322–7.

137. Pachulski RT, Chan KL. Progression of aortic valve dysfunction in 51 adult patients with congenital bicuspid aortic valve: assessment and follow up by Doppler echocardiography. Br Heart J 1993;69:237–40.

138. Roberts WC, Ko JM. Frequency by decades of unicuspid, bicuspid, and tricuspid aortic valves in adults having isolated aortic valve replacement for aortic stenosis, with or without associated aortic regurgitation. Circulation 2005;111:920–5.

139. Lund O, Nielsen TT, Pilegaard HK, et al. The influence of coronary artery disease and bypass grafting on early and late survival after valve replacement for aortic stenosis. J Thorac Cardiovasc Surg 1990;100:327–37.

140. Kelly TA, Rothbart RM, Cooper CM, et al. Comparison of outcome of asymptomatic to symptomatic patients older than 20 years of age with valvular aortic stenosis. Am J Cardiol 1988;61:123–30.

141. Faggiano P, Ghizzoni G, Sorgato A, et al. Rate of progression of valvular aortic stenosis in adults. Am J Cardiol 1992;70:229–33.

142. Pellikka PA, Nishimura RA, Bailey KR, et al. The natural history of adults with asymptomatic, hemodynamically significant aortic stenosis. J Am Coll Cardiol 1990;15:1012–7.

143. Pellikka PA, Sarano ME, Nishimura RA, et al. Outcome of 622 adults with asymptomatic, hemodynamically significant aortic stenosis during prolonged follow-up. Circulation 2005;111:3290–5.

144. Rosenhek R, Binder T, Porenta G, et al. Predictors of outcome in severe, asymptomatic aortic stenosis. N Engl J Med 2000;343:611–7.

145. Rosenhek R, Zilberszac R, Schemper M, et al. Natural history of very severe aortic stenosis. Circulation 2010;121:151–6.

146. Easterling TR, Chadwick HS, Otto CM, et al. Aortic stenosis in pregnancy. Obstet Gynecol 1988;72:113–8.

147. Keane JF, Driscoll DJ, Gersony WM, et al. Second natural history study of congenital heart defects. Results of treatment of patients with aortic valvar stenosis. Circulation 1993;87:I16-27.

148. Rosenhek R, Klaar U, Schemper M, et al. Mild and moderate aortic stenosis; Natural history and risk stratification by echocardiography. Eur Heart J 2004;25:199–205.

149. Antonini-Canterin F, Faggiano P, Zanuttini D, et al. Is aortic valve resistance more clinically meaningful than valve area in aortic stenosis? Heart 1999;82:9–10.

150. Bahler RC, Desser DR, Finkelhor RS, et al. Factors leading to progression of valvular aortic stenosis. Am J Cardiol 1999;84:1044–8.

151. Vaturi M, Porter A, Adler Y, et al. The natural history of aortic valve disease after mitral valve surgery. J Am Coll Cardiol 1999;33:2003–8.

152. Messika-Zeitoun D, Aubry MC, Detaint D, et al. Evaluation and clinical implications of aortic valve calcification measured by electron-beam computed tomography. Circulation 2004;110:356–62.

153. Monin JL, Lancellotti P, Monchi M, et al. Risk Score for Predicting Outcome in Patients With Asymptomatic Aortic Stenosis. Circulation 2009;120:69–75.

154. Bergler-Klein J, Klaar U, Heger M, et al. Natriuretic peptides predict symptom-free survival and postoperative outcome in severe aortic stenosis. Circulation 2004;109:2302–8.

155. Lancellotti P, Donal E, Magne J, et al. Risk stratification in asymptomatic moderate to severe aortic stenosis: the importance of the valvular, arterial and ventricular interplay. Heart 2010;96:1364–71.

156. Rajani R, Rimington H, Chambers J. B-type natriuretic peptide and tissue doppler for predicting symptoms on treadmill exercise in apparently asymptomatic aortic stenosis. The Journal of heart valve disease 2009;18:565–71.

157. Delgado V, Tops LF, van Bommel RJ, et al. Strain analysis in patients with severe aortic stenosis and preserved left ventricular ejection fraction undergoing surgical valve replacement. European heart journal 2009;30:3037–47.

158. Cioffi G, Faggiano P, Vizzardi E, et al. Prognostic effect of inappropriately high left ventricular mass in asymptomatic severe aortic stenosis. Heart 2011;97:301–7.

159. Stewart RA, Kerr AJ, Whalley GA, et al. Left ventricular systolic and diastolic function assessed by tissue Doppler imaging and outcome in asymptomatic aortic stenosis. European heart journal 2010;31:2216–22.

160. Archer SL, Mike DK, Hetland MB, et al. Usefulness of mean aortic valve gradient and left ventricular diastolic filling pattern for distinguishing symptomatic from asymptomatic patients. Am J Cardiol 1994;73:275–81.

161. Turina J, Hess O, Sepulcri F, et al. Spontaneous course of aortic valve disease. Eur Heart J 1987;8:471–83.

162. Otto CM, Mickel MC, Kennedy JW, et al. Three-year outcome after balloon aortic valvuloplasty. Insights into prognosis of valvular aortic stenosis. Circulation 1994;89:642–50.

163. Leon MB, Smith CR, Mack M, et al. Transcatheter aortic-valve implantation for aortic stenosis in patients who cannot undergo surgery. The New England journal of medicine 2010;363:1597–607.

164. Nessmith MG, Fukuta H, Brucks S, et al. Usefulness of an elevated B-type natriuretic peptide in predicting survival in patients with aortic stenosis treated without surgery. Am J Cardiol 2005;96:1445–8.

165. Herrmann S, Stork S, Niemann M, et al. Low-gradient aortic valve stenosis myocardial fibrosis and its influence on function and outcome. J Am Coll Cardiol 2011;58:402–12.

166. Otto CM, Lind BK, Kitzman DW, et al. Association of aortic-valve sclerosis with cardiovascular mortality and morbidity in the elderly. N Engl J Med 1999;341:142–7.

167. Novaro GM, Katz R, Aviles RJ, et al. Clinical factors, but not C-reactive protein, predict progression of calcific aortic-valve disease: the Cardiovascular Health Study. J Am Coll Cardiol 2007;50:1992–8.

168. Faggiano P, Antonini-Canterin F, Erlicher A, et al. Progression of aortic valve sclerosis to aortic stenosis. Am J Cardiol 2003;91:99–101.

169. Brener SJ, Duffy CI, Thomas JD, et al. Progression of aortic stenosis in 394 patients: relation to changes in myocardial and mitral valve dysfunction. J Am Coll Cardiol 1995;25:305–10.

170. Otto CM, Pearlman AS, Gardner CL. Hemodynamic progression of aortic stenosis in adults assessed by Doppler echocardiography. J Am Coll Cardiol 1989;13:545–50.

171. Palta S, Pai AM, Gill KS, et al. New insights into the progression of aortic stenosis: implications for secondary prevention. Circulation 2000;101:2497–502.

172. Peter M, Hoffmann A, Parker C, et al. Progression of aortic stenosis. Role of age and concomitant coronary artery disease. Chest 1993;103:1715–19.

173. Roger VL, Tajik AJ, Bailey KR, et al. Progression of aortic stenosis in adults: new appraisal using Doppler echocardiography. Am Heart J 1990;119:331–8.

174. Aronow WS, Ahn C, Kronzon I, et al. Association of coronary risk factors and use of statins with progression of mild valvular aortic stenosis in older persons. Am J Cardiol 2001;88:693–5.

175. Bellamy MF, Pellikka PA, Klarich KW, et al. Association of cholesterol levels, hydroxymethylglutaryl coenzyme-A reductase inhibitor treatment, and progression of aortic stenosis in the community. J Am Coll Cardiol 2002;40:1723–30.

176. Cowell SJ, Newby DE, Prescott RJ, et al. A randomized trial of intensive lipid lowering therapy in calcific aortic stenosis. N Engl J Med 2005;352(23):2389–97

177. Novaro GM, Tiong IY, Pearce GL, et al. Effect of hydroxymethylglutaryl coenzyme a reductase inhibitors on the progression of calcific aortic stenosis. Circulation 2001;104:2205–9.

178. Rosenhek R, Rader F, Loho N, et al. Statins but not angiotensin-converting enzyme inhibitors delay progression of aortic stenosis. Circulation 2004;110:1291–5.

179. Moura LM, Ramos SF, Zamorano JL, et al. Rosuvastatin affecting aortic valve endothelium to slow the progression of aortic stenosis. J Am Coll Cardiol 2007;49:554–61.

180. Rossebo AB, Pedersen TR, Boman K, et al. Intensive lipid lowering with simvastatin and ezetimibe in aortic stenosis. N Engl J Med 2008;359:1343–56.

181. Chan KL, Teo K, Dumesnil JG, et al. Effect of Lipid lowering with rosuvastatin on progression of aortic stenosis: results of the aortic stenosis progression observation: measuring effects of rosuvastatin (ASTRONOMER) trial. Circulation 2010;121:306–14.

182. Georgeson S, Meyer KB, Pauker SG. Decision analysis in clinical cardiology: when is coronary angiography required in aortic stenosis? J Am Coll Cardiol 1990;15:751–62.

183. Alcalai R, Viola N, Mosseri M, et al. The value of percutaneous coronary intervention in aortic valve stenosis with coronary artery disease. Am J Med 2007;120:185 e187–113.

184. Iung B, Drissi MF, Michel PL, et al. Prognosis of valve replacement for aortic stenosis with or without coexisting coronary heart disease: a comparative study. J Heart Valve Dis 1993;2:430–9.

185. Carabello BA. Timing of valve replacement in aortic stenosis. Moving closer to perfection. Circulation 1997;95:2241–3.

186. Faggiano P, Aurigemma GP, Rusconi C, et al. Progression of valvular aortic stenosis in adults: literature review and clinical implications. Am Heart J 1996;132:408–17.

187. Kaleschke G, Baumgartner H. Asymptomatic aortic stenosis: when to operate? Curr Cardiol Rep 2011;13:220–5.

188. Rosenhek R, Maurer G, Baumgartner H. Should early elective surgery be performed in patients with severe but asymptomatic aortic stenosis? Eur Heart J 2002;23:1417–21.

189. Kang DH, Park SJ, Rim JH, et al. Early surgery versus conventional treatment in asymptomatic very severe aortic stenosis. Circulation 2010;121:1502–9.

190. Brown ML, Pellikka PA, Schaff HV, et al. The benefits of early valve replacement in asymptomatic patients with severe aortic stenosis. J Thorac Cardiovasc Surg 2008; 135:308–15.

191. Society of Thoracic Surgeons. STS national database: STS US. cardiac surgery database: 1997 Aortic valve replacement patients: preoperative risk variables. Available at: http://www.ctsnet.org/doc/3031. Accessed March 20th 2008.

192. Weidemann F, Herrmann S, Stork S, et al. Impact of myocardial fibrosis in patients with symptomatic severe aortic stenosis. Circulation 2009;120:577–84.

193. Lim P, Monin JL, Monchi M, et al. Predictors of outcome in patients with severe aortic stenosis and normal left ventricular function: role of B-type natriuretic peptide. Eur Heart J 2004;25:2048–53.

194. Antonini-Canterin F, Popescu BA, Popescu AC, et al. Heart failure in patients with aortic stenosis: clinical and prognostic significance of carbohydrate antigen 125 and brain natriuretic peptide measurement. Int J Cardiol 2008;128:406–12.

195. Rosenhek R, Iung B, Tornos P, et al. ESC Working Group on Valvular Heart Disease Position Paper: assessing the risk of interventions in patients with valvular heart disease. Eur Heart J 2012;33:822–8.

196. Osswald BR, Gegouskov V, Badowski-Zyla D, et al. Overestimation of aortic valve replacement risk by EuroSCORE: implications for percutaneous valve replacement. Eur Heart J 2009;30:74–80.

197. Likosky DS, Sorensen MJ, Dacey LJ, et al. Long-term survival of the very elderly undergoing aortic valve surgery. Circulation 2009;120:S127–133.

198. Makkar RR, Fontana GP, Jilaihawi H, et al. Transcatheter aortic-valve replacement for inoperable severe aortic stenosis. N Engl J Med 2012;366:1696–704.

199. Kodali SK, Williams MR, Smith CR, et al. Two-year outcomes after transcatheter or surgical aortic-valve replacement. N Engl J Med 2012;366:1686–95.

200. Smith CR, Leon MB, Mack MJ, et al. Transcatheter versus surgical aortic-valve replacement in high-risk patients. N Engl J Med 2011;364:2187–98.

201. Iung B, Cachier A, Baron G, et al. Decision-making in elderly patients with severe aortic stenosis: why are so many denied surgery? Eur Heart J 2005;26:2714–20.

202. Fighali SF, Avendano A, Elayda MA, et al. Early and late mortality of patients undergoing aortic valve replacement after previous coronary artery bypass graft surgery. Circulation 1995;92:II163–168.

203. Sethi GK, Miller DC, Souchek J, et al. Clinical, hemodynamic, and angiographic predictors of operative mortality in patients undergoing single valve replacement. Veterans Administration Cooperative Study on Valvular Heart Disease. J Thorac Cardiovasc Surg 1987;93:884–97.

204. Collins JJ Jr, Aranki SF. Management of mild aortic stenosis during coronary artery bypass graft surgery. J Card Surg 1994;9:145–7.

205. Fremes SE, Goldman BS, Ivanov J, et al. Valvular surgery in the elderly. Circulation 1989;80:I77–90.

206. Thibault GE. Too old for what? N Engl J Med 1993;328:946–50.

207. Connolly HM, Oh JK, Schaff HV, et al. Severe aortic stenosis with low transvalvular gradient and severe left ventricular dysfunction:result of aortic valve replacement in 52 patients. Circulation 2000;101:1940–6.

208. Pereira JJ, Lauer MS, Bashir M, et al. Survival after aortic valve replacement for severe aortic stenosis with low transvalvular gradients and severe left ventricular dysfunction. J Am Coll Cardiol 2002;39:1356–63.

209. Aurigemma G, Battista S, Orsinelli D, et al. Abnormal left ventricular intracavitary flow acceleration in patients undergoing aortic valve replacement for aortic stenosis. A marker for high postoperative morbidity and mortality. Circulation 1992;86:926–36.

210. Bartunek J, Sys SU, Rodrigues AC, et al. Abnormal systolic intraventricular flow velocities after valve replacement for aortic stenosis. Mechanisms, predictive factors, and prognostic significance. Circulation 1996;93:712–9.

211. Wiseth R, Samstad S, Rossvoll O, et al. Cross-sectional left ventricular outflow tract velocities before and after aortic valve replacement: a comparative study with two-dimensional Doppler ultrasound. J Am Soc Echocardiogr 1993;6:279–85.

212. Orsinelli DA, Aurigemma GP, Battista S, et al. Left ventricular hypertrophy and mortality after aortic valve replacement for aortic stenosis. A high risk subgroup identified by preoperative relative wall thickness. J Am Coll Cardiol 1993;22:1679–83.

213. Harpole DH, Jones RH. Serial assessment of ventricular performance after valve replacement for aortic stenosis. J Thorac Cardiovasc Surg 1990;99:645–50.

214. Munt BI, Legget ME, Healy NL, et al. Effects of aortic valve replacement on exercise duration and functional status in adults with valvular aortic stenosis. Can J Cardiol 1997;13:346–50.

215. Hwang MH, Hammermeister KE, Oprian C, et al. Preoperative identification of patients likely to have left ventricular dysfunction after aortic valve replacement. Participants in the Veterans Administration Cooperative Study on Valvular Heart Disease. Circulation 1989;80:I65–76.

216. Jin XY, Pepper JR, Brecker SJ, et al. Early changes in left ventricular function after aortic valve replacement for isolated aortic stenosis. Am J Cardiol 1994;74:1142–6.

217. Monrad ES, Hess OM, Murakami T, et al. Time course of regression of left ventricular hypertrophy after aortic valve replacement. Circulation 1988;77:1345–55.

218. Lund O, Erlandsen M. Changes in left ventricular function and mass during serial investigations after valve replacement for aortic stenosis. J Heart Valve Dis 2000;9:583–93.

219. Gilchrist IC, Waxman HL, Kurnik PB. Improvement in early diastolic filling dynamics after aortic valve replacement. Am J Cardiol 1990;66:1124–9.

220. Villari B, Vassalli G, Betocchi S, et al. Normalization of left ventricular nonuniformity late after valve replacement for aortic stenosis. Am J Cardiol 1996;78:66–71.

221. Olsson M, Granstrom L, Lindblom D, et al. Aortic valve replacement in octogenarians with aortic stenosis: a case-control study. J Am Coll Cardiol 1992;20:1512–16.

222. Bauer F, Zghal F, Dervaux N, et al. Pre-operative tissue Doppler imaging differentiates beneficial from detrimental left ventricular hypertrophy in patients with surgical aortic stenosis. A postoperative morbidity study. Heart 2008;94(11):1440–5

223. Otto CM. Aortic stenosis—listen to the patient, look at the valve. N Engl J Med 2000;343:652–4.

224. Carabello BA, Stewart WJ, Crawford FA. Aortic valve disease. In: Topol E, editor. Textbook of Cardiovascular Medicine. Philadelphia: Lippincott Williams & Wilkins; 1998. p. 533–55.

225. O'Brien KD, Zhao XQ, Shavelle DM, et al. Hemodynamic effects of the angiotensin-converting enzyme inhibitor, ramipril, in patients with mild to moderate aortic stenosis and preserved left ventricular function. J Investig Med 2004;52:185–91.

226. Chockalingam A, Venkatesan S, Subramaniam T, et al. Safety and efficacy of angiotensin-converting enzyme inhibitors in symptomatic severe aortic stenosis: Symptomatic Cardiac Obstruction-Pilot Study of Enalapril in Aortic Stenosis (SCOPE-AS). Am Heart J 2004;147:E19.

227. Jimenez-Candil J, Bermejo J, Yotti R, et al. Effects of angiotensin converting enzyme inhibitors in hypertensive patients with aortic valve stenosis: a drug withdrawal study. Heart 2005;91:1311–18.

228. Stout KK, Otto CM. Pregnancy in women with valvular heart disease. Heart 2007;93:552–8.

229. Regitz-Zagrosek V, Blomstrom Lundqvist C, Borghi C, et al. ESC Guidelines on the management of cardiovascular diseases during pregnancy: the Task Force on the Management of Cardiovascular Diseases during Pregnancy of the European Society of Cardiology (ESC). Eur Heart J 2011;32:3147–97.

230. Elkayam U, Bitar F. Valvular heart disease and pregnancy part I: native valves. J Am Coll Cardiol 2005;46:223–30.

231. Hameed A, Karaalp IS, Tummala PP, et al. The effect of valvular heart disease on maternal and fetal outcome of pregnancy. J Am Coll Cardiol 2001;37:893–9.

232. Silversides CK, Colman JM, Sermer M, et al. Early and intermediate-term outcomes of pregnancy with congenital aortic stenosis. Am J Cardiol 2003;91:1386–9.

233. Raymer K, Yang H. Patients with aortic stenosis: cardiac complications in non-cardiac surgery. Can J Anaesth 1998;45:855–9.

234. Torsher LC, Shub C, Rettke SR, et al. Risk of patients with severe aortic stenosis undergoing noncardiac surgery. Am J Cardiol 1998;81:448–52.

235. Kertai MD, Bountioukos M, Boersma E, et al. Aortic stenosis: an underestimated risk factor for perioperative complications in patients undergoing noncardiac surgery. Am J Med 2004;116:8–13.

236. O'Keefe JH Jr, Shub C, Rettke SR. Risk of noncardiac surgical procedures in patients with aortic stenosis. Mayo Clin Proc 1989;64:400–5.

237. Ben-Ami M, Battino S, Rosenfeld T, et al. Aortic valve replacement during pregnancy. A case report and review of the literature. Acta Obstet Gynecol Scand 1990;69:651–3.

238. Rosenhek R. Statins for aortic stenosis. N Engl J Med 2005;352:2441–3.

239. Shah SJ, Ristow B, Ali S, et al. Acute myocardial infarction in patients with versus without aortic valve sclerosis and effect of statin therapy (from the Heart and Soul Study). Am J Cardiol 2007;99:1128–33.

240. O'Brien KD, Shavelle DM, Caulfield MT, et al. Association of angiotensin-converting enzyme with low-density lipoprotein in aortic valvular lesions and in human plasma. Circulation 2002;106:2224–30.

241. O'Brien KD, Probstfield JL, Caulfield MT, et al. Angiotensin-converting enzyme inhibitors and change in aortic valve calcium. Arch Intern Med 2005;165:858–62.

242. Nadir MA, Wei L, Elder DH, et al. Impact of renin-angiotensin system blockade therapy on outcome in aortic stenosis. J Am Coll Cardiol 2011;58:570–6.

243. Kennedy KD, Nishimura RA, Holmes DR Jr, et al. Natural history of moderate aortic stenosis. J Am Coll Cardiol 1991;17:313–19.

244. Bonow RO, Carabello BA, Chatterjee K, et al. 2008 focused update incorporated into the ACC/AHA 2006 guidelines for the management of patients with valvular heart disease: a report of the American College of Cardiology/American Heart Association Task Force on Practice Guidelines (Writing Committee to revise the 1998 guidelines for the management of patients with valvular heart disease). Endorsed by the Society of Cardiovascular Anesthesiologists, Society for Cardiovascular Angiography and Interventions, and Society of Thoracic Surgeons. J Am Coll Cardiol 2008;52:e1–142.

CHAPTER 12 Aortic Regurgitation

Pilar Tornos, Arturo Evangelista, and Robert O. Bonow

Key Points

- The majority of causes of aortic regurgitation produce chronic volume overload with slow indolent left ventricular dilation and a prolonged asymptomatic phase.
- Severe acute aortic regurgitation manifests as hypotension and tachycardia, and many of the characteristic clinical findings of volume overload are absent.
- In chronic aortic regurgitation excessive preload and excessive afterload may overcome the ability of the left ventricle to compensate via hypertrophy and recruitment of preload reserve, leading to left ventricular systolic dysfunction. This may occur in the absence of symptoms.
- Left ventricular systolic function (ejection fraction) and end-systolic dimension or volume are the most important predictors of survival and functional recovery after aortic valve replacement.
- Indications for aortic valve replacement include development of (1) symptoms, (2) left ventricular systolic dysfunction, (3) excessive left ventricular dilation, and/or (4) severe dilation of the aortic root or ascending aorta.
- In patients with aortic regurgitation due to enlargement of the ascending aorta or aortic root, the natural history of the disease and thus the timing and choice of surgical intervention are often based on the degree and rate of aortic dilation rather than on the left ventricular response to it.

Etiology

Pure aortic regurgitation (AR) has multiple causes involving abnormalities of the aortic valve leaflets, aortic root, or both (Table 12-1). The most frequent causes are congenital abnormalities of the aortic valve (most notably bicuspid valves [Figure 12-1] but also unicuspid, tricuspid, and quadricuspid valves), rheumatic disease, infective endocarditis, calcific degeneration, and myxomatous degeneration. Other common causes of AR represent diseases of the aorta without direct involvement of the aortic valve, as in ascending aorta dilation secondary to atherosclerosis or systemic hypertension, idiopathic annuloaortic ectasia, aortic dissection, and Marfan syndrome.[1,2] Less common causes of AR include traumatic injuries to the aortic valve, aortitis occurring in ankylosing spondylitis, syphilitic infection, rheumatoid arthritis, osteogenesis imperfecta, giant cell aortitis, Takayasu disease, Ehlers-Danlos syndrome and Reiter syndrome. AR can also occur in cases of discrete subaortic stenosis and ventricular septal defect with prolapse of an aortic cusp, in ruptured aneurysms of the sinuses of Valsalva, and in cases of fenestrated aortic cusps.[3] AR has also been described as a complication of balloon aortic valvuloplasty and transcatheter aortic valve implantation,[4,5] and anorectic drugs and dopamine agonist have also been reported to cause AR.[6,7] However, in many cases of AR the precise etiology is unclear. In a pathologic study of a surgical series of excised aortic valves, up to 34% cases of pure AR were considered of unclear etiology.[2] In the Euro Heart Survey on Valvular Disease,

AR represented 13.3% of patients with single native left-sided disease: 15.2% of cases were considered of congenital origin, and the same percentage was observed for rheumatic origin.[8]

The majority of these lesions produce chronic AR, with slow, insidious left ventricular (LV) dilation and a prolonged asymptomatic phase. Other lesions, in particular infective endocarditis, aortic dissection, and trauma more often produce acute severe AR with sudden elevation of LV filling pressures, pulmonary edema, and reduction in cardiac output.

Acute Aortic Regurgitation

Pathophysiology

In acute severe AR the sudden large regurgitant volume is imposed on a left ventricle of normal size that has not had time to adjust to the volume overload. Thus, the acute increase in diastolic flow into the nondilated left ventricle leads to a marked elevation in end-diastolic pressure owing to a rightward shift along the normal LV diastolic pressure-volume curve. In severe cases, the increased ventricular pressures during the diastolic filling period in conjunction with the decrease in the aortic diastolic pressure leads to a rapid equalization of aortic and LV pressures at end-diastole[9] (Figure 12-2).

With acute regurgitation, forward cardiac output is decreased because the total stroke volume of the nondilated ventricle now includes both regurgitant and forward stroke volumes. Compensatory tachycardia may partially correct this decline in forward stroke volume, but it is often insufficient to maintain cardiac output, and hence patients may be in cardiogenic shock. Pulmonary edema results from the markedly elevated LV end-diastolic pressure and concomitant elevation of pulmonary venous pressure. In addition, coronary flow reserve is acutely diminished, possibly leading to subendocardial ischemia. As the LV end-diastolic pressure approaches the diastolic aortic and coronary artery pressures, myocardial perfusion pressure in the subendocardium is diminished, whereas myocardial oxygen demand is increased by the effects of greater afterload and tachycardia.[10]

Diagnosis

Many of the characteristic physical findings in chronic volume overload are modified or absent when valvular regurgitation is acute. Therefore, the severity of AR can be underestimated. Because of the acute hemodynamic deterioration, patients with acute AR are often tachycardic and tachypneic and have pulmonary edema. However, LV size may be normal on physical examination, and chest radiography may not demonstrate cardiomegaly. In addition, pulse pressure may not be increased because systolic pressure is reduced in relation to the decrease in forward stroke volume and because diastolic pressure equilibrates with the elevated LV diastolic pressure. In the absence of a widened pulse pressure, the characteristic peripheral signs of AR are absent. Although a diastolic murmur is usually present, it can be soft and short because the rapidly rising LV diastolic pressure reduces the aortic-ventricular pressure gradient. The murmur is thus often poorly heard.[11]

Echocardiography is indispensable in confirming the presence and severity of AR, assessing its cause, and determining whether there is a rapid equilibration of aortic and LV diastolic pressure. Evidence for rapid pressure equilibration includes a short AR diastolic half-time (<300 ms) (see Figure 12-2), a short mitral deceleration time (<150 ms), and premature closure of the mitral valve (Figure 12-3).

Transesophageal echocardiography is indicated when aortic dissection (Figure 12-4), acute endocarditis (Figure 12-5), or trauma is suspected or when the mechanism of acute AR is uncertain. Computed tomography (CT) or cardiac magnetic resonance imaging (CMR) can be used in some settings if it will lead to a more rapid diagnosis than can be achieved by transesophageal echocardiography.[12-14]

Management

Death due to pulmonary edema, ventricular arrhythmias, electromechanical dissociation, or circulatory collapse is common in acute, severe AR. Thus, patients require emergency or urgent surgery for correction of the underlying disease process and relief of the acute volume overload. Intraaortic balloon counterpulsation is contraindicated. In patients with acute AR due to an ascending aortic dissection, prompt surgical intervention is needed, including a composite replacement of the aorta along with aortic valve or a valve-sparing reimplantation technique.[15-17] Patients with severe acute AR due to infective endocarditis need immediate initiation of antibiotics and aggressive medical treatment. If the hemodynamic situation does not immediately improve, emergency valve replacement may be life saving. If the clinical situation stabilizes, surgery can be postponed for a few days with the patient under strict medical supervision in order to allow antibiotic treatment to become effective before surgical correction.[18-20]

Chronic Aortic Regurgitation

Pathophysiology

The left ventricle responds to the volume load of chronic AR with a series of compensatory mechanisms, including an increase in

TABLE 12-1	Causes of Aortic Regurgitation
Leaflet abnormalities	Rheumatic disease
	Aortic valve sclerosis and calcification
	Congenital abnormalities (bicuspid, unicuspid, and quadricuspid valves, and AR associated with discrete subaortic stenosis and ventricular septal defect)
	Infective endocarditis
	Myxomatous valve disease
	Complicating balloon valvuloplasty and transcatheter aortic valve implantation
	Rare causes (drugs, leaflet fenestration, irradiation, nonbacterial endocarditis, trauma)
Aortic root abnormalities	Chronic hypertension
	Marfan syndrome
	Annuloaortic ectasia
	Aortic dissection
	Ehlers-Danlos syndrome
	Osteogenesis imperfecta
	Atherosclerotic aneurysm
	Syphilitic aortitis
	Other systemic inflammatory disorders (giant cell aortitis, Takayasu disease, Reiter syndrome)
Combined valve and aortic root abnormalities	Bicuspid aortic valve
	Ankylosing spondylitis

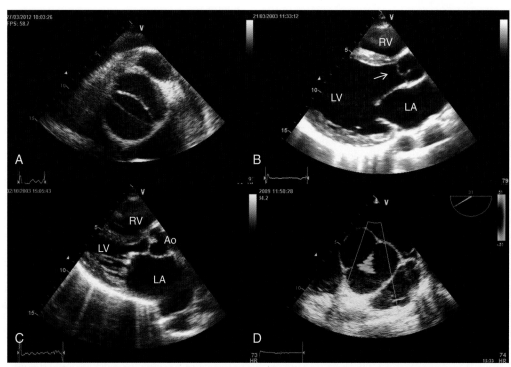

FIGURE 12-1   Role of echocardiography in the diagnosis of aortic regurgitation etiology. A, Transthoracic parasternal short-axis view showing a bicuspid aortic valve. **B,** Myxomatous aortic valve with a prolapse of the right coronary cusp (*arrow*). **C,** Rheumatic valvular disease with mitral and aortic involvement. **D,** Transesophageal echocardiography showing a central regurgitant orifice secondary to an annuloaortic ectasia defined by color Doppler (*green triangular area*) during diastole. *Ao,* aorta; *LA,* left atrium; *LV,* left ventricle; *RV,* right ventricle.

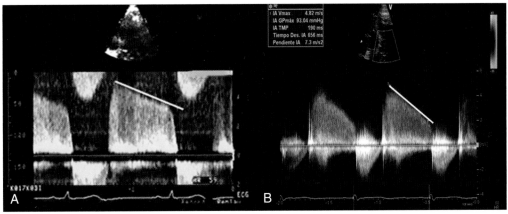

FIGURE 12-2 Continuous-wave Doppler curves. A, Chronic severe aortic regurgitation. **B,** Acute severe aortic regurgitation. Note the steeper deceleration slope in the acute case, which is due to the equalization of left ventricular and aortic diastolic pressures.

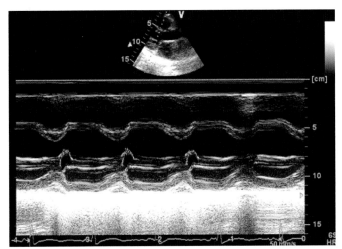

FIGURE 12-3 Transthoracic parasternal long-axis view echocardiogram in a patient with acute aortic regurgitation due to infective endocarditis. The M-mode images show early closure of the mitral valve.

end-diastolic volume, an increase in chamber compliance that accommodates the increased volume without a rise in filling pressures, and a combination of eccentric and concentric hypertrophy. The central hemodynamic feature of chronic AR is combined volume and pressure overload of the left ventricle.[21-23] Because total LV stroke volume equals forward plus regurgitant stroke volumes, normal cardiac output is maintained by an increase in

total stroke volume corresponding to the severity of regurgitation. This increase in total stroke volume is achieved by progressive ventricular dilation, with increased end-diastolic and end-systolic volumes. The greater diastolic volume permits the ventricle to eject a large total stroke volume, thus keeping forward stroke volume in the normal range. This is accomplished through rearrangement of myocardial fibers with the addition of new sarcomeres and development of eccentric LV hypertrophy.[24] As a result, preload at the sarcomere level remains normal or near normal and the ventricle retains its preload reserve. The enhanced total stroke volume is achieved through normal performance of each contractile unit along the enlarged circumference.[25] Thus LV ejection performance is normal, and ejection phase indices such as ejection fraction (EF) and fractional shortening remain in the normal range. However, the enlarged chamber size and the associated increase in systolic wall stress also result in a stimulus for further hypertrophy.[26]

Despite an increase in end-systolic dimension and pressure early in the course of the disease, end-systolic wall stress is maintained in the normal range by a compensatory increase in wall thickness. Thus, patients with compensated chronic AR have substantial increases in LV mass as well as LV volumes, and EF and end-systolic elastance tend to be normal. As the disease progresses, recruitment of preload reserve and compensatory hypertrophy permit the left ventricle to maintain normal ejection performance despite the elevated afterload.[22,27,28] The majority of patients remain asymptomatic during this compensated phase, which may last for decades. During this compensated phase, ejection phase indices of LV systolic function at rest are normal. It is recognized, however, that other indices of LV

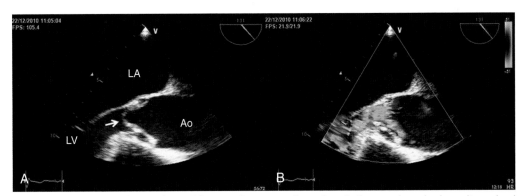

FIGURE 12-4 Acute aortic regurgitation in a patient with ascending aorta dissection. A, Transesophageal echocardiography shows an intimal flap prolapsing through the aortic valve (*arrow*). **B,** Severe aortic regurgitation is observed by color Doppler (*green area* corresponds to regurgitant jet). *Ao,* aorta; *LA,* left atrium; *LV,* left ventricle.

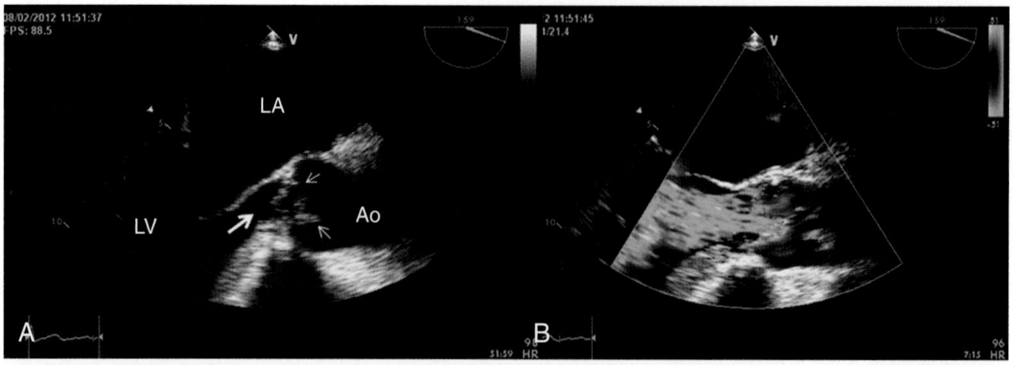

FIGURE 12-5 **Transesophageal echocardiography in a patient with infective endocarditis. A,** Eversion of the left coronary cusp (*large arrow*) and vegetations in the left and right coronary sigmoids (*small arrows*). **B,** Jet of severe aortic regurgitation defined by color Doppler (*green area*). *Ao,* aorta; *LA,* left atrium; *LV,* left ventricle.

function may not be normal. It is further recognized that the transition to LV dysfunction represents a continuum and that no single hemodynamic measurement represents the absolute boundary between normal LV systolic function and LV systolic dysfunction.

In a large subset of patients, the balance among afterload excess, preload reserve, and hypertrophy cannot be maintained indefinitely. Preload reserve may be exhausted and/or the hypertrophic response may be inadequate,[29] so that further increases in afterload result in a reduction in EF, first into the low-normal range and then below normal. Impaired contractility may also contribute to this process. Dyspnea often develops at this point in the natural history. In addition, diminished coronary blood flow reserve in the hypertrophied myocardium may result in exertional angina.[30] However, this transition may be more insidious, and it is possible for patients to remain asymptomatic even after severe LV dysfunction has developed.

LV systolic dysfunction (defined as an EF below normal at rest) is initially a reversible phenomenon related predominantly to afterload excess, and full recovery of LV size and function is possible with aortic valve replacement (AVR).[31-42] With time, during which the left ventricle develops progressive chamber enlargement and a more spherical geometry, depressed myocardial contractility predominates over excessive loading as the cause of progressive dysfunction. This process can progress to the extent that the full benefit of surgical correction of the regurgitant lesion, in terms of recovery of LV function and improved survival, can no longer be achieved. A number of studies have identified LV systolic function and end-systolic size as the most important determinants of survival and postoperative recovery of LV function in patients undergoing valve replacement for chronic AR.[43-64] Studies of predictors of surgical outcome are listed in Table 12-2.

Among patients undergoing valve replacement for chronic AR with preoperative LV systolic dysfunction, several factors are associated with worse functional and survival results after the operation. They are listed in Table 12-3.

Clinical Presentation

CLINICAL HISTORY

Many patients with AR are diagnosed before symptom onset, on the basis of the finding of a diastolic murmur on physical examination, the discovery of an enlarged cardiac silhouette on chest radiography, or evidence of LV hypertrophy on electrocardiography. The most common initial symptom in patients with chronic severe AR is exertional dyspnea, most likely due to an elevated LV end-diastolic pressure with exercise.[65] Because chronic AR has a slowly progressive course, the gradual decrease in exercise capacity may not be recognized as abnormal by the patient, and therefore very careful questioning is often needed to elicit evidence of a subtle decrease in functional status. In cases in which

symptoms are doubtful or equivocal, exercise testing may be valuable in assessing functional capacity. In more advanced cases, with severe LV dysfunction, patients can have symptoms of overt heart failure, including dyspnea at rest, orthopnea, and pulmonary edema. The acute onset of heart failure symptoms can occur in patients with chronic disease as a result of an acute increase in the severity of regurgitation, for example, in patients with infective endocarditis or aortic dissection.

In some patients, an uncomfortable awareness of the heartbeat, or palpitations, related to the increased pulse pressure, is the earliest complaint that leads to the diagnosis of AR.

Angina may occur, even in the absence of atherosclerotic coronary artery disease, because of a decreased myocardial perfusion pressure, increased myocardial oxygen demand, and a decreased ratio of coronary artery size to myocardial mass. Syncope or sudden death, although rare, can occur in AR. Sudden death has been reported in association with extreme degrees of LV dilation.[66]

PHYSICAL EXAMINATION

In patients with mild or moderate AR, the only finding on physical examination may be the diastolic murmur, but in many patients there is also a systolic outflow murmur related to the increased stroke volume, and often the systolic murmur is more apparent than the diastolic murmur. Most cases of severe AR are detectable through physical examination with the combination of cardiac murmur, widened pulse pressure on blood pressure measurement, and peripheral findings related to this widened pulse pressure (Table 12-4). Classically in severe AR systolic arterial pressure is elevated and diastolic pressure is abnormally low, but the blood pressure may remain normal in many patients with severe AR.[67] The apical impulse is diffuse and hyperdynamic and is displaced laterally and inferiorly because of the LV dilation. The carotid pulse is bounding with a more rapid rate of pressure rise in early systole as well as an increase in the amplitude of the systolic pressure curve. A bisferiens carotid pulse may be present.[68] In very severe cases, the head may bob forward with each heart beat (De Musset sign). The classic peripheral signs of AR are present only in cases of severe and chronic regurgitation and reflect the increased pulse pressure. They include the water-hammer or collapsing pulse (Corrigan pulse),[69] systolic pulsation of the fingernail bed on gentle pressure (Quincke pulse),[70] and a systolic and diastolic bruit over the femoral arteries on gentle compression by the stethoscope (Duroziez sign), a manifestation of the reversal of flow in the descending aorta.

A short midsystolic murmur related to the increased ejection rate and stroke volume may be audible at the base of the heart and transmitted to the carotid vessels. The aortic regurgitant murmur is one of high frequency that begins immediately after S2, continues to S1, and has a decrescendo intensity. With valve leaflet abnormalities, the murmur is best heard along the left

TABLE 12-2 Preoperative Predictors of Surgical Outcome in Aortic Regurgitation

STUDY (AUTHOR[S], YEAR)	STUDY DESIGN	NUMBER OF PATIENTS	OUTCOME ASSESSED	FINDINGS
Cunha et al, 1980[46]	Retrospective	86	Survival	High-risk group identified by preoperative echocardiographic LV FS <0.30 Mortality also significantly associated with preoperative ESD Among patients with FS <0.30, mortality higher in NYHA FC III-IV than in FC I-II
Forman et al, 1980[47]	Retrospective	90	Survival	High-risk group identified by preoperative angiographic LV EF <0.50
Henry et al, 1980[53]	Prospective	50	Survival	High-risk group identified by preoperative echocardiographic LV FS <0.25 and/or ESD >55 mm
Greves et al, 1981[48]	Retrospective	45	Survival	High-risk group identified by preoperative angiographic LV EF <0.45 and/or CI <2.5 L/mm Among patients with EF <0.45, mortality higher in NYHA FC III-IV than in FC I-II
Kumpuris et al, 1982[54]	Prospective	43	Survival, heart failure, LV function	Persistent LV dilation after AVR predicted by preoperative echocardiographic LV ESD, RTR mean, and end-systolic wall stress All deaths occurred in patients with persistent LV dilation
Fioretti et al, 1983[55]	Retrospective	47	LV function	Persistent LV dysfunction predicted by preoperative EDD ≥75 mm and/or ESD ≥55 mm
Gaasch et al, 1983[49]	Prospective	32	Symptoms, LV function	Persistent LV dilation after AVR predicted by echocardiographic LV ESD >2.6 cm/m² and RTR >3.8. Trend toward worse survival in patients with persistent LV dilation
Stone et al, 1984[56]	Prospective	113	LV function	Normal LV function after AVR predicted by preoperative LV FS g >0.26, ESD <55 mm, and EDD <80 mm No preoperative variable predicted postoperative LV function
Bonow et al, 1985, 1988[41,50]	Prospective	80	Survival, LV function	Postoperative survival and LV function predicted by preoperative LV EF, FS, ESD High-risk group identified by subnormal EF at rest Among patients with subnormal EF, poor exercise tolerance and prolonged duration of LV dysfunction identified the highest-risk group
Daniel et al, 1985[57]	Retrospective	84	Survival, symptoms, LV function	Outcome after AVR predicted by preoperative LV FS and ESD Survival at 2.5 years was 90.5% with FS >0.25 and ESD ≤55 mm but only 70% with ESD >55 mm and FS ≤25%
Cormier et al, 1986[58]	Prospective	73	Survival	High-risk group identified by preoperative LV EF <0.40 and ESD ≥55 mm
Sheiban et al, 1986[59]	Retrospective	84	Survival	High-risk group identified by preoperative LV EF <0.50 and ESD >55 mm
Carabello et al, 1987[39]	Retrospective	14	LV function	Postoperative LV EF predicted by preoperative ESD, FS, EDD, and RTR
Taniguchi et al, 1987[40]	Retrospective	62	Survival	High-risk group identified by preoperative ESV >200 mL/m² and/or EF <0.40
Michel et al, 1995[52]	Retrospective	286	LV function	Postoperative LV dysfunction predicted by preoperative LV EF, FS, ESD, and EDD
Klodas et al, 1996,[60] 1997[61]	Retrospective	289	Survival	High-risk group identified by symptom severity and preoperative EF <0.50
Turina et al, 1998[62]	Retrospective	192	Survival	High-risk group identified by symptom severity, low EF, and elevated end-diastolic volume
Tornos et al, 2006[63]	Prospective	170	Survival	High risk identified by symptom severity, low EF, and elevated EDD and ESD

AVR, aortic valve replacement; *CI,* cardiac index; *EDD,* end-diastolic dimension; *EF,* ejection fraction; *ESD,* end-systolic dimension; *ESV,* end-systolic volume; *FS,* fractional shortening; *LV,* left ventricular; *NYHA FC,* New York Heart Association functional class; *R/TR,* radius/thickness ratio.
Modified from Bonow R, Carabello BA, Chatterjee K, et al. ACC/AHA 2006 guidelines for the management of patients with valvular heart disease: a report of the American College of Cardiology/American Heart Association Task Force on Practice Guidelines. Circulation 2006;114:e84–231.

TABLE 12-3 Factors Predictive of Reduced Postoperative Survival and Recovery of Left Ventricular (LV) Function in Patients with Aortic Regurgitation and Preoperative LV Systolic Dysfunction

Severity of preoperative symptoms or reduced exercise tolerance

Severity of depression of LV ejection fraction

Duration of preoperative LV systolic dysfunction

From Bonow R, Carabello BA, Chatterjee K, et al. ACC/AHA 2006 guidelines for the management of patients with valvular heart disease: a report of the American College of Cardiology/American Heart Association Task Force on Practice Guidelines. Circulation 2006;114:e84–231.

sternal border in the third or fourth intercostal space, whereas with aortic root disease, a selective radiation along the right sternal border is common.[71] However, the diastolic murmur is often not appreciated on physical examination. In comparison with Doppler echocardiography and aortic angiography, the sensitivity of auscultation for detection of AR is 37% to 73%, and the specificity is 85% to 92%.[72-74] The loudness of the murmur correlates with disease severity to some extent.[75] Another classic finding in patients with severe chronic AR is the Austin Flint murmur, a low-pitched middiastolic rumble that mimics the murmur of mitral stenosis.[76] Comparisons of Doppler echocardiographic findings with physical findings suggest that this diastolic murmur is related to the severity of AR, with a jet directed toward

TABLE 12-4   Chronic Compensated, Chronic Decompensated, and Acute Aortic Regurgitation

CHARACTERISTICS	CHRONIC COMPENSATED	CHRONIC DECOMPENSATED	ACUTE
Etiology	Valvular or aortic root abnormalities	Valvular or aortic root abnormalities	Dissection, endocarditis, trauma
Physiology			
LV volume	Increased (ESD <55 mm)	Increased (ESD >55 mm)	Normal
Ejection fraction	Normal (>55%)	Normal or decreased	Normal or decreased
LV EDP	Normal	Normal or increased	Increased
Physical examination			
Diastolic murmur	High-pitched, decrescendo, holodiastolic	High-pitched, decrescendo, holodiastolic	Low-pitched, harsh, early diastolic
Pulse pressure	Wide	Wide	Normal
LV impulse	Enlarged	Enlarged	Normal
Peripheral signs of AR	Present	Present	Absent
Clinical presentation	Asymptomatic	Gradual onset of symptoms, typically exertional	Sudden onset, pulmonary edema, and hypotension

AR, aortic regurgitation; *EDP,* end-diastolic pressure; *ESD,* end-systolic dimension; *LV,* left ventricular.
From Otto CM, Aortic regurgitation. In: Otto CM, editor. Valvular heart disease. 2nd ed. Philadelphia: Saunders, 2004.

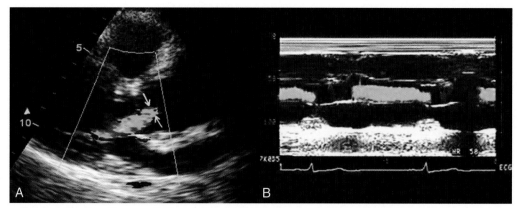

FIGURE 12-6   Assessing severity of aortic regurgitation. A, Parasternal long-axis view Doppler echocardiogram showing the vena contracta of the regurgitant flow in a patient with severe aortic regurgitation. **B,** Color M-mode echocardiogram in the same patient, showing the width of the regurgitant jet.

the anterior mitral leaflet or LV free wall causing vibrations appreciated on auscultation as a low-pitched diastolic rumble.[77-79]

The physical findings in acute AR differ from those in chronic regurgitation, in parallel with the different hemodynamics of acute and chronic disease (see Table 12-4).

ELECTROCARDIOGRAM AND CHEST RADIOGRAPHY

The electrocardiogram (ECG) findings in patients with AR include voltage criteria for LV hypertrophy and associated repolarization abnormalities. A strain pattern on the resting ECG correlates strongly with abnormal LV dimensions, mass, and wall stress.[80-82] However, some cases of severe AR and pathologic LV hypertrophy do not meet ECG criteria for LV hypertrophy.[83] When the ECG is normal at rest, flat and/or downsloping ST depression may develop with exercise, even in the absence of coronary artery disease, and is associated with an increased LV systolic dimension.[84] Ventricular ectopic beats and nonsustained ventricular arrhythmias are also relatively common in AR, and have a significant correlation with LV hypertrophy and function.[85]

The chest radiograph shows an enlarged silhouette due to LV dilation. Aortic root enlargement is also frequently present as a result of primary diseases of the aorta or of dilation secondary to the increased flow. Both evidence of LV hypertrophy on ECG and cardiac size on radiography have been shown to be predictors of outcome after valve replacement.[86-90] However, neither the ECG nor the chest radiograph offers sufficiently precise data to be useful in clinical decision making or sequential follow-up of patients with AR.

ECHOCARDIOGRAPHY

After the history and physical examination, echocardiography is the most important examination in patients with AR. Echocardiography is used to diagnose and estimate the severity of regurgitation using color Doppler flow imaging (vena contracta of regurgitant jet) (Figure 12-6) and pulsed-wave tissue Doppler imaging (holodiastolic flow reversal in the descending thoracic and abdominal aorta)[91,92] (Figure 12-7). These indices are influenced by loading conditions and the compliance of the ascending aorta and the left ventricle. Quantitative Doppler echocardiography, using the continuity equation or analysis of proximal isovelocity surface area, is less sensitive to loading conditions[93] and provides measures of regurgitant volume, regurgitant fraction, and effective regurgitant orifice. The criteria for defining severe AR are shown in Table 12-5.

Echocardiography is also performed to identify the mechanisms of regurgitation, describe the valve anatomy, and determine the feasibility of valve repair. An important role of echocardiography is to provide precise and reproducible measures of LV dimensions, volumes, and systolic performance, and therefore it is the cornerstone for clinical decision making and serial follow-up in patients with chronic AR (Figure 12-8). Indexing for body surface area (BSA) is especially recommended in women and in men of small body size.[61,94] Although LV EF is the fundamental parameter for evaluating LV contractility, new parameters obtained by tissue Doppler imaging and strain rate imaging may be useful in patients with borderline EF measurements. Two studies have shown peak systolic wave velocity less than 9 cm/s at the mitral annulus to be a predictor of complications and to be related to LV contractile reserve.[95,96] Serial echocardiographic evaluations of LV size and function should take into account the potential of confounding factors, such as interval changes in instrumentation, variability in recording and measuring the data, variability in loading condition, and physiologic variability. When a change is detected, it is prudent to repeat the examination to confirm the magnitude and direction of the change. Good-quality echocardiograms and data confirmation are essential before surgery can be recommended to asymptomatic patients. Echocardiography should also image the aorta at four different levels: annulus, sinuses of Valsalva, sinotubular junction, and ascending aorta (Figure 12-9). Transesophageal echocardiography may be performed to better define the anatomy of the valve and ascending aorta, especially when aortic pathology is suspected or a valve-sparing intervention is considered.[97] Studies have also demonstrated the feasibility and accuracy of three-dimensional transthoracic echocardiography (3D TTE) in quantifying AR.[98]

OTHER IMAGING MODALITIES

CARDIAC MAGNETIC RESONANCE. In patients with indeterminant echocardiographic findings, CMR is a reliable tool for assessment of the severity of AR.[98a,99] Magnetic resonance *phase-contrast sequences* perpendicular to the aortic valve allow accurate antegrade and retrograde blood flow measurements in the ascending aorta,[100] so that the severity of AR by calculation of regurgitant volume, peak velocity, and regurgitant fraction can be assessed.[101,102] Additionally, cine CMR sequences, such as steady-state free precession techniques, permit visualization of the aortic valve in a chosen plane with excellent image quality. Cine CMR also aids in determination of the morphology of the valve, and valve area can be measured by planimetry methods[101-106] (Figure 12-10). Moreover, with the use of serial short axis slices of the left ventricle, it is possible to calculate LV volumes, mass, and EF very accurately. Several studies have shown that CMR is an excellent technique to monitor LV volumes and EF with a high degree of interobserver reproducibility ($r = 0.96$-0.99).[107] Finally,

TABLE 12-5	Criteria for the Definition of Severe Aortic Regurgitation
Specific signs	Central jet, width ≥ 65% of left ventricular outflow tract Vena contracta > 0.6 cm
Supportive signs	Pressure half-time < 200 ms Holodiastolic aortic flow reversal in descending aorta Moderate or greater LV enlargement
Quantitative parameters	Regurgitant volume ≥ 60 mL/beat Regurgitant fraction ≥ 50% Effective regurgitant orifice area ≥ 0.30 cm²

Modified from Zoghbi WA, Enriquez-Sarano M, Foster E et al. Recommendations for evaluation of the severity of native valvular regurgitation with two-dimensional and Doppler echocardiography. J Am Soc Echocardiogr 2003;16:777–8.

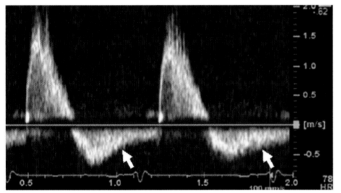

FIGURE 12-7   Assessing severity of aortic regurgitation. Pulsed Doppler echocardiogram in the abdominal aorta showing pandiastolic regurgitant flow (*arrows*).

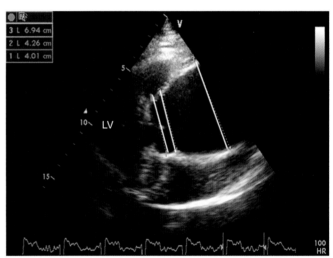

FIGURE 12-9   Parasternal long-axis view echocardiogram in a patient with aortic regurgitation. There is enlargement of the aortic root and ascending aorta. *From left to right,* lines identify the aortic diameter at the level of sinuses of Valsalva, sinotubular junction, and ascending aorta. *LV,* left ventricle.

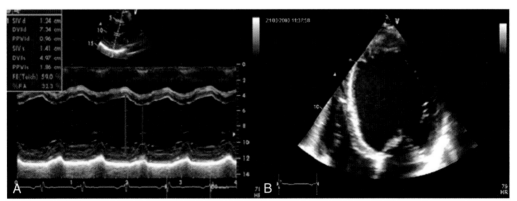

FIGURE 12-8   Left ventricular dilation in aortic regurgitation. A, Transthoracic parasternal long-axis view echocardiogram showing enlargement of left ventricular parameters in a patient with severe chronic aortic regurgitation. **B,** Apical four-chamber view of the same patient showing a spherical enlargement of the left ventricle.

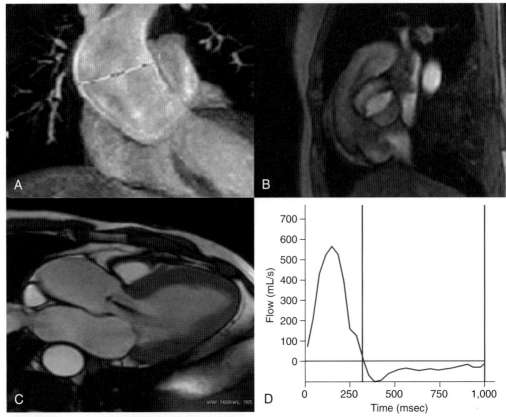

FIGURE 12-10 **Cardiac magnetic resonance imaging showing a bicuspid aortic valve with aortic regurgitation and ascending aorta dilation.** **A,** Fast single-shot steady-state free precession (SSFP) image in a coronal view. **B,** Retrospectively reconstructed magnitude image from a phase-contrast sequence showing a bicuspid aortic valve. **C,** Balanced SSFP image. Oblique axial left ventricle inflow/outflow view, showing grade 2 aortic regurgitation. **D,** Flow-versus-time plot for the ascending aorta. Antegrade flow calculated at 140 mL/beat, retrograde flow 40 mL/beat, and aortic regurgitant fraction 33%.

the use of contrast agents (gadolinium-DTPA) and different magnetic resonance angiography sequences or three-dimensional whole chest steady-state free precession sequences (without contrast agent) enables determination of the aortic root and ascending aortic anatomy and diameters.

Therefore, CMR is a useful technique to obtain a global evaluation of patients with AR, to determine the evolution of the regurgitation and its impact on LV volume and function, and to choose the optimum time for surgery.[108]

CARDIAC COMPUTED TOMOGRAPHY. The utility of 64-slice multidetector CT has been investigated in patients with AR. Aortic root and LV parameters determined by CT correlate well with corresponding measurements by transthoracic echocardiography.[109] Direct planimetry of the aortic valve anatomic regurgitant orifice accurately detects and quantifies AR.[110] CT coronary angiography is also useful for the detection of coronary artery disease in patients with AR.[111]

RADIONUCLIDE VENTRICULOGRAPHY. Radionuclide ventriculography can provide accurate measurements of LV volumes and function and can also be used as an alternative to echocardiography in patients with suboptimal echocardiograms or in patients showing discrepancies between clinical and echocardiographic data.[112]

EXERCISE TESTING

Exercise stress testing and stress echocardiography are useful for assessing functional capacity and symptomatic responses in patients with equivocal symptoms and to assist the early detection of latent systolic failure.[113,114] Exercise testing is also useful in patients with AR before participation in athletic activities.[114] Several investigators have suggested that exercise testing, with or without concurrent imaging, may help identify patients with early

systolic LV dysfunction. On exercise electrocardiography, the finding of at least 1.0 mm of ST segment depression is associated with lower resting and exercise EFs, higher wall stress, and greater end-systolic dimension in comparison with no ST segment changes with exercise.[115,116]

Echocardiography can be used to measure the incremental change in LV dimensions and EF with exercise in patients with AR.[117] Measurements of the change in EF with exercise echocardiography reflect contractile reserve and may be more predictive of clinical outcome than resting EF,[118] although the main limitation is measurement accuracy of EF during exercise. Similarly, an increase in radionuclide EF with exercise of at least 5 EF units correlates with preserved LV systolic function, whereas any decrease or increase of less than 5 units indicates an elevated end-systolic wall stress, increased end-systolic dimension, and impaired systolic function.[112] At present the role of exercise testing must be individualized. It may be helpful when there is a discrepancy between the clinical presentation and the resting echocardiographic findings. However, clinical decisions should not be based solely on changes in EF with exercise, nor on data from stress echocardiography, because these indices have not been adequately validated in large-scale prospective, randomized studies focusing on patient outcomes.

Natural History

There is no information regarding the natural history of mild AR. There is also little information in the literature regarding the progression from mild to moderate or severe regurgitation. It has been postulated that decreased aortic distensibility with age contributes to progressive AR as a result of the increase in LV afterload.[119] Doppler echocardiography measures of jet width and regurgitant orifice area suggest that there is progressive enlargement of the regurgitant orifice over time.[120] One echocardiographic study showed that the severity of regurgitation increased in 30% of patients who had undergone at least two echocardiographic studies, in association with increases in severity of LV dilation, the greatest increases in LV volumes and mass being observed in those with severe AR.[121]

PATIENTS WITH NORMAL LEFT VENTRICULAR SYSTOLIC FUNCTION

The data regarding the natural history of asymptomatic patients with severe AR and normal LV systolic function was analyzed by the American College of Cardiology/American Heart Association (ACC/AHA) Task Force on Practice Guidelines for the management of valvular heart disease,[122] which reviewed nine published series involving a total of 593 such patients[66,123-130] (Table 12-6).

These studies consistently show that patients can remain asymptomatic with preserved LV function for a long time. The rate of progression to symptoms and/or LV dysfunction averaged 4.3% per year. Sudden death occurred in 7 of the 593 patients, for an average mortality rate of less than 0.2% per year. The information available also shows that the rate of development of LV dysfunction, defined as EF at rest below normal, occurs at a rate of 1.2% per year.

Despite the low likelihood of the development of asymptomatic LV dysfunction in patients with severe AR, it should be emphasized that more than one fourth of patients in these series developed LV dysfunction before the onset of warning symptoms. Thus, in the serial evaluation of patients, quantitative assessment of LV function is indispensable. The natural history studies have also defined predictors of unfavorable outcomes. These variables are age, LV end-systolic dimension or volume, and LV EF during

TABLE 12-6	Studies of the Natural History of Asymptomatic Patients With Aortic Regurgitation						
STUDY (AUTHOR[S], YEAR)	NUMBER OF PATIENTS	MEAN FOLLOW-UP, Y	PROGRESSION TO SYMPTOMS, DEATH, OR LV DYSFUNCTION (RATE/YEAR, %)	Progression to Asymptomatic LV Dysfunction		MORTALITY (NO. OF PATIENTS)	COMMENTS
				(N)	RATE PER YEAR (%)		
Bonow et al, 1983, 1991[66,123]	104	8.0	3.8	4	0.5	2	Outcome predicted by LV ESD, EDD, change in EF with exercise, and rate of change in ESD and EF at rest with time
Scognamiglio et al, 1986*[124]	30	4.7	2.1	3	2.1	0	3 patients in whom asymptomatic LV dysfunction developed initially had lower PAP/ESV ratios and trend toward higher LV ESD and EDD and lower FS
Siemienczuk et al, 1989[125]	50	3.7	4.0	1	0.5	0	Patients included those receiving placebo and medical dropouts in a randomized drug trial, as well as some patients with NYHA FC II symptoms; outcome predicted by LV ESV, EDV, change in EF with exercise, and end-systolic wall stress
Scognamiglio et al, 1994*[126]	74	6.0	5.7	15	3.4	0	All patients received digoxin as part of a randomized trial
Tornos et al, 1995[127]	101	4.6	3.0	6	1.3	0	Outcome predicted by pulse pressure, LV ESD, EDD, and EF at rest
Ishii et al, 1996[128]	27	14.2	3.6	—	—	0	Development of symptoms predicted by systolic BP, LV ESD, EDD, mass index, and wall thickness LV function not reported in all patients
Borer et al, 1998[129]	104	7.3	6.2	7	0.9	4	20% of patients in NYHA FC II; outcome predicted by initial FC II symptoms, change in LV EF with exercise, LV ESD, and LV FS
Tarasoutchi et al, 2003[130]	72	10	4.7	1	0.1	0	Development of symptoms predicted by LV ESD and EDD LV function not reported in all patients
Evangelista et al, 2005[67]	31	7	3.6	—	—	1	Placebo control group in 7-year vasodilator clinical trial
Average	593	6.6	4.3	37	1.2	(0.18%/yr)	

BP, blood pressure; EDD, end-diastolic dimension; EDV, end-diastolic volume; EF, ejection fraction; ESD, end-systolic dimension; ESV, end-systolic volume; FC, functional class; FS, fractional shortening; LV, left ventricular; NYHA, New York Heart Association; PAP, pulmonary artery pressure.
*Two studies by same authors involved separate patient groups.
From Bonow R, Carabello BA, Chatterjee K, et al. ACC/AHA 2006 guidelines for the management of patients with valvular heart disease: a report of the American College of Cardiology/American Heart Association Task Force on Practice Guidelines. Circulation 2006;114:e84–231.

exercise.[66,125,126,129] In two multivariate analyses only age and end-systolic dimensions were independent predictors of outcome on the initial study, as were the rate of increase in end-systolic dimension and decrease in resting EF in longitudinal studies.[66,130] During a mean follow-up period of 8 years, in patients with initial end-systolic dimensions greater than 50 mm, the likelihood of death, symptoms, and/or LV dysfunction was 19% per year. In those with initial end-systolic dimensions of 40 to 50 mm, the likelihood was 6% per year, and in those with dimensions less than 40 mm, it was zero.

A tenth study of asymptomatic patients with normal LV systolic function, published after the 2006 ACC/AHA guidelines, reported a higher clinical event rate and also a higher mortality rate.[131] This study, in which quantitative measurement of severity of AR was obtained with Doppler echocardiography, reported that patients with severe AR (using the definitions shown in Table 12-5) had a much higher mortality risk and a higher likelihood of AVR than patients with less severe AR. The measures of AR severity were stronger predictors of outcome than LV EF or any of the measures of LV dilation. Importantly, the annual mortality rate in this tenth study of patients with initially normal EFs was 2.2%,[131] tenfold higher than the average 0.2% per year mortality rate found in the previous nine studies.[122,131a] This higher mortality rate may be explained by the older age of the patients in the last study (60 years), which is more than 20 years higher than the average age in the other studies (39 years). This difference suggests that severe AR in older patients, who have stiffer arteries and stiffer left ventricles, may be more poorly tolerated than in younger patients.[131a]

PATIENTS WITH LEFT VENTRICULAR SYSTOLIC DYSFUNCTION

There are very limited data in asymptomatic patients with depressed LV function, but it has been estimated that the average rate of symptom onset in such patients is more than 25% per year.[132-134] Symptoms due to AR are a strong predictor of clinical outcome.[135] The data developed in the presurgical era indicate that patients with dyspnea, angina, or overt heart failure have a poor outcome with medical therapy, with mortality rates higher than 10% in those with angina and higher than 20% in those with heart failure.[90,136,137]

Medical Management

The aims of medical management in patients with significant AR are to carefully follow the clinical course in order to identify the best timing for surgical indication and to prevent complications.

ROLE OF VASODILATOR THERAPY

Vasodilator therapy has been designed to reduce regurgitant volume overload, LV volumes, and wall stress. These effects could theoretically be beneficial in AR through preservation of LV function and reduction in LV mass. Vasodilators are useful in patients with severe AR and symptoms and/or LV dysfunction who are considered poor candidates for surgery because of severe comorbidities. Vasodilators are also useful for improving the hemodynamic profile in patients with severe heart failure symptoms before AVR. The most controversial effect of vasodilators is their use in the absence of systemic hypertension to alter the natural history in asymptomatic patients with AR and preserved LV systolic function and to prolong the compensated phase of the disease. If vasodilator therapy successfully delays decompensation of the left ventricle, surgery can be postponed. Several studies with small numbers of patients and short-term follow-up periods found different beneficial effects of vasodilators on hemodynamic and echocardiographic parameters of LV function.[138-145] Regarding long-term effects, only one study reported that long-acting nifedipine therapy produced a reduction in LV dimensions and an increase in EF,[126] and two studies demonstrated

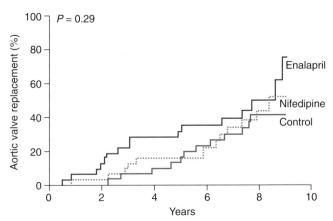

FIGURE 12-11 Progression to aortic valve replacement in initially asymptomatic patients with aortic regurgitation. Patients were randomly assigned to treatment with enalapril, nifedipine, or placebo (*Control*). *(From Evangelista A, Tornos P, Sambola A, et al. Long-term vasodilator therapy in patients with severe aortic regurgitation. N Engl J Med 2005;353:1342–9.)*

improvement in hemodynamic parameters with enalapril and quinapril, particularly when this effect was accompanied by a drop in blood pressure.[139,145] A clinical trial using nifedipine, enalapril, or no treatment in asymptomatic patients with severe AR and normal LV function did not, however, demonstrate any significant benefit of such therapy; vasodilators did not delay the need for AVR after an extended follow-up period and did not result in a reduction in regurgitant volume or a beneficial effect on LV size or function (Figure 12-11).[67] If vasodilator therapy is used in asymptomatic patients with severe AR, the goal should be to reduce systolic blood pressure, and drug dosage should be increased until a measurable decrease in blood pressure is achieved. The role of angiotensin-converting enzyme (ACE) inhibitors in chronic AR has been reassessed; in a retrospective analysis of 2266 patients with moderate to severe AR, treatment with angiotensin-converting enzyme inhibitors was associated with significantly lower all-cause and cardiovascular mortality.[146] This observation requires further confirmation in prospectively designed clinical trials.

ROLE OF BETA-BLOCKERS

In chronic AR, treatment with beta-adrenergic blockers has been controversial, because lowering heart rate may increase the regurgitant volume. A retrospective observational study reported that beta-blocker therapy was associated with better survival in patients with chronic AR, mainly in the subgroup with higher heart rates.[147] However, this was not an asymptomatic population; 70% had heart failure, 25% had atrial fibrillation, and many had LV systolic dysfunction (the mean EF was 54%). Thus, these data do not necessarily pertain to the long-term management of asymptomatic patients with preserved LV systolic function.

PREVENTION OF ENDOCARDITIS

Patients with AR should be instructed in the importance of good oral hygiene and regular dental cleaning and examinations. Patients should also be instructed on early reporting of unexplained fever lasting for more than 1 week and on the importance of refraining from self-medication with antibiotics in the case of fever. According to the 2007 American Heart Association guidelines on endocarditis prevention, antibiotic prophylaxis before dental work or other invasive procedures is no longer recommended in patients with AR or other forms of native valve disease; antibiotic prophylaxis is recommended only in those patients with AR who have a previous history of endocarditis.[148]

Serial Evaluations

The aim of serial evaluation of asymptomatic patients with chronic AR is to detect the onset of clinical symptoms and to objectively assess changes in LV function and size that can occur in the absence of symptoms, in order to determine the optimal time for surgery. Patients with mild to moderate AR can be seen on a yearly basis, and echocardiography performed every 2 years. The patient who has severe AR when first seen and in whom the chronic nature of the regurgitation is uncertain should be reevaluated within 2 to 3 months in order to be certain that the patient is stable and that a subacute process with rapid progression is not under way. Once the chronicity and stability of the regurgitation has been established, the frequency of the clinical reevaluation and interval between echocardiographic examinations depend on the severity of the regurgitation, the extent of LV dilation, and the level of systolic function at rest.

Patients with severe AR, normal EF at rest (>50%), and moderate LV dilation (end-diastolic dimension 60 to 65 mm) may be seen every 6 months. During every visit a careful clinical history should be obtained. An exercise test is useful in case of equivocal symptoms. Echocardiographic measurements should also be obtained yearly or whenever there is a suspected change in the clinical situation. In patients with more severe dilation, with end-diastolic dimensions approaching 70 mm, it is wise to recommend clinical evaluations and echocardiographic measurements every 6 months, or even more frequently if a progressive dilation or decline in EF is detected. In those patients stress echocardiography can be used to detect earlier signs of LV dysfunction.[113,114] Brain natriuretic peptide (BNP) measurements have been used as a biomarkers for the monitoring of the disease[149,150]; and Pizarro et al,[151] in a prospective evaluation of a cohort of 294 asymptomatic patients with chronic severe AR and normal EF (>55%), determined that a brain natriuretic peptide value higher than 130 pg/mL could identify a subgroup of patients at higher risk for development of symptoms, LV dysfunction, or death during follow-up.

CMR or radionuclide ventriculography can be used in the serial assessment as an alternative to echocardiography, particularly in patients with technically suboptimal echocardiograms.

In patients with aortic root dilation, serial echocardiograms should include accurate measurements of the aorta. Indexing for body surface area could be recommended, especially in patients of small body size and in women.[152,153] CMR and CT are also good alternatives for following the severity of aortic dilation, mainly if dilation occurs in the upper part of the sinotubular junction.

Indications for Surgery

The surgical management in AR usually requires AVR. In highly selected patients and in surgical centers of excellence, there is growing experience in aortic valve repair.[154-156] Some surgical groups use the pulmonic autograft procedure (the Ross procedure) in younger patients.[157,158] The indications for surgery on the aortic valve are the same irrespective of the surgical technique used.

The goals of operation are to improve outcome, to diminish symptoms, to prevent the development of postoperative heart failure and cardiac death, and to avoid aortic complications in patients who present with aortic aneurysms. Several investigators have identified preoperative predictors of patient outcome and LV function after valve replacement for chronic AR.[39-41,43,46,48-50,52-60,62,63] The most consistent of these measures have been the functional class, EF and end-systolic dimension. On the basis of robust observational evidence, the recommended indications for surgical intervention for severe AR are similar in both the ACC/AHA and the European guidelines (Figures 12-12 and 12-13).[122,159]

Symptom onset is an indication for surgery irrespective of LV function. When the LV systolic function is normal and the patient experiences symptoms, every effort should be made to clearly relate the symptoms to the AR. Especially when the symptoms are mild, such as New York Heart Association (NYHA) functional class II dyspnea, clinical judgment is necessary, and in this setting the role of exercise testing is valuable. However, in patients with LV dilation and progressive enlargement in chamber size or decline in EF on serial studies, the beginning of mild symptoms is a clear indication for valve replacement.

In symptomatic patients with decreased LV systolic function (subnormal EF), surgery is clearly indicated. Several studies have shown that the long-term outcome is excellent if such patients undergo AVR when asymptomatic or only mildly symptomatic or with mild LV dysfunction[41,50,61,63] (Figure 12-14). Therefore, every effort should be made to refer patients to surgery at this stage. Postoperative survival and the likelihood of recovery of systolic function is worse in patients with preoperative NYHA functional class IV symptoms[160] or with extremely enlarged ventricles (>55 mm at end-systole) and/or very poor EF (<30%)[63,161] (see Table 12-3). However, even in those very ill patients, AVR with subsequent medical treatment is a better alternative than long-term medical therapy alone or cardiac transplantation. Recent data demonstrating a significant decrease in operative mortality in patients with AR and severe LV dysfunction reinforce this opinion (see Table 12-6).[64]

Surgery should also be considered in asymptomatic patients with severe AR and impaired LV function at rest, defined as resting EF less than 50%, and/or extreme degrees of LV dilation (end-diastolic diameter ≥70-75 mm and end-systolic diameter ≥50-55 mm).[162-168] In these patients, the likelihood that symptoms will develop in the short term is high, perioperative mortality is very low, and the postoperative long-term results are excellent. Good-quality echocardiograms and data confirmation with repeated measurements are necessary before surgery is recommended to asymptomatic patients.

In patients with AR undergoing other cardiac operations, such as coronary bypass surgery and mitral valve surgery, the decision to replace the aortic valve should be individualized according to the severity of AR, age, and overall clinical situation. If the AR is severe, replacement of the aortic valve is almost always indicated,[122] whereas AVR can be postponed when the AR is mild.

Concomitant Aortic Root Disease

In patients with AR secondary to enlargement of the ascending aorta or aortic root, the natural history of the disease and thus the timing and choice of surgical intervention are often based on the extent and rate of aortic or aortic root dilation rather than the LV response to AR. These considerations are particularly important in patients with Marfan syndrome, patients with bicuspid aortic valves, and patients with annuloaortic ectasia. When the severity of AR is mild or moderate in such patients, management decisions may depend on treating the underlying aortic and aortic root disease. In those with severe AR, decisions may need to be based on both conditions.

In patients with Marfan syndrome, beta-blockers slow the progression of aortic dilation.[169] Enalapril has also been used to delay aortic dilation in patients with Marfan syndrome.[170] Animal models of Marfan syndrome have shown a beneficial effect of the angiotensin-receptor blocker losartan in normalizing the aortic root growth and aortic wall architecture,[171] and a clinical trial comparing the effects of atenolol and losartan is currently underway.[172,173] Whether the same beneficial effect of beta-blockers or other drugs occurs in patients with bicuspid aortic valves and aortic dilation is unknown.

The rationale for an aggressive surgical approach in patients with aortic dilation and only mild AR is better defined in patients with Marfan syndrome than in patients with bicuspid aortic valves or annuloaortic ectasia.[152] Aortic root dilation greater than 55 mm should be considered a surgical indication irrespective of the

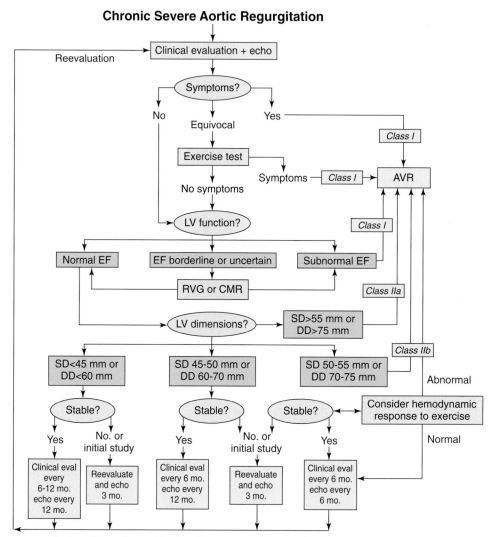

Chronic Severe Aortic Regurgitation

FIGURE 12-12   Management strategy for patients with chronic severe aortic regurgitation. Preoperative coronary angiography should be performed routinely as determined by age, symptoms, and coronary risk factors. Cardiac catheterization and angiography may also be helpful when there is discordance between clinical echocardiographic findings and. "Stable" refers to stable echocardiographic measurements. In some centers, serial follow-up evaluations (eval) may be performed with radionuclide ventriculography or cardiac magnetic resonance rather than echocardiography (echo) to assess left ventricular (LV) volume and systolic function. *AVR*, aortic valve replacement; *class*, New York Heart Association functional class; *DD*, end-diastolic dimension; *EF*, ejection fraction; *CMR*, cardiac magnetic resonance; *RVG*, radionuclide ventriculography; *SD*, end-systolic dimension. *(From Bonow R, Carabello BA, Chatterjee K, et al. ACC/AHA 2006 guidelines for the management of patients with valvular heart disease. A report of the American College of Cardiology/American Heart Association Task Force on Practice Guidelines. Circulation 2006;114:e84–231.)*

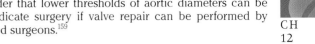

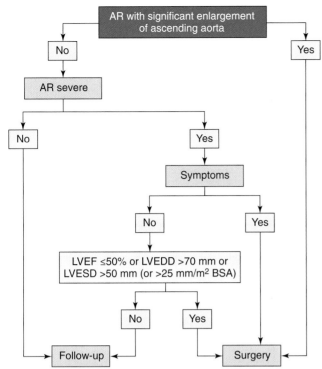

FIGURE 12-13   Management of aortic regurgitation. *AR,* aortic regurgitation; *BSA,* body surface area; *EDD,* end-diastolic dimension; *EF,* ejection fraction; *ESD,* end-systolic dimension; *LV,* left ventricular. *(From Vahanian A, Alfieri O, Andreotti F, et al. Guidelines on the management of valvular heart disease (version 2012). Joint Task Force on the Management of Valvular Heart Disease of the European Society of Cardiology and the European Association for Cardio-Thoracic Surgery. Eur Heart J 2012;33:2451–96.)*

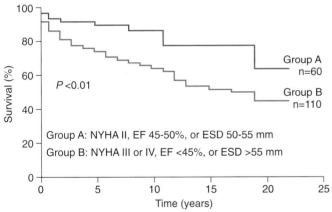

FIGURE 12-14   Long-term survival after valve replacement for aortic regurgitation. These data demonstrate improved outcome with early surgery. *EF,* ejection fraction; *ESD,* end-systolic dimension; *NYHA,* New York Heart Association functional class. *(From Tornos P, Sambola A, Permanyer-Miralda G, et al. Long term outcome of surgically treated aortic regurgitation: influence of guidelines adherence toward early surgery. J Am Coll Cardiol 2006;47:1012–17.)*

ascending aorta.[122] In borderline cases, the decision to replace the ascending aorta also relies on perioperative surgical findings as regards the thickness of the aortic valve and the status of the rest of the aorta. In the European Guidelines, the recommendations also consider that lower thresholds of aortic diameters can be used to indicate surgery if valve repair can be performed by experienced surgeons.[159]

REFERENCES

1. Olson LJ, Subramanian R, Edwards WD. Surgical pathology of pure aortic insufficiency: a study of 255 cases. Mayo Clin Proc 1984;59:835–41.
2. Roberts WC, KO JM, Moore TR, et al. Causes of pure aortic regurgitation in patients having isolated aortic valve replacement in a single US tertiary hospital (1993-2005). Circulation 2006;114:422–9.
3. Baszyk H, Witkiewicz AJ, Edwards WD. Acute aortic regurgitation due to spontaneous rupture of a fenestrated cusp: report in a 65-year-old man and review of seven additional cases. Cardiovasc Pathol 1999;8:213–6.
4. Maskatia SA, Ing FF, Justino H, et al. Twenty-five year experience with balloon aortic valvuloplasty for congenital aortic stenosis. Am J cardiol 2011;108:1024–8.
5. Abdel-Wahab M, Zahn R, Horack M, et al. German transcatheter aortic valve interventions registry investigators. Aortic regurgitation after transcatheter aortic valve implantation: incidence and early outcome. Results from the German transcatheter aortic valve interventions registry. Heart 2011, 97:899–906.
6. Connolly HM, Crary JL, McGoon MD, et al. Valvular heart disease associated with fenfluramine-phentermine. N Engl J Med 1997;337;581–8.
7. Zanettini R, Antonini A, Gatto G, et al. Valvular heart disease and the use of dopamine agonists for Parkinson's disease. N Engl J Med 2007;356:39–46.
8. Iung B, Baron G, Butchart EG. A prospective survey of patients with valvular heart disease in Europe: The Euro Heart Survey on Valvular Heart Disease. Eur Heart J 2003;24:1231–43.
9. Morganroth J, Perloff JK, Zeldis SM, et al. Acute severe aortic regurgitation: pathophysiology, clinical recognition and management. Ann Intern Med 1977;87:223–32.
10. Ardehali A, Segal J, Cheitlin MD. Coronary blood flow reserve in acute aortic regurgitation. J Am Coll Cardiol 1995;25:1387–92.
11. Mann T, McLaurin L, Grossman W, et al. Assessing the hemodynamic severity of acute aortic regurgitation due to infective endocarditis. N Engl J Med 1975;293:108–13.
12. Cigarroa JE, Isselbacher EM, DeSanctis RW, et al. Diagnostic imaging in the evaluation of suspected aortic dissection: old standards and new directions. N Engl J Med 1993;328:35–43.
13. Nienaber CA, von KY, Nicholas V, et al. The diagnosis of thoracic aortic dissection by noninvasive imaging procedures. N Engl J Med 1993;328:1–9.
14. Mith MD, Cassidy JM, Souther S, et al. Transesophageal echocardiography in the diagnosis of traumatic rupture of the aorta. N Engl J Med 1995;332;356–62.
15. David TE, Feindel CM. An aortic valve–sparing operation for patients with aortic incompetence and aneurysm of the ascending aorta. J Thorac Cardiovasc Surg 1992;103:617–22.
16. Graeter TP, Langer F, Nikoloudakis N, et al. Valve-preserving operations in acute aortic dissection type A. Ann Thorac Surg 2000;70:1460–5.
17. Kallenbach K, Oelze T, Salcher R, et al. Evolving strategies for treatment of acute aortic dissection type A. Circulation 2004;110 (suppl II) II-243–II-249.
18. Habib G, Avierinos JF, Thuny F. Aortic valve endocarditis: is there an optimal surgical timing? Curr Opin Cardiol 2007;22:77–83.
19. Cabell CH, Abrutyn E, Fowler VG, et al. Use of surgery in patients with native valve endocarditis: results from the international collaboration on endocarditis merged database. Am Heart J 2005;150:1092–8.
20. Aksoy O, Sexton DJ, Wang A et al. Early surgery in patients with infective endocarditis: a propensity score analysis. Clin Infect Dis 2007;44:364–72.
21. Carabello BA. Aortic regurgitation: a lesion with similarities to both aortic stenosis and mitral regurgitation. Circulation 1990;82:1051–3.
22. Ross J Jr. Afterload mismatch in aortic and mitral valve disease: implications for surgical therapy. J Am Coll Cardiol 1985;5:811–26.
23. Borow KM. Surgical outcome in chronic aortic regurgitation: a physiologic framework for assessing preoperative predictors. J Am Coll Cardiol 1987:10:1165–70.
24. Grossman W, Jones D, McLaurin LP. Wall stress and patterns of hypertrophy in the human left ventricle. J Clin Invest 1975;56:56–64.
25. Ross J Jr, McCullagh WH. Nature of enhanced performance of the dilated left ventricle in the dog during chronic volume overloading. Circ Res 1972;30:549–56.
26. Wisenbaugh T, Spann JF, Carabello BA. Differences in myocardial performance and load between patients with similar amounts of chronic aortic versus chronic mitral regurgitation. J Am Coll Cardiol 1984;3:916–23.
27. Ricci DR. Afterload mismatch and preload reserve in chronic aortic regurgitation. Circulation 1982;66:826–34.
28. Rigolin VH, Bonow RO. Hemodynamic characteristics and progression to heart failure in regurgitant lesions. Heart Failure Clin 2007;2:453–60.
29. Gaasch WH. Left ventricular radius to wall thickness ratio. Am J Cardiol 1979;43:1189–94.
30. Nitenberg A, Foult JM, Blanchet F, et al. Coronary flow and resistance reserve in patients with chronic aortic regurgitation, angina pectoris and normal coronary arteries. J Am Coll Cardiol 1988;11:478–86.
31. Gaasch WH, Andrias CW, Levine HJ. Chronic aortic regurgitation: the effect of aortic valve replacement on left ventricular volume, mass and function. Circulation 1978;58:825–36.

severity and etiology of AR. In cases of Marfan syndrome or bicuspid valves, a smaller diameter of root dilation (>50 mm) has been proposed as an indicator for surgery. However, even smaller diameters (<45 mm) can be considered in patients with high-risk factors for dissection, such as a rapid increase in aortic diameter between serial measurements (5 mm per year) or family history of aortic dissection.[122,159,174-177] For patients who have reached the recommended indications for surgery on the basis severity of AR, a lower threshold can be used for combining surgery on the

32. Schwarz F, Flameng W, Langebartels F, et al. Impaired left ventricular function in chronic aortic valve disease: survival and function after replacement by Bjork Shiley prosthesis. Circulation 1979;60:48–58.
33. Borer JS, Rosing DR, Kent KM, et al. Left ventricular function at rest and during exercise after aortic valve replacement in patients with aortic regurgitation. Am J Cardiol 1979;44:1297–305.
34. Clark DG, McAnulty JH, Rahimtoola SH. Valve replacement in aortic insufficiency with left ventricular dysfunction. Circulation 1980;61:411–21.
35. Toussaint C, Cribier A, Cazor JL, et al. Hemodynamic and angiographic evaluation of aortic regurgitation 8 and 27 months after aortic valve replacement. Circulation 1981;64:456–63.
36. Carroll JD, Gaasch WH, Zile MR, et al. Serial changes in left ventricular function after correction of chronic aortic regurgitation: dependence on early changes in preload and subsequent regression of hypertrophy. Am J Cardiol 1983;51:476–82.
37. Bonow RO, Rosing DR, Maron BJ, et al. Reversal of left ventricular dysfunction after aortic valve replacement for chronic aortic regurgitation: influence of duration of preoperative left ventricular dysfunction. Circulation 1984;70:570–9.
38. Fioretti P, Roclandt J, Sclavo M, et al. Postoperative regression of left ventricular dimensions in aortic insufficiency: a long term echocardiographic study. J Am Coll Cardiol 1985;5:856–61.
39. Carabello BA, Usher BW, Hendrix GH, et al. Predictors of outcome for aortic valve replacement in patients with aortic regurgitation and left ventricular dysfunction: a change in the measuring stick. J Am Coll Cardiol 1987;10:991–7.
40. Taniguchi K, Nakano S, Hirose H, et al. Preoperative left ventricular function: minimal requirement for successful late results of valve replacement for aortic regurgitation. J Am Coll Cardiol 1987;10:510–18.
41. Bonow RO, Dodd JT, Maron BJ, et al. Long term serial changes in left ventricular function and reversal of ventricular dilatation after valve replacement for chronic aortic regurgitation. Circulation 1988;78:1108–20.
42. Borer JS, Herrold EM, Hochreiter C, et al. Natural history of left ventricular performance at rest and during exercise after aortic valve replacement for aortic regurgitation. Circulation 1991;84 (suppl III):III-133–III-139.
43. Cohn PF, Gorlin R, Cohn LH, et al. Left ventricular ejection fraction as a prognostic guide in surgical treatment of coronary and valvular disease. Am J Cardiol 1974;34: 136–41.
44. Copeland JG, Grepp RB, Stinson EB, et al. Long term follow-up after isolated aortic valve replacement. J Thorac Cardivasc Surg 1977;74:875–89.
45. Herreman F, Amcur A, de Vernejoul F, et al. Pre and postoperative hemodynamic and cineangiographic assessment of left ventricular function in patients with aortic regurgitation. Am Heart J 1979;98:63–72.
46. Cuhna CL, Giuliani ER, Fuster V, et al. Preoperative M mode echocardiography as predictor of surgical results in chronic aortic insufficiency. J Thorac Cardiovasc Surg 1980;79;256–65.
47. Forman R, Firth BG, Barnard MS. Prognostic significance of preoperative left ventricular ejection fraction and valve lesion in patients with aortic valve replacement. Am J Cardiol 1980;45:1120–5.
48. Greves J, Rahimtoola SH, McAnulty JH, et al. Preoperative criteria predictive of late survival following valve replacement for severe aortic regurgitation. Am Heart J 1981;101:300–8.
49. Gaasch WH, Carroll JD, Levine H, et al. Chronic aortic regurgitation: prognostic value of left ventricular end-systolic dimension and end-diastolic radius/thickness ratio. J Am Coll Cardiol 1983;1:775–82.
50. Bonow RO, Picone AL, McIntosh CL, et al. Survival and functional results after valve replacement for aortic regurgitation from 1976 to 1983: impact of preoperative left ventricular function. Circulation 1985;72:1244–56.
51. Carabello BA, Williams H, Gaasch AK, et al. Hemodynamic predictors of outcome in patients undergoing valve replacement. Circulation 1986;72:1244–56.
52. Michel PL, Iung B, Abou JS, et al. The effect of left ventricular systolic function on long term survival in mitral and aortic regurgitation. J Heart Valve Dis 1995;4(suppl 2):S160–8.
53. Henry WL, Bonow RO, Borer JS, et al. Observations on the optimum time for operative intervention for aortic regurgitation. I. Evaluation of the results of aortic valve replacement in symptomatic patients. Circulation 1980;61:471–83.
54. Kumpuris AG, Quinones MA, Waggoner AD, et al. Importance of preoperative hypertrophy, wall stress and end-systolic dimension as echocardiographic predictors of normalization of left ventricular dilatation after valve replacement in symptomatic patients. Am J Cardiol 1982;49:1091–100.
55. Fioretti P, Roelandt J, Bos RJ, et al. Echocardiography in chronic aortic insufficiency: is valve replacement too late when left ventricular end systolic dimension reaches 55 mm? Circulation 1983;67:216–21.
56. Stone PH, Clark RD, Goldschlager N, et al. Determinants of prognosis of patients with aortic regurgitation who undergo aortic valve replacement. J Am Coll Cardiol 1984;3:1118–26.
57. Daniel WG, Hood WP Jr, Siart A, et al. Chronic aortic regurgitation: reassessment of the prognostic value of preoperative left ventricular end systolic dimension and fractional shortening. Circulation 1985;7:669–80.
58. Cormier B, Vahanian A, Luxereaux P, et al. Should asymptomatic or mildly symptomatic aortic regurgitation be operated on? Z Kardiol 1986;75(suppl 2):141–5.
59. Sheiban I, Trevi GP, Carassotto D, et al. Aortic valve replacement in patients with aortic incompetence: preoperative parameters influencing long term results. Z Kardiol 1986;75 (suppl 2):146–54.
60. Klodas E, Enriquez-Sarano M, Tajik AJ, et al. Aortic regurgitation complicated by extreme left ventricular dilation: long-term outcome after surgical correction. J Am Coll Cardiol 1996;27:670–7.
61. Klodas E, Enriquez-Sarano M, Tajik AJ, et al. Optimizing timing of surgical correction in patients with severe aortic regurgitation: role of symptoms. J Am Coll Cardiol 1997;30:746–52.
62. Turina J, Milinic J, Seifert B, et al. Valve replacement in chronic aortic regurgitation: true predictors of survival after extended follow-up. Circulation 1998;98 (suppl II): II-100–II-106.
63. Tornos P, Sambola A, Permanyer-Miralda G, et al. Long term outcome of surgically treated aortic regurgitation: influence of guidelines adherence toward early surgery. J Am Coll Cardiol 2006;47:1012–7.
64. Bhudia SK, McCarthy PM, Kumpati GS, et al. Improved outcomes after aortic valve surgery for chronic aortic regurgitation with severe left ventricular dysfunction. J Am Coll Cardiol 2007;49:1465–71.
65. Kawanishi DT, McKay CR, Chandraratna PA, et al. Cardiovascular response to dynamic exercise in patients with chronic symptomatic mild to moderate and severe aortic regurgitation. Circulation 1986;73:62–72.
66. Bonow RO, Lakatos E, Maron BJ, et al. Serial long-term assessment of the natural history of asymptomatic patients with chronic aortic regurgitation and normal left ventricular systolic function. Circulation 1991;84:1625–35.
67. Evangelista A, Tornos P, Sambola A, et al. Long-term vasodilator therapy in patients with severe aortic regurgitation. N Engl J Med 2005;353:1342–9.
68. Perloff JK. Physical examination of the heart and circulation. Philadelphia: Saunders; 1982.
69. Corrigan DJ. On permanent patency of the mouth of the aorta, or inadequacy of the aortic valve. Edinburgh Med Surg 1832;37:225.
70. Quincke H. Observations on capillary and venous pulse. Berl Klin Wochenschr 1868;5:357 (translated in Willius FA, Keys TE eds: Classics of Cardiology. New York: Dover 1961).
71. Harvey WP, Corrado MA, Perloff JK. Right sided murmurs of aortic insufficiency (diastolic murmurs better heard to the right of the sternum than to the left). Am J Med Sci 1963;245:533.
72. Grayburn PA, Smith MD, Handshoe R, et al. Detection of aortic insufficiency by standard echocardiography, pulsed Doppler echocardiography and auscultation. A comparison of accuracies. Ann Intern Med 1986;104:599–605.
73. Kinney EL. Causes of false-negative auscultation of regurgitant lesions: a Doppler echocardiographic study of 294 patients. J Gen Intern Med 1988;3:429–34.
74. Aronow WS, Krozon I. Correlation of prevalence and severity of aortic regurgitation detected by pulsed Doppler echocardiography with the murmur of aortic regurgitation in elderly patients in a long term health facility. Am J Cardiol 1989;63:128–9.
75. Desjardin VA, Enriquez Sarano M, Tajik AJ, et al. Intensity of murmurs correlates with severity of valvular regurgitation. Am J Med 1996;100:149–56.
76. Flint A. On cardiac murmurs. Am J Med Sci 1862;44:29–55.
77. Emi S, Fukuda N, Oki T, et al. Genesis of the Austin Flint murmur: relation to mitral flow and aortic regurgitant flow dynamics. J Am Coll Cardiol 1993;21:1399–405.
78. Rahko PS. Doppler and echocardiography characteristics of patients having an Austin Flint murmur. Circulation 1991;83:1940–50.
79. Landzberg JS, Pflugfelder PW, Cassidy MM, et al. Etiology of the Austin Flint murmur. J Am Coll Cardiol 1992;20:408–13.
80. Roman MJ, Kligfield P, Devereux RB, et al. Geometric and functional correlates of electrocardiographic repolarization and voltage abnormalities in aortic regurgitation. J Am Coll Cardiol 1987;9:500–8.
81. Chen J, Okin PM, Roman MJ, et al. Combined rest and exercise electrocardiographic repolarization findings in relation to structural and functional abnormalities in symptomatic aortic regurgitation. Am Heart J 1996;132:343–7.
82. Kligfield P, Ameisen O, Okin PM, et al. Relationship of the electrocardiographic response to exercise to geometric and functional findings in aortic regurgitation. Am Heart J 1987;113:1097–102.
83. Reichek N, Devereux RB. Left ventricular hypertrophy: relationship of anatomic, echocardiographic and electrocardiographic findings. Circulation 1981;63:1391–8.
84. Bishop N, Boyle R, Watson DA, et al. Aortic valve disease and the ST/heart rate relationship: a longitudinal study before and after aortic valve replacement. J Electrocardiol 1988;21:31–7.
85 Martinez Useros C, Tornos P, Montoyo J, et al. Ventricular arrhythmias in aortic valve disease: a further marker of impaired ventricular function. Int J Cardiol 1992;34: 49–56.
86. Samuels DA, Curfman GD, Friedlich AL, et al. Valve replacement for aortic regurgitation: long term follow up with factors that influence the results. Circulation 1979;60: 647–54.
87. Acar J, Luxereau P, Ducimetiere P, et al. Prognosis of surgically treated chronic aortic valve disease: predictive indicators of early postoperative risk and long term survival based on 439 cases. J Thorac Cardiovasc Surg 1981;82:114–26.
88. Isom OW, Dembrow JM, Glassman E, et al. Factors influencing long-term survival after isolated aortic valve replacement. Circulation 1974;50:154–62.
89. Hirshfield JW, Epstein SE, Roberts AJ, et al. Indices predicting long-term survival after valve replacement in patients with aortic regurgitation and patients with aortic stenosis. Circulation 1974;50:1190–9.
90. Spagnuolo M, Kloth H, Taranta A, et al. Natural history of rheumatic aortic regurgitation: criteria predictive of death, congestive heart failure and angina in young patients. Circulation 1971:44:368–80.
91. Lancellotti P, Tribouilloy C, Hagendorff A, et al. European Association of Echocardiography recommendations for the assessment of valvular regurgitation. Part 1: aortic and pulmonary regurgitation (native valve disease). Eur J Echocardiogr 2010;11:223–44.
92. Evangelista A, Garcia del Castillo H, Calvo F, et al. Strategy for optimal aortic regurgitation quantification by Doppler echocardiography: agreement among different methods. Am Heart J 2000;139:773–81.
93. Xic GY, Berk MR, Smith MD, et al. A simplified method for determining regurgitant fraction by Doppler echocardiography in patients with aortic regurgitation. J Am Coll Cardiol 1994;24:1041–5.
94. Sambola A, Tornos P, Ferreira I, et al. Prognostic value of preoperative indexed end-systolic left ventricular diameter in the outcome after surgery in patients with chronic aortic regurgitation. Am Heart J 2008;155:1114–20.

95. Vinereanu D, Ionescu AA, Fraser G. Assessment of left ventricular long axis contraction can detect early myocardial dysfunction in asymptomatic patients with severe aortic regurgitation. Heart 2001;85:30–6.

96. Paraskevaidis IA, Kyrzopoulos S, Farmakis D et al. Ventricular long-axis contraction as an earlier predictor of outcome in asymptomatic aortic regurgitation. Am J Cardiol 2007;100:1677–82.

97. deWaroux JB, Pouleur AC, Goffinet C, et al. Functional anatomy of aortic regurgitation: accuracy, prediction of surgical reparability and outcome implications of transesophageal echocardiography. Circulation 2007;116(suppl I):I-264–I-269.

98. Perez de Isla L, Zamorano J, Fernandez-Golfin C, et al. 3D color-Doppler echocardiography and chronic aortic regurgitation: a novel approach for severity assessment. Int J Cardiol 2011 Dec 20 [epub ahead of print].

98a. Debl K, Djavidani B, Buchner S, et al. Assessment of the anatomic regurgitant orifice in aortic regurgitation: a clinical magnetic resonance imaging study. Heart 2007; 94:e8.

99. Gentchos GE, Tischler MD, Christian TF. Imaging and quantifying valvular heart disease using magnetic resonance techniques. Curr Treatment Options Cardiovasc Med 2006;8:453–60.

100. Chatzimavroudis GP, Oshinski JN, Franch RH, et al. Evaluation of the precision of magnetic resonance phase velocity mapping for blood flow measurements. J Cardiovasc Magn Reson 2001;3:11–19.

101. Kozerke S, Schwitter J, Pedersen EM, et al. Aortic and mitral regurgitation: quantification using moving slice velocity mapping. J Magn Reson Imaging 2001;14: 106–12.

102. Chatzimavroudis GP, Oshinski JN, Franch RH, et al. Quantification of the aortic regurgitant volume with magnetic resonance phase velocity mapping: a clinical investigation of the importance of imaging slice location. J Heart Valve Dis 1998;7:94–101.

103. Friedrich MG, Schulz-Menger J, Poetsch T, et al. Quantification of valvular aortic stenosis by magnetic resonance imaging. Am Heart J 2002;144:329–34.

104. John AS, Dill T, Brandt RR, et al. Magnetic resonance to assess the aortic valve area in aortic stenosis. How does it compare to current diagnostic standards? J Am Coll Cardiol 2003;42:519–26.

105. Kupfahl C, Honold M, Meinhardt G, et al. Evaluation of aortic stenosis by cardiovascular magnetic resonance imaging: comparison with established routine clinical techniques. Heart 2004;90:893–901.

106. Debl K, Djavidani B, Seitz J, et al. Planimetry of aortic valve area in aortic stenosis by magnetic resonance imaging. Invest Radiol 2005;40:631–6.

107. Doherty NE 3rd, Seelos KC, Sazuki J, et al. Application of cine MR imaging for sequential evaluation of response to angiotensin converting enzyme inhibitor therapy in dilated cardiomyopathy. J Am Coll Cardiol 1992;19:1294–302.

108. Masci PG, Dymarkowski S, Bogaert J. Valvular heart disease: what does cardiovascular MRI add? Eur Radiol 2008;18:197–208.

109. Alkadhi H, Desbioller L, Husmann L, et al. Aortic regurgitation: assessment with 64 section CT. Radiology 2007;245:111–21.

110. Jassae DS, Shapiro MD, Neilan Th, et al. 64-slice multidetector computed tomography (MDTC) for detection of aortic regurgitation and quantification of severity. Invest Radiol 2007;42:507–12.

111. Scheffeld H, Leschkas S, Plass A, et al. Accuracy of 64-slice computed tomography for the preoperative detection of coronary artery disease in patients with chronic aortic regurgitation. Am J Cardiol 2007;100:701–6.

112. Iskandrian AS, Heo J. Radionuclide angiographic evaluation of left ventricular performance at rest and exercise response in aortic regurgitation. Am J Cardiol 1985;55: 428–31.

113. Bonow RO, Carabello BA, Chaterjee K et al. 2008 Focused update incorporated into the ACC/AHA 2006. Guidelines for the management of patients with valvular heart disease. Circulation 2008;118:e-523–e-661.

114. Pierard LA, Lancellotti P. Stress testing in valve disease. Hear 2007;93:766–72.

115. Misra M, Thakur R, Bhandari K, et al. Value of treadmill exercise test in asymptomatic and minimally symptomatic patients with chronic severe aortic regurgitation. Int J Cardiol 1987;15:309–16.

116. Scriven AJ, Lipkin DP, Fox KM, et al. Maximal oxygen uptake in severe aortic regurgitation: a different view of left ventricular function. Am Heart J 1990;120:902–9.

117. Wahi S, Haluska B, Pasquet A, et al. Exercise echocardiography predicts development of left ventricular dysfunction in medically and surgically treated patients with asymptomatic aortic regurgitation. Heart 2000;84:606–14.

118. Wu WC. Evaluation of aortic valve disorders using stress echocardiography. Echocardiography 2004;21:459–66.

119. Wilson RA, McDonald RW, Bristow JD, et al. Correlates of aortic distensibility in chronic aortic regurgitation and relation to progression to surgery. J Am Coll Cardiol 1992; 19:259–65.

120. Reimold SC, Orav EJ, Come PC, et al. Progressive enlargement of the regurgitant orifice in patients with chronic aortic regurgitation. J Am Soc Echocardiogr 1998;11: 259–65.

121. Padial LR, Oliver A, Vivaldi M, et al. Doppler echocardiographic assessment of progression of aortic regurgitation. Am J Cardiol 1997;80:306–14.

122. Bonow R, Carabello BA, Chatterjee K, et al. ACC/AHA 2006 guidelines for the management of patients with valvular heart disease. A report of the American College of Cardiology/American Heart Association Task Force on Practice Guidelines (writing committee to revise the 1998 Guidelines for the Management of Patients With Valvular Heart Disease). Circulation 2006;114:e84–e231.

123. Bonow RO, Rosing DR, McIntosh CL, et al. The natural history of asymptomatic patients with aortic regurgitation and normal left ventricular function. Circulation 1983;68:509–15.

124. Scognamiglio R, Fasoli G, Dalla Volta S. Progression of myocardial dysfunction in asymptomatic patients with severe aortic insufficiency. Clin Cardiol 1986;9:151–6.

125. Siemienczuk D, Greenberg B, Morris C, et al. Chronic aortic insufficiency: factors associated with progression to aortic valve replacement. Ann Intern Med 1989;110:587–92.

126. Scognamiglio R, Rahimtoola SH, Fasoli G, et al. Nifedipine in asymptomatic patients with severe aortic regurgitation and normal left ventricular function. N Engl J Med 1994;331:689–94.

127. Tornos MP, Olona M, Permanyer-Miralda G, et al. Clinical outcome of severe asymptomatic chronic aortic regurgitation: a long term prospective follow up study. Am Heart J 1995;130:333–9.

128. Ishii K, Hirota Y, Suwa M, et al. Natural history and left ventricular response in chronic aortic regurgitation. Am J Cardiol 1996;78:357–61.

129. Borer JS, Hochreiter C, Herrold E, et al. Prediction of indications for valve replacement among asymptomatic or minimally symptomatic patients with chronic aortic regurgitation and normal left ventricular performance. Circulation 1998;97:525–34.

130. Tarasoutchi F, Grinberg M, Spina GS, et al. Ten year clinical laboratory follow up after application of a symptom-based therapeutic strategy to patients with severe aortic regurgitation of predominant rheumatic etiology. J Am Coll Cardiol 2003;41:1316–24.

131. Detaint D, Messika-Zeitoun D, Maalouf J, et al. Quantitative echocardiographic determinants of clinical outcome in asymptomatic patients with aortic regurgitation: a prospective study. J Am Coll Cardiol Imaging 2008;1:1–11.

131a. Bonow RO. Chronic mitral regurgitation and aortic regurgitation: have indications for surgery changed? J Am Coll Cardiol 2013;61:693–701.

132. Henry WL, Bonow RO, Rosing DR, et al. Observations on the optimum time for operative intervention for aortic regurgitation. II. Serial echocardiographic evaluation of asymptomatic patients. Circulation 1980;61:484–92.

133. McDonald IG, Jelinck VM. Serial M mode echocardiography in severe aortic regurgitation. Circulation 1980;62:1291–6.

134. Bonow RO. Radionuclide angiography in the management of asymptomatic aortic regurgitation. Circulation 1991;84(suppl I):I-296–I-302.

135. Dujardin KS, Enriquez-Sarano M, Schaff HV, et al. Mortality and morbidity of aortic regurgitation in clinical practice. A long-term follow up study. Circulation 1999;99: 1851–7.

136. Hegglin R, Scheu H, Rothlin M. Aortic insufficiency. Circulation 1968;38:77–92.

137. Rapaport E. Natural history of aortic and mitral valve disease. Am J Cardiol 1975; 35:221–7.

138. Greenberg BH, Massie B, Bristow JD, et al. Long term vasodilator therapy of chronic aortic insufficiency: a randomized double-blinded, placebo controlled clinical trial. Circulation 1988;78:92–103.

139. Schon HR, Dorn R, Barthel P, et al. Effects of 12 month quinapril therapy in asymptomatic patients with chronic aortic regurgitation. J Heart Valve Dis 1994;3:500–9.

140. Sondegaard L, Aldershvile J, Hildebrant P, et al. Vasodilatation with felodipine in chronic asymptomatic aortic regurgitation. Am Heart J 2000;139:667–74.

141. Greenberg BH, DeMots H, Murphy E, et al. Mechanism for improved cardiac performance with arteriolar dilators in aortic insufficiency. Circulation 1981;63:263–8.

142. Greenberg BH, DeMots H, Murphy E, et al. Beneficial effects of hydralazine on rest and exercise hemodynamics in patients with chronic severe aortic insufficiency. Circulation 1980:62:49–55.

143. Fioretti P, Benussi B, Scardi S, et al. Afterload reduction with nifedipine in aortic insufficiency. Am J Cardiol 1982;49:1728–32.

144. Scognamiglio R, Fasoli G, Ponchia A, et al. Long term nifedipine unloading therapy in asymptomatic patients with chronic severe aortic regurgitation. J Am Coll Cardiol 1990;1:424–9.

145. Lin M, Chiang H, Lin S, et al. Vasodilator therapy in chronic asymptomatic aortic regurgitation: enalapril versus hydralazine therapy. J Am Coll Cardiol 1994;24:1046–53.

146. Elder DH, Wei L, Szwejkowski BR, et al. The impact of renin-angiotensin-aldosterone system blockade on heart failure outcomes and mortality in patients identified to have aortic regurgitation: a large population cohort study. J Am Coll Cardiol 2011;58: 2084–91.

147. Sampat U, Varadarajan P, Turk R, et al. Effect of beta-blocker therapy on survival in patients with severe aortic regurgitation results from a cohort of 756 patients. J Am Coll Cardiol 2009;54:452–7.

148. Wilson W, Taubert KA, Gewitz M, et al. Prevention of infective endocarditis. A guideline from the American Heart Association Rheumatic Fever, Endocarditis, and Kawasaki Disease Committee, Council on Cardiovascular Disease in the Young, and the Council on Clinical Cardiology, Council on Cardiovascular Surgery and Anesthesia, and the Quality of Care and Outcomes Research Interdisciplinary Working Group. Circulation 2007;116:1736–54.

149. Weber M, Arnold R, Rau M, et al. Relation of N Terminal pro-B-type natriuretic peptide to progression of aortic valve disease. Eur Heart J 2005;26:1023–30.

150. Eimer MJ, Ekery DL, Rigolin VH, et al. Elevated B type natriuretic peptide in asymptomatic men with chronic aortic regurgitation and preserved left ventricular function. Am J Cardiol 2004;94:676–8.

151. Pizarro R, Bazzino OO, Oberti PF, et al. Prospective validation of the prognostic usefulness of B-type natriuretic peptide in asymptomatic patients with chronic aortic regurgitation. J Am Coll Cardiol 2011;58:1705–14.

152. Jude DP, Dietz HC. Marfan's syndrome. Lancet 2005;366:1965–76.

153. Davies RR, Goldstein LJ, Coady MA, et al. Yearly rupture or dissection rates for thoracic aneurysms: simple prediction based on size. Ann Thorac Surg 2002;73: 1–27.

154. El Khoury G, Vanoverschelde JL, Glineur D, et al. Repair of bicuspid aortic valves in patients with aortic regurgitation. Circulation 2006;114(suppl I):I-610–I-616.

155. Izumoto H, Kawazoe K, Oka T, et al. Aortic valve repair for aortic regurgitation: intermediate-term results in patients with tricuspid morphology. J Heart Valve Dis 2006;15:163–73.

156. Boodhwani M, de Kerchove L, Glineur D, et al. Repair-oriented classification of aortic insufficiency: impact on surgical techniques and clinical outcomes. J Thorac Cardiovasc Surg 2009;137:286–94.

157. Hanke T, Stierle U, Boehm JO, et al. Autograft regurgitation and aortic root dimensions after the Ross procedure: the German Ross Registry experience. Circulation 2007;116 (suppl I):I-251–I-258.

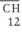

CH
12

158. Chiappini B, Absil B, Rubay J, et al. The Ross procedure: clinical and echocardiographic follow up in 219 consecutive patients. Ann Thorac Surg 2007;83:1285–9.

159. Vahanian A, Alfieri O, Andreotti F, et al. Guidelines on the management of valvular heart disease (version 2012). Joint Task Force on the Management of Valvular Heart Disease of the European Society of Cardiology and the European Association for Cardio-Thoracic Surgery. Eur Heart J 2012;33:2451–96.

160. Dujardin KS, Enriquez-Sarano M, Schaff HV, et al. Mortality and morbidity of aortic regurgitation in clinical practice: a long term follow up study. Circulation 1999;99:1851–7.

161. Bonow RO, Nikas D, Elefteriades JA. Valve replacement for regurgitant lesions of the aortic or mitral valve in advanced left ventricular dysfunction. Cardiol Clin 1995;13:73–83.

162. Nishimura RA, McGoon MD, Schaff HV, et al. Chronic aortic regurgitation: indications for operation 1988. Mayo Clin Proc 1988;63:270–80.

163. Carabello BA. The changing unnatural history of valvular regurgitation. Ann Thorac surg 1992;53:191–9.

164. Gaasch WH, Sundaram M, Meyer TE. Managing asymptomatic patients with chronic aortic regurgitation. Chest 1997;111:1702–9.

165. Bonow RO. Chronic aortic regurgitation: role of medical therapy and optimal timing for surgery. Cardiol Clin 1998;16:449–61.

166. Borer JS, Bonow RO. Contemporary approach to aortic and mitral regurgitation. Circulation 2003;108:2432–8.

167. Enriquez-Sarano M, Tajik AJ. Clinical practice: aortic regurgitation. N Engl J Med 2004;351:1539–46.

168. Bonow RO. Chronic mitral regurgitation and aortic regurgitation: have indications for surgery changed? J Am Coll Cardiol 2012 Dec 13. doi:pii: S0735-1097(12)05519-2.

169. Shores J, Berger KR, Murphy EA, et al. Progression of aortic dilatation and the benefit of long term beta-adrenergic blockade in Marfan's Syndrome. N Engl J Med 1994;330:1335–41.

170. Yetman AT, Bornemeier RA, McCrindle BW. Usefulness of enalapril versus propranolol or atenolol for prevention of aortic dilatation in patients with Marfan syndrome. Am J Cardiol 2005;95:1125–7.

171. Habashi JP, Judge DP, Holm TM, et al. Losartan, an AT1 antagonist, prevents aortic aneurysm in a mouse model of Marfan syndrome. Science 2006;312:117–21.

172. Lacro R, Dietz HC, Wruck LM, et al. Rationale and design of a randomized clinical trial of beta-blocker therapy (atenolol) versus angiotensin II receptor blocker therapy (losartan) in individuals with Marfan syndrome. Am Heart J 2007;154:624–31.

173. Radonic T, de Witte P, Baars MJH, et al; and COMPARE study group. Losartan therapy in adults with Marfan syndrome: study protocol of the multicenter randomized controlled COMPARE trial. Trials 2010;11:1–3.

174. Silverman DI, Gray J, Roman MJ, et al. Family history of severe cardiovascular disease in Marfan syndrome associated with increased aortic diameter and decreased survival. J Am Coll Cardiol 1995;26:1062–7.

175. Davies RR, Gallo A, Coady MA, et al. Novel measurements of relative aortic size predicts rupture of thoracic aortic aneurysm. Ann Thorac Surg 2006;81:169–77.

176. Davies RR, Goldstein LJ, Coady MA, et al. Yearly rupture or dissection rates for thoracic aortic aneurysms: simple prediction based on size. Ann Thorac Surg 2002;73:17–27.

177. Bonow RO. Bicuspid aortic valves and dilated aortas: a critical review of the critical review of the ACC/AHA guidelines recommendations. Am J Cardiol 2008;102:111–14.

CHAPTER 13

The Bicuspid Aortic Valve and Associated Aortic Disease

Alan C. Braverman

Key Points

- The bicuspid valve is one of the most common congenital heart conditions affecting about 1% of the population.
- Familial occurrence of a bicuspid aortic valve is noted in 9% of first-degree relatives. Familial aortic aneurysm with or without a bicuspid aortic valve may occur in certain families.
- Bicuspid aortic valve may accompany other congenital cardiovascular defects. Individuals with bicuspid valve and coarctation of the aorta are at increased risk of aortic complications.
- When transthoracic echocardiography is not diagnostic, transesophageal echocardiography, cardiac magnetic resonance imaging, or cardiac computed tomography may be useful in diagnosing bicuspid aortic valve disease.
- Approximately 50% of severe aortic stenosis in adults is related to the bicuspid aortic valve.
- Ascending aortic dilation occurs frequently in bicuspid aortic valve disease, even in the absence of aortic stenosis or regurgitation.
- The aortopathy of bicuspid aortic valve disease is associated with cystic medial degeneration, alternations in signaling pathways and matrix metalloproteinase activity, and apoptosis, placing the patient with bicuspid aortic valve (BAV) at increased risk for aortic aneurysm and aortic dissection.
- Abnormal aortic systolic blood flow patterns and aortic wall stress may contribute to the aortopathy in bicuspid aortic valve disease.
- Most patients with bicuspid aortic valves will require surgical therapy on the valve and/or aorta during their lifetime.
- After bicuspid aortic valve replacement, the patient remains at risk for late ascending aortic complications including aneurysm formation and dissection. Surveillance of the aortic valve late after bicuspid aortic valve replacement is necessary.

The bicuspid aortic valve (BAV) is one of the most common congenital heart disorders, affecting approximately 1% of the population and occurring either in isolation or in association with complex congenital heart defects. BAV disease may be sporadic, inherited as an autosomal dominant condition with incomplete penetrance, or associated with aortic aneurysm syndromes. BAV disease often leads to aortic stenosis and regurgitation at variable intervals and is associated with an increased risk for infective endocarditis. Aortopathy may accompany BAV disease, leading to ascending aortic enlargement, aneurysm formation, and aortic dissection. In the majority of people with a BAV, complications from the valve and/or ascending aorta develop during their lifetimes, so lifelong surveillance of the aortic valve and aorta is required, along with surgical intervention for many of them. Discoveries in gene expression and signaling pathways, advances in imaging, and improvements in aortic and valve surgery have dramatically improved the understanding and management of BAV and associated aortic disease, as summarized in this chapter.

History of the Bicuspid Aortic Valve

The BAV has been long recognized as an important cause of valvular heart disease. Leonardo da Vinci sketched the bicuspid variant of the aortic valve more than 400 years ago.[1] The clinical and valvular sequelae of the BAV were realized more than 150 years ago.[1,2] Osler's landmark report of 18 cases of BAV in 1886 emphasized the frequent complication of infective endocarditis in this lesion.[1,2] The fact that aortic stenosis occurred in BAV as a result of a primary valve pathology rather than rheumatic disease was realized in the 1950s.[1,2] Autopsy studies established BAV as the most common congenital anomaly of the heart. The association of congenital BAV with diseases of the aorta was first recorded by Abbott[3] in 1927. In 1984, Larson and Edwards[4] highlighted the relationship between the BAV and aortic root disease, noting a ninefold greater risk of aortic dissection in patients with BAV.[4]

Widespread performance of cardiac imaging has clarified the prevalence of BAV in the general population. Discoveries in molecular genetics and vascular biology have begun to elucidate basic mechanisms of BAV and the aortopathy associated with it.

Embryology

The semilunar valves originate from the mesenchymal outgrowths (cardiac cushions) along the ventricular outflow tract of the primary heart tube. Endocardial cushion formation has been studied in many different species, and several molecular signaling pathways have been implicated in the development of the atrioventricular and outflow tract regions, including transforming growth factor-beta (TGF-β), Ras, Wnt/B-catenin, vascular endothelial growth factor (VEGF), and *NOTCH* signaling.[5,6]

The pathogenesis of BAV is unknown. In a Syrian hamster model of BAV, fusion of the right and the left valve cushions appears to be a key factor, and BAV is not the consequence of improper development of the conotruncal ridges, conotruncal malseptation, or valve cushion agenesis.[7] Anomalous behavior of cells derived from the neural crest has been implicated as a possible etiology because BAV is often associated with congenital malformations of the aortic arch and other neural crest-derived systems.[1,8,9] A primary molecular abnormality of the extracellular matrix may trigger abnormal valvulogenesis, given that matrix proteins help direct cell differentiation and cusp formation during valvulogenesis.[10] Endothelial nitric oxide (eNOS) signaling may be important in BAV pathogenesis and possibly in the associated aortic disease.[11,12]

Different molecular and biologic pathways may be responsible for leaflet orientation among animal species with BAV (Figure 13-1). In knockout mice, fused right and noncoronary leaflet BAVs result from a defective development of the cardiac outflow tract endocardial cushions that may rely on a nitric oxide–dependent epithelial-to-mesenchymal transformation.[9] In inbred Syrian hamsters, fused right and left coronary leaflet BAVs are due to an extrafusion of the septal and parietal outflow tract ridges likely caused by a distorted behavior of neural crest cells.[9]

The GATA family of zinc finger proteins may be important in cardiac development. *Gata5* expression is restricted to endocardial cushions, and targeted inactivation of *Gata5* in mice leads to development of BAV, involving several signaling pathways (including Notch).[13] The ubiquitin fusion degradation 1–like gene is expressed in the developing embryonic outflow tract and is downregulated in BAV tissue.[14]

NOTCH1 encodes for a transmembrane protein that activates a signaling pathway important in cardiac embryogenesis, including the aortic and pulmonary valve and aorta. *NOTCH1* mutations (9q34.3) have been found in a small number of families with BAV and ascending aortic aneurysms.[5]

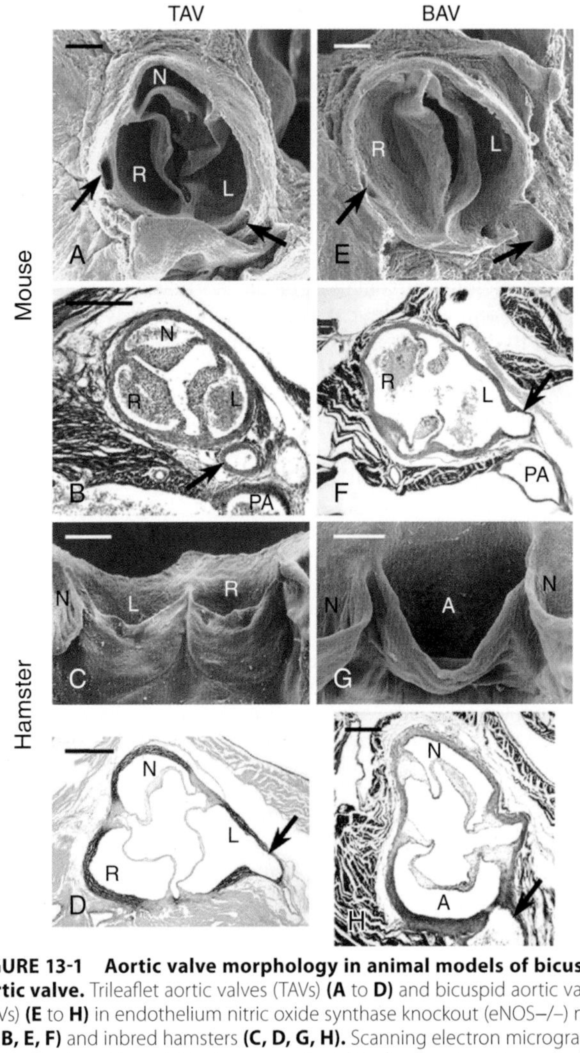

Anatomy, Pathology, and Classification Schemes

The anatomy of the BAV includes unequal cusp size (due to fusion of two cusps leading to one larger cusp), a raphe (usually in the center of the larger of the two cusps), and smooth cusp margins (Figure 13-2). The raphe or fibrous ridge is the site of congenital fusion of the two components of the conjoined cusps and is identifiable in most cases.[15] There is a wide spectrum of BAV, from completely missing one commissure—leading to two cusps, sinuses, and commissures only—to an underdevelopment of one or two commissures and the adjacent cusps, which occurs in the majority of cases with one or two raphes.[16] Fusion may occur between any of the leaflets, most commonly between the right and left coronary leaflets (70% to 86%), although also between the right and noncoronary leaflets (12%), and least commonly between the left and noncoronary leaflets (3%).[1] With right and left coronary leaflet fusion, the leaflets are oriented right and left and the true commissures are oriented in an anterior and posterior manner.[17] The coronary arteries tend to arise from the front

FIGURE 13-1 Aortic valve morphology in animal models of bicuspid aortic valve. Trileaflet aortic valves (TAVs) **(A** to **D)** and bicuspid valves (BAVs) **(E** to **H)** in endothelium nitric oxide synthase knockout (eNOS–/–) mice **(A, B, E, F)** and inbred hamsters **(C, D, G, H)**. Scanning electron micrographs, cranial **(A, E)** and frontal **(C, G)** views. In **C** and **G,** the specimens were opened through the noncoronary aortic sinus to show the anterior aspect of the valve. Transverse sections stained with Mallory trichrome **(B, F),** Masson-Goldner trichrome **(H),** and orcein-picrofuchsin **(D)** stains. The *arrows* point to the coronary arteries. In the mouse BAVs, *R* indicates the right aortic sinus supporting the fused right and noncoronary leaflets. Bars = 200 µm **(A, B, E, F)** and 400 µm **(C, D, G, H).** *A*, Aortic sinus supporting the fused right and left coronary leaflets; *L*, left aortic sinus; *N*, noncoronary sinus; *PA*, pulmonary artery; *R*, right aortic sinus. *(Reproduced with permission from Fernandez B, Duran AC, Fernandez-Gallego T, et al. Bicuspid aortic valves with different spatial orientations of the leaflets are distinct etiological entities. J Am Coll Cardiol 2009;54:2312–18.)*

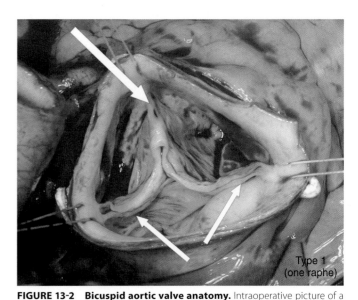

FIGURE 13-2 Bicuspid aortic valve anatomy. Intraoperative picture of a bicuspid aortic valve type 1 (left-right cusp fusion) with one completely developed noncoronary cusp, two completely developed commissures *(small arrows)*, and one raphe between the underdeveloped left and right coronary cusps extending to the corresponding malformed commissures *(large arrow)*, with hemodynamic signs of regurgitation due to prolapse of the conjoint cusps. *(Reproduced with permission from Sievers HH, Schmidtke C. A classification system for the bicuspid aortic valve from 304 surgical specimens. J Thorac Cardiovasc Surg 2007;133:1226–33.)*

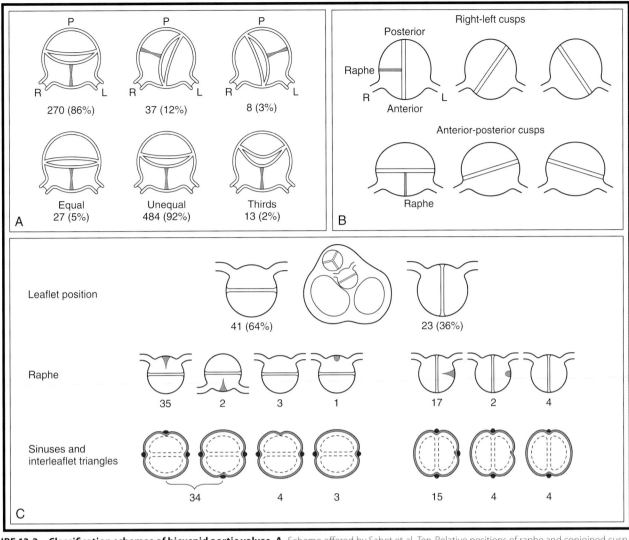

FIGURE 13-3 **Classification schemes of bicuspid aortic valves. A,** Scheme offered by Sabet et al. *Top,* Relative positions of raphe and conjoined cusp in 315 bicuspid aortic valves. *Bottom,* Relative cusp sizes in 524 valves (data not available in 18 of 542 cases). *L,* Left; *P,* posterior; *R,* right. **B,** Classification from Roberts,[2] based on 85 autopsy cases. **C,** Angelini et al (Angelini A, Ho SY, Anderson RH, et al. The morphology of the normal aortic valve as compared with the aortic valve having two leaflets. J Thorac Cardiovasc Surg 1989;98:362-367.) The positions of the raphe and cusps, the relative sizes of cusps, as well as the number of sinuses and interleaflet triangles as described from the left ventricular outflow were main but not uniform determinants for classifying bicuspid aortic valves. *(From Sievers HH, Schmidtke C. A classification system for the bicuspid aortic valve from 304 surgical specimens. J Thorac Cardiovasc Surg 2007;133:1226–33.)*

of the cusps, in which a raphe is present. BAVs without any redundant tissue tend to develop stenosis, whereas valves with more redundant tissue usually develop valvular incompetence.[1]

Various classification schemes have been used to characterize the BAV[16,18] (Figure 13-3). A review of echocardiograms of 1135 children with BAV revealed that in 70% of cases, right coronary and left coronary leaflet fusion was the most common morphologic variant (pattern A).[19] Pattern B, or the fusion of the right coronary and noncoronary leaflet, was more likely to be associated with aortic stenosis or regurgitation in this pediatric series. Pattern C (fusion of the left coronary and noncoronary cusps) was the least common morphologic variant. In a surgical pathology study of 542 cases of BAV, 86% were noted to have pattern A, 12% pattern B, and 3% pattern C.[15]

The valve orientation of a BAV may be predictive of clinical outcomes.[19,20] Fusion of the right and noncoronary valve leaflets has been associated with more rapid progression of aortic stenosis and regurgitation than fusion of the right and left coronary leaflets,[20] although later population studies did not demonstrate an association of leaflet orientation with valvular degeneration.[21,22] In addition, leaflet orientation in BAV may also be predictive of aortic elastic properties.[23]

Calcium deposition and the development of fibrosis of the BAV increases with age and is largely confined to the raphe and base of the cusp[2,24] (Figure 13-4). The calcification process occurring in patients with BAV is similar to that in those with trileaflet aortic valve but occurs at an accelerated rate and includes lipid deposition, neoangiogenesis, and inflammatory cell infiltration.[1,25] BAVs demonstrate folding or wrinkling of the valve tissue, increased doming of the leaflets during the cardiac cycle, and abnormal currents of turbulence, even when the leaflets are not stenotic.[26] These factors may increase susceptibility to BAV degeneration. As a result of multiple mechanisms, most patients with BAV require valve surgery during their lifetimes.[24,27]

Prevalence

The prevalence of BAV is approximately 1% of the population with a male/female ratio of between 2:1 and 3:1.[1,2,28-31] (Table 13-1). In the largest reported necropsy series involving 21,417 consecutive cases, 293 subjects were noted to have BAV, for a prevalence rate of 1.37%.[31]

Echocardiography screening has improved understanding of the prevalence of BAV in the general population. In an

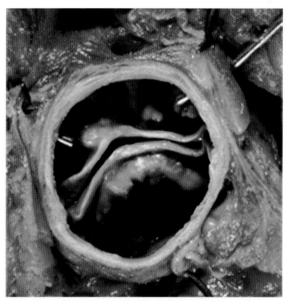

FIGURE 13-4 Pathologic specimen of a bicuspid aortic valve with calcification of the leaflets. Probes are present in the coronary arteries. *(Photograph courtesy Dr. Jeffrey Saffitz.)*

TABLE 13-1	Prevalence of Bicuspid Aortic Valve (BAV) in Reported Necropsy Studies		
AUTHOR(S)	**YEAR**	**STUDY POPULATION (N)**	**BAV PREVALENCE (%)**
Olser	1886	800	1.2
Lewis and Grant	1923	215	1.39
Wauchope	1928	9,966	0.5
Grant et al	1928	1,350	0.89
Gross	1937	5,000	0.56
Roberts	1970	1,440	0.9
Larson and Edwards	1984	21,417	1.37
Datta et al	1988	8,800	0.59
Pauperio et al	1999	2,000	0.65

Adapted from Basso C, Boschello M, Perrone C, et al. An echocardiographic survey of primary school children for bicuspid aortic valve. Am J Cardiol 2004;93:661–3. See the paper by Basso et al for the full citations for the studies listed in this table.

echocardiography study of 817 asymptomatic children, a BAV was found in 4 of the 817 children (0.5%), 3 of 4 being found in males.[29] In an echocardiography study of 1075 neonates, the prevalence of BAV was 4.6 per 1000 live births (7.1 per 1000 males and 1.9 per 1000 females).[32] Of 20,946 military recruits in Italy, the prevalence of BAV was 0.8%.[33] This may be an underestimation, as only those with an abnormal history, physical examination, or ECG underwent screening echocardiograms.[33]

Certain patients have a much higher prevalence of BAV than the general population, including approximately 50% of patients with coarctation of the aorta[1] and 30% of females with Turner syndrome.[34,35]

Genetics

Case reports describing the familial clustering of BAV and reports of BAVs in monozygotic twins underscored the genetic predisposition for BAV.[36-39] In a study of 41 families with surgically proven BAV in one member, 15% of the families were noted to have more than one member with BAV.[39] In families in which more than one member had aortic valve disease, 24% of relatives had evidence of aortic valve disease, likely secondary to a BAV.[40] Echocardiographic studies in families of patients with BAV report the prevalence of BAV in first-degree relatives of an individual with BAV to be about 9%.[41,42] With the use of variance component analysis, the heritability (h^2) of BAV was calculated to be 89%.[42] The inheritance of BAV is consistent with an autosomal dominant pattern with reduced penetrance.[41,42] Diverse genes with dissimilar inheritance patterns in families are considered responsible.[42]

The specific gene loci or products, whether structural proteins or ones with vital roles in cardiac development, that are responsible for the development of BAVs have yet to be discovered. Nongenetic factors also play an important role in this development.[43] In animal models with BAV, potential mechanisms and pathways have been reported in eNOS, NKX2.5, and *NOTCH* signaling.[5]

Human studies have demonstrated the genetic influences on left-sided outflow lesions, including hypoplastic left heart syndrome (HLHS) and BAV.[5] An increased prevalence of BAV in probands and family members of patients with HLHS is recognized, and linkage analysis demonstrates that some cases of HLHS and BAV are genetically related.[44,45] In a study evaluating the first-degree relatives of pediatric patients with left ventricular outflow tract obstruction, 20% of families had another individual with a cardiac anomaly, most commonly a BAV.[46] DiGeorge and velocardiofacial syndromes, involving deletions within chromosome 22q11.2, have been associated with concomitant BAV. Gene network analysis techniques have identified $AXIN_1$-$PDIA_2$ and endoglin haplotypes associated with BAV.[47] Anderson syndrome, due to a mutation in *KCNJ2* and associated with abnormal potassium signaling, is associated with an increased prevalence of BAV.[48]

NOTCH1 mutations have been found in a small number of families with nonsyndromic BAV or with BAV and ascending aortic aneurysms[5] (see later section Familial Bicuspid Aortic Valve and Ascending Aortic Aneurysm). Because of the familial nature of BAV, screening of first-degree relatives for BAV has been recommended in the 2008 American College of Cardiology/American Heart Association (ACC/AHA) guidelines for the management of adults with congenital heart disease.[49]

Associated Cardiovascular Lesions

In most instances, BAV is an isolated cardiovascular finding. However, BAV may coexist with a number of other congenital cardiovascular defects or syndromes (Table 13-2). The presence of a BAV may account for significant morbidity associated with these syndromes and should trigger an evaluation for related cardiovascular disorders. Conversely, the presence of any of the lesions discussed here should also prompt further search for the presence of BAV.

Coarctation of the Aorta

Coarctation of the aorta (CoA) can be either "simple" (isolated defect) or "complex" (associated with other intracardiac or extracardiac defects). A BAV occurs in 25-75% of complex aortic coarctation. The BAV accompanying CoA has been described as "equally bicuspid" with two symmetric sinuses of Valsalva.[1] Morphologic analysis of the BAV has demonstrated an increased frequency of fusion of the left and right coronary cusps in the presence of CoA.[50] Identification of BAV in patients with coarctation is vital because its presence confers a substantially increased risk for aortic aneurysm and dissection[3,25,51,52] (Figure 13-5). In addition, valvular complications from the BAV such as aortic stenosis and regurgitation are more prevalent in subjects with both CoA and BAV.[51]

Individuals with BAV require long-term follow-up not only of the coarctation repair but also of the BAV and ascending aorta.[51-53] In one large series of patients with surgical coarctation repair, 41%

TABLE 13-2	Bicuspid Aortic Valve (BAV) and Associated Cardiovascular Conditions	
CONDITION	**INCIDENCE OF BAV (%)**	**COMMENTS**
Coarctation of the aorta (CoA)	50	BAV confers increased risk of aortic complications
Turner syndrome	30	Most frequent cardiac abnormality Right-left cusp fusion most common
Supravalvular aortic stenosis	30	Usually part of William syndrome BAV associated with higher risk of reoperation
Subvalvular aortic stenosis	23	May result in significant aortic regurgitation
Patent ductus arteriosus	Unknown	Usually diagnosed in childhood/infancy
Sinus of Valsalva aneurysm	15-20	Frequently asymptomatic Most commonly involves right coronary sinus
Ventricular septal defect	30	May result in significant aortic regurgitation
Shone complex	60-85	Series of left-sided obstructive lesions (supravalvular mitral ring, parachute mitral valve, subaortic stenosis, CoA)
Ascending aortic dilation	Common	BAV is one of the most common associates of a dilated ascending aorta
Aortic aneurysm syndromes:		
Loeys-Dietz syndrome	2.5-17	*TGFBR1* or *TGFBR2* mutations
Familial thoracic aortic aneurysm syndrome	3	*ACTA2* mutations

of those who needed reoperation did so primarily for valvular indications.[53] Such patients should undergo meticulous follow-up with routine echocardiographic and radiographic assessment.

Turner Syndrome

Turner syndrome is characterized by complete or partial absence of one X chromosome. About 50% of cases are due to the 45,XO karyotype, and the remainder are due to 45,XO/XX mosaicism or other X chromosomal abnormalities.[35] Cardiovascular defects occur in up to 75% of patients with Turner syndrome.[54] BAV is present in about 30% of cases,[35,54,55] and associated defects include ascending aortic dilation, aortic coarctation, pseudocoarctation and elongated aortic arch.[54-56]

In patients with Turner syndrome, BAV is most commonly due to fusion of right and left coronary cusps. The presence of BAV is associated with larger aortic dimensions at the annulus, sinuses, sinotubular junction, and ascending aorta.[35] Patients with Turner syndrome may have a shortened life expectancy, death most commonly occurring from cardiovascular causes.[1,56] Because patients with Turner syndrome have short stature, ascending aortic dimensions may be significantly dilated relative to body surface area. Because of the small stature of such patients, prophylactic aortic surgery is recommended at smaller aortic dimensions, and the aortic size should be indexed to body surface area.[56,57] Screening for BAV and other cardiovascular abnormalities as well as serial echocardiographic and radiographic follow-up evaluations is necessary in patients with Turner syndrome.

Associated Congenital Heart Malformations

Other congenital heart diseases and syndromes commonly associated with BAV are listed in Table 13-2.[1]

Coronary Artery Anomalies

Congenital coronary anomalies have been described in association with BAV, with left coronary artery dominance in 24% to

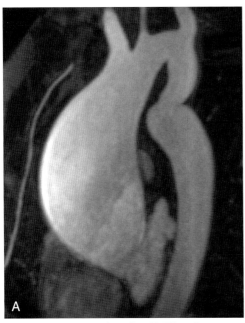 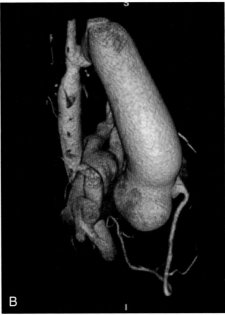

FIGURE 13-5 **Cardiac magnetic resonance imaging (CMR) and computed tomography (CT) of the aorta in patients with a bicuspid aortic valve and coarctation of the aorta (CoA). A,** CMR of ascending aortic aneurysm in patient with unrepaired mild CoA who died suddenly from an aortic wall rupture. **B,** Three-dimensional image on multidetector CT scan of posterior sinus of Valsalva aneurysm in patient with stented CoA. *(From Oliver JM, Alonso-Gonzalez R, Gonzalez AE, et al. Risk of aortic root or ascending aorta complications in patients with bicuspid aortic valve with and without coarctation of the aorta. Am J Cardiol 2009;104:1001–6.)*

57%.[1,14,58] Additionally, patients with BAV have shorter left main coronary arteries than patients with a trileaflet aortic valve.[58] Isolated congenital coronary artery anomalies have also been reported with BAV.[1,59] These features should lead one to consider evaluation of the coronary anatomy prior to elective valve surgery with either catheter-based or computed tomography (CT) coronary angiography to prevent coronary injury and provide for adequate intraoperative myocardial protection.

Clinical Presentation and Imaging

Physical Examination

The clinical examination of the patient with BAV is variable and depends on the function of the valve and any associated lesions. The majority of young patients with isolated BAV are asymptomatic and are diagnosed incidentally when a systolic ejection sound or murmur is noted or on echocardiography. A functionally normal BAV has an ejection sound or "click" and is often followed by an early peaking systolic flow murmur. The ejection sound is a reflection of the sudden cephalad movement of the dome-shaped bicuspid valve in systole and generally correlates with valve leaflet mobility.[1]

In the setting of progressive aortic stenosis, the ejection murmur becomes harsher and later peaking. It is accompanied by a displaced and sustained left ventricular (LV) impulse and decreased arterial pulses. The ejection sound diminishes as the valve cusps become more immobile. In the setting of an incompetent BAV, the findings vary with the severity of lesion. An ejection sound typically is present with mild to moderate aortic regurgitation (AR) and absent when regurgitation is severe.[1,60] With significant AR, a typical early diastolic decrescendo murmur is best heard at the left lower sternal border. When the murmur of AR is heard loudest at the right midsternal border, concern should arise about the presence of a dilated ascending aorta complicating the BAV.

Give the frequent association of BAV with other cardiovascular lesions, routine physical examination should include auscultation for the presence of ventricular septal defect (VSD) and CoA, including a careful vascular examination.

Chest Radiography

The chest radiograph may provide significant clues as to the presence of BAV and any sequelae related to valvular complications or associated vascular lesions. However, the findings may be entirely unremarkable. Aortic valve calcification may be detected on the plain film and is best seen on the lateral projection.[61] A complete or partial ring with or without a calcified central raphe characterizes the distinctive pattern of calcification of the BAV. In general, LV size remains normal unless advanced heart failure is present.[60,61] In the setting of chronically regurgitant BAV, an enlarged cardiac silhouette may be noted. The chest radiograph is notoriously inadequate to detect dilation of the aortic root. On occasion, a dilated aortic shadow may be present. When aortic coarctation is associated with BAV, rib notching and convexity of the proximal descending aorta are often seen.[60]

Transthoracic Echocardiography

In light of the clinical significance of BAV, echocardiographic identification and characterization are imperative. A number of distinct features of the BAV seen on transthoracic echocardiography (TTE) assist in making this diagnosis[1,18] (Table 13-3). Care must be taken to assess the valve in both systole and diastole (see Chapter 6). In patients with a prominent raphe, the valve may appear trileaflet in diastole, but the distinct elliptical or "football-shaped" orifice is visualized in systole, indicating that the raphe is not a functional commissure (Figure 13-6A and 6B).

TABLE 13-3	Echocardiographic Features of the Bicuspid Aortic Valve
Systolic doming	
Eccentric valve closure	
Leaflet redundancy	
Presence of raphe (often calcified)	
Elliptical ("football"-shaped) systolic orifice	
Distinct opening pattern: opens from the center and separates at the commissures in a curvilinear fashion	
Eccentric jets of aortic regurgitation	
Dilated ascending aorta	

The leaflets of a BAV are often thickened and calcified out of proportion to the patient's age. Prominent systolic doming of the leaflets and eccentric valve closure are often noted on the parasternal long-axis view[1,18] (Figure 13-6C and 6E). It is noteworthy that up to 25% of BAVs may not demonstrate eccentric closure, and conversely, trileaflet valves may infrequently have eccentric closure. The presence of leaflet redundancy on parasternal and apical long-axis views should suggest the presence of a BAV. Unexplained eccentric jets of AR may also suggest an underlying BAV.

Valvular calcification is a function of age, increasing significantly after age 40 years. It is important to note that significant calcification may limit the degree of systolic doming and additionally give the appearance of a stenotic trileaflet valve on short-axis views.

When poor acoustic windows or technical limitations prohibit adequate leaflet visualization, the opening pattern of the valve may aid in the diagnosis. The BAV tends to open from the center and separate at the commissures in a curvilinear fashion, like a rope going slack from the center,[62] whereas the leaflets of a normal aortic valve maintain a straighter shape in diastole, pivoting from their point of annular insertion.

In the diagnosis of BAV, TTE has a sensitivity of 78% to 92% and a specificity of 96%,[18,63] but the accuracy depends on image quality, valve calcification, and the experience of the interpreter. Heavy calcification limits the ability to discern leaflet number accurately. A prominent raphe may often give the appearance of a third coaptation line, suggesting a trileaflet valve. Conversely, the aortic valve may appear bicuspid when one of the cusps is diminutive.[62] Ascending aortic enlargement should trigger a careful evaluation for a BAV[54,64] (Figure 13-7). Because aortic dilation is frequently largest in the ascending aorta, the entire aspect of the aortic root and proximal ascending aorta should be imaged to insure accurate assessment of the aortic dimensions.[1,57,65]

VALVULAR COMPLICATIONS

Once BAV is detected, the echocardiogram should include a formal assessment for valvular complications. Aortic stenosis tends to occur at a younger age than trileaflet valve, particularly when the aortic cusps are asymmetric or there is fusion of the right and left cusps.[24] Because of the eccentric nature of the systolic jet, interrogation of the jet via the right parasternal window may yield the highest gradients. Patients with BAV often have larger LV outflow tracts. Therefore, use of the continuity equation may yield larger calculated valve areas, potentially underestimating the hemodynamic severity. The use of serial gradients and velocity time integral ratios may more accurately reflect the hemodynamic burden in these patients.[66]

AR may be the main clinical manifestation of BAV in the adolescent or young adult. The jets of BAV AR may be highly eccentric, making severity more difficult to assess. Multiple mechanisms may lead to AR in BAV (see Aortic Regurgitation).

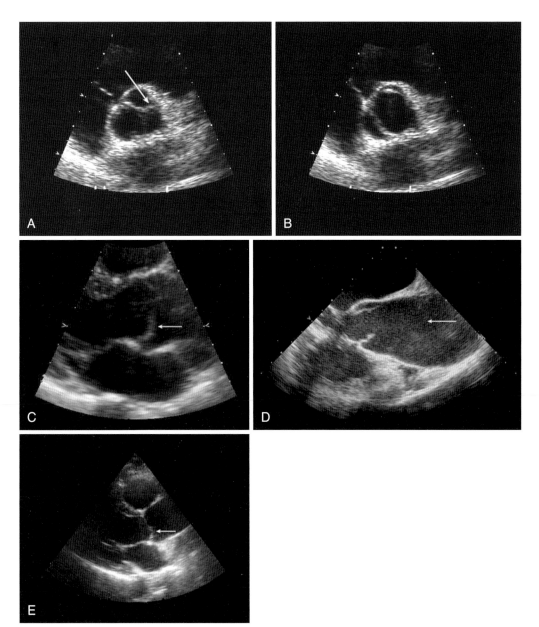

FIGURE 13-6 **Transthoracic echocardiography of bicuspid aortic valve. A,** Short-axis view of the bicuspid aortic valve in diastole, demonstrating asymmetrical sinuses and a raphe *(arrow)*. **B,** Bicuspid aortic valve in systole with elliptical opening pattern. **C,** Long axis view showing prominent systolic doming of the aortic valve leaflets *(arrow)*. **D,** Dilated ascending aorta *(arrow)*, **E,** Eccentric closure of the aortic valve *(arrow* denotes coaptation point).

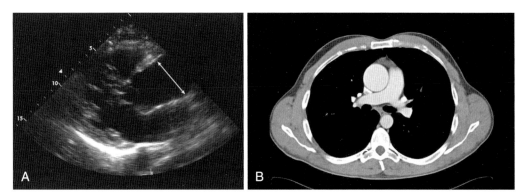

FIGURE 13-7 **Aortic root aneurysm complicating a "functionally normal" bicuspid aortic valve. A,** Transthoracic echocardiogram of a 4.9-cm ascending aorta *(line* denotes ascending aortic aneurysm). **B,** Corresponding computed tomography (CT) scan of the aortic root aneurysm.

ASSOCIATED LESIONS

When a BAV is present, the echocardiographic examination should include a routine evaluation for the presence of coexisting cardiovascular lesions (see Table 13-2). Care should be taken to assess for the presence of VSD, aortic coarctation, and aortic root and ascending aortic pathology (sinus of Valsalva aneurysm, supravalvular aortic stenosis, aneurysm, aortic dissection), and LV outflow tract abnormalities. The standard examination should include an interrogation of the distal aortic arch via suprasternal notch views to assess for the presence of coarctation.

Transesophageal Echocardiography

In a subset of patients the morphology of the aortic valve cannot be accurately determined by transthoracic echocardiogram. Transesophageal echocardiography (TEE) is useful in such cases for diagnosis of BAV. Multiplane TEE is highly accurate at detecting BAV, with reported sensitivity of 87% and specificity of 91%[67] (Figure 13-8). The sensitivity of TEE approaches 100% when little valvular calcification is present. In the presence of moderate to severe valvular calcification, sensitivity is lower.[68]

TEE also provides vital information in patients with BAV with coexisting cardiovascular malformations, including aortic abnormalities (ascending aortic aneurysm and dissection, sinus of Valsalva aneurysm, supravalvular stenosis), outflow tract defects (subvalvular stenosis, membranous VSD), and valvular complications (aortic stenosis, regurgitation, and endocarditis).

Other Imaging Approaches

Cardiovascular magnetic resonance (CMR) and CT imaging represent vital noninvasive modalities in addition to standard echocardiography in the diagnosis and management of BAV. CT has a high sensitivity (94%) and specificity (100%) for detecting BAVs.[69] CMR is also highly accurate in diagnosing BAV, with a sensitivity of 100% and specificity of 95%[70] (Figure 13-9).

In a study comparing CT, CMR, and TTE in patients undergoing valve surgery, both CT and CMR were highly accurate for identifying aortic valve morphology.[71] Sensitivities, specificities, and positive and negative predictive values for aortic valve morphology assessment (trileaflet versus bicuspid) were: 97%, 95%, 98%, and 94% for CT angiography; 98%, 96%, 98%, and 95% for CMR; and 98%, 88%, 95%, and 96% for TTE.[71] CT has been shown to accurately identify BAV and assess aortic valve area via planimetry when compared with CMR, TEE, and TTE.[72,73] CMR correlates well with both echocardiographic and invasive catheter-based techniques for evaluation of stenotic and regurgitant valvular lesions.[72] CMR may also accurately assess BAV morphology on the basis of the orientation of leaflets and raphes.[74]

CT angiography and CMR are also important diagnostic modalities in the assessment of associated vascular complications and congenital lesions, many of which are suboptimally visualized and defined by standard echocardiography. Routine CMR or CT follow-up is warranted in the presence of aortic root aneurysm and coarctation.

Disease Course and Outcomes

Complications will develop in the majority of patients with BAV during their lifetimes,[1,21,22,24] including aortic valve dysfunction,

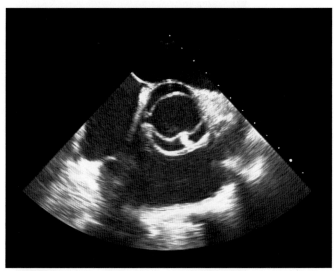

FIGURE 13-8 Transesophageal echocardiogram of a bicuspid aortic valve with a raphe.

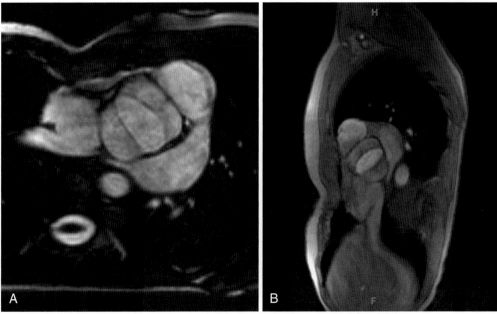

FIGURE 13-9 Cardiac magnetic resonance angiography demonstrating a bicuspid aortic valve. **A,** Short-axis view; **B,** sagittal view.

TABLE 13-4 Late Outcomes in Adults with Bicuspid Aortic Valve (BAV) Disease

	PATIENTS WITH BAV AND NO SIGNIFICANT AORTIC VALVE DYSFUNCTION (N = 212)*	PATIENTS WITH BAV WITH A SPECTRUM OF VALVE FUNCTION (N = 642)†
Mean follow-up, yrs (range)	15 ± 6 (0.4-25)	9 ± 5 (2-26)
Mean age at baseline, yrs	32 ± 20	35 ± 16
Outcomes:		
Overall survival	90 ± 3% at 20 yrs	96 ± 1% at 10 yrs
Cardiac deaths	6.6%	3 ± 1%
Aortic valve or ascending aorta surgery	27 ± 4%	22 ± 2%
Cardiovascular medical events	33 ± 5%	Not available
Aortic dissection	0	2 ± 1%
Hospital admission for heart failure	7 ± 2%	2 ± 1%
Endocarditis	2%	2%
Predictors of outcomes		
Predictors of cardiac events (medical and surgical)	Age ≥50 yrs Valve degeneration	Age >30 yrs Moderate or severe AS or AR

AS, aortic stenosis; AR, aortic regurgitation.
Adapted with permission from Siu SA, Silversides CK. Bicuspid aortic valve disease. J Am Coll Cardiol 2010;55:2789–2800.
*Data from Michelena HI, Desjardins VA, Avierinos JF, et al. Natural history of asymptomatic patients with normally functioning or minimally dysfunctional bicuspid aortic valve in the community. Circulation 2008;117:2776–84. *Cardiovascular medical events* = cardiac death, congestive heart failure, new cardiovascular symptoms (dyspnea, syncope, anginal pain), stroke, and endocarditis. *Surgical events* = aortic valve surgery (aortic valve replacement, repair, or valvotomy) and surgery of the thoracic aorta (for aneurysms, dissection, or coarctation).
†Data from Tzemos N, Therrien J, Yip J, et al. Outcomes in adults with bicuspid aortic valves. JAMA 2008;300:1317–25. *Primary cardiac events* = surgery on the aortic valve or ascending aorta, percutaneous aortic valvotomy, aortic complications (dissection or aneurysm development), congestive heart failure requiring hospital admission or cardiac death.

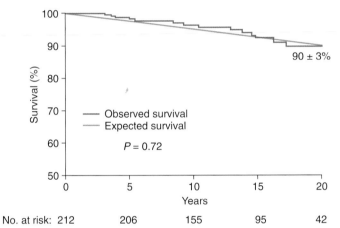

No. at risk: 212   206   155   95   42

FIGURE 13-10 Survival in asymptomatic adults with bicuspid aortic valve with no significant aortic valve dysfunction. *Blue line* represents subjects with bicuspid aortic valve disease compared with an age- and sex-matched control population (*yellow line*). The numbers at the bottom indicate the patients at risk for each interval. The survival (+SE) is indicated 20 years after diagnosis. *(From Michelena HI, Desjardins VA, Avierinos JF, et al. Natural history of asymptomatic patients with normally functioning or minimally dysfunctional bicuspid aortic valve in the community. Circulation 2008;117:2776–84.)*

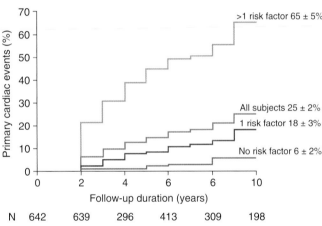

N   642   639   296   413   309   198

FIGURE 13-11 Frequency of adverse cardiac events in adults with bicuspid aortic valve disease stratified according to risk profile. Risk factors included: age >30 years, moderate or severe aortic regurgitation, and moderate or severe aortic stenosis. *(From Tzemos N, Therrien J, Yip J, et al. Outcomes in adults with bicuspid aortic valves. JAMA 2008;300:1317–25 [original content]; and Siu SA, Silversides CK. Bicuspid aortic valve disease. J Am Coll Cardiol 2010;55:2789–2800.)*

endocarditis, and aortic aneurysm or dissection. For some patients the BAV functions nearly normally for much of their lives, whereas for others, a valve disorder or aortic complication occurs early in life[21,22] (Table 13-4). In a population-based study of 212 initially asymptomatic patients with minimally dysfunctional BAV, survival values were 97% ± 1% and 90% ± 3%, 10 and 20 years after diagnosis, respectively, and were identical to expected survival values in the age- and sex-matched population (Figure 13-10).[21] However, the 20-year rate for surgical events (aortic valve or aorta) was 27% ± 4% and the rate for any cardiovascular event was 42% ± 5%.[21] As expected, cardiac events were more common in those with increasing age (>30 years) and moderate to severe valvular dysfunction.

In another study of the natural history of BAV, survival rates in a cohort of 642 adults in a referral-based population were not significantly different from those in the general population (see Table 13-4).[22] Vascular risk factors such as hypertension, cigarette smoking, and hyperlipidemia were associated with worse outcomes among patients with BAV.[21] The age of the patient and presence of valvular dysfunction and aortic aneurysm also predicted adverse clinical outcomes[21,22,75] (Figure 13-11).

Aortic Stenosis

The reported incidence of aortic stenosis complicating BAV in autopsy series has ranged from 15% to 75%.[2,28] Surgical pathology series report the incidence of aortic stenosis for BAV as between 5% and 50%[24,76-78] (see Figure 13-4). In a series of 932 adults with isolated nonrheumatic aortic stenosis, the incidence of BAVs leading to aortic valve replacement (AVR) depended on the age of the patient.[76] Among the 7% of patients undergoing AVR who were younger than 50 years, approximately two thirds had BAV and the other third had a unicuspid aortic valve. Of the 40% of patients undergoing AVR between 50 and 70 years old, two thirds had BAV and one third had TAV. Among the 53% of patients older than 70 years, 40% had BAV.[76] Among octogenarians and nonagenarians undergoing AVR, 22% and 18%, respectively were found to have BAV.[79]

Progression of BAV stenosis is age-related, with fibrosis beginning in the second decade and calcification progressing significantly after the fourth decade.[1,24] The morphology of the BAV as well as traditional risk factors for atherosclerotic disease and gender may play a role in the progression of aortic stenosis in BAV.[1,21]

The valve orientation may be predictive of subsequent valvular pathology. In children and adolescents, fusion of the right and noncoronary cusps (right-left morphology) have been found to be highly correlated with both aortic stenosis and regurgitation, whereas fusion of the right and left cusps (anteroposterior morphology) correlated strongly with presence of aortic coarctation.[20,24] Interestingly, in adults, fusion of right and left coronary cusps may predispose to more rapid progression of aortic stenosis.[24,80] This discrepancy may be due in part to selection bias, in that fewer children with fusion of right and noncoronary cusps reach adulthood without prior surgical correction. However, two later population studies of BAV did not demonstrate any effect of valve leaflet orientation on subsequent valve degeneration.[21,22]

Traditional risk factors for atherosclerosis may play a role in the progression of aortic stenosis in patients with BAV.[21] Valvular calcification, once thought to be a function solely of aging, shares the histologic features of atherosclerotic lesions, namely lipid deposits, neoangiogenesis, and inflammatory cells.[81] Cigarette smoking and hypercholesterolemia are risk factors for progression to severe aortic stenosis.[81,82] Currently there are no studies demonstrating that pharmacologic therapy, with statins or other drugs, alters the natural history of BAV aortic stenosis. The Aortic Stenosis Progression Observation: Measuring Effects of Rosuvastatin (ASTRONOMER) study, in which patients with aortic stenosis underwent statin therapy, did not find any improvement in trileaflet or bicuspid aortic valve stenosis with such therapy.[83] However, a nonrandomized, uncontrolled study using a catheterization laboratory database observed that patients with BAV who were receiving statin therapy had smaller aortic dimensions than patients who were not not.[84]

Stenosis of a bicuspid aortic valve progresses more rapidly than that of a trileaflet valve. Patients with BAV generally undergo surgery for aortic stenosis 5 to 10 years earlier than those with trileaflet valves. Early observational studies showed that one third of initially asymptomatic patients with BAV experience significant valvular deterioration during 2 to 11 years of follow-up.[1,85] Approximately one quarter of patients with BAV without significant valvular stenosis at initial presentation have progressive disease and have undergone valve replacement at 20-year follow-up.[21] Age greater than 50 years and valve degeneration at diagnosis were independent predictors of subsequent aortic valve surgery.

Aortic Regurgitation

Isolated AR in patients with BAV is less common than aortic stenosis, affecting 2% to 10% of patients.[1] Isolated AR may be more common in the child or adolescent. In adults, AR may coexist with stenosis but is often only mild to moderate in severity. While BAV is more common in men than women, isolated AR due to BAV has an even greater male predominance.[15] BAV is considered to be the most common cause of primary aortic valve regurgitation in the developed world.[21]

Multiple mechanisms may lead to AR in BAV disease (Table 13-5). It may be a result of leaflet fibrosis with retraction of the commissural margins of the leaflets, cusp prolapse, aneurysmal root enlargement, aortic dissection, or valvular destruction from endocarditis. Additionally, the presence of a VSD, subaortic membrane, or sinus of Valsalva aneurysm may lead to AR. Prior balloon aortic valvuloplasty in childhood BAV aortic stenosis may lead to AR. Endocarditis accounts for up to 60% of cases of severe BAV

TABLE 13-5	Mechanisms of Aortic Regurgitation in Bicuspid Aortic Valve Disease
Leaflet fibrosis	
Cusp prolapse	
Endocarditis	
Aortic root dilation	
Aortic dissection	
Coexisting congenital defects (ventricular septal defect, subaortic membrane, sinus of Valsalva aneurysm)	
Prior balloon valvotomy	

regurgitation and may be the presenting symptom in patients with previously undiagnosed BAV.[1,86]

Aortic valve replacement for BAV regurgitation occurs much earlier in life (typically at 20 to 50 years of age) than for BAV stenosis. Population studies report AVR for AR in 3% to 6% of patients with BAV.[21,22] In surgical series of patients undergoing AVR because of AR, 15% to 20% are due to BAV-related AR.[15]

Infective Endocarditis

The bicuspid aortic valve, whether related to abnormal leaflet structure and function or turbulent flow across the leaflets, is at risk for infective endocarditis. *Staphylococcus* and *Streptococcus* are the most common microorganisms. Older pathologic studies reported more than one third of aortic valve specimens with endocarditis were BAVs.[30] Although the exact incidence and prevalence are unknown, selected case series reported a 10% to 30% incidence of endocarditis in patients with BAV.[28] The true incidence is likely to be less, and more contemporary estimates place the population risk for endocarditis closer to 3%.[27] Later population studies report an endocarditis incidence of 2% to 3% among patients with BAV.[21,22]

In children, the BAV is one of the most common underlying valve lesions associated with endocarditis. Acute endocarditis may be the initial diagnosis of BAV in previously asymptomatic patients. Endocarditis accounts for up to 60% of cases of severe AR in patients with BAV, most commonly occurring from cusp perforation.[24] BAV endocarditis has a very high complication rate, requiring surgical correction more often than TAV endocarditis.[87] An increased frequency of periannular complications (perivalvular abscess) has been reported in BAV endocarditis than in TAV endocarditis.[88,89] Whether this complication in BAV endocarditis is related to the underlying aortopathy is unknown.

The overall risk of infective endocarditis in BAV is difficult to quantify. Of 642 patients with BAV in one study, endocarditis occurred in 13 patients (2%) over a 9-year follow-up.[22] In an Olmsted County population study, endocarditis occurred in 4 of 212 patients (1.9%) with BAV over a 20-year interval.[21] The lifetime risk for development of endocarditis in patients with congenital aortic stenosis has been estimated at 271 in 100,000 patient-years, whereas the risk in the general population is 5 per 100,000 patient-years.[90] The highest-risk population (patients who have undergone replacement of infected prosthetic valves) have an estimated risk of 2160 per 100,000 patient-years.[90] The ACC/AHA guidelines for the prevention of endocarditis no longer endorse preprocedural antibiotic prophylaxis in the setting of isolated BAV, instead recommending a focus on improved dental care and oral health in patients predisposed to the development of infective endocarditis.[91]

Pregnancy

In general, severe left heart obstruction (symptomatic or not) is poorly tolerated in pregnancy (see Chapter 27). Likewise, severely regurgitant left-sided valve lesions with New York Heart

Association (NYHA) functional class III or IV symptoms are associated with significant peripartal risk.[92]

In the presence of severe congenital aortic stenosis, clinical deterioration and cardiovascular complications have been found in one study to occur in 10% to 30% of pregnancies, accompanied by a high rate of therapeutic abortions, but with a relatively low complication rate among women with only mild to moderate aortic stenosis.[93] Later studies report an overall mortality rate less than 1%.[14] Despite the low to moderate complication rate during pregnancy, up to 40% of mothers with severe aortic stenosis required surgical intervention during short-term follow-up.[93] Sudden clinical deterioration during pregnancy, including worsening heart failure, angina, and arrhythmias, require prompt intervention and are associated with increases in both maternal and fetal risk. Therefore, in women at high risk (severe valvular stenosis or NYHA class III/IV symptoms), pregnancy should be proscribed until surgical correction is achieved.[91] Interventions during pregnancy in the form of balloon aortic valvuloplasty and valve replacement have been reported. Cardiac surgery requiring cardiopulmonary bypass during pregnancy carries a significant risk to the fetus. Pregnancy may also accelerate the need for postpartum surgery in women with significant aortic stenosis.[14]

Women with mild to moderate aortic stenosis or NYHA class I/II symptoms with AR generally tolerate pregnancy well. Parents should be counseled regarding the risk of congenital cardiac defects in their offspring (6% to 7 %).[94]

Pregnancy may predispose to increased risk for aortic pathology as a result of hormone-induced histologic changes in the aortic wall coupled with the hemodynamic stress of pregnancy. The presence of BAV and its concomitant risk for aortic pathology may put some women at risk for aortic complications during pregnancy. In a series of 50 women with aortic dissection during pregnancy, 5 women had BAVs.[95] However, the absolute risk of aortic dissection for women with BAV is very low.[96] There is very little information about the absolute risk of pregnancy in patients with BAV with aortic dilation to guide the patient or physician.[14] Surgery before pregnancy is recommended when the aortic diameter is 5 cm or greater.[49] In the guidelines for adults with congenital heart disease, it has been recommended that women with BAV and aortic diameters larger than 4.5 cm be "counseled about the high risk of pregnancy."[14,49] For those woman with aortic dimension larger than 4 cm or increase in aortic root size during pregnancy, close monitoring is recommended, especially during and up to 3 months after pregnancy. Use of beta-blockers may be beneficial but can result in low birth weight, therefore requiring close monitoring of fetal development. Cesarean section may be warranted in women with significantly dilated aortas.[57] Unfortunately, outcome data are lacking in this area. The presence of CoA may further raise peripartal risk for dissection. In later series, maternal outcomes were satisfactory, with only one dissection reported in a patient with Turner syndrome.[97,98] Nevertheless, pre-pregnancy counseling in addition to thorough evaluation of the coarctation (repaired or not) is warranted.

Associated Abnormalities of the Aortic Wall

Hemodynamics and Flow

The BAV is associated with various disorders of the thoracic aorta, including aortic coarctation and aortic dissection.[1,54] Aortic root dilation has been recognized to be a frequent complication of the BAV, even in the absence of aortic stenosis and regurgitation. The aortic wall abnormality complicating the BAV may occur independently of any hemodynamically significant valvular stenosis or regurgitation.[1,54] However, the relative role of intrinsic aortic wall defects and hemodynamic stress on aortic dilation in BAV has been debated.[26,99] Hemodynamic factors may contribute to the ascending aortic pathology in patients with BAV.[26,99-102] It is recognized that the BAV exhibits abnormal leaflet folding and wrinkling and increased leaflet doming, resulting in turbulence in the absence of any valve stenosis.[99] In a computer simulation model, the BAV is intrinsically stenotic, with turbulent flow even in the absence of a transvalvular gradient.[26,99] Evidence of markedly abnormal helical flow has been demonstrated in the ascending aorta of patients with BAV, including those without aortic aneurysm and aortic stenosis[100,102] (Figure 13-12). Increased mid-ascending aortic wall shear stress related to asymmetric and higher-flow velocity has been demonstrated in BAV than in normal trileaflet valve[102] (Figure 13-13). Leaflet orientation also influenced areas of maximum aortic wall stress.[102] In these models of BAV disease, the orientation of the BAV openings with respect to the plane of aortic curvature results in different jet shapes and different distributions of wall stress on the aorta.[101,102] An asymmetric spatial pattern of extracellular matrix protein expression and smooth muscle cell changes in the convexity, in comparison with the concavity of the dilated ascending aorta, in patients with BAV has been demonstrated.[99,103] Abnormal patterns of systolic

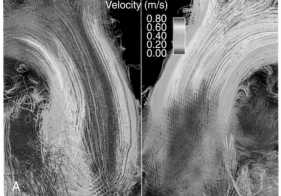
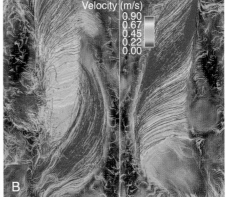

FIGURE 13-12   Four-dimensional flow cardiac magnetic resonance imaging (CMR) of the ascending thoracic aorta during peak systole. A, Normal systolic flow in a patient with a trileaflet aortic valve and normal thoracic aorta dimensions. Four-dimensional flow CMR data in an oblique-sagittal orientation with three-dimensional streamlines (color-coded for velocity during peak systole. *Left*, From right side of thoracic aorta; *right*, from left side of thoracic aorta. Note the smooth trajectory and the absence of substantial secondary flow features. **B**, Right-handed nested helical flow in a patient with normal aortic dimensions and a bicuspid aortic involving right-left leaflet fusion. Streamline analysis shows greater than 180-degree curvature of peak systolic streamlines in a right-handed twist around the slower central helical flow. *Left*, From right side of ascending thoracic aorta; *right*, from left side of ascending thoracic aorta. *(From Hope MD, Hope TA, Meadows AK, et al. Bicuspid aortic valve: four-dimensional MR evaluation of ascending aortic systolic flow patterns. Radiology 2010;255:53–61.)*

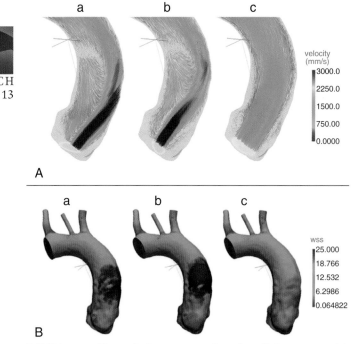

FIGURE 13-13 **Flow velocity vectors and aortic wall shear stress with two types of bicuspid aortic valve (BAV) and a normal trileaflet aortic valve. A,** Vectors of the velocity field plotted in a longitudinal section at time *t* = 0.098 s (early systole). On each of the selected points, a vector with length proportional to the magnitude of the velocity field and with the same direction of the field is plotted. The three valve models are presented: *a*, type 1 BAV (anteroposterior commissures); *b*, type 2 BAV (laterolateral commissures; *c*, trileaflet aortic valve. Greater flow asymmetry is seen in *a*, then in *b*, whereas *c* shows no flow asymmetry. **B,** Aortic wall shear stress is plotted (in dyne/cm²). The three valve models are presented: *a*, type 1 BAV; *b*, type 2 BAV; *c*, trileaflet aortic valve. The precise localization of maximum shear stress for BAV configurations (corresponding to the *red area*) is similarly plotted at the convexity of the mid-ascending aorta. *(From Viscardi F, Vergara C, Antiga L, et al. Comparative finite element model analysis of ascending aortic flow in bicuspid and tricuspid aortic valve. Artif Organs 2010;34:1114–20.)*

flow and abnormal distribution of wall stress may underlie vascular remodeling and aneurysm formation in certain patients with BAV.[26,99-102]

The term "post-stenotic" dilation has often been used for an enlarged aortic root associated with aortic valve disease (especially AS). However, an alternative explanation underlies this process.[54,64] Few patients with trileaflet aortic valve disease have an enlarged aortic root or ascending aorta. In contrast, the BAV is commonly associated with a dilated proximal aorta and must be considered one of the most common etiologies of aortic root enlargement.[54,64] In a survey of aortic root size in severe AS, patients with severe BAV stenosis had significantly larger aortic root and ascending aortic diameters than those with stenosis of a trileaflet valve.[104] Thus, the notion of "post-stenotic" dilation should be dispelled.

Coarctation of the Aorta

Approximately 50% of patients with CoA also have BAV.[3,24,34,51] Aortic coarctation is associated with an increased risk of dissection. In the presurgical era, aortic dissection was the cause of death in 19% to 27% of patients with CoA, but was the cause of death in 50% of patients with CoA and coexistant BAV.[3] Importantly, in one study of patients with BAV and coarctation of the aorta, aortic dissection occurred in approximately 50% of patients.[61] In another series of 235 patients with aortic coarctation, the presence of BAV was the strongest clinical predictor of subsequent aortic wall complications (ascending aortic aneurysm, descending aortic aneurysm, aortic dissection, and aortic

rupture)[51,52] (see Figure 13-5). Moreover, the aortic abnormalities were not confined to the ascending aorta, suggesting that the aortopathy involves the thoracic aorta more diffusely.[51]

Aortic Dissection

BAV disease is a well-recognized risk factor for aortic dissection, independent of hypertension and aortic coarctation. In both autopsy and clinical series of aortic dissection, between 7% and 15% of patients also have BAV.[1,4,24,105] Aortic dissection occurs 5 to 10 times more commonly in patients with BAV than in those with trileaflet valve.[4] Among 416 patients with BAV from Olmsted County, Minnesota, the age-adjusted risk for aortic dissection was 8.4 for patients with a BAV in comparison with the general population.[75] Age greater than 50 years and ascending aortic aneurysm larger than 4.5 cm were risk factors for aortic dissection.

Two studies of individuals younger than 40 years who sustained an aortic dissection found that 9% to 28% had BAV.[54,106] In the International Registry of Aortic Dissection (IRAD), BAV was present in 9% of the 68 patients younger than 40 years compared with only 1% of older patients,[106] with an average ascending aortic diameter at the time of dissection of 5.4 ± 1.8 cm.[106] In the Yale experience of 70 ascending aortic aneurysms associated with BAV, 6 patients (8.6%) suffered aortic dissection or rupture in follow-up, with the average size of the ascending aorta at the time of dissection measuring 5.2 cm.[107] Aortic dissection occurs at a younger age in patients with BAV, and that average age at the time of dissection was 54 years with a BAV but 62 years for patients with trileaflet aortic valve.[108]

Despite the association of BAV and aortic dissection, the absolute risk of aortic dissection for the patient with BAV is low and depends on many factors, most significantly the size of the aortic root or ascending aorta and the age of the patient.[21,22,75] In the series from Olmsted County, Minnesota, no aortic dissections occurred among 212 patients monitored for 20 years.[21] In a report from Toronto, 5 of 642 patients with BAV suffered aortic dissection during 9-year follow-up.[22] Only 2 of 416 patients with BAV suffered aortic dissection over a 16-year follow in another Olmsted County study; the incidence was 3.1 cases (95% confidence interval [CI], 2.1-33.5) per 10,000 patient-years.[75] Incidences for patients older than 50 years and bearers of aortic aneurysms at baseline were 17.4 (95% CI, 2.9-53.6) and 44.9 (95% CI 7.5-138.5) cases per 10,000 patient-years, respectively.[75]

When aortic dissection occurs in the presence of BAV, the valve is usually functionally normal.[24] Aortic dissection may also occur with BAV stenosis or regurgitation and may occur late AVR.[109] BAV has also been associated with spontaneous cervicocephalic arterial dissection, extending the association of arterial medial abnormalities to the cervical arteries.[110]

Aortic Medial Disease and Ascending Aortic Dilation

The aortic wall abnormalities that complicate BAV have led many to theorize the presence of a common underlying developmental defect involving the aortic valve and aortic wall in patients with BAV, which includes cystic medial degeneration.[1,3,36] Hemodynamic factors may also be important in pathogenesis.[26,99,100] To investigate whether aortic wall structural abnormalities underlie the aortopathy of BAV disease, any study must demonstrate the presence of a pathologic or clinical correlate of aortic wall fragility.[111] Noninvasive imaging studies and histopathologic examinations using tissue samples have been performed to address these issues.

Echocardiograms have demonstrated significantly greater aortic root and ascending aortic diameters compared in patients with functionally normal BAVs than in control subjects[111-114] (see Figure 13-6D and 13-7). The degree of aortic enlargement is greater in those with AR than in those with stenotic or functionally

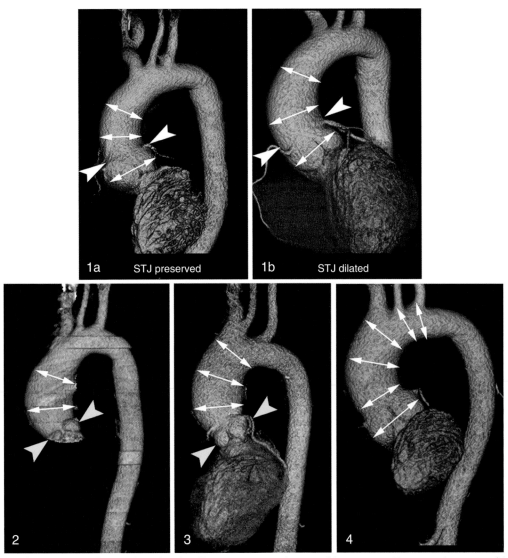

FIGURE 13-14   Types of aortopathy in bicuspid aortic valve disease. Type 1: involvement of the aortic root; **Type 1a:** enlargement of the sinuses of Valsalva and tubular aortic segment; **Type 1b:** sinotubular junction is effaced and tubular aorta is dilated. **Type 2:** Involvement of the tubular aorta. **Type 3:** Involvement of tubular portion of ascending aorta and transverse aortic arch. **Type 4:** Diffuse aortic enlargement (aortic root, ascending aorta, proximal arch). *White double arrows* indicate dilated aortic segments. *White arrowheads* indicate the sinotubular junction (STJ), which is preserved/dilated in *types 1a and 1b. Yellow arrowheads* indicate normal sinuses in *types 2 and 3. (From Kari FA, Fazel SS, Mitchell RS, et al. Bicuspid aortic valve configuration and aortopathy pattern might represent different pathophysiologic substrates. J Thorac Cardiovasc Surg 2012 144(2):516–7; and Fazel SS, Mallidi HR, Lee RS, et al. The aortopathy of bicuspid aortic valve disease has distinctive patterns and usually involves the transverse aortic arch. J Thorac Cardiovasc Surg 2008;135:901–907.e2.)*

normal BAVs.[112] Distinct types of aortic enlargement may be present in the patient with BAV[115] (Figure 13-14). Differing from the aortic enlargement pattern in Marfan syndrome (which typically involves the sinuses of Valsalva), the enlargement in BAV may arise in the sinuses, the proximal ascending aorta, or the mid-ascending aorta.[113,114] In some patients, the aortic arch is also enlarged.[115] In patients with BAV, aortic root dilation is more prevalent in older age groups, and the aortic dimension is usually largest in the mid-ascending aorta.[54,115]

Depending on the definition of dilation, about 50% of patients with BAV younger than 30 years and about 90% of those older than 80 years have aortic dilation.[116] Even young children with BAV have enlarged aortas.[115,117-119] The dilation is most pronounced in the tubular portion of the ascending aorta, is larger than normal at all measured levels, and is independent of any functional abnormality of the BAV.[117] In a series of 333 children with BAV (mean age 13.5 years, range 0-30 years), the aortic root was dilated (z score >2) in 22% of patients and the ascending aorta was dilated in 49%.[119]

In a population study of BAV, 15% of patients had ascending aortic diameters greater than 40 mm, and in those who underwent repeated measurements longitudinally, the prevalence of aortic dilation (>40 mm) increased to 40%.[21] In a cohort study, 32 of 416 (7.7%) patients with BAV had an ascending aortic aneurysm (mean size 48 ± 6 mm) at a mean age of 55 ± 17 years.[75] Of 304 patient undergoing BAV operations at a single tertiary referral institution, 90 (30%) had ascending aortic aneurysms of at least 5 cm.[16] Another large tertiary center reported that proactive aortic repair of a dilated aorta (≥4.5 cm) accounted for 20% of all operations on patients with BAV.[120]

Leaflet orientation in the BAV may play a role in the various aortic root shapes/phenotypes in the patient with BAV.[119,121] Right-left coronary leaflet fusion was associated with larger aortic root diameters than right-noncoronary BAVs in one study, whereas right-noncoronary leaflet fusion was associated with larger ascending aortic diameter.[119] This finding may be related to differing orientation of the eccentric flow jets among cusp fusion phenotypes.[121] Other studies have not demonstrated a relationship between cusp orientation and aortic dilation[115] or between cusp orientation and type of aortic dilation.[116]

In an echocardiographic investigation, 20% of these patients in whom a dilated aortic root was discovered were also found to have BAV.[121a] Variables related to the presence of BAV included age less than 65 years, aortic stenosis, and normotension.[122]

Thus, careful assessment of the entire thoracic aorta is important in the evaluation of each patient with BAV.[1,57,65] In many, this assessment involves imaging with CT or CMR to better visualize the ascending aorta[57] (see Figures 13-7 and 13-14). These data support the view that BAV and aortic root dilation may reflect a common developmental defect.[1,36]

Noninvasive evaluation of aortic wall elastic properties using CMR has demonstrated reduced aortic elasticity and aortic root distensibility in patients with BAV but without stenosis.[122] Measures of aortic wall strain, including aortic wall distension and recoil, differ in patients with BAV and those with trileaflet valves, and this finding has been demonstrated in nondilated aortas.[123] The elastic tissues properties of the aorta in BAV may be related to cusp orientation. Compared with those with right-left leaflet orientation, patients with anterior-posterior leaflet orientation had larger aortic diameters, higher aortic stiffness indices, and lower distensibility.[23] Relatives of patients with BAV have also been demonstrated to exhibit abnormal aortic elastic properties.[124]

The rate of aortic growth among patients with BAV is variable, with reports from about 0.2 to 1.0 mm/year.[125] The patient's age, underlying valve disease, location of the dilation, original size of the aorta, and other factors all play a role in the rate of progression of dilation. In a study of children with BAV, more than one third were found to have significant aortic enlargement during follow-up.[126] Elevated aortic valve gradients or right-noncoronary commissural fusion were associated with accelerated growth.[126] In one study of children with BAV, the mean rate of ascending aortic growth was 1.2 mm/year, but the rate of growth must be correlated with age, body surface area, and linear growth rate.[127] In a report of 333 pediatric patients with BAV, 221 underwent serial echocardiographic examinations.[119] The ascending aortic diameter z score demonstrated only a minimal change (0.063 SD per year) during a 6-year median follow-up. Only 3 patients required aortic surgery for aortic dilation (>4.9 cm). In this study, dilation of the ascending aorta occurred more rapidly in right-noncoronary leaflet fusion BAV than in right-left leaflet fusion BAV.[119]

In a retrospective study of adult patients with BAV evaluated by echocardiogram, the mean rate of aortic diameter dilation was 0.5 mm/year at the sinuses of Valsalva and 0.9 mm/year at the ascending aorta.[128] The prevalence of aortic root dilation also increased during the study. Other studies have reported the growth of the ascending aorta in adults with BAV to be from 0.2 mm/year[129] to 0.86 mm/year.[130]

In a series of 384 patients with BAV without aortic aneurysm at the time of initial study, 49 (13%) had an aortic aneurysm (>45 mm) at a mean interval of 14 ± 6 years after diagnosis.[75] The 25-year risk for development of an aneurysm (>45 mm) was 26% in this BAV population.[75]

One group of investigators have reported that BAV aortic aneurysms grow faster than aneurysms associated with TAV and even more so when aortic stenosis is present.[107] Others have not been able to demonstrate any difference in aortic aneurysm growth between patients with BAV and those with TAV.[131]

Pathophysiology and Molecular Biology of Bicuspid Aortic Valve Aortopathy

The histologic abnormality underlying aortic root complications in BAV is cystic medial degeneration, which has been demonstrated in the aortic walls of patients with BAV even without significant aneurysm formation.[131-133]

The pulmonary autograft has been noted in one study to dilate in some patients with BAV in whom the aortic root was dilated before performance of the Ross procedure.[132] Because the pulmonary trunk and aorta have a common embryologic origin, the trunk has been theorized to be similarly affected. Cystic medial degeneration in both the aorta and pulmonary trunk has been demonstrated to be much more severe in patients with BAV than in patients with TAV. Although other investigators have not reported late autograft dilation after Ross procedure for BAV disease,[134] concerns have been raised about the appropriateness of the Ross procedure for patients with BAV disease and ascending aortic enlargement.[132,135]

Cystic medial degeneration has been demonstrated in multiple types of congenital heart disease, including BAV.[136,137] In many patients with BAV requiring surgery, moderate or severe medial degeneration is present.[136] When the para-coarctation aorta of patients with coarctation of the aorta and BAV was evaluated histologically, the medial abnormalities proximal and distal to the coarctation were identical, implying that the abnormalities were not hemodynamically mediated.[136] The type of valve lesion present (stenosis versus regurgitation) may predict underlying cystic medial degeneration. In a series of patients with BAV undergoing AVR and aneurysm (>4.5 cm) resection, almost half of patients with pure AR had cystic medial degeneration, whereas only the minority of those with aortic stenosis had these changes (Figure 13-15).[137]

Apoptosis is a mechanism that may underlie aortic medial layer smooth muscle cell loss, leading to aneurysm formation in patients with BAV.[138-142] Massive focal apoptosis has been observed in the medial layers of patients with BAV, whether or not aortic dilation was present.[138] In comparison with TAV-associated aneurysms, BAV-associated aneurysms exhibit a distinct pattern of medial destruction, elastic fragmentation, and increased apoptosis.[139]

Differences or imbalances in the proteolytic matrix metalloproteinases (MMP) and their endogenous inhibitors are observed to be slightly different in the ascending aortic aneurysms of patients with BAVs and of those with TAVs.[131,140-144] Elevated MMP-2 expression has been demonstrated in the BAV aorta, whereas MMP-9 activity is normal.[140,145] Differing cusp morphology of BAVs has also been associated with unique ratios of MMPs and their endogenous inhibitors.[144] Altered tissue expression of members of the protein kinase C signaling pathways and decreased expression of metallotheionein in smooth muscle cells has been demonstrated in patients with BAV.[146,147] It has been theorized that the abnormal elastic properties, dilation and fragmentation of elastic components within the aortic walls of patients with BAV may be associated with the greater expression of matrix-degrading proteins.[142]

Fibrillin-1 content is lower in BAV aortas (and pulmonary arteries) than in TAV aortas.[140] In the mouse model of Marfan syndrome (fibrillin-1–deficient mouse), abnormal fibrillin-1 is associated with increased MMP levels, matrix fragmentation, and reduced structural integrity of the aorta.[148] In BAV disease, the abnormal fibrillin content may be related to greater degradation by tissue enzymes or to a defect in smooth muscle protein secretion.[140] Matrix proteins have been examined in aortic aneurysms in patients with BAV and those with Marfan syndrome.[141] Reduced extracellular deposition and altered quantity of matrix proteins are associated with a similar degree of increased apoptosis in vascular smooth muscle cells from BAV aneurysms and aneurysms in Marfan syndrome.[141] These studies suggest that the extracellular matrix proteolytic cascade within the aortas of patients with BAV and ascending aortic aneurysm differs from that in patients with TAV and aneurysm.

Abnormalities in TGF-β signaling pathways have been implicated as underlying aneurysm syndromes, including Marfan syndrome and Loeys-Dietz syndrome.[149] Higher TGF-β levels and greater TGB-β signaling have been demonstrated in the aortic walls of patients with BAV aortic aneurysms,[150] and abnormalities

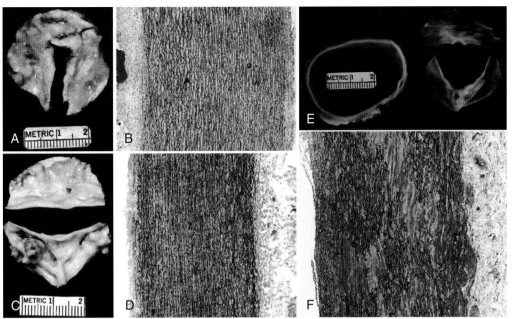

FIGURE 13-15 Bicuspid aortic morphology and aortic wall pathology. Photograph of an operatively excised unicommissural unicuspid stenotic (and regurgitant) aortic valve **(A)** and histologic section of the histologically normal aorta **(B)** in a 41-year-old woman. Photograph of operatively excised congenitally bicuspid stenotic aortic valve **(C)** and histologic section of ascending aorta **(D)** in a 77-year-old man showing 1+/4+ loss of medial elastic fibers. **E,** Photograph of operatively excised purely regurgitant congenitally bicuspid aortic valve and portion of resected aorta in a 54-year-old man. **F,** Histologic section of ascending aorta (maximal diameter = 6.7 cm) shows a 3+/4+ loss of medial elastic fibers. (Figures **B, D,** and **F** are Movat stain preparations, ×100). *(From Roberts WC, Voiwel TJ, Ko J, et al. Comparison of the structure of the aortic valve and ascending aorta in adults having aortic valve replacement for aortic stenosis versus for pure aortic regurgitation and resection of the ascending aorta for aneurysm. Circulation 2011;123:886–903.)*

in TGF-β signaling have been hypothesized to play a role in BAV aneurysm disease.[149,150] Defective TGF-β splicing of fibronectin messenger RNA, which potentially could contribute to defective vascular repair, has been demonstrated in patients with BAV.[151]

Late Aortic Complications Following Bicuspid Aortic Valve Replacement

The aortic root and ascending aorta may continue to dilate after valve surgery for BAV.[109,152] Thus, it is important to continue to survey the aortic root and ascending aorta in patients with BAV after aortic valve surgery. In comparison with patients with TAV, those with BAV have a higher number of aortic complications years after AVR, including aortic dissection, late aneurysm formation, and sudden death.[109,152,153] Additionally, late echocardiography surveillance demonstrates significantly larger ascending aortas in patients with BAV.[109]

Borger et al[153] reported on a 10-year follow-up in 201 patients who underwent AVR for BAV without ascending aortic aneurysm replacement.[153] Ascending aortic size was less than 4.0 cm in 57%, 4.0 to 4.4 cm in 32%, and 4.5 to 4.9 cm in 11% of patients. All aortas larger than 5.0 cm were replaced at the primary operation, which occurred in 17% of all the patients with BAV. During follow-up, 18 patients (9%) required late ascending aortic replacement, with a mean aortic diameter of 58 ± 9 mm. The rates of freedom from ascending aortic complications, including late aneurysm repair, dissection, and sudden death, were 78% ± 6%, 81% ± 6%, and 43% ± 15% in the three aortic size groups, respectively (Figure 13-16).[153]

Other researchers have reported a much lower risk of aortic complications after AVR for BAV disease.[154,155] In a series of 1286 patients (mean age 58 ± 14 years) undergoing AVR for BAV stenosis or regurgitation who were followed up for a median of 12 years (range 0 to 38), there were 13 aortic dissections (1%), 11 ascending aortic replacements (1%), and 127 cases of progressive ascending aortic dilation (>5 cm or >1 cm from time of AVR) (10%).[155] The

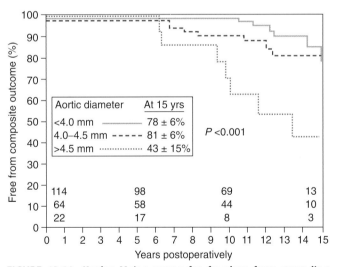

FIGURE 13-16 Kaplan-Meier curves for freedom from ascending aortic complications for the three groups of patients with bicuspid aortic valves undergoing valve replacement surgery. Patients with an ascending aortic diameter of 4.5 cm or greater had a significantly increased risk of future aortic complications (aneurysm, dissection, or sudden death) (P < 0.001). *(From Borger MA, Preston M, Ivanov J, et al. Should the ascending aorta be replaced more frequently in patients with bicuspid aortic valve disease? J Thorac Cardiovasc Surg 2004;128:677–83.)*

rate of 15-year freedom from these aortic complications was 89% in this population.

In a series of 1449 patients with BAV who underwent AVR between 1993 and 2003, only 3 patients (0.2%) had late aortic events after valve operation if their aortic diameter had been smaller than 4.5 cm at the time of valve surgery.[120]

TABLE 13-6	ACC/AHA Guidelines for Managing Bicuspid Aortic Valve with Dilated Ascending Aorta

Class I

1. Patients with known bicuspid aortic valves should undergo an initial transthoracic echocardiogram to assess the diameters of the aortic root and ascending aorta. (Level of Evidence: B)
2. Cardiac magnetic resonance imaging or cardiac computed tomography is indicated in patients with bicuspid aortic valves when morphology of the aortic root or ascending aorta cannot be assessed accurately by echocardiography. (Level of Evidence: C)
3. Patients with bicuspid aortic valves and dilation of the aortic root or ascending aorta (diameter greater than 4.0 cm*) should undergo serial evaluation of aortic root/ascending aorta size and morphology by echocardiography, cardiac magnetic resonance, or computed tomography on a yearly basis. (Level of Evidence: C)
4. Surgery to repair the aortic root or replace the ascending aorta is indicated in patients with bicuspid aortic valves if the diameter of the aortic root or ascending aorta is greater than 5.0 cm* or if the rate of increase in diameter is 0.5 cm per year or more. (Level of Evidence: C)
5. In patients with bicuspid aortic valves undergoing aortic valve replacement because of severe aortic stenosis or aortic regurgitation, repair of the aortic root or replacement of the ascending aorta is indicated if the diameter of the aortic root or ascending aorta is greater than 4.5 cm.* (Level of Evidence: C)

Class IIa

1. It is reasonable to give β-adrenergic blocking agents to patients with bicuspid valves and dilated aortic roots (diameter greater than 4.0 cm*) who are not candidates for surgical correction and who do not have moderate to severe aortic regurgitation. (Level of Evidence: C)
2. Cardiac magnetic resonance imaging or cardiac computed tomography is reasonable in patients with bicuspid aortic valves when aortic root dilation is detected by echocardiography to further quantify severity of dilation and involvement of the ascending aorta. (Level of Evidence: B)

From Bonow RO, Carabello B, Chatterjee K, et al. ACC/AHA 2006 Guidelines for the Management of Patients With Valvular Heart Disease: a report of the American College of Cardiology/ American Heart Association Task Force on Practice Guidelines (Writing Committee to Revise the 1998 Guidelines for the Management of Patients with Valvular Heart Disease). J Am Coll Cardiol 2006;48:e1-e148.
*Consider lower threshold values for patients of small stature of either gender.

A series of 153 patients with BAV (mean age 54 ± 10.5 years) with BAV stenosis and concomitant ascending aortic dilation of 40 to 50 mm who underwent isolated AVR were followed up for a mean of 11.5 ± 3.2 years to evaluate for late aortic complications.[156] Ascending aortic surgery for progressive aneurysm was required in 5 patients (3%). No documented late aortic dissection or rupture occurred, and the rates of freedom from aortic events at 10 and 15 years postoperatively were 95% and 93%, respectively. A separate subgroup of 21 patients with BAV (mean age 41 ± 7 years) with predominant *aortic root* dilation (mean diameter 44 ± 3 mm) who underwent AVR for AR had a much higher rate of aortic complications. Five adverse aortic events (24% of patients) occurred after a mean follow-up of 10.3 ± 4.6 years, including aortic root replacement, aortic dissection, and sudden death.[156] Patients with predominantly aortic regurgitation and BAV may have a different prognosis related to aortic disease, and this difference may be explained by a greater degree of aortic medial degeneration.[157]

The potential fate of the aorta has implications for the management of the aortic root and ascending aorta in patients with BAV undergoing valve surgery and for the timing of prophylactic root replacement.[1,109,120,152,153,155,157] Current AHA/ACC guidelines for the management of the aortic root in BAV disease are listed in Table 13-6.[91] Because concomitant aortic surgery increases the operative risk of AVR, many factors must be considered before the decision is made to resect the ascending aorta at the time of aortic valve surgery.[157,158]

Familial Bicuspid Aortic Valve and Ascending Aortic Aneurysms

The BAV may be hereditary or familial, and studies demonstrate the occurrence of a BAV in approximately 9% of first-degree relatives of individuals with the disease.[41,42] Aneurysms associated with BAV may also be familial.[57,159,160] A comprehensive evaluation of multiple pedigrees segregating BAV with ascending aortic aneurysm revealed a high incidence of individuals with ascending aneurysm alone, suggesting that BAV and ascending aortic aneurysm are both primary manifestations of a single gene defect with variable expression. Potential loci at 5q, 13q, 15q, and 18q have also been reported for BAV and aortic aneurysm.[159,160] Abnormal aortic elastic properties have been demonstrated in relatives of patients with BAV disease, even without overt aortic dilation.[124] Aortic dimensions in patients with BAV may be independently influenced by both genetics and BAV.[161]

In a prospective evaluation of 13 families with BAV and ascending aortic aneurysm, almost half of families had at least two family members with both BAV and thoracic aortic aneurysm, often in successive generations.[1,159] Either partial penetrance (BAV alone) or complete nonpenetrance was observed in obligate carriers. Importantly, thoracic aortic aneurysm may occur in these families independent of BAV. The aortic dilation was maximal above the sinotubular junction in most patients. Aortic dissection was observed in 7 of 13 families and occurred in individuals with or without BAV. These data are consistent with consideration of BAV as an autosomal dominant disorder with variable expressivity and incomplete penetrance.[159] Careful evaluation of the aortic valve and ascending aorta is important for first-degree relatives of the patient with BAV and ascending aortic aneurysm.[54,57,159]

NOTCH1 mutations have been found in a small number of families with BAV or BAV with ascending aortic aneurysm.[5,162] In the families with *NOTCH1* mutations, the BAV is stenotic and calcified. However, most families with BAV and aortic aneurysm do not have associated calcific aortic stenosis, raising the possibility of alternative genetic explanations for the majority with BAV and associated aortic aneurysm.[163]

The BAV may also be present in syndromes associated with aortic or vascular disease. Patients with Turner syndrome have an increased prevalence of ascending aortic aneurysm and BAV. Loeys-Dietz syndrome, which is due to mutations in *TGFBR1* and *TGFBR2*, has the characteristic triad consisting of craniofacial defects (hypertelorism, bifid uvula, craniosynostosis), arterial tortuosity, and aortic aneurysms and dissections.[164] BAV has been reported in 2.5% to 17% of patients with Loeys-Dietz syndrome or *TGFBR2* mutations.[165] Familial thoracic aortic aneurysm (FTAA) syndrome, due to *ACTA2* mutations, is associated with patent ductus arteriosus, cerebral aneurysms, livedo reticularis, premature coronary artery disease, and moyamoya (a progressive cerebrovascular disease typically with bilateral stenosis of the arteries around the circle of Willis).[57,166] BAV has been reported in about 3% of cases of FTAA due to *ACTA2* mutations.[166] An increased frequency of intracranial aneurysms was reported in a small case-control study of BAV, but this finding has not been verified in larger population studies.[167]

Therefore, in the assessment of the patient with BAV and aortic aneurysm, it is important to perform a detailed family history and careful physical examination to evaluate for an underlying disorder or aneurysm syndrome.

Surgical Treatment of the Bicuspid Aortic Valve and Ascending Aorta

The indications for replacement of a BAV with stenosis or regurgitation are well established.[91] However, patients undergoing

AVR for BAV are often young, making the decision to implant a mechanical or a bioprosthetic valve more complex.[1,91] Valve repair for the regurgitant BAV may be performed in carefully selected cases, but durability of the repair remains a concern.[167-169] In a large series of BAV repair for AR, the rate of 10-year freedom from reoperation for BAV repair is about 80% for valve-alone procedures and about 90% for combined valve-aorta procedures.[170] The decision as to when to perform prophylactic aortic root replacement is also complex.[1,109,152,153,157,158] Although experienced centers report a very low operative risk,[170] large databases report that aortic root replacement increases the risk ratio by 2.78 in comparison with isolated AVR.[171] It is recommended that patients with BAV with ascending aortic aneurysms exceeding 4.5 cm undergo simultaneous aortic replacement at the time of AVR.[57,91,153,170] Outstanding long-term results from experienced centers have been reported using this strategy.[170] In patients with BAVs and normal valve function, aortic aneurysm resection is recommended if the aorta exceeds 5 cm or is associated with rapid growth.[57,91] Gender and body surface area may also be important factors in the timing of ascending aortic surgery,[57,170,172] and some authorities advocate using an aortic cross-sectional area/height ratio higher than 10 cm/m^2 to indicate when surgery is required for patients with BAV.[57,170,172]

For patients who require simultaneous valve repair or replacement and ascending aortic replacement for BAV, multiple surgical options are available, and the procedure chosen should be tailored to the specific patient, aortic valve lesion, and aortic characteristics.[170,173-175] Surgical options include: (1) valve replacement (or repair) and separate supracoronary graft replacement of the ascending aorta, leaving the sinuses intact, (2) aortic valve and root replacement with a composite valve-graft conduit and coronary reimplantation, (3) valve-sparing root replacement, and (4) reduction aortoplasty.[1,86] When the aortic sinuses are not significantly dilated, separate AVR and ascending aortic grafting have satisfactory long-term outcome and low risk of significant late sinus dilation.[171] Reduction aortoplasty is controversial in the management of BAV and aortic dilation because of concerns about risk for recurrent dilation and is not recommended.[86] Five percent of patients undergoing ascending aortic aortoplasty required reoperation for progressive dilation a mean of 10 years after initial surgery in one series.[175] The Ross procedure (pulmonary autograft) is an alternative to prosthetic valve replacement in BAV disease.[134] Initial reports of late autograft dilation after this procedure raised concerns about its appropriateness for adult patients, especially those with significant annular or aortic dilation.[1,86,134,176,177] Other studies have not reported a relationship between BAV and pulmonary autograft failure.[134] A dilated aortic annulus, mismatch in annular diameters, and AR are all associated with late pulmonary autograft failure.[178]

BAV has been considered an exclusion criterion for trials of transcatheter aortic valve replacement (TAVR) because of concerns about the risks of paravalvular regurgitation, poor valve seating, and aortic characteristics. Initial experience of TAVR in a small series of selected patients with BAV demonstrated acceptable outcomes.[179] Because 20% of cases of aortic stenosis in patients older than 80 years are due to BAV, and because it may be difficult to correctly identify the leaflet morphology in severe aortic stenosis, outcomes of TAVR in BAV will be an important area of investigation.[79]

Recommendations for Management

There are significant relationships between BAV and its valvular lesions as well as an intrinsic aortopathy that may lead to significant morbidity and mortality. The long-term management of the patient with BAV involves several important steps. First, a patient must be correctly identified as having this lesion by echocardiogram or other imaging modality. Once recognized, the patient must be educated about the potential for progressive valve dysfunction, risk of infective endocarditis, and the possibility of aortic aneurysm formation and risk of aortic dissection (when appropriate). The importance of good dental hygiene should be emphasized.

Because BAV may be familial, one should strongly consider screening all first-degree relatives of the patient with BAV for the disease. This issue is especially important when an ascending aortic aneurysm or aortic dissection complicates the BAV. The patient with BAV should undergo serial clinical and imaging assessments over his or her lifetime for detection of complications from the valve and aortic root/ascending aorta and appropriate timing of surgical intervention. The frequency of imaging depends on the size of the aorta at initial assessment: an aorta smaller than 40 mm should be reimaged approximately every 2 years, and the aorta 40 mm or larger should be reimaged yearly or more often as progression of aortic dilation warrants, or whenever there is a change in clinical symptoms or findings.[49,57,59] CT or CMR is indicated in patients with BAV when morphology of the aortic root or ascending aorta cannot be assessed accurately by echocardiography and to evaluate further the dilated aorta visualized on echocardiography.[57,91] Because the aortic valve lesion may potentially respond favorably to "risk factor modification," the patient with BAV should follow a sensible diet, avoid cigarette smoking, and treat hypertension and hyperlipidemia. There are no data to date demonstrating that pharmacologic therapy to lower cholesterol alters the natural history of BAV stenosis.

BAV is associated with abnormal aortic elastic properties and risk for aneurysm formation. Patients should be counseled about this possibility and, in many instances, given guidelines to avoid strenuous isometric activities, such as weightlifting and other competitive athletics.[180] Patients with BAV aortic aneurysm may participate only in low static or low dynamic sports and should not participate in sports with potential for bodily collision.[180] Although prophylactic β-adrenergic blockade is often recommended when aortic root dilation is present, there is no long-term data on its use in the treatment of bicuspid valve aortic root enlargement.[54,57,91] The ACC/AHA guidelines propose beta-blocker therapy for patients with BAV and dilated aortic roots (>4.0 cm) who are not candidates for surgical correction and who do not have moderate to severe AR (NYHA functional class IIa; level of evidence C).[91]

The TGF-β signaling pathway may be involved in BAV aortic disease.[149] Angiotensin-receptor blocker (ARB) therapy has been demonstrated to reduce plasma levels of free TGF-β, diminish tissue expression of TGF-β-responsive genes, and decrease levels of intracellular mediators within the TGF-β signaling cascade.[181] Data regarding the use of ARB therapy in BAV disease are lacking. The BAV Study (Beta Blockers and Angiotensin Receptor Blockers in Bicuspid Aortic Valve Disease Aortopathy [BAV Study NCT01202721]) will compare the rate of ascending aortic growth in patients with BAV by CMR over 60 months in patients randomly allocated to receive ARB (telmisartan) therapy, beta-blocker (atenolol) therapy, or placebo. Whether therapy such as ARB, which is aimed at blocking TGF-β, or novel agents affecting other pathways will affect the aneurysm disease in patients with BAV is as yet unknown.

In carefully followed adults with BAV, the survival rates were not significantly different from those in the general population.[21,22,75] However, timely surgical treatment of valve lesions and aortic aneurysm is critical to the longevity of the patient with BAV. Finally, even after surgical replacement of the BAV, the patient is at risk for future aortic dilation, aneurysm formation, and dissection and must undergo long-term imaging surveillance.

ACKNOWLEDGEMENT

The author gratefully acknowledges the outstanding contribution of Dr. Michael Beardslee to the previous version of this chapter in the last edition of this text.

REFERENCES

1. Braverman AC, Guven H, Beardslee MA, et al. The bicuspid aortic valve. Curr Prob Cardiol 2005;30:470–522.

2. Roberts W. The congenitally bicuspid aortic valve: a study of 85 autopsy cases. Am J Cardiol 1970;26:72–83.

3. Abbott ME. Coarctation of the aorta of adult type; statistical study and historical retrospect of 200 recorded cases with autopsy; of stenosis or obliteration of descending arch in subjects above age of two years. Am Heart J 1928;3:574.

4. Larson EW, Edwards WD. Risk factors for aortic dissection: a necropsy study of 161 cases. Am J Cardiol 1984;53:849–55.

5. Garg V. Molecular genetics of aortic valve disease. Curr Opin Cardiol 2006;21:180–4.

6. Markwald RR, Norris RA, Moreno-Rodriguez R, et al. Developmental basis of adult cardiovascular diseases: valvular heart diseases. Ann N Y Acad Sci 2010;1188:177–83.

7. Sans-Coma V, Fernandez B, Duran AC, et al. Fusion of valve cushions as a key factor in the formation of congenital bicuspid aortic valves in Syrian hamsters. Anat Rec 1996;244:490–8.

8. Fernández B, Fernandez MC, Durán AC, et al. Anatomy and formation of congenital bicuspid and quadricuspid pulmonary valves in Syrian hamsters. Anat Rec 1998; 250:70–9.

9. Fernandez B, Duran AC, Fernandez-Gallego T, et al. Bicuspid aortic valves with different spatial orientations of the leaflets are distinct etiological entities. J Am Coll Cardiol 2009;54:2312–8.

10. Fedak PW, Verma S, David TE, et al. Clinical and pathophysiological implications of a bicuspid aortic valve. Circulation 2002;106:900–4.

11. Lee TC, Zhao YD, Courtman DW, et al. Abnormal aortic valve development in mice lacking endothelial nitric oxide synthase. Circulation 2000;101:2345–8.

12. Aicher D, Urbich C, Zeiher A, et al. Endothelial nitric oxide synthase in bicuspid aortic valve disease. Ann Thorac Surg 2007;83:1290–4.

13. Laforest B, Andelfinger G, Nemer M. Loss of Gata5 in mice leads to bicuspid aortic valve. J Clin Invest 2011;121:2876–87.

14. Siu SA, Silversides CK. Bicuspid aortic valve disease. J Am Coll Cardiol 2010; 55:2789–800.

15. Sabet HY, Edwards WD, Tazelaar HD, et al. Congenitally bicuspid aortic valves: a surgical pathology study of 542 cases and a literature review of 2,715 additional cases. Mayo Clin Proc 1999;74:14–26.

16. Sievers HH, Schmidtke C. A classification system for the bicuspid aortic valve from 304 surgical specimens. J Thorac Cardiovasc Surg 2007;133:1226–33.

17. Yener N, Oktar GL, Erer D, et al. Bicuspid aortic valve. Ann Thorac Cardiovasc Surg 2002;8:264–7.

18. Brandenburg RO, Tajik AJ, Edwards WD, et al. Accuracy of 2 dimensional echocardiographic diagnosis of congenitally bicuspid aortic valve: Echocardiographic-anatomic correlation in 115 patients. Am J Cardiol 1983;51:1469–73.

19. Fernandes SM, Sanders SP, Khairy P, et al. Morphology of bicuspid aortic valve in children and adolescents. J Am Coll Cardiol 2004;44:1648–51.

20. Fernandes SM, Khairy P, Sanders SP, et al. Bicuspid Aortic Valve Morphology and interventions in the Young. J Am Coll Cardiol 2007;49:2211–4.

21. Michelena HI, Desjardins VA, Avierinos JF, et al. Natural history of asymptomatic patients with normally functioning or minimally dysfunctional bicuspid aortic valve in the community. Circulation 2008;117(21):2776–84.

22. Tzemos N, Therrien J, Yip J, et al. Outcomes in adults with bicuspid aortic valves. JAMA 2008;300:1317–25.

23. Schaefer BM, Lewin MB, Stout KK, et al. Usefulness of bicuspid aortic valve phenotype to predict elastic properties of the ascending aorta. Am J Cardiol 2007;99:686–90.

24. Ward C. Clinical significance of the bicuspid aortic valve. Heart 2000;83:81–5.

25. Wallby L, Janerot-Sjoberg B, Steffensen T, et al. T lymphocyte infiltration in non-rheumatic aortic stenosis: a comparative descriptive study between tricuspid and bicuspid aortic valves. Heart 2002;88:348–51.

26. Robiscsek F, Thubrikar MJ, Cook JW, et al. The congenitally bicuspid aortic valve: How does it function? Why does it fail? Ann Thor Surg 2004;77:177–85.

27. Lewin MB, Otto CM. The Bicuspid aortic valve: adverse outcomes from infancy to old age. Circulation 2005;111:832–34.

28. Osler W. On the condition of fusion of two segments of the semilunar valves. Montreal Gen Hosp Reports 1880;1:233.

29. Basso C, Boschello M, Perrone C, et al. An echocardiographic survey of primary school children for bicuspid aortic valve. Am J Cardiol 2004;93:661–3.

30. Lewis T, Grant RT. Observations relating to subacute infective endocarditis. Heart 1923;10:21–9.

31. Larson EW, Edwards WD. Risk factors for aortic dissection: a necropsy study of 161 cases. Am J Cardiol 1984;53:849–55.

32. Tutar E, Ekicki F, Atalay S, et al. The prevalence of bicuspid aortic valve in newborns by echocardiographic screening. Am Heart J 2005;150:513–5.

33. Nistri S, Basso C, Marzari C, et al. Frequency of bicuspid aortic valve in young male conscripts by echocardiogram. Am J Cardiol 2005;96:718–21.

34. Roos-Hesselink JW, Scholzel BE, Heijdra RJ, et al. Aortic valve and aortic arch pathology after coarctation repair. Heart 2003;89:1074–77.

35. Sachdev V, Matura LA, Sidenko S, et al. Aortic valve disease in Turner syndrome. J Am Coll Cardiol 2008;51:1904–9.

36. McKusick V. Association of congenital bicuspid aortic valve and Erdheim's cystic medial necrosis. Lancet 1972;1:1026–7.

37. Gale AN, McKusick VA, Hutchins GH, et al. Familial congenital bicuspid aortic valve. Chest 1977;72:668–70.

38. Brown C, Sane DC, Kitzman DW. Bicuspid aortic valves in monozygotic twins. Echocardiography 2003;20:183–4.

39. Emanuel R, Withers R, O'Brien K, et al. Congenitally bicuspid aortic valves, clinicogenetic study of 41 families. Br Heart J 1978;40:1402–7.

40. Glick BN, Roberts WC. Congenitally bicuspid aortic valve in multiple family members. Am J Cardiol 1994;73:400–4.

41. Huntington K, Hunter A, Chan K. A prospective study to assess the frequency of familial clustering of congenital bicuspid aortic valve. J Am Coll Cardiol 1997;30:1809–12.

42. Cripe L, Andelfinger G, Martin LJ, et al. Bicuspid aortic valve is heritable. J Am Coll Cardiol 2004;44:138–43.

43. Fernandez B, Duran AC, Fernandez MC, et al. Genetic contribution of bicuspid aortic valve morphology. Am J Med Genet Part A 2011;155:2897–8.

44. Hinton RB, Martin LJ, Tabangin ME, et al. Hypoplastic left heart syndrome is heritable. J Am Coll Cardiol 2007;50:1590–5.

45. Hinton RB, Martin LJ, Rame-Gowda S, et al. Hypoplastic left heart syndrome links to chromosomes 10q and 6q and is genetically related to bicuspid aortic valve. J Am Coll Cardiol 2009;53:1065–71.

46. Kerstjens-Frederikse WS, Du Marchie Sarvaas GJ, Ruiter JS, et al. Left ventricular outflow tract obstruction: should cardiac screening be offered to first-degree relatives? Heart 2011;97:1228–32.

47. Wooten EC, Iyer LK, Montefusco MC, et al. Application of gene network analysis techniques identifies AXIN1/PDIA2 and endoglin haplotypes associated with bicuspid aortic valve. PloS One 2010;5:1–10.

48. McBride KL, Varg V. Heredity of bicuspid aortic valve: is family screening indicated? Heart 2011;97:1193–5.

49. Warnes CA, Williams RG, Bashore TM, et al. ACC/AHA 2008 Guidelines for the Management of Adults with Congenital Heart Disease: a report of the American College of Cardiology/American Heart Association Task Force on Practice Guidelines (writing committee to develop guidelines on the management of adults with congenital heart disease). Circulation 2008; 118:e714–833.

50. Fernandes SM, Sanders SP, Khairy P, et al. Morphology of bicuspid aortic valve in children and adolescents. J Am Coll Cardiol 2004; 44:1648–51.

51. Oliver JM, Gallego P, Gonzalez A, et al. Risk factors for aortic complications in adults with coarctation of the aorta. J Am Coll Cardiol 2004;44:1641–7.

52. Oliver JM, Alonso-Gonzalez R, Gonzalez AE, et al. Risk of aortic root or ascending aorta complications in patients with bicuspid aortic valve with and without coarctation of the aorta. Am J Cardiol 2009;104:1001–6.

53. Cohen M, Fuster V, Steele PM, et al. Coarctation of the aorta. Long-term follow-up and prediction of outcome after surgical correction. Circulation 1989;80: 840–5.

54. Braverman AC. Aortic involvement in patients with a bicuspid aortic valve. Heart 2011;97:506–13.

55. Ho VB, Bakalov VK, Cooley M, et al . Major Vascular Anomalies in Turner Syndrome: Prevalence and Magnetic Resonance Angiographic Features. Circulation 2004;110: 1694–700.

56. Matura LA, Ho VB, Rosing D, et al. Aortic dilation and dissection in Turner Syndrome. Circulation 2007;116:1–7.

57. Hiratzka LF, Bakris GL, Beckman JA, et al. 2010 ACCF/AHA/AATS/ACR/ASA/SCA/SCAI/SIR/STS/SVM Guidelines for the Diagnosis and Management of Patients with Thoracic Aortic Disease. Circulation 2010;121:e266–369.

58. Lerer PK, Edwards WD. Coronary arterial anatomy in bicuspid aortic valve. Necropsy study of 100 hearts. Br Heart J 1981;45:142–7.

59. Doty DB. Anomalous origin of the left circumflex coronary artery associated with bicuspid aortic valve. J Thorac Cardiovasc Surg 2001;122:842–3.

60. Brickner ME, Hillis LD, Lange RA. Congenital heart disease in adults. N Engl J Med 2000;342:334–42.

61. Steiner RM, Reddy GP, Flicker S. Congenital cardiovascular disease in the adult patient: imaging update. J Thorac Imaging 2002;17:1–17.

62. Weyman AE, Griffin BP. Left ventricular outflow tract: the aortic valve, aorta and subvalvular outflow tract. In: Weyman AE ed.; Principles and Practice of Echocardiography, 2nd ed. Philadelphia: Lea & Febiger, 1994; pp 505–8.

63. Chan KL, Stinson WA, Veinot JP. Reliability of transthoracic echocardiography in the assessment of aortic valve morphology; pathological correlation in 178 patients. Can J Cardiol 1999;15:48–52.

64. Boyer J, Guittierez F, Braverman AC. Approach to the dilated aortic root. Curr Opin Cardiol 2004;19:563–9.

65. Albano AJ, Mitchell E, Pape LA. Standardizing the method of measuring by echocardiogram the diameter of the ascending aorta in patients with a bicuspid aortic valve. Am J Cardiol 2010;105:1000–4.

66. Ahmed S, Honos GN, Walling AD, et al. Clinical outcome and echocardiographic predictors of aortic valve replacement in patients with bicuspid aortic valve. J Am Soc Echocardiogr 2007;20:998–1003.

67. Espinal M, Fuisz AR, Nanda NC, et al. Sensitivity and specificity of transesophageal echocardiography for determination of aortic valve morphology. Am Heart J 2000; 139:1071–6.

68. Makkar A, Siddiqui TS, Stoddard MF, et al. Impact of valvular calcification on the diagnostic accuracy of transesophageal echocardiography for the detection of congenital aortic valve malformation. Echocardiography 2007;24:745–9.

69. Tanaka R, Yoshioka K, Niinuma H, et al. Diagnostic value of cardiac CT in the evaluation of bicuspid aortic valve stenosis: comparison with echocardiography and operative findings. AJR Am J Roentgenol 2010;195:895–9.

70. Gleeson TG, Mwangi I, Horgan SJ, et al. Steady-state free-precession (SSFP) cine MRI in distinguishing normal and bicuspid aortic valves. J Magn Reson Imaging 2008;28: 873–8.

71. Lee SC, Ko SM, Song MG, et al. Morphological assessment of the aortic valve using coronary computed tomography angiography, cardiovascular magnetic resonance, and transthoracic echocardiography: comparison with intraoperative findings. Int J Cardiovasc Imag 2012;28(Suppl 1):33–44. DOI 10.1007/s10554-012-0066-9.

72. Caruthers SD, Shiow JL, Brown P, et al. Practical value of cardiac magnetic resonance imaging for clinical quantification of aortic valve stenosis—comparison with echocardiography. Circulation 2003;108:2236–43.

73. Pouler AC, le Polain de Waroux JB, et al. Aortic valve area assessment: multidetector CT compared with cine MR imaging and transthoracic and transesophageal echocardiography. Radiology 2007;244: 745–54.
74. Buchner S, Hulsmann M, Poschenrieder F, et al. Variable phenotypes of bicuspid aortic valve disease: classification by cardiovascular magnetic resonance. Heart 2010;96: 1233–40.
75. Michelena HI, Khanna AD, Mahoney D, et al. Incidence of aortic complications in patients with bicuspid aortic valves. JAMA 2011;306:1104–13.
76. Roberts WC, Ko JM. Frequency of unicuspid, bicuspid and tricuspid aortic valves by decade in adults having aortic valve replacement for isolated aortic stenosis. Circulation 2005;111:920–5.
77. Subramanian R, Olson LJ, Edwards WD. Surgical pathology of pure aortic stenosis: a study of 374 Cases. Mayo Clin Proc 1984;59:683–90.
78. Turri M, Thiene G, Bortolotti U, et al. Surgical pathology of aortic valve disease: a study based on 602 specimens. Eur J Cardiothorac Surg 1990; 4:556–60.
79. Roberts WC, Janning KG, Ko JM, et al. Frequency of congenital bicuspid aortic valves in patients >80 years of age undergoing aortic valve replacement for aortic stenosis (with or without aortic regurgitation) and implications for transcatheter aortic valve implantation. Am J Cardiol 2012;109:1632–6.
80. Novaro GM, Tiong IY, Pearce GL, et al. Features and predictors of ascending aortic dilatation in association with a congenital bicuspid aortic valve. Am J Cardiol 2003;92: 99–101.
81. Mohler ER. Are atherosclerotic processes involved in aortic-valve calcification? Lancet 2000;356:524–5.
82. Chan KL, Ghani M, Woodend K, et al. Case-controlled study to assess risk factors for aortic stenosis in congenitally bicuspid aortic valve. Am J Cardiol 2001;88:690–3.
83. Chan KL, Teo K, Dumesnil JG, et al. Effect of lipid lowering with rosuvastatin on progression of aortic stenosis. Results of the Aortic Stenosis Progression Observation: Measuring Effects of Rosuvastatin (ASTRONOMER) trial. Circulation 2010;121:306–14.
84. Goel SS, Tuzcu EM, Agarwal S, et al. Comparison of ascending aortic size in patients with severe bicuspid aortic valve stenosis treated with versus treated without a statin drug. Am J Cardiol 2011;108:1458–62.
85. Pachulski RT, Chan KL. Progression of aortic valve dysfunction in 51 adult patients with congenital bicuspid aortic valve. Br Heart J 1993;69:237–40.
86. Fedak PWM, David TE, Borger M, et al. Bicuspid aortic valve disease: Recent insights in pathophysiology and treatment. Expert Rev Cardiovasc Ther 2005;3:295–308.
87. Lamas CC, Eykyn SJ. Bicuspid aortic valve – A silent danger: analysis of 50 cases of infective endocarditis. Clin Inf Dis 2000;30:336–41.
88. Tribouilloy C, Rusinaru D, Sorel C, et al. Clinical characteristics and outcome of infective endocarditis in adults with bicuspid aortic valves: a multicentre observational study. Heart 2010;96:1723–9.
89. Kahveci G, Bayrak F, Pala S, et al. Impact of bicuspid aortic valve on complications and death in infective endocarditis of native aortic valves. Tex Heart Inst J 2009; 36:111–6.
90. Wilson W, Taubert KA, Gewitz M, et al. Prevention of infective endocarditis: Guidelines from the American Heart Association Rheumatic Fever, Endocarditis, and Kawasaki Disease Committee, Council on Cardiovascular Disease in the Young, and the Council on Clinical Cardiology, Council on Cardiovascular Surgery and Anesthesia, and the Quality of Care and Outcomes Research Interdisciplinary Working Group. Circulation 2007;116:1736–54.
91. Bonow RO, Carabello B, Chatterjee K, et al. ACC/AHA 2006 Guidelines for the Management of Patients With Valvular Heart Disease: A Report of the American College of Cardiology/ American Heart Association Task Force on Practice Guidelines (Writing Committee to Revise the 1998 Guidelines for the Management of Patients with Valvular Heart Disease). J Am Coll Cardiol 2006:48:e1–e148.
92. Siu SC, Sermer M, Colman JM, et al. Prospective multicenter study of pregnancy outcomes in women with heart disease. Circulation 2001;104:515–52.
93. Silversides C, Colman JM, Sermer M, et al. Early and intermediate – term outcomes of pregnancy with congenital aortic stenosis. Am J Cardiol 2003;91:1386–9.
94. Brickner ME. Valvar aortic stenosis. In: Diagnosis and Management of Adult Congenital Heart Disease. Ed: Gatzoulis MA, Webb GD, Daubeney PE. Philadelphia: Churchill Livingstone 2003.
95. Immer FF, Bansi AG, Alexsandra S, et al. Aortic dissection in pregnancy: analysis of risk factors and outcome. Ann Thorac Surg 2003;76:309–14.
96. McKellar SH, MacDonald RJ, Michelena H, et al. Frequency of cardiovascular events in women with a congenitally bicuspid aortic valve in a single community and effect of pregnancy on events. Am J Cardiol 2011;107:96–9.
97. Beauchesne LM, Connolly HM, Ammash NM, et al. Coarctation of the aorta: outcome of pregnancy. J Am Coll Cardiol 2001;38:1728–33.
98. Vriend JW, Drenthen W, Pieper PG, et al. on behalf of the ZAHARA investigators. Outcome of pregnancy in patients after repair of aortic coarctation. Eur Heart J 2005;26:2173–8.
99. Girdauskas E, Borger MA, Secknus MA, et al. Is aortopathy in bicuspid aortic valve disease a congenital defect or a result of abnormal hemodynamics? A critical reappraisal of a one-sided argument. Eur J Cardiothorac Surg 2011;39:809–14.
100. Hope MD, Hope TA, Meadows AK, et al. Bicuspid aortic valve: four-dimensional MR evaluation of ascending aortic systolic flow patterns. Radiology 2010;255:53–61.
101. Viscardi F, Vergara C, Antiga L, et al. Comparative finite element model analysis of ascending aortic flow in bicuspid and tricuspid aortic valve. Artif Organs 2010;34: 1114–20.
102. Vergara C, Viscardi F, Antiga L, et al. Influences of bicuspid aortic valve geometry on ascending aortic fluid dynamics: A parametric study. Artif Organs 2012;36:368–78.
103. Cotrufo M, Della Corte A. The association of bicuspid aortic valve disease with asymmetric dilatation of the tubular ascending aorta: identification of a definite syndrome. J Cardiovasc Med (Hagerstown) 2009;10:291–7.
104. Morgan-Hughes GJ, Roobottom CA, et al. Dilatation of the aorta in pure, severe bicuspid aortic valve stenosis. Am Heart J 2004;147:736–40.
105. Gore I. Dissecting aneurysm of the aorta in persons under forty years of age. Arch Pathol 1953;55:1–13.
106. Januzzi JL, Isselbacher EM, Fattori R et al. Characterizing the young patient with aortic dissection: results from the International Registry of Aortic Dissection (IRAD). J Am Coll Cardiol 2004;43:665–9.
107. Davies RR, Kaple RK, Mandapati D, et al. Natural history of ascending aortic aneurysms in the setting of an unreplaced bicuspid aortic valve. Ann Thorac Surg 2007;83: 1338–44.
108. Roberts CS, Roberts WC. Dissection of the aorta associated with congenital malformation of the aortic valve. J Am Coll Cardiol 1991;17:712–6.
109. Russo CF, Mazzetti S, Garatti A, et al. Aortic complications after bicuspid aortic valve replacement: long-term results. Ann Thorac Surg 2002;74:S1773–6.
110. Schievink WI, Mikri B. Familial aorto-cervicocephalic arterial dissections and congenitally bicuspid aortic valve. Stroke 1995;26:1935–40.
111. Pachulski RT, Winberg AL, Chan KL. Aortic aneurysm in patients with functionally normal or minimally stenotic bicuspid aortic valve. Am J Cardiol 1991;67:781–2.
112. Hahn RT, Roman MJ, Mogtader AH, et al. Association of aortic dilation with regurgitant, stenotic and functionally normal bicuspid aortic valves. J Am Coll Cardiol 1992;19: 283–8.
113. Nkomo VT, Enrique-Sarano M, Ammash NM, et al. Bicuspid aortic valve associated with aortic dilatation: a community-based study. Arterioscler Thromb Vasc Biol 2003;23: 351–6.
114. Cecconi M, Manfrin M, Moraca A, et al. Aortic dimensions in patients with bicuspid aortic valve without significant valve dysfunction. Am J Cardiol 2005;95:292–4.
115. Kari FA, Fazel SS, Mitchell RS, et al. Bicuspid aortic valve configuration and aortopathy pattern might represent different pathophysiologic substrates. J Thorac Cardiovasc Surg 2012; (Available online 13 June 2012) http://dx.doi.org/10.1016/j.jtcvs.2012.05.035.
116. Della Corte A, Bancone C, Quarto C, et al. Predictors of ascending aortic dilatation with bicuspid aortic valve: a wide spectrum of clinical expression. Eur J Cardiothorac Surg 2007;31:397–404; discussion 404-405.
117. Gurvitz M, Chang RK, Drant S, et al. Frequency of aortic root dilation in children with a bicuspid aortic valve. Am J Cardiol 2004;94:1337–40.
118. Basso C, Boschello M, Perrone C, et al. An echocardiographic survey of primary school children for bicuspid aortic valve. Am J Cardiol 2004;93:661–3.
119. Fernandes S, Khairy P, Graham DA, et al. Bicuspid aortic valve and associated aortic dilatation in the young. Heart 2012;98:1014–19.
120. Svensson LG, Kim KH, Blackstone EH, et al. Bicuspid aortic valve surgery with proactive ascending aorta repair. J Thor Cardiovasc Surg 2011;142:622–9.
121. Schaefer BM, Lewin MB, Stout KK, et al. The bicuspid aortic valve: An integrated phenotypic classification of leaflet morphology and aortic root shape. Heart 2008;94: 1634–8.
121a. Alegret JM, Duran I, Palazon O, et al. Prevalence of and predictors of bicuspid aortic valves in patients with dilated aortic roots. Am J Cardiol 2003;91:619–22.
122. Grotenhuis HB, Ottenkamp J, Westenberg JJM, et al. Reduced aortic elasticity and dilatation are associated with aortic regurgitation and left ventricular hypertrophy in nonstenotic bicuspid aortic valve patients. J Am Coll Cardiol 2007;49:1660–5.
123. Aquaro GD, Ait-Ali L, Basso ML, et al. Elastic properties of aortic wall in patients with bicuspid aortic valve by magnetic resonance imaging. Am J Cardiol 2011;108: 81–7.
124. Biner S, Rafique AM, Ray I, et al. Aortopathy is prevalent in relatives of bicuspid aortic valve patients. J Am Coll Cardiol 2009;53:2288–95.
125. Tadros TM, Klein MD, Shapira OM. Ascending aortic dilatation associated with bicuspid aortic valve. Pathology, molecular biology, and clinical implications. Circulation 2009;119:880–90.
126. Holmes KW, Lehmann CU, Dalal D, et al. Progressive dilation of the ascending aorta in children with isolated bicuspid aortic valve. Am J Cardiol 2007;99:978–83.
127. Beroukhim BS, Kruzick TL, Taylor AL, et al. Progression of aortic dilation in children with a functionally normal bicuspid aortic valve. Am J Cardiol 2006;98:828–30.
128. Ferencik M, Pape LA. Changes in size of the ascending aorta and aortic valve function with time in patients with congenitally bicuspid aortic valves. Am J Cardiol 2003;92: 43–6.
129. Novaro GM, Griffin BP. Congenital bicuspid aortic valve and rate of ascending aortic dilatation. Am J Cardiol 2003;92:525–6.
130. La Canna G, Ficarra E, Tsagalau E, et al. Progression rate of ascending aortic dilation in patients with normally functioning bicuspid and tricuspid aortic valves. Am J Cardiol 2006;98:249–53).
131. LeMaire SA, Wang X, Wilks JA, et al. Matrix metalloproteinases in ascending aortic aneurysms: bicuspid versus trileaflet aortic valves. J Surg Res 2005;123:40–8.
132. de Sa M, Moshkovitz Y, Butany J, et al. Histologic abnormalities of the ascending aorta and pulmonary trunk in patients with bicuspid aortic valve disease: clinical relevance to the Ross procedure. J Thorac Cardiovasc Surg 1999;118:588–94.
133. Fedak PWM, Verma S, David TE, et al. Clinical and pathophysiological implications of a bicuspid aortic valve. Circulation 2002;106:900–4.
134. Luciani GB, Mazzucco A. Aortic root disease after the Ross procedure. Curr Opin Cardiol 2006;21:555–60.
135. Hanke T, Charitos EI, Stierle U, et al. The Ross operation—a feasible and safe option in the setting of a bicuspid aortic valve? Eur J Cardiothorac Surg 2010;38:338–9.
136. Niwa K, Perloff JK, Bhuta SM, et al. Structural abnormalities of great arterial walls in congenital heart disease. Circulation 2001;103:393–400.
137. Roberts WC, Voiwel TJ, Ko J, et al. Comparison of the structure of the aortic valve and ascending aorta in adults having aortic valve replacement for aortic stenosis versus for pure aortic regurgitation and resection of the ascending aorta for aneurysm. Circulation 2011;123:986–03.
138. Bonderman D, Gharehbaghi-Schell E, Wollenek G, et al. Mechanisms underlying aortic dilatation in congenital aortic valve malformation. Circulation 1999;99:2138–43.
139. Schmid FX, Bielenberg K, Schneider A, et al. Ascending aortic aneurysm associated with bicuspid and tricuspid aortic valve: involvement and clinical relevance of smooth

muscle cell apoptosis and expression of cell death-initiating proteins. Eur J Cardiothorac Surg 2003;23:537–43.

140. Fedak PWM, de Sa MPL, Verma S, et al. Vascular matrix remodeling in patients with bicuspid aortic valve malformations: implications for aortic dilatation. J Thorac Cardiovasc Surg 2003;126:797–806.

141. Nataatmadja M, West M, West J, et al. Abnormal extracellular matrix protein transport associated with increased apoptosis of vascular smooth muscle cells in Marfan syndrome and bicuspid aortic valve thoracic aortic aneurysm. Circulation 2003;108[suppl II]:II-329–334.

142. Boyum J, Fellinger EK, Schmoker JD, et al. Matrix metalloproteinase activity in thoracic aortic aneurysms associated with bicuspid and tricuspid aortic valves. J Thorac Cardiovasc Surg 2004;127:686–91.

143. Ikonomidis JS, Jones JA, Barbour JR, et al. Expression of matrix metalloproteinases and endogenous inhibitors within ascending aortic aneurysms of patients with bicuspid or tricuspid aortic valves. J Thorac Cardiovasc Surg 2007;133:1028–36.

144. Ikonomidis JS, Ruddy MM, Benton SM, et al. Aortic dilatation with bicuspid aortic valves: cusp fusion correlates to MMPs and inhibitors. Ann Thorac Surg 2012;93:457–64.

145. Tzemos N, Lyseggen E, Silversides C, et al. Endothelial function, carotid-femoral stiffness, and plasma matrix metalloproteinase-2 in men with bicuspid aortic valve and dilated aorta. J Am Coll Cardiol 2010;55:660–8.

146. Jones JA, Stroud RE, Kaplan BS, et al. Differential protein kinase C isoform abundance in ascending aortic aneurysms from bicuspid versus tricuspid aortic valves. Circulation 2007;116(11Suppl):I144–I149.

147. Phillippi JA, Eskay MA, Kubala AA, et al. Altered oxidative stress responses and increased type I collagen expression in bicuspid aortic valve patients. Ann Thorac Surg 2010;90:1893–8.

148. Pereira L, Lee SY, Gayraud B, et al. Pathogenetic sequence for aneurysm revealed in mice underexpressing fibrillin-1. Proc Natl Acad Sci 1999;96:3819–23.

149. Lindsay M, Dietz H. Lessons on the pathogenesis of aneurysm from heritable conditions. Nature 2011;473:308–16.

150. Gomez D, Al Haj Zen A, Borges LF, et al. Syndromic and non-syndromic aneurysms of the human ascending aorta share activation of the Smad2 pathway. J Pathol 2009;218:131–42.

151. Kurtovic S, Paloschi V, Folkersen L, et al. Diverging alternative splicing fingerprints in TGF-beta signaling pathway identified in thoracic aortic aneurysms. Mol Med 2011;17:665–75.

152. Yasuda H, Nakatani S, Stugaard M, et al. Failure to prevent progressive dilation of ascending aorta by aortic valve replacement in patients with bicuspid aortic valve: comparison with tricuspid aortic valve. Circulation 2003;108:[suppl II]:II-291–294.

153. Borger MA, Preston M, Ivanov J, et al. Should the ascending aorta be replaced more frequently in patients with bicuspid aortic valve disease? J Thorac Cardiovasc Surg 2004;128:677–83.

154. Roberts WC. Prophylactic replacement of a dilated aorta at the time of aortic valve replacement of a dysfunctioning congenitally unicuspid or bicuspid aortic valve. Am J Cardiol 2011;108:1371–2.

155. McKeller SH, Michelena HI, Li Z, et al. Long-term risk of aortic events following aortic valve replacement in patients with bicuspid aortic valves. Am J Cardiol 2010;106:1626–33.

156. Girdauskas E, Disha K, Raisin HH, et al. Risk of late aortic events after an isolated aortic valve replacement for bicuspid aortic valve stenosis with concomitant ascending aortic dilation. Eur J Cardiothorac Surg 2012;42(5):832–7; discussion 837-8. doi:10.1093/ejcts/ezs137.

157. Roberts WC, Vowel TJ, Ko JM, et al. Comparison of the structure of the aortic valve and ascending aorta in adults having aortic valve replacement for aortic stenosis verus for pure aortic regurgitation and resection of the ascending aorta for aneurysm. Circulation 2011;123:896–903.

158. Sundt TM. Replacement of the ascending aorta in bicuspid aortic valve disease: where do we draw the line? J Thorac Cardiovasc Surg 2010;140:S41–4.

159. Loscalzo ML, Goh D, Loeys B, et al. Familial thoracic aortic dilation and bicommissural aortic valve: A prospective analysis of the Natural History and Inheritance. Am J Med Genet Part A 2007;143A:1960–7.

160. Martin L, Ramachandran V, Cripe L, et al. Evidence in favor of linkage to human chromosomal regions 18q, 5q, and 13q for bicuspid aortic valve and associated cardiovascular malformations. Hum Genet 2007;121:275–84.

161. Martin LJ, Hinton RB, Zhang X, et al. Aorta measurements are heritable and influenced by bicuspid aortic valve. Frontiers in Genetics 2011;2:1–9.

162. McKeller SH, Tester DJ, Yagubyan M, et al. Novel NOTCH1 mutations in patients with bicuspid aortic valve disease and thoracic aortic aneurysms. J Thorac Cardiovasc Surg 2007;134:290–6.

163. Kent KC, Loscalzo ML, Goh DLM, et al. Genotype-phenotype correlation in patients with bicuspid aortic valve and aneurysm. J Thorac Cardiovasc Surg 2012 doi:10.1016/j.jtcvs.2012.09.060 [epub ahead of print].

164. Loeys BL, Chen J, Neptune ER, et al. A syndrome of altered cardiovascular, craniofacial, neurocognitive and skeletal development caused by mutations in TGFBR1 or TGFBR2. Nat Genet 2005;37(3):275–81.

165. Cedars A, Braverman AC. The many faces of bicuspid aortic valve disease. Prog Ped Cardiol 2012;34:91–96.

166. Milewicz DM, Guo DC, Tran-Fadulu V, et al. Genetic basis of thoracic aortic aneurysms and dissections: focus on smooth muscle cell contractile dysfunction. Annu Rev Genomics Hum Genet 2008;9:283–302.

167. Schievink WI, Raissi SS, Maya MM, et al. Screening for intracranial aneurysms in patients with bicuspid aortic valve. Neurology 2010;74:1430–3.

168. Minakata K, Schaff HV, Zehr KJ, et al. Is repair of aortic valve regurgitation a safe alternative to valve replacement? J Thorac Cardiovasc Surg 2004;127:645–53.

169. Davierwala PM, David TE, Armstrong S, et al. Aortic valve repair versus replacement in bicuspid aortic valve disease. J Heart Valve Dis 2003;12:679–86.

170. Svensson LG, Batizy LH, Blackstone EH, et al. Results of matching valve and root repair to aortic valve and root pathology. J Thorac Cardiovasc Surg 2011;142:1491–8.

171. Park CB, Greason KL, Suri RM, et al. Fate of nonreplaced sinuses of Valsalva in bicuspid aortic valve disease. J Thorac Cardiovasc Surg 2011;142:602–7.

172. Svensson LG, Lim KH, Lytle BW, et al. Relationship of aortic cross-sectional area to height ratio and the risk of aortic dissection in patients with bicuspid aortic valves. J Thorac Cardiovasc Surg 2003;126:892–3.

173. Razel SS, Mallidi HR, Lee RS, et al. The aortopathy of bicuspid aortic valve disease has distinctive patterns and usually involves the transverse aortic arch. J Thorac Cardiothorac Surg 2008;135:901–7, 907.e1-2.

174. Nazer RI, Elhenawy AM, Fazel SS, et al. The influence of operative techniques on the outcomes of bicuspid aortic valve disease and aortic dilatation. Ann Thorac Surg 2010;89:1918–24.

175. Park CB, Greason KL, Suri RM, et al. Should the proximal arch be routinely replaced in patients with bicuspid aortic valve disease and ascending aortic aneurysm? J Thorac Cardiovasc Surg 2011;142:602–7.

176. Kouchoukos NT, Masetti P, Nickerson NJ, et al. The Ross procedure. Long-term clinical and echocardiographic follow-up. Ann Thorac Surg 2004;78:773–81.

177. David TE, Omran A, Ivanov J, et al. Dilation of the pulmonary autograft after the Ross procedure. J Thorac Cardiovasc Surg 2000;119:210–20.

178. David TE. Reoperations after the Ross procedure. Circulation 2010;122:1139–40.

179. Wijesinghe N, Ye J, Rodes-Cabau J, et al. Transcatheter aortic valve implantation in patients with bicuspid aortic valve stenosis. J Am Coll Cardiol Intv 2010;3:1122–5.

180. Maron BJ, Ackerman MJ, Nishimura RA, et al. Task Force 4: HCM and other cardiomyopathies, mitral valve prolapse, myocarditis, and Marfan syndrome. J Am Coll Cardiol 2005;45:1340–5.

181. Brooke BS, Habashi JP, Judge DP, et al. Angiotensin II blockade and aortic-root dilation in Marfan's syndrome. N Engl J Med 2008;358:2787–95.

CHAPTER 14

Surgical Approach to Diseases of the Aortic Valve and the Aortic Root

S. Chris Malaisrie and Patrick M. McCarthy

Key Points

- Aortic valve replacement (AVR) has become increasingly safe even though an older population of patients is now being treated, with the best outcomes achieved at high-volume centers.
- More stented bioprosthetic valves are being used than mechanical valves, homografts, and pulmonary autografts combined, reflecting advances in valve technology.
- Aortic root replacement with a composite valve-graft (Bentall procedure) is the gold standard operation for aortic root aneurysm; however, the valve-sparing aortic root replacement (David or Yacoub procedures) is a good option for patients who want to avoid the long-term oral anticoagulation required with mechanical valves and structural valve deterioration associated with bioprosthetic valves in younger patients.
- A complete primary median sternotomy is the standard approach for aortic valve and aortic root replacement, but minimally invasive approaches, including the upper hemisternotomy and right anterior thoracotomy, can be performed with equivalent safety and better outcomes.
- Sutureless valves combine the advantages of a surgical AVR procedure (control of aortic atheroemboli, resection of diseased native valve) with transcatheter technology (decreased procedure time, improved valve hemodynamic function).
- Porcelain aorta, which can prevent safe central cannulation and aortic cross-clamping, can be managed with peripheral cannulation and hypothermic circulatory arrest.
- Aortic regurgitation from acute type A aortic dissections is life-threatening and is commonly managed with valve resuspension, with aortic root replacement being reserved for patients with intrinsic root pathology.
- Reoperative aortic valve and aortic root surgery can be performed safely through utilization of preoperative imaging, advanced techniques for myocardial protection, and safe management of existing bypass grafts.

The past decade has shown historic change in the surgical approach to patients with aortic valve disease. During this time, transcatheter aortic valve implantation (TAVI) was developed and tested, leading to a new treatment option approved by the U.S. Food and Drug Administration (FDA) for patients who previously would have been managed by medical therapy or for patients for whom conventional aortic valve replacement (AVR) poses a very high risk (Society of Thoracic Surgeons [STS] predicted risk of mortality [PROM] ≥8).[1,2] Additional testing is ongoing in randomized clinical trials to determine the proper use of TAVI in patients for whom AVR poses an intermediate surgical

risk (STS score ≥4).[3,4] Also, late freedom from structural valve deterioration (SVD) is now available for patients receiving stented bovine pericardial valves and stented porcine valves. The field has been influenced by new valve guidelines regarding the choice of bioprosthetic versus mechanical valve with an emphasis on the patient's role in decision making as well as expanded indications for treatment of aortic aneurysm in patients with a bicuspid aortic valve (BAV).

The impact of these changes has led to the most dramatic change in the clinical practice of aortic valve surgery in decades. Figure 14-1 demonstrates, by year, the changing pattern of valve replacement choices. The graph shows a striking shift in choice of prosthesis. In 2001, 63.6% of aortic valve replacements were bioprostheses, a figure that steadily rose to 81.8% in 2011. The rate of mechanical valve use dropped by more than half, from 30.8% to 14%. The rage of homograft replacement fell from 2.9% to 0.5%, and the Ross procedure has nearly vanished, dropping in rate from 1.0% to 0.1%, a tenfold decrease.

This chapter explores the data that led to the change in valve prosthesis choice, and review the surgical techniques that are appropriate in a variety of clinical settings.

Aortic Valve Replacement/Repair

Tissue Valves: Stented

The valve most commonly used to replace the aortic valve is a stented bioprosthetic valve, either bovine pericardium or porcine (Figures 14-2 and 14-3). The advantages to such a valve are: (1) ease of implantation and the rare occurrence of clinically significant patient prosthesis mismatch due to improving valve hemodynamics, (2) no lifelong need for anticoagulation with warfarin (unless the patient requires it for a different reason), (3) a relatively straightforward future reoperation for SVD, if necessary, and (4) the potential for a valve-in-valve procedure using a transcatheter heart valve for SVD. The most important disadvantage to tissue valves is the occurrence of SVD, which is primarily age dependent.

The technical aspects of AVR with a stented bioprosthetic valve are straightforward. The aortic valve can be exposed through a variety of aortotomies, including a hockey-stick, transverse, and oblique incisions. The aortic valve is excised and the annulus is extensively débrided of calcific plaques with care taken in the area of the conduction system (below the commissure between the noncoronary and right coronary cusps). Calcific extensions on the anterior leaflet of the mitral valve are removed. With

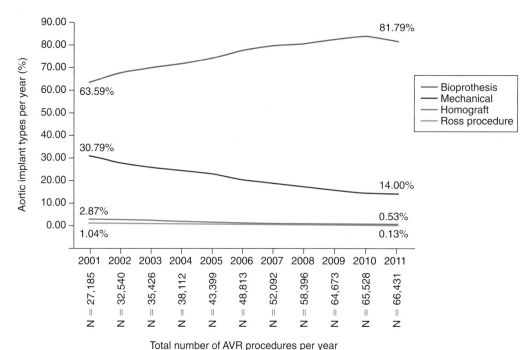

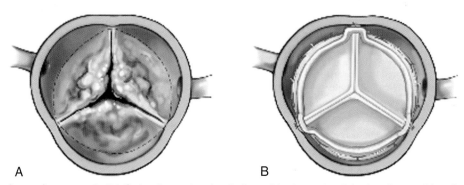

FIGURE 14-1   Trend in valve choice in aortic valve replacement in the Society of Thoracic Surgeons National Database. Bioprosthetic valves are most commonly implanted in the current era. Mechanical valves, homografts, and pulmonary autografts are all declining in use over time. *AVR,* Aortic valve replacement.

FIGURE 14-2   Aortic valve replacement. A, Calcified native aortic valve. **B,** Stented bovine pericardial valve. *(Reprinted from Stelzer P, Adams DH. Surgical approach to aortic valve disease. In: Otto CM, Bonow RO, editors. Valvular heart disease: a companion to Braunwald's heart disease. 3rd ed. Philadelphia: Elsevier Science; 2009. p. 187–208.)*

adequate débridement of annular calcification, perivalvular leak is rare, and with current-generation bioprostheses, clinically significant patient-prosthesis mismatch is uncommon.

Bioprosthetic Valves: Stentless

In the 1990s, "stentless" bioprosthetic valves made from porcine aortic valves became available. The advantages of this type of valve versus stented bioprosthetic valves were thought to be: (1) avoiding anticoagulation with a low risk for stroke and (2) improved hemodynamics compared to stented and mechanical valves.[5-7] The disadvantages to stentless valves were: (1) more complex operation requiring either a "mini-root" with reimplantation of the coronary ostia (Figure 14-4) or subcoronary implantation (Figure 14-5) and (2) data indicating concerns about freedom from SVD.[8]

Some surgeons use stentless porcine valves primarily in patients with BAVs with aneurysms. In this case, the aortic valve, root, and a portion of the tubular ascending aorta are replaced. Current American College of Cardiology/American Heart Association (ACC/AHA) indicate that if a patient with a BAV requires AVR and

has an ascending aortic diameter greater than 4.5 cm, then aortic replacement should be undertaken.[9] When this operation is performed with a bioprosthetic valve, current-generation stented valve must be sewn into a separate vascular graft, adding a few minutes to the procedure. With a stentless porcine valve, that step is not required because the porcine valve is packaged as a complete root.

Mechanical Valves

Mechanical valves have the advantages of long-term durability and a long track record with designs that have been durable for decades.[10,11] The major disadvantages are: (1) the need for lifelong anticoagulation, currently with warfarin, (2) a higher risk of thromboembolism than with bioprosthetic valves, and (3) audible clicking in some patients with several of the mechanical valve types that may be troublesome.

A newer model of mechanical valve, the On-X prosthetic heart valve (On-X Life Technologies, Inc., Austin, Texas), first implanted in 1996, has been shown to have low adverse clinical event rates, including 0.6% thromboembolism per patient-year, 0.4% bleeding

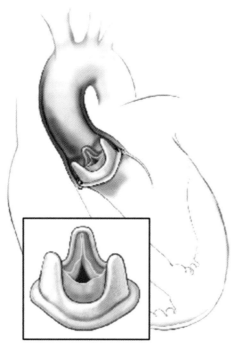

FIGURE 14-3   Stented porcine valve. The heterologous porcine tissue leaflets are attached to the supporting frame with an incorporated sewing ring. *(Reprinted from Stelzer P, Adams DH. Surgical approach to aortic valve disease. In: Otto CM, Bonow RO, editors. Valvular heart disease: a companion to Braunwald's heart disease. 3rd ed. Philadelphia: Elsevier Science; 2009. p. 187–208).*

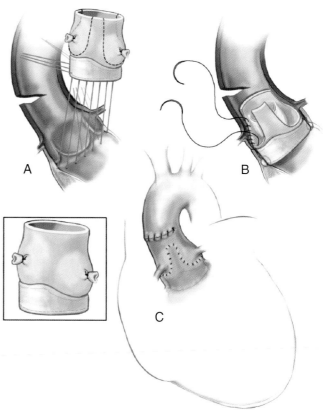

FIGURE 14-5   Stentless porcine root *(inset)* implanted with a modified subcoronary technique. A, Proximal interrupted suture line in a circular plan at or below annulus. **B,** Distal, continuous polypropylene suture line attaching residual aortic wall to native aortic wall, running below the coronary ostia and preserving the porcine noncoronary sinus. **C,** Aortotomy closed showing relationship of distal suture line to coronary ostia. *(Reprinted from Stelzer P, Adams DH. Surgical approach to aortic valve disease. In: Otto CM, Bonow RO, editors. Valvular heart disease: a companion to Braunwald's heart disease. 3rd ed. Philadelphia: Elsevier Science; 2009. p. 187–208.)*

Aortic Homografts

The first successful orthotopic placement of an aortic homograft was performed in 1962 by Donald Ross.[14] Much like the procedure for stentless bioprosthetic valves, the operation is more complex than straightforward implantation of a stented tissue valve, because a mini-root may be performed (Figure 14-6) or the valve may be sewn in the subcoronary position, as with aortic homografts.

The perceived advantages to the homograft were: (1) freedom from anticoagulation and a low risk for thromboembolic events typical for bioprosthetic valves, (2) perception that the durability may be higher than that for stented or stentless tissue valves, and (3) belief that homografts are more resistant to reinfection. As to the last advantage, in the setting of endocarditis, most surgeons consider the homograft the valve of choice, although the data for this belief is not very robust. The disadvantages to a homograft are: (1) the increased complexity of implantation, (2) difficulty of reoperation in many patients because of calcification that develops in the wall,[15] and (3) a higher rate of SVD than originally hoped.[15,16]

Ross Procedure

Donald Ross also developed the Ross procedure using the pulmonic valve and root autograft with homograft replacement of the patient's own pulmonic valve (Figure 14-7). The perceived advantages of this technique were freedom from anticoagulation

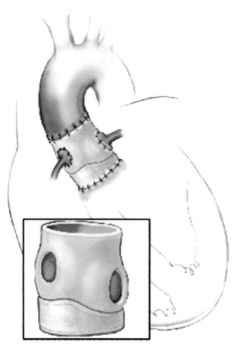

FIGURE 14-4   Stentless porcine root for aortic root replacement. The porcine root completely replaces the native aortic root, and coronaries are reimplanted. *(Reprinted from Stelzer P, Adams DH. Surgical approach to aortic valve disease. In: Otto CM, Bonow RO, editors. Valvular heart disease: a companion to Braunwald's heart disease. 3rd ed. Philadelphia: Elsevier Science; 2009. p. 187–208.)*

rate per patient-year, and 0% thrombosis rate when used in the aortic position.[12] An ongoing clinical trial (Prospective Randomized On-X Anticoagulation Clinical Trial [PROACT]) is studying the safety of lower doses of warfarin in patients with high-risk for thromboembolism and antiplatelet drugs only (aspirin/clopidogrel) in patients with low-risk for thromboembolism.[13]

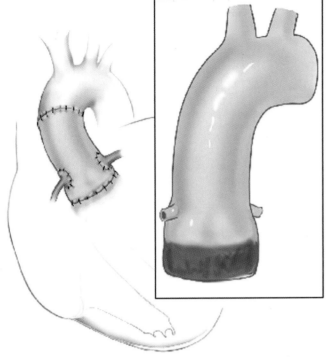

FIGURE 14-6 Aortic homograft. The root replacement configuration using the cryopreserved aortic homograft with reimplantation of coronary ostia is shown. *(Reprinted from Stelzer P, Adams DH. Surgical approach to aortic valve disease. In: Otto CM, Bonow RO, editors. Valvular heart disease: a companion to Braunwald's heart disease. 3rd ed. Philadelphia: Elsevier Science; 2009. p. 187–208.)*

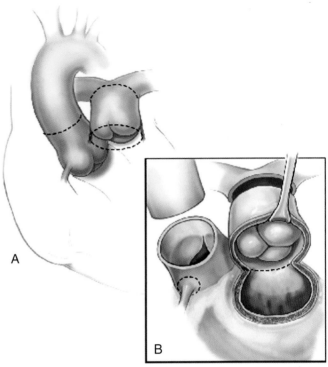

FIGURE 14-7 Ross procedure. Incision lines are illustrated *(dotted lines)* for aortic (transverse and distal) and pulmonary roots. The distal pulmonary incision is made first to allow inspection of the valve and to enable accurate placement of the proximal incision below the annulus. *(Reprinted from Stelzer P, Adams DH. Surgical approach to aortic valve disease. In: Otto CM, Bonow RO, editors. Valvular heart disease: a companion to Braunwald's heart disease. 3rd ed. Philadelphia: Elsevier Science; 2009. p. 187–208.)*

and decreased risk of stroke. Also, in children, unlike with homografts and bioprosthetic valves, the tissue continues to grow with the patient. The disadvantages are: (1) much more complex operation than other procedures that simply replace the pathologic aortic valve, (2) the potential for dysfunction of two valves, the pulmonic homograft and the autograft, (3) the development of late aneurysms requiring reoperation, and (4) the potential for injury to the first septal perforator when mobilizing the pulmonary autograft.[17]

Guidelines for Valve Choice

Choosing a valve according to the patient's age is controversial. Findings of two major randomized clinical trials have not been consistent regarding difference in long-term survival between bioprosthetic and mechanical valves.[18,19] Although both trials compared first-generation porcine valves and single-tilting disk Bjork-Shiley valves (neither valve is currently in use), the Veterans Affairs Cooperative Study[19] showed improved 15-year survival with mechanical valves than with bioprosthetic valves, but the Edinburgh Heart Valve Trial[18] showed no difference in 20-year survival. Regarding age threshold for valve choice, both the U.S.[9] and European[20] guidelines recommend bioprosthetic valves for patients 65 years and older when only age is considered (Table 14-1). The European guidelines, however, have a class I recommendation for mechanical valve in patients younger than 40 years and a class IIa recommendation for patients younger than 60 years, recognizing that in patients between 60 and 65 years, other factors impact valve choice.[20] Guidelines for mechanical valves show that requirement for anticoagulation due to a mechanical valve in another position and a condition associated with high risk of thromboembolism are factors favoring the use of mechanical valves (Table 14-2). On the other hand, contraindication to anticoagulation and planned pregnancy favors the use

TABLE 14-1	Age Thresholds for Valve Choice	
	ACC/AHA 2006 GUIDELINES	**ESC/EACTS 2012 GUIDELINES**
Mechanical valve	<65 years (class IIaC)	<60 years (class IIaC)
		<40 years (class IC)
Bioprosthetic valve	≥65 years (class IIaC) <65 years (class IIaC)*	>65 years (class IIaC)

ACC/AHA, American College of Cardiology/American Heart Association; *ESC/EACTS*, European Society of Cardiology/European Association of Cardio-Thoracic Surgery.
*A bioprosthesis is reasonable for aortic valve replacement (AVR) in patients less than 65 years of age who elect to receive this valve for lifestyle considerations after detailed discussions of the risks of anticoagulation versus the likelihood that a second AVR may be necessary in the future.

of bioprosthetic valves (Table 14-3). Both guidelines acknowledge patient preference after informed consent, balancing the risk of long-term anticoagulation required for mechanical valves and the risk of SVD requiring re-intervention that is associated with bioprosthetic valves.

Long-term follow-up of commonly used bioprosthetic valves for the aortic position show good durability to more than 15 years in several large series (Table 14-4). Freedom from SVD for stented bovine pericardial valves has been reported to be 82.3% at 15 years for the Carpentier-Edwards bovine pericardial valve (Edwards Lifesciences Corporation, Irvine, California)[21] and 62.3% at 20 years for the Mitroflow aortic pericardial heart valve (Sorin Group, Milan).[22] For stented porcine valves, the freedom from SVD has been reported to be 63.4% at 20 years for the Hancock II valve (Medtronic, Inc., Minneapolis, Minnesota)[23] and the freedom from reoperation for SVD to be 61.1% for the Biocor valve (St. Jude Medical, Inc., St. Paul, Minnesota).[24] All of these

TABLE 14-2 Guidelines Favoring Mechanical Valves

	ACC/AHA 2006 GUIDELINES	ESC/EACTS 2012 GUIDELINES
Patient already undergoing anticoagulation for mechanical prosthesis in another position	Class IC	Class IC
Patient preference	Class IIaC	Class IC
Accelerated risk of structural valve deterioration (Age <40 years, hyperparathyroidism)	None	Class IC
Patient already undergoing anticoagulation due to high risk of thromboembolism (atrial fibrillation, venous thromboembolism, thrombophilia, severe left ventricular dysfunction)	Class IIaC	Class IIbC
Reasonable life expectancy (>10 years) and high risk for future "repeat" aortic valve replacement	None	Class IIac

ACC/AHA, American College of Cardiology/American Heart Association; *ESC/EACTS*, European Society of Cardiology/European Association of Cardio-Thoracic Surgery.

TABLE 14-3 Guidelines Favoring Bioprosthetic Valves

	ACC/AHA 2006 GUIDELINES	ESC/EACTS 2012 GUIDELINES
Anticoagulation contraindicated	Class IC	Class IC
Patient preference	Class IIaC	Class IC
Reoperation of mechanical valve thrombosis despite good long-term anticoagulation	None	Class IC
Woman of child-bearing age contemplating pregnancy	Class IIbC	Class IIaC
Low risk for future "repeat" aortic valve replacement	None	Class IIaC

ACC/AHA, American College of Cardiology/American Heart Association; *ESC/EACTS*, European Society of Cardiology/European Association of Cardio-Thoracic Surgery.

TABLE 14-4 Structural Valve Deterioration of Bioprosthetic Valves

AUTHOR (YEAR)	Mean Follow-Up AVR	Mean Follow-Up MVR	Number of Valves AVR	Number of Valves MVR	TIME OF SVD ESTIMATE (YR)	AGE (YR)	Actuarial Freedom from Reoperation for Structural Valve Deterioration (%) AVR	Actuarial Freedom from Reoperation for Structural Valve Deterioration (%) MVR	VALVE
Yankah et al (2008)[22]	—	—	1513	—	20	>65 >70	71.8 ± 6.0 84.8 ± 0.7	— —	Mitroflow aortic pericardial bioprosthesis (Sorin Group)
Mykén et al (2009)[24]	6.0 ± 4.5	6.2 ± 5.6	1518	194	20	≤50 51-60 61-70 71-80 >80	37.7 ± 8.6 60.7 ± 10.3 81.0 ± 5.1 97.8 ± 1.2 100	57.6 ± 1.5 80.0 ± 1.9 86.3 ± 0.7 100 (>70 yr) 100 (>70 yr)	Biocor porcine bioprosthesis (St. Jude Medical, Inc.)
David et al (2009)[25]	12.2	—	1134	—	20	<60 60-70 >70	32.6 ± 6.2 89.8 ± 3.2 100	— — —	Hancock II aortic porcine bioprosthesis (Medtronic, Inc.)
McClure et al (2010)[21]	6.0 ± 3.6	—	1000	—	15	<65 65-75 >75	34.7 (CI 6-67) 89.4 (CI 63-97) 99.5 (CI 97-99.9)	— — —	Carpentier-Edwards pericardial aortic bioprosthesis (Edwards Lifesciences Corporation)

AVR, Aortic valve replacement; *CI*, 95% confidence interval; *MVR*, mitral valve replacement.

series stratified their results by patient age, which is the major determinant of durability, and found that 20-year freedom from reoperation for SVD in patients 70 years and older to be between 84.8% (Mitroflow)[22] and 100% (Hancock II).[25]

Controversy exists for valve choice in younger patients who would like to avoid the risk of complications associated with the use of long-term warfarin therapy required for mechanical valves. Even in patients as young as 45 years, freedom from SVD was about 85% at 10 years and 55% at 15 years with the Carpentier-Edwards pericardial valve in a study from the Cleveland Clinic.[26] Also in a review of very young patients (mean age 22.7 ± 6.8 yrs), freedom from all bioprosthetic valve-related complications was 85.8% at 8 years.[27] El Oakley et al[28] calculated that for a 50-year-old patient, the risk of valve-related morbidity over the projected life expectancy of the patient was 108% with a mechanical valve,

compared with 48% with a bioprosthesis. Different types of bioprosthetic valves also have been compared, and results may not be uniform. Rahimtoola[29] compared reports of SVD with the use of bovine pericardial valves and porcine valves and found a much lower rate of SVD with pericardial valves.

For young patients who eventually develop SVD requiring intervention in the future, repeat AVR may not be mandatory. The possibility of TAVI for failed bioprosthetic valves (valve-in-valve procedure) has the potential of making AVR with a bioprosthetic valve more attractive to the patient (see Chapter 15). The feasibility of the valve-in-valve procedure has been demonstrated in single-center series.[30-33] Procedural success was 100% in one series of 23 patients, and another report of 47 patients noted one intraoperative death.[30,34] An international registry of 202 patients demonstrated 30-day mortality after valve-in-valve procedure of

8.4% and 1-year survival of 85.8%.[35] Procedural concerns, however, included device malposition in 15.3% of patients, coronary ostial obstruction in 3.5%, and relatively high mean gradients, 15.9 ± 8.6 mm Hg.

Reintervention for failed bioprosthetic valves can, therefore, be performed as either an open surgical procedure or a transcatheter procedure. The safety of reoperative AVR is discussed later. Although currently considered an "off-label" use of transcatheter heart valves, the valve-in-valve procedure for failed bioprosthetic valves offers a potential application for future transcatheter technology. Safer future reinterventions may justify use of bioprosthetic valves in younger patients. Ultimately, the patient makes the decision after discussion with the surgeon and cardiologist about the risks and benefits as well as the perceived future of TAVI versus standard reoperation valve surgery.

Aortic Valve Repair

Aortic valve repair can be performed in selected patients with aortic regurgitation (AR). Unfortunately, valve repair in patients with aortic stenosis (AS) involving leaflet decalcification is not a feasible treatment option and has been associated with early postoperative AR due to leaflet scarring and late restenosis due to recalcification. As with mitral valve repair, the benefit of aortic valve repair over AVR is avoidance of prosthetic valve-related complications such as thromboembolism and infective endocarditis. Data on aortic valve repair durability are limited to experienced centers, but 10-year freedom from reoperation can be as high as 93% in tricuspid aortic valves.[36-38] The durability of BAV repair, however, is less than that of tricuspid aortic valves, and repair for these patients with BAV remains controversial. No guidelines exist for aortic valve repair.

Repair of a normal, but regurgitant tricuspid aortic valve uses a combination of cusp repair and annuloplasty. Typically, one or more cusps are redundant which causes cusp prolapse. Central free margin plication at the nodulus of Arantius effectively shortens the cusp, resulting in a higher zone of coaptation with the other cusps (Figure 14-8).[39] An alternative method of cusp shortening is free margin resuspension with a continuous over-and-over suture from commissure to commissure (Figure 14-9). This technique is also useful for closing cusp fenestrations, which are typically located near the commissures, where cusp stress is highest. The least common technique of cusp repair is cusp extension with pericardium in cases of inadequate cusp tissue (Figure 14-10). Occasionally, leaflet perforations such as those that occur after healed endocarditis can be simply repaired with

a pericardial patch (Figure 14-11). A reduction annuloplasty may also be required in cases of annuloaortic ectasia. The simplest technique is the commissural plication (Figure 14-12). This technique achieves narrowing of the interleaflet triangle below the commissure and reduces the diameter of the aortic root, thereby increasing coaptation of the cusp surfaces. Novel techniques utilizing an external aortic annulus ring for the purpose of downsizing the aortic annulus have been described, but these rings are not currently available in the United States.[40]

Repair of the BAV can be performed with similar techniques of cusp repair and reduction annuloplasty. The goal of BAV repair is to restore a competent BAV rather than to create a tricuspid

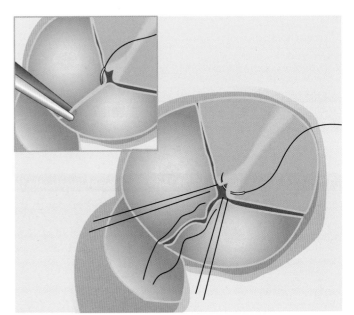

FIGURE 14-8   Free margin plication. After the prolapsing leaflets are identified, the free margin is plicated at the nodulus of Arantius with a simple, interrupted 5-0 polypropylene stitch. Shortening the free margin brings the leaflet coaptation surface higher in the aortic root. *(From Schafers HJ, Langer F, Glombitza P, et al. Aortic valve reconstruction in myxomatous degeneration of aortic valves: are fenestrations a risk factor for repair failure? J Thorac Cardiovasc Surg 2010;139:660–4.)*

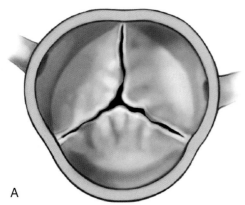

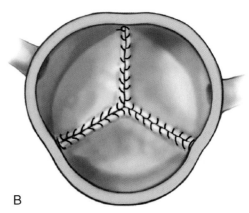

A   B

FIGURE 14-9   Leaflet shortening. A and **B,** Continuous over-and-over suture from commissure to commissure is one method of shortening leaflets; 6-0 expanded polytetrafluoroethylene (GORE-TEX) is suggested for this maneuver, with the knots placed outside the aorta. *(Reprinted from Stelzer P, Adams DH. Surgical approach to aortic valve disease. In: Otto CM, Bonow RO, editors. Valvular heart disease: a companion to Braunwald's heart disease. 3rd ed. Philadelphia: Elsevier Science; 2009. p. 187–208.)*

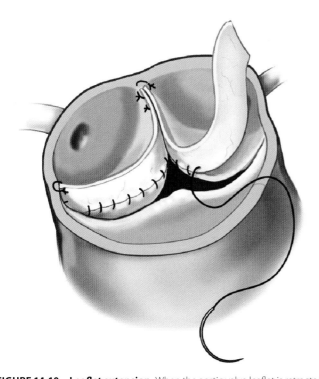

FIGURE 14-10   Leaflet extension. When the aortic valve leaflet is retracted or shortened, the cusp can be extended using pericardium. The pericardium is sewn from commissure to commissure, along the free margin of the leaflet, thereby enlarging the coaptation surface. *(Reprinted from Stelzer P, Adams DH. Surgical approach to aortic valve disease. In: Otto CM, Bonow RO, editors. Valvular heart disease: a companion to Braunwald's heart disease. 3rd ed. Philadelphia: Elsevier Science; 2009. p. 187–208.)*

aortic valve. In cases with equal-size cusps and commissure oriented at 180 degrees to each other, repair can be performed readily as with a tricuspid aortic valve. However, in the more common type of BAV involving a conjoint (fused) cusp (Figure 14-13), the raphe may be sclerosed and immobile, requiring additional techniques. In these cases, a triangular resection of the raphe can be performed with reapproximation of the edges to create a shortened and pliable cusp (Figure 14-14). When tissue the conjoint cusp is inadequate, the raphe can be released from the commissure and shaved to improve cusp mobility. Judgment must be used in cases with severely sclerosed valves, because the durability of a repair of a diseased BAV may be less than even that of a bioprosthetic valve.

Risks of Aortic Valve Replacement

The risks of surgery can be quantitatively estimated by several models (see Chapter 10), including The STS Predicted Risk of Mortality (STS PROM),[41] European System for Cardiac Operative Risk Evaluation (EuroSCORE) II,[42] and Ambler scores.[43] In addition to operative mortality, the STS PROM score provides an estimate of important complications such as prolonged hospitalization, stroke, respiratory failure, mediastinitis, renal failure, and reoperation. These risk calculators are important for surgical decision making and require informed consent from the patient prior to the planned operation.

Data from the STS indicates that the operative mortality for patients 70 years of age or older who underwent isolated AVR or AVR with coronary artery bypass grafting surgery (CABG) between 1994 and 2003 fell from 10% to less than 6%.[44] In the most recent analysis using the STS database on 108,687 patients from 1997 to 2006 with a mean age of 68 years undergoing isolated AVR, the in-hospital mortality was 2.6% with an observed stroke

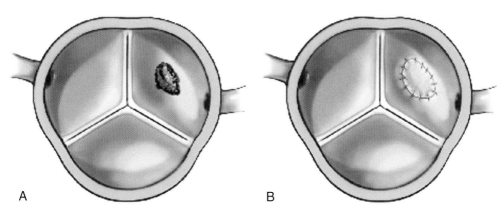

FIGURE 14-11   Repair of healed endocarditis. A simple leaflet perforation **(A)** can be repaired with an autologous pericardial patch **(B)**. *(Reprinted from Stelzer P, Adams DH. Surgical approach to aortic valve disease. In: Otto CM, Bonow RO, editors. Valvular heart disease: a companion to Braunwald's heart disease. 3rd ed. Philadelphia: Elsevier Science; 2009. p. 187–208.)*

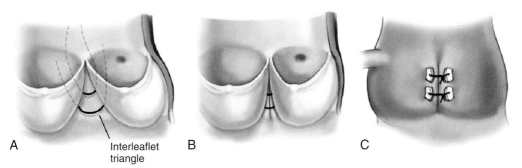

Interleaflet triangle

FIGURE 14-12   Aortic commissuroplasty. The wide interleaflet triangle **(A)** is narrowed with sutures that plicate this area to increase coaptation. **B,** View from inside the aorta; **C,** External view. *(Reprinted from Stelzer P, Adams DH. Surgical approach to aortic valve disease. In: Otto CM, Bonow RO, editors. Valvular heart disease: a companion to Braunwald's heart disease. 3rd ed. Philadelphia: Elsevier Science; 2009. p. 187–208.)*

rate of 1.3% and length of stay of 7.8 days for the year 2006.[45] Among patients 80 to 85 years of age, 30-day mortality was 4.9% with an observed stroke rate of 2.0%.[45]

Experience at centers of excellence within the last 5 years have demonstrated significantly improved operative mortality, less than 1%, after isolated AVR.[46-50] The incidence of perioperative stroke in these contemporary series ranged from 0% to 1.9%, and the length of stay was as short as 5 days.[47] Di Eusanio et al[49] reported a 3-year survival rate, comparable to the life expectancy of an age- and gender-matched 2006 population (82% vs. 81%; P = 0.157).[49] Overall, the reported patient survival rates at 1 and 3 years in these series were 94% to 97% and 88% to 94%, respectively.

In the prospective, randomized, multicenter Placement of Aortic Transcatheter Valves (PARTNER) trial comparing high-risk patients (mean STS score 11.8%) receiving TAVI or AVR for severe, symptomatic AS, outcomes for both procedures were excellent.[2]

Patients undergoing AVR (n = 351, mean age 85 years) had a 30-day mortality of 6.5%, setting a new benchmark for operative outcomes in a high-risk cohort of patients treated at centers of excellence. Moreover, comparative results showed that early and late strokes and transient ischemic attacks were significantly lower in the AVR group than the TAVI group (30 days, 2.4% vs. 5.5%, respectively, P = 0.04; 1 year, 4.3% vs. 8.3%, respectively, P = 0.04).[2]

Aortic Root Surgery

Indications

Indications for aortic root replacement include aneurysms of the ascending aorta, aortic valve endocarditis with annular abscess, and acute type A aortic dissection. The most common indication is aneurysm of the aortic root or ascending aorta. The size threshold for aneurysm repair depends on whether the aneurysm is the primary indication for surgery or whether it coexists in a patient already requiring cardiac surgery.

Primary aneurysms of the aortic root are secondary to either genetically mediated disorders or acquired disorders. The acquired disorders include degenerative thoracic aortic aneurysm, chronic aortic dissection, intramural hematoma, penetrating atherosclerotic ulcer, mycotic aneurysm, and pseudoaneurysm. Size threshold for surgical repair in this group of patients is 5.5 cm for both the aortic root and ascending aorta according to class I recommendations by the 2010 ACC/AHA Guidelines for the Diagnosis and management of Patients with Thoracic Aortic Disease developed by a multigroup-sponsored task force.[51] The genetically mediated disorders include Marfan syndrome, vascular Ehlers-Danlos syndrome, Turner syndrome, BAV, familial thoracic aortic aneurysm and dissection, and Loeys-Dietz syndrome. These disorders are associated with a greater risk of rupture, dissection, and death, in particular Loeys-Dietz syndrome. Size threshold for operative intervention in this group of patients is 5.0 cm according to the same guidelines.[51] This recommendation is consistent with a size threshold of 5.0 cm in patients with BAV in the 2006 ACC/AHA Guidelines for for the Management of Patients with Valvular Heart Disease.[9] Surgical repair may be considered in patients with Loeys-Dietz syndrome and aortic diameters as small as 4.2 cm, depending on imaging modality.[51]

When aortic root aneurysm or aneurysm of the ascending aorta coexists in a patient already requiring cardiac surgery, the threshold for concomitant aortic replacement is an aortic diameter of 4.5 cm (class IC in the thoracic aortic disease guidelines).[51] In the most common clinical scenario involving patients with BAV requiring aortic valve surgery, the size threshold is similarly 4.5 cm (class IC in the valvular heart disease guidelines).[9] The

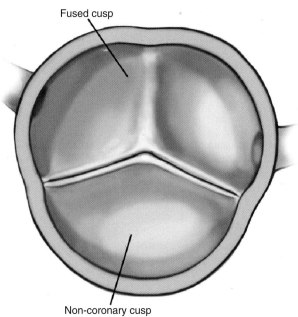

FIGURE 14-13 Bicuspid valve. The most common configuration is really a fusion of two leaflets (most often right and left coronary leaflets) with a rudimentary commissure of raphe where the normal commissure would be. *(Reprinted from Stelzer P, Adams DH. Surgical approach to aortic valve disease. In: Otto CM, Bonow RO, editors. Valvular heart disease: a companion to Braunwald's heart disease. 3rd ed. Philadelphia: Elsevier Science; 2009. p. 187–208.)*

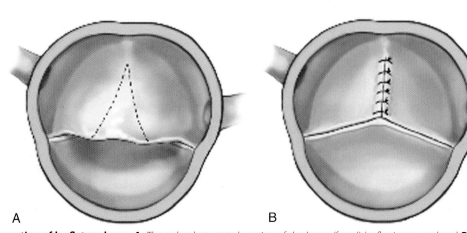

FIGURE 14-14 Resection of leaflet prolapse. A, The redundant central portion of the larger (fused) leaflet is resected and **B,** is closed primarily to restore normal coaptation level. *(Reprinted from Stelzer P, Adams DH. Surgical approach to aortic valve disease. In: Otto CM, Bonow RO, editors. Valvular heart disease: a companion to Braunwald's heart disease. 3rd ed. Philadelphia: Elsevier Science; 2009. p. 187–208.)*

rationale for prophylactic repair at a smaller size is to prevent future aneurysmal degeneration requiring later reoperative cardiac surgery.[23]

These guidelines are predicated on an operative risk for aortic root replacement of less than 5%. Currently, no risk model is available to predict the risk of operative mortality for aortic root replacement. However, results from two national registries demonstrate that elective aortic root replacement is associated with an operative mortality of 4.5% to 5.8%.[52,53] The United Kingdom registry (1962 patients undergoing any first-time aortic root replacement from 1986 to 2004) identified concomitant CABG (odds ratio [OR] 3.38), nonelective surgery (OR 3.20), left ventricular ejection fraction less than 50% (OR 2.63), valve size less than 23 mm (OR 1.97), hospital volume 8 cases or fewer per year (OR 1.53), and age more than 70 years (OR 1.20) as independent risk factors for early death.[53] The STS database (13,358 patients undergoing either elective aortic root replacement or AVR/ ascending aortic procedure from 2004 to 2007) demonstrated a 58% difference in operative mortality between high-volume and low-volume centers, with the most pronounced difference in centers performing fewer than 30 cases per year ($P = 0.001$).[52] Moreover, when complicating factors such as reoperative cardiac surgery, emergency operations for aortic dissections, and complex infective endocarditis are involved, differences between outcomes of procedures performed in high-volume and low-volume centers may be even more pronounced.

Aortic Root Replacement with Composite Valve-Graft (Modified Bentall Procedure)

The replacement of the entire aortic root, including both the aortic wall and the aortic valve, was first described in 1968 by Bentall and De Bono.[54] In this procedure, a mechanical valve was attached to the end of a Dacron tube graft to construct a composite valve-graft. The composite valve-graft was then implanted inside the native aortic root at the level of the aortic annulus. Holes were made in the side of the Dacron graft, and the two coronary ostia were reattached to the graft by sewing of the graft to the aortic wall around the ostia. The distal end of the graft was sewn inside the distal aorta, and the native aortic wall was completely closed over the Dacron graft. The "classic" Bentall procedure was performed to control bleeding from the coronary artery suture lines and porous graft material used in that era; however, long-term follow-up showed that this procedure was prone to pseudoaneurysm formation. This classic Bentall procedure is no longer performed in modern-day practice.

Current technique of aortic root replacement with composite valve-graft is a modification of the Bentall procedure (Figure 14-15).[55] In this modification, the composite valve-graft is implanted at the aortic annulus in a similar fashion; however, coronary reconstruction is performed by reattaching the coronary ostia as "buttons" rather than using the classic "inclusion" technique. Other, less common techniques of coronary reconstruction include creation of a Dacron bypass graft to the coronary ostia (Cabrol technique, Figure 14-16),[56] interposition of a saphenous vein graft to the coronary ostia (Kay-Zubiate technique, Figure 14-17),[57] and traditional CABG to the epicardial arteries. These advanced techniques for coronary reconstruction are typically used during reoperative aortic root surgery in which the coronary arteries are "frozen" and cannot be mobilized from the surrounding scar tissue.

The modified Bentall procedure using a mechanical valve has been used extensively in young patients with Marfan syndrome. In 2002, the Johns Hopkins group reported 24 years of experience with this operation in 271 patients with Marfan syndrome.[58] The results show an operative mortality of 0% with 84% actual overall survival at 24 years. Actuarial rates of 20-year freedom from thromboembolism, endocarditis, and reoperation were 93%, 90%, and 74%, respectively.

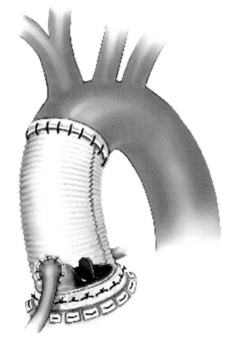

FIGURE 14-15 Modified Bentall procedure. The current configuration of freestanding complete aortic root replacement with a mechanical valved conduit, with coronary buttons reimplanted into the conduit. *(Reprinted from Stelzer P, Adams DH. Surgical approach to aortic valve disease. In: Otto CM, Bonow RO, editors. Valvular heart disease: a companion to Braunwald's heart disease. 3rd ed. Philadelphia: Elsevier Science; 2009. p. 187–208.)*

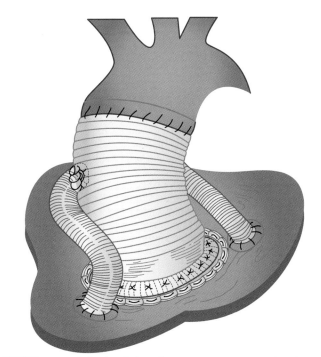

FIGURE 14-16 Cabrol technique for coronary reconstruction. In cases in which the coronary arteries cannot be safely mobilized for reimplantation in the conduit, coronary reconstruction can be accomplished by sewing a synthetic polyester (Dacron) tube graft from coronary os to os, followed by a side-to-side anastomosis to the conduit.

Similarly, the modified Bentall procedure using a bioprosthetic valve has been shown to have excellent outcomes. In 2007, the Mount Sinai group reported 12 years of experience with 275 patients.[59] The results showed an operative mortality of 6.2% with 75% overall survival at 5 years. The rates of stroke and significant

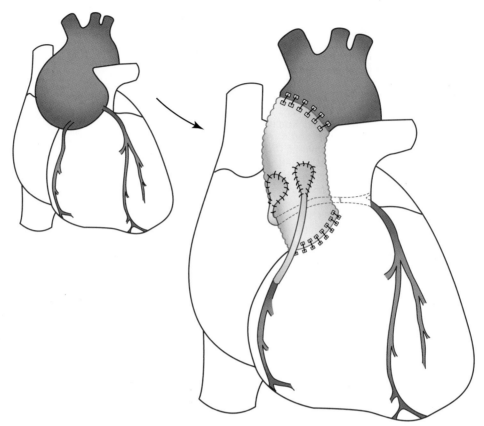

FIGURE 14-17 Kay-Zubiate technique. An alternative technique for coronary reconstruction during aortic root replacement is performed with use of saphenous vein as interposition grafts between the aortic graft and native origins of the coronary arteries. *(Reprinted with permission from Weldon, SC, Conners, JP, Martz, MN. Use of saphenous vein to extend and relocate coronary arteries: clinical experience during extensive reconstructive operations of the aortic root. Arch Surg 2003;114:1330–5.)*

hemorrhage were 0.85 and 0.3 per 100 patient-years, respectively. Only one patient required a reoperation. Impregnated Dacron grafts cannot be stored with bioprosthetic valves; therefore, composite valve-grafts are not typically premanufactured. Construction of a composite valve-graft at the time of operation allows for greater versatility in bioprosthetic valve type and size while adding little time to the operation (Figure 14-18).

Overall, the modified Bentall procedure with replacement of both the ascending aorta and aortic valve is the gold standard operation for aortic root replacement. The technique is reproducible and safe. Proven durability of more than 20 years is the benchmark for the many alternative techniques.

Valve-Sparing Aortic Root Replacement (David and Yacoub Procedures)

Aortic root replacement with preservation of the native aortic valve was first described in the early 1990s by Sir Magdi Yacoub and Tirone David. Both the remodeling technique (Yacoub procedure) and the reimplantation technique (David procedure) have the common advantage of sparing the native aortic valve, thereby eliminating the need for a prosthetic valve and preserving the flow characteristics of a normal aortic valve. Theoretical disadvantages of the valve-sparing aortic root replacement include abnormal eddy currents within the neoroot, which can increase stress during leaflet closure and contribute to abnormal coronary flow reserve.[60] The possibility of leaflet trauma on the Dacron graft may be mitigated by recreating pseudo-sinuses with the Dacron graft.[61]

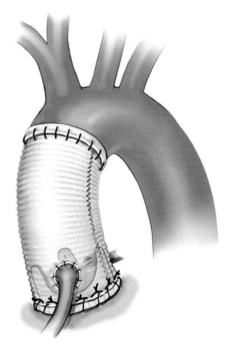

FIGURE 14-18 Bio-Bentall procedure. The biological valve is first attached to the conduit, and then the composite is attached to the aortic root. Coronary arteries are reimplanted into the graft. *(Reprinted from Stelzer P, Adams DH. Surgical approach to aortic valve disease. In: Otto CM, Bonow RO, editors. Valvular heart disease: a companion to Braunwald's heart disease. 3rd ed. Philadelphia: Elsevier Science; 2009. p. 187–208.)*

Successful preservation of the native aortic valve is more likely in patients with normal or near-normal leaflets. Thinning of the cusps secondary to severely enlarged roots can cause stress fenestrations toward the commissures. When more than one cusp is involved, repair is not advised.[25] Valves with AR are typically secondary to cusp prolapse and can be repaired with techniques described earlier in this chapter. Preventing leaflet prolapse during the procedure has been shown to improve durability.[36] Results of the valve-sparing aortic root replacement have been reported for both procedures, and long-term follow-up has shown that reintervention rates are lower with the David procedure than with the Yacoub procedure.[62]

YACOUB PROCEDURE

The remodeling technique for valve-sparing aortic root replacement (Yacoub procedure) involves resection of the sinus tissue and construction of neo-sinuses using a tailored Dacron graft (Figure 14-19). The coronary arteries are reimplanted in their corresponding neo-sinuses as buttons, as in the modified Bentall procedure. In this procedure, however, the aortic annulus is not supported by the Dacron graft and is best suited for patients without annular dilation or a predisposition to future annular dilation.

DAVID PROCEDURE

The reimplantation technique for valve-sparing aortic root replacement (David technique) involves resection of the sinus tissue and reimplantation of the native aortic valve within a Dacron graft (Figure 14-20). The coronary arteries are reconstructed as coronary buttons for the corresponding neo-sinus. Because the annulus is enclosed with the Dacron graft, the size of the annulus can be reduced, and further dilation prevented. Several modifications of the David procedure have been described, with newer modifications attempting to construct bulging neo-sinuses to mimic the natural aortic root.[63,64]

Aortic Root Enlargement

The aortic root can be enlarged by dividing the annulus and augmenting the root with a patch. The most common technique involves enlarging the posterior annulus of the aortic root at the noncoronary cusp as described by Nicks et al[65] (posterior root enlargement; Figure 14-21). The division of the aortic root can be extended through the aortic annulus into the anterior leaflet of the mitral valve as described by Manougian et al.[66] Both procedures require repair of the defect with a patch of bovine pericardium, autologous pericardium, or synthetic graft, which effectively enlarges the aortic annulus. The latter procedure allows for placement of a larger patch but also requires repair of the dome of the left atrium and the anterior leaflet of the mitral valve.[66] Anterior annulus enlargement (Konno procedure)[67] is more commonly used in a pediatric patient when the left ventricular outflow tract itself requires enlargement for subvalvular stenosis. This technique enlarges the anterior aortic annulus just to the left of the right coronary os, through the ventricular septum, into the right ventricular outflow tract. The resulting defect is closed with a pericardial or synthetic patch. Both posterior and anterior aortic root enlargement techniques allow for implantation of a larger aortic prosthesis.

The indication for a root enlargement procedure is the presence of a small aortic annulus that would accommodate an aortic prosthesis that is too small relative to patient size, resulting in patient-prosthesis mismatch (PPM). The concept of PPM can be quantified using the indexed effective orifice area (EOAi). Current guidelines published by the Association Society of Echocardiography defines PPM as absent if EOAi is 0.85 cm^2/m^2 or higher, moderate if it is lower than 0.85 cm^2/m^2 but higher than 0.60 cm^2/m^2, and severe if it is 0.60 cm^2/m^2 or lower.[68] Moreover, the guidelines suggest that PPM should not be considered unless corroborated by additional echocardiographic evidence, such as aortic jet velocity higher than 3 m/s, acceleration time less than 100 msec, and dimensionless velocity index less than 0.25.

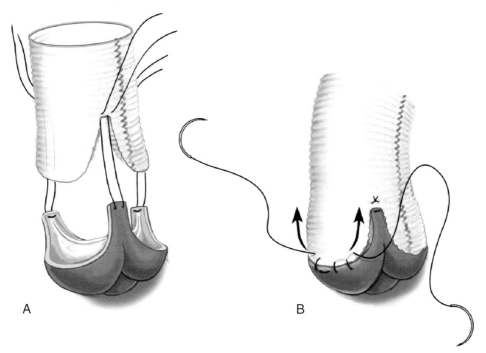

A   B

FIGURE 14-19 Yacoub procedure. A, The sinuses are cut out, and the commissures are carefully suspended to maintain root height. **B,** The sinuses are effectively replaced with tailored "tongues" of vascular graft, with the longest parts of the graft placed at the depth of each sinus. *(Reprinted from Stelzer P, Adams DH. Surgical approach to aortic valve disease. In: Otto CM, Bonow RO, editors. Valvular heart disease: a companion to Braunwald's heart disease. 3rd ed. Philadelphia: Elsevier Science; 2009. p. 187–208.)*

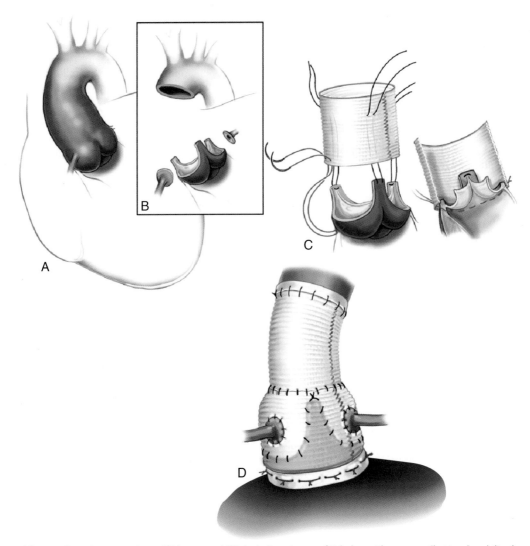

FIGURE 14-20 David procedure. Aneurysmal root **(A)** is resected **(B),** including sinuses of Valsalva, with coronary "buttons" mobilized away. **C,** Subannular sutures (six to eight) are placed. Commissural posts are drawn up inside the valve, and the annular sutures are passed through the proximal end of the graft. **D,** Annular sutures are tied gently. Then the valve is reimplanted with continuous 5-0 polypropylene suture inside the graft. Aortic continuity is reestablished with another graft of a size appropriate to the desired sinotubular junction and proximal arch. *(Reprinted from Stelzer P, Adams DH. Surgical approach to aortic valve disease. In: Otto CM, Bonow RO, editors. Valvular heart disease: a companion to Braunwald's heart disease. 3rd ed. Philadelphia: Elsevier Science; 2009. p. 187–208.)*

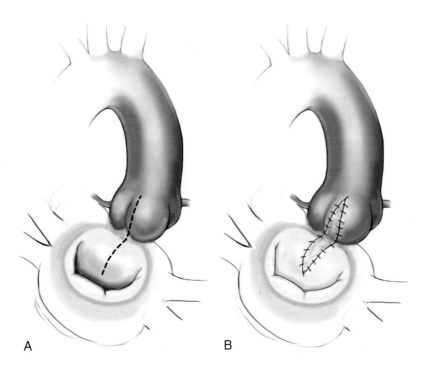

FIGURE 14-21 Root enlargement. A, Incision in the non-coronary sinus is carried down into the anterior mitral leaflet. **B,** A patch of pericardium is used to expand the leaflet, annulus, and aortic wall to allow implantation of a larger aortic valve. *(Reprinted from Stelzer P, Adams DH. Surgical approach to aortic valve disease. In: Otto CM, Bonow RO, editors. Valvular heart disease: a companion to Braunwald's heart disease. 3rd ed. Philadelphia: Elsevier Science; 2009. p. 187–208.)*

The significance of PPM remains controversial in terms of both incidence and clinical relevance. Pibarot et al[69] have shown that PPM is seen in up to 70% of AVRs, but other studies have reported a prevalence of severe PPM of less than 1%.[70] Several large studies have provided evidence that PPM has a significant negative impact on postoperative survival,[71-74] although other studies have suggested that PPM has no impact on short-term or long-term mortality.[75,76]

The prevention of PPM by means of aortic root enlargement during AVR has declined as a result of improved hemodynamics of both mechanical and bioprosthetic valves. An alternative strategy to prevent PPM includes aortic root replacement (described previously). The possibility of a valve-in-valve procedure for failed bioprostheses is another consideration when one is performing AVR in a small aortic root. The patient with a small bioprosthetic valve, such as those 19 or 21 mm, may not be a candidate for a future valve-in-valve procedure because the rigid stent of the bioprosthetic valve limits the size of the intended transcatheter heart valve.

Special Challenges

Aortic Dissection

Acute type A aortic dissections are associated with significant AR in approximately one half of patients which is typically caused by prolapse of detached commissures from the aortic wall.[77] The intraoperative management of the aortic valve and root remains controversial. Correction of the AR can be performed with resuspension of the aortic valve via suture fixation of the commissure to the aortic adventitia (Figure 14-22). Reattachment of the dissected layers can be supplemented with biological glue, felt, or fabric graft reinforcement.

Alternatively, an aortic root replacement with composite valve-graft or a valve-sparing technique can be employed. Patients with intrinsic root abnormality (such as patients with Marfan syndrome, preexisting annuloaortic ectasia prone to future root

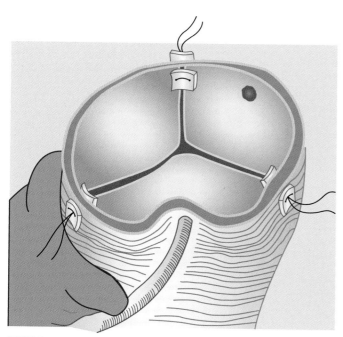

FIGURE 14-22 Aortic valve resuspension. When an aortic dissection extends into the aortic root, valve competency can be restored by resuspension of the commissures to aortic adventitia using polytetrafluoroethylene (Teflon) felt pledgeted sutures. The dissected layers can then by reapproximated with surgical adhesives or fabrics. *(Reprinted with permission from Arom KV, Grover FL. Adult cardiac surgery during the first 50 years of the Southern Thoracic Surgical Association. Ann Thorac Surg 2003;76:517–46.)*

enlargement, or progression of AR) are ideal candidates for aortic root replacement. To avoid future aortic root surgery, some centers favor an aggressive approach to aortic root replacement for acute type A aortic dissection.[78]

In patients with normal aortic sinuses, an AVR can be performed when the aortic valve has intrinsic pathology such as sclerosis, calcifications, or stenosis. The technique of AVR with a separate supracoronary graft has limited utility in acute type A aortic dissection because of the combined disadvantage of retaining abnormal aortic sinus tissue and exposing the patient to risks of a prosthetic valve.

The use of intraoperative transesophageal echocardiogram is mandatory in the evaluation of the aortic root in order to assist the surgeon with management of the aortic root. The conservative approach using valve resuspension is expeditious and effectively addresses acute AR during an emergency operation. Nevertheless, patients undergoing valve resuspension have a 20% to 25% risk of late aortic root enlargement or significant AR requiring reoperation[79] and should be carefully monitored during long-term follow-up.

Aortic Valve Replacement after Coronary Artery Bypass Grafting Surgery

AS and coronary artery disease (CAD) frequently coexist because of common pathophysiology.[80] A significant subset of patients with AS requiring AVR has had previous CABG (43% in the PARTNER Trial).[2] Often AS is recognized at the time of the index CABG, and currently guidelines recommend AVR at the time of CABG in patients with AS that is severe (class I) or moderate (class IIa).[9] Moreover, a class IIb guideline recommendation exists for concomitant AVR in patients who have mild AS but who are at risk for rapid progression, such as those with moderate to severe valve calcification.[9]

Reoperative cardiac surgery can be complicated by injury to cardiovascular structures during sternal reentry, in particular, injury to patent bypass grafts in patients with previous CABG. AVR after prior CABG was previously associated with an operative mortality as high as 14%.[81] However, current series show that operative mortality is approximately 3.8% even in patients with patent bypass grafts.[82] Reoperative cardiac surgery has therefore become safer with appropriate perioperative planning and is not a contraindication to AVR.

The management of a patent internal mammary artery graft during AVR after CABG requires attention to preoperative planning and operative management. Some surgeons consider the presence of a patent internal mammary artery graft crossing the midline and directly adherent to the sternum to be a high-risk factor, because injury to the internal mammary artery graft during reoperation is associated with increased operative mortality. Routine preoperative high-resolution computed tomography is indispensable in identifying patients with cardiovascular structures at risk for injury during sternal reentry.[83] Exposure of peripheral vessels (axillary or femoral) for cardiopulmonary bypass and institution of cardiopulmonary bypass prior to sternal reentry are useful strategies when injury to underlying structures is imminent.[84] Injury to the internal mammary artery graft is, nevertheless, associated with an operative mortality in current large series of 12% to 17.9%.[83,84]

Myocardial protection in patients with a patent left internal mammary artery grafts to the left anterior descending coronary artery poses another challenge during AVR. The traditional strategy of clamping the left internal mammary artery graft during cardioplegic arrest of the heart can risk injury to the graft itself during the initial identification and exposure. The alternative strategy, of leaving the left internal mammary artery graft unclamped, can safely be performed by including moderate systemic hypothermia and delivery of retrograde cardioplegia during cardioplegic arrest. This alternative strategy has been associated with comparable operative mortality and avoids the risk of injury to the graft.[85,86]

Second Aortic Valve Replacement Procedure

SVD of bioprosthetic valves is the most common indication for repeat AVR. Other indications are prosthetic valve endocarditis, pannus formation, and valve thrombosis with either bioprosthetic or mechanical valves. Increasing use of bioprosthetic valves in younger populations may lead to future need for interventions secondary to SVD. Fortunately, repeat AVR remains a safe procedure, with an operative mortality of 5%.[87]

A special concern with repeat AVR involves the management of new ascending aortic aneurysms after previous AVR. Preoperatively, the use of contrast-enhanced imaging to determine the relationship of the aneurysm to the sternum can significantly change the operative technique. For patients with an aneurysm adherent to the sternum, cardiopulmonary bypass via peripheral cannulation should be instituted prior to sternal reentry. The use of the axillary artery for arterial cannulation is preferred over the femoral artery in these cases because of the lower risk of stroke and operative mortality.[88] This technique can allow for temporary decompression of the aneurysm by inducing low pump flows to allow for safe division of the sternum. In addition, rapid institution of cardiopulmonary bypass with hypothermia can avert major neurologic injury if catastrophic arterial injury to the aneurysm occurs during reentry.

A patent saphenous vein bypass graft arising from new ascending aortic aneurysm is managed according to the amount of disease present in the graft. For a vein graft with no significant atherosclerotic disease, a patch of aorta containing the proximal anastomoses can be reimplanted on the Dacron graft (Figure 14-23). Alternatively, a new saphenous vein graft can be used to replace part or all of the old diseased graft with construction of a separate proximal anastomosis.

Failed Aortic Root Replacements

Patients who have had previous aortic root replacements, particularly younger patients, may require reoperation for SVD leading to AS or AR. Reoperation may also be required because of aneurysm of the unresected native aorta or because of a pseudoaneurysm of the replaced root at the anastomotic lines. Common clinical scenarios include patients with failed pulmonary autografts (Ross procedure) and failed aortic homografts. The challenge in reoperative aortic root replacement is the management of the native coronary arteries as they arise from the replaced root. Unlike in primary operations, the coronary arteries can be difficult to mobilize from the surrounding scar tissue, resulting in the inability to fashion a reliable coronary button for reimplantation ("frozen button"). Alternative techniques to manage frozen buttons include construction of a Dacron tube connecting the ostia of both coronary arteries (see Figure 14-16, Cabrol technique) and construction of an interposition vein graft (see Figure 14-17; Kay-Zubiate technique).[56,57] If the coronary arteries cannot be reconstructed, then ligation with standard CABG is a less desirable but viable option.

In some circumstances after failed aortic root replacement, only the aortic valve requires replacement. This option is attractive because the coronary arteries can be left in place without the need for complex reconstruction. The outcomes after reoperative aortic root replacements are understandably less favorable than those after primary aortic root replacements but are acceptable. The largest series of repeat aortic root replacement demonstrated an operative mortality of 7%.[89] Factors associated with poor outcome include age, chronic obstructive pulmonary disease, and ejection fraction less than 30%.[89] The option of a valve-in-valve procedure using a transcatheter heart valve may be an acceptable option for failed aortic root replacement with SVD, although it does not address the often coexisting ascending aortic pathology.

Porcelain Aorta

Porcelain aorta is the presence of concentric calcification of the entire ascending aorta (Figure 14-24). During standard AVR, the ascending aorta is typically cannulated and cross-clamped. Therefore, the presence of porcelain aorta prevents standard approaches to AVR. Alternative sites of cannulation for cardiopulmonary can easily be used, the most common peripheral site

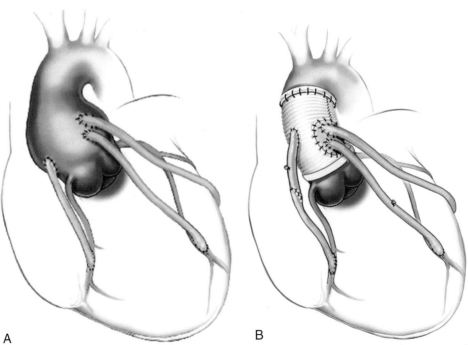

A   B

FIGURE 14-23 Aneurysm after bypass grafting. A, Patent grafts arise from a new ascending aneurysm. **B,** The right coronary graft is extended with a new segment of saphenous vein. The left-sided grafts are reimplanted as a single island of native aorta.

being the right axillary artery. The porcelain aorta cannot be clamped; therefore, hypothermic circulatory arrest must be utilized in order to open the ascending aorta in a bloodless fashion. During hypothermic circulatory arrest, three procedures can be performed. The first procedure is to open the aorta (without cross-clamping) and complete the entire valve replacement during hypothermic circulatory arrest. The second is to perform an aortic endarterectomy, clamp the decalcified ascending aorta, resume cardiopulmonary bypass, and perform the valve replacement in the standard fashion. The third is to replace the ascending aorta during hypothermic circulatory arrest with a synthetic graft (typically Dacron), clamp the synthetic graft, resume cardiopulmonary bypass, and complete the valve

replacement in standard fashion. Results of these approaches are shown in Table 14-5.

Another surgical approach to porcelain aorta is the apico-aortic conduit (or aortic valve bypass).[90] In this approach, a left thoracotomy is performed and the ascending aorta is avoided altogether. A valved-conduit is then constructed from the left

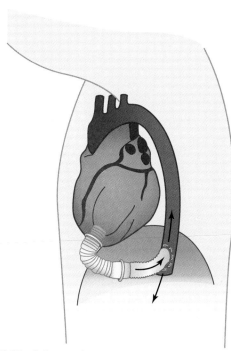

FIGURE 14-25 Apico-aortic conduit. A valved-conduit is attached to the left ventricular apex and the descending thoracic aorta via a left thoracotomy (*Arrows* indicate direction of blood flow).

TABLE 14-5	Results of Hypothermic Circulatory Arrest for Patient with Porcelain Aorta		
AUTHOR (YEAR)*	**METHOD(S) (n)**	**STROKE (%)**	**MORTALITY (%)**
Gillinov et al (2000)	Inspect and cross-clamp (n = 6)	0	0
	AVR, HCA (n = 24)	17	12
	AVR, aortic endarterectomy, HCA (n = 16)	12	19
	AVR, aortic replacement, HCA (n = 12)	0	25
Aranki et al (2005)	AVR, HCA (n = 13)	15	0
	AVR, aortic endarterectomy, HCA (n = 13)	7.6	0
	AVR, aortic replacement, HCA (n = 44)	11.3	6.8

AVR, Aortic valve replacement; *HCA,* hypothermic circulatory arrest.
*Data from Gillinov AM, Lytle BW, Hoang V, et al. The atherosclerotic aorta at aortic valve replacement: surgical strategies and results. J Thorac Cardiovasc Surg 2000;120:957-65, and Aranki SF, Nathan M, Shekar P, et al. Hypothermic circulatory arrest enables aortic valve replacement in patients with unclampable aorta. Ann Thorac Surg 2005;80:1679–87.

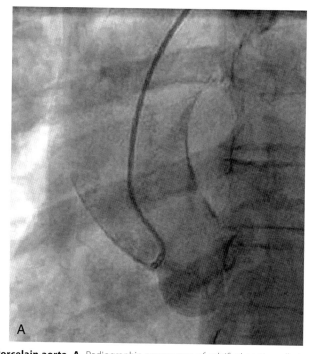

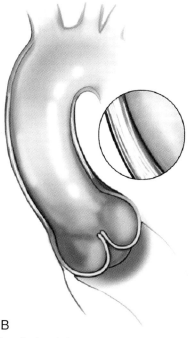

FIGURE 14-24 Porcelain aorta. A, Radiographic appearance of calcified aortic wall at catheterization. A dense strip of calcification can be seen in both the greater and lesser curvatures in this left anterior oblique aortogram. **B,** Artist's conception of the calcified wall seen in cutaway view with close-up *(inset)*.

ventricular apex to the descending thoracic aorta (Figure 14-25). The stenosed native aortic valve is left in place, and blood is passed extra-anatomically through the valved-conduit. Outcomes of the apico-aortic conduit are limited but have demonstrated 13% perioperative mortality in a high-risk cohort (average age 81 years, 16% with porcelain aorta).[91] A disadvantage of this procedure is that the procedure cannot be performed in patients with significant AR or with a severely calcified descending aorta.

Current Controversies

Minimally Invasive Approaches

The complete median sternotomy is the standard approach for AVR. Minimally invasive approaches to AVR include any incision that does not involve a complete median sternotomy. The upper hemisternotomy and the right anterior thoracotomy are the two most common minimally invasive approaches. Cosmesis has been the driving factor associated with the development of minimally invasive approaches, but the approaches have not been shown to compromise safety or outcomes.[92]

UPPER HEMISTERNOTOMY

The upper hemisternotomy is performed through a vertical skin incision measuring 5 to 8 cm below the angle of Louis (Figure 14-26). The sternotomy is extended into the right third or fourth interspace. Cannulation for cardiopulmonary bypass and cardioplegic arrest can be performed through the incision or through peripheral sites. Exposure of the aortic valve is comparable to the complete sternotomy and does not require the use of special instruments. In a meta-analysis of 26 studies comparing AVR through a partial sternotomy (n = 2054) and AVR through a full sternotomy (n = 2532), no significant difference in operative mortality was found between the two groups (OR 0.71, 95% CI 0.49-1.02) despite a longer mean cross-clamp time (8-minute longer in partial sternotomy) and cardiopulmonary bypass time (12-minute

longer in partial sternotomy).[92] Benefits of the partial sternotomy approach included a shorter in-hospital stay (weighted mean difference [WMD] 0.9 days), less ventilator time (WMD 2.1 hours), and less blood loss within 24 hours (WMD 79 mL).[92]

RIGHT ANTERIOR THORACOTOMY

The right anterior thoracotomy is performed through a horizontal skin incision measuring 4 to 7 cm lateral to the sternum (Figure 14-27). The chest cavity is entered in either the second or third interspace, often with division of the right internal thoracic vessels. Cannulation for cardiopulmonary bypass and cardioplegic arrest is performed peripherally. The aortic valve is adequately visualized, but specialized long-handled instruments are required to complete the valve replacement. Less data regarding outcomes of this approach are available; however, single-center series have demonstrated outcomes comparable to those of the complete sternotomy.[93]

AVR with Sutureless Prosthetic Valve

A sutureless valve is a bioprosthetic valve mounted on a metallic frame similar to a transcatheter heart valve. The first sutureless valve was implanted in a human in 2005 (Figure 14-28).[94] Sutureless valves are implanted with use of cardiopulmonary bypass and cardioplegic arrest after complete excision of the native aortic valve. Benefits of sutureless valve include rapid deployment and implantation under direct vision. Initial results show that these technical benefits can translate into shorter aortic cross-clamp times[95,96] and facilitate minimally invasive approaches (Figure 14-29).[97] Whether sutureless valves will be comparable in hemodynamics to standard bioprosthetic valves, including low transvalvular gradients and absence of perivalvular regurgitation, remains to be proven (Table 14-6).[97-99] As with all new valve technology, the long-term durability of sutureless valves has not been proven, except for those incorporating existing valve design (Figure 14-30). As of this writing, the Sorin Perceval S, Medtronic

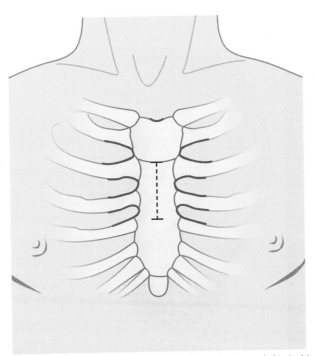

FIGURE 14-26   Upper hemisternotomy. Through a vertical skin incision *(dashed line)*, the upper sternotomy is divided and extended into either the third or fourth interspace, typically to the right.

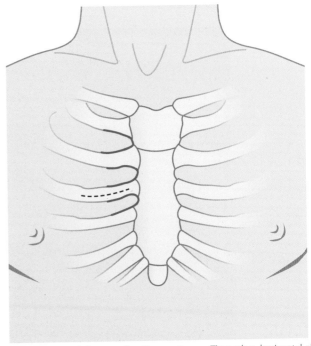

FIGURE 14-27   Right anterior thoracotomy. Through a horizontal skin incision *(dashed line)*, the right pleural cavity is entered through either the second or third interspace, directly lateral to the sternal border.

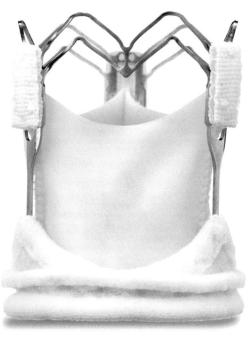

FIGURE 14-28 Medtronic 3F Enable aortic bioprosthesis. This sutureless valve (Medtronic, Inc., Minneapolis, Minnesota) incorporates equine pericardial leaflets on a nitinol frame.

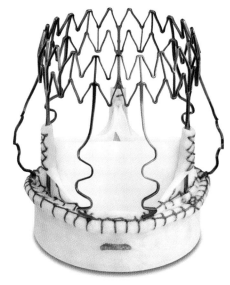

FIGURE 14-29 Sorin PERCEVAL S valve. This sutureless valve (Sorin Group, Milan) incorporates bovine pericardial leaflets on a nitinol frame.

TABLE 14-6	Sutureless Aortic Valves		
	MEDTRONIC 3F ENABLE	**SORIN PERCEVAL S**	**EDWARDS INTUITY**
Leaflet material	Equine pericardium	Bovine pericardium	Bovine pericardium
Metal frame	Nitinol	Nitinol	Stainless steel
Metal at inflow	Yes	Yes	Yes
Metal at outflow	Yes	Yes	No
Sizes (mm)	19, 21, 23, 25, 27, 29	21, 23, 25	19, 21, 23, 25, 27
Initial clinical experience (Author, year)	Martens et al (2011)[98]	Folliguet et al (2012)[97]	Kocher et al (2013)[98]
Patients (n)	140	208	146
Minimally invasive approach (%)	20	22	30
Cross-clamp time (minutes)*	37	30	41
Operative mortality (%)	3.6	2.4	2.1
Mean gradient (mm Hg)	9.0	10.4	8.8
Significant perivalvular regurgitation (%)	2.1	4	1.4
Implantation of permanent pacemaker (%)	7	7	7
CE Mark obtained	2009	2011	2012
U.S. Food and Drug Administration investigational device exemption trial	No	No	Yes

*Isolated aortic valve replacement.

3f Enable, and Edwards Intuity have CE mark and are commercially available only in Europe.

Aortic Valve Replacement in the Elderly

Increased life expectancy has led to the growing elderly population frequently presenting with AS.[100] Age has been perceived as a major deterrent to AVR, despite well-published reports on the success of isolated AVR in elderly patients.[46,47,49,50,101] The 2006 ACC/AHA guidelines state that age itself is not a contraindication to AVR because of the excellent results with AVR in patients with advanced age.[9] Operative mortality in previous single-center series have ranged from 2.4% to 11.6% in the octogenarian group. In the largest sample of patients, involving 2945 octogenarians, the 2006 STS database reported a 4.7% mortality risk after isolated AVR in patients 80 to 90 years of age.[45] Results from the PARTNER trial have established a benchmark for AVR in elderly patients.[2] In the group randomly assigned to AVR, 351 patients had an average age of 84 years with an STS PROM score of 12%. Observed 30-day mortality was 6.5%, giving an impressive observed-to-expected ratio of 0.54.

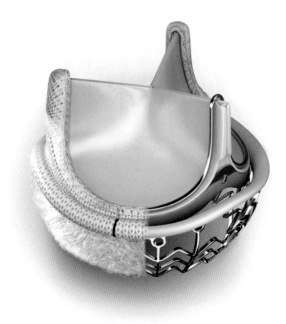

FIGURE 14-30 Edwards INTUITY valve. This sutureless valve (Edwards Lifesciences Corporation, Irvine, California) incorporates bovine pericardial leaflets on a stainless steel frame.

Recovery is an equally important factor for patients with advanced age and a deterrent to AVR in the elderly. Despite improvement in patient survival, patients with advanced age undergoing cardiac surgery are at greater risk for prolonged recovery and poor functional outcome. Compared with patients less than 80 years, octogenarians are more likely to have a prolonged hospital stay after cardiac surgery, and approximately 50% of octogenarian are discharged to home directly from the hospital.[47,102] Functional outcome and quality of life in patients with advanced age after cardiac surgery has not been well-studied. Frailty scoring (see Chapter 10) may emerge as a tool to predict poor functional outcome for octogenarians.[9,103] The identification of frail patients may allow better patient selection for less invasive procedures, including TAVI.

Conclusion

Surgery of the aortic valve can now be accomplished with greater safety and efficacy in the majority of patients. In patients with higher operative risks, TAVI is already a proven acceptable alternative to AVR. The choice of valve prosthesis is guided by patient preference, life expectancy, and comorbidities relevant to SVD and anticoagulation. Aortic valve repair in the young patient with AR avoids the risks associated with valve prostheses, but long-term durability is unknown. Aortic root surgery similarly can be performed with replacement of both the aortic valve and aortic wall, but valve-sparing techniques may offer the advantage of durability equivalent to that of normal native aortic valves with avoidance of prosthetic valve-related complications. Reoperative aortic valve and aortic root surgery, like isolated AVR, can be performed safely with best outcomes at high-volume centers.

REFERENCES

1. Leon MB, Smith CR, Mack M, et al. Transcatheter aortic-valve implantation for aortic stenosis in patients who cannot undergo surgery. N Engl J Med 2010;363:1597–607.
2. Smith CR, Leon MB, Mack MJ, et al. Transcatheter versus surgical aortic-valve replacement in high-risk patients. N Engl J Med 2011;364:2187–98.
3. Edwards Lifesciences. The PARTNER II Trial: placement of AoRTic TraNscathetER Valves. In: National Library of Medicine. <http://clinicaltrials.gov/ct2/show/NCT01314313>. NLM Identifier: NCT01314313.
4. Medtronic Cardiovascular. Safety and efficacy study of the Medtronic CoreValve® system in the treatment of severe, symptomatic aortic stenosis in intermediate risk subjects who need aortic valve replacement (SURTAVI). <http://clinicaltrials.gov/show/NCT01586910> NLM Identifier: NCT01586910.
5. Ali A, Halstead JC, Cafferty F, et al. Early clinical and hemodynamic outcomes after stented and stentless aortic valve replacement: results from a randomized controlled trial. Ann Thorac Surg 2007;83:2162–8.
6. Cohen G, Christakis GT, Joyner CD, et al. Are stentless valves hemodynamically superior to stented valves? A prospective randomized trial. Ann Thorac Surg 2002;73:767–75; discussion 775–768.
7. Cohen G, Zagorski B, Christakis GT, et al. Are stentless valves hemodynamically superior to stented valves? Long-term follow-up of a randomized trial comparing Carpentier-Edwards pericardial valve with the Toronto stentless porcine valve. J Thorac Cardiovasc Surg 2010;139:848–59.
8. Desai ND, Merin O, Cohen GN, et al. Long-term results of aortic valve replacement with the St. Jude Toronto stentless porcine valve. Ann Thorac Surg 2004;78:2076–83; discussion 2076–83.
9. Bonow RO, Carabello BA, Kanu C, et al. ACC/AHA 2006 guidelines for the management of patients with valvular heart disease: a report of the American College of Cardiology/American Heart Association Task Force on Practice Guidelines (writing committee to revise the 1998 Guidelines for the Management of Patients With Valvular Heart Disease): developed in collaboration with the Society of Cardiovascular Anesthesiologists: endorsed by the Society for Cardiovascular Angiography and Interventions and the Society of Thoracic Surgeons. Circulation 2006;114:e84–231.
10. Lehmann S, Walther T, Leontyev S, et al. Eight-year follow-up after prospectively randomized implantation of different mechanical aortic valves. Clin Res Cardiol 2008;97:376–82.
11. Bryan AJ, Rogers CA, Bayliss K, et al. Prospective randomized comparison of Carbo-Medics and St. Jude Medical bileaflet mechanical heart valve prostheses: ten-year follow-up. J Thorac Cardiovasc Surg 2007;133:614–22.
12. Chambers JB, Pomar JL, Mestres CA, et al. Clinical event rates with the On-X bileaflet mechanical heart valve: a multicenter experience with follow-up to 12 years. J Thorac Cardiovasc Surg 2013;145:420–4.
13. Medical Carbon Research Institute, LLC. Prospective randomized On-X Anticoagulation Clinical Trial (PROACT). <http://clinicaltrials.gov/show/NCT00291525> NLM Identifier: NCT00291525.
14. Ross DN. Homograft replacement of the aortic valve. Lancet 1962;2:487.
15. Sales VL, McCarthy PM, Carr JC, et al. Near-complete obstruction of an aortic homograft. Circulation 2012;125:e392–4.
16. Nowicki ER, Pettersson GB, Smedira NG, et al. Aortic allograft valve reoperation: surgical challenges and patient risks. Ann Thorac Surg 2008;86:761–8.
17. Ross D. The Ross operation. J Card Surg 2002;17:188–93.
18. Oxenham H, Bloomfield P, Wheatley DJ, et al. Twenty year comparison of a Bjork-Shiley mechanical heart valve with porcine bioprostheses. Heart 2003;89:715–21.
19. Hammermeister K, Sethi GK, Henderson WG, et al. Outcomes 15 years after valve replacement with a mechanical versus a bioprosthetic valve: final report of the Veterans Affairs randomized trial. J Am Coll Cardiol 2000;36:1152–8.
20. Vahanian A, Alfieri O, Andreotti F, et al. Guidelines on the management of valvular heart disease (version 2012). Eur Heart J 2012;33:2451–96.
21. McClure RS, Narayanasamy N, Wiegerinck E, et al. Late outcomes for aortic valve replacement with the Carpentier-Edwards pericardial bioprosthesis: up to 17-year follow-up in 1,000 patients. Ann Thorac Surg 2010;89:1410–6.
22. Yankah CA, Pasic M, Musci M, et al. Aortic valve replacement with the Mitroflow pericardial bioprosthesis: durability results up to 21 years. J Thorac Cardiovasc Surg 2008;136:688–96.
23. Borger MA, Preston M, Ivanov J, et al. Should the ascending aorta be replaced more frequently in patients with bicuspid aortic valve disease? J Thorac Cardiovasc Surg 2004;128:677–83.
24. Mykén PS, Bech-Hansen O. A 20-year experience of 1712 patients with the Biocor porcine bioprosthesis. J Thorac Cardiovasc Surg 2009;137:76–81.
25. David TE, Armstrong S, Maganti M, et al. Long-term results of aortic valve-sparing operations in patients with Marfan syndrome. J Thorac Cardiovasc Surg 2009;138:859–64; discussion 863–854.
26. Banbury MK, Cosgrove 3rd DM, White JA, et al. Age and valve size effect on the long-term durability of the Carpentier-Edwards aortic pericardial bioprosthesis. Ann Thorac Surg 2001;72:753–7.
27. Berrebi AJ, Carpentier SM, Phan KP, et al. Results of up to 9 years of high-temperature-fixed valvular bioprostheses in a young population. Ann Thorac Surg 2001;71(Suppl):S353–5.
28. El Oakley R, Kleine P, Bach DS. Choice of prosthetic heart valve in today's practice. Circulation 2008;117:253–6.
29. Rahimtoola SH. Choice of prosthetic heart valve in adults an update. J Am Coll Cardiol 2010;55:2413–26.
30. Bapat V, Attia R, Redwood S, et al. Use of transcatheter heart valves for a valve-in-valve implantation in patients with degenerated aortic bioprosthesis: technical considerations and results. J Thorac Cardiovasc Surg 2012;144:1372–9; discussion 1379–80.
31. Eggebrecht H, Schafer U, Treede H, et al. Valve-in-valve transcatheter aortic valve implantation for degenerated bioprosthetic heart valves. JACC Cardiovasc Interv 2011;4:1218–27.
32. Webb JG, Wood DA, Ye J, et al. Transcatheter valve-in-valve implantation for failed bioprosthetic heart valves. Circulation 2010;121:1848–57.
33. Khawaja MZ, Haworth P, Ghuran A, et al. Transcatheter aortic valve implantation for stenosed and regurgitant aortic valve bioprostheses CoreValve for failed bioprosthetic aortic valve replacements. J Am Coll Cardiol 2010;55:97–101.
34. Eggebrecht H, Schafer U, Treede H, et al. Valve-in-valve transcatheter aortic valve implantation for degenerated bioprosthetic heart valves. JACC Cardiovasc Interv 2011;4:1218–27.

35. Dvir D, Webb J, Brecker S, et al. Transcatheter aortic valve replacement for degenerative bioprosthetic surgical valves: results from the global valve-in-valve registry. Circulation 2012;126:2335–44.
36. Aicher D, Fries R, Rodionycheva S, et al. Aortic valve repair leads to a low incidence of valve-related complications. Eur J Cardiothorac Surg 2010;37:127–32.
37. El Khoury G, Vanoverschelde JL, Glineur D, et al. Repair of aortic valve prolapse: experience with 44 patients. Eur J Cardiothorac Surg 2004;26:628–33.
38. El Khoury G, de Kerchove L. Principles of aortic valve repair. J Thorac Cardiovasc Surg 2013;145(Suppl. 3):S26–29.
39. Schafers HJ, Langer F, Glombitza P, et al. Aortic valve reconstruction in myxomatous degeneration of aortic valves: are fenestrations a risk factor for repair failure? J Thorac Cardiovasc Surg 2010;139:660–4.
40. Lansac E, Di Centa I, Bonnet N, et al. Aortic prosthetic ring annuloplasty: a useful adjunct to a standardized aortic valve-sparing procedure? Eur J Cardiothorac Surg 2006;29:537–44.
41. Shroyer AL, Coombs LP, Peterson ED, et al. The Society of Thoracic Surgeons: 30-day operative mortality and morbidity risk models. Ann Thorac Surg 2003;75:1856–64; discussion 1864–55.
42. Nashef SA, Roques F, Sharples LD, et al. EuroSCORE II. Eur J Cardiothorac Surg 2012;41:734–45.
43. Ambler G, Omar RZ, Royston P, et al. Generic, simple risk stratification model for heart valve surgery. Circulation 2005;112:224–31.
44. Rankin JS, Hammill BG, Ferguson TB Jr, et al. Determinants of operative mortality in valvular heart surgery. J Thorac Cardiovasc Surg 2006;131:547–57.
45. Brown JM, O'Brien SM, Wu C, et al. Isolated aortic valve replacement in North America comprising 108,687 patients in 10 years: changes in risks, valve types, and outcomes in the Society of Thoracic Surgeons National Database. J Thorac Cardiovasc Surg 2009;137:82–90.
46. Filsoufi F, Rahmanian PB, Castillo JG, et al. Excellent early and late outcomes of aortic valve replacement in people aged 80 and older. J Am Geriatr Soc 2008; 56:255–61.
47. Malaisrie SC, McCarthy PM, McGee EC, et al. Contemporary perioperative results of isolated aortic valve replacement for aortic stenosis. Ann Thorac Surg 2010; 89:751–6.
48. Bakaeen FG, Chu D, Huh J, et al. Is an age of 80 years or greater an important predictor of short-term outcomes of isolated aortic valve replacement in veterans? Ann Thorac Surg 2010;90:769–74.
49. Di Eusanio M, Fortuna D, De Palma R, et al. Aortic valve replacement: results and predictors of mortality from a contemporary series of 2256 patients. J Thorac Cardiovasc Surg 2011;141:940–7.
50. Thourani VH, Myung R, Kilgo P, et al. Long-term outcomes after isolated aortic valve replacement in octogenarians: a modern perspective. Ann Thorac Surg 2008;86:1458–1464; discussion 1464–55.
51. Hiratzka LF, Bakris GL, Beckman JA, et al. 2010 ACCF/AHA/AATS/ACR/ASA/SCA/SCAI/SIR/STS/SVM guidelines for the diagnosis and management of patients with Thoracic Aortic Disease: a report of the American College of Cardiology Foundation/American Heart Association Task Force on Practice Guidelines, American Association for Thoracic Surgery, American College of Radiology, American Stroke Association, Society of Cardiovascular Anesthesiologists, Society for Cardiovascular Angiography and Interventions, Society of Interventional Radiology, Society of Thoracic Surgeons, and Society for Vascular Medicine. Circulation 2010;121:e266–369.
52. Hughes GC, Zhao Y, Rankin JS, et al. Effects of institutional volumes on operative outcomes for aortic root replacement in North America. J Thorac Cardiovasc Surg 2013;145:166–71.
53. Kalkat MS, Edwards MB, Taylor KM, et al. Composite aortic valve graft replacement: mortality outcomes in a national registry. Circulation 2007;116(Suppl. I): I-301–6.
54. Bentall H, De Bono A. A technique for complete replacement of the ascending aorta. Thorax 1968;23:338–9.
55. Kouchoukos NT, Karp RB. Resection of ascending aortic aneurysm and replacement of aortic valve. J Thorac Cardiovasc Surg 1981;81:142–3.
56. Cabrol C, Pavie A, Gandjbakhch I, et al. Complete replacement of the ascending aorta with reimplantation of the coronary arteries: new surgical approach. J Thorac Cardiovasc Surg 1981;81:309–15.
57. Zubiate P, Kay JH. Surgical treatment of aneurysm of the ascending aorta with aortic insufficiency and marked displacement of the coronary ostia. J Thorac Cardiovasc Surg 1976;71:415–21.
58. Gott VL, Cameron DE, Alejo DE, et al. Aortic root replacement in 271 Marfan patients: a 24-year experience. Ann Thorac Surg 2002;73:438–43.
59. Etz CD, Homann TM, Rane N, et al. Aortic root reconstruction with a bioprosthetic valved conduit: a consecutive series of 275 procedures. J Thorac Cardiovasc Surg 2007;133:1455–63.
60. Kvitting JP, Kari FA, Fischbein MP, et al. David valve-sparing aortic root replacement: equivalent mid-term outcome for different valve types with or without connective tissue disorder. J Thorac Cardiovasc Surg 2013;145:117–26, 127; e111–e115; discussion 126–117.
61. De Paulis R, Scaffa R, Nardella S, et al. Use of the Valsalva graft and long-term follow-up. J Thorac Cardiovasc Surg 2010;140(Suppl):S23–7; discussion S45–S51.
62. Benedetto U, Melina G, Takkenberg JJ, et al. Surgical management of aortic root disease in Marfan syndrome: a systematic review and meta-analysis. Heart 2011;97:955–8.
63. Demers P, Miller DC. Simple modification of "T. David-V" valve-sparing aortic root replacement to create graft pseudosinuses. Ann Thorac Surg 2004;78:1479–81.
64. De Paulis R, De Matteis GM, Nardi P, et al. One-year appraisal of a new aortic root conduit with sinuses of Valsalva. J Thorac Cardiovasc Surg 2002;123:33–9.
65. Nicks R, Cartmill T, Bernstein L. Hypoplasia of the aortic root: the problem of aortic valve replacement. Thorax 1970;25:339–46.
66. Manouguian S, Seybold-Epting W. Patch enlargement of the aortic valve ring by extending the aortic incision into the anterior mitral leaflet: new operative technique. J Thorac Cardiovasc Surg 1979;78:402–12.
67. Konno S, Imai Y, Iida Y, et al. A new method for prosthetic valve replacement in congenital aortic stenosis associated with hypoplasia of the aortic valve ring. J Thorac Cardiovasc Surg 1975;70:909–17.
68. Zoghbi WA, Chambers JB, Dumesnil JG, et al. Recommendations for evaluation of prosthetic valves with echocardiography and doppler ultrasound: a report From the American Society of Echocardiography's Guidelines and Standards Committee and the Task Force on Prosthetic Valves, developed in conjunction with the American College of Cardiology Cardiovascular Imaging Committee, Cardiac Imaging Committee of the American Heart Association, the European Association of Echocardiography, a registered branch of the European Society of Cardiology, the Japanese Society of Echocardiography and the Canadian Society of Echocardiography, endorsed by the American College of Cardiology Foundation, American Heart Association, European Association of Echocardiography, a registered branch of the European Society of Cardiology, the Japanese Society of Echocardiography, and Canadian Society of Echocardiography. J Am Soc Echocardiogr 2009;22:975–1014.
69. Pibarot P, Dumesnil JG. Prosthesis-patient mismatch: definition, clinical impact, and prevention. Heart 2006;92:1022–9.
70. Flameng W, Meuris B, Herijgers P, et al. Prosthesis-patient mismatch is not clinically relevant in aortic valve replacement using the Carpentier-Edwards Perimount valve. AnnThorac Surg 2006;82:530–536.
71. Blackstone EH, Cosgrove DM, Jamieson WR, et al. Prosthesis size and long-term survival after aortic valve replacement. J Thorac Cardiovasc Surg 2003;126:783–96.
72. Blais C, Dumesnil JG, Baillot R, et al. Impact of valve prosthesis-patient mismatch on short-term mortality after aortic valve replacement. Circulation 2003;108:983–8.
73. Hanayama N, Christakis GT, Mallidi HR, et al. Patient prosthesis mismatch is rare after aortic valve replacement: valve size may be irrelevant. Ann Thorac Surg 2002;73:1822–1829; discussion 1829.
74. Rao V, Jamieson WR, Ivanov J, et al. Prosthesis-patient mismatch affects survival after aortic valve replacement. Circulation 2000;102(Suppl. 3):III5–III9.
75. Howell NJ, Keogh BE, Ray D, et al. Patient-prosthesis mismatch in patients with aortic stenosis undergoing isolated aortic valve replacement does not affect survival. Ann Thorac Surg 2010;89:60–4.
76. Mascherbauer J, Rosenhek R, Fuchs C, et al. Moderate patient-prosthesis mismatch after valve replacement for severe aortic stenosis has no impact on short-term and long-term mortality. Heart 2008;94:1639–45.
77. Movsowitz HD, Levine RA, Hilgenberg AD, et al. Transesophageal echocardiographic description of the mechanisms of aortic regurgitation in acute type A aortic dissection: implications for aortic valve repair. J Am Coll Cardiol 2000;36:884–90.
78. Halstead JC, Spielvogel D, Meier DM, et al. Composite aortic root replacement in acute type A dissection: time to rethink the indications? Eur J Cardiothorac Surg 2005;27:626–32; discussion 632–623.
79. Bonser RS, Ranasinghe AM, Loubani M, et al. Evidence, lack of evidence, controversy, and debate in the provision and performance of the surgery of acute type A aortic dissection. J Am Coll Cardiol 2011;58:2455–74.
80. Stewart BF, Siscovick D, Lind BK, et al. Clinical factors associated with calcific aortic valve disease: Cardiovascular Health Study. J Am Coll Cardiol 1997;29:630–4.
81. Fighali SF, Avendano A, Elayda MA, et al. Early and late mortality of patients undergoing aortic valve replacement after previous coronary artery bypass graft surgery. Circulation 1995;92(Suppl):II163–II168.
82. Dobrilovic N, Fingleton JG, Maslow A, et al. Midterm outcomes of patients undergoing aortic valve replacement after previous coronary artery bypass grafting. Eur J Cardiothorac Surg 2012;42:819–25.
83. Park CB, Suri RM, Burkhart HM, et al. Identifying patients at particular risk of injury during repeat sternotomy: analysis of 2555 cardiac reoperations. J Thorac Cardiovasc Surg 2010;140:1028–35.
84. Roselli EE, Pettersson GB, Blackstone EH, et al. Adverse events during reoperative cardiac surgery: frequency, characterization, and rescue. J Thorac Cardiovasc Surg 2008;135:316–23, 323 e311–e316.
85. Park CB, Suri RM, Burkhart HM, et al. What is the optimal myocardial preservation strategy at re-operation for aortic valve replacement in the presence of a patent internal thoracic artery? Eur J Cardiothorac Surg 2011;39:861–5.
86. Smith RL, Ellman PI, Thompson PW, et al. Do you need to clamp a patent left internal thoracic artery-left anterior descending graft in reoperative cardiac surgery? Ann Thorac Surg 2009;87:742–7.
87. Potter DD, Sundt 3rd TM, Zehr KJ, et al. Operative risk of reoperative aortic valve replacement. J Thorac Cardiovasc Surg 2005;129:94–103.
88. Svensson LG, Blackstone EH, Rajeswaran J, et al. Does the arterial cannulation site for circulatory arrest influence stroke risk? Ann Thorac Surg 2004;78:1274–84; discussion 1274–84.
89. Etz CD, Plestis KA, Homann TM, et al. Reoperative aortic root and transverse arch procedures: a comparison with contemporaneous primary operations. J Thorac Cardiovasc Surg 2008;136:860–7, 867.e1-3.
90. Gammie JS, Brown JW, Brown JM, et al. Aortic valve bypass for the high-risk patient with aortic stenosis. Ann Thorac Surg 2006;81:1605–10.
91. Gammie JS, Krowsoski LS, Brown JM, et al. Aortic valve bypass surgery: midterm clinical outcomes in a high-risk aortic stenosis population. Circulation 2008;118:1460–6.
92. Brown ML, McKellar SH, Sundt TM, et al. Ministernotomy versus conventional sternotomy for aortic valve replacement: a systematic review and meta-analysis. J Thorac Cardiovasc Surg 2009;137:670–679.e5.
93. Ruttmann E, Gilhofer TS, Ulmer H, et al. Propensity score-matched analysis of aortic valve replacement by mini-thoracotomy. J Heart Valve Dis 2010;19:606–14.
94. Sadowski J, Kapelak B, Pfitzner R, et al. Sutureless aortic valve bioprothesis "3F/ATS Enable"—4.5 years of a single-centre experience. Kardiologia Polska 2009;67: 956–63.

CH
14

95. Flameng W, Herregods MC, Hermans H, et al. Effect of sutureless implantation of the Perceval S aortic valve bioprosthesis on intraoperative and early postoperative outcomes. J Thorac Cardiovasc Surg 2011;142:1453–7.

96. Shrestha M, Folliguet T, Meuris B, et al. Sutureless Perceval S aortic valve replacement: a multicenter, prospective pilot trial. J Heart Valve Dis 2009;18:698–702.

97. Folliguet TA, Laborde F, Zannis K, et al. Sutureless Perceval aortic valve replacement: results of two European centers. Ann Thorac Surg 2012;93:1483–8.

98. Kocher AA, Laufer G, Haverich A, et al. One-year outcomes of the Surgical Treatment of Aortic Stenosis With a Next Generation Surgical Aortic Valve (TRITON) trial: a prospective multicenter study of rapid-deployment aortic valve replacement with the EDWARDS INTUITY Valve System. J Thorac Cardiovasc Surg 2013;145:110–16.

99. Martens S, Sadowski J, Eckstein FS, et al. Clinical experience with the ATS 3f Enable(R) sutureless bioprosthesis. Eur J Cardiothorac Surg 2011;40:749–55.

100. Cohn LH, Narayanasamy N. Aortic valve replacement in elderly patients: what are the limits? Curr Opin Cardiol 2007;22:92–5.

101. Huber CH, Goeber V, Berdat P, et al. Benefits of cardiac surgery in octogenarians—a postoperative quality of life assessment. Eur J Cardiothorac Surg 2007;31:1099–105.

102. Bardakci H, Cheema FH, Topkara VK, et al. Discharge to home rates are significantly lower for octogenarians undergoing coronary artery bypass graft surgery. Ann Thorac Surg 2007;83:483–9.

103. Freiheit EA, Hogan DB, Eliasziw M, et al. Development of a frailty index for patients with coronary artery disease. J Am Geriatr Soc 2010;58:1526–31.

CHAPTER 15

Transcatheter Aortic Valve Implantation

Brad Munt and John G. Webb

Key Points

- The outlook for patients with symptomatic valvular aortic stenosis is grave, with death rates of 50.7% at 1 year and 68% at 2 years in a series of high-risk patients deemed not to be surgical candidates and treated with standard medical (including balloon aortic valvuloplasty) therapy.
- Two types of aortic valves for percutaneous transcatheter aortic valve implantation (TAVI) have been used in a significant number of patients: balloon-expandable and self-expanding. Many new valve technologies are in development.
- Data from randomized trials indicate that TAVI is superior to medical therapy in patients who cannot undergo surgery, and it is not inferior to surgical aortic valve replacement in high-risk surgical patients with aortic stenosis.
- TAVI is technically feasible in most patients with aortic stenosis. The larger question is when should TAVI be offered? Evaluation should identify patients in whom a significant improvement in quality and duration of life is likely and avoid unnecessary intervention in patients in whom the procedure can be performed but benefit is unlikely. For this reason evaluation of neurocognitive functioning, frailty, functional status, mobility, and social support is important in patient selection.
- Transthoracic and transesophageal echocardiography, cardiac computed tomography, and invasive angiography are all used to perform anatomic evaluations specific to TAVI.
- Evaluation of appropriate candidates for TAVI requires a noncompetitive team approach involving interventional cardiologists with expertise in structural heart disease, cardiac and vascular surgeons, anesthesiologists, imaging specialists, and specialized nurses. The proper equipment and a minimum volume of TAVI procedures performed per operator are required.
- Randomized trials and large registries of TAVI indicate procedural success rates of more than 95%, 30-day survival of more than 90%, meaningful improvement in quality of life, and acceptable complication rates (procedure-related stroke <2%, vascular access site complications <5%, permanent pacemaker rates <5%).
- Experience with TAVI within failed bioprostheses (valve-in-valve procedures) has been reported. Critical issues in achieving a successful valve-in-valve procedure include an understanding of the manufacturer sizing and labeling of surgical bioprostheses and correct positioning of the valve in valve. Early experience suggests that TAVI will be an important option for treatment of patients with failed bioprostheses.
- More than 100,000 TAVI procedures have been performed to date. Alternatives to TAVI include surgical aortic valve replacement, balloon aortic valvuloplasty (with or without external beam radiation), and apical-to-aortic conduits.

The outlook for patients with symptomatic valvular aortic stenosis (AS) is grave, with death rates of 51% at 1 year and 68% at 2 years in one series of patients who were deemed not to be surgical candidates and were treated with standard medical therapy (including balloon aortic valvuloplasty).[1]

Definitive therapy of valvular AS requires relief of obstruction to left ventricular ejection. Currently, open surgical aortic valve replacement (or repair in rare instances) (AVR) is the most commonly used modality and offers excellent long-term results.[2] However, given the aging of the population, the frequency of patients presenting for reoperation, and medical advances that have allowed patients with comorbidities to survive and present with valvular AS, a significant number of patients are deemed to have excessive risk for traditional surgery.[3] Percutaneous techniques, therefore, were developed initially to offer relief of obstruction to left ventricular ejection in patients who were not candidates for surgery.

Initial results with balloon aortic valvuloplasty were disappointing, with neither hemodynamic nor clinical improvement over the long term.[4] The need for alternative treatment options, including transcatheter aortic valve implantation (TAVI), is demonstrated by the Euro Heart Survey on Valvular Heart Disease, in which up to one third of patients with symptomatic AS were denied traditional surgery.[3,5]

Interest in TAVI started with work of Andersen et al[6] in animals, followed by the work of a number of groups. Cribier et al[7] are credited with the first implantation in humans. Webb et al[8] popularized the retrograde arterial approach (initially from the femoral artery), which is now the standard for TAVI. These pioneers led the development of percutaneous techniques for aortic valve implantation and have begun a new era in the therapy of patients with valvular AS.

TAVI is the only intervention for AS shown to prolong life in a randomized trial.[1,9] In many experienced centers this procedure is now the standard of care for extremely high-risk or "inoperable" patients, and it is a valid alternative to surgery for many high-risk but "operable" patients. More than 100,000 TAVI procedures have been performed to date. In this chapter we present our current views on the valve designs, findings from randomized trials and registries, and implantation techniques for TAVI.

Percutaneous Aortic Valve Designs

Two types of aortic valves for percutaneous implantation have been used in a significant number of patients: balloon-expandable and self-expanding (Figure 15-1).

Balloon-Expandable Percutaneous Aortic Valves

Balloon-expandable prostheses for which there is extensive published data for human implantation include the first-generation

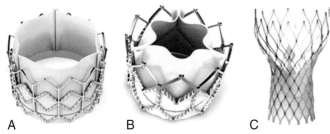

FIGURE 15-1 Current widely available transcatheter valves. A, The Edwards SAPIEN THV balloon-expandable valve (Edwards Lifesciences Corporation, Irvine, California) incorporates a stainless steel frame, bovine pericardial leaflets, and a fabric sealing cuff. **B,** The SAPIEN XT THV (Edwards Lifesciences) utilizes a cobalt chromium alloy frame and is compatible with lower-profile delivery catheters. **C,** The Medtronic CoreValve (Medtronic, Inc, Minneapolis, Minnesota) incorporates a self-expandable frame, porcine pericardial leaflets, and a pericardial seal. *(From Webb JG, Wood DA. Current status of transcatheter aortic valve replacement. J Am Coll Cardiol 2012;60:483–92.)*

Cribier-Edwards valve and the modified second-generation SAPIEN (SAPIEN and SAPIEN XT) series of valves (both from Edwards Lifesciences Corporation, Irvine, California) (see Figure 15-1).

On September 5, 2007, Edwards Lifesciences announced that it had received CE Mark approval for European commercial sales of its Edwards SAPIEN transcatheter aortic heart valve technology with the RetroFlex transfemoral delivery system. On March 5, 2008, Edwards announced that the first three human implants of a next-generation SAPIEN XT Edwards transcatheter aortic heart valve had been performed at St. Paul's Hospital in Vancouver, British Columbia, Canada.

This state-of-the-art Edwards SAPIEN XT transcatheter heart valve is a balloon-expandable cobalt chromium alloy tubular frame within which are sewn bovine pericardium leaflets. The inflow of the frame is covered with a fabric cuff to provide an annular seal (see Figure 15-1). For transarterial implantation, the transcatheter valve is compressed onto a low-profile NovaFlex (Edwards Lifesciences) delivery catheter (Figure 15-2) and introduced through a sheath placed in the femoral artery. Alternatively a sheath can be placed surgically in the left ventricular apex or ascending aorta. The SAPIEN XT valve is balloon-expanded within the diseased native valve, displacing the diseased native leaflets. A low-profile (16F to 19F) SAPIEN XT/NovaFlex trans-femoral system is in widespread clinical use in many countries. The first Placement of AoRTic TraNscathetER Valve (PARTNER I) trial (see The PARTNER Trial) used the earlier SAPIEN valve, which requires the use of larger-diameter (22F to 24F) sheaths; this is the current system used clinically in the United States (see Figure 15-2).

Self-Expanding Valves

The self-expanding valve with the most published human implantation data is the CoreValve ReValving System (Medtronic, Inc, Minneapolis, Minnesota) (see Figure 15-1). Currently, 23-, 26-, 29-, and 31-mm devices allow treatment of patients with annulus diameters from 20 to 29 mm. The CoreValve technology features a multilevel frame with porcine pericardial leaflets. The term "frame" is used rather than "stent" because by engineering definition, a stent exhibits the same radial force at every point of its peripheral circumference; the CoreValve frame exhibits three entirely different radial and hoop strength levels at different parts of its peripheral circumference.

The CoreValve is compressed within an Accutrak delivery catheter (Medtronic) (see Figure 15-2) and introduced through an 18F sheath into the common femoral or subclavian artery. Once the CoreValve is positioned correctly within the diseased native valve, the delivery catheter is withdrawn, releasing the valve. The multistage frame is anchored within the aortic annulus, but owing

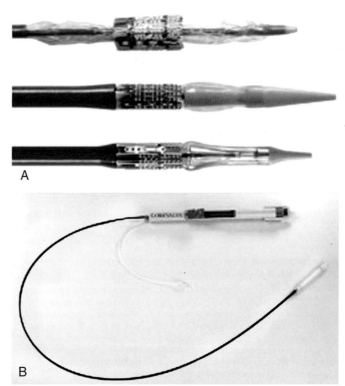

FIGURE 15-2 Valve delivery catheters. A, *Top,* the RetroFlex 1 delivery system for the Edwards SAPIEN THV (Edwards Lifesciences Corporation, Irvine, California) as used in the PARTNER 1 (Placement of AoRTic TraNscathetER Valve 1) trials (8-mm diameter). *Middle,* the RetroFlex 3 system (Edwards Lifesciences). *Bottom,* the NovaFlex/SAPIEN XT system (6-mm diameter; Edwards Lifesciences). **B,** The Accutrak delivery system with the Medtronic CoreValve (6-mm diameter, also with a tapered nose cone; Medtronic, Inc, Minneapolis, Minnesota). The prosthesis is enclosed within an outer sheath. *(From Webb JG, Wood DA. Current status of transcatheter aortic valve replacement. J Am Coll Cardiol 2012;60:483–92.)*

to its length also extends superiorly to anchor in the supracoronary aorta.

"Next-Generation" Valves

The ACURATE TA (Symetis Inc., Ecublens, Switzerland) (Figure 15-3) is a nitinol-based valve that incorporate features that facilitate positioning and anatomic orientation in relation to the native valve commissures and coronaries. The valve is currently implanted only transapically. The system received CE Mark approval on September 30, 2011, on the basis of studies conducted at 6 sites in Germany enrolling 90 high-risk patients with severe AS.[10] The mean logistic EuroSCORE (European System for Cardiac Operative Risk Evaluation) was 20.4 ± 8.7% and the Society of Thoracic Surgeons (STS) risk score was 8.4 ± 6.4%. All patients had New York Heart Association (NYHA) functional class III or IV heart failure symptoms, the average age was 84 ± 4 years, and 69% were female. The procedural success rate was 94.4% (n = 85), with 2 patients requiring a valve-in-valve procedure and 3 patients requiring conversion to open surgery.

Thirty-day data included a 92.2% survival rate, a stroke rate of 3.3%, and a myocardial infarction (MI) rate of 2.2%.

In an effort to reduce delivery catheter diameter, improve ease of positioning and sealing, or facilitate repositioning or removal, a number of newer transcatheter valves (see Figure 15-3) are in early clinical evaluation. Mostly nitinol based, the valves offer the following advantages:

- Lotus valve (Boston Scientific Inc., Natick, Massachusetts) is designed to expand laterally as longitudinal nitinol wires are retracted

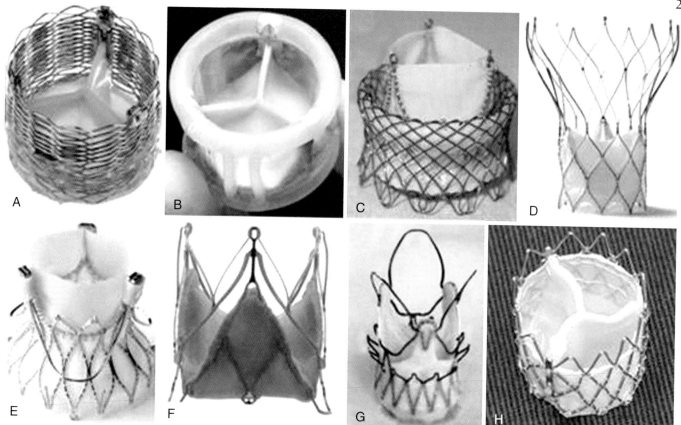

FIGURE 15-3 **Valves undergoing early evaluation. A,** Lotus (Boston Scientific Inc., Natick, Massachusetts); **B,** Direct Flow (Direct Flow Medical Inc., Santa Rosa, California); **C,** HLT (Bracco Inc., Princeton, New Jersey); **D,** Portico (St. Jude Medical Inc., St. Paul, Minnesota), **E,** Engager (Medtronic, Inc, Minneapolis, Minnesota); **F,** JenaValve (JenaValve Technology, Munich); **G,** ACURATE TA(Symetis Inc., Ecublens, Switzerland); and **H,** Inovare (Braile Biomedica Inc., São José do Rio Preto, Brazil). *(From Webb JG, Wood DA. Current status of transcatheter aortic valve replacement. J Am Coll Cardiol 2012;60:483–92.)*

- Direct Flow valve (Direct Flow Medical Inc., Santa Rosa, California) has a tubular fabric frame that is inflated with a rapidly setting polymerizing agent
- ACURATE TA, already described, and Portico (St. Jude Medical, Inc., St. Paul, Minnesota) valves extend from the annulus to the supracoronary aorta to assist in coaxial alignment and fixation (like CoreValve)
- Engager (Medtronic) and JenaValve (JenaValve Technology, Munich) valves incorporate features that facilitate positioning and anatomic orientation in relation to the native valve commissures and coronaries.

Experience with these newer valve technologies is limited. Whether clinical outcomes will be equivalent or superior to those of currently available TAVI systems is unknown.

Randomized TAVI Trials

The PARTNER Trial

The main 1- and 2-year results of the PARTNER trial[1,9,11,12] are presented in Table 15-1. The following points deserve emphasis when one considers the results of the trial. The trial used early-generation TAVI systems (SAPIEN 23-mm and 26-mm valves with 22F and 24F femoral delivery catheters) in centers with minimal operator experience with TAVI.

PARTNER part B compared transfemoral TAVI with standard therapy (including balloon aortic valvuloplasty).[9] At 1-year follow-up, the rates of death were 50.7% in the standard therapy group and 30.7% in the TAVI group; only five patients needed to be treated with TAVI to prevent one death at 1 year. TAVI was associated with a significant reduction in symptoms at 1 year as assessed by NYHA functional class (74.8% of surviving patients

who had undergone TAVI were in NYHA class II or lower, versus 42.0% of those treated with standard therapy) and 6-minute walk test. The rate of major stroke was numerically (but not statistically) higher with TAVI, whereas those of vascular complications and major bleeding were significantly higher (see Table 15-1). The SAPIEN valve demonstrated good hemodynamic performance.

In the 2-year follow-up of PARTNER part B, mortality remained lower in the TAVI group that in the standard therapy group (43.3% versus 68%), and the TAVI group had lower mortality between years 1 and 2 (18.2% mortality in patients alive at 1 year in the TAVI group versus 35.1% mortality in patients alive at 1 year in the standard therapy group).[1] It was noted that TAVI did not improve mortality in patients with an STS risk score higher than 14.9% upon entry into the trial. Rates of all strokes were higher in the TAVI group (13.8% versus 5.5%), the excess driven primarily by hemorrhagic events.

PARTNER part A compared transfemoral and transapical TAVI with surgical AVR.[11] One-year data showed the non-inferiority of TAVI (death from all causes 24.2% with TAVI versus 26.8% with standard surgery). Of the 699 patients undergoing random allocation, 42 did not undergo the assigned procedure (4 in the TAVI group and 38 in the surgical group). Rates of major strokes were numerically (but not significantly) higher in the TAVI group. Subgroup analysis indicated that women and patients who had not undergone previous coronary artery bypass grafting (CABG) may benefit more from TAVI than from standard surgical AVR.

The 2-year follow-up of PARTNER part A showed that the rates of death from any cause were not different between TAVI and surgical AVR (33.9% versus 35%), and the rate of stroke remained numerically (but not statistically significantly) higher in the TAVI group.[12] Multivariate predictors of mortality in the TAVI group included a higher body mass index (BMI) and higher preprocedure transvalvular gradient predicting lower risk, and reduced

TABLE 15-1   Design and Results of the PARTNER and STACCATO Trials

TRIAL AND DESCRIPTION	INCLUSION CRITERIA	EXCLUSION CRITERIA	BASELINE DEMOGRAPHICS	RESULTS
PARTNER Part B: TAVI vs. standard therapy in "nonoperable" patients	Cardiac symptoms (NYHA II, III, or IV) Severe AS (AVA <0.8 cm² *plus* mean gradient ≥40 mm Hg or peak jet velocity ≥4.0 m/s Not suitable candidates for traditional surgical AVR	Bicuspid or noncalcified aortic valve Acute MI CAD requiring revascularization LVEF <20% Aortic annulus diameter <18 mm or >25 mm Severe (4+) aortic or mitral regurgitation Stroke or TIA within past 6 months Severe renal insufficiency	Mean age 83 years 46% male Mean STS score 11.6% NYHA III or IV 93% CAD 71%, COPD 47% (O_2-dependent 23%), extensively calcified aorta (15%), chest wall deformity or deleterious effects of chest wall irradiation (13%), frailty according to prespecified criteria (23%)	*1-year follow-up:* Primary end point: all-cause mortality: 30.7% TAVI 50.7% standard therapy (P <0.001) Co-primary end point: composite of all-cause mortality or repeat hospitalization: 42.5% TAVI 71.6% standard therapy (P <0.001) Major strokes: 7.8% TAVI 3.9% standard therapy (P = 0.18) Composite of all-cause mortality or stroke: 33.0% TAVI 51.3% standard therapy (P <0.001) *2-year follow-up:* All-cause mortality: 43.3% TAVI 68.0% standard therapy (P <0.001)
PARTNER Part A: TAVI vs. surgical AVR in high-risk patients	Cardiac symptoms (NYHA II, III, or IV) Severe AS (AVA <0.8 cm² plus mean gradient ≥40 mm Hg or peak jet velocity ≥4.0 m/s Candidates for traditional surgical AVR but deemed to be at high risk STS score ≥10%	Bicuspid or noncalcified aortic valve Acute MI CAD requiring revascularization LVEF <20% Aortic annulus diameter <18 mm or >25 mm Severe (4+) aortic or mitral regurgitation Stroke or TIA within past 6 months Severe renal insufficiency	Mean age 84 years 57% male Mean STS score 11.8%, NYHA III or IV 94%, CAD 76%, COPD 43% (O_2 dependent 8%), frailty according to prespecified criteria (17%)	*1-year follow-up:* Primary end point: all-cause mortality: 24.2% TAVI 26.8% surgical AVR (P = 0.44); (P = 0.001 for noninferiority) Major strokes: 5.1% TAVI 2.4% surgical AVR (P = 0.18) Composite of all-cause mortality or stroke: 26.5% TAVI 28.0% surgical AVR (P = 0.68) *2-year follow-up:* All-cause mortality: 33.9% TAVI 35.0% surgical AVR (P = 0.78)
STACCATO Trial: Transapical TAVI vs. surgical AVR in "operable" elderly patients	Severe AS (AVA <1 cm²) Initially age >69 years; after 11 patients enrolled, age cutoff increased to >74 years Surgical and apical TAVI candidates Expected survival >1 year after successful treatment	CAD requiring revascularization Previous MI, cardiac surgery, or PCI within 12 months Need for emergency surgery Unstable cardiac condition (assist device or inotropic agents) Stroke within 1 month Reduced pulmonary function Renal failure requiring hemodialysis	Of 525 patients screened, 34 patients received apical TAVI and 36 patients surgical AVR Study terminated early (planned enrollment was 200 patients) on advice of the data safety monitoring board	Composite of 30-day all-cause mortality, major stroke, or renal failure: 14.7% apical TAVI 2.8% surgical AVR (P = 0.07)

AS, Aortic stenosis; *AVA,* aortic valve area; *AVR,* aortic valve replacement; *CAD,* coronary artery disease; *COPD,* chronic obstructive pulmonary disease; *LVEF,* left ventricular ejection fraction; *MI,* myocardial infarction; *NYHA,* New York Heart Association; *PCI,* percutaneous coronary intervention; *STS,* Society of Thoracic Surgeons; *TAVI,* transcatheter aortic valve implantation; *TIA,* transient ischemic attack.

renal function and prior vascular surgery or stent predicting higher risk. Prior CABG was protective in the surgical group, whereas higher STS score, liver disease, or more than mild mitral regurgitation was detrimental. Stroke and major bleeding raised mortality in both groups.

The STACCATO Trial

The STACCATO trial was a prospective, randomized trial of transapical transcatheter aortic valve implantation versus surgical aortic valve replacement in operable elderly patients with aortic stenosis. In the STACCATO trial, the composite of 30-day all-cause mortality, major stroke, or renal failure was numerically (but not significantly) higher in the transapical TAVI than traditional surgical group.[13] On the basis of historic primary event rates of 13.5% with traditional surgery and 2.5% in a nonrandomized TAVI group, a planned enrollment of 200 patients was proposed (randomized 1:1 to standard surgery or TAVI at three hospitals in Denmark). The trial was stopped by the data safety monitoring board after 70 patients had received valves. Five patients suffered primary events in the TAVI group (1 death of a patient on the waiting list, 2 major strokes, 1 renal failure requiring dialysis,1 left main occlusion; there were a total of 3 deaths) and 1 patient in the traditional surgical group had a primary event (major stroke). Average aortic valve area (AVA) increased equally in the two groups (from approximately 0.6 cm^2 to 1.3 cm^2). Four patients (13%) in the TAVI arm had moderate or severe aortic regurgitation, but no patient in the traditional surgery arm had more that minimal aortic regurgitation. The investigators acknowledge the limitation that the low number of patients enrolled raises the possibility that the play of chance accounts for the results. They also acknowledge that the study used older-generation valves for TAVI for which limited valve sizes were available.

Findings from TAVI Registries

ADVANCE Registry

The ADVANCE registry enrolled 1015 patients undergoing CoreValve implantation in experienced centers (at least 40 prior procedures) between March 2010 and July 2011.[14] The average age was 81 years, the mean logistic EuroSCORE was more than 19, and the patients were frail. At 30 days, the rate of major adverse cardiac and cerebrovascular events (MACCEs) was 8.3%; total mortality was 4.5% (cardiac mortality 3.4%), major strokes occurred in 2.9% of patients, major bleeding in 9.7%, and life threatening or disabling bleeds in 4%. At 6 months, all-cause mortality was 12.8% (cardiovascular mortality 8.4%). In patients with a EuroSCORE exceeding 20, the 6-month death rate was 17.3%.

Canadian Registry

We have contributed data to a Canadian registry of TAVI[14,15] performed with the Edwards SAPIEN series of valves. In 396 patients treated between January 2005 and June 2009, data for up to 4 years (median 3 years) are available. Mortality was approximately 50% at 4 years, with similar rates in patients undergoing transfemoral and transapical procedures. Strokes led to approximately 8% of deaths, but major causes were pulmonary or renal. The 30-day stroke rate (including the first patients treated in Canada at our center) was 2.3%. The rate of heart block requiring pacemaker implantation was 4.9% at 30 days.

United Kingdom Transcatheter Aortic Valve Implantation Registry

The United Kingdom Transcatheter Aortic Valve Implantation (UK TAVI) registry reported data on 1600 patients treated between January 2007 and December 2009 and followed up to December 31, 2010.[16] Baseline demographics of the patients are presented in Table 15-2, main outcomes in Table 15-3, and the predictors of outcomes in Table 15-4.

Approximately 50% of patients received CoreValves and the remainder SAPIEN valves. The SAPIEN is approved in Europe for implantation via the transfemoral and transapical approaches, whereas the CoreValve is generally inserted via the transfemoral or subclavian route. In the registry, the CoreValve was inserted transfemorally in more than 85% of patients, and the SAPIEN

TABLE 15-2 **Demographics of Patients in the United Kingdom Transcatheter Aortic Valve Implantation Registry***

VARIABLES	ALL PATIENTS (N = 870)	TRANSFEMORAL ROUTE (N = 599)	OTHER ROUTES (N = 271)	P VALUE	MEDTRONIC COREVALVE (N = 452)	EDWARDS SAPIEN (N = 410)	P VALUE
Male gender	456/870 (52.4)	311/599 (51.9)	145/271 (53.5)	0.66	235/452 (52.0)	217/410 (52.9)	0.78
Age, years	81.9 ± 7.1	81.7 ± 7.4	82.3 ± 6.6	0.32	81.3 ± 7.4	82.6 ± 6.7	0.007
Aortic valve peak gradient	80.9 ± 27.2	82.1 ± 27.8	77.9 ± 25.7	0.05	83.4 ± 28.5	77.5 ± 25.0	0.003
Left ventricular ejection fraction: ≥50% 30%-49% <30%	553/865 (64.0) 238/865 (27.0) 74/865 (9.0)	382/597 (64.0) 166/597 (28.0) 49/597 (8.0)	171/268 (63.8) 72/268 (26.9) 25/268 (9.3)	0.85	288/452 (63.7) 123/452 (27.2) 41/452 (9.1)	262/406 (64.5) 112/406 (7.9) 32/406 (7.9)	0.82
NYHA functional class: I/II III/IV	199/866 (23.0) 667/866 (77.0)	156/597 (26.1) 441/597 (73.9)	43/269 (16.0) 226/269 (84.0)	0.001	118/452 (26.1) 334/452 (73.9)	80/406 (19.7) 326/406 (80.3)	0.03
Coronary artery disease	394/828 (47.6)	249/574 (43.4)	145/254 (57.1)	<0.001	194/436 (44.5)	198/384 (51.6)	0.04
Any previous cardiac surgery	259/853 (30.4)	160/586 (27.3)	99/267 (37.1)	0.004	129/439 (29.4)	126/406 (31.0)	0.60
Peripheral vascular disease	241/832 (29.0)	110/563 (19.5)	131/269 (48.7)	<0.001	109/423 (25.8)	130/401 (32.4)	0.04
Diabetes mellitus	196/861 (22.8)	137/595 (23.0)	59/266 (22.2)	0.79	101/450 (22.4)	92/403 (22.8)	0.89
Chronic obstructive pulmonary disease	239/834 (28.7)	158/574 (27.5)	81/260 (31.2)	0.28	120/438 (27.4)	115/388 (29.6)	0.48
Creatinine >200 mmol/L	55/863 (6.7)	32/588 (5.4)	25/265 (9.4)	0.03	28/444 (6.3)	28/401 (7.0)	0.69
Logistic EuroSCORE	18.5 (11.7-27.9)	17.1 (11.0-25.5)	21.4 (14.4-33.6)	<0.001	18.1 (11.1-27.9)	18.5 (12.4-27.7)	0.34

NYHA, New York Heart Association; EuroSCORE, European System for Cardiac Operative Risk Evaluation.
From Moat NE, Ludman P, de Belder MA, et al. Long-term outcomes after transcatheter aortic valve implantation in high-risk patients with severe aortic stenosis: the U.K. TAVI (United Kingdom Transcatheter Aortic Valve Implantation) Registry. J Am Coll Cardiol 2011;58:2130–8.
*Values are n/N (%), mean ± SD, or median (interquartile range).

TABLE 15-3 Outcomes of Patients by Implantation Route and Valve Type in the United Kingdom Transcatheter Aortic Valve Implantation Registry

VARIABLES	ALL PATIENTS (N = 870)	TRANSFEMORAL ROUTE (N = 599)	OTHER ROUTES (N = 271)	P VALUE	MEDTRONIC COREVALVE (N = 452)	EDWARDS (N = 410)	P VALUE
Procedural success	846/870 (97.2)	583/599 (97.3)	263/271 (97.1)	0.82	444/452 (98.2)	402/410 (98.1)	0.84
All-cause mortality at end of follow-up	249/870 (28.6)	153/599 (25.5)	96/271 (35.4)	0.003	122/452 (27.0)	122/410 (29.8)	0.37
30-day mortality (% dead)	62/870 (7.1)	33/599 (5.5)	29/271 (10.7)	0.006	26/452 (5.8)	35/410 (8.5)	0.11
1-year mortality (% dead)	186/870 (26.3)	111/599 (18.5)	75/271 (27.7)	0.002	93/452 (21.7)	89/410 (20.6)	0.68
2-year mortality (% dead)	229/870 (26.3)	135/599 (22.5)	94/271 (36.7)	<0.001	108/452 (23.9)	116/410 (28.3)	0.14
Major adverse cardiovascular and cerebrovascular events in hospital	90/870 (10.3)	56/599 (9.4)	34/271 (12.6)	0.15	42/452 (9.3)	48/410 (11.7)	0.25
Stroke, in hospital	35/864 (4.1)	24/594 (4.0)	11/270 (4.1)	0.98	18/448 (4.0)	17/408 (4.2)	0.91
Myocardial infarction	11/864 (1.3)	6/594 (1.0)	5/270 (1.9)	0.31	5/447 (1.1)	6/409 (1.5)	0.65
Aortic regurgitation moderate/severe	115/849 (13.6)	91/585 (15.6)	24/264 (9.1)	0.01	76/439 (17.3)	39/405 (9.6)	0.001
Surgical conversion	6/850 (0.7)	0/592 (0)	6/268 (2.2)	0.001*	0/450 (0)	6/402 (1.5)	0.01*
Major vascular complication	55/869 (6.3)	50/598 (8.4)	5/271 (1.9)	<0.001	28/451 (6.2)	26/410 (6.3)	0.94
Repeat procedure	7/870 (0.8)	7/599 (1.2)	0/271 (0)	0.11*	7/452 (1.6)	0/410 (0)	0.02*
Pacemaker	141/867 (16.3)				110/451 (24.4)	30/408 (7.4)	<0.001

Values are n/N (%).
From Moat NE, Ludman P, de Belder MA, et al. Long-term outcomes after transcatheter aortic valve implantation in high-risk patients with severe aortic stenosis: the U.K. TAVI (United Kingdom Transcatheter Aortic Valve Implantation) Registry. J Am Coll Cardiol 2011;58:2130–8.
*Fisher exact test.

TABLE 15-4 Predictors of Mortality at One Year of Patients the United Kingdom Transcatheter Aortic Valve Implantation Registry

VARIABLES	ALIVE (N = 684)	DEAD (N = 186)	Univariate Model RESULT	P VALUE	Multivariate Model RESULT	P VALUE
Valve:						
Edwards SAPIEN	321/680 (47.2)	89/182 (48.9)	1.00			
Medtronic CoreValve	359/680 (52.8)	93/182 (51.1)	0.95 (0.70-1.29)	0.75		
Route:						
Other	196/684 (28.7)	75/186 (40.3)	1.00			
Transfemoral	488/684 (71.3)	111/186 (59.7)	0.65 (0.48-0.88)	0.006	0.73 (0.52-1.04)	0.08
Aortic regurgitation moderate/severe	83/674 (12.3)	32/175 (18.3)	1.49 (1.00-2.21)	0.048	1.66 (1.10-2.51)	0.016
Major vascular complication	39/684 (5.7)	16/185 (8.7)	1.42 (0.82-2.45)	0.21		
Permanent pacemaker	108/683 (15.8)	33/184 (17.9)	1.21 (0.83-1.77)	0.32		
Male gender	355/684 (59.9)	101/186 (54.3)	1.19 (0.88-1.61)	0.25		
Age, years	81.8 ± 7.3	82.3 ± 6.4	1.01 (0.99-1.03)	0.52		
Aortic valve gradient	81.1 ± 27.1	79.9 ± 27.8	0.996 (0.990-1.002)	0.20		
Left ventricular ejection fraction:						
≥50%	459/680 (67.5)	94/185 (50.8)	1.00		1.00	
30%-49%	169/680 (24.9)	69/185 (37.3)	1.93 (1.40-2.66)	<0.001	1.49 (1.03-2.16)	0.03
30%	52/680 (7.6)	22/185 (11.9)	1.89 (1.16-3.07)	0.01	1.65 (0.98-2.79)	0.06
NYHA class:						
I/II	160/680 (23.5)	39/186 (21.0)	1.00			
III/IV	520/680 (76.5)	147/186 (79.0)	1.14 (0.79-1.63)	0.50		
Coronary artery disease	301/653 (46.1)	93/175 (53.1)	1.38 (1.01-1.87)	0.04	1.23 (0.88-1.73)	0.23
Any previous cardiac surgery	202/667 (30.3)	57/186 (30.7)	1.04 (0.75-1.43)	0.83		
Peripheral vascular disease	179/654 (27.4)	62/178 (34.8)	1.28 (0.91-1.75)	0.16		
Diabetes mellitus	146/675 (21.6)	50/136 (26.9)	1.36 (0.98-1.89)	0.07		
Chronic obstructive pulmonary disease	176/654 (26.9)	63/180 (35.0)	1.40 (1.02-1.93)	0.04	1.41 (1.00-1.98)	0.05
Creatinine >200 mmol/L	38/668 (5.7)	19/185 (10.3)	1.84 (1.14-2.97)	0.012	1.55 (0.90-2.68)	0.11

NYHA, New York Heart Association.
Values are n/N (%), mean ± SD, or hazard ratio (95% confidence interval).
From Moat NE, Ludman P, de Belder MA, et al. Long-term outcomes after transcatheter aortic valve implantation in high-risk patients with severe aortic stenosis: the U.K. TAVI (United Kingdom Transcatheter Aortic Valve Implantation) Registry. J Am Coll Cardiol 2011;58:2130–8.

valves were inserted equally via the transfemoral and transapical routes.

The results showed no difference in 30-day or 12-month mortality between the two patient groups (CoreValve and SAPIEN) receiving valves via the transfemoral route and no significant differences in terms of stroke, myocardial infarction, or major access-site complications.

The 30-day and 12-month mortality rates were significantly higher in patients receiving a SAPIEN valve via the transapical route than in patients undergoing TAVI with either valve via the transfemoral route. In the CoreValve subclavian access group, the 30-day mortality was similar to, but the 12-month mortality higher than, that in the CoreValve transfemoral access group.

The FRench Aortic National CoreValve and Edwards (FRANCE 2) Registry

Data from all patients undergoing TAVI in France (and one center in Monaco) since 2010 contribute to the FRANCE 2 registry.[17] SAPIEN and CoreValve prostheses were used. All patients had severe AS with NYHA functional class II, III, or IV symptoms and were not candidates for surgical AVR because of coexisting illnesses. Severe AS was defined as an AVA less than 0.8 cm[2], a mean aortic valve gradient of 40 mm Hg or more, or a peak aortic jet velocity of 4.0 m/s or more. Most centers had performed more than five procedures prior to enrolling patients, and centers that had not performed five procedures were proctored until they gained sufficient experience. At each center, a multidisciplinary team determined eligibility for TAVI (with a clinical evaluation, echocardiography, angiographic assessment, and multidetector CT [MDCT]). The transfemoral approach was used if feasible. SAPIEN devices were implanted by the transfemoral or transapical route, and CoreValve devices by the transfemoral or subclavian route. The characteristics of the patients at baseline are presented in Table 15-5. Characteristics of the patients according to TAVI approach are presented in Table 15-6. The outcomes according to TAVI approach and device are presented in Tables 15-7 and 15-8, respectively, and the main results are presented in Figure 15-4.

Of the 3195 TAVIs that were performed, 80.4% were percutaneous and 19.6% were surgical (17.6% transapical approach, 1.8% transaortic or transcarotid approach). A SAPIEN device was used in 66.9% of patients and a CoreValve device in 33.1%. Mortality was 9.7% at 30 days. On multivariate analysis, the independent predictors of 1-year mortality were increased logistic EuroSCORE, NYHA functional class III or IV, the use of a transapical approach, and post-TAVI periprosthetic regurgitation grade of 2 or more (on a scale of 0 to 4).

Patient Selection

TAVI is technically feasible in most patients with AS. A larger question, we believe, is when TAVI should be offered. The answer has been expressed multiple ways, including: "Treat patients dying from AS, not diagnosed with AS;" "Avoid patients who could be classified as PARTNER Cohort C;" and "Avoid extreme comorbidities that overwhelm the benefit of TAVI and render the intervention futile."[18] Increasingly, evaluation is directed at identifying patients in whom a significant improvement in quality and duration of life is likely and avoiding unnecessary intervention in

TABLE 15-5	**FRANCE 2 Registry Patient Characteristics at Baseline According to Valve Type**		
CHARACTERISTIC	**ALL PATIENTS (N = 3195)**	**THOSE RECEIVING EDWARDS SAPIEN (N = 2107)**	**THOSE RECEIVING MEDTRONIC COREVALVE (N = 1043)**
Age, year	82.7 ± 7.2	82.9 ± 7.2	82.3 ± 7.2
Male gender, no. (%)	1630 (51.0)	981 (46.6)	626 (60.0)
Society of Thoracic Surgeons Score, %	14.4 ± 11.9	15.6 ± 12.4	14.2 ± 11.2
Logistic EuroSCORE, %	21.9 ± 14.3	22.2 ± 14.3	21.3 ± 14.3
New York Heart Association functional class III or IV, no./total no. (%)	2376/3132 (75.9)	1565/2072 (75.5)	788/1035 (76.1)
Clinical history, no./total no. (%):			
Coronary artery disease	1483/3093 (47.9)	997/2046 (48.7)	474/1025 (46.2)
Previous myocardial infarction	508/3093 (16.4)	347/2046 (17.0)	158/1025 (15.4)
Previous coronary artery bypass graft	564/3093 (18.2)	373/2046 (18.2)	188/1025 (18.3)
Cerebrovascular disease	308/3093 (10.0)	205/2046 (10.0)	101/1025 (9.9)
Aortic abdominal aneurysm	148/3093 (10.0)	98/2046 (4.8)	50/1025 (4.9)
Peripheral vascular disease	643/3093 (20.8)	447/2046 (21.8)	191/1025 (18.6)
Chronic obstructive pulmonary disease	790/3093 (25.5)	518/2046 (25.3)	269/1025 (26.2)
Renal dialysis	82/3093 (2.7)	47/2046 (2.3)	32/1025 (3.1)
Atrial fibrillation	820/3083 (26.6)	514/2038 (25.2)	303/1024 (29.6)
Permanent pacemaker	447/3135 (14.3)	280/2073 (13.5)	160/1034 (15.5)
Pulmonary hypertension	478/2435 (19.6)	324/1635 (19.8)	151/787 (19.2)
Echocardiographic findings			
Aortic valve area, cm[2]	0.7 ± 0.2	0.7 ± 0.2	0.7 ± 0.2
Mean aortic valve gradient, mm Hg	48.1 ± 16.5	48.6 ± 16.5	47.1 ± 16.4
Left ventricular ejection fraction, %	53.2 ± 14.1	53.8 ± 14.0	52.0 ± 14.0
Moderate or severe mitral regurgitation, no./total no. (%)	58/2966 (2.0)	37/1974 (1.9)	21/972 (2.2)
Previous surgical aortic-valve replacement, no./total no. (%)	49/3093 (1.6)	18/2046 (0.9)	31/1025 (3.0)
Life expectancy <1 year, no./total no. (%)	102/3093 (3.3)	40/2046 (2.0)	41/1025 (4.0)
Patient's decision to undergo transcatheter aortic valve implantation, no./total no. (%)	499/3165 (15.8)	358/2096 (17.1)	136/1039 (13.1)

From Gilard M, Eltchaninoff H, Iung B, et al. Registry of transcatheter aortic-valve implantation in high-risk patients. N Engl J Med 2012;366:1705–15.

TABLE 15-6   FRANCE 2 Registry Patient Characteristics at Baseline According to TAVI Approach

CHARACTERISTIC	ALL PATIENTS (N = 2361)	TRANSAPICAL APPROACH (N = 567)	SUBCLAVIAN APPROACH (N = 184)	P VALUE
Age, years	83.0 ± 7.2	81.5 ± 7.4	82.2 ± 6.7	<0.001
Male gender, no. (%)	1120 (47.4)	332 (58.6)	131 (71.2)	<0.001
Logistic EuroSCORE (%)	21.2 ± (14.7)	24.8 ± 14.7	20.3 ± 15.2	<0.001
Society of Thoracic Surgeons Score (%)	14.5 ± 11.9	15.1 ± 13.8	16.6 ± 13.4	0.15
NYHA functional class III or IV, no./total no. (%)	1808/2323 (77.8)	388/554 (70.0)	130/182 (71.4)	<0.001
Clinical history, no./total no. (%):				
Coronary artery disease	1018/2293 (44.4)	325/547 (59.4)	104/178 (58.4)	<0.001
Previous myocardial infarction	333/2293 (14.5)	137/547 (25.0)	33/178 (18.5)	<0.001
Previous coronary artery bypass graft	348/2293 (15.2)	164/547 (30.0)	43/178 (24.2)	<0.001
Previous balloon aortic valvuloplasty	389/2293 (17.0)	106/547 (19.4)	39/178 (21.9)	0.13
Cerebrovascular disease	219/2293 (9.6)	60/547 (11.0)	20/178 (11.2)	0.50
Aortic abdominal aneurysm	59/2293 (2.6)	54/547 (9.9)	28/178 (15.7)	<0.001
Peripheral vascular disease	286/2293 (12.5)	263/547 (48.1)	74/178 (41.6)	<0.001
Chronic obstructive pulmonary disease	580/2293 (25.3)	124/547 (22.7)	63/178 (35.4)	0.003
Renal dialysis	60/2293 (2.6)	17/547 (3.1)	4/178 (2.2)	0.80
Atrial fibrillation	638/2287 (27.9)	114/544 (21.0)	56/178 (31.5)	0.002
Pulmonary hypertension	364/1820 (20.0)	72/429 (16.8)	31/132 (23.5)	0.16
Severe aortic calcification	127/2314 (5.5)	10/556 (1.8)	21/177 (11.9)	<0.001
Harmful chest wall irradiation	144/2320 (6.2)	29/553 (5.2)	3/177 (1.7)	0.02
Chest wall deformity	62/2326 (2.7)	6/557 (1.1)	6/179 (3.4)	0.06
Previous surgical aortic valve replacement	37/2293 (1.6)	8/547 (1.5)	4/178 (2.2)	0.72
Life expectancy <1 year, no./total no. (%)	64/2293 (2.8)	8/547 (1.5)	8/178 (4.5)	0.06
Patient's decision to undergo TAVI, no./total no. (%)	356/2349 (15.2)	82/559 (14.7)	23/182 (12.6)	0.64

NYHA, New York Heart Association.

From Gilard M, Eltchaninoff H, Iung B, et al. Registry of transcatheter aortic-valve implantation in high-risk patients. N Engl J Med 2012;366:1705–15.

TABLE 15-7   FRANCE 2 Registry Outcomes According to TAVI Approach and Device

OUTCOME	ALL PATIENTS (N = 3195)	Approach			P VALUE	Valve	
		TRANSFEMORAL (N = 2361)	TRANSAPICAL (N = 567)	SUBCLAVIAN (N = 184)		EDWARDS SAPIEN (N = 2107)	MEDTRONIC COREVALVE (N = 1043)
Procedural success, no. (%)	3095 (96.9)	2293 (97.1)	544 (95.9)	178 (96.7)	0.35	2044 (97.0)	1018 (97.6)
Hospital stay, days	11.1 ± 8.0	10.5 ± 8.1	13.3 ± 7.8	11.6 ± 6.0	<0.001	10.9 ± 7.5	11.3 ± 8.9
Death, no. (%):							
At 30 days:							
From any cause	293 (9.7)	190 (8.5)	77 (13.9)	19 (10.1)	<0.001	195 (9.6)	91 (9.4)
From cardiovascular cause	212 (7.0)	132 (5.9)	59 (10.8)	15 (8.7)	0.73	141 (7.0)	64 (6.7)
At 6 months:							
From any cause	474 (18.6)	321 (17.2)	110 (22.4)	32 (23.3)	0.002	312 (18.1)	155 (19.6)
From cardiovascular cause	301 (11.7)	197 (10.5)	77 (15.7)	18 (12.1)	0.81	201 (11.5)	93 (11.7)
At 1 year:							
From any cause	528 (24.0)	355 (21.7)	129 (32.3)	33 (25.1)	<0.001	352 (24.0)	168 (23.7)
From cardiovascular cause	324 (14.3)	212 (12.7)	84 (19.8)	19 (14.4)	0.79	217 (14.2)	100 (14.3)

From Gilard M, Eltchaninoff H, Iung B, et al. Registry of transcatheter aortic-valve implantation in high-risk patients. N Engl J Med 2012;366:1705–15.

patients in whom the procedure can be performed but benefit is unlikely. For this reason, evaluation of neurocognitive functioning, frailty, functional status, mobility, and social support is increasingly being recognized as important in patient selection.

Although we evaluate each patient individually and we do not have (or advocate) a strict cutoff for TAVI candidacy, the following points merit consideration. In the PARTNER IB cohort, patients with an STS score higher than 14.9% did no better with TAVI than with standard medical therapy.[1,9] In the FRANCE 2 and other registries, similar themes have emerged: higher logistic EuroSCORE, NYHA functional class III or IV symptoms, the use of a transapical approach, and periprosthetic regurgitation grade of 2 or more (on a scale of 0 to 4) are independent predictors of mortality after TAVI.[14,17] As noted previously, multivariate predictors of higher mortality in the TAVI group at 2 years in PARTNER part A

included a lower body mass index, lower preprocedure transvalvular gradient, reduced renal function, and prior vascular surgery or stent.[12] In PARTNER B, multivariate risk predictors of death at 2 years were lower body mass index, prior stroke, and chronic obstructive pulmonary disease (COPD) requiring supplemental oxygen.

Both the logistic EuroSCORE and the STS score incorporate many comorbidities, so before a patient is offered TAVI, they should be calculated and considered along with NYHA functional class, the preprocedure transvalvular gradient, renal function, prior vascular surgery or stent, prior stroke, COPD requiring supplemental oxygen, and whether TAVI can be performed transfemorally. TAVI should be offered to patients who are likely to benefit and in whom standard AVR would pose equivalent or greater risk.

TABLE 15-8 FRANCE 2 Registry Complications According to TAVI Approach and Device

COMPLICATION	ALL PATIENTS (N = 3195)	Approach			P VALUE	Device	
		TRANSFEMORAL (N = 2361)	TRANSAPICAL (N = 567)	SUBCLAVIAN (N = 184)		EDWARDS SAPIEN (N = 2107)	MEDTRONIC COREVALVE (N = 1043)
Periprosthetic regurgitation at 30 days, no./total no. (%):							
Grade 0	724/1915 (37.8)	483/1418 (34.1)	173/334 (51.8)	37/112 (33.0)		515/1256 (41.0)	203/642 (31.6)
Grade 1	875/1915 (45.7)	671/1418 (47.3)	131/334 (39.2)	58/112 (51.8)		567/1256 (45.1)	301/642 (46.9)
Grade 2	301/1915 (15.7)	251/1418 (17.7)	30/334 (9.0)	15/112 (13.4)		169/1256 (13.5)	128/642 (19.9)
Grade 3	15/1915 (0.8)	13/1418 (0.9)	0	2/112 (1.8)		5/1256 (0.4)	10/642 (1.6)
Complications at 1 year, no. (%):							
Stroke							
Major	72 (2.3)	51 (2.2)	12 (2.1)	5 (2.7)	0.88	41 (1.9)	27 (2.6)
Minor	59 (1.8)	36 (1.5)	13 (2.3)	8 (4.3)	0.07	41 (1.9)	18 (1.7)
Myocardial infarction	37 (1.2)	20 (0.8)	10 (1.8)	6 (3.3)	0.004	16 (0.8)	20 (1.9)
Bleeding:							
Life-threatening	39 (1.2)	29 (1.2)	8 (1.4)	1 (0.5)	0.76	32 (1.5)	6 (0.6)
Major	144 (4.5)	26 (1.5)	19 (3.4)	6 (3.3)	<0.001	42 (2.0)	16 (1.5)
Minor	236 (7.4)	161 (6.8)	54 (9.5)	13 (7.1)	0.08	166 (7.9)	70 (6.7)
Vascular complication:							
Major	150 (4.7)	129 (5.5)	11 (1.9)	8 (4.3)	0.002	57 (2.7)	47 (4.5)
Minor	160 (5.0)	139 (5.9)	9 (1.6)	12 (6.5)	<0.001	60 (2.8)	49 (4.7)
New pacemaker	497 (15.6)	359 (15.2)	77 (13.6)	47 (25.5)	<0.001	243 (11.5)	252 (24.2)
Valve migration	40 (1.3)	28 (1.2)	8 (1.4)	2 (1.1)	0.91	23 (1.1)	17 (1.6)

From Gilard M, Eltchaninoff H, Iung B, et al. Registry of transcatheter aortic-valve implantation in high-risk patients. N Engl J Med 2012;366:1705–15.

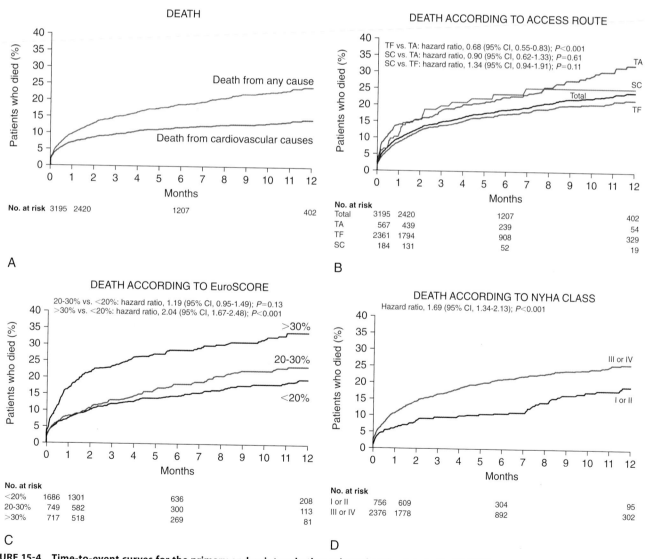

FIGURE 15-4 Time-to-event curves for the primary end point and other selected end points in the FRANCE 2 Registry. **A,** Rate of death from any cause (the primary end point) and from cardiovascular causes. **B,** Rates of death from any cause according to the TAVI access route: transapical (TA) transfemoral (TF), or subclavian (SC). **C,** Rates of death from any cause according to the logistic EuroSCORE (with a score >20% indicating very high surgical risk). **D,** Rates of death from any cause according to New York Heart Association (NYHA) functional class. Event rates were calculated with the use of Kaplan-Meier methods and were compared by means of the log-rank test. Deaths from unknown causes were assumed to be from cardiovascular causes. CI, confidence interval. (From Gilard M, Eltchaninoff H, Iung B, et al. Registry of transcatheter aortic-valve implantation in high-risk patients. N Engl J Med 2012;366:1705–15.)

Transthoracic echocardiography (TTE), transesophageal echocardiography (TEE),[19] MDCT,[20] and invasive angiography are all used to perform anatomic evaluations specific to TAVI. TTE, TEE or MDCT is commonly used to measure the dimensions of the aortic annulus, which determines valve size (Figures 15-5, 15-6, and 15-7). Arterial access is generally assessed with invasive angiography or contrast MDCT.[21] The aorta can be evaluated with invasive angiography or contrast MDCT to assess technical issues related to the delivery and implantation of the specific valve type, the aortic root and valvular calcification, and the risk of coronary obstruction.[21]

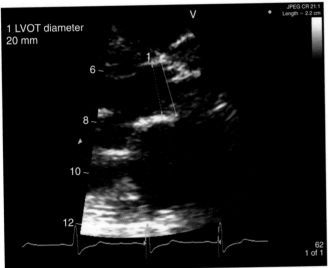

FIGURE 15-5   Measurement of the aortic annulus diameter at the cusp insertion on transthoracic echocardiography. The annulus measures 22 mm, and the left ventricular outflow tract (LVOT) measures 20 mm.

Current TAVI "State of the Art"

Around 100,000 TAVI procedures have been performed in more than 40 countries, yet TAVI remains a procedure in constant evolution. We advocate surgical AVR as the standard of care for most patients with symptomatic severe AS. We consider TAVI the procedure of choice for patients for whom surgical risk is prohibitive (PARTNER part B patients) and AVR is indicated. TAVI is an increasingly reasonable alternative for selected "operable" patients in whom the high risk of either mortality or of morbidity is high (PARTNER part A patients).

Work is ongoing and continues to be needed in patient evaluation. TAVI is technically feasible in the majority of patients, but the onus is on the physicians to identify patients in whom a significant improvement is quality of life will occur after the procedure. We believe this identification requires a noncompetitive team approach involving interventional cardiologists with expertise in structural heart disease, cardiac and vascular surgeons, anesthesiologists, imaging specialists, and specialized nurses. The proper equipment and a minimum volume of TAVI procedures performed are required for optimal outcomes.[3] Although controversial, the data on procedural volumes indicate to us that with transfemoral SAPIEN and CoreValve implants, centers should aim for a minimum of 50 procedures per year per operator for optimal outcome.[3,22] Improved success with transapical TAVI with experience and volume has also been suggested.[23]

This improvement will require establishment of centers of excellence for TAVI. With this infrastructure we believe procedural success of more than 95%, 30-day survival more than 90%, meaningful improvement in quality of life and acceptable complication rates (including procedure related stroke <2%, vascular access site complications <5%, permanent pacemaker rates <5% with higher pacemaker rates expected with CoreValve than with SAPIEN) can be achieved in properly selected patients.[14,21]

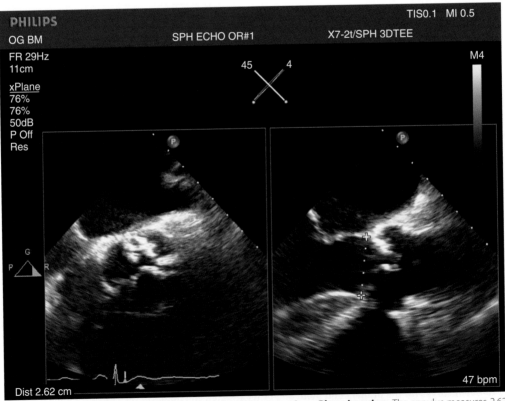

FIGURE 15-6   Transesophageal measurement of the aortic annulus diameter using xPlane imaging. The annulus measures 2.62 cm, as indicated by plus signs and dotted line on xPlane images obtained with the Philips iE33 xMATRIX Multimedia system (Philips Healthcare, Andover, Massachusetts).

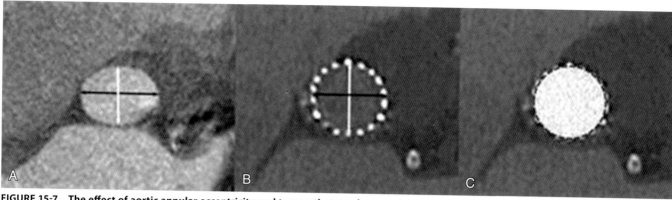

FIGURE 15-7 **The effect of aortic annular eccentricity and transcatheter valve oversizing on valve expansion and eccentricity.** This effect is demonstrated by matched multidector computed tomography scans obtained before and after transcatheter aortic valve implantation of an Edwards SAPIEN THV (Edwards Lifesciences Corporation, Irvine, California). **A,** At baseline, the aortic annulus is eccentric (29%) with a mean diameter of 20.5 mm (17.0 mm × 24.1 mm) and an area of 3.45 cm². **B,** Following implantation of a 23-mm transcatheter valve, imaging shows a circular implant (23.2 mm × 23.5 mm, eccentricity 1.3%). **C,** Even though it is oversized relative to the annular area by 20%, the valve is fully expanded with an expansion ratio of 103.6% (area of THV, 4.30 cm²). *(From Willson AB, Webb JG, LaBounty TM, et al. 3-dimensional aortic annular assessment by multidetector computed tomography predicts moderate or severe paravalvular regurgitation after transcatheter aortic valve replacement: a multicenter retrospective analysis. J Am Coll Cardiol 2012;59:1287–94.)*

Valve-in-Valve Procedures

Experience with implantation of transcatheter valves within failed bioprostheses (valve-in-valve procedures) has been reported.[24] Factors that make this a potentially preferable option include a higher risk of reoperation in many patients and the rigid frame of most bioprostheses, which facilitates transcatheter valve positioning and paravalvular sealing while reducing the risk of atrioventricular block, annular rupture, and coronary obstruction. However, not all bioprostheses have radiopaque stents; some are stentless, and all (with perhaps higher risk in prostheses with externally mounted leaflets) have the potential for coronary ostial obstruction if diseased bioprosthetic leaflets are in close proximity to the coronary ostia. Small-diameter surgical bioprostheses may not allow for optimal expansion of current transcatheter implants. Durability data are limited owing to a relative low number of procedures reported with adequate follow-up.

Critically important issues in a achieving a successful valve-in-valve procedure include understanding the manufacturer sizing and labeling of surgical bioprostheses (Figure 15-8) and correct positioning of the valve in valve (Figures 15-9 and 15-10). We believe early experience suggests that TAVI will be an important option for treatment of patients with failed bioprostheses.[25-27]

Alternatives to TAVI

Surgical Aortic Valve Replacement

Surgical AVR should be considered in all patients regardless of age. One-, two-, and five-year survival rates among selected patients older than 80 years undergoing surgical AVR have been reported as 87%, 78%, and 68%, respectively.[28] We advocate assessment of all patients considered for TAVI by a multidisciplinary team that includes cardiovascular surgeons to make sure that surgical AVR is one of the options considered.

Balloon Aortic Valvuloplasty

Historically, suggested indications for balloon aortic valvuloplasty have included hemodynamically significant AS and any of the following: as a bridge to surgical AVR in hemodynamically unstable patients; increased perioperative risk (STS score >15); anticipated survival less than 3 years; age in the late 80s or 90s and patient preference for an aortic valvuloplasty over surgical AVR; severe comorbidities such as porcelain aorta, severe lung

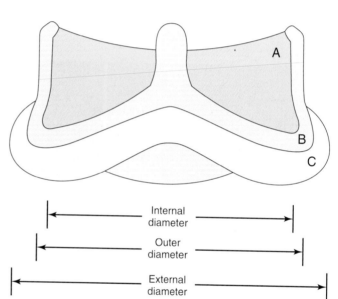

FIGURE 15-8 **Schematic diagram of stented bioprosthetic valves.** Valve leaflet **(A),** stent frame **(B),** and external sewing ring **(C).** The internal, outer, and external diameters all represent different dimensions of surgical bioprostheses. *(From Gurvitch R, Cheung A, Ye J, et al. Transcatheter valve-in-valve implantation for failed surgical bioprosthetic valves. J Am Coll Cardiol 2011;58: 2196–209.)*

disease, and others for which the surgeon prefers not to operate; and severe neuromuscular or arthritic conditions that would limit the patient's ability to undergo postoperative rehabilitation.[29] In general, we now perform TAVI in the majority of patients with these conditions.

Currently we reserve balloon aortic valvuloplasty for the rare hemodynamically unstable patient as a bridge to a decision to provide more definitive therapy of the AS, for the patient with a predicted survival from noncardiac causes measured in weeks to a few months, and for the patient who has a contraindication to TAVI in whom we believe that relief of the aortic obstruction will improve quality of life, such as a patient with severe AS and a metastatic gastrointestinal malignancy who requires a palliative abdominal operative procedure for symptom relief that can be safely performed only if the AS gradient is reduced.

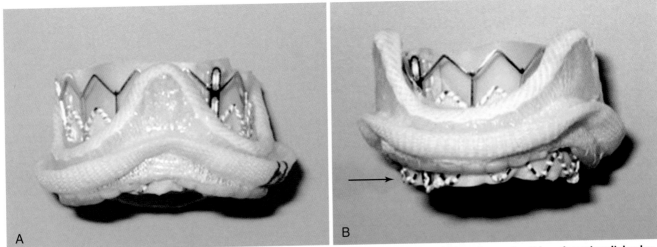

FIGURE 15-9   In vitro demonstration of a transcatheter valve (Edwards SAPIEN) implanted within a Carpentier-Edwards pericardial valve. A,
Incorrect positioning: The transcatheter valve (Edwards SAPIEN, Edward Lifesciences Corporation, Irvine, California) is implanted too high within the outflow tract of the surgical valve (Carpentier-Edwards valve, Edward Lifesciences). This error may result in splaying of the surgical valve posts and transcatheter valve emboliza-tion. **B,** Correct valve positioning: The transcatheter valve (*arrow*) is implanted so that it overlaps the surgical valve sewing ring, allowing better anchoring and a more secure position. *(From Webb JG, Wood DA, Ye J, et al. Transcatheter valve-in-valve implantation for failed bioprosthetic heart valves. Circulation 2010;121:1848–57.)*

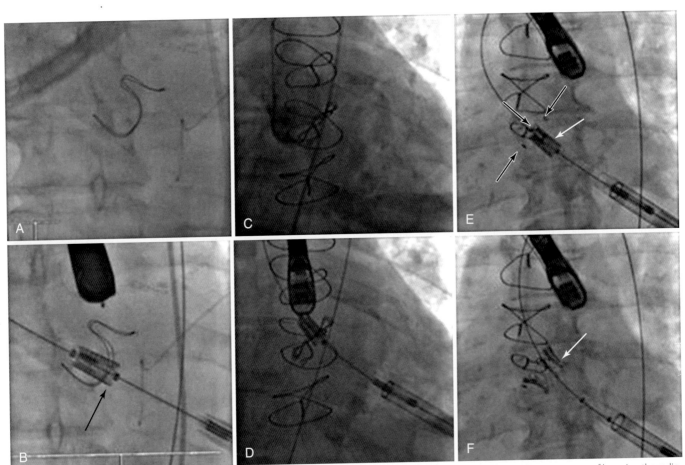

FIGURE 15-10   Fluoroscopic positioning for valve-in-valve implantation for bioprosthetic aortic valve failure. The importance of knowing the radio-graphic appearance of the surgical valve treated. **A,** Carpentier-Edwards Pericardial Valve (Edwards Lifesciences Corporation, Irvine, California). The wire frame within the valve posts is visible, although the rigid sewing ring below it required for valve-in-valve fixation is radiolucent in this model. **B,** Positioning of the Edwards SAPIEN valve (Edwards Lifesciences Corporation) just below the lowest radiopaque portion (*arrow* indicates lowest portion of the SAPIEN valve). **C,** Mitroflow Aortic Pericardial Heart Valve (Sorin Group, Milan). **D,** Positioning the Edwards SAPIEN just below the lowest radiopaque portion. **E,** Medtronic Mosaic valve (Medtronic, Inc, Minneapolis, Minnesota): The radiopaque markers are near the top of the surgical stent posts (*black arrows*); hence the valve is positioned completely below these markers (*white arrow*). **F,** Deployed Edwards SAPIEN valve. The "waist" at the lower part of the implanted valve demonstrates the narrowest location of the surgical valve (*white arrow*). In the procedure shown here, the SAPIEN valve remained slightly underexpanded, and the residual mean gradient was 30 mm Hg. *(From Gurvitch R, Cheung A, Ye J, et al. Transcatheter valve-in-valve implantation for failed surgical bioprosthetic valves. J Am Coll Cardiol 2011;58:2196–209.)*

Balloon Aortic Valvuloplasty Followed by External-Beam Irradiation

Balloon aortic valvuloplasty for calcific AS has been largely abandoned because of high restenosis rates.[30] Radiation therapy has been used for preventing restenosis after vascular interventions.[31,32] A 20-patient study evaluating external-beam irradiation to prevent restenosis after balloon aortic valvuloplasty in elderly patients (age 89 ± 4 years) with calcific AS has been reported (RADAR pilot trial).[33] Total radiation doses of 12 to 18 Gy were delivered in fractions over 3 to 5 days after balloon aortic valvuloplasty. There were no complications related to external-beam irradiation. Twelve patients survived to 1 year (60%). One patient underwent surgical AVR; no patient had a second balloon aortic valvuloplasty. Four of the survivors had restenosis (defined as loss of >50% of the initial increase in AVA).

Apical-to-Aortic Conduit

Several small series have reported on the use of a valved conduit between the left ventricular apex and the aorta for treatment of patients in whom a standard surgical AVR was contraindicated.

In one series conducted from 2002 through 2005, 13 patients (mean age, 75 ± 8.7 years; 8 men) with severe calcific AS underwent insertion of an apical aortic valved conduit because of a porcelain aorta ($n = 4$), previous coronary bypass grafting ($n = 6$), or both ($n = 3$).[34] An off-pump technique was used in 9 patients; a mini-extracorporeal circulation system was used in 4 patients. Mean intensive care unit stay was 2 ± 2.7 days, and mean hospital stay was 12 ± 8 days. The 30-day mortality was 15%. Mortality later than 30 days postoperatively was 23% (follow-up from 6 to 33 months). The remaining 8 patients are reported to have NYHA class I or II symptoms at follow-up. Echocardiography shows a low gradient over the valved conduit in survivors.

Another series reported results from procedures performed between 1995 and 2003.[35] Thirteen patients (mean age 71 years) underwent insertion of an apical aortic conduit for severe symptomatic AS (mean valve area 0.65 ± 0.02 cm²). Indications for apical aortic conduit were heavily calcified ascending aorta and aortic root, patent retrosternal mammary grafts, calcified ascending aorta and aortic root plus patent retrosternal mammary graft, retrosternal colonic interposition, and multiple previous sternotomies. The procedures were performed with use of cardiopulmonary bypass through a left thoracotomy (n = 10), median sternotomy (n = 2), or bilateral thoracotomy (n = 1). Hearts were kept beating (n = 5) or fibrillated (n = 7). Circulatory arrest was used in one patient. Three patients (23%) died in the hospital; the mean hospital stay was 26 days. At a mean follow-up of 2.1 years, four (31%) late deaths have been reported.

ACKNOWLEDGMENT AND DISCLOSURE

Brad Munt has been a consultant for and has honoraria from Edwards Lifesciences Corporation, Irvine, California. He would like to thank Stephanie, Duncan, Lucy, Benjamin, and Oliver for keeping him interested in expanding his horizons, and the members of the heart team and echocardiography laboratory at St. Paul's Hospital for their support and encouragement.

REFERENCES

1. Makkar RR, Fontana GP, Jilaihawi H, et al. Transcatheter aortic-valve replacement for inoperable severe aortic stenosis. N Engl J Med 2012;366:1696–704.

2. Bonow RO, Carabello B, Chatterjee K, et al. ACC/AHA 2006 guidelines for the management of patients with valvular heart disease: a report of the American College of Cardiology/American Heart Association Task Force on Practice Guidelines (writing Committee to Revise the 1998 guidelines for the management of patients with valvular heart disease) developed in collaboration with the Society of Cardiovascular Anesthesiologists endorsed by the Society for Cardiovascular Angiography and Interventions and the Society of Thoracic Surgeons. J Am Coll Cardiol 2006;48: e1–148.

3. Holmes DR Jr, Mack MJ. Transcatheter valve therapy: a professional society overview from the American College of Cardiology Foundation and the Society of Thoracic Surgeons. Ann Thorac Surg 2011;92:380–9.

4. Otto CM, Mickel MC, Kennedy JW, et al. Three-year outcome after balloon aortic valvuloplasty: insights into prognosis of valvular aortic stenosis. Circulation 1994;89: 642–50.

5. Iung B, Cachier A, Baron G, et al. Decision-making in elderly patients with severe aortic stenosis: why are so many denied surgery? Eur Heart J 2005;26:704–8.

6. Andersen HR, Knudsen JL, Hasenkam JM. Transluminal implantation of artificial heart valves: description of a new expandable aortic valve and initial results with implantation by catheter technique in closed chest pigs. Eur Heart J 1992;13:704–8.

7. Cribier A, Eltchaninoff H, Bash A, et al. Percutaneous transcatheter implantation of an aortic valve prosthesis for calcific aortic stenosis: first human case description. Circulation 2002;106:3006–8.

8. Webb JG, Chandavimol M, Thompson CR, et al. Percutaneous aortic valve implantation retrograde from the femoral artery. Circulation 2006;113:842–50.

9. Leon MB, Smith CR, Mack M, et al. Transcatheter aortic-valve implantation for aortic stenosis in patients who cannot undergo surgery. N Engl J Med 2010;363: 1597–607.

10. Nainggolan L. Two new TAVI devices debut at surgery meeting. October 4, 2011 [accessed 2013 3 February]; Available from: www.theheart.org/article/1290089.

11. Smith CR, Leon MB, Mack MJ, et al. Transcatheter versus surgical aortic-valve replacement in high-risk patients. N Engl J Med 2011;364:2187–98.

12. Kodali SK, Williams MR, Smith CR, et al. Two-year outcomes after transcatheter or surgical aortic-valve replacement. N Engl J Med 2012;366:1686–95.

13. O'Riordan M. STACCATO: Transapical TAVI in surgery-eligible patients stopped due to adverse events. November 10, 2011 [accessed 2013 3 February]; Available from: www.theheart.org/article/1307437.

14. Wood S. TAVI registry updates ADVANCE the field, raise hope for lower stroke rates. March 24, 2012 [accessed 2013 3 February]; Available from: www.theheart.org/article/1374163.

15. Rodes-Cabau J, Webb JG, Cheung A, et al. Transcatheter aortic valve implantation for the treatment of severe symptomatic aortic stenosis in patients at very high or prohibitive surgical risk: acute and late outcomes of the multicenter Canadian experience. J Am Coll Cardiol 2010;55:1080–90.

16. Moat NE, Ludman P, de Belder MA, et al. Long-term outcomes after transcatheter aortic valve implantation in high-risk patients with severe aortic stenosis: the U.K. TAVI (United Kingdom Transcatheter Aortic Valve Implantation) Registry. J Am Coll Cardiol 2011;58: 2130–8.

17. Gilard M, Eltchaninoff H, Iung B, et al. Registry of transcatheter aortic-valve implantation in high-risk patients. N Engl J Med 2012;366:1705–15.

18. Miller R. Some valve patients are too sick for TAVI or surgery. May 3, 2012 [accessed 2013 3 February]; Available from: www.theheart.org/article/1393457.

19. Moss RR, Ivens E, Pasupati S, et al. Role of echocardiography in percutaneous aortic valve implantation. JACC Cardiovasc Imaging 2008;1:15–24.

20. Leipsic J, Gurvitch R, LaBounty TM, et al. Multidetector computed tomography in transcatheter aortic valve implantation. JACC Cardiovasc Imaging 2011;4: 416–29.

21. Webb JG, Wood DA. Current status of transcatheter aortic valve replacement. J Am Coll Cardiol 2012;60:483–92.

22. Alli OO, Booker JD, Lennon RJ, et al. Transcatheter aortic valve implantation: assessing the learning curve. JACC Cardiovasc Interv 2012;5:72–9.

23. Miller R. PARTNER CAP data show transapical outcomes improve with practice. January 31, 2012 [accessed 2012 3 April]; Available from: www.theheart.org/article/1348117.

24. Gurvitch R, Cheung A, Ye J, et al. Transcatheter valve-in-valve implantation for failed surgical bioprosthetic valves. J Am Coll Cardiol 2011;58:2196–209.

25. Piazza N, Bleiziffer S, Brockmann G, et al. Transcatheter aortic valve implantation for failing surgical aortic bioprosthetic valve: from concept to clinical application and evaluation (part 2). JACC Cardiovasc Interv 2011;4:733–42.

26. Piazza N, Bleiziffer S, Brockmann G, et al. Transcatheter aortic valve implantation for failing surgical aortic bioprosthetic valve: from concept to clinical application and evaluation (part 1). JACC Cardiovasc Interv 2011;4:721–32.

27. Webb JG, Wood DA, Ye J, et al. Transcatheter valve-in-valve implantation for failed bioprosthetic heart valves. Circulation 2010;121:1848–57.

28. Varadarajan P, Kapoor N, Bansal RC, et al. Survival in elderly patients with severe aortic stenosis is dramatically improved by aortic valve replacement: results from a cohort of 277 patients aged greater than or equal to 80 years. Eur J Cardiothorac Surg 2006;30: 722–7.

29. Hara H, Pedersen WR, Ladich E, et al. Percutaneous balloon aortic valvuloplasty revisited: time for a renaissance? Circulation 2007;115:e334–8.

30. Hashimoto H, Tamura T, Ikari Y, et al. Comparison of aortic valve replacement and percutaneous aortic balloon valvuloplasty for elderly patients with aortic stenosis. Jpn Circ J 1996;60:142–8.

31. Verin V, Popowski Y, de Bruyne B, et al. Endoluminal beta-radiation therapy for the prevention of coronary restenosis after balloon angioplasty. The Dose-Finding Study Group. N Engl J Med 2001;344:243–9.

32. Hagenaars T, Po IF, Sambeek R, et al. Gamma radiation induces positive vascular remodeling after balloon angioplasty: a prospective, randomized intravascular ultrasound scan study. J Vasc Surg 2002;36:318–24.

33. Pedersen WR, Van Tassel RA, Pierce TA, et al. Radiation following percutaneous balloon aortic valvuloplasty to prevent restenosis (RADAR pilot trial). Catheter Cardiovasc Interv 2006;68:183–92.

34. Lockowandt U. Apicoaortic valved conduit: potential for progress? J Thorac Cardiovasc Surg 2006;132:796–801.

35. Crestanello J, Zehr KG, Daly RC, et al. Is there a role for the left ventricle apical-aortic conduit for acquired aortic stenosis? J Heart Valve Dis 2004;13:57–62; discussion 62–3.

CHAPTER 16 | Imaging Guidance of Transcatheter Valve Procedures

Ernesto E. Salcedo and John D. Carroll

> ## Key Points

- In industrialized countries the etiology of valvular heart disease has shifted from rheumatic heart disease, a disease of the young, to calcific valve disease, a disease of the elderly.
- Comorbidities and frailty in the elderly significantly increase surgical morbidity and mortality, so alternatives to surgery have been developed to provide less invasive forms of therapy in this aging population.
- The interventional field has moved forward not only in the invention of new devices, but also because of breakthroughs, refinements, and implementation of imaging guidance that enable the interventionalist to perform these new treatments.
- The choice of imaging guidance is based on specific differences between modalities as well as other variables, including cost, clinical scenario, operator expertise, and complexity of procedure.
- Fluoroscopy and cineangiography have traditionally been used in the catheterization laboratory to guide coronary interventional procedures; today they are the central guidance tools for noncoronary interventions.
- Computed tomography is being used in both aortic and mitral transcatheter-based interventions. It provides a comprehensive anatomic assessment of the aortic valve complex and, to a lesser degree, of the mitral valve apparatus, aiding the selection of the most appropriate procedural approach, decreasing complications, and improving outcomes.
- Cardiac magnetic resonance is a comprehensive noninvasive imaging tool capable of evaluating all aspects of valvular heart disease. Its main advantages include direct quantification of regurgitant lesions, accurate assessment of ventricular size, mass, and function, and visualization of myocardial scar.
- Intracardiac echocardiography provides procedural guidance for valvular interventions, although it has several limitations including, its current two-dimensional character, restricted location of the imaging catheter, and lack of standardization of imaging protocols. On the other hand, its very high spatial and temporal resolutions of valve structures is a major strength.
- Because of its universal availability, portability, and capability to provide high quality, reliable physiologic and morphologic information, echocardiography has been embraced with enthusiasm in the catheterization laboratory to provide guidance for transcatheter valve procedures.

Valvular Heart Disease in the Era of Transcatheter Valve Procedures

In population-based studies the overall age-adjusted prevalence of valvular disease has been estimated to be 2.5% of the population. The prevalence according to the type of valvular disease is 1.7% for mitral regurgitation, 0.5% for aortic regurgitation, 0.4% for aortic stenosis, and 0.1% for mitral stenosis. Importantly, and relevant to this chapter, the prevalence of valvular heart disease increases significantly with age, from less than 2% in persons younger than 65 years, to 8.5% of those between 65 and 75 years, to 13.2% of those older than 75 years.[1]

Although rheumatic heart disease remains common in developing countries, where its prevalence is estimated at 2% to 3%, the etiology and epidemiology of valvular heart disease have shifted in industrialized countries from rheumatic heart disease, a disease of the young, to calcific valve disease, a disease of the elderly.[2,3] The decrease in the prevalence of rheumatic heart disease has been outweighed by an increase in age-related valve diseases.[2,4,5] Calcific valve disease is characterized by the formation of cartilaginous deposits in the mitral valves and bone formation in the calcified aortic valves;[6] the main characteristic of this valvular pathology is an increase in its prevalence with age (see Chapters 3 and 4). In addition to aortic stenosis, mitral regurgitation is increasingly common in the elderly due to age-related degenerative changes of the valve leaflets or due to secondary mitral regurgitation with ischemic or myocardial disease.[7] Furthermore, given the increase in life expectancy, the burden of valvular disease in the elderly is expected to rise.

Over the past decade, valvular procedures have increased not only in number (accounting now for more than 20% of all cardiac surgeries) but also in complexity. A third of patients referred for the management of valvular disease have previously undergone open heart surgery.[5]

Comorbidities and frailty in the elderly significantly raise surgical morbidity and mortality,[8] so alternatives to surgery have been developed to provide less invasive forms of therapy in this aging population. Guidelines from Europe[9] and the United States[10] for the management of valvular heart disease now include recommendations for transcatheter valve procedures. The high level of interest in transcatheter valve procedures is apparent from the number of new publications and reviews that address this topic.[11,12]

Tables 16-1 and 16-2 summarize the established mechanical interventions used in advanced valvular heart disease.

TABLE 16-1   Established Mechanical Interventions in Valvular Heart Disease

LESION	VALVE REPLACEMENT	VALVE REPAIR	PERCUTANEOUS INTERVENTION
Aortic stenosis	Yes +++	Yes +	Yes ++
Aortic regurgitation	Yes +++	Yes +	No
Bicuspid aortic valve	Yes +++	Yes ++	No
Mitral stenosis	Yes ++	Yes +	Yes +++
Degenerative mitral regurgitation	Yes ++	Yes +++	Yes ++
Functional mitral regurgitation	Yes +++	Yes +++	Yes ++
Pulmonic stenosis	Yes +++	Yes +++	Yes +++
Pulmonic regurgitation	Yes +++	Yes +++	Yes ++
Tricuspid stenosis	Yes +++	Yes ++	Yes ++
Tricuspid regurgitation	Yes ++	Yes +++	No
Multiple valve disease	Yes +++	Yes ++	No
Prosthetic stenosis	Yes +++	No	Yes +
Prosthetic regurgitation	Yes +++	No	Yes +
Paraprosthetic leak	Yes ++	Yes ++	Yes +++
Infective endocarditis	Yes +++	Yes ++	No

Yes, Used; *No,* not used; +++, favored use; ++, common use; +, occasional use.

TABLE 16-2   Transcatheter Valve Procedures

TRANSCATHETER VALVE PROCEDURES	VALVE DISEASE
Balloon valvuloplasty	Aortic stenosis Mitral stenosis Pulmonic stenosis Tricuspid stenosis Bioprosthesis stenosis
Transcatheter valve implantation	Aortic stenosis Pulmonic stenosis Mitral valve disease (experimental) Tricuspid valve disease (experimental)
Transcatheter transapical valve implantation	Aortic stenosis

Leaflet repair:
    MitraClip (Abbott Laboratories, Abbott Park, Illinois)
    Mobius (Edwards Lifesciences Corporation, Irvine, California)
	Mitral regurgitation

Coronary sinus annuloplasty: experimental
    Monarch Annuloplasty System (Edwards Lifesciences, Irvine, California)
    CARILLON Mitral Control System (Cardiac Dimensions, Inc., Kirkland, Washington)
    PTMA (Viacor, Wilmington, Massachussetts)
	Mitral regurgitation

Direct annuloplasty: experimental
    QuantumCor (QuantumCor, Inc., Lake Forest, California)
    Accucinch (Guided Delivery Systems, Inc., Santa Clara, California)
    Percutaneous restrictive ring annuloplasty-Cardioband (Valtech Cardio Ltd., Tel Aviv, Israel)
	Mitral regurgitation

Ventricular remodelling (experimental): iCoapsys Repair System (Myocor, Inc., Maple Grove, Minnesota)	Mitral regurgitation
Percutaneous transcatheter repair of paravalvular regurgitation	Paraprosthetic leak
Valve-in-valve implantation	Prosthetic valve dysfunction

TABLE 16-3   Value of Imaging Modalities in Valvular Heart Disease Interventions

	PREPROCEDURE PLANNING	INTRAPROCEDURE GUIDANCE	ASSESSMENT OF RESULTS	LONG-TERM FOLLOW-UP
Fluoroscopy and angiography	0	+++	+++	0
Computed tomography	+++	0	0	++
Cardiac magnetic resonance	+	0	0	+
Intracardiac echocardiography	0	+	++	0
Transthoracic echocardiography	+++	+	+	+++
Transesophageal echocardiography	++	+++	+++	+++

0, No value; +, little value; ++, moderate value; +++, best value.

TABLE 16-4   Role and Relative Value of Different Cardiac Imaging Modalities on Common Transcatheter Valve Procedures

VALVULAR INTERVENTION	FLUOROSCOPY ANGIOGRAPHY	COMPUTED TOMOGRAPHY	MAGNETIC RESONANCE	ICE	TTE	TEE
Aortic balloon valvuloplasty	++++	++++	+	+	+++	++
Transcatheter aortic valve implantation	++++	++++	+	++	+++	+++
Balloon mitral valvotomy	++++	+	+	++	+++	++++
Edge-to-edge transcatheter mitral valve repair	+++	+	+	+	+++	++++
Pulmonic valve balloon valvuloplasty	++++	+++	+++	++	++++	++
Transcatheter pulmonic valve replacement	++++	+++	+++	++	+++	++
Transcatheter periprosthetic leak repair	+++	++++		++	++	++++

+, Little value, ++, mild value; +++, moderate value; ++++, most value.
ICE, intracardiac echocadiography; TEE, transesophageal echocardiography; TTE, transthoracic echocardiography.

Approaches to Imaging Guidance

The interventional field has moved forward not only in the invention of new devices but also because of breakthroughs, refinements, and implementation of imaging guidance that enable the interventionalist to perform these new treatments.[13]

Cardiovascular imaging, including fluoroscopy and angiography, computed tomography (CT), cardiac magnetic resonance (CMR) imaging, and echocardiography, have played a central role in the development of transcatheter valve procedures.[14] Periprocedural imaging for patient selection and procedural planning and guidance are critical for the success of a structural heart disease program and constitute one of the cornerstones for the new paradigm in the management of valvular heart disease by a multidisciplinary heart team.[15,16]

Fluoroscopy, angiography, and two-dimensional echocardiography maintain a central role in procedural guidance. Novel three-dimensional (3D) imaging modalities are gaining importance; these include CT, CMR, 3D echocardiography, and rotational angiography.[17,18]

The choice of imaging guidance modality is based on specific differences between imaging systems as well as other variables, such as cost, clinical scenario, operator expertise, and complexity of procedure.[19]

The roles and relative values of different cardiac imaging modalities in common transcatheter valve procedures are outlined on Tables 16-3 And 16-4.

Fluoroscopy and Angiography

Fluoroscopy and cineangiography have traditionally been used in the catheterization laboratory to guide coronary interventional procedures; today they are the central guidance tools for noncoronary interventions.[14] Because only radiopaque objects are visible with these modalities, radiopaque dye has to be injected to visualize chambers, great vessels, and outlines of valves; nevertheless, fluoroscopy is an integral part of all cardiac catheterization laboratories, and all of the catheters and devices are radiopaque, having been engineered for their use and deployment in the catheterization laboratory.

The major advantages of image guidance with fluoroscopy and cineangiography are well exemplified in patients undergoing transcatheter aortic valve replacement, as illustrated in Figure 16-1. The major disadvantages of fluoroscopy and cineangiography include radiation exposure, lack of visualization of the myocardium and valvular tissue, and the need to inject radiopaque and potentially nephrotoxic contrast agents.

New radiography-based imaging techniques under development, referred to as three-dimensional rotational angiography and C-arm CT, hold great promise for improving current device implantation and the understanding of cardiovascular anatomy. A variety of anatomic targets, from the aortic root and pulmonary arteries (for percutaneous aortic and pulmonic valve implantation) to general visualization and assessment of the whole heart, are being explored[20,21] (Figure 16-2A). Fluoroscopy has been fused to 3D transesophageal echocardiography (TEE), providing simultaneous imaging with both techniques and allowing for similar anatomic perspective (Figure 16-2B).

Multidetector Computed Tomography

Multidetector CT (MDCT) provides 3D volumetric data sets, allowing multiplane reconstructions of the heart and great vessels. It plays an important role in preprocedural screening for and planning of several transcatheter valve interventions, thereby improving procedural outcomes and minimizing procedure-related

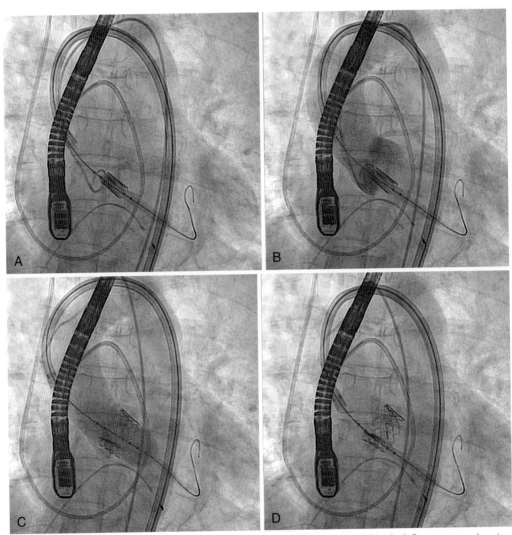

FIGURE 16-1 **Fluoroscopy and angiography in guidance of transcatheter aortic valve implantation.** Both fluoroscopy and angiography are extensively used during this procedure. The gantry position is critically important to provide a view for valve deployment. **A** shows such a view, in which the undeployed stent-valve is perpendicular to a line drawn at the base of all three aortic sinuses. **B,** Aortography to document that the undeployed valve is approximately 50/50 below and above the valve plane. **C,** Balloon inflation with stent expansion and deployment of a SAPIEN valve (Edwards Lifesciences Corporation, Irvine, California). **D,** Immediately after deployment, a well-expanded stent-valve with the calcified aortic cusps pushed to the side can be seen.

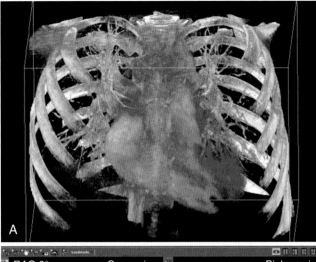

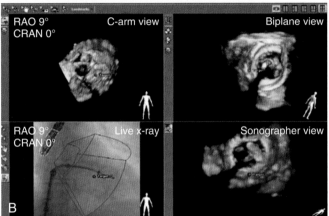

FIGURE 16-2 **Next-generation image guidance systems for valvular interventions.** Innovations in image guidance of valvular heart disease interventions are developing new technologies that are integrated in the procedure room. **A,** A three-dimensional (3D) reconstruction from a rotational angiographic acquisition with the flat x-ray detector making a 180-degree arc around the patient. Like a computed tomography scan, it can be segmented to show chambers and valves and can be used for fluoroscopic registration with image overlay. **B,** The combination of 3D transesophageal echocardiographic imaging with fluoroscopy is being used here to guide a MitraClip implantation (Abbott Laboratories, Abbott Park, Illinois). The radiographic and 3D ultrasound images are registered to provide a similar perspective.

complications.[22,23] In patients being considered for percutaneous transcatheter aortic valve implantation (TAVI), MDCT can provide detailed information on the shape and size of the aortic annulus and the relation between the annulus and the ostia of the coronary arteries[24-26] (Figures 16-3 and 16-4).

Aortic valve calcification as assessed by MDCT has been shown to be well correlated to aortic valve area (AVA) and may be a useful adjunct for the evaluation of the severity of aortic stenosis severity, especially in difficult cases such as patients with low ejection fraction (EF).[27]

As described later, MDCT enables an accurate sizing of the aortic valve annulus and constitutes a valuable imaging tool to evaluate prosthesis location and deployment for TAVI. MDCT also facilitates the understanding of the underlying mechanisms of postprocedural aortic regurgitation.[28] In addition, preprocedural MDCT can be used to predict optimal angiographic deployment projections for implantation of transcatheter valves.[29]

In patients being considered for TAVI, MDCT is used as the "gold standard" for determining of the appropriateness of

the peripheral vasculature for percutaneous femoral access (Figure 16-5).

MDCT is being used in both aortic and mitral transcatheter-based interventions. It provides a comprehensive anatomic assessment of the aortic valve complex and, to a lesser degree, of the mitral valve apparatus, helping in selection of the most appropriate procedural approach, decreasing complications, and improving outcomes.

Cardiac Magnetic Resonance

Cardiac magnetic resonance (CMR) is a comprehensive noninvasive tool capable of evaluating all aspects of valvular heart disease. Its main advantages include direct quantification of regurgitant lesions, accurate assessment of ventricular size mass and function, and visualization of myocardial scar.[30] A system for x-ray fused with magnetic resonance imaging, has been developed and validated; this will be of value to guide catheter procedures with high spatial precision.[31] Interventional magnetic resonance imaging to guide procedures is evolving slowly, however, because it requires considerable capital investment and special compatible instruments.[14] Patients are imaged in the CMR imaging suite and then transported to fluoroscopic laboratories capable of some type of image fusion.

CMR has been used to guide transcatheter valve implantation in the aortic valve position in experimental animals. CMR enables assessment of cardiovascular anatomy and function. During and after implantation, the position and function of the prosthetic valve is easy to determine. In addition, CMR provides immediate post-intervention physiologic parameters of cardiac function and proximal coronary artery perfusion.[32]

Use of CMR to assess the aortic valve area and aortic root dimensions has been compared with a multimodality imaging approach including Doppler ultrasonography, 2-dimensional (2D) transthoracic echocardiography (TTE), 3D TTE and TEE, and catheterization. CMR and TEE provided similar assessments of the aortic valve annulus dimensions, especially at the limits of the TAVI range.[33]

Intracardiac Echocardiography

Intracardiac echocardiography (ICE) has been used for septal defect closure but also may be used for some valvular interventions.[34-39] As seen in Figure 16-6, all four cardiac valves can be assessed with ICE, and the clarity of the structures is as good as and sometimes better than that with TEE. Yet because of the 2D aspect of ICE images, it is generally not used for interventional treatments such as MitraClip insertion (Abbott Laboratories, Abbott Park, Illinois) and TAVI. The tip of the ICE catheter must be placed in a location to allow accurate Doppler assessment of valvular lesions, both stenotic and regurgitant. ICE is expected to improve and to be better integrated into the procedure room. Unlike with TEE there is no potential compromise of the airway or need for general anesthesia for long interventions with ICE. Currently ICE can be quite useful for performing transseptal puncture, which is often needed for mitral interventions such as balloon valvuloplasty and MitraClip therapy. On the other hand, the 2D format of ICE images may make guiding transseptal puncture to a certain location on the septum difficult. Figure 16-7 shows how ICE complements fluoroscopy for standard transseptal puncture.

Transthoracic and Transesophageal Echocardiography

Echocardiography is widely recognized as the preferred imaging tool for the evaluation and management of patients with stenotic,[40] regurgitant,[41] and prosthetic valves.[42] The development

Short axis   Long axis   3D Vol

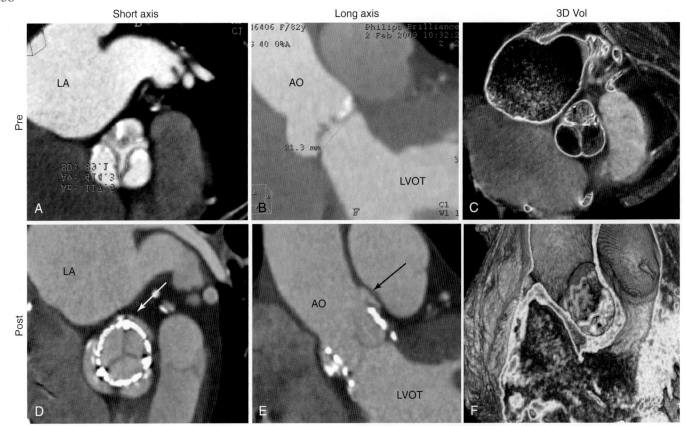

FIGURE 16-3 **Cardiac computed tomography before and after transcatheter aortic valve implantation.** CT images illustrating short- and long-axis views and three-dimensional (3D) volumetric reconstructions before (**A** to **C**)and after (**D** to **F**) transcatheter aortic valve implantation. In short-axis views, **A** illustrates the traced aortic valve area, and **D** the deployed valve *(arrow)*. In long-axis views, **B** shows the aortic annular dimension, and **E** the deployed prosthesis in relation to the left main coronary artery *(arrow)*. The 3D volumetric reconstructions panel C illustrate the stenotic aortic valve seen in short axis **(C)** and the stent of the deployed valve **(F)**. *AO,* Aorta; *LA,* left atrium; *LVOT,* left ventricular outflow tract. *(Images courtesy Dr. Robert Quaife, University of Colorado Denver.)*

of real-time 3D echocardiography has resulted in improved spatial resolution on images and enhanced visualization of the morphologic features of the cardiac valves.[43,44] Because of its universal availability, portability, and capacity to provide high-quality, reliable physiologic and morphologic information, echocardiography has been embraced with enthusiasm in the catheterization laboratory to provide guidance for transcatheter interventions for structural heart disease.[45-50]

In addition to helping with patient selection, procedure guidance, and prevention and recognition of procedure complications, echocardiography can enable a clearer understanding of the hemodynamic and physiologic consequences of the devices being deployed.[51]

Both transthoracic and transesophageal echocardiography play a role in the management of patients undergoing transcatheter valve interventions, and all modalities of ultrasound, including 2D, 3D, and Doppler techniques, are being used in interventional suites and in the hybrid operating rooms dealing with valvular heart disease transcatheter interventions. Figure 16-8 illustrates the use of 3D TEE for TAVI guidance.

Transcatheter Treatment of Valve Disease

Because of the aging of the population, with the consequent greater complexity of and higher surgical risk of potential candidates, surgical valve replacement and valve repair, traditionally the only viable options to treat advanced valvular heart disease, are being supplemented by newly developed transcatheter valve procedures[52-54] (see Tables 16-1 and 16-2).

Cardiac imaging has played an important role in the development and implementation of these new procedures; in the next

section we discuss the most common transcatheter valve procedures with emphasis on the central role cardiac imaging plays in their clinical use.

Transcatheter Balloon Valve Procedures

Balloon Aortic Valvuloplasty

Percutaneous balloon aortic valvuloplasty was first described by Cribier et al[55] in 1986. The procedure was carried out in three elderly patients with acquired severe aortic stenosis. Transvalvular systolic pressure gradient was considerably decreased at the end of the procedures, during which there were no complications. Cardiac imaging, in the form angiography and echocardiography, confirmed increased valve opening. The initial enthusiasm for this technique[56-62] was tempered by the recognition that the hemodynamic and clinical improvement was short lived. During follow-up, Doppler echocardiographic results demonstrated a trend toward the preprocedural severity of the aortic stenosis. Progression of restenosis assessed by Doppler echocardiography was accelerated in the patients who subsequently died or underwent repeat balloon valvuloplasty or aortic valve replacement (AVR).[63] Restenosis after balloon aortic valvuloplasty is common, occurring in as many as 50% or more of patients during the first year; histologic changes in restenosed valves differ from those seen in calcific aortic stenosis, with granulation tissue, fibrosis, and ossification being present.[64] An encouraging factor was the demonstration that AVR could be performed with a low mortality rate, excellent palliation of symptoms, and prolongation of survival in selected high-risk patients with a history of previous balloon aortic valvuloplasty.[65] One center has reported that repeat

LVOT₁   Aortic valve   LM orifice

LVOT₂   LVOT   RCA orifice

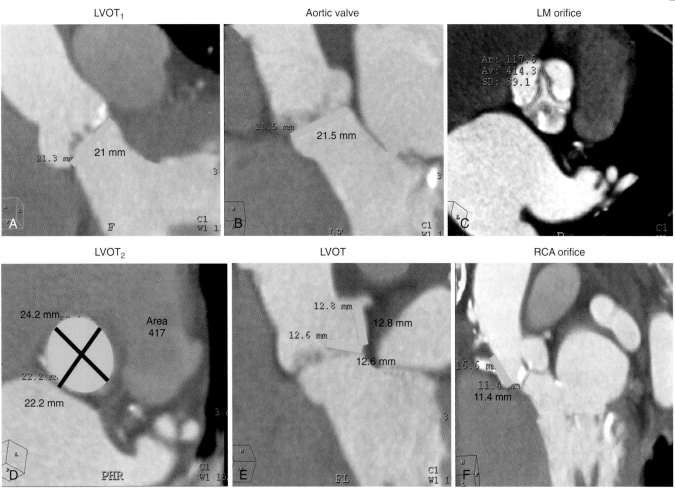

FIGURE 16-4   Cardiac computed tomography key measurements for transcatheter aortic valve implantation. A and **B** illustrate the two orthogonal measurements of the aortic annulus that are used for prosthesis sizing (LVOT₁ and LVOT₂). In **A,** the *blue bar* corresponds to a annular dimension of 21 mm; in **B,** the annular dimension is 21.5 mm. **C,** The aortic valve area measured in short axis. **D,** The area at the level of the aortic annulus is depicted as a *blue ellipse.* The maximal and minimal orthogonal diameters at this level are also noted (*black lines*). **E,** *Blue bars* represent the distance from the aortic valve plane to the orifice of the left main trunk, 12.8 mm, and the left coronary leaflet length, 12.6 mm. **F,** The distance from the valve to the right coronary ostium (RCA) is measured at 11.4 mm (*blue bar*). *(Images courtesy Dr Robert Quaife, University of Colorado Denver.)*

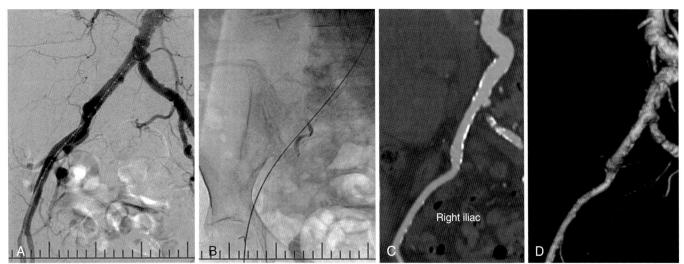

FIGURE 16-5   Digital angiography and computed tomography angiography for assessment of vascular access before transcatheter aortic valve implantation. This procedure involves large delivery catheters and requires assessment of potential vascular access routes. Different modalities are used, including digital angiography **(A),** fluoroscopy with rigid guide wire to assess whether straightening of the vessel is needed **(B),** CT angiography with multiplanar reformatting to allow coaxial assessment of vessel diameter **(C),** and CT angiography three-dimensional reconstruction to assess tortuosity **(D).**

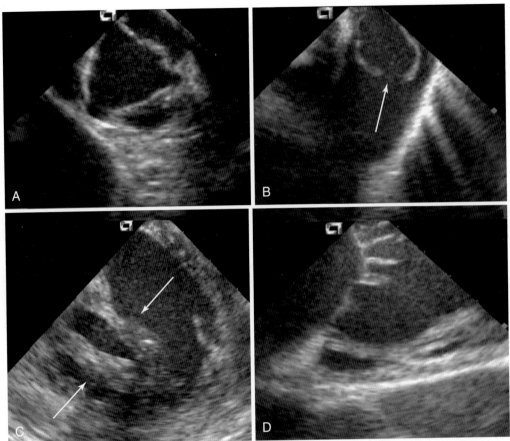

FIGURE 16-6 Visualization of all valves on intracardiac echocardiography (ICE). ICE provides detailed visual assessment of all valves, including valve leaflets and subvalvular apparatus. **A,** Normal aortic valve. **B,** Congenital pulmonic valve stenosis with doming (*arrow*). **C,** Rheumatic mitral stenosis with extensive chordae thickening and shortening (*arrows*). **D,** Normal tricuspid valve. Catheter positions in **A** through **C** were various locations within the right ventricle; in **D,** catheter was in the right atrium.

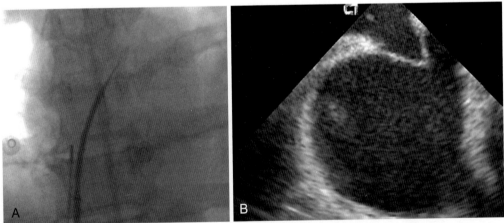

FIGURE 16-7 Imaging guidance of transseptal puncture with intracardiac echocardiography (ICE). The safety and precision of transseptal catheterization have been greatly improved by the use of ultrasound, including ICE. **A** shows a fluoroscopic image of the transseptal needle extending past the tip of the dilator of the transseptal sheath. **B** shows the corresponding ICE image that reveals the tenting of the septum but no crossing of the needle into the left atrium. With this knowledge from imaging, the operator can safely push with more force to complete the puncture.

balloon valvuloplasty is a viable treatment strategy in patients who have severe calcific aortic stenosis and are not candidates for surgery, because it provides a median survival rate of approximately 3 years and maintains clinical improvement,[66] although this is not the experience at most centers.

Aortic balloon valvuloplasty has enjoyed a revival thanks to the interest in and development of TAVI. As discussed later, balloon valvuloplasty is used during TAVI to facilitate the passage of the crimped aortic valve through the narrow aortic valve orifice. Aortic balloon valvuloplasty can also be used to improve hemodynamics in some patients who are not surgical candidates and have severe AS, and a proportion of these patients improve to a point at which AVR can be performed. Use of balloon valvuloplasty as a bridge to TAVI will provide further options to high-risk patients who cannot be "bridged" to conventional AVR.[67-70]

The key uses of imaging for aortic balloon valvuloplasty are summarized on Table 16-5.

Volume rendition | Multiplane reconstruction

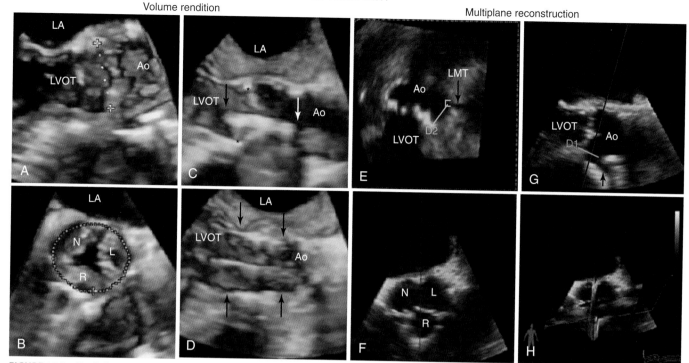

FIGURE 16-8 **Real-time three-dimensional transesophageal echocardiography guidance for transcatheter aortic valve implantation. A** to **D,** The use of volume rendition mode three-dimensional (3D) transesophageal echocardiography guidance of the implantation procedure. **A,** The *dotted line* represents a 3D "measurement on glass" of the aortic annulus. **B,** The measurement on glass of the circumference of the aortic annulus **C,** The crimped prosthesis (*arrows*) is being centered to the aortic annulus (*asterisks*). **D,** The deployed prosthesis is delineated by the *arrows*. **E** to **H,** The multiplane reconstruction mode being used in this case to delineate the distance from the left main trunk (LMT, *black arrow*) to the aortic leaflets. **E,** The *green line* marks the distance (D$_2$) from the base of the left coronary cusp to the LMT. In **G,** the *line* (D$_1$) marks the same distance in an orthogonal plane. **F** illustrates the 3D short-axis view of the aortic valve depicting the right (R), left (L), and noncoronary (N) cusps. **H** shows the three orthogonal planes used to obtain these views. *Ao,* Aorta; *LA,* left atrium; *LVOT,* left ventricular outflow tract.

Balloon Mitral Valvotomy

In 1984 Inoue et al[71] reported a new balloon catheter technique that allows mitral commissurotomy without thoracotomy. The procedure was successful in five of the six patients with mitral stenosis so treated. Two-dimensional echocardiography showed a marked to moderate degree of dilation of the mitral orifice in each patient. Balloon mitral valvotomy (BMV) was rapidly accepted, refined, and expanded as an effective nonsurgical procedure to treat patients with mitral stenosis, including those with pliable valves, those with previous commissurotomy, and even those with mitral calcification.[72]

In patients with rheumatic mitral stenosis, transcatheter mitral valve balloon valvotomy has virtually replaced surgery as the preferred method to improve mitral valve area.[73-77]

The central role of echocardiography in patient selection for BMV was initially described by Wilkins et al.[78] The appearance of the mitral valve on the predilation echocardiogram was scored for leaflet mobility, leaflet thickening, subvalvular thickening, and calcification. A high score, indicating advanced leaflet deformity, on predilation imaging had a suboptimal outcome, whereas a low score (a mobile valve with limited thickening) was associated with an optimal outcome. In addition, the presence of commissural calcium has been found to be a strong predictor of outcome after percutaneous mitral balloon valvotomy. Patients with evidence of calcium in a commissure have a lower survival rate and a higher rate of later mitral valve replacement.[79]

BMV can be performed with fluoroscopic guidance alone with the self-centering Inoue balloon catheter (Figure 16-9); however, even an experienced operator can be misled by radiographic tissue landmarks. The addition of real-time TEE during BMV facilitates the success and safety of this procedure by guiding the transseptal puncture and assisting with navigation of the dilating

balloon catheters across the stenotic mitral valve.[80] In addition to guiding the manipulation of catheters, real-time TEE is useful for confirming the efficacy of valvotomy and for detecting and managing complications. Severe mitral regurgitation is a relatively infrequent complication of Inoue balloon valvotomy; it results from disruption of valve integrity (Figure 16-10), including chordal rupture and leaflet tearing.[81] TEE facilitates careful balloon positioning so as to avoid chordal rupture. The additional value of 3D echocardiography in patients with mitral valve stenosis undergoing balloon valvuloplasty is now well recognized.[82,83] The 3D TEE method enables a better description of the mitral valvular anatomy, especially after BMV.[84]

The key uses of imaging for BMV are summarized in Table 16-6 and Figure 16-11.

Pulmonic Valve Balloon Valvuloplasty

Since the initial 1982 description by Pepine et al[85] of successful percutaneous balloon valvuloplasty for pulmonic valve stenosis in the adult, this procedure has essentially superseded surgical pulmonic valve replacement as the treatment of choice for this condition.[86]

Mullins et al[87] evaluated the efficacy, technique, and follow-up results for balloon dilation angioplasty in 63 patients with valvular pulmonic stenosis (ages 3 months to 76 years). The pressure gradient across the pulmonic valve was determined with right ventricular and main pulmonary artery catheters and simultaneously by continuous-wave Doppler echocardiography. There was excellent linear correlation between the simultaneous catheter pressure gradient and the pressure gradient estimated by Doppler echocardiography. These data confirmed that balloon dilation angioplasty for valvular pulmonic stenosis is safe and effective. Patients with congenital pulmonic stenosis who present in late

TABLE 16-5 Aortic Balloon Valvuloplasty

TASK	IMAGING
Patient Selection	
Severe calcific aortic stenosis	Echocardiography: aortic valve area (AVA) < 1 cm², mean gradient 40 mm Hg, peak velocity 4 m/sec
Procedural Guidance	
Crossing the aortic valve	Fluoroscopy
Balloon positioning and inflation	Fluoroscopy and angiography Two-dimensional (2D) and 3D echocardiography
Evaluation of Results	
Increase aortic valve area	Echocardiography: improved AVA by planimetry or continuity equation
Fracture calcium deposits	Echocardiography: improved leaflet mobility
Late restenosis (several months)	Echocardiography: serial AVA measurements
Early restenosis	Fluoroscopy: insufficient balloon inflation
Evaluation of Potential Complications	
Cardiac perforation and tamponade	2D echocardiography and Doppler hemodynamics
Leaflet damage resulting in aortic regurgitation	2D and 3D echocardiography, color Doppler, aortography
Left ventricular failure and low cardiac output	2D and 3D echocardiography

TABLE 16-6 Mitral Balloon Valvotomy

TASK	IMAGING
Patient Selection	
Severe mitral stenosis	Mitral valve area (MVA) <1cm² Mean gradient >10 mm Hg Pulmonic pressure >50 mm Hg
Suitable valve	• Valve score: leaflet mobility, leaflet thickening, subvalvar thickening, and leaflet calcification • Absence of significant mitral regurgitation • Absence of left atrial thrombus • Absence of commissural calcium
Procedural Guidance	
Septal puncture catheter navigation	Fluoroscopy Two-dimensional (2D) and 3D transesophageal echocardiography (TEE)
Balloon positioning and inflation	2D and 3D TEE
Evaluation of Results	
Increased mitral valve area	2D and 3D echocardiography of MVA
Decreased gradient	Doppler mean gradient
Commissural splitting	2D and 3D echocardiography
Evaluation of Potential Complications	
Cardiac perforation and tamponade	2D echocardiography and Doppler hemodynamics
Severe mitral regurgitation	Color Doppler
Embolism	2D 3D echocardiography
Large interatrial shunt	Color Doppler

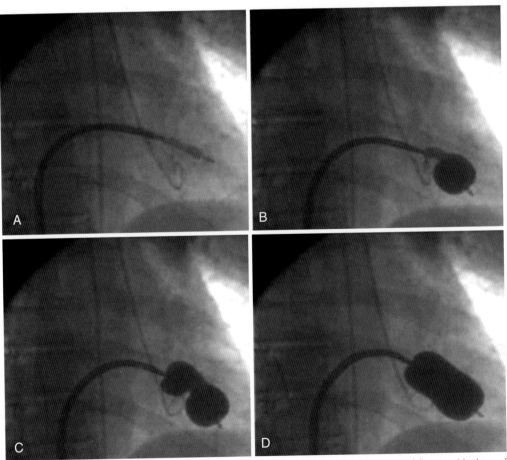

FIGURE 16-9 **Fluoroscopic Guidance of balloon mitral valvotomy.** Fluoroscopy can be the main imaging modality to guide the performance of the procedure using the Inoue balloon catheter. **A,** Crossing of the catheter from the left atrium into the left ventricle is often straightforward. **B,** Inflation of the balloon first occurs in the distal balloon, allowing the catheter to be pulled back to engage the valve orifice. **C,** Further inflation enlarges the proximal part of the balloon, which "locks" the mitral valve orifice, and the stenotic orifice accentuates a "dog-balloon" appearance. **D,** The final full inflation straightens the midportion of the balloon, providing the force to split the fused commissures.

LA view	LV view	Color doppler

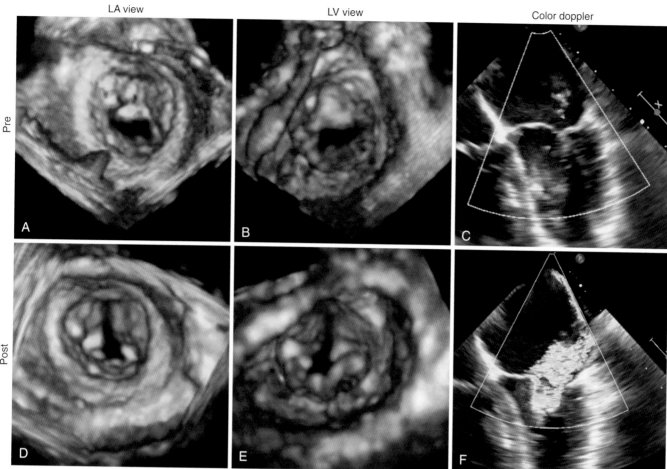

FIGURE 16-10 Complication during balloon mitral valvotomy. Transesophageal echocardiographic images in a patient with mitral stenosis (**A** and **B**) who underwent BMV and in whom the balloon dilation caused anterior mitral leaflet rupture. **D** and **E,** A cleft has occurred along the middle of the anterior leaflet. Trace mitral regurgitation seen before the procedure (**C**) changed to severe mitral regurgitation after balloon dilation (**F**).

PRE	POST	During

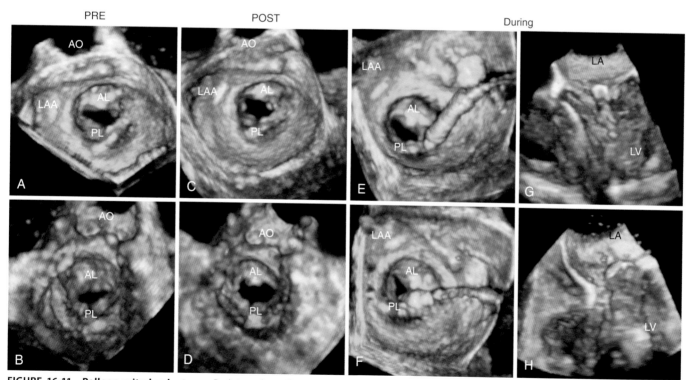

FIGURE 16-11 Balloon mitral valvotomy. Real-time three-dimensional transesophageal echocardiographic images obtained before, during, and after balloon mitral valvotomy in a patient with mitral stenosis. **A** and **B** illustrate the stenotic mitral orifice as seen from the left atrium (**A**) and from the left ventricle (**B**) immediately prior to the procedure. **C** and **D,** obtained immediately after the procedure, show the commissure splitting and the larger mitral valve orifice. **E** to **H,** obtained during the procedure, illustrate the catheter approximating the narrow mitral orifice (**E**), the catheter being advanced through the mitral orifice (**F**), the catheter being aligned with the long axis of the left ventricle (LV) (**G**), and the balloon after inflation (**H**). *AL,* anterior leaflet; *AO,* aorta; *LA,* left atrium; *LAA,* left atrial appendix; *PL,* posterior leaflet.

adolescence or adult life can now be treated with percutaneous balloon valvuloplasty with excellent short-term and long-term results that are similar to those in young children.[88]

TTE is the imaging modality of choice in the diagnosis, evaluation, and follow-up of patients with pulmonic stenosis (PS). Valvular PS is usually diagnosed by 2D imaging, and Doppler echocardiography allows for the quantification of severity of the valvular lesion.[88] CT and CMR provide complementary anatomic characterization of the pulmonic annulus and valve prior to percutaneous balloon valvuloplasty.

Imaging guidance during pulmonic balloon valvuloplasty usually entails the use of fluoroscopy and cineangiography. Echocardiography can be of assistance in the detection and management of the rare complications from pulmonic balloon valvuloplasty, such as valve and annulus disruption, injury to the pulmonary artery, and tricuspid valve injury.

Bioprosthetic Valve Balloon Valvuloplasty

Dejam et al[89] reported on a patient with prosthetic aortic valve stenosis who was treated with valvuloplasty using intracardiac and fluoroscopic guidance and in whom recurrence was treated with repeat valvuloplasty with promising intermediate-term outcome. Yunoki et al[90] reported the successful use of percutaneous transcatheter balloon valvuloplasty in a patient with bioprosthetic tricuspid valve stenosis. However, these are isolated reports and the effectiveness of this approach is yet to be proven in a large number of patients.[91] Fluoroscopy and sometimes TEE are the imaging tools favored for guidance in these procedures.

Transcatheter Valve Implantation

Although the incidence of severe mitral or aortic valve disease in the elderly is relatively high, many patients who are potential candidates for valve repair or replacement are undiagnosed, are not referred for surgery, or are too sick or unwilling to undergo the required surgery. In addition, the management of patients with previous surgery for congenital heart disease with postoperative right ventricular (RV) outflow tract dysfunction is difficult and complex. As a response, transcatheter heart valves for the aortic, pulmonic, and mitral positions have been developed and are in clinical use in many countries or in clinical trials throughout the United States.[92,93]

Transcatheter Aortic Valve Implantation

In 2002, Cribier et al[94] described the first human implantation of a transcatheter aortic valve bioprosthesis; it was performed in a 57-year-old man with calcific aortic stenosis, cardiogenic shock, subacute leg ischemia, and other associated noncardiac diseases. Since then there has been an explosion of interest in the percutaneous deployment of aortic valve prostheses; standardized end point definitions for TAVI clinical trials have been published,[95] and large clinical trials have demonstrated its efficacy.[96-98] In addition transfemoral and transapical TAVI approaches have been reported.[99-103]

A central theme in the successful clinical implementation of transcatheter valve procedures has been the development of "heart teams" composed of multiple cardiovascular specialists, including cardiac imagers, interventionalists, cardiac anesthesiologists, cardiovascular surgeons, and support personnel.

In this section we describe the most important aspects of TAVI cardiovascular imaging for patient evaluation and selection, prosthetic choice and sizing, procedural guidance, recognition and management of complications, and evaluation of results (Table 16-7; Figures 16-12 and 16-13).

One of the initial steps in identification of candidates for TAVI is the evaluation of vascular access.[104] This is critical because the delivery catheters are rather large and require a target artery of acceptable size. Patients without adequate peripheral arteries

TABLE 16-7	Transcatheter Aortic Valve Implantation: SAPIEN* Valve—Transarterial Retrograde Approach	
TASK	**IMAGING**
Patient Selection	
Severe aortic stenosis	Echocardiography: aortic valve area ≤0.8 cm², mean gradient ≥40 mm Hg, peak aortic valve velocity ≥4 m/sec
Aortic annulus size	TTE, TEE, CT: >17 mm and <26 mm
Femoral artery size	CT angiography: >7 mm
Valve Size Selection	• Echocardiography: aortic annulus size • CT: aortic annulus size and annulus-to-LMT distance • CT angiography and descending aortography: femoral artery size
Procedural Guidance	
Crossing the aortic valve	Fluoroscopy, 2D and 3D echocardiography
Balloon valvuloplasty	Fluoroscopy, angiography, 2D and 3D echocardiography
Valve implantation	• CT 3D reconstruction: to select best fluoroscopy plane • Aortography: for plane selection • Fluoroscopy: placement of prosthesis at mid valve level • TEE: placement of prosthesis at mid valve level
Recognition of Complications	• Right or left ventricular perforation: echocardiographic effusion-tamponade • Prosthesis misplacement/embolization: fluoroscopy, TEE • Aortic regurgitation: TEE color Doppler, aortography • Annular dissection: TEE, aortography • Arterial perforation: descending aortography • LMT obstruction: coronary arteriography, TEE • Aortic dissection: TEE • Mitral regurgitation from prosthesis impingement: TEE • Thrombus formation: TEE
Evaluation of Results	• Correct valve placement and stability: fluoroscopy, TEE • Origin and severity of aortic regurgitation: TEE, color Doppler, aortography • Transvalvular gradients: TEE, spectral Doppler

2D, Two-dimensional; *CT*, computed tomography; *Doppler*, Doppler echocardiography; *LMT*, left main trunk; *TEE*, transesophageal echocardiography; *TTE*, transthoracic echocardiography.
*Edwards Lifesciences Corporation, Irvine, California.

may be candidates for the transapical approach. Arteriography and CT angiography are now routinely used for this purpose, as illustrated in Figure 16-5.

The inclusion criteria for TAVI require echocardiographic demonstration of severe calcific trileaflet aortic stenosis with a valve area of less than 0.8 cm², a mean transvalvular gradient of at least 40 mm Hg, and a peak transaortic velocity of 4 m/sec or more (see Chapter 15).[96] Exclusion criteria, which are mainly evaluated by echocardiography, include a bicuspid or noncalcified aortic valve, a left ventricular ejection fraction of less than 20%, an aortic annulus diameter of less than 18 mm or more than 25 mm, and severe (>3+) mitral or aortic regurgitation.[96] Patients with left ventricular dysfunction who are thought to have a low-gradient, (mean aortic valve gradient <40 mm Hg) severe aortic stenosis may undergo dobutamine stress echocardiography; if the mean transaortic gradient becomes higher than 40 mm Hg with dobutamine, they may be considered for TAVI.

At this time there is only a very limited choice of valve sizes for TAVI, so determination of the correct replacement valve requires

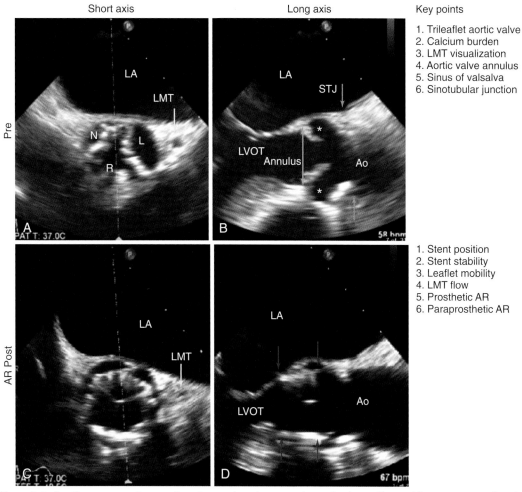

Short axis | Long axis | Key points

Key points
1. Trileaflet aortic valve
2. Calcium burden
3. LMT visualization
4. Aortic valve annulus
5. Sinus of valsalva
6. Sinotubular junction

1. Stent position
2. Stent stability
3. Leaflet mobility
4. LMT flow
5. Prosthetic AR
6. Paraprosthetic AR

FIGURE 16-12 **Key points for the preprocedure and postprocedure transesophageal echocardiographic assessment of patients undergoing transcatheter aortic valve implantation.** The key points to consider during the preprocedure evaluation include demonstration of the presence of three aortic leaflets as seen in **A;** and evaluation of the calcium burden (in this case small), visualization of the left main trunk (LMT), and characterization and sizing of the aortic annulus (*blue arrow*), sinus of Valsalva (*asterisks*), and sinotubular junction (STJ, *orange arrows*), as illustrated in **B. C** and **D,** Immediately after implantation, the key points to consider include stent position and stability (*red arrows*), proper leaflet motility, normal LMT flow, and presence and severity of aortic regurgitation. *Ao,* Aorta; *L,* left coronary cusp; *LA,* left atrium; *LVOT,* left ventricular outflow tract; *N,* noncoronary cusp; *R,* right coronary cusp.

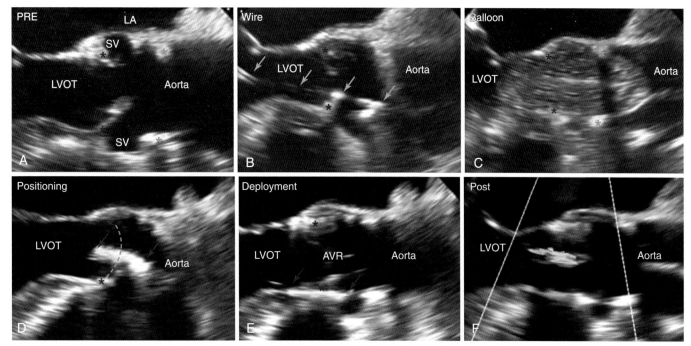

FIGURE 16-13 **Transesophageal echocardiographic guidance for transcatheter aortic valve implantation.** Imaging guidance by TEE for the implantation procedure includes **A,** preprocedural evaluation of the aortic annular dimension (*red asterisks*), sinus of Valsalva (SV), and sinotubular junction (*orange asterisks*). In images obtained during the procedure, **B** depicts the guide wire (*blue arrows*) being advanced through the stenotic aortic valve; **C** shows the the balloon inflated, extending from the left ventricular outflow tract (LVOT) to the aorta; **D** shows the crimped prosthesis (*red arrows*) being positioned in the center of the aortic annulus (*dotted green line*); and **E** illustrates the deployed (*red arrows*) aortic prosthesis (AVR). **F,** a color Doppler image obtained immediately after deployment, illustrates mild central prosthetic aortic regurgitation.

246

precise understanding of the shape and size of the aortic valve complex[105] and the most accurate measure of the aortic annulus. Both echocardiography (transthoracic and transesophageal) and CT are currently used for this purpose.[106-110]

In addition to the aortic valve annulus size, a successful TAVI procedure depends on diminishing the chances of coronary ostia occlusion by accurately measuring the aortic leaflets length and aortic annulus–to–left coronary ostium distance. Both echocardiography[111] and CT[28] are being used for this purpose.

During the TAVI procedure, catheter and device navigation and valve deployment are guided mainly with fluoroscopy and cineangiography (see Figure 16-1). TEE plays a secondary role during catheter navigation and device deployment, but a central role in the immediate postdeployment period. The key points at this time are the demonstration of a well-placed and stable prosthesis, appropriate function of the three leaflets, and absence of significant prosthetic and periprosthetic regurgitation (see Figure 16-12). Another important facet of the echocardiographic evaluation during and after aortic valve implantation is the search for and recognition of potential complications,[112] as summarized in Table 16-7.

Transcatheter Pulmonic Valve Implantation

In 2000, Bonhoeffer reported the first case of transcatheter pulmonic valve implantation in a 12-year-old boy with stenosis and regurgitation of a prosthetic conduit from the right ventricle to the pulmonary artery. In 2002 and 2005, the same group reported their expanded experience and concluded that transcatheter pulmonic valve implantation is feasible, has low risk, and results in quantifiable improvement in CMR-defined ventricular parameters and pulmonary regurgitation as well as in subjective and objective improvement in exercise capacity.[113,114] Since then about 1500 valves have been implanted worldwide, several groups have reported their experiences,[115-121] and this procedure is becoming the preferred therapeutic option for patients with RV outflow stenosis or regurgitation dysfunction after previous surgery or stent placement.

In such patients, echocardiography is the main imaging technique to evaluate for the presence and severity of both RV outflow obstruction and pulmonic regurgitation. CMR is better suited for the evaluation of RV and outflow tract size and RV systolic function. Intraprocedure guidance is usually done with fluoroscopy and cineangiography (Figure 16-14).

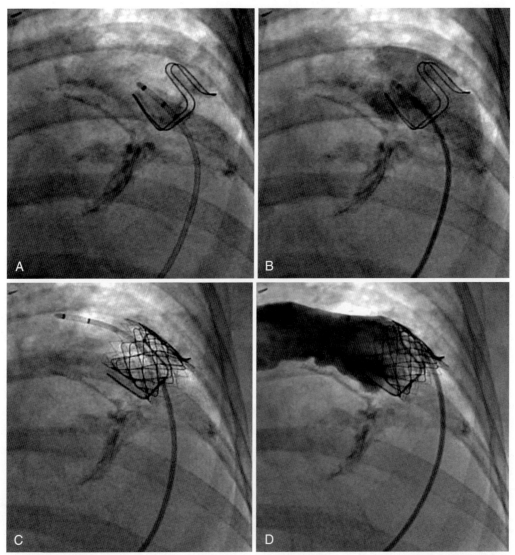

FIGURE 16-14 **Radiographic guidance for implantation of a Melody Valve (Medtronic, Inc, Minneapolis, Minnesota).** Transcatheter implantation of the pulmonic valve is carried out using fluoroscopy and angiography. **A,** Degenerated bioprosthesis in the pulmonary position is shown before and **B,** after angiography demonstrating severe regurgitation. **C,** After placement of a Melody valve **D,** angiography shows a competent valve with no regurgitation. *(Images courtesy Drs. Joseph Kay and Thomas Fagan, University of Colorado Denver.)*

Transcatheter Mitral Valve Implantation

As of today transcatheter implantation of mitral valves has not reached clinical applications. Several groups have demonstrated the potential of this approach in experimental animals,[122-124] and it is likely that in the near future it will be applied in clinical trials. Echocardiography and 3D TTE in particular are likely to play a central role in patient selection and device deployment in patients undergoing the procedure.

Transcatheter Procedures for Mitral Regurgitation

Edge-to-Edge Mitral Valve Repair

Surgical repair of the mitral valve consisting of anchoring the free edge of a prolapsing leaflet to the corresponding free edge of the facing leaflet—the edge-to-edge technique—was described by Maisano et al[125] in 1998. on the basis of this concept, a percutaneous approach for edge-to-edge mitral valve report was developed, and the results of a multicenter trial (Everest Phase I clinical trial) involving 27 patients was reported by Feldman et al[126] in 2005. General anesthesia, fluoroscopy, and echocardiographic guidance are used. A guide is positioned in the left atrium. A clip (MitraClip) is centered over the mitral orifice, passed into the left ventricle, and pulled back to grasp the mitral leaflets. After verification that mitral regurgitation (MR) is reduced, the clip is released.[126] In 2009 Feldman et al[127] reported on the safety and midterm durability of this procedure in the initial EVEREST cohort of the Percutaneous repair with the MitraClip system; this trial, involving 107 patients, demonstrated that percutaneous edge-to-edge mitral repair can be accomplished with low rates of morbidity and mortality and with acute reduction in MR severity to less than 2+ in the majority of patients, and with sustained freedom from death, surgery, and recurrent MR in a substantial proportion of patients.[127]

From an imaging perspective, this trial was commendable in that it used a core echocardiography laboratory.[128] On reporting on the use of echocardiography for the MitraClip device, Foster et al[128] concluded that quantitative assessment of MR is feasible in a multicenter trial, and percutaneous mitral repair with the MitraClip produces a sustained decrease in MR severity to moderate or less for at least 6 months. Echocardiography plays a central role in procedural guidance and evaluation of results. TEE is used as the primary imaging modality to guide this procedure and is essential to its success. A streamlined approach to echocardiographic guidance, using predetermined standardized views and a common anatomically based vocabulary, shortens the procedure time and allows for efficient percutaneous repair.[129] Table 16-8 summarizes, and Figures 16-15 and 16-16 illustrate the key uses of imaging in percutaneous edge-to-edge mitral valve repair.

Other Procedures

Other transcatheter procedures for the treatment of mitral regurgitation being investigated include coronary sinus annuloplasty,[130-136] direct annuloplasty,[137] and ventricular remodeling.[138] None of these procedures has reached clinical utilization so they are not detailed here.

Transcatheter Repair of Paravalvular Regurgitation

Of the approximately 60,000 prosthetic valve replacements done in the United States every year, paravalvular regurgitation develops in 5% to 17%.[139] Affected patients frequently have hemolysis or heart failure, and because of underlying tissue friability,

TABLE 16-8	Transcatheter Edge-to-Edge Mitral Valve Repair
TASK	**IMAGING**
Patient Selection	
Moderate or severe MR	Quantitative echocardiography[129]: 1. Color-flow jet may be central and large (>6 cm² or >30% of the left atrial area as measured in all apical four-chamber or a long-axis view) or smaller if eccentric, encircling the left atrium. 2. Pulmonary vein flow may show systolic blunting or systolic flow reversal. 3. Vena contracta width >0.3 cm measured in the parasternal long-axis view. 4. Regurgitant volume of >45 mL/beat. 5. Regurgitant fraction >40%. 6. Regurgitant orifice area >0.30 cm.
Degenerative MR	2D TEE: Flail gap and flail width
Functional MR	2D TEE: Tethering height and coaptation length
Procedural Guidance	
Transseptal puncture	Fluoroscopy, 2D and 3D TEE Superior and posterior puncture points
Advancing the clip delivery system	2D and 3D TEE
Positioning and orienting the clip	2D and 3D TEE
Grasping the leaflets	2D and 3D TEE
Recognizing Complications	
Right, left ventricular perforation	Echocardiography effusion-tamponade
Partial clip detachment	Echocardiography, fluoroscopy
Evaluation of Results	
MR reduction	2D, 3D TEE, color Doppler
Stable and adequately placed clip	2D, 3D TEE

2D, Two dimensional; *Doppler,* Doppler echocardiography; *MR,* mitral regurgitation; *TEE,* transesophageal echocardiography.

scarring, or calcification, reoperation is associated with increased morbidity and mortality. Transthoracic and real-time 3D TEE is key for characterizing the number of defects, defect location, size, and shape[140-142] (Figures 16-17 and 16-18). MDCT can further characterize the size, location, and shape of the leak.[143] Paramitral defects are usually approached with an antegrade transseptal approach guided by fluoroscopy and real-time 3D TEE. Closure devices such as vascular plugs, guide wires, and catheters are clearly visible on fluoroscopy, so fluoroscopic guidance may be used extensively (Figure 16-19). Retrograde transaortic cannulation and transapical access with retrograde cannulation are potential alternative approaches. For oblong or crescentic defects, the simultaneous or sequential deployment of two smaller devices, as opposed to one large device, results in a higher rate of procedural success and safety because the risk of impingement on the prosthetic leaflets is minimized. Most paraaortic defects are approached in a retrograde manner and closed with a single device.[139]

With detailed imaging guidance, meticulous anatomic assessment, and careful planning, and procedural execution, successful closure rates of 90% or more can be attained, as reported in

Pre   Post   During

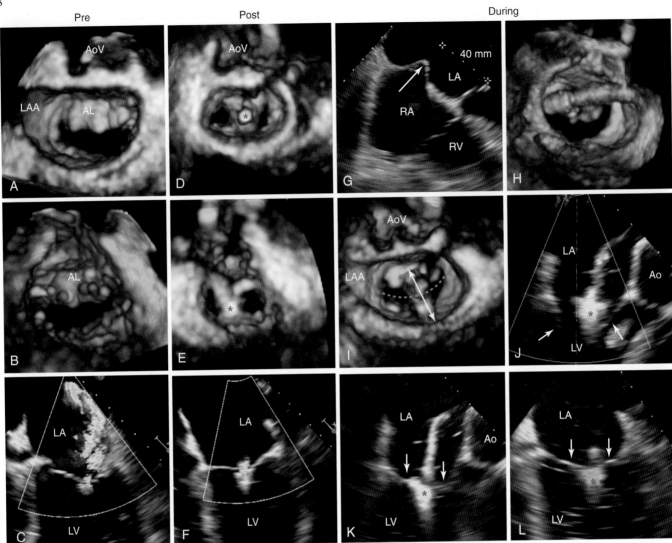

FIGURE 16-15 **Transesophageal echocardiographic guidance of edge-to-edge mitral valve repair.** Transesophageal echocardiography (TEE) in a patient with severe secondary mitral regurgitation undergoing edge-to-edge mitral valve repair. **A** to **C,** Preprocedure images illustrate the presence of severe mitral regurgitation **(C)** in a structurally normal mitral valve as seen from the left atrium (LA) **(A)** and from the left ventricle (LV) **(B). D** and **E,** Postprocedure images showing the clip in place *(green asterisk),* creating a double-orifice *(red asterisks)* mitral valve. **F,** The presence of only mild mitral regurgitation at the end of the procedure. **G** to **L** illustrate the complementary role that two-dimensional and three-dimensional TEE plays during the deployment of the mitral clip. **G,** The "tenting" that occurs during the septal puncture *(arrow).* A precise postero-superior puncture site is required to provide maneuverability of the delivery catheter in the left atrium. The *white dotted line* marks an appropriate 40-mm distance from the puncture site to the mitral valve plane. **H,** The delivery catheter is advanced into the left atrium and toward the mitral valve orifice. **I,** The clip with extended arms *(double-headed arrow)* is oriented perpendicularly to the line of coaptation of the mitral valve *(doted green line).* **J,** The clip *(green asterisk)* is advanced through the mitral valve *(arrows)* into the inflow tract of the left ventricle. **K** and **L** are simultaneously obtained orthogonal biplane views of the mitral valve. **K** represents the left ventricular outflow view, and **L** the bicommissural view. These views are ideal for guiding leaflet grasping *(red arrows)* during the clip procedure. *AL,* anterior leaflet of the mitral valve; *Ao,* aorta; *AoV,* aortic valve; *LAA,* left atrial appendage.

a series of 115 patients by Sorajja et al.[144] Table 16-9 summarizes the imaging aspects of transcatheter repair of paravalvular regurgitation.

Transcatheter Valve-in-Valve Implantation

Because of a lower risk of thrombotic and bleeding events and the desire to avoid anticoagulation, bioprosthetic heart valves are often favored over more durable mechanical valves. With time, however, bioprosthetic valves tend to deteriorate and eventually fail. The significant risks carried by reoperations have led to the development of alternative percutaneous prosthetic "valve-in-valve" implantation. In single-center[145] and multicenter[146] trials, this alternative been found to be a reproducible option for the

management of bioprosthetic valve failure. Several reports have documented the validity of this approach for bioprostheses in pulmonic,[147] tricuspid,[148] mitral,[149-151] and aortic[152] positions. The majority of these reports describe using the Edwards SAPIEN valve (Edwards Lifesciences Corporation, Irvine, California), and the imaging guidance is commonly based on fluoroscopy, angiography, and TEE.

Summary

The landscape of valvular heart disease is significantly changing as a consequence of the aging of the affected patients and the resulting switch in management to less invasive procedures. No longer is rheumatic heart disease, a disease of the young, the main valvular pathology requiring a mechanical solution. In industrialized countries, calcific valvular disease, a disease of the

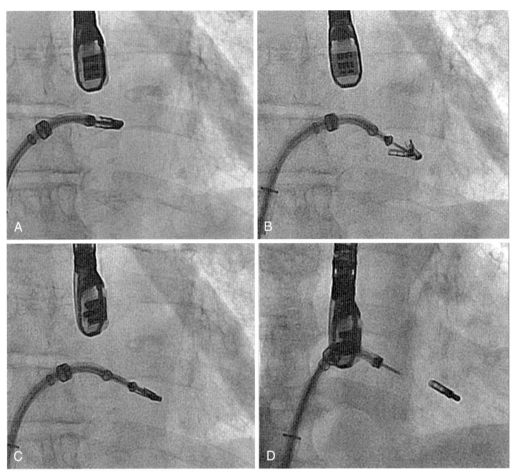

FIGURE 16-16   Placement of a MitraClip (Abbott Laboratories, Abbott Park, Illinois) with fluoroscopic imaging. Placement of the MitraClip uses both echocardiography and fluoroscopy for guidance. Four steps in the procedure are shown in these fluoroscopic images. **A,** Clip-on-clip delivery system exiting the guiding catheter in the left atrium; **B,** Clip opened in the left ventricle and ready for leaflet grasping; **C,** Leaflets grasped and clip still attached if repositioning needed; **D,** Release of clip.

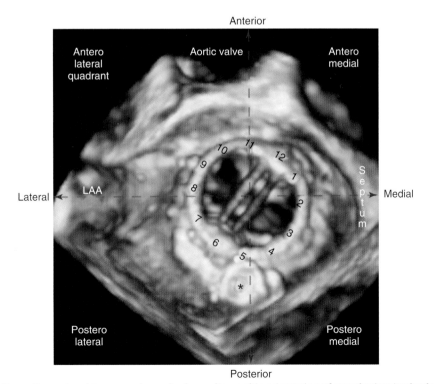

FIGURE 16-17   Real-time three-dimensional transesophageal echocardiographic orientation of prosthetic mitral valve paravalvular plug location. Real-time image of a bileaflet mitral valve mechanical prosthesis with a plug *(red asterisk)* to remedy paraprosthetic leak. Localization of the leak is facilitated by first determining in what quadrant the leak is (in this case, posterolateral). The *red dotted arrows* are perpendicular to each other, and by using the anatomic landmarks of the aorta, left atrial appendage, and interatrial septum, one can deduce what are anterior, posterior, lateral, and medial, and from this knowledge create the four quadrants described. One can then fine-tune the location by using the circumference of the suture ring as the face of a clock (in this case, the plug is at 5 o'clock). *LAA*, left atrial appendage.

Pre

Post

During

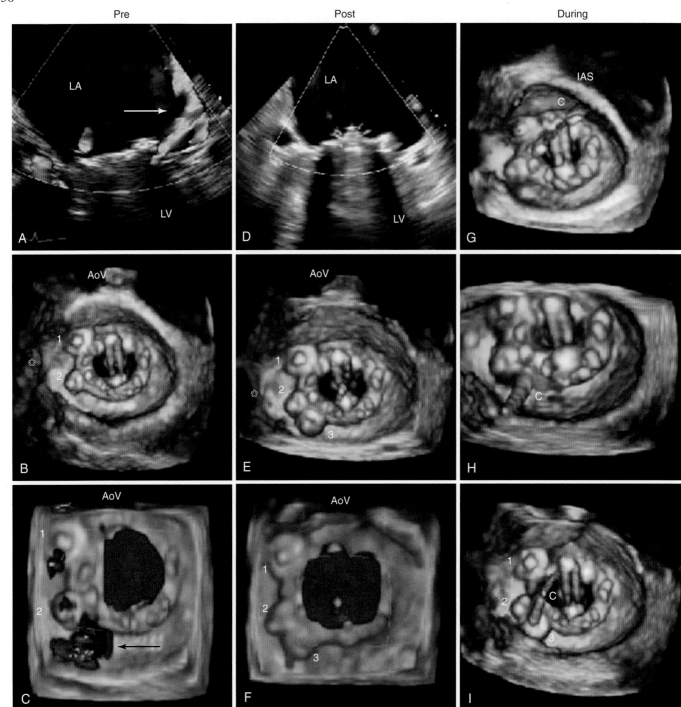

FIGURE 16-18 **Real-time three-dimensional transesophageal echocardiographic guidance of paraprosthetic leak closure in a patient with two prior plugs. A** to **C,** Preprocedure images. In **A** and **C,** the presence of a significant residual paraprosthetic leak is indicated by the *arrow.* The location of the leak is unclear on the two-dimensional color Doppler image **(A),** whereas it is distinctly localized in the posterolateral quadrant at 7 o'clock on the three-dimensional (3D) color image **(C).** In **B,** the location of prior plugs (*1* and *2*) at 9 o'clock and 11 o'clock are clearly determined. **D** to **F,** Postprocedure panels. **D** and **F,** The absence of significant residual paravalvular regurgitation. **E,** The three plugs in place (*1, 2,* and *3*). **G** to **I** illustrate the use of 3D transesophageal echocardiography for intraprocedure guidance of the paraprosthetic leak closure. **G,** The delivery catheter (C) has been advanced through the septal puncture into the left atrium. **H,** The catheter has been advanced into the paravalvular leak orifice. **I,** The third (*3*) plug has been deployed. *AoV,* aortic valve; *IAS,* interatrial septum; *LA,* left atrium; *LV,* left ventricle; *Red asterisk,* left atrial appendage.

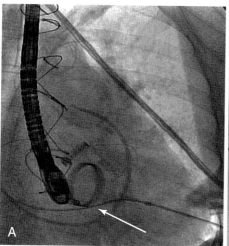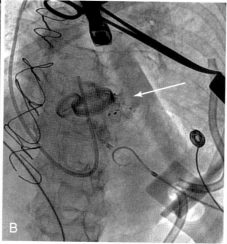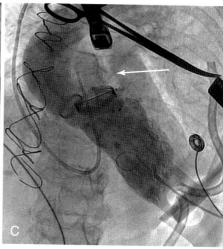

FIGURE 16-19 **Closure of paravalvular leak using transapical access and fluoroscopic guidance.** Patients undergoing transcatheter closure of paraprosthetic leaks often have high surgical risks and have undergone multiple prior operations, as shown here. **A,** Transapical approach to a mitral paravalvular leak was used, and the guide wire crossing from left ventricle to left atrium is clearly outside the valve ring (*arrow*). **B,** A cranial gantry angulation helped deploy two vascular plugs in an area with marked calcification (*arrow*) likely to have contributed to partial valve dehiscence. **D,** Completion left ventricular angiography shows no contrast agent regurgitating into the left atrium (*arrow*).

TABLE 16-9	Transcatheter Repair of Paravalvular Regurgitation
TASK	**IMAGING**
Patient Selection	
Mitral Paravalvular Defects	
Size: <25% of circumference Leak severity: mild, moderate, severe Shape: crescentic, oblong, serpiginous tracks Number: single, multiple Location: use anatomic land marks; relation to tilting or hemi-discs or bioprosthetic leaflets	TEE Color Doppler: assessment of leak severity, valvular vs. paravalvular leak 3D TEE particularly helpful for detailed anatomic characterization of defects Multislice computed tomography
Aortic Paravalvular Defects	
Size: usually small Leak severity: mild, moderate, severe Shape: usually round Number: usually single Location: use anatomic land marks; relation to tilting or hemi-discs or bioprosthetic leaflets	Consider TTE or ICE for anterior leaks TEE for posterior leaks Color Doppler: assessment of leak severity, valvular vs. paravalvular leak Paravalvular leak severity difficult to assess by color Doppler; Consider aortogram
Procedural Guidance	
Mitral Paravalvular Defects	
Antegrade transseptal approach Retrograde transapical approach Retrograde transaortic approach	Fluoroscopy, biplane recommended TEE 3D TEE recommended
Aortic Paravalvular Defects	
Retrograde approach	TTE (anterior defects) Fluoroscopy (all defects) ICE (anterior defects, ICE catheter placed in right ventricular outflow tract) TEE (posterior defects)
Recognition of Complications	
Obstruction of mechanical tilting-disk valve Device tilting after deployment, blocking the prosthetic leaflet Device embolization Coronary artery obstruction Thromboembolism, stroke	Fluoroscopy 2D and 3D TEE Aortography Coronary angiography
Evaluation of Results	

Determine therapeutic end point before initiating procedure:
  For heart failure: substantial reduction of leak required
  For hemolysis: no residual leak required
	Color Doppler
	Pulsed Doppler of pulmonary veins
	Aortography

2D, Two-dimensional; *Doppler,* Doppler echocardiography; *ICE,* intracardiac echocardiography; *TEE,* transesophageal echocardiography; *TTE,* transtracheal echocardiography;

252

elderly, causes most of the severe forms of valvular pathology. The development of transcatheter procedures to effectively treat advanced valvular heart disease has changed the way patients with valvular heart disease are being treated. Cardiac imaging plays a central role in patient selection, procedural guidance, recognition and management of complications, and evaluation of results and follow-up of patients undergoing transcatheter valve procedures.

CH
16

REFERENCES

1. Nkomo VT, Gardin JM, Skelton TN, et al. Burden of valvular heart diseases: a population-based study. Lancet 2006;368:1005–11.
2. Vahanian A, Iung B, Himbert D, et al. Changing demographics of valvular heart disease and impact on surgical and transcatheter valve therapies. Int J Cardiovasc Imaging 2011;27:1115–22.
3. Iung B, Vahanian A. Epidemiology of valvular heart disease in the adult. Nat Rev Cardiol 2011;8:162–72.
4. Soler-Soler J, Galve E. Worldwide perspective of valve disease. Heart 2000;83:721–5.
5. d'Arcy JL, Prendergast BD, Chambers JB, et al. Valvular heart disease: the next cardiac epidemic. Heart 2011;97:91–3.
6. Caira FC, Stock SR, Gleason TG, et al. Human degenerative valve disease is associated with up-regulation of low-density lipoprotein receptor-related protein 5 receptor-mediated bone formation. J Am Coll Cardiol 2006;47:1707–12.
7. Iung B, Baron G, Butchart EG, et al. A prospective survey of patients with valvular heart disease in Europe: The Euro Heart Survey on Valvular Heart Disease. Eur Heart J 2003;24:1231–43.
8. Mack MJ. Risk scores for predicting outcomes in valvular heart disease: how useful? Curr Cardiol Rep 2011;13:107–12.
9. Vahanian A, Baumgartner H, Bax J, et al. Guidelines on the management of valvular heart disease: The Task Force on the Management of Valvular Heart Disease of the European Society of Cardiology. Eur Heart J 2007;28:230–68.
10. Bonow RO, Carabello BA, Chatterjee K, et al. 2008 focused update incorporated into the ACC/AHA 2006 guidelines for the management of patients with valvular heart disease: a report of the American College of Cardiology/American Heart Association Task Force on Practice Guidelines (Writing Committee to revise the 1998 guidelines for the management of patients with valvular heart disease). Endorsed by the Society of Cardiovascular Anesthesiologists, Society for Cardiovascular Angiography and Interventions, and Society of Thoracic Surgeons. J Am Coll Cardiol 2008;52:e1–142.
11. Rosenhek R. Almanac 2011: valvular heart disease. The national society journals present selected research that has driven recent advances in clinical cardiology. Heart 2011;97:2007–17.
12. Rahimtoola SH. The year in valvular heart disease. J Am Coll Cardiol 2011;58:1197–207.
13. Carroll JD. The future of image guidance of cardiac interventions. Catheter Cardiovasc Interv 2007;70:783.
14. Kapadia SR, Schoenhagen P, Stewart W, et al. Imaging for transcatheter valve procedures. Curr Probl Cardiol 2010;35:228–76.
15. Hahn RT. The new paradigm for the management of valvular heart disease: the multidisciplinary heart team. J Am Soc Echocardiogr 2011;24:A28.
16. Hilliard AA, Nishimura RA. The interventional cardiologist and structural heart disease: the need for a team approach. JACC Cardiovasc Imaging 2009;2:8–10.
17. Bateman MG, Iaizzo PA. Comparative imaging of cardiac structures and function for the optimization of transcatheter approaches for valvular and structural heart disease. Int J Cardiovasc Imaging 2011;27:1223–34.
18. Schoenhagen P, Bax J. Transcatheter repair of valvular heart disease and periprocedural imaging. Int J Cardiovasc Imaging 2011;27:1113.
19. Hudson PA, Eng MH, Kim MS, et al. A comparison of echocardiographic modalities to guide structural heart disease interventions. J Interv Cardiol 2008;21:535–46.
20. Schwartz JG, Neubauer AM, Fagan TE, et al. Potential role of three-dimensional rotational angiography and C-arm CT for valvular repair and implantation. Int J Cardiovasc Imaging 2011;27:1205–22.
21. Wallace MJ, Kuo MD, Glaiberman C, et al. Three-dimensional C-arm cone-beam CT: applications in the interventional suite. J Vasc Interv Radiol 2008;19:799–813.
22. Ewe SH, Klautz RJ, Schalij MJ, et al. Role of computed tomography imaging for transcatheter valvular repair/insertion. Int J Cardiovasc Imaging 2011;27:1179–93.
23. Leipsic J, Wood D, Manders D, et al. The evolving role of MDCT in transcatheter aortic valve replacement: a radiologists' perspective. AJR Am J Roentgenol 2009;193:W214–9.
24. Tops LF, Wood DA, Delgado V, et al. Noninvasive evaluation of the aortic root with multislice computed tomography implications for transcatheter aortic valve replacement. JACC Cardiovasc Imaging 2008;1:321–30.
25. Wood DA, Tops LF, Mayo JR, et al. Role of multislice computed tomography in transcatheter aortic valve replacement. Am J Cardiol 2009;103:1295–301.
26. del Valle-Fernandez R, Jelnin V, Panagopoulos G, et al. A method for standardized computed tomography angiography-based measurement of aortic valvar structures. Eur Heart J 2010;31:2170–8.
27. Cueff C, Serfaty JM, Cimadevilla C, et al. Measurement of aortic valve calcification using multislice computed tomography: correlation with haemodynamic severity of aortic stenosis and clinical implication for patients with low ejection fraction. Heart 2011;97:721–6.
28. Delgado V, Ng AC, van de Veire NR, et al. Transcatheter aortic valve implantation: role of multi-detector row computed tomography to evaluate prosthesis positioning and deployment in relation to valve function. Eur Heart J 2010;31:1114–23.
29. Gurvitch R, Wood DA, Leipsic J, et al. Multislice computed tomography for prediction of optimal angiographic deployment projections during transcatheter aortic valve implantation. JACC Cardiovasc Interv 2010;3:1157–65.
30. Christiansen JP, Karamitsos TD, Myerson SG. Assessment of valvular heart disease by cardiovascular magnetic resonance imaging: a review. Heart Lung Circ 2011;20:73–82.
31. Gutierrez LF, Silva R, Ozturk C, et al. Technology preview: X-ray fused with magnetic resonance during invasive cardiovascular procedures. Catheter Cardiovasc Interv 2007;70:773–82.
32. Kuehne T, Yilmaz S, Meinus C, et al. Magnetic resonance imaging-guided transcatheter implantation of a prosthetic valve in aortic valve position: Feasibility study in swine. J Am Coll Cardiol 2004;44:2247–9.
33. Paelinck BP, Van Herck PL, Rodrigus I, et al. Comparison of magnetic resonance imaging of aortic valve stenosis and aortic root to multimodality imaging for selection of transcatheter aortic valve implantation candidates. Am J Cardiol 2011;108:92–8.
34. Ussia GP, Barbanti M, Sarkar K, et al. Accuracy of intracardiac echocardiography for aortic root assessment in patients undergoing transcatheter aortic valve implantation. Am Heart J 2012;163:684–9.
35. Chessa M, Butera G, Carminati M. Intracardiac echocardiography during percutaneous pulmonary valve replacement. Eur Heart J 2008;29:2908.
36. Deftereos S, Giannopoulos G, Raisakis K, et al. Intracardiac echocardiography imaging of periprosthetic valvular regurgitation. Eur J Echocardiogr 2010;11:E20.
37. Kim SS, Hijazi ZM, Lang RM, et al. The use of intracardiac echocardiography and other intracardiac imaging tools to guide noncoronary cardiac interventions. J Am Coll Cardiol 2009;53:2117–28.
38. Bartel T, Bonaros N, Muller L, et al. Intracardiac echocardiography: a new guiding tool for transcatheter aortic valve replacement. J Am Soc Echocardiogr 2011;24:966–75.
39. de Sousa L. Intracardiac echocardiography in structural heart disease: current prospects. Rev Port Cardiol 2012;31(6):413–4.
40. Baumgartner H, Hung J, Bermejo J, et al. Echocardiographic assessment of valve stenosis: EAE/ASE recommendations for clinical practice. J Am Soc Echocardiogr 2009;22:1–23; quiz 101–2.
41. Zoghbi WA, Enriquez-Sarano M, Foster E, et al. Recommendations for evaluation of the severity of native valvular regurgitation with two-dimensional and Doppler echocardiography. J Am Soc Echocardiogr 2003;16:777–802.
42. Zoghbi WA, Chambers JB, Dumesnil JG, et al. Recommendations for evaluation of prosthetic valves with echocardiography and Doppler ultrasound. J Am Soc Echocardiogr 2009;22:975–1014.
43. Lang RM, Tsang W, Weinert L, et al. Valvular heart disease. The value of 3-dimensional echocardiography. J Am Coll Cardiol 2011;58:1933–44.
44. Salcedo EE, Quaife RA, Seres T, et al. A framework for systematic characterization of the mitral valve by real-time three-dimensional transesophageal echocardiography. J Am Soc Echocardiogr 2009;22:1087–99.
45. Moss RR, Ivens E, Pasupati S, et al. Role of echocardiography in percutaneous aortic valve implantation. JACC Cardiovasc Imaging 2008;1:15–24.
46. Naqvi TZ. Echocardiography in percutaneous valve therapy. JACC Cardiovasc Imaging 2009;2:1226–37.
47. Perk G, Lang RM, Garcia-Fernandez MA, et al. Use of real time three-dimensional transesophageal echocardiography in intracardiac catheter based interventions. J Am Soc Echocardiogr 2009;22:865–82.
48. Silvestry FE, Kerber RE, Brook MM, et al. Echocardiography-guided interventions. J Am Soc Echocardiogr 2009;22:213–31; quiz 316–7.
49. Goncalves A, Marcos-Alberca P, Zamorano JL. Echocardiography: guidance during valve implantation. EuroIntervention 2010;6(Suppl G):G14–9.
50. Siegel RJ, Luo H, Biner S. Transcatheter valve repair/implantation. Int J Cardiovasc Imaging 2011;27:1165–77.
51. Shames S, Koczo A, Hahn R, et al. Flow Characteristics of the SAPIEN Aortic Valve: The Importance of Recognizing In-Stent Flow Acceleration for the Echocardiographic Assessment of Valve Function. J Am Soc Echocardiogr 2012;25:603–9.
52. Rosenhek R, Iung B, Tornos P, et al. ESC Working Group on Valvular Heart Disease Position Paper: assessing the risk of interventions in patients with valvular heart disease. Eur Heart J 2012;33:822–8.
53. Blumenstein J, Van Linden A, Arsalan M, et al. Transapical access: current status and future directions. Expert Rev Med Devices 2012;9:15–22.
54. Holmes DR Jr, Mack MJ. Transcatheter valve therapy a professional society overview from the american college of cardiology foundation and the society of thoracic surgeons. J Am Coll Cardiol 2011;58:445–55.
55. Cribier A, Savin T, Saoudi N, et al. Percutaneous transluminal valvuloplasty of acquired aortic stenosis in elderly patients: an alternative to valve replacement? Lancet 1986;1:63–7.
56. Cribier A, Berland J, Koning R, et al. Percutaneous transluminal aortic valvuloplasty: indications and results in adult aortic stenosis. Eur Heart J 1988;9(Suppl E):149–54.
57. Cribier A, Letac B. Two years' experience of percutaneous balloon valvuloplasty in aortic stenosis. Herz 1988;13:110–8.
58. Letac B, Cribier A. Personal answer to a personal view on balloon aortic valvuloplasty. Eur Heart J 1988;9:195–7.
59. Letac B, Cribier A, Berland J. [Percutaneous valvuloplasty using a balloon catheter in acquired mitral and aortic stenosis in adults]. Schweiz Med Wochenschr Suppl 1988;118:1673–80.
60. Letac B, Cribier A, Koning R, et al. Results of percutaneous transluminal valvuloplasty in 218 adults with valvular aortic stenosis. Am J Cardiol 1988;62:598–605.
61. Letac B, Gerber LI, Koning R. Insights on the mechanism of balloon valvuloplasty in aortic stenosis. Am J Cardiol 1988;62:1241–7.
62. Percutaneous balloon aortic valvuloplasty. Acute and 30-day follow-up results in 674 patients from the NHLBI Balloon Valvuloplasty Registry. Circulation 1991;84:2383–97.

63. Geibel A, Kasper W, Reifart N, et al. Clinical and Doppler echocardiographic follow-up after percutaneous balloon valvuloplasty for aortic valve stenosis. Am J Cardiol 1991;67:616–21.
64. Feldman T, Glagov S, Carroll JD. Restenosis following successful balloon valvuloplasty: bone formation in aortic valve leaflets. Cathet Cardiovasc Diagn 1993;29:1–7.
65. Lieberman EB, Wilson JS, Harrison JK, et al. Aortic valve replacement in adults after balloon aortic valvuloplasty. Circulation 1994;90:II205–8.
66. Agarwal A, Kini AS, Attanti S, et al. Results of repeat balloon valvuloplasty for treatment of aortic stenosis in patients aged 59 to 104 years. Am J Cardiol 2005;95: 43–7.
67. Kapadia SR, Goel SS, Yuksel U, et al. Lessons learned from balloon aortic valvuloplasty experience from the pre-transcatheter aortic valve implantation era. J Interv Cardiol 2010;23:499–508.
68. Ussia GP, Capodanno D, Barbanti M, et al. Balloon aortic valvuloplasty for severe aortic stenosis as a bridge to high-risk transcatheter aortic valve implantation. J Invasive Cardiol 2010;22:161–6.
69. Saia F, Marrozzini C, Moretti C, et al. The role of percutaneous balloon aortic valvuloplasty as a bridge for transcatheter aortic valve implantation. EuroIntervention 2011;7:723–9.
70. Tissot CM, Attias D, Himbert D, et al. Reappraisal of percutaneous aortic balloon valvuloplasty as a preliminary treatment strategy in the transcatheter aortic valve implantation era. EuroIntervention 2011;7:49–56.
71. Inoue K, Owaki T, Nakamura T, et al. Clinical application of transvenous mitral commissurotomy by a new balloon catheter. J Thorac Cardiovasc Surg 1984;87: 394–402.
72. Palacios I, Block PC, Brandi S, et al. Percutaneous balloon valvotomy for patients with severe mitral stenosis. Circulation 1987;75:778–84.
73. Ben Farhat M, Ayari M, Maatouk F, et al. Percutaneous balloon versus surgical closed and open mitral commissurotomy: seven-year follow-up results of a randomized trial. Circulation 1998;97:245–50.
74. Iung B, Garbarz E, Michaud P, et al. Late results of percutaneous mitral commissurotomy in a series of 1024 patients. Analysis of late clinical deterioration: frequency, anatomic findings, and predictive factors. Circulation 1999;99:3272–8.
75. de Souza JA, Martinez EE Jr, Ambrose JA, et al. Percutaneous balloon mitral valvuloplasty in comparison with open mitral valve commissurotomy for mitral stenosis during pregnancy. J Am Coll Cardiol 2001;37:900–3.
76. Palacios IF, Sanchez PL, Harrell LC, et al. Which patients benefit from percutaneous mitral balloon valvuloplasty? Prevalvuloplasty and postvalvuloplasty variables that predict long-term outcome. Circulation 2002;105:1465–71.
77. Iung B, Nicoud-Houel A, Fondard O, et al. Temporal trends in percutaneous mitral commissurotomy over a 15-year period. Eur Heart J 2004;25:701–7.
78. Wilkins GT, Weyman AE, Abascal VM, et al. Percutaneous balloon dilatation of the mitral valve: an analysis of echocardiographic variables related to outcome and the mechanism of dilatation. Br Heart J 1988;60:299–308.
79. Cannan CR, Nishimura RA, Reeder GS, et al. Echocardiographic assessment of commissural calcium: a simple predictor of outcome after percutaneous mitral balloon valvotomy. J Am Coll Cardiol 1997;29:175–80.
80. Goldstein SA, Campbell AN. Mitral stenosis. Evaluation and guidance of valvuloplasty by transesophageal echocardiography. Cardiology clinics 1993;11:409–25.
81. Herrmann HC, Lima JA, Feldman T, et al. Mechanisms and outcome of severe mitral regurgitation after Inoue balloon valvuloplasty. North American Inoue Balloon Investigators. J Am Coll Cardiol 1993;22:783–9.
82. Zamorano J, Perez de Isla L, Sugeng L, et al. Non-invasive assessment of mitral valve area during percutaneous balloon mitral valvuloplasty: role of real-time 3D echocardiography. Eur Heart J 2004;25:2086–91.
83. Eng MH, Salcedo EE, Quaife RA, et al. Implementation of real time three-dimensional transesophageal echocardiography in percutaneous mitral balloon valvuloplasty and structural heart disease interventions. Echocardiography 2009;26:958–66.
84. Langerveld J, Valocik G, Plokker HW, et al. Additional value of three-dimensional transesophageal echocardiography for patients with mitral valve stenosis undergoing balloon valvuloplasty. J Am Soc Echocardiogr 2003;16:841–9.
85. Pepine CJ, Gessner IH, Feldman RL. Percutaneous balloon valvuloplasty for pulmonic valve stenosis in the adult. Am J Cardiol 1982;50:1442–5.
86. Herrmann HC, Hill JA, Krol J, et al. Effectiveness of percutaneous balloon valvuloplasty in adults with pulmonic valve stenosis. Am J Cardiol 1991;68:1111–3.
87. Mullins CE, Ludomirsky A, O'Laughlin MP, et al. Balloon valvuloplasty for pulmonic valve stenosis–two-year follow-up: hemodynamic and Doppler evaluation. Cathet Cardiovasc Diagn 1988;14:76–81.
88. Chen CR, Cheng TO, Huang T, et al. Percutaneous balloon valvuloplasty for pulmonic stenosis in adolescents and adults. New Engl J Med 1996;335:21–5.
89. Dejam A, Hokinson M, Laham R. Repeated successful balloon valvuloplasty of a bioprosthetic aortic valve in a nonagenerian. Catheter Cardiovasc Interv 2011;77:589–92.
90. Yunoki K, Naruko T, Itoh A, et al. Images in cardiovascular medicine. Percutaneous transcatheter balloon valvuloplasty for bioprosthetic tricuspid valve stenosis. Circulation 2006;114:e558–9.
91. Webb J. Balloon valvuloplasty for stenotic bioprosthetic aortic valves. Catheter Cardiovasc Interv 2011;77:593.
92. Laske T, Denton M, Eberhardt C. The development of transcatheter heart valves: opportunities and challenges. Conf Proc IEEE Eng Med Biol Soc 2009;2009:163–5.
93. Dworakowski R, Maccarthy P. Where should transcatheter aortic valve implantation go beyond 2012? J Cardiovasc Med (Hagerstown) 2012;13(8):516–23.
94. Cribier A, Eltchaninoff H, Bash A, et al. Percutaneous transcatheter implantation of an aortic valve prosthesis for calcific aortic stenosis: first human case description. Circulation 2002;106:3006–8.
95. Leon MB, Piazza N, Nikolsky E, et al. Standardized endpoint definitions for Transcatheter Aortic Valve Implantation clinical trials: a consensus report from the Valve Academic Research Consortium. J Am Coll Cardiol 2011;57:253–69.
96. Leon MB, Smith CR, Mack M, et al. Transcatheter aortic-valve implantation for aortic stenosis in patients who cannot undergo surgery. New Engl J Med 2010;363:1597–607.
97. Smith CR, Leon MB, Mack MJ, et al. Transcatheter versus surgical aortic-valve replacement in high-risk patients. New Engl J Med 2011;364:2187–98.
98. Makkar RR, Fontana GP, Jilaihawi H, et al. Transcatheter aortic-valve replacement for inoperable severe aortic stenosis. New Engl J Med 2012;366:1696–704.
99. Cribier A, Eltchaninoff H, Tron C, et al. Early experience with percutaneous transcatheter implantation of heart valve prosthesis for the treatment of end-stage inoperable patients with calcific aortic stenosis. J Am Coll Cardiol 2004;43:698–703.
100. Lichtenstein SV, Cheung A, Ye J, et al. Transapical transcatheter aortic valve implantation in humans: initial clinical experience. Circulation 2006;114:591–6.
101. Webb JG, Chandavimol M, Thompson CR, et al. Percutaneous aortic valve implantation retrograde from the femoral artery. Circulation 2006;113:842–50.
102. Ye J, Cheung A, Lichtenstein SV, et al. Transapical aortic valve implantation in humans. J Thorac Cardiovasc Surg 2006;131:1194–6.
103. Webb JG, Pasupati S, Humphries K, et al. Percutaneous transarterial aortic valve replacement in selected high-risk patients with aortic stenosis. Circulation 2007;116: 755–63.
104. da Gama Ribeiro V, Vouga L, Markowitz A, et al. Vascular access in transcatheter aortic valve implantation. Int J Cardiovasc Imaging 2011;27:1235–43.
105. Piazza N, de Jaegere P, Schultz C, et al. Anatomy of the aortic valvar complex and its implications for transcatheter implantation of the aortic valve. Circ Cardiovasc Interv 2008;1:74–81.
106. Bagur R, Rodes-Cabau J, Doyle D, et al. Usefulness of TEE as the primary imaging technique to guide transcatheter transapical aortic valve implantation. JACC Cardiovasc Imaging 2011;4:115–24.
107. Jabbour A, Ismail TF, Moat N, et al. Multimodality imaging in transcatheter aortic valve implantation and post-procedural aortic regurgitation: comparison among cardiovascular magnetic resonance, cardiac computed tomography, and echocardiography. J Am Coll Cardiol 2011;58:2165–73.
108. Svensson LG, Kapadia S, Rodriguez L, et al. Percutaneous aortic valves and imaging. JACC Cardiovasc Imaging 2011;4:125–7.
109. Jilaihawi H, Kashif M, Fontana G, et al. Cross-sectional computed tomographic assessment improves accuracy of aortic annular sizing for transcatheter aortic valve replacement and reduces the incidence of paravalvular aortic regurgitation. J Am Coll Cardiol 2012;59:1275–86.
110. Kempfert J, Van Linden A, Lehmkuhl L, et al. Aortic annulus sizing: echocardiographic vs. computed tomography derived measurements in comparison with direct surgical sizing. Eur J Cardiothorac Surg 2012;42(4):627–33.
111. Tamborini G, Fusini L, Gripari P, et al. Feasibility and Accuracy of 3DTEE Versus CT for the Evaluation of Aortic Valve Annulus to Left Main Ostium Distance Before Transcatheter Aortic Valve Implantation. JACC Cardiovasc Imaging 2012;5:579–88.
112. Masson JB, Kovac J, Schuler G, et al. Transcatheter aortic valve implantation: review of the nature, management, and avoidance of procedural complications. JACC Cardiovasc Interv 2009;2:811–20.
113. Khambadkone S, Coats L, Taylor A, et al. Percutaneous pulmonary valve implantation in humans: results in 59 consecutive patients. Circulation 2005;112:1189–97.
114. Bonhoeffer P, Boudjemline Y, Qureshi SA, et al. Percutaneous insertion of the pulmonary valve. J Am Coll Cardiol 2002;39:1664–9.
115. Lurz P, Bonhoeffer P. Percutaneous implantation of pulmonary valves for treatment of right ventricular outflow tract dysfunction. Cardiol Young 2008;18:260–7.
116. Lurz P, Coats L, Khambadkone S, et al. Percutaneous pulmonary valve implantation: impact of evolving technology and learning curve on clinical outcome. Circulation 2008;117:1964–72.
117. Lurz P, Nordmeyer J, Muthurangu V, et al. Comparison of bare metal stenting and percutaneous pulmonary valve implantation for treatment of right ventricular outflow tract obstruction: use of an x-ray/magnetic resonance hybrid laboratory for acute physiological assessment. Circulation 2009;119:2995–3001.
118. Boone RH, Webb JG, Horlick E, et al. Transcatheter pulmonary valve implantation using the Edwards SAPIEN transcatheter heart valve. Catheter Cardiovasc Interv 2010;75: 286–94.
119. McElhinney DB, Hellenbrand WE, Zahn EM, et al. Short- and medium-term outcomes after transcatheter pulmonary valve placement in the expanded multicenter US melody valve trial. Circulation 2010;122:507–16.
120. Demkow M, Biernacka EK, Spiewak M, et al. Percutaneous pulmonary valve implantation preceded by routine prestenting with a bare metal stent. Catheter Cardiovasc Interv 2011;77:381–9.
121. Ewert P, Horlick E, Berger F. First implantation of the CE-marked transcatheter Sapien pulmonic valve in Europe. Clin Res Cardiol 2011;100:85–7.
122. Ma L, Tozzi P, Huber CH, et al. Double-crowned valved stents for off-pump mitral valve replacement. Eur J Cardiothorac Surg 2005;28:194–8; discussion 8–9.
123. Goetzenich A, Dohmen G, Hatam N, et al. A new approach to interventional atrioventricular valve therapy. J Thorac Cardiovasc Surg 2010;140:97–102.
124. Lozonschi L, Bombien R, Osaki S, et al. Transapical mitral valved stent implantation: a survival series in swine. J Thorac Cardiovasc Surg 2010;140:422–6 e1.
125. Maisano F, Torracca L, Oppizzi M, et al. The edge-to-edge technique: a simplified method to correct mitral insufficiency. Eur J Cardiothorac Surg 1998;13:240–5; discussion 5–6.
126. Feldman T, Wasserman HS, Herrmann HC, et al. Percutaneous mitral valve repair using the edge-to-edge technique: six-month results of the EVEREST Phase I Clinical Trial. J Am Coll Cardiol 2005;46:2134–40.
127. Feldman T, Kar S, Rinaldi M, et al. Percutaneous mitral repair with the MitraClip system: safety and midterm durability in the initial EVEREST (Endovascular Valve Edge-to-Edge REpair Study) cohort. J Am Coll Cardiol 2009;54:686–94.
128. Foster E, Wasserman HS, Gray W, et al. Quantitative assessment of severity of mitral regurgitation by serial echocardiography in a multicenter clinical trial of percutaneous mitral valve repair. Am J Cardiol 2007;100:1577–83.

129. Silvestry FE, Rodriguez LL, Herrmann HC, et al. Echocardiographic guidance and assessment of percutaneous repair for mitral regurgitation with the Evalve MitraClip: lessons learned from EVEREST I. J Am Soc Echocardiogr 2007;20:1131–40.

130. Duffy SJ, Federman J, Farrington C, et al. Feasibility and short-term efficacy of percutaneous mitral annular reduction for the therapy of functional mitral regurgitation in patients with heart failure. Catheter Cardiovasc Interv 2006;68:205–10.

131. Sack S, Kahlert P, Bilodeau L, et al. Percutaneous transvenous mitral annuloplasty: initial human experience with a novel coronary sinus implant device. Circ Cardiovasc Interv 2009;2:277–84.

132. Kaye DM, Byrne M, Alferness C, et al. Feasibility and short-term efficacy of percutaneous mitral annular reduction for the therapy of heart failure-induced mitral regurgitation. Circulation 2003;108:1795–7.

133. Schofer J, Siminiak T, Haude M, et al. Percutaneous mitral annuloplasty for functional mitral regurgitation: results of the CARILLON Mitral Annuloplasty Device European Union Study. Circulation 2009;120:326–33.

134. Tops LF, Van de Veire NR, Schuijf JD, et al. Noninvasive evaluation of coronary sinus anatomy and its relation to the mitral valve annulus: implications for percutaneous mitral annuloplasty. Circulation 2007;115:1426–32.

135. Webb JG, Harnek J, Munt BI, et al. Percutaneous transvenous mitral annuloplasty: initial human experience with device implantation in the coronary sinus. Circulation 2006;113:851–5.

136. Choure AJ, Garcia MJ, Hesse B, et al. In vivo analysis of the anatomical relationship of coronary sinus to mitral annulus and left circumflex coronary artery using cardiac multidetector computed tomography: implications for percutaneous coronary sinus mitral annuloplasty. J Am Coll Cardiol 2006;48:1938–45.

137. Tibayan FA, Rodriguez F, Liang D, et al. Paneth suture annuloplasty abolishes acute ischemic mitral regurgitation but preserves annular and leaflet dynamics. Circulation 2003;108(Suppl 1):II128–33.

138. Grossi EA, Patel N, Woo YJ, et al. Outcomes of the RESTOR-MV Trial (Randomized Evaluation of a Surgical Treatment for Off-Pump Repair of the Mitral Valve). J Am Coll Cardiol 2010;56:1984–93.

139. Rihal CS, Sorajja P, Booker JD, et al. Principles of percutaneous paravalvular leak closure. JACC Cardiovasc Interv 2012;5:121–30.

140. Kronzon I, Sugeng L, Perk G, et al. Real-time 3-dimensional transesophageal echocardiography in the evaluation of post-operative mitral annuloplasty ring and prosthetic valve dehiscence. J Am Coll Cardiol 2009;53:1543–7.

141. Hamilton-Craig C, Boga T, Platts D, et al. The role of 3D transesophageal echocardiography during percutaneous closure of paravalvular mitral regurgitation. JACC Cardiovasc Imaging 2009;2:771–3.

142. Garcia-Fernandez MA, Cortes M, Garcia-Robles JA, et al. Utility of real-time three-dimensional transesophageal echocardiography in evaluating the success of percutaneous transcatheter closure of mitral paravalvular leaks. J Am Soc Echocardiogr 2010;23:26–32.

143. Ruiz CE, Jelnin V, Kronzon I, et al. Clinical outcomes in patients undergoing percutaneous closure of periprosthetic paravalvular leaks. J Am Coll Cardiol 2011;58:2210–7.

144. Sorajja P, Cabalka AK, Hagler DJ, et al. Percutaneous repair of paravalvular prosthetic regurgitation: acute and 30-day outcomes in 115 patients. Circ Cardiovasc Interv 2011;4:314–21.

145. Latib A, Ielasi A, Montorfano M, et al. Transcatheter valve-in-valve implantation with the Edwards SAPIEN in patients with bioprosthetic heart valve failure: the Milan experience. EuroIntervention 2012;7:1275–84.

146. Webb JG, Wood DA, Ye J, et al. Transcatheter valve-in-valve implantation for failed bioprosthetic heart valves. Circulation 2010;121:1848–57.

147. Nordmeyer J, Coats L, Lurz P, et al. Percutaneous pulmonary valve-in-valve implantation: a successful treatment concept for early device failure. Eur Heart J 2008;29:810–5.

148. Hon JK, Cheung A, Ye J, et al. Transatrial transcatheter tricuspid valve-in-valve implantation of balloon expandable bioprosthesis. Ann Thorac Surg 2010;90:1696–7.

149. Elmariah S, Arzamendi D, Llanos A, et al. First experience with transcatheter valve-in-valve implantation for a stenotic mitral prosthesis within the United States. JACC Cardiovasc Interv 2012;5:e13–4.

150. Michelena HI, Alli O, Cabalka AK, et al. Successful percutaneous transvenous antegrade mitral valve-in-valve implantation. Catheter Cardiovasc Interv 2012.

151. Seiffert M, Conradi L, Baldus S, et al. Transcatheter mitral valve-in-valve implantation in patients with degenerated bioprostheses. JACC Cardiovasc Interv 2012;5:341–9.

152. De Vroey F, Legget M, Ormiston J, et al. "Valve in valve" percutaneous aortic valve implantation for severe mixed bioprosthetic aortic valve disease. N Z Med J 2012;125:146–8.

CHAPTER 17

Rheumatic Mitral Valve Disease

Bernard Iung and Alec Vahanian

Key Points

- Despite the decrease in the incidence of rheumatic heart diseases, mitral stenosis (MS) remains prevalent in industrialized countries. It is frequent and underdiagnosed in developing countries.
- Clinical assessment is paramount to detect MS in asymptomatic patients and to evaluate symptoms.
- Planimetry using two-dimensional echocardiography is the reference measurement for valve area.
- Intervention is needed in symptomatic patients who have MS with a valve area <1.5 cm^2.
- Balloon mitral valvotomy can be considered in selected asymptomatic patients who have MS with a valve area <1.5 cm^2, in particular those who have a high risk for thromboembolism.
- The choice between balloon mitral valvotomy and surgery should be individualized and based not only on valve anatomy but also on other clinical and echocardiographic characteristics.
- Balloon mitral valvotomy and surgery are complementary techniques, which should be used at different times of the evolution of MS.

Despite the decrease in the incidence of rheumatic heart disease, MS remains prevalent, even in industrialized countries. The main purpose of investigation of MS is to determine the optimal timing of intervention as well as the most appropriate treatment—percutaneous technique or surgery. The treatment of this disease has been reoriented with the development of balloon mitral valvotomy. Large series reporting long-term follow-up after the procedure have contributed to improvement in the level of evidence of decision making for interventions in MS, as attested by contemporary guidelines.

Pathophysiology

Mechanisms of Valve Obstruction

Unlike other heart valve diseases, mitral stenosis (MS) remains, in most cases, a consequence of rheumatic fever.[1] The main mechanism of stenosis is commissural fusion. Posterior leaflet thickening and restriction are almost constant but have limited hemodynamic consequences. Thickening and rigidity of the anterior leaflet and/or the subvalvular apparatus can also contribute to stenosis (Figure 17-1).[2] Commissural fusion explains why the area of the mitral orifice is relatively constant in severe stenosis, whereas it may vary according to flow conditions once commissures have been opened after balloon mitral valvotomy (BMV).[3]

Degenerative mitral annular calcification occurs frequently in the elderly. It has few or no hemodynamic consequences in most

patients, but obstruction may appear over time.[4] Significant stenosis seldom occurs and is related to restriction of both leaflets due to extensive calcification, without commissural fusion.

Other etiologies are rare. Congenital MS is mainly the consequence of abnormalities of the subvalvular apparatus. Inflammatory diseases (e.g., systemic lupus erythematosus), infiltrative diseases, carcinoid heart disease, and drug-induced valve diseases are characterized by a predominance of leaflet thickening and restriction but seldom with fusion of commissures.

The predominance of rheumatic etiology explains why the prevalence of MS has decreased in industrialized countries.[1] However, it still accounts for approximately 10% of native valve diseases and affects young immigrants or old patients.[5] Conversely, the prevalence of rheumatic heart disease remains sustained in developing countries, being estimated as between 1 and 7 per 1000 in children according to clinical data, and 10 times higher with systematic echocardiographic screening.[6,7]

Hemodynamic Consequences of Mitral Stenosis

MITRAL GRADIENT

The first consequence of MS is the increase in diastolic mitral pressure gradient, which depends on mitral valve area but also on other factors such as transvalvular flow and heart rate.[8] For a given valve area, mean mitral gradient increases when cardiac output increases or when tachycardia reduces the length of the diastolic filling period. Atrial contraction contributes to the increase of transmitral flow in end-diastole and, therefore, of mitral gradient. Severe MS may thus be associated with low mitral gradient in patients with low cardiac output, in particular those who are in chronic atrial fibrillation.

LEFT ATRIUM

Mitral gradient causes an increase in left atrial pressure. Chronic left atrial pressure overload leads to enlargement of the left atrium, according to the severity and chronicity of MS, although it is subject to important interpatient variability. Atrial enlargement favors the occurrence of atrial fibrillation.

The other consequences of MS are blood stasis in the left atrium and, upstream, the decrease in systolic pulmonary vein flow. The severity of blood stasis can be assessed with the use of Doppler echocardiography from the intensity of left atrial spontaneous echo contrast and the decrease in flow velocities in the left atrial appendage in patients in sinus rhythm. Blood stasis and left atrial appendage flow velocities are considerably impaired when

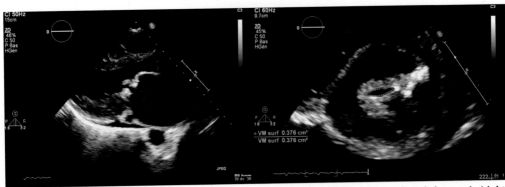

FIGURE 17-1   Severe mitral stenosis. Transthoracic echocardiography: parasternal long-axis *(left panel)* and short-axis *(right panel)* views. Valve area is 0.4 cm². Leaflet tips are thickened but anterior leaflet is pliable. Subvalvular apparatus is severely impaired with shortened and fused chordae. Both leaflets are moderately thickened with a pliable anterior leaflet on the long-axis view and fusion of both commissures on the short-axis view. There is a dense nodule of the internal commissure.

atrial fibrillation occurs, thereby increasing the risk of thrombosis. The left atrial appendage is the most common location of left atrial thrombus.[9]

Thrombus formation may also be favored by local abnormalities of hemostasis, in particular the increase in fibrinopeptide A and thrombin–antithrombin III complex.[10]

PULMONARY CIRCULATION

A constant mechanism of pulmonary hypertension in MS is the passive rise in pulmonary artery pressure following the increase in left atrial pressure. In addition, pulmonary hypertension can be worsened in certain patients by an increase in pulmonary vascular resistance, which determines a gradient larger than 10 mm Hg between diastolic pulmonary pressure and left atrial pressure. Increased pulmonary vascular resistance involves vasoconstriction and structural changes of the pulmonary arterial wall and explains the possibility of persistent pulmonary hypertension after intervention in MS.[11]

Vasoconstriction seems to involve endothelium-dependent vascular tone regulation, as shown by the decrease in pulmonary vascular resistance after inhaled nitric oxide and the probable synthesis of endothelin-1 in the pulmonary circulation.[11,12]

The sequence of histologic changes in pulmonary hypertension due to MS is characterized initially by medial thickening in muscular arteries and arterioles, followed by intimal thickening.[13] These changes are likely to be reversible with a decrease in pulmonary pressures. More severe pulmonary hypertension is associated with fibrinoid necrosis and arteritis, loss of smooth muscle cell nuclei, fibrin deposition in the arterial wall, and the presence of inflammatory cells. The pathologic hallmark of end-stage, irreversible pulmonary hypertension is the plexiform lesion, which consists of aneurysmal dilation of the arterial wall with a plexus of glomus-like, thin-walled channels branching to join with adjacent capillaries. Nonspecific parenchymal changes in severe pulmonary hypertension include pulmonary hemosiderosis and cholesterol granuloma formation.

In a multivariate analysis comprising 744 patients with severe MS, factors associated with pulmonary vascular bed gradient were mitral gradient, left ventricular end-diastolic pressure, mitral valve area, and a history of chronic pulmonary disease.[14] These numerous factors explain the wide range in pulmonary pressures for any given degree of MS.

RIGHT HEART

Chronic pulmonary hypertension leads to right ventricular hypertrophy, right ventricular dilation, and right heart failure. This process may be exacerbated by significant tricuspid regurgitation due either to rheumatic involvement of the tricuspid valve or to annular dilation secondary to right ventricular enlargement. Although pulmonary hypertension presumably is the cause of right heart dysfunction, there is a poor correlation between pulmonary pressures and right ventricular failure in patients with MS.

LEFT VENTRICLE

Left ventricular size is generally normal or moderately reduced in MS.

The main consequence of MS in the left ventricle is impaired diastolic filling. In comparison with normal subjects, patients with MS have a prolongation of early diastolic filling and an increased contribution of left atrial contraction. This finding explains why hemodynamics are severely impaired when atrial fibrillation occurs with loss of atrial contraction. Left ventricular filling may also be impaired by abnormal septal motion due to RV pressure or volume overload.

Although left ventricular contractility typically is normal in isolated MS, forward stroke volume may be reduced because of low filling volumes across the stenotic mitral valve. In addition, left ventricular ejection fraction is impaired in 5% to 10% of patients with MS in the absence of another cause, in particular other valve or coronary artery disease.[15] This impairment does not seem to be explained by abnormal loading conditions because left ventricular dysfunction generally persists after the relief of MS.

Early diastolic filling is prolonged with the slow rate of increase in ventricular volumes. Atrial fibrillation further alters diastolic filling through loss of effective atrial contraction.

Exercise Physiology

Hemodynamic changes during exercise provide additional insights into the multiple factors interacting with the severity of the stenosis to determine its repercussions. The increase in transmitral gradient at exercise is the consequence of the shortening of the diastolic filling period, and it causes an upstream increase in pulmonary artery pressure. However, changes in mitral gradient and pulmonary artery pressure are highly variable for a given degree of stenosis.[16] This heterogeneity may be explained by differences in the evolution of stroke volume during exercise and by differences in atrioventricular compliance.[17,18]

An increase in stroke volume at exercise, as also occurs in normal patients, is associated with an increase in mitral valve area during exercise in patients who have a moderate impairment of valve anatomy. Conversely, in patients with a severe impairment of valve anatomy, stroke volume does not increase or even decreases during exercise. Net atrioventricular compliance is the strongest determinant of left atrial and pulmonary artery pressures at rest, stronger than valve area, gradient, and pulmonary vascular resistance.[19] A low net compliance is mainly the consequence of a low compliance of the left atrium and is also associated, even more than at rest, with a higher pulmonary artery pressure at exercise and more severe symptoms.[18]

Clinical Presentation

History

Dyspnea, the most frequent symptom of MS, also has a prognostic value. It may be difficult to assess given the progressive course of the disease. Patients frequently adapt their level of activity to their functional capacity and do not complain of dyspnea despite objective effort limitation. This fact underlines the need for a careful discussion with the patient and relatives, taking into account the patient's lifestyle and comparing the evolution of activity levels over time. Paroxysmal dyspnea should always be looked for because it could be triggered not only by paroxysmal atrial fibrillation, but also by emotional stress, sexual intercourse, or fever, even in patients with few or no symptoms at exercise. Paroxysmal cough or hemoptysis occurs more seldom but should be sought particularly in the young during effort.

Patients sometimes complain more of fatigue rather than of dyspnea, in particular older patients and/or those who have advanced heart disease with chronic atrial fibrillation. Asthenia and abdominal pain are suspicious for right heart failure. It is now unusual to observe hoarseness due to compression of the left recurrent laryngeal nerve by the enlarged left atrium.

Complications, such as atrial fibrillation, or embolic events may reveal MS in previously asymptomatic patients. Pregnancy is a common cause of decompensation of a previously well-tolerated MS, because the increases in cardiac output and tachycardia cause sharp increases in mitral gradient and pulmonary artery pressure during the second trimester.

The search for comorbidity is important in elderly patients, who account for a growing proportion of patients with MS in developed countries.[20,21]

Physical Examination

Auscultation reveals a loud first heart sound, an opening snap in early diastole just after the second heart sound, followed by a holodiastolic rumbling murmur that decreases in intensity with time and increases in end-diastole in patients in sinus rhythm (Figure 17-2). The murmur is often difficult to identify because it is localized and of low acoustic frequency. Thus, careful auscultation is needed, using the bell of the stethoscope in different points around the apex with the patient in the left lateral decubitus position.

The loudness of the murmur depends on the intensity of the transmitral gradient. A loud murmur with a thrill suggests severe stenosis. Conversely, a low-intensity murmur does not exclude severe stenosis in patients with low cardiac output. The duration of the interval between the second aortic sound and the opening snap is shortened in severe stenosis because increased left atrial pressure causes earlier opening of the mitral valve.[8] The intensity of the first sound and the opening snap may be diminished in cases of extensive calcification that limits leaflet motion.

Auscultation should also search for a holosystolic murmur at the apex, which suggests combined mitral regurgitation (MR) and MS. The holosystolic murmur of tricuspid regurgitation is usually located at the xiphoid but may be heard near the apex when the right ventricle is enlarged. It is differentiated from a murmur of MR by its respiratory variation. It is of importance to pay attention even to low-intensity midsystolic murmur attesting to associated aortic stenosis, the severity of which tends to be underestimated in combined MS and MR.

A diastolic murmur at the left sternal border is more likely to be the consequence of aortic rather than pulmonic regurgitation. The second pulmonary sound is louder in pulmonary hypertension.

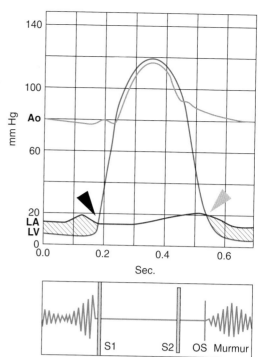

FIGURE 17-2 Correspondence between hemodynamics and auscultation of mitral stenosis. The diastolic rumbling murmur corresponds to the pressure gradient between the left atrium and left ventricle (in *gray*). Murmur intensity decreases progressively and is reinforced in end-diastole with atrial contraction. Intensity of the first heart sound (S1) is increased. The interval between the second heart sound (S2) and the opening snap (OS) decreases as mitral stenosis becomes more severe. *Black arrowhead* indicates mitral valve closure and *gray arrowhead* indicates mitral valve opening. *Ao,* Aortic pressure; *LA,* left atrial pressure; *LV,* left ventricular pressure.

Auscultation is also the first means of detecting arrhythmias, which should be confirmed by electrocardiogram.

Clinical signs of left-sided heart failure, in particular pulmonary rales, are present in patients with severe symptoms. Signs of right heart failure are observed in patients with severe and, often, long-standing disease, including hepatomegaly, which may be expansive in cases of severe tricuspid regurgitation; peripheral edema; and jugular distention, which is the most specific sign. "Mitral facies" is characterized by patchy flushing of the cheeks and has become rare because it is encountered in patients with long-standing untreated MS.

Chest Radiography and Electrocardiography

The first abnormality of the cardiac silhouette on chest radiography is left atrial enlargement, characterized by left atrial double density and prominence of the left atrial appendage. Pulmonary hypertension causes dilation of the pulmonary artery trunk and branches. Heart size is normal at this stage. Severe chronic MS leads to right ventricular and right atrial enlargement and cardiomegaly. Pulmonary vascular redistribution and, later, interstitial edema are radiographic signs of elevated left atrial pressure (Figure 17-3), which are often seen even in patients with moderate symptoms and without clinical signs of heart failure. Alveolar edema is a sign of acute hemodynamic decompensation. Transverse chest radiograph is useful to diagnose right ventricular enlargement, mild pleural effusion, and mitral valve calcification, which is detected by fluoroscopy with a higher sensitivity.

Left atrial enlargement is the only electrocardiographic abnormality at an early stage. Right atrial and right ventricular enlargements with right axis deviation and right bundle branch block are observed in more advanced diseases with severe and/or long-standing pulmonary hypertension. Electrocardiography plays a

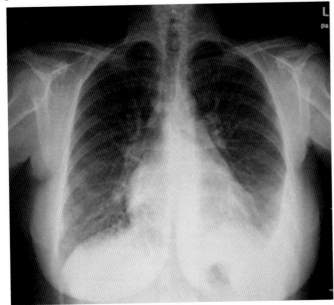

FIGURE 17-3   Chest radiograph in a patient with mitral stenosis. Left atrium and pulmonary trunk are enlarged. There is marked pulmonary congestion with interstitial pulmonary edema and left pleural effusion.

TABLE 17-1	Classification of Mitral Stenosis Severity: European Association of Echocardiography/ American Society of Echocardiography Recommendations for Clinical Practice		
		Significant	
	MILD	**MODERATE**	**SEVERE**
Specific findings: Valve area (cm²)	>1.5	1.0-1.5	<1.0
Supportive findings: Mean gradient (mm Hg)* Systolic pulmonary artery pressure (mm Hg)	<5 <30	5-10 30-50	>10 >50

Adapted from Baumgartner H, Hung J, Bermejo J, et al. Echocardiographic assessment of valve stenosis: EAE/ASE recommendations for clinical practice. J Am Soc Echocardiogr 2009;22:1-23.
*At heart rates between 60 and 80 beats/min and in sinus rhythm.

major role in the detection of atrial arrhythmias; that is, frequent atrial premature beats and transient or persistent atrial fibrillation or, less frequently, atrial flutter or atrial tachycardia.

Echocardiography

Echocardiography is the cornerstone in the evaluation of suspected or known MS and is used to confirm the diagnosis, evaluate the severity and consequences of valve lesions, and assess valve anatomy and associated diseases.[22] Echocardiographic techniques are detailed in Chapter 6.

The diagnostic features are leaflet thickening and decreased mobility, commissural fusion, and involvement of the subvalvular apparatus.

ASSESSMENT OF SEVERITY

A parasternal short-axis view enables planimetry to be performed, which is the reference measurement of mitral valve area.[23] Its advantage is that it is the only direct measurement of valve area, thereby being independent of loading conditions and associated heart diseases. However, technical expertise is needed to scan the mitral valve apparatus to position the measurement plan on the leaflet tip. Positioning the measurement plan can be facilitated with the use of three-dimensional (3D) echocardiography, which improves reproducibility in this setting, particularly when performed by less experienced echocardiographers.[24-26] Planimetry is also useful during balloon mitral valvotomy to monitor the procedure and immediately after balloon mitral valvotomy, when it is the most reliable technique. However, planimetry may be difficult, even not feasible, in the case of an irregular and heavily calcified orifice or in patients with poor echogenicity.

Besides planimetry, the parasternal short-axis view assesses commissural fusion. This assessment is of particular importance to differentiate rheumatic MS from MS of other etiologies, in particular degenerative MS, in which commissures are not fused, and to determine the feasibility of balloon or surgical valvotomy. The assessment of commissural opening is also an additional indication of the efficacy of balloon mitral valvotomy during and after the procedure as well as during late follow-up. The assessment of commissural opening is more accurate with 3D than with two-dimensional (2D) echocardiography.[26]

The pressure half-time method is generally easier to perform and is therefore widely used. However, it may be misleading in cases of aortic regurgitation, in abnormal compliance of cardiac chambers, and immediately after balloon mitral valvotomy.[23] The most important discrepancies with planimetry are observed in patients older than 60 years and in those in atrial fibrillation.[27]

The use of the continuity equation to assess valve area is not valid in cases of associated significant mitral or aortic regurgitation. The method's accuracy and reproducibility are limited given the number of measurements involved.[23]

The proximal isovelocity surface area is technically demanding and requires multiple measurements. Its accuracy can be improved with the use of M-mode echocardiography.[28]

Mean mitral gradient, as assessed by pulsed or continuous wave Doppler echocardiography, is not a reliable means to assess the severity of MS because it is highly dependent on flow conditions. However, the gradient value should be consistent with the valve area value, and it has prognostic value after balloon mitral valvotomy.

The consistency of results of planimetry, pressure half-time method, and gradient should always be checked, with the limitations of the different measurements kept in mind.[23,29,30] The continuity equation and proximal isovelocity surface area are not used routinely but may be useful when other methods lead to uncertain or discordant findings.

Mitral valve area is considered significant when valve area is less than 1.5 cm² and severe when it is 1 cm².[23,29,30] A valve area of 1.5 cm² corresponds to the value above which hemodynamics are not affected at rest. The interpretation of valve area should take body size into account, even if no definite value indexed on body surface area is advised in guidelines (Table 17-1).

Mitral valve resistance has been proposed as an alternative measurement of the severity of valve obstruction.[23,31] Although it is a good predictor of pulmonary artery pressure, mitral valve resistance has not superceded valve area as the marker of MS severity.

ASSESSMENT OF VALVE MORPHOLOGY

The analysis of the morphology of valve leaflets and subvalvular apparatus using two-dimensional echocardiography is a key feature of diagnosis of MS and has important implications for the potential of progression and, in particular, the choice of the most appropriate intervention when needed.[23]

Echocardiographic evaluation assesses leaflet thickening (significant if greater than or equal to 5 mm), leaflet mobility on the long-axis parasternal view, and calcification, which is best confirmed by fluoroscopic examination. The parasternal short-axis view is paramount not only for planimetry, but also to evaluate the homogeneity of the impairment of the mitral orifice, with

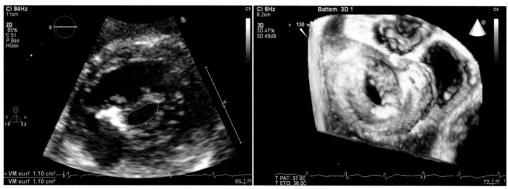

FIGURE 17-4   Mitral stenosis with calcification of the external commissure. *Left panel,* Two-dimensional echocardiography, parasternal short-axis view. *Right panel,* Three-dimensional echocardiography, view from the left atrium.

TABLE 17-2   Assessment of Mitral Valve Anatomy According to the Wilkins Score*

GRADE	MOBILITY	THICKENING	CALCIFICATION	SUBVALVULAR THICKENING
1	Highly mobile valve with only leaflet tips restricted	Leaflets near normal in thickness (4-5 mm)	A single area of increased echocardiographic brightness	Minimal thickening just below the mitral leaflets
2	Leaflet mid and base portions have normal mobility	Mid-leaflets normal, considerable thickening of margins (5-8 mm)	Scattered areas of brightness confined to leaflet margins	Thickening of chordal structures extending to one of the chordal length
3	Valve continues to move forward in diastole, mainly from the base	Thickening extending through the entire leaflet (5-8 mm)	Brightness extending into the mid-portions of the leaflets	Thickening extended to distal third of the chords
4	No or minimal forward movement of the leaflets in diastole	Considerable thickening of all leaflet tissue (>8-10 mm)	Extensive brightness throughout much of the leaflet tissue	Extensive thickening and shortening of all chordal structures extending down to the papillary muscles

From Wilkins GT, Weyman AE, Abascal VM, et al. Percutaneous balloon dilatation of the mitral valve: an analysis of echocardiographic variables related to outcome and the mechanism of dilatation. Br Heart J 1988;60:299–308.
*The total score is the sum of the four items and ranges between 4 and 16.

focus on commissural areas (Figure 17-4). Long-axis parasternal and apical views enable impairment of subvalvular apparatus (thickening and/or shortening of chordae) to be assessed, although it tends to be underestimated in comparison with anatomic findings.

The severity of valvular and subvalvular involvement usually is described by a combined score. The Wilkins score grades each of the following components of mitral apparatus from 1 to 4: leaflet mobility, thickness, calcification, and impairment of subvalvular apparatus (Table 17-2).[32] The final scores range from 4 to 16. An alternative approach, described by Cormier et al,[33,34] is to assess the whole mitral valve anatomy according to the best surgical alternative, which leads to classification in one of three groups (Table 17-3).

These two scoring systems share limitations related to the lack of a detailed location of calcification and leaflet thickening, particularly particular in relation to commissural areas, which are likely to influence the results of balloon mitral valvotomy.[35-39] In addition, they both tend to underestimate the weight of subvalvular apparatus impairment.[40] Other scoring systems include a more detailed approach, some of which aim to achieve a better prediction of the results of balloon mitral valvotomy.[23,41] However, in addition to concerns related to their reproducibility, they still lack validation in large prospective series and so are not widely used in current practice. Thus, no comparative evaluation of different scoring systems enables a particular one to be recommended.[42] In addition, it is unlikely that a single scoring system could combine reproducibility and accurate prediction of the results of mitral valvotomy. It is advised that the echocardiographer use a method with which he or she is familiar and include the assessment of valve morphology among other clinical and echocardiographic findings.

TABLE 17-3   Assessment of Mitral Valve Anatomy According to the Cormier Score

ECHOCARDIOGRAPHIC GROUP	MITRAL VALVE ANATOMY
1	Pliable noncalcified anterior mitral leaflet and mild subvalvular disease (i.e., thin chordae ≥10 mm long)
2	Pliable noncalcified anterior mitral leaflet and severe subvalvular disease (i.e., thickened chordae <10 mm long)
3	Calcification of mitral valve of any extent, as assessed by fluoroscopy, whatever the state of subvalvular apparatus

Data from Cormier B, Vahanian A, Michel PL, et al. Evaluation by two-dimensional and Doppler echocardiography of the results of percutaneous mitral valvuloplasty. Arch Mal Coeur Vaiss 1989;82:185-191; and Vahanian A, Michel PL, Cormier B, et al. Results of percutaneous mitral commissurotomy in 200 patients. Am J Cardiol 1989;63:847–52.

CONSEQUENCES OF MITRAL STENOSIS

The quantitation of left atrial enlargement using time-motion measurement is the most widely used but lacks accuracy. The estimation of left atrial area or, better, volume using two-dimensional echocardiography is preferred (Figure 17-5).[43,44]

Systolic pulmonary artery pressure is estimated from the velocity of Doppler echocardiograph measurement of tricuspid flow. Diastolic and mean pulmonary artery pressures can be derived from pulmonary flow.

CH
17

MITRAL REGURGITATION

The quantitation of associated MR should combine different semiquantitative and quantitative measurements and check their consistency. An accurate evaluation using quantitative methods is of particular importance for moderate regurgitation because it may have important implications in the choice of the type of intervention.[45]

ASSOCIATED LESIONS

Rheumatic aortic valve disease is frequently associated with MS. Decreased stroke volume due to MS may lead to underestimation of aortic stenosis because of a low gradient. Valve area should be quantitated with the continuity equation and/or planimetry of the aortic valve.

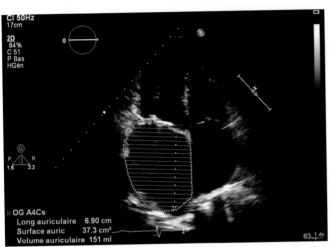

FIGURE 17-5 Left atrial volume measurement. Apical four-chamber view of the left atrium with traced contour to determine left atrial area and volume. Left atrial area is 37 cm², and volume is 151 mL.

Functional tricuspid regurgitation is caused by enlargement of right cavities secondary to pulmonary hypertension without rheumatic lesions of the valve. The quantitation of tricuspid regurgitation is less well established than that of left-sided heart valve regurgitation and is highly dependent on loading conditions. The diameter of the tricuspid annulus seems to be a better marker of the persistence of severe tricuspid regurgitation after the treatment of MS.[45,46] However, further standardization of its measurement is needed. Rheumatic tricuspid disease is less frequent. It is characterized by thickening and decreased mobility of tricuspid leaflets and may combine stenosis and regurgitation.

THROMBOEMBOLIC RISK

Transesophageal echocardiography (TEE) has a much higher sensitivity than transthoracic echocardiography to detect left atrial thrombus, in particular that located in the left atrial appendage. TEE is therefore mandatory before BMV. TEE is also useful to assess left atrial spontaneous echo contrast, which is a strong predictor of thromboembolic risk in patients with MS.[47]

Stress Testing

Semisupine bicycle ergometry enables hemodynamic changes to be sequentially assessed for increasing workload, in particular mean mitral gradient and estimated systolic pulmonary artery pressure (Figure 17-6). It is useful in patients whose symptoms are equivocal or are discordant with the severity of MS. However, thresholds of mitral gradient and pulmonary artery pressure, as stated in guidelines to consider intervention in asymptomatic patients, rely on low levels of evidence and are frequently achieved in practice.[23]

Dobutamine stress echocardiography, although less physiologic than exercise echocardiography, increases mean gradient and systolic pulmonary artery pressure.[23] It has been shown to have a prognostic value in one study.[48]

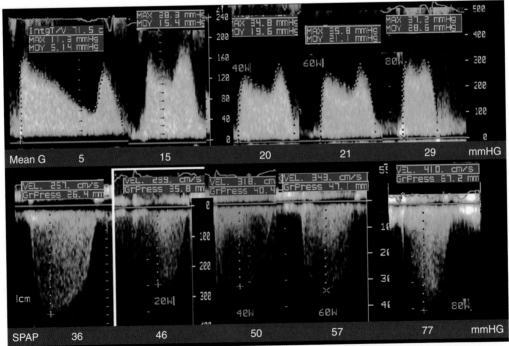

FIGURE 17-6 Exercise echocardiography in mitral stenosis. Monitoring of mitral gradient *(upper panel)* and pulmonary artery pressure *(lower panel)* at rest and at *(from left to right)* 20, 40, 60, and 80 watts with bicycle exercise in a semisupine position. *Mean G,* Mean mitral gradient; *SPAP,* systolic pulmonary artery pressure. *(Courtesy Dr Brochet.)*

Other Noninvasive Investigations

Preliminary reports suggest that cardiac magnetic resonance and multislice computed tomography are reliable alternate techniques for performing planimetry of the mitral valve.[49,50] Although the availability of such techniques is limited, they may be helpful when echocardiographic imaging is of poor quality.

Cardiac Catheterization

There is now little interest in the use of right and left heart cardiac catheterization to calculate mitral valve area using the Gorlin formula. The validity of the Gorlin formula is questionable when cardiac output is decreased and immediately after balloon mitral valvotomy.[51] Thus, invasive evaluation of the severity of MS is justified in only cases in which echocardiography results are inconclusive.[23,29,30]

Cardiac catheterization remains, however, the only technique for calculating pulmonary vascular resistance, which may be useful to assess the risk of surgery in patients with severe pulmonary hypertension. In current practice, the main indication for invasive investigations is the assessment of associated coronary disease with coronary angiography. Monitoring of the results of balloon mitral valvotomy now relies mainly on per-procedure echocardiography, in particular when the Inoue stepwise technique is used.

Natural History

Onset and Progression of Valvular Lesions

The development of MS takes many years following acute rheumatic fever. It is difficult to evaluate the course of the disease because rheumatic fever is not always diagnosed, is often subject to recurrences, and is subject to highly variable evolution according to the country considered. A majority of patients with initial rheumatic carditis eventually have chronic rheumatic valve disease. A prospective study using echocardiography identified three risk factors for progression toward chronic rheumatic valve disease: the severity of carditis, recurrences of acute rheumatic fever, and mother's low educational level.[52] The course of the disease is particularly rapid in countries where rheumatic fever is endemic, leading to severe MS in young adults, adolescents, and even children. Conversely, MS frequently occurs in adults older than 50 years in western countries. This is illustrated by series of balloon mitral valvotomy, in which mean patient age is around 30 years in Asia and North Africa but between 40 and 60 years in series from Europe and the United States.[53]

The progression of MS has been evaluated in series involving serial hemodynamic or echocardiographic evaluations.[54-56] They are subject to bias because all of them were retrospective and included a limited number of patients. They reported an average decrease of 0.01 cm²/year, although this figure reflects a mix between patients in whom valve area remains stable, accounting for between one and two thirds, and patients experiencing progression with an annual decrease in valve area ranging between 0.1 and 0.3 cm². Impairment of valve anatomy (Wilkins score ≥8) and a peak mitral gradient of 10 mm Hg or greater were identified as predictors of a more rapid progression of MS.[55] A nonrandomized study suggested that the use of statin drugs may slow the progression of MS.[57]

Clinical Outcome without Intervention

As in other valve diseases, studies on the natural history of MS are frequently old, retrospective, and subject to inclusion bias. Despite these limitations, which may explain differences in estimations, there is an agreement on the poor prognosis of MS when patients become symptomatic, with 10-year survival rates ranging from 34% to 61% and 20-year rates between 14% and 21%.[58,59] A later series reported 44% survival at 5 years in patients refusing intervention.[60] Survival is highly influenced by the evolutionary stage of the disease, in particular symptoms and atrial fibrillation. Asymptomatic patients have a 20-year survival exceeding 80%, but approximately half of them become symptomatic after 10 years.[58] Clinical deterioration is sudden in approximately half of patients.

The leading cause of death is heart failure, in about 60% of patients, followed by thromboembolic complications in about 20%.[58]

Complications

Atrial fibrillation is a frequent complication of MS and it is largely related to left atrial enlargement. However, its frequency is only partly related to the severity of stenosis.[61] As in the general population, the frequency of atrial fibrillation is also strongly dependent on patient age.[20]

The use of systematic Holter electrocardiogram (ECG) monitoring in one study showed that half of patients with MS in sinus rhythm had atrial arrhythmias although 95% were asymptomatic; 14% of them presented embolic complications. The three predictive factors of atrial arrhythmias were age, left atrial diameter, and valve calcification.[62]

Atrial fibrillation considerably worsens the consequences of MS. The lack of atrial contraction and the shortening of the diastolic filling period further impair hemodynamics and may cause acute decompensation such as pulmonary edema. The other consequence is the increase in blood stasis in the left atrium, which increases the thromboembolic risk. The Framingham Heart Study[62a] estimated a 17-fold increase in the risk of stroke in patients with atrial fibrillation and MS, compared with a 5-fold increase in risk for atrial fibrillation in the absence of mitral valve disease.

Annual linearized risk of thromboembolism in atrial fibrillation without anticoagulant therapy has been estimated to 3.6% for moderate MS and 5.7% for severe MS. The corresponding figures in patients in sinus rhythm were estimated to be 0.25% for moderate MS and 0.85% for severe MS.[60] In cases of atrial fibrillation, most embolic complications originate from left atrial thrombosis, which is located in the left atrial appendage. Embolic events are cerebral in location in 60% to 70% of cases, leave sequelae in 30% to 45% of cases, and are prone to recurrence.[63] Left atrial spontaneous echo contrast as assessed by TEE plays a particularly important role in risk stratification for thromboembolic risk in MS.[64]

Medical Therapy

The goals of medical therapy are to prevent rheumatic fever, to improve symptoms, and to decrease the thromboembolic risk. Medical therapy should be considered in conjunction with a close follow-up, enabling a timely intervention when needed.

Prevention of Rheumatic Fever

Primary prevention relies on adapted antibiotic treatment of streptococcal pharyngitis. Secondary prevention is based on the use of continuous antibiotic therapy.[65] Although painful, intramuscular injection of benzathine penicillin every 3 weeks has the advantage of a better compliance than daily oral treatment, in particular in young patients and in developing countries. Antibiotic prophylaxis of rheumatic fever treatment is advised for up to 25 years in patients with rheumatic carditis (see Chapter 9). Once rheumatic valve disease has occurred, no medical treatment has been shown to be able to slow the progression of MS.

The prevention of infective endocarditis has been recently reoriented toward reduced indications for antibiotic prophylaxis, which is no longer advised in native heart valve diseases. On the other hand, the importance of general hygiene measures is stressed, particularly dental and cutaneous hygiene.[66,67]

Treatment of Symptoms

The occurrence of dyspnea in a patient with MS should first lead to consideration of intervention. Medical treatment of symptomatic MS relies on diuretics to relieve congestion and beta-blockers to lengthen the diastolic filling period.

Beta-blockers are particularly useful in pregnant women, enabling a dramatic decrease in mean gradient and pulmonary artery pressure in most cases. However, beta-blockers do not seem to improve exercise tolerance in MS.[68,69]

In patients with MS and atrial fibrillation, restoration of sinus rhythm is superior to rate control as regards indices of functional capacity and quality of life.[70] When atrial fibrillation cannot be converted in sinus rhythm, rate control is obtained using digitalis and/or beta-blockers.

Prevention of Thromboembolism

Unlike in patients with nonvalvular atrial fibrillation, there are no randomized trials on the efficacy of anticoagulant therapy in patients with MS with or without atrial arrhythmias. Permanent or paroxysmal atrial fibrillation is a class I indication for oral anticoagulation, regardless of stenosis severity, in American College of Cardiology/American Heart Association (ACC/AHA) as well as European Society of Cardiology/European Association for Cardio-Thoracic Surgery (ESC/EACTS) guidelines.[29,30] In a retrospective study, oral anticoagulation decreased the annual risk of thromboembolism in patients with MS and atrial fibrillation from 5.7% to 1.0% for severe MS and from 3.6% to 0.9% for moderate MS.[60]

In patients with MS in sinus rhythm, the annual risk of thromboembolism decreased from 0.85% to 0.10% for severe MS and from 0.25% to 0.10% for moderate MS.[60] Given the risk of bleeding inherent to oral anticoagulation, the analysis of risk and benefits does not support systematic anticoagulant therapy in patients with MS in sinus rhythm. Anticoagulant therapy using vitamin K antagonists is advised in selected patients with MS in sinus rhythm who are at high risk for thromboembolic events according to the following criteria. Prior embolism and left atrial thrombus are class I recommendations for oral anticoagulation in ACC/AHA and ESC/EACTS guidelines. Dense spontaneous echo contrast and enlargement of the left atrium are class IIa recommendations in ESC/EACTS guidelines and class IIb recommendations in ACC/AHA guidelines. Target international normalized ratio is 2.5 (i.e., a range between 2.0 and 3.0). Aspirin or other antiplatelet drugs alone are not valid alternatives to decrease thromboembolic risk in patients with MS. Newer anticoagulants, such as dabigatran, rivaroxaban, and apixaban, cannot be recommended at present because patients with MS were excluded from trials comparing these drugs with warfarin for the prevention of embolism in atrial fibrillation.

A randomized trial found benefit in a combination of an antiplatelet drug with low-dose oral anticoagulation over conventional anticoagulation, but this finding requires further confirmation.[71]

Pharmacologic or electric cardioversion should be attempted in patients with nonsevere MS who have persistent atrial fibrillation. In patients with severe MS, cardioversion should be postponed after the intervention on the mitral valve, in most cases, because restoration of sinus rhythm is unlikely to be sustained in the absence of intervention.[30]

Modalities of Follow-Up

Follow-up timing should be adapted to the severity of MS, symptoms, and potential complications.

Clinical follow-up should search for symptoms and clinical signs of examination suggesting complications, in particular transient ischemic attacks, which may not be spontaneously reported by the patient. Auscultation may signal an increase in the severity of MS or arrhythmia.

In asymptomatic patients with significant MS in whom intervention is not planned, systematic clinical and echocardiographic follow-up is performed yearly. In patients with moderate MS, follow-up intervals can be longer, in particular as regards echocardiography, which may be performed at 2- or 3-year intervals.

The patient should be educated to identify interim changes in symptoms, which should lead to a prompt visit. Women should be informed of the risks inherent to pregnancy. Appropriate contraception is indicated, and balloon mitral valvotomy can be offered to patients who desire pregnancy and have MS and a valve area less than 1.5 cm^2, even without symptoms (see Chapter 27).

Follow-up should be adapted to circumstances that raise the risk of complications, such as pregnancy and infections. Repeated monthly echocardiographic examination intervals are useful during the second and third trimesters of pregnancy to monitor mean gradient and pulmonary artery pressure.[72]

Follow-up after successful balloon mitral valvotomy is the same as in asymptomatic patients. Its periodicity can be adapted through the use of a simple scoring system to estimate the probability of long-term event-free survival according to baseline patient characteristics and the results of balloon mitral valvotomy.[73] The intervals should be shorter when restenosis occurs.

Closed Surgical Commissurotomy

The initial surgical approach for the relief of MS, introduced in 1948, was "closed" commissurotomy—that is, dilation of the stenotic valve via the left atrium, without direct visualization of the valve. This procedure does not visualize the valve but also does not require cardiopulmonary bypass. The valve is dilated by the surgeon's finger or with a transventricular dilator inserted through the left atrial appendage and across the mitral valve. Disadvantages of this procedure are the risk of embolic events due to dislodging atrial thrombi, incomplete relief of MS, and induction of excessive MR due to tearing of the leaflets rather than opening of the fused commissures.

Closed mitral commissurotomy results in excellent relief of MS symptoms with an operative mortality averaging 3% to 4%.[74-77] Most patients have significant improvement in symptoms after closed mitral commissurotomy and have an average increase of 1.0 cm^2 in valve area.[74] Extensive calcification of the valve is associated with suboptimal hemodynamic results and poor clinical outcome.

Long-term outcome after closed commissurotomy is quite good, with 31% to 50% of patients requiring reoperation within 15 years of the initial procedure, and 76% within 20 years.[74-77] Recurrent symptoms most often are due to incomplete relief of MS at the initial procedure or a combination of worsened MR and residual MS, with restenosis after an initially successful procedure being the least common indication for reoperation.[78]

Predictors of late death after closed commissurotomy are age, male gender, and the presence of atrial fibrillation. Multivariate predictors of the need for subsequent valve replacement are functional class, mitral valve calcification and subvalvular fusion, and the adequacy of the initial surgical procedure.

This operation is effective and easily accessible, features that explain its widespread use until very recently in developing countries.

Open Surgical Commissurotomy

Open mitral commissurotomy is usually performed via a median sternotomy with the patient on full cardiopulmonary bypass. The mitral valve apparatus is directly visualized from the left atrium, with careful sharp dissection of the fused commissures under direct vision. In addition, the degree of valve opening can be further improved by release of fused chordae or correction of chordal shortening. If needed, an annuloplasty ring can be used to decrease the severity of coexisting MR.

Compared with closed commissurotomy, the advantages of the open procedure are the abilities to visualize the valve structure in detail and to perform a more directed surgical repair. The left atrium also can be evaluated more fully, allowing detection and removal of left atrial thrombus. As with the closed approach, the best hemodynamic results and long-term outcome are seen in patients with little valve calcification, flexible and mobile leaflets, and only minimal MR.

With appropriate patient selection and in experienced hands, open commissurotomy is feasible in 80% to 90% of referred subjects with an operative mortality of about 1%.[79] The hemodynamic results of open commissurotomy are at least equivalent to those of the closed technique, with valve area increasing by about 1.0 cm^2 on average. Long-term outcome after open surgical commissurotomy has been excellent, with survival rates of 80% to 90% at 10 years and around 40% at 20 years.[79,80]

Mitral Valve Replacement

Valve replacement uses mostly mechanical valves because of their greater durability in the mitral position and because most patients require long-term anticoagulation for atrial fibrillation.

Most studies reporting the operative mortality for mitral valve replacement include patients with both MS and regurgitation. Operative mortality ranges between 3% and 10% and correlates with age, functional class, pulmonary hypertension, and presence of coronary artery disease.[81,82]

Long-term outcome after valve replacement for MS depends on the durability, hemodynamics, and complications of the prosthetic valve; the risks of chronic anticoagulation; any residual anatomic or hemodynamic abnormalities secondary to MS, such as pulmonary hypertension, left atrial enlargement, atrial fibrillation, and right ventricular enlargement and dysfunction; and involvement of other valves by the rheumatic process.

Balloon Mitral Valvotomy

Balloon mitral valvotomy acts similarly to surgical commissurotomy by splitting the closed commissures.[83] Although the term "commissurotomy" may be appropriate, "valvotomy" is most often used for percutaneous balloon procedures. Sometimes the fracturing of calcification may play a role in specific circumstances.

Patient Selection

The application of balloon mitral valvotomy depends on three major factors: the patient's clinical condition, valve anatomy, and the experience of the medical and surgical teams of the institution concerned.

Evaluation of patient's clinical condition must take into account the degree of functional disability, the presence of contraindications to transseptal catheterization, and the alternative risk of surgery as a function of the underlying cardiac and noncardiac status. Exercise testing is recommended to show symptoms in asymptomatic patients or in those with doubtful symptoms.

Contraindications to transseptal catheterization include suspected left atrial thrombosis severe hemorrhagic disorder, and severe cardiothoracic deformity. Increased surgical risk could be of cardiac origin (previous surgical commissurotomy or aortic valve replacement) or extracardiac origin (comorbidity such as respiratory insufficiency, old age).

The first step in the evaluation of valve anatomy is to establish the severity of MS. The performance of balloon mitral valvotomy is usually restricted to patients with moderate to severe MS (valve area <1.5 cm^2).[29,30] However, to define a threshold of valve area above which balloon mitral valvotomy should not be performed is somewhat arbitrary because, in addition to measuring valve area, one must take into account body surface area, functional disability, and pulmonary pressures at rest and with exercise.

The assessment of anatomy also aims at establishing indications and prognostic considerations. It is critical to ensure that there are no anatomic contraindications to the technique. The first of these is the presence of left atrial thrombosis, which must be excluded by systematic performance of TEE a few days before the procedure. The second is the degree of MR. The third, the coexistence of another valve disease in the aorta or tricuspid valve, should be looked for.

For prognostic considerations, echocardiographic assessment allows the classification of patients into anatomic groups with a view to predicting the results. Most investigators use the Wilkins score,[32] whereas others, such as Cormier et al,[33,34] use a more general assessment of valve anatomy.[23,84] Controversy exists regarding the most effective echocardiography scoring system in the prediction of results of balloon mitral valvotomy. In fact, none of the scores available today has been shown to be superior to the others, and all echocardiographic classifications have the same limitations regarding the weight given the estimation of each lesion, their reproducibility, and the lack of assessment of localized changes in specific portions of the valve apparatus (leaflets, commissures), which may increase the risk of severe MR.[23] Other scores taking into account the uneven distribution of the anatomic deformities of the leaflets or the commissural area are promising, but their exact value needs to be validated in large series.[41,85]

Experience of the Medical and Surgical Teams

The incidence of technical failures and complications, particularly those related to transseptal catheterization, is clearly related to the operator's experience.[86] In addition to improvements in the management of the interventional procedure, experience improves the selection of patients by means of clinical evaluation and echocardiographic assessment.[87,88]

Even though the considerable simplification resulting from the use of the Inoue balloon may lead to a false sense of security during application of the technique, balloon mitral valvotomy clearly should be restricted to teams that have extensive experience with transseptal catheterization and are able to perform an adequate number of procedures. The interventionists who perform balloon mitral valvotomy must also be able to perform emergency pericardiocentesis. Immediate surgical backup does not seem to be necessary.

Technique

The transvenous or antegrade approach is the most widely used. Transseptal catheterization, which allows access to the left atrium, is the first step in the procedure and one of the most crucial. The retrograde technique without transseptal catheterization, whereby the balloon is introduced through the femoral artery, is currently very seldom used.[89]

The Inoue technique (Figure 17-7), the first to be developed, is now almost exclusively used. The Inoue balloon, which is made of nylon and rubber micromesh, is self-positioning and pressure extensible. The balloon has three distinct parts, each with a specific elasticity, which can be inflated sequentially. The Inoue balloon comes in four sizes, ranging from 24 to 30 mm, and each is pressure dependent, so that its diameter can be varied by up to 4 mm as required by circumstances. Balloon size is usually chosen according to the patient characteristics of height and body surface area.[90] The use of a stepwise dilation technique under echocardiographic guidance is recommended (Figure 17-8). The first inflation is performed to the minimum diameter of the balloon chosen. The balloon is then deflated and withdrawn into the left atrium. If MR has not increased and valve area is insufficient, the balloon is readvanced across the mitral valve, and inflation is repeated with the balloon diameter increased by 1 to 2 mm.

The other techniques, such as the double-balloon technique and its variant the multitrack balloons, are very seldom used in developing countries, where economic constraints lead to

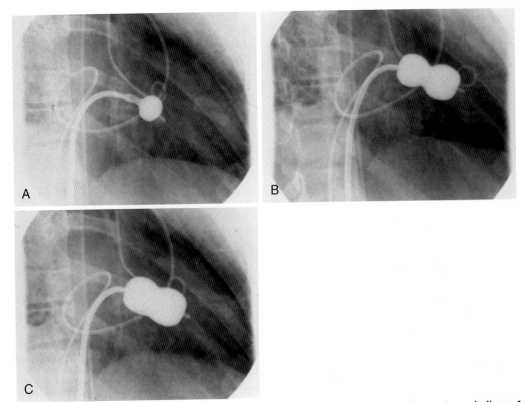

FIGURE 17-7   Balloon valvotomy. Fluoroscopic images recorded during a balloon mitral valvotomy using an Inoue balloon. A, The distal balloon has been inflated to secure the position at the valvular level. **B,** The proximal segment also has been inflated. **C,** The dilating segment is briefly inflated.

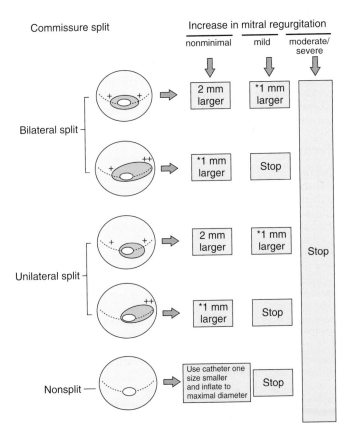

FIGURE 17-8   Algorithm for decision making during balloon valvotomy. The stepwise dilation technique using the Inoue balloon is modified according to echocardiographic findings after each balloon inflation. +, Incomplete split; ++, complete split; *, stop in cases of severely diseased valve or age >65 years. (*From Topol E. Textbook of interventional cardiology. 5th ed. Philadelphia: WB Saunders; 2008.*)

reuse of the balloons.[91] The metallic commissurotome is not largely used.[92]

In experienced teams, the use of TEE or intracardiac echocardiography is limited to the rare cases in which difficulty is encountered during transseptal catheterization or in particularly high-risk circumstances, such as severe cardiothoracic deformity or pregnancy.[93,94]

Monitoring of the Procedure and Assessment of Immediate Results

Two methods are used to assess immediate results in the catheterization laboratory: hemodynamics and echocardiography. Although echocardiography may be difficult to perform in the catheterization laboratory for logistic reasons, it provides essential information on the efficacy of the procedure and also enables early detection of complications. The evaluation of the results necessitates a combined analysis of the following:[23]

- Commissural opening shown by parasternal short-axis echocardiographic view; this can be done with two-dimensional transthoracic echocardiography or the newer three-dimensional real-time echocardiography.
- Measurement of valve area using planimetry, because pressure half-time measurement is not adequate in the acute setting.
- Measurement of the mean gradient.
- Evaluation of the presence and degree of MR assessed in several views with special attention to MR originating in the commissural areas.

The following criteria have been proposed for the desired end point of the procedure: (1) mitral valve area greater than 1 cm^2/m^2 of body surface area, (2) complete opening of at least one commissure, or (3) appearance or increment of regurgitation greater than a grade one classification in a four-grade system.[90] Tailoring the strategy to the individual circumstances is important; clinical factors as well as anatomic factors and the cumulative data of periprocedural monitoring should be taken into account. For example, balloon size, increments of size, and expected final valve area are smaller in elderly patients; in patients with very tight MS or extensive valve and subvalvular disease; and in patients with nodular calcification.

Immediately after the procedure, the most accurate evaluation of valve area is provided by planimetry using echocardiography (Figure 17-9).[23] To allow for the slight loss in valve area that occurs during the first 24 hours, echocardiography should be performed 1 or 2 days after balloon mitral valvotomy, when calculation of the valve area may be done using planimetry, the pressure half-time method, or the continuity equation. Despite its dependence on flow conditions, mean mitral gradient should be assessed because it has a prognostic value. The final assessment

of the degree of regurgitation may be made with the use of angiography or color-flow Doppler imaging. Transesophageal examination is recommended in cases of severe MR to determine the mechanisms involved (Figure 17-10). The most sensitive method for the assessment of shunting is color-flow Doppler imaging, especially when TEE is used, which shows the severity of the defect and detects shunting in a more sensitive way than the assessment of hemodynamics.

Immediate Results

The technique of balloon mitral valvotomy has now been evaluated in several thousand patients with different clinical conditions and valve anatomy.

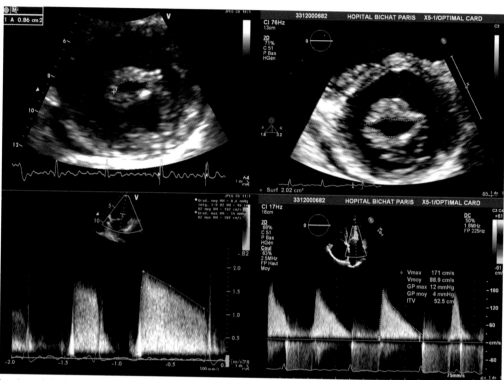

FIGURE 17-9   Evaluation of the immediate results of balloon mitral valvotomy. *Upper panel,* Two-dimensional echocardiography (parasternal short-axis view) shows opening of both commissures and an increase in valve area from 0.86 cm² *(left panel)* to 2.02 cm² *(right panel). Lower panel,* Doppler echocardiography of transmitral flow shows a decrease in mean mitral gradient from 9 to 4 mm Hg.

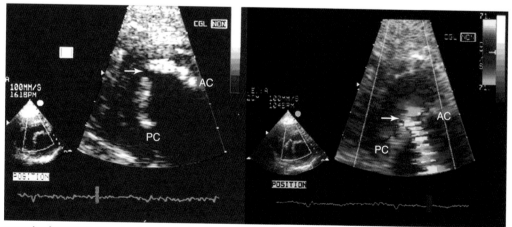

FIGURE 17-10   Severe mitral regurgitation due to anterior leaflet tear following balloon mitral valvotomy. *Left panel,* Transesophageal two-dimensional echocardiography shows a leaflet tear *(arrow). Right panel,* Color-flow Doppler imaging shows severe mitral regurgitation originating from leaflet tear *(arrow). AC,* Anterior commissure; *PC,* posterior commissure. *(Courtesy Dr. Cormier.)*

EFFICACY

The results shown in Table 17-4 demonstrate that balloon mitral valvotomy usually provides an increase of more than 100% in valve area.[21,89,95-104] Overall good immediate results, defined as a final valve area greater than 1.5 cm[2] without MR more severe than grade 2 in a four-grade system, are observed in more than 80% of cases and in patients with diverse characteristics.[53]

The improvement in valve function results in an immediate decrease in left atrial pressure and a slight increase in cardiac index. Gradual decreases in pulmonary arterial pressure and pulmonary vascular resistance are seen. High pulmonary vascular resistance continues to decrease in the absence of restenosis.[105]

Balloon mitral valvotomy has a beneficial effect on exercise capacity.[106] In addition, studies have shown that this technique improves left atrial and left atrial appendage pump function and decreases left atrial stiffness.

FAILURES

The failure rates range from 1% to 17%.[21,86,89,95-102,104] Most failures occur in the early part of the investigators' experience. Others are due to unfavorable anatomy.

RISKS

Procedural mortality ranges from 0 to 3% (Table 17-5).[21,86,89,95-102,104] The main causes of death are left ventricular perforation and the poor general condition of the patient. The incidence of hemopericardium varies from 0.5% to 12%. Pericardial hemorrhage may be related to transseptal catheterization or to apex perforation by the guidewires or the balloon itself when using the double-balloon technique. Embolism is encountered in 0.5% to 5% of cases.

The frequency of severe MR ranges from 2% to 19%. Surgical findings have shown that it is mostly related to non-commissural

TABLE 17-4	Immediate Results of Balloon Mitral Valvotomy (BMV): Increase in Mitral Valve Area				
			Mitral Valve Area (cm²)		
	PATIENTS (n)	AGE (YEARS)	BEFORE BMV	AFTER BMV	TECHNIQUE
Arora et al[95]	4850	27	0.7	1.9	Inoue or double-balloon or metallic commissurotome
Chen and Cheng[96]	4832	37	1.1	2.1	Inoue balloon
Iung et al[21]	2773	47	1.0	1.9	Inoue, single-, or double-balloon
Neumayer et al[97]	1123	57	1.1	1.8	Inoue balloon
Palacios et al[98]	879	55	0.9	1.9	Inoue or double-balloon
Ben-Farhat et al[99]	654	33	1.0	2.1	Inoue or double-balloon
Hernandez et al[100]	561	53	1.0	1.8	Inoue balloon
Meneveau et al[101]	532	54	1.0	1.7	Double- or Inoue ballon
Fawzy et al[102]	520	31	0.9	2.0	Inoue balloon
Eltchaninoff et al[103]	500	34	0.9	2.1	Metallic commissurotome
Stefanadis et al[89]	441	44	1.0	2.1	Modified single-, double-, or Inoue ballon (Retrograde)
Kang et al[104] (randomized comparison)	152	42	0.9	1.8	Inoue balloon
	150	40	0.9	1.9	Double-balloon

TABLE 17-5	Severe Complications of Balloon Mitral Valvotomy					
	n	AGE (YEARS)	IN-HOSPITAL DEATH (%)	TAMPONADE (%)	EMBOLIC EVENTS (%)	SEVERE MITRAL REGURGITATION (%)
Arora et al[95] (1987-2000)	4850	27	0.2	0.2	0.1	1.4
Chen and Cheng*[96] (1985-1994)	4832	37	0.1	0.8	0.5	1.4
Iung et al[21] (1986-2001)	2773	47	0.4	0.2	0.4	4.1
Neumayer et al[97] (1989-2000)	1123	57	0.4	0.9	0.9	6.0
National Heart, Lung, and Blood Institute Registry*[86] (1987-1989)	738	54				
n < 25			2	6	4	4
25 ≤ n < 100			1	4	2	3
n ≥ 100			0.3	2	1	3
Palacios et al[98] (1986-2000)	879	55	0.6	1.0	1.8	9.4
Ben-Farhat et al[99] (1987-1998)	654	33	0.5	0.6	1.5	4.6
Hernandez et al[100] (1989-1995)	620	53	0.5	0.6	—	4.0
Meneveau et al[101] (1986-1996)	532	54	0.2	1.1	—	3.9
Fawzy et al[102] (1989-2004)	520	31	0	0.7	0.5	1.6
Stefanadis et al*[89] (1988-1996)	441	44	0.2	0	0	3.4

*Multicenter series Larger study size (n) was associated with lower complication rates.

TABLE 17-6　Late Results after Balloon Mitral Valvotomy

	n	AGE (YEARS)	MAXIMUM FOLLOW-UP (YEARS)	EVENT-FREE SURVIVAL (%)	PREDICTIVE FACTORS OF EVENT-FREE SURVIVAL
Bouleti et al[73]	1024	49	20	30[†]	Age, sex, NYHA class, rhythm, anatomy, MVA post, gradient post
Palacios et al[98]	879	55	12	33[†]	Age, NYHA IV, prior comm., anatomy, MR, MR post, PAP post
Dean et al[116] (NHLBI registry)	736	54	4	60[*]	NYHA class, MVA post, PAP post, gradient decrease
Ben Farhat et al[99]	654	34	10	72[†]	Anatomy, LA pressure post, gradient post, MR post
Song et al[117]	402	44	9	90[*]	Age, MVA post, commissural opening, MR post
Hernandez et al[100]	561	53	7	69[†]	MVA post, MR post
Meneveau et al[101]	532	54	7.5	52[†]	Age, anatomy, CTI, gradient post, PAP post
Fawzy et al[‡118]	547	31	19	28[†]	Anatomy, rhythm
Stefanadis et al[89]	441	44	9	75[†]	NYHA class, anatomy, MVA post
Wang et al[119]	310	53	6	80	Age, anatomy, NYHA class, gradient post
Cohen et al[172]	146	59	5	51[*]	Anatomy, MVA post, LVED pressure post
Orrange et al[120]	132	44	7	65[*]	MVA post, capillary wedge pressure post

CTI, cardiothoracic index; *LVED,* left ventricular end-diastolic; *MR,* mitral regurgitation; *MVA,* mitral valve area; *NYHA,* New York Heart Association; *NHLBI,* National Heart, Lung, and Blood Institute; *PAP,* pulmonary artery pressure; *post,* after balloon mitral valvotomy.
*Survival without intervention
†Survival without intervention and in New York Heart Association class I or II.
‡Patients with good immediate results.

leaflet tearing, which could be associated with chordal rupture.[88,100,107-110] The development of severe MR depends more on the distribution of the morphologic changes of the valve than on their severity.[41,111] Severe MR may be well tolerated, but more often it is not, and scheduled surgery is necessary. In most cases, valve replacement is required because of the severity of the underlying valve disease. Conservative surgery has been successfully performed in selected young patients with less severe valve deformity.[107]

The frequency of atrial septal defect after balloon mitral valvotomy varies from 10% to 90%, depending on the technique used for its detection.[112] The shunt with this defect is usually small and without clinical consequences.

Although urgent surgery (within 24 hours) is seldom needed for complications, it may be required for massive hemopericardium resulting from left ventricular perforation intractable to treatment by pericardiocentesis or, less frequently, for severe MR with poor hemodynamic tolerance.[88,108-110]

PREDICTORS OF IMMEDIATE RESULTS

The prediction of results is multifactorial.[88,113-115] Several studies have shown that, in addition to morphologic factors, preoperative variables, such as age, history of surgical commissurotomy, functional class, small mitral valve area, presence of MR before balloon mitral valvotomy, atrial fibrillation, high pulmonary artery pressure, and presence of severe tricuspid regurgitation, as well as procedural factors, such as balloon type and size, are all independent predictors of the immediate results.

Two multivariate models derived from large series and validated on different populations show that older age, higher New York Heart Association (NYHA) functional class, impaired valve anatomy as assessed by echocardiography, and smaller mitral valve area are the most important predictive factors of poor immediate results of balloon mitral valvotomy.[88,115] The sensitivity of predictive models is high but the specificity is low.[88] Low specificity indicates insufficient prediction of poor immediate results, which is particularly true for the prediction of severe MR. This low specificity is related to the intrinsic limitations of the prediction of immediate results, that is to say, to the possibility of good results in patients who are at high risk for poor results. The possibility of

good results in theoretically unsuitable cases has been demonstrated in experimental studies and confirmed clinically.

Long-Term Results

Data from follow-up of up to 20 years can now be analyzed. In clinical terms the overall long-term results of balloon mitral valvotomy are good (Table 17-6).[73,89,98-101,116-120] Late outcome after balloon mitral valvotomy differs according to the quality of the immediate results and depends on patient characteristics (Figures 17-11 and 17-12).

When the immediate results are unsatisfactory, patients experience only transient or no functional improvement, and delayed surgery is usually performed when the extracardiac conditions allow.

Conversely, if balloon mitral valvotomy is initially successful, then survival rates are excellent, functional improvement occurs in the majority of cases, and the need for secondary surgery is infrequent. When clinical deterioration occurs in these patients, it is late and mainly related to mitral restenosis. Determining the incidence of restenosis with echocardiography is compromised by the absence of a uniform definition. It has generally been defined as a loss of more than 50% of the initial gain with a valve area becoming less than 1.5 cm². After a successful procedure, the incidence of restenosis is usually low, ranging from 2% to 40% at time intervals of 3 to 9 years (Figure 17-13).[100,117,119] The possibility of repeating balloon mitral valvotomy in cases of recurrent MS is one of the potential advantages of this nonsurgical procedure. Repeated balloon mitral valvotomy can be proposed if recurrent stenosis leads to symptoms, occurs several years after an initially successful procedure, and the predominant mechanism of restenosis is commissural refusion.[38,121-125] At the moment, results of only a small number of series on repeat balloon mitral valvotomy are available; these show good immediate and mid-term outcomes in patients with favorable characteristics. Although the results are less favorable in patients presenting with worse characteristics, repeat balloon mitral valvotomy has a palliative role in patients who are not surgical candidates.[121,123] These preliminary results are encouraging; however, defining the exact role of repeat balloon mitral valvotomy must await the results of larger series with longer follow-up.

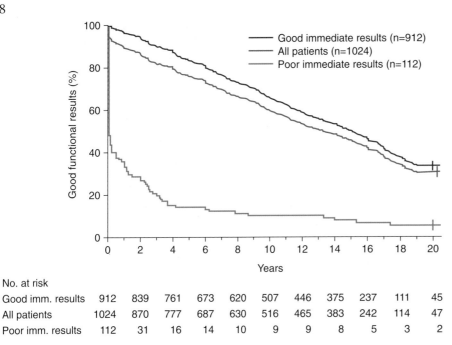

No. at risk

Good imm. results	912	839	761	673	620	507	446	375	237	111	45
All patients	1024	870	777	687	630	516	465	383	242	114	47
Poor imm. results	112	31	16	14	10	9	9	8	5	3	2

FIGURE 17-11 Functional results after balloon valvotomy for mitral stenosis. Good functional results (survival considering cardiovascular-related deaths with no need for mitral surgery or repeat dilation and in New York Heart Association functional class I or II) after balloon mitral valvotomy in 1024 patients. *(From Bouleti C, Iung B, Laouénan C, et al. Late results of percutaneous mitral commissurotomy up to 20 years: development and validation of a risk score predicting late functional results from a series of 912 patients. Circulation 2012;125:2119–27.)*

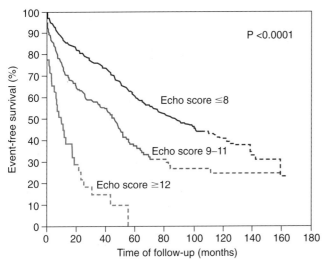

FIGURE 17-12 Outcomes after balloon mitral valvotomy stratified by echocardiography morphology score. Event-free survival (alive and free of mitral valve replacement or repeat balloon mitral valvotomy) after balloon mitral valvotomy according to echocardiography score. *(From Palacios IF, Sanchez PL, Harrell LC, et al. Which patients benefit from percutaneous mitral balloon valvuloplasty? Prevalvuloplasty and postvalvuloplasty variables that predict long-term outcome. Circulation 2002;105:1465–71.)*

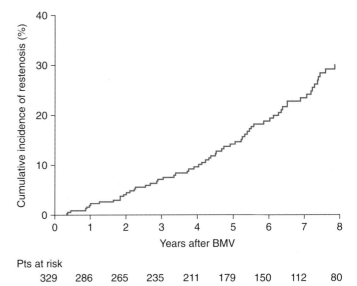

Pts at risk

329	286	265	235	211	179	150	112	80

FIGURE 17-13 Restenosis after balloon mitral valvotomy. Cumulative incidence of restenosis after successful balloon mitral valvotomy (BMV). *Pts,* Patients. *(From Song JK, Song JM, Kang DH, et al. Restenosis and adverse clinical events after successful percutaneous mitral valvuloplasty: immediate post-procedural mitral valve area as an important prognosticator. Eur Heart J 2009; 30:1254–62.)*

The degree of MR generally remains stable or slightly decreases during follow-up. Atrial septal defects are likely to close over time in the majority of cases because of reduction in the interatrial pressure gradient. The persistence of shunts is related to their magnitude or to unsatisfactory relief of the valve obstruction. They very seldom require treatment on their own. Finally, clinical series of surgical commissurotomy and balloon commissurotomy suggest that intervention reduces markers of the risk of embolism, such as intensity of left atrial echocardiographic contrast, size, and function.[126-130] Two nonrandomized comparative series suggested that the incidence of thromboembolic events in MS was lower after balloon mitral valvotomy than with medical management.[131,132] No direct evidence exists that balloon mitral

valvotomy reduces the incidence of atrial fibrillation, even if its favorable influence on predictors of atrial fibrillation, such as atrial size and degree of obstruction, seems to indicate that this is indeed the case.[133-136] If atrial fibrillation after successful balloon mitral valvotomy is of recent onset, and in the absence of severe left atrial enlargement, electric shock cardioversion is recommended.[70]

Several randomized studies have compared surgical commissurotomy with balloon mitral valvotomy, mostly in patients with favorable characteristics. They consistently showed that balloon mitral valvotomy is at least comparable to surgical commissurotomy as regards short- and mid-term follow-up up to 15 years.[137-140] A nonrandomized series comparing balloon mitral valvotomy with mitral surgery showed no difference in overall survival but a lower event-free survival after balloon mitral valvotomy in patients who had unfavorable valve anatomy or were in atrial fibrillation.[141]

PREDICTORS OF LONG-TERM RESULTS

Prediction of long-term results is multifactorial.[73,98,101,110,116,135,138,142] It is based on clinical variables such as age; valve anatomy as assessed by different echocardiographic scores or the presence of valve calcification; factors related to the evolutional stage of the disease, that is, a higher New York Heart Association class before balloon mitral valvotomy; history of previous commissurotomy; severe tricuspid regurgitation; cardiomegaly; atrial fibrillation; high pulmonary vascular resistances; and the results of the procedure (see Table 17-6). Among the results of the procedure, moderate MR is not consistently identified as predictive of poor late outcome.[143,144] On the other hand, postprocedural valve area and gradients are strong independent determinants of late functional results. Mitral gradient should therefore systematically be taken into account in conjunction with valve area in the assessment of the results of balloon mitral valvotomy.[73]

The quality of the late results is generally considered independent of the technique used.

The identification of these predictors provides important information for patient selection and is relevant to follow-up: patients who have good immediate results but who are at high risk for further events must be carefully followed to detect deterioration and allow for timely intervention. A score combining seven variables enables risk stratification to be easily performed, which is useful for patient information and planning follow-up (Table 17-7; Figure 17-14).[73]

Applications of Balloon Mitral Valvotomy in Special Patient Groups

AFTER SURGICAL COMMISSUROTOMY

Patients who have undergone surgical commissurotomy are of interest because in western countries recurrent MS is becoming more frequent than primary MS, and reoperation in this context is associated with a higher risk of morbidity and mortality and requires valve replacement in most cases.[145-147] Balloon mitral valvotomy is feasible in this setting and significantly improves valve function. On the whole, the results are good, even if slightly less satisfactory than those obtained in patients without previous commissurotomy; this difference probably can be attributed to less favorable characteristics observed in patients previously subjected to operation. These encouraging preliminary data suggest that balloon mitral valvotomy may well postpone reoperation in selected patients with restenosis after commissurotomy. The indications for balloon mitral valvotomy in this subgroup of patients are similar to those for "primary balloon mitral valvotomy," but echocardiographic examination must exclude any patients in whom restenosis is due mainly to valve rigidity without significant commissural refusion (Figure 17-15). The latter mechanism could be responsible for the exceptional cases of MS that develop in patients who have undergone mitral ring annuloplasty for correction of MR.

PATIENTS FOR WHOM SURGERY POSES HIGH RISK

Preliminary series have suggested that balloon mitral valvotomy can be performed safely and effectively in patients with severe pulmonary hypertension.[148,149]

In Western countries, patients with MS are older and may have concomitant noncardiac disease, which may also increase the risk of surgery.[4,21,25,150,151] Balloon mitral valvotomy can be performed as a life-saving procedure in critically ill patients,[152,153] as

the sole treatment when there is an absolute contraindication to surgery, or as a "bridge" to surgery in other cases.[154] In this context dramatic improvement has been observed in young patients; however, the outcome is very bad in elderly patients presenting with "end-stage" disease who should be treated conservatively.

In elderly patients, balloon mitral valvotomy results in moderate but significant improvement in valve function at an acceptable risk, although subsequent functional deterioration is frequent.[155-158] Therefore, balloon mitral valvotomy is a valid, if only a palliative, treatment for these patients, in particular when the alternative of surgery carries a high risk because of age, comorbidities, and the evolutionary stage of the disease.

During pregnancy, symptomatic MS carries a high risk of maternal and fetal complications in the absence of intervention[159] (see Chapter 27). Surgery with the use of extracorporeal circulation is harmful for the fetus, carrying 20% to 30% mortality rates. Balloon mitral valvotomy can be performed safely during pregnancy; the procedure is effective and results in normal delivery in most cases.[160] As regards radiation exposure, balloon mitral valvotomy is safe for the fetus, provided that protection is given by a shield that completely surrounds the patient's abdomen and that the procedure is performed after the 20th week.[161] Preliminary series have shown a satisfactory development of the infants over 5 to 10 years of follow-up. Nevertheless, it must be borne in mind that, in addition to radiation, balloon mitral valvotomy carries the potential risk of related hypotension and the ever-present risk of complications that require urgent surgery. These data, which now represent several hundreds of cases, suggest that balloon mitral valvotomy can be a useful technique in the treatment of pregnant patients with MS and refractory heart failure despite medical treatment.[72]

Treatment Strategy

An image of the current practice can be derived from the Euro Heart Survey on Valvular Heart Disease, which was performed prospectively in 92 centers throughout Europe during a 4-month period in 2001.[5] It showed that balloon mitral valvotomy is now used in more than a third of cases of MS, the other patients being treated by valve replacement mostly using mechanical prostheses. Thus, in current practice, percutaneous intervention has almost replaced surgical commissurotomy. This development is due to the good results of the interventional techniques and also to the fact that most surgeons have lost experience with the conservative techniques in the treatment of MS owing to the limited number of cases performed.

Intervention should be performed only in patients with significant MS (valve area <1.5 cm^2) because before this threshold the risks probably outweigh the benefits, and patients with less severe MS can usually be managed well with medical treatment.[29,30] There may be rare cases in which the procedure may be offered to patients with slightly larger valve areas if they have a large stature, are highly symptomatic, and have favorable presenting characteristics.

Surgery is the only alternative when balloon mitral valvotomy is contraindicated. The most important contraindication being left atrial thrombosis, the recommendation is self-evident if the thrombus is free-floating or is situated in the left atrial cavity; this also applies when it is located on the interatrial septum. Small series have suggested that balloon mitral valvotomy can be performed when the thrombus is located in the left atrial appendage; however, it has not been shown to our satisfaction that the Inoue technique with transesophageal guidance precludes a risk of embolism.[162] Thrombus in this location is considered a contraindication to the technique under the current guidelines. If the patient is clinically stable, as is the case for most patients with MS, vitamin K antagonists can be given for 2 to 6 months; and if a new transesophageal examination shows that the thrombus has disappeared, balloon mitral valvotomy can be attempted.[29,30,163]

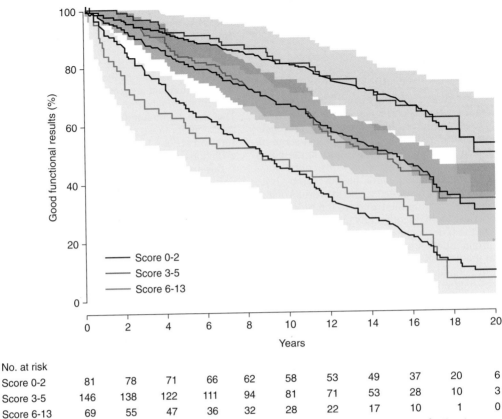

FIGURE 17-14 **Prediction of long-term success after balloon mitral valvotomy.** Assessment of the performance of a 13-point score predicting good late functional results of balloon mitral valvotomy (survival with no cardiovascular death or intervention, and in New York Heart Association functional class I or II). The 13-point additive score is calculated from Table 17-7. Observed rates with their 95% confidence intervals *(red, score 0-2; blue, score 3-5; green, score 6-13)* and corresponding predicted rates *(black lines). (From Bouleti C, Iung B, Laouénan C, et al. Late results of percutaneous mitral commissurotomy up to 20 years: development and validation of a risk score predicting late functional results from a series of 912 patients. Circulation 2012;125:2119-27.)*

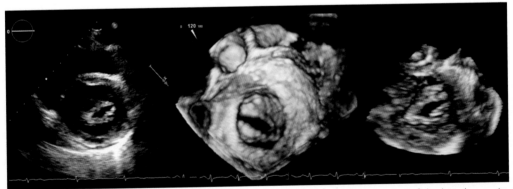

FIGURE 17-15 **Example of restenosis after prior commissurotomy.** The images show persistent opening of the lateral commissure. *Left panel,* Two-dimensional (2D) echocardiography, parasternal short-axis view. *Middle panel,* 3D echocardiography, view from the left atrium. *Right panel,* 3D echocardiography, view from the left ventricle.

Other contraindications to balloon mitral valvotomy are as follows (Table 17-8):[29-30]
- MR more than mild; balloon mitral valvotomy can, however, be considered in selected patients with moderate MR if the surgical risk is high or even prohibitive.
- Severe calcification.
- Absence of commissural fusion.
- Combined MS and severe aortic disease, in which surgery is obviously indicated in the absence of contraindications.

On the other hand, the coexistence of moderate aortic valve disease and severe MS is another situation in which balloon mitral valvotomy is preferable in order to postpone the inevitable subsequent surgical treatment of both valves. This is particularly the case for associated aortic regurgitation, which worsens slowly over time.[164] Combined severe tricuspid stenosis and tricuspid regurgitation with clinical signs of heart failure is an indication for surgery on both valves. The existence of tricuspid regurgitation is not a contraindication to the procedure even though it represents a negative prognostic factor.[165] Less frequently, coronary disease may favor surgical therapy. In such patients, valve replacement is preferred in most cases, although open commissurotomy may be performed by experienced teams in young

TABLE 17-7	**Predictive Factors of Poor Late Functional Results after Good Immediate Results of Balloon Mitral Valvotomy:* Multivariable Analysis and Definition of a 13-Point Predictive Score**		
	ADJUSTED HAZARD RATIO (95% CI)	P	POINTS FOR SCORE (/13)
Age (yrs) and final mitral valve area (cm²):			
<50 and MVA ≥2.00	1		0
<50 and MVA 1.50-2.00 **OR** 50-70 and MVA >1.75	2.1 (1.6-2.9)	<0.0001	2
50-70 and MVA 1.50-1.75 **OR** ≥70 and MVA ≥1.50	5.1 (3.5-7.5)	<0.0001	5
Valve anatomy and sex:			
No valve calcification	1		0
Valve calcification:			
Female	1.2 (0.9-1.6)	0.18	0
Male	2.3 (1.6-3.2)	<0.0001	3
Rhythm and NYHA class:			
Sinus rhythm **OR** Atrial fibrillation and NYHA class I-II	1		0
Atrial fibrillation and NYHA class III-IV	1.8 (1.4-2.3)	<0.0001	2
Final mean mitral gradient (mm Hg):			
≤3	1		0
3-6	1.1 (1.0-1.8)	0.05	1
≥6	2.5 (1.8-3.5)	<0.0001	3

CI, Confidence interval; *MVA*, mitral valve area; *NYHA*, New York Heart Association.
From Bouleti C, Iung B, Laouenan C, et al. Late results of percutaneous mitral commissurotomy up to 20 years: development and validation of a risk score predicting late functional results from a series of 912 patients. Circulation 2012;125:2119–27.
*Valve area ≥1.5 cm² with no regurgitation > grade 2/4.

patients who are in sinus rhythm and have no or mild calcification and mild to moderate MR.

Regarding indications, balloon mitral valvotomy is clearly recommended in cases in which surgery is contraindicated or for "ideal candidates." Balloon mitral valvotomy is the only solution when surgery is contraindicated. It is also preferable to surgery, at least as a first attempt, in patients with an increased risk with surgery.

Surgery may pose higher risks in patients with cardiac conditions such as restenosis after surgical commissurotomy, previous aortic valve replacement, or severe pulmonary hypertension. Balloon mitral valvotomy can be performed as a lifesaving procedure in critically ill patients, as the sole treatment in cases of absolute contraindication to surgery, or as a bridge to surgery in other cases. It can also be performed in elderly patients as a palliative procedure or in pregnant patients who remain symptomatic despite medical treatment.

In symptomatic patients with favorable characteristics, such as young patients with good anatomy—that is, pliable valves and moderate subvalvular disease (echocardiographic score ≤8), who are often seen in countries where rheumatic fever is still present, results of balloon mitral valvotomy are generally excellent (Table 17-9; Figures 17-16 and 17-17).[152,153,166] In addition, if

TABLE 17-8	**Contraindications to Balloon Mitral Valvotomy**

Mitral valve area >1.5 cm²
Left atrial thrombus
More than mild mitral regurgitation
Severe or bicommissural calcification
Absence of commissural fusion
Severe concomitant aortic valve disease OR severe combined tricuspid stenosis and regurgitation
Concomitant coronary artery disease requiring bypass surgery

From Vahanian A, Alfieri O, Andreotti F, et al. Guidelines on the management of valvular heart disease (version 2012). Eur Heart J 2012;33:2451–396.

TABLE 17-9	**Recommendations for Balloon Mitral Valvotomy in Symptomatic Patients with Mitral Stenosis**

ACC/AHA GUIDELINES[29]		ESC/EACTS GUIDELINES[30]	
Symptomatic patients (NYHA functional class II, III, or IV) with moderate or severe mitral stenosis* and valve morphology favorable for percutaneous balloon valvotomy in the absence of left atrial thrombus and of moderate to severe mitral regurgitation	(IA)	Patients with mitral stenosis and valve area <1.5 cm²:	
		Symptomatic patients with favorable characteristics† for percutaneous mitral commissurotomy	(IB)
Patients with moderate or severe mitral stenosis* who have a nonpliable calcified valve, are in NYHA functional class III-IV, and are either not candidates for surgery or would be at high risk with surgery	(IIaC)	Symptomatic patients with contraindications to or high risk with surgery	(IC)
		As initial treatment in symptomatic patients with unfavorable anatomy but without unfavorable clinical characteristics†	(IIaC)
Symptomatic patients (NYHA functional class II, III, or IV), with mitral valve area >1.5 cm² if there is evidence of hemodynamically significant mitral stenosis based on pulmonary artery systolic pressure >60 mm Hg, pulmonary artery wedge pressure ≥25 mm Hg, or mean mitral valve gradient >15 mm Hg during exercise	(IIbC)		
As an alternative to surgery for patients with moderate or severe mitral stenosis* who have a nonpliable calcified valve and are in NYHA functional class III-IV	(IIbC)		

ACC, American College of Cardiology; *AHA*, American Heart Association; *ESC*, European Society of Cardiology; *EACTS*, European Association for Cardio-Thoracic Surgery; *NYHA*, New York Heart Association.
*See Table 17-1. Numbers in parentheses indicate level of recommendation (I, IIa, or IIb) and level of evidence (A, B, or C). See appendix for definitions.
†Unfavorable characteristics for percutaneous mitral commissurotomy can be defined by the presence of several of the following characteristics:
• Clinical characteristics: old age, history of commissurotomy, NYHA class IV, permanent atrial fibrillation, severe pulmonary hypertension.
• Anatomic characteristics: echocardiography score >8, Cormier score 3 (calcification of mitral valve of any extent, as assessed by fluoroscopy), very small mitral valve area, severe tricuspid regurgitation.

CH
17

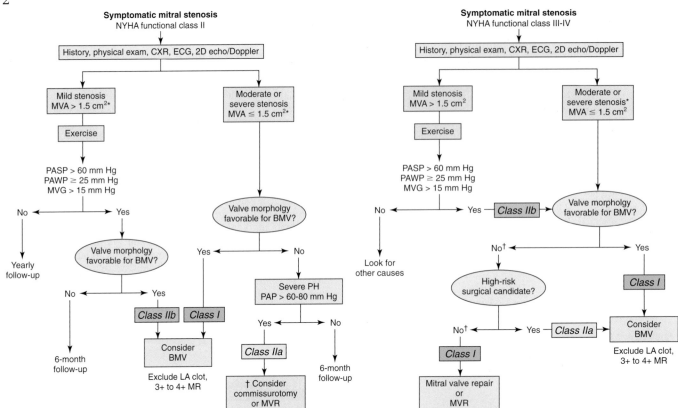

FIGURE 17-16 **American College of Cardiology/American Heart Association guidelines for balloon mitral valvotomy in symptomatic patients with mitral stenosis.** *2D,* Two-dimensional; *BMV,* balloon mitral valvotomy; *CXR,* chest radiograph; *ECG,* electrocardiogram; *echo,* echocardiography; *LA,* left atrial; *MR,* mitral regurgitation; *MVA,* mitral valve area; *MVG,* mean valve gradient; *MVR,* mitral valve replacement; *NYHA,* New York Heart Association; *PAP,* pulmonary artery pressure; *PASP,* pulmonary artery systolic pressure; *PAWP,* pulmonary artery wedge pressure; *PH,* pulmonary hypertension. *(From Bonow RO, Carabello BA, Chatterjee K, et al. Focused update incorporated into the ACC/AHA 2006 guidelines for the management of patients with valvular heart disease. Circulation 2008;118:e523–661.)*

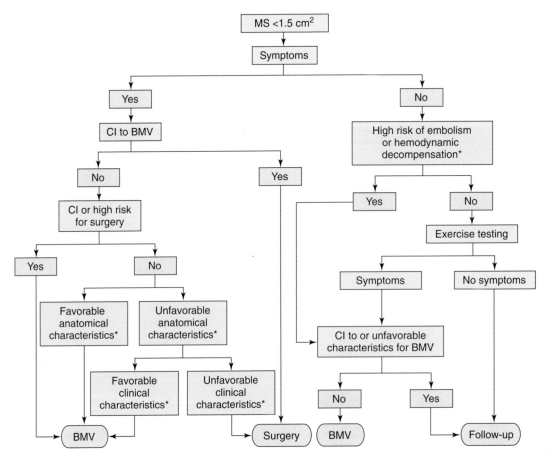

FIGURE 17-17 **European Society of Cardiology guidelines for balloon mitral valvotomy in patients with mitral stenosis.** *BMV,* Balloon mitral valvotomy; *CI,* contraindication; *MS,* mitral stenosis. *(From Vahanian A, Alfieri O, Andreotti F, et al. Guidelines on the management of valvular heart disease [version 2012]. Eur Heart J 2012; 33:2451–96.)* *For the definitions of favorable and unfavorable characteristics, see Table 17-10.

TABLE 17-10 Recommendations for Balloon Mitral Valvotomy in Asymptomatic Patients with Mitral Stenosis

ACC/AHA GUIDELINES[29]		ESC/EACTS GUIDELINES[30]	
Asymptomatic patients with moderate or severe mitral stenosis* and valve morphology favorable for balloon mitral valvotomy who have pulmonary hypertension (pulmonary artery systolic pressure >50 mm Hg at rest or >60 mm Hg with exercise) in the absence of left atrial thrombus and of moderate to severe mitral regurgitation	(IC)	Asymptomatic patients with mitral stenosis with valve area <1.5 cm², without unfavorable characteristics† for percutaneous mitral commissurotomy and:	
		High thromboembolic risk (previous history of embolism, dense spontaneous echocardiographic contrast in the left atrium, recent or paroxysmal atrial fibrillation)	(IIaC)
Asymptomatic patients with moderate or severe mitral stenosis* and valve morphology favorable for balloon mitral valvotomy who have new onset of atrial fibrillation in the absence of left atrial thrombus and of moderate to severe mitral regurgitation	(IIbC)	**AND/OR**	
		High risk of hemodynamic decompensation (systolic pulmonary artery pressure >50 mm Hg at rest, need for major noncardiac surgery, desire for pregnancy)	(IIaC)

ACC, American College of Cardiology; *AHA,* American Heart Association; *ESC,* European Society of Cardiology; *EACTS,* European Association for Cardio-Thoracic Surgery; *NYHA,* New York Heart Association.
*See Table 17-1. Numbers in parentheses indicate level of recommendation (I, IIa or IIb) and level of evidence (A, B or C). See appendix for definitions.
†Unfavorable characteristics for percutaneous mitral commissurotomy can be defined by the presence of several of the following characteristics:
  • Clinical characteristics: old age, history of commissurotomy, NYHA functional class IV, permanent atrial fibrillation, severe pulmonary hypertension.
  • Anatomic characteristics: echocardiography score >8, Cormier score 3 (calcification of mitral valve of any extent, as assessed by fluoroscopy), very small mitral valve area, severe tricuspid regurgitation.

restenosis occurs, patients treated with balloon mitral valvotomy could undergo repeat balloon mitral valvotomy or surgery without the difficulties and inherent risk resulting from the pericardial adhesions and chest wall scarring that often occur with surgery. Balloon mitral valvotomy would thus appear to be the procedure of choice for these patients in whom we may expect to further delay surgery, enabling, for example, pregnancy to occur.

Controversy remains as regards the performance of balloon mitral valvotomy in asymptomatic patients and in those with unfavorable anatomy.

The level of evidence for performing balloon mitral valvotomy in asymptomatic patients is low because no randomized comparison between the results of balloon mitral valvotomy and medical therapy for such patients has been performed (Table 17-10, Figures 17-17 and 17-18). For these patients, the goal is not to prolong life or to decrease symptoms, but rather to prevent thromboembolism.[131,132] Truly asymptomatic patients, however, are not usually candidates for the procedure because of the small but definite risk inherent in the technique. For truly asymptomatic patients, balloon mitral valvotomy may be considered in selected cases such as the following: patients at high risk of thromboembolism (previous history of embolism or heavy spontaneous echo contrast in the left atrium); recurrent atrial arrhythmias; and pulmonary hypertension. A comparative nonrandomized study suggested that asymptomatic patients benefit from balloon mitral valvotomy in particular when they are in atrial fibrillation or have prior embolic events.[167] Balloon mitral valvotomy can also be performed when systolic pulmonary pressure is higher than 50 mm Hg at rest. In the U.S. guidelines, the procedure can be recommended if systolic pulmonary pressure exceeds 60 mm Hg with exercise.[29] However, this latter threshold should be refined by the increasing experience gained in exercise echocardiography. The European guidelines do not fix a threshold for systolic pulmonary pressure with exercise but recommend performing balloon mitral valvotomy if symptoms appear during exercise.[30] Finally, balloon mitral valvotomy can be considered for asymptomatic patients requiring major extracardiac surgery or to allow for pregnancy.

In asymptomatic patients, balloon mitral valvotomy should be performed only by experienced interventionists and when valve anatomy is favorable, in which case a safe and successful procedure can be expected. In the future, balloon mitral valvotomy could be combined with percutaneous closure of the left atrial appendage or catheter ablation of atrial fibrillation to further reduce the embolic risk.[168,169]

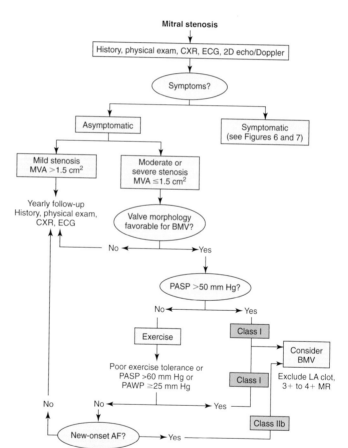

FIGURE 17-18 American College of Cardiology/American Heart Association guidelines for balloon mitral valvotomy in asymptomatic patients with mitral stenosis. *2D,* Two-dimensional; *AF,* atrial fibrillation; *BMV,* balloon mitral valvotomy; *CXR,* chest radiograph; *Doppler,* Doppler echocardiography; *ECG,* electrocardiography; *echo,* echocardiography; *LA,* left atrial; *MR,* mitral regurgitation; *MVA,* mitral valve area; *PASP,* pulmonary artery systolic pressure; *PAWP,* pulmonary artery wedge pressure. *(From Bonow RO, Carabello BA, Chatterjee K, et al. Focused update incorporated into the ACC/AHA 2006 guidelines for the management of patients with valvular heart disease. Circulation 2008;118:e523–661.)*

Much remains to be done in refining the indications for balloon mitral valvotomy in patients with unfavorable anatomy.[170,171] For this group, some authorities favor immediate surgery because of the less satisfying results of balloon mitral valvotomy, whereas others prefer balloon mitral valvotomy as an initial treatment for selected candidates and reserve surgery for cases in which this treatment fails.

Among patients with less favorable valve anatomy, the comparison between the results of balloon mitral valvotomy and of surgery is also difficult. Unfortunately, no randomized study has been performed examining this issue. Indications in this subgroup of patients must take into account their heterogeneity with respect to anatomy and clinical status. An individualistic approach is favored that allows for the multifactorial nature of prediction. Current opinion is that surgery can be considered the treatment of choice in patients with bicommissural or heavy calcification. On the other hand, balloon mitral valvotomy can be attempted as a first step in patients with extensive lesions of the subvalvular apparatus or moderate or unicommissural calcification, the more so because their clinical status argues in favor of this approach, such as in young patients with the expectation of further delaying valve replacement, with its inherent mortality and morbidity. Surgery should be considered reasonably early after unsatisfactory results or secondary deterioration.[29,30] The use of scoring systems derived from multivariate models is helpful for decision making based on a multifactorial approach (see Figure 17-14).[73,115] The development of new anatomic scores using, in particular, three-dimensional imaging is theoretically promising but limited in practice by issues linked to complexity and reproducibility.

In conclusion, the good results that have been obtained with balloon mitral valvotomy in large populations with long-term follow-up enable us to say that, currently, this technique has an important place in the treatment of MS and has virtually replaced surgical commissurotomy. In the treatment of MS, balloon mitral valvotomy and valve replacement must be regarded not as rivals but as complementary techniques, each applicable at the appropriate stage of the disease.

REFERENCES

1. Iung B, Vahanian A. Epidemiology of valvular heart disease in the adult. Nat Rev Cardiol 2011;8:162–72.
2. Roberts WC, Virmani R. Aschoff bodies at necropsy in valvular heart disease. Evidence from an analysis of 543 patients over 14 years of age that rheumatic heart disease, at least anatomically, is a disease of the mitral valve. Circulation 1978;57:803–7.
3. Okay T, Deligonul U, Sancaktar O, et al. Contribution of mitral valve reserve capacity to sustained symptomatic improvement after balloon valvulotomy in mitral stenosis: implications for restenosis. J Am Coll Cardiol 1993;22:1691–6.
4. Pressman GS, Agarwal A, Braitman LE, et al. Mitral annular calcium causing mitral stenosis. Am J Cardiol 2010;105:389–91.
5. Iung B, Baron G, Butchart EG, et al. A prospective survey of patients with valvular heart disease in Europe: The Euro Heart Survey on Valvular Heart Disease. Eur Heart J 2003;24:1231–43.
6. Carapetis JR. Rheumatic heart disease in Asia. Circulation 2008;118:2748–53.
7. Marijon E, Ou P, Celermajer DS, et al. Prevalence of rheumatic heart disease detected by echocardiographic screening. N Engl J Med 2007;357:470–6.
8. Rahimtoola SH, Durairaj A, Mehra A, et al. Current evaluation and management of patients with mitral stenosis. Circulation 2002;106:1183–8.
9. Shaw TR, Northridge DB, Sutaria N. Mitral balloon valvotomy and left atrial thrombus. Heart 2005;91:1088–9.
10. Peverill RE, Harper RW, Gelman J, et al. Determinants of increased regional left atrial coagulation activity in patients with mitral stenosis. Circulation 1996;94:331–9.
11. Fernandes JL, Sampaio RO, Brandao CM, et al. Comparison of inhaled nitric oxide versus oxygen on hemodynamics in patients with mitral stenosis and severe pulmonary hypertension after mitral valve surgery. Am J Cardiol 2011;107:1040–5.
12. Yamamoto K, Ikeda U, Mito H, et al. Endothelin production in pulmonary circulation of patients with mitral stenosis. Circulation 1994;89:2093–8.
13. Remetz MS, Cleman MW, Cabin HS. Pulmonary and pleural complications of cardiac disease. Clin Chest Med 1989;10:545–92.
14. Otto CM, Davis KB, Reid CL, et al. Relation between pulmonary artery pressure and mitral stenosis severity in patients undergoing balloon mitral commissurotomy. Am J Cardiol 1993;71:874–8.
15. Gaasch WH, Folland ED. Left ventricular function in rheumatic mitral stenosis. Eur Heart J 1991;12(Suppl B):66–9.
16. Brochet E, Détaint D, Fondard O, et al. Early hemodynamic changes versus peak values: what is more useful to predict occurrence of dyspnea during stress echocardiography in patients with asymptomatic mitral stenosis? J Am Soc Echocardiogr 2011;24:392–8.
17. Dahan M, Paillole C, Martin D, et al. Determinants of stroke volume response to exercise in patients with mitral stenosis: a Doppler echocardiographic study. J Am Coll Cardiol 1993;21:384–9.
18. Schwammenthal E, Vered Z, Agranat O, et al. Impact of atrioventricular compliance on pulmonary artery pressure in mitral stenosis: an exercise echocardiographic study. Circulation 2000;102:2378–84.
19. Li M, Dery JP, Dumesnil JG, et al. Usefulness of measuring net atrioventricular compliance by Doppler echocardiography in patients with mitral stenosis. Am J Cardiol 2005;96:432–5.
20. Shaw TR, Sutaria N, Prendergast B. Clinical and haemodynamic profiles of young, middle aged, and elderly patients with mitral stenosis undergoing mitral balloon valvotomy. Heart 2003;89:1430–6.
21. Iung B, Nicoud-Houel A, Fondard O, et al. Temporal trends in percutaneous mitral commissurotomy over a 15-year period. Eur Heart J 2004;25:701–7.
22. Iung B, Vahanian A. Echocardiography in the patient undergoing catheter balloon mitral valvotomy: patient selection, hemodynamic results, complications and long-term outcome. In: Otto CM, editor. The practice of clinical echocardiography. 4th ed. Philadelphia: Saunders; 2012. p. 389–407.
23. Baumgartner H, Hung J, Bermejo J, et al. Echocardiographic assessment of valve stenosis: EAE/ASE recommendations for clinical practice. J Am Soc Echocardiogr 2009;22:1–23; quiz 101–2.
24. Zamorano J, Cordeiro P, Sugeng L, et al. Real-time three-dimensional echocardiography for rheumatic mitral valve stenosis evaluation: an accurate and novel approach. J Am Coll Cardiol 2004;43:2091–6.
25. Sebag IA, Morgan JG, Handschumacher MD, et al. Usefulness of three-dimensionally guided assessment of mitral stenosis using matrix-array ultrasound. Am J Cardiol 2005;96:1151–6.
26. Messika-Zeitoun D, Brochet E, Holmin C, et al. Three-dimensional evaluation of the mitral valve area and commissural opening before and after percutaneous mitral commissurotomy in patients with mitral stenosis. Eur Heart J 2007;28:72–9.
27. Messika-Zeitoun D, Meizels A, Cachier A, et al. Echocardiographic evaluation of the mitral valve area before and after percutaneous mitral commissurotomy: the pressure half-time method revisited. J Am Soc Echocardiogr 2005;18:1409–14.
28. Messika-Zeitoun D, Fung Yiu S, Cormier B, et al. Sequential assessment of mitral valve area during diastole using colour M-mode flow convergence analysis: new insights into mitral stenosis physiology. Eur Heart J 2003;24:1244–53.
29. Bonow RO, Carabello BA, Chatterjee K, et al. 2008 Focused update incorporated into the ACC/AHA 2006 guidelines for the management of patients with valvular heart disease: a report of the American College of Cardiology/American Heart Association Task Force on Practice Guidelines (Writing Committee to Revise the 1998 Guidelines for the Management of Patients With Valvular Heart Disease): endorsed by the Society of Cardiovascular Anesthesiologists, Society for Cardiovascular Angiography and Interventions, and Society of Thoracic Surgeons. Circulation 2008;118:e523–661.
30. Vahanian A, Alfieri O, Andreotti F, et al. Guidelines on the management of valvular heart disease (version 2012). Eur Heart J 2012;33:2451–96.
31. Izgi C, Ozdemir N, Cevik C, et al. Mitral valve resistance as a determinant of resting and stress pulmonary artery pressure in patients with mitral stenosis: a dobutamine stress study. J Am Soc Echocardiogr 2007;20:1160–6.
32. Wilkins GT, Weyman AE, Abascal VM, et al. Percutaneous balloon dilatation of the mitral valve: an analysis of echocardiographic variables related to outcome and the mechanism of dilatation. Br Heart J 1988;60:299–308.
33. Cormier B, Vahanian A, Michel PL, et al. Evaluation by two-dimensional and doppler echocardiography of the results of percutaneous mitral valvuloplasty. Arch Mal Coeur Vaiss 1989;82:185–91.
34. Vahanian A, Michel PL, Cormier B, et al. Results of percutaneous mitral commissurotomy in 200 patients. Am J Cardiol 1989;63:847–52.
35. Fatkin D, Roy P, Morgan JJ, et al. Percutaneous balloon mitral valvotomy with the Inoue single-balloon catheter: commissural morphology as a determinant of outcome. J Am Coll Cardiol 1993;21:390–7.
36. Cannan CR, Nishimura RA, Reeder GS, et al. Echocardiographic assessment of commissural calcium: a simple predictor of outcome after percutaneous mitral balloon valvotomy. J Am Coll Cardiol 1997;29:175–80.
37. Sutaria N, Shaw TR, Prendergast B, et al. Transoesophageal echocardiographic assessment of mitral valve commissural morphology predicts outcome after balloon mitral valvotomy. Heart 2006;92:52–7.
38. Turgeman Y, Atar S, Suleiman K, et al. Feasibility, safety, and morphologic predictors of outcome of repeat percutaneous balloon mitral commissurotomy. Am J Cardiol 2005;95:989–91.
39. Rifaie O, Esmat I, Abdel-Rahman M, et al. Can a novel echocardiographic score better predict outcome after percutaneous balloon mitral valvuloplasty? Echocardiography 2009;26:119–27.
40. Turgeman Y, Atar S, Rosenfeld T. The subvalvular apparatus in rheumatic mitral stenosis: methods of assessment and therapeutic implications. Chest 2003;124:1929–36.
41. Padial LR, Freitas N, Sagie A, et al. Echocardiography can predict which patients will develop severe mitral regurgitation after percutaneous mitral valvulotomy. J Am Coll Cardiol 1996;27:1225–31.
42. Vahanian A, Palacios IF. Percutaneous approaches to valvular disease. Circulation 2004;109:1572–9.

43. Messika-Zeitoun D, Bellamy M, Avierinos JF, et al. Left atrial remodelling in mitral regurgitation–methodologic approach, physiological determinants, and outcome implications: a prospective quantitative Doppler-echocardiographic and electron beam-computed tomographic study. Eur Heart J 2007;28:1773–81.

44. Keenan NG, Cueff C, Cimadevilla C, et al. Usefulness of left atrial volume versus diameter to assess thromboembolic risk in mitral stenosis. Am J Cardiol 2010;106:1152–6.

45. Lancellotti P, Moura L, Pierard LA, et al. European Association of Echocardiography recommendations for the assessment of valvular regurgitation. Part 2: mitral and tricuspid regurgitation (native valve disease). Eur J Echocardiogr 2010;11:307–32.

46. Dreyfus GD, Corbi PJ, Chan KM, et al. Secondary tricuspid regurgitation or dilatation: which should be the criteria for surgical repair? Ann Thorac Surg 2005;79:127–32.

47. Black IW, Hopkins AP, Lee LC, et al. Left atrial spontaneous echo contrast: a clinical and echocardiographic analysis. J Am Coll Cardiol 1991;18:398–404.

48. Reis G, Motta MS, Barbosa MM, et al. Dobutamine stress echocardiography for noninvasive assessment and risk stratification of patients with rheumatic mitral stenosis. J Am Coll Cardiol 2004;43:393–401.

49. Lin SJ, Brown PA, Watkins MP, et al. Quantification of stenotic mitral valve area with magnetic resonance imaging and comparison with Doppler ultrasound. J Am Coll Cardiol 2004;44:133–7.

50. Messika-Zeitoun D, Serfaty JM, Laissy JP, et al. Assessment of the mitral valve area in patients with mitral stenosis by multislice computed tomography. J Am Coll Cardiol 2006;48:411–3.

51. Segal J, Lerner DJ, Miller DC, et al. When should Doppler-determined valve area be better than the Gorlin formula?: Variation in hydraulic constants in low flow states. J Am Coll Cardiol 1987;9:1294–305.

52. Meira ZM, Goulart EM, Colosimo EA, et al. Long term follow up of rheumatic fever and predictors of severe rheumatic valvar disease in Brazilian children and adolescents. Heart 2005;91:1019–22.

53. Marijon E, Iung B, Mocumbi AO, et al. What are the differences in presentation of candidates for percutaneous mitral commissurotomy across the world and do they influence the results of the procedure? Arch Cardiovasc Dis 2008;101:611–7.

54. Dubin AA, March HW, Cohn K, et al. Longitudinal hemodynamic and clinical study of mitral stenosis. Circulation 1971;44:381–9.

55. Gordon SP, Douglas PS, Come PC, et al. Two-dimensional and Doppler echocardiographic determinants of the natural history of mitral valve narrowing in patients with rheumatic mitral stenosis: implications for follow-up. J Am Coll Cardiol 1992;19:968–73.

56. Sagie A, Freitas N, Padial LR, et al. Doppler echocardiographic assessment of long-term progression of mitral stenosis in 103 patients: valve area and right heart disease. J Am Coll Cardiol 1996;28:472–9.

57. Antonini-Canterin F, Moura LM, Enache R, et al. Effect of hydroxymethylglutaryl coenzyme-a reductase inhibitors on the long-term progression of rheumatic mitral valve disease. Circulation 2010;121:2130–6.

58. Rowe JC, Bland EF, Sprague HB, et al. The course of mitral stenosis without surgery: ten- and twenty-year perspectives. Ann Intern Med 1960;52:741–9.

59. Olesen KH. The natural history of 271 patients with mitral stenosis under medical treatment. Br Heart J 1962;24:349–57.

60. Horstkotte D, Niehues R, Strauer BE. Pathomorphological aspects, aetiology and natural history of acquired mitral valve stenosis. Eur Heart J 1991;12(Suppl B):55–60.

61. Moreyra AE, Wilson AC, Deac R, et al. Factors associated with atrial fibrillation in patients with mitral stenosis: a cardiac catheterization study. Am Heart J 1998;135:138–45.

62. Ramsdale DR, Arumugam N, Singh SS, et al. Holter monitoring in patients with mitral stenosis and sinus rhythm. Eur Heart J 1987;8:164–70.

62a. Wolf PA, Dawber TR, Thomas HE Jr., et al. Epidemiologic assessment of chronic atrial fibrillation and risk of stroke: the Framingham study. Neurology 1978;28(10):973–7.

63. Selzer A, Cohn KE. Natural history of mitral stenosis: a review. Circulation 1972;45:878–90.

64. Fatkin D, Feneley M. Stratification of thromboembolic risk of atrial fibrillation by transthoracic echocardiography and transesophageal echocardiography: the relative role of left atrial appendage function, mitral valve disease, and spontaneous echocardiographic contrast. Prog Cardiovasc Dis 1996;39:57–68.

65. Gerber MA, Baltimore RS, Eaton CB, et al. Prevention of rheumatic fever and diagnosis and treatment of acute Streptococcal pharyngitis: a scientific statement from the American Heart Association Rheumatic Fever, Endocarditis, and Kawasaki Disease Committee of the Council on Cardiovascular Disease in the Young, the Interdisciplinary Council on Functional Genomics and Translational Biology, and the Interdisciplinary Council on Quality of Care and Outcomes Research: endorsed by the American Academy of Pediatrics. Circulation 2009;119:1541–51.

66. Wilson W, Taubert KA, Gewitz M, et al. Prevention of infective endocarditis: guidelines from the American Heart Association: a guideline from the American Heart Association Rheumatic Fever, Endocarditis, and Kawasaki Disease Committee, Council on Cardiovascular Disease in the Young, and the Council on Clinical Cardiology, Council on Cardiovascular Surgery and Anesthesia, and the Quality of Care and Outcomes Research Interdisciplinary Working Group. Circulation 2007;116:1736–54.

67. Habib G, Hoen B, Tornos P, et al. Guidelines on the prevention, diagnosis, and treatment of infective endocarditis (new version 2009): the Task Force on the Prevention, Diagnosis, and Treatment of Infective Endocarditis of the European Society of Cardiology (ESC). Eur Heart J 2009;30:2369–413.

68. Patel JJ, Dyer RB, Mitha AS. Beta adrenergic blockade does not improve effort tolerance in patients with mitral stenosis in sinus rhythm. Eur Heart J 1995;16:1264–8.

69. Stoll BC, Ashcom TL, Johns JP, et al. Effects of atenolol on rest and exercise hemodynamics in patients with mitral stenosis. Am J Cardiol 1995;75:482–4.

70. Hu CL, Jiang H, Tang QZ, et al. Comparison of rate control and rhythm control in patients with atrial fibrillation after percutaneous mitral balloon valvotomy: a randomised controlled study. Heart 2006;92:1096–101.

71. Perez-Gomez F, Alegria E, Berjon J, et al. Comparative effects of antiplatelet, anticoagulant, or combined therapy in patients with valvular and nonvalvular atrial fibrillation: a randomized multicenter study. J Am Coll Cardiol 2004;44:1557–66.

72. Regitz-Zagrosek V, Blomstrom Lundqvist C, Borghi C, et al. ESC Guidelines on the management of cardiovascular diseases during pregnancy: The Task Force on the Management of Cardiovascular Diseases during Pregnancy of the European Society of Cardiology (ESC). Eur Heart J 2011;32:3147–97.

73. Bouleti C, Iung B, Laouenan C, et al. Late Results of Percutaneous Mitral Commissurotomy up to 20 Years: Development and Validation of a Risk Score Predicting Late Functional Results from a Series of 912 Patients. Circulation 2012;125:2119–27.

74. Ellis LB, Singh JB, Morales DD, et al. Fifteen-to twenty-year study of one thousand patients undergoing closed mitral valvuloplasty. Circulation 1973;48:357–64.

75. John S, Bashi VV, Jairaj PS, et al. Closed mitral valvotomy: early results and long-term follow-up of 3724 consecutive patients. Circulation 1983;68:891–6.

76. Rihal CS, Schaff HV, Frye RL, et al. Long-term follow-up of patients undergoing closed transventricular mitral commissurotomy: a useful surrogate for percutaneous balloon mitral valvuloplasty? J Am Coll Cardiol 1992;20:781–6.

77. Detter C, Fischlein T, Feldmeier C, et al. Mitral commissurotomy, a technique outdated? Long-term follow-up over a period of 35 years. Ann Thorac Surg 1999;68:2112–8.

78. Higgs LM, Glancy DL, O'Brien KP, et al. Mitral restenosis: an uncommon cause of recurrent symptoms following mitral commissurotomy. Am J Cardiol 1970;26:34–7.

79. Smith WM, Neutze JM, Barratt-Boyes BG, et al. Open mitral valvotomy. Effect of preoperative factors on result. J Thorac Cardiovasc Surg 1981;82:738–51.

80. Reichart DT, Sodian R, Zenker R, et al. Long-term (</=50 years) results of patients after mitral valve commissurotomy-a single-center experience. J Thorac Cardiovasc Surg 2012;143:S96–98.

81. O'Brien SM, Shahian DM, Filardo G, et al. The Society of Thoracic Surgeons 2008 cardiac surgery risk models: part 2–isolated valve surgery. Ann Thorac Surg 2009;88:S23–42.

82. Rankin JS, Hammill BG, Ferguson TB Jr, et al. Determinants of operative mortality in valvular heart surgery. J Thorac Cardiovasc Surg 2006;131:547–57.

83. Inoue K, Owaki T, Nakamura T, et al. Clinical application of transvenous mitral commissurotomy by a new balloon catheter. J Thorac Cardiovasc Surg 1984;87:394–402.

84. Messika-Zeitoun D, Iung B, Brochet E, et al. Evaluation of mitral stenosis in 2008. Arch Cardiovasc Dis 2008;101:653–63.

85. Mezilis NE, Salame MY, Oakley GD. Predicting mitral regurgitation following percutaneous mitral valvotomy with the Inoue balloon: comparison of two echocardiographic scoring systems. Clin Cardiol 1999;22:453–8.

86. Complications and mortality of percutaneous balloon mitral commissurotomy. A report from the National Heart, Lung, and Blood Institute Balloon Valvuloplasty Registry. Circulation 1992;85:2014–24.

87. Tuzcu EM, Block PC, Palacios IF. Comparison of early versus late experience with percutaneous mitral balloon valvuloplasty. J Am Coll Cardiol 1991;17:1121–4.

88. Iung B, Cormier B, Ducimetiere P, et al. Immediate results of percutaneous mitral commissurotomy. A predictive model on a series of 1514 patients. Circulation 1996;94:2124–30.

89. Stefanadis CI, Stratos CG, Lambrou SG, et al. Retrograde nontransseptal balloon mitral valvuloplasty: immediate results and intermediate long-term outcome in 441 cases–a multicenter experience. J Am Coll Cardiol 1998;32:1009–16.

90. Vahanian A, Cormier B, Iung B. Mitral valvuloplasty In: Topol EJ, editor. Textbook of interventional cardiology 5th ed. Philadelphia: Saunders Elsevier; 2008. p. 879–93.

91. Bonhoeffer P, Esteves C, Casal U, et al. Percutaneous mitral valve dilatation with the Multi-Track System. Catheter Cardiovasc Interv 1999;48:178–83.

92. Cribier A, Eltchaninoff H, Koning R, et al. Percutaneous mechanical mitral commissurotomy with a newly designed metallic valvulotome: immediate results of the initial experience in 153 patients. Circulation 1999;99:793–9.

93. Park SH, Kim MA, Hyon MS. The advantages of On-line transesophageal echocardiography guide during percutaneous balloon mitral valvuloplasty. J Am Soc Echocardiogr 2000;13:26–34.

94. Liang KW, Fu YC, Lee WL, et al. Intra-cardiac echocardiography guided trans-septal puncture in patients with dilated left atrium undergoing percutaneous transvenous mitral commissurotomy. Int J Cardiol 2007;117:418–21.

95. Arora R, Kalra GS, Singh S, et al. Percutaneous transvenous mitral commissurotomy: immediate and long-term follow-up results. Catheter Cardiovasc Interv 2002;55:450–6.

96. Chen CR, Cheng TO. Percutaneous balloon mitral valvuloplasty by the Inoue technique: a multicenter study of 4832 patients in China. Am Heart J 1995;129:1197–203.

97. Neumayer U, Schmidt HK, Fassbender D, et al. Early (three-month) results of percutaneous mitral valvotomy with the Inoue balloon in 1,123 consecutive patients comparing various age groups. Am J Cardiol 2002;90:190–3.

98. Palacios IF, Sanchez PL, Harrell LC, et al. Which patients benefit from percutaneous mitral balloon valvuloplasty? Prevalvuloplasty and postvalvuloplasty variables that predict long-term outcome. Circulation 2002;105:1465–71.

99. Ben-Farhat M, Betbout F, Gamra H, et al. Predictors of long-term event-free survival and of freedom from restenosis after percutaneous balloon mitral commissurotomy. Am Heart J 2001;142:1072–9.

100. Hernandez R, Banuelos C, Alfonso F, et al. Long-term clinical and echocardiographic follow-up after percutaneous mitral valvuloplasty with the Inoue balloon. Circulation 1999;99:1580–6.

101. Meneveau N, Schiele F, Seronde MF, et al. Predictors of event-free survival after percutaneous mitral commissurotomy. Heart 1998;80:359–64.

102. Fawzy ME, Shoukri M, Al Buraiki J, et al. Seventeen years' clinical and echocardiographic follow up of mitral balloon valvuloplasty in 520 patients, and predictors of long-term outcome. J Heart Valve Dis 2007;16:454–60.

103. Eltchaninoff H, Koning R, Derumeaux G, et al. Percutaneous mitral commissurotomy by metallic dilator. Multicenter experience with 500 patients. Arch Mal Coeur Vaiss 2000;93:685–92.

104. Kang DH, Park SW, Song JK, et al. Long-term clinical and echocardiographic outcome of percutaneous mitral valvuloplasty: randomized comparison of Inoue and double-balloon techniques. J Am Coll Cardiol 2000;35:169–75.

105. Krishnamoorthy KM, Dash PK, Radhakrishnan S, et al. Response of different grades of pulmonary artery hypertension to balloon mitral valvuloplasty. Am J Cardiol 2002;90:1170–3.

106. Tanabe Y, Oshima M, Suzuki M, et al. Determinants of delayed improvement in exercise capacity after percutaneous transvenous mitral commissurotomy. Am Heart J 2000;139:889–94.

107. Acar C, Jebara VA, Grare P, et al. Traumatic mitral insufficiency following percutaneous mitral dilation: anatomic lesions and surgical implications. Eur J Cardiothorac Surg 1992;6:660–3; discussion 663–4.

108. Choudhary SK, Talwar S, Venugopal P. Severe mitral regurgitation after percutaneous transmitral commissurotomy: underestimated subvalvular disease. J Thorac Cardiovasc Surg 2006;131:927; author reply 927–8.

109. Varma PK, Theodore S, Neema PK, et al. Emergency surgery after percutaneous transmitral commissurotomy: operative versus echocardiographic findings, mechanisms of complications, and outcomes. J Thorac Cardiovasc Surg 2005;130:772–6.

110. Zimmet AD, Almeida AA, Harper RW, et al. Predictors of surgery after percutaneous mitral valvuloplasty. Ann Thorac Surg 2006;82:828–33.

111. Reifart N, Nowak B, Baykut D, et al. Experimental balloon valvuloplasty of fibrotic and calcific mitral valves. Circulation 1990;81:1005–11.

112. Cequier A, Bonan R, Serra A, et al. Left-to-right atrial shunting after percutaneous mitral valvuloplasty. Incidence and long-term hemodynamic follow-up. Circulation 1990;81:1190–7.

113. Herrmann HC, Ramaswamy K, Isner JM, et al. Factors influencing immediate results, complications, and short-term follow-up status after Inoue balloon mitral valvotomy: a North American multicenter study. Am Heart J 1992;124:160–6.

114. Feldman T, Carroll JD, Isner JM, et al. Effect of valve deformity on results and mitral regurgitation after Inoue balloon commissurotomy. Circulation 1992;85:180–7.

115. Cruz-Gonzalez I, Sanchez-Ledesma M, Sanchez PL, et al. Predicting success and long-term outcomes of percutaneous mitral valvuloplasty: a multifactorial score. Am J Med 2009;122:581 e511-589.

116. Dean LS, Mickel M, Bonan R, et al. Four-year follow-up of patients undergoing percutaneous balloon mitral commissurotomy. A report from the National Heart, Lung, and Blood Institute Balloon Valvuloplasty Registry. J Am Coll Cardiol 1996;28:1452–7.

117. Song JK, Song JM, Kang DH, et al. Restenosis and adverse clinical events after successful percutaneous mitral valvuloplasty: immediate post-procedural mitral valve area as an important prognosticator. Eur Heart J 2009;30:1254–62.

118. Fawzy ME. Long-term results up to 19 years of mitral balloon valvuloplasty. Asian Cardiovasc Thorac Ann 2009;17:627–33.

119. Wang A, Krasuski RA, Warner JJ, et al. Serial echocardiographic evaluation of restenosis after successful percutaneous mitral commissurotomy. J Am Coll Cardiol 2002;39:328–34.

120. Orrange SE, Kawanishi DT, Lopez BM, et al. Actuarial outcome after catheter balloon commissurotomy in patients with mitral stenosis. Circulation 1997;95:382–9.

121. Pathan AZ, Mahdi NA, Leon MN, et al. Is redo percutaneous mitral balloon valvuloplasty (PMV) indicated in patients with post-PMV mitral restenosis? J Am Coll Cardiol 1999;34:49–54.

122. Iung B, Garbarz E, Michaud P, et al. Immediate and mid-term results of repeat percutaneous mitral commissurotomy for restenosis following earlier percutaneous mitral commissurotomy. Eur Heart J 2000;21:1683–9.

123. Kim JB, Ha JW, Kim JS, et al. Comparison of long-term outcome after mitral valve replacement or repeated balloon mitral valvotomy in patients with restenosis after previous balloon valvotomy. Am J Cardiol 2007;99:1571–4.

124. Chmielak Z, Klopotowski M, Kruk M, et al. Repeat percutaneous mitral balloon valvuloplasty for patients with mitral valve restenosis. Catheter Cardiovasc Interv 2010;76:986–92.

125. Yazicioglu N, Arat Ozkan A, Orta Kilickesmez K, et al. Immediate and follow-up results of repeat percutaneous mitral balloon commissurotomy for restenosis after a successful first procedure. Echocardiography 2010;27:765–9.

126. Stefanadis C, Dernellis J, Stratos C, et al. Effects of balloon mitral valvuloplasty on left atrial function in mitral stenosis as assessed by pressure-area relation. J Am Coll Cardiol 1998;32:159–68.

127. Cormier B, Vahanian A, Iung B, et al. Influence of percutaneous mitral commissurotomy on left atrial spontaneous contrast of mitral stenosis. Am J Cardiol 1993;71:842–7.

128. Porte JM, Cormier B, Iung B, et al. Early assessment by transesophageal echocardiography of left atrial appendage function after percutaneous mitral commissurotomy. Am J Cardiol 1996;77:72–6.

129. Zaki A, Salama M, El Masry M, et al. Immediate effect of balloon valvuloplasty on hemostatic changes in mitral stenosis. Am J Cardiol 2000;85:370–5.

130. Chen MC, Wu CJ, Chang HW, et al. Mechanism of reducing platelet activity by percutaneous transluminal mitral valvuloplasty in patients with rheumatic mitral stenosis. Chest 2004;125:1629–34.

131. Chiang CW, Lo SK, Ko YS, et al. Predictors of systemic embolism in patients with mitral stenosis. A prospective study. Ann Intern Med 1998;128:885–9.

132. Liu TJ, Lai HC, Lee WL, et al. Percutaneous balloon commissurotomy reduces incidence of ischemic cerebral stroke in patients with symptomatic rheumatic mitral stenosis. Int J Cardiol 2008;123:189–90.

133. Krasuski RA, Assar MD, Wang A, et al. Usefulness of percutaneous balloon mitral commissurotomy in preventing the development of atrial fibrillation in patients with mitral stenosis. Am J Cardiol 2004;93:936–9.

134. Leon MN, Harrell LC, Simosa HF, et al. Mitral balloon valvotomy for patients with mitral stenosis in atrial fibrillation: immediate and long-term results. J Am Coll Cardiol 1999;34:1145–52.

135. Fan K, Lee KL, Chow WH, et al. Internal cardioversion of chronic atrial fibrillation during percutaneous mitral commissurotomy: insight into reversal of chronic stretch-induced atrial remodeling. Circulation 2002;105:2746–52.

136. Krittayaphong R, Chotinaiwatarakul C, Phankingthongkum R, et al. One-year outcome of cardioversion of atrial fibrillation in patients with mitral stenosis after percutaneous balloon mitral valvuloplasty. Am J Cardiol 2006;97:1045–50.

137. Turi ZG, Reyes VP, Raju BS, et al. Percutaneous balloon versus surgical closed commissurotomy for mitral stenosis. A prospective, randomized trial. Circulation 1991;83:1179–85.

138. Reyes VP, Raju BS, Wynne J, et al. Percutaneous balloon valvuloplasty compared with open surgical commissurotomy for mitral stenosis. N Engl J Med 1994;331:961–7.

139. Ben Farhat M, Ayari M, Maatouk F, et al. Percutaneous balloon versus surgical closed and open mitral commissurotomy: seven-year follow-up results of a randomized trial. Circulation 1998;97:245–50.

140. Rifaie O, Abdel-Dayem MK, Ramzy A, et al. Percutaneous mitral valvotomy versus closed surgical commissurotomy. Up to 15 years of follow-up of a prospective randomized study. J Cardiol 2009;53:28–34.

141. Song JK, Kim MJ, Yun SC, et al. Long-term outcomes of percutaneous mitral balloon valvuloplasty versus open cardiac surgery. J Thorac Cardiovasc Surg 2010;139:103–10.

142. Langerveld J, Thijs Plokker HW, Ernst SM, et al. Predictors of clinical events or restenosis during follow-up after percutaneous mitral balloon valvotomy. Eur Heart J 1999;20:519–26.

143. Jneid H, Cruz-Gonzalez I, Sanchez-Ledesma M, et al. Impact of pre- and postprocedural mitral regurgitation on outcomes after percutaneous mitral valvuloplasty for mitral stenosis. Am J Cardiol 2009;104:1122–7.

144. Iung B, Garbarz E, Michaud P, et al. Late results of percutaneous mitral commissurotomy in a series of 1024 patients. Analysis of late clinical deterioration: frequency, anatomic findings, and predictive factors. Circulation 1999;99:3272–8.

145. Jang IK, Block PC, Newell JB, et al. Percutaneous mitral balloon valvotomy for recurrent mitral stenosis after surgical commissurotomy. Am J Cardiol 1995;75:601–5.

146. Iung B, Garbarz E, Michaud P, et al. Percutaneous mitral commissurotomy for restenosis after surgical commissurotomy: late efficacy and implications for patient selection. J Am Coll Cardiol 2000;35:1295–302.

147. Fawzy ME, Hassan W, Shoukri M, et al. Immediate and long-term results of mitral balloon valvotomy for restenosis following previous surgical or balloon mitral commissurotomy. Am J Cardiol 2005;96:971–5.

148. Umesan CV, Kapoor A, Sinha N, et al. Effect of Inoue balloon mitral valvotomy on severe pulmonary arterial hypertension in 315 patients with rheumatic mitral stenosis: immediate and long-term results. J Heart Valve Dis 2000;9:609–15.

149. Maoqin S, Guoxiang H, Zhiyuan S, et al. The clinical and hemodynamic results of mitral balloon valvuloplasty for patients with mitral stenosis complicated by severe pulmonary hypertension. Eur J Intern Med 2005;16:413–8.

150. Carroll JD, Feldman T. Percutaneous mitral balloon valvotomy and the new demographics of mitral stenosis. JAMA 1993;270:1731–6.

151. Iung B, Baron G, Tornos P, et al. Valvular heart disease in the community: a European experience. Curr Probl Cardiol 2007;32:609–61.

152. Gamra H, Betbout F, Ben Hamda K, et al. Balloon mitral commissurotomy in juvenile rheumatic mitral stenosis: a ten-year clinical and echocardiographic actuarial results. Eur Heart J 2003;24:1349–56.

153. Fawzy ME, Stefadouros MA, Hegazy H, et al. Long term clinical and echocardiographic results of mitral balloon valvotomy in children and adolescents. Heart 2005;91:743–8.

154. Goldman JH, Slade A, Clague J. Cardiogenic shock secondary to mitral stenosis treated by balloon mitral valvuloplasty. Cathet Cardiovasc Diagn 1998;43:195–7.

155. Tuzcu EM, Block PC, Griffin BP, et al. Immediate and long-term outcome of percutaneous mitral valvotomy in patients 65 years and older. Circulation 1992;85:963–71.

156. Iung B, Cormier B, Farah B, et al. Percutaneous mitral commissurotomy in the elderly. Eur Heart J 1995;16:1092–9.

157. Hildick-Smith DJ, Taylor GJ, Shapiro LM. Inoue balloon mitral valvuloplasty: long-term clinical and echocardiographic follow-up of a predominantly unfavourable population. Eur Heart J 2000;21:1690–7.

158. Sutaria N, Elder AT, Shaw TR. Long term outcome of percutaneous mitral balloon valvotomy in patients aged 70 and over. Heart 2000;83:433–8.

159. Diao M, Kane A, Ndiaye MB, et al. Pregnancy in women with heart disease in sub-Saharan Africa. Arch Cardiovasc Dis 2011;104:370–4.

160. Hameed AB, Mehra A, Rahimtoola SH. The role of catheter balloon commissurotomy for severe mitral stenosis in pregnancy. Obstet Gynecol 2009;114:1336–40.

161. Iung B, Cormier B, Elias J, et al. Usefulness of percutaneous balloon commissurotomy for mitral stenosis during pregnancy. Am J Cardiol 1994;73:398–400.

162. Chen WJ, Chen MF, Liau CS, et al. Safety of percutaneous transvenous balloon mitral commissurotomy in patients with mitral stenosis and thrombus in the left atrial appendage. Am J Cardiol 1992;70:117–9.

163. Silaruks S, Thinkhamrop B, Kiatchoosakun S, et al. Resolution of left atrial thrombus after 6 months of anticoagulation in candidates for percutaneous transvenous mitral commissurotomy. Ann Intern Med 2004;140:101–5.

164. Vaturi M, Porter A, Adler Y, et al. The natural history of aortic valve disease after mitral valve surgery. J Am Coll Cardiol 1999;33:2003–8.

165. Song H, Kang DH, Kim JH, et al. Percutaneous mitral valvuloplasty versus surgical treatment in mitral stenosis with severe tricuspid regurgitation. Circulation 2007;116:I246–250.

166. Kothari SS, Ramakrishnan S, Kumar CK, et al. Intermediate-term results of percutaneous transvenous mitral commissurotomy in children less than 12 years of age. Catheter Cardiovasc Interv 2005;64:487–90.

167. Kang DH, Lee CH, Kim DH, et al. Early percutaneous mitral commissurotomy vs. conventional management in asymptomatic moderate mitral stenosis. Eur Heart J 2012;33:1511–7.

168. Reddy VY, Holmes D, Doshi SK, et al. Safety of percutaneous left atrial appendage closure: results from the Watchman Left Atrial Appendage System for Embolic Protection in Patients with AF (PROTECT AF) clinical trial and the Continued Access Registry. Circulation 2011;123:417–24.

169. Adragao P, Machado FP, Aguiar C, et al. Ablation of atrial fibrillation in mitral valve disease patients: five year follow-up after percutaneous pulmonary vein isolation and mitral balloon valvuloplasty. Rev Port Cardiol 2003;22:1025–36.

170. Post JR, Feldman T, Isner J, et al. Inoue balloon mitral valvotomy in patients with severe valvular and subvalvular deformity. J Am Coll Cardiol 1995;25:1129–36.

171. Iung B, Garbarz E, Doutrelant L, et al. Late results of percutaneous mitral commissurotomy for calcific mitral stenosis. Am J Cardiol 2000;85:1308–14.

172. Cohen DJ, Kuntz RE, Gordon SP, et al. Predictors of long-term outcome after percutaneous balloon mitral valvuloplasty. N Engl J Med 1992;327:1329–35.

RHEUMATIC MITRAL VALVE DISEASE

CHAPTER 18

Myxomatous Mitral Valve Disease

Amar Krishnaswamy and Brian P. Griffin

> ### Key Points
>
> - Mitral valve prolapse (MVP) occurs in 2.4% of the population and is the leading cause of mitral regurgitation in developed countries.
> - Tensile strength is seriously compromised in myxomatous chordae despite an increase in thickness and extensibility. Myxomatous chordae fail at 25% of the load that it takes to rupture a normal chord.
> - On two-dimensional echocardiography, MVP is diagnosed when either or both of the mitral leaflets are displaced 2 mm or more in systole above a line connecting the annular hinge points in the parasternal or apical long-axis view.
> - Mitral regurgitation from MVP is often eccentric in nature, and the color display may underestimate the true severity. It is important to examine the left atrium in multiple views, including off-axis views, to fully define the jet. Transesophageal imaging is helpful in this situation to characterize the jet.
> - Although MVP is equally prevalent in men and women, men are much more likely to experience significant complications. Risk factors for development of progressively severe mitral regurgitation include male gender, hypertension, increased body mass index, and increasing age. Echocardiographic factors associated with increased risk of severe mitral regurgitation include redundant thickened leaflets, prolapse involving the posterior leaflet, and increased left ventricular size.

Mitral valve prolapse is a common disorder that has been recognized as a specific condition since the 1960s, when Barlow and Bosman[1] used cineangiography to delineate the cause of systolic clicks and murmurs. Previously, myxomatous change in mitral valve tissue had been recognized pathologically. However, it was only with the arrival of two-dimensional (2D) echocardiography in the 1970s and subsequently that the natural history and pathophysiology of the condition and its complications became manifest. Mitral valve prolapse (MVP), a term originally coined by Criley et al,[2] is now recognized as the major cause of mitral regurgitation (MR) in developed countries and a cause of premature mortality and considerable morbidity if not diagnosed and appropriately managed.[3,4] In this chapter, we outline the pathogenesis of myxomatous mitral valve disease, its natural history and clinical manifestations, and the current approach to diagnosis and management of the disease and its complications.

Definition

One of the difficulties in diagnosing and managing patients with MVP is appropriate patient classification. Myxomatous mitral valve disease and MVP are conditions that occur together but are not necessarily synonymous (Figure 18-1).[5,6] Understanding the interplay between these entities is essential. Myxomatous mitral valve disease is a pathologic condition in which the mitral valve leaflets and chordae are thickened, there is hooding of the leaflets, and abnormal accumulations of mucopolysaccharides are seen in chordae and leaflets.[3,7] The valve abnormalities and especially the chordal elongation produce prolapse of the leaflets recognized echocardiographically that, in some cases, leads to MR.[8] A systolic click and murmur are characteristic clinical findings.[9] This condition is associated with complications in a substantial minority of patients affected and may eventually lead to the need for valve surgery.[10-12] However, myxomatous mitral valve disease may exist in a preclinical phase without any overt echocardiographic or clinical manifestations. *Barlow disease* defines the situation of significant and diffuse myxomatous degeneration leading to bileaflet redundancy and broad bileaflet prolapse.

Observation of superior displacement of part of a mitral valve leaflet in systole on 2D echocardiography is common even in normal people. Before the refinement of echocardiographic criteria, prolapse was diagnosed in a substantial portion of the population.[13] Even with stricter echocardiographic criteria for diagnosis, superior displacement of the mitral valve leaflets is seen in the absence of leaflet thickening or MR in some normal people. This form of prolapse appears to arise in many instances from a disproportion between mitral leaflet size and left ventricular (LV) size. For example, it can be seen in patients with a small left ventricle and may subsequently disappear with volume loading.[14-16] It can also be seen in patients with an atrial septal defect, and may disappear on closure of the septal defect.[17,18] This subtle type of prolapse is not a precursor of myxomatous changes in the mitral valve and appears to have a very benign prognosis.

Anatomy of the Normal and Myxomatous Mitral Valve

A basic knowledge of the anatomy of the normal mitral valve is important to understanding and recognizing the variable presentation of myxomatous mitral valve disease.[19,20] The mitral valve consists of anterior and posterior leaflets attached at their bases to a fibrous or fibromuscular ring, the mitral annulus (Figure 18-2). The leaflets in turn are attached to the two papillary muscles (anterolateral and posteromedial) by chordae tendineae, one of whose functions is to prevent eversion or prolapse of the leaflets in systole.

The anterior leaflet is generally larger than the posterior leaflet and is triangular. The anterior area leaflet has two distinct portions, a thin translucent area at the base and a more opaque thicker area at the free edge (the rough zone) where coaptation with the posterior leaflet occurs. The posterior leaflet is smaller, has a longer attachment to the annulus, and is generally segmented by clefts at the free edge into three segments or scallops. The anterior and posterior leaflets meet at the two commissures (posteromedial and anterolateral) and are fused there by a rim of valve tissue of variable (<1 cm) width. Carpentier[21] has provided a surgical classification of mitral valve anatomy that is widely used. In this classification, the mitral valve has six segments, three

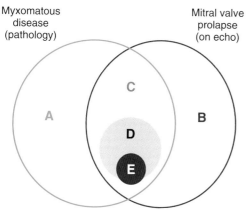

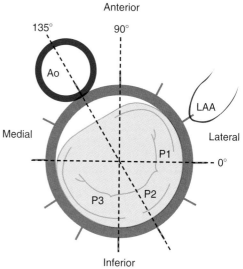

FIGURE 18-1   Interaction of myxomatous disease of the mitral valve, which is diagnosed on pathologic examination, and mitral valve prolapse, which is diagnosed on an echocardiogram. A, Myxomatous disease can exist in a preclinical state before the onset of prolapse. **B,** Mitral valve prolapse may occur on echocardiography as a benign condition without myxomatous change mainly due to valve-ventricle disproportion. **C,** Myxomatous valve disease is a major cause of mitral valve prolapse. **D,** A subset of patients with myxomatous disease and MVP have high-risk clinical and echocardiographic features that make them more prone to the development of complications **(E),** such as severe mitral regurgitation requiring surgery and endocarditis.

FIGURE 18-3   Mitral valve as viewed from the left ventricle. Angles correspond to the transesophageal echocardiography planes that cut the mitral valve as demonstrated. The exact location of the plane depends on the height of the probe in the esophagus and the extent of anteflexion or retroflexion. *Ao,* Aorta; *LAA,* left atrial appendage; *P,* posterior; *P1, P2, P3,* the three scallops of the posterior leaflet.

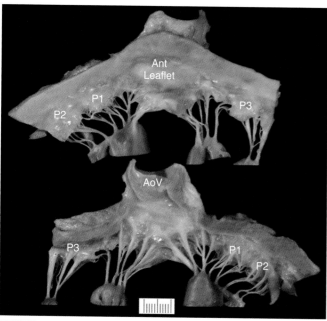

FIGURE 18-2   Normal mitral valve. The thin translucent leaflets and chordae and papillary muscles are visualized from the atrial side *(top)* and the ventricular side *(bottom).* The two leaflets (*Ant,* anterior) and the three scallops of the posterior leaflet (*P1, P2,* and *P3*) are shown. *AoV,* Aortic valve.

mitral valve replacement techniques). Of note, the secondary chords that attach to the anterior leaflet are more prominent than those attaching to the posterior leaflet. The tertiary chords arise directly from the ventricular trabeculae and attach to the posterior leaflet annulus. Additional chordae are attached at the commissures and at each cleft of the posterior mitral leaflet. The chordae to the posterior leaflet are inserted into each of the scallops, explaining why chordal rupture may lead to prolapse or flail of an individual scallop. On average, 25 major chordal trunks attach the leaflets to the papillary muscles, equally divided between anterior and posterior; an additional 100 smaller chords also attach to the leaflets.[23]

The coaptation area of the two leaflets is much greater than that of the mitral orifice, and that of the anterior leaflet may be sufficient in itself to cover the entire orifice in systole. Mitral valve repair takes advantage of this property when resection of a prolapsing portion of the posterior leaflet is necessary: The anterior leaflet provides most of the coverage of the mitral orifice without allowing significant leakage. In many instances, the posterior leaflet provides an anchor or keystone against which the anterior leaflet abuts to maintain a stable and competent coaptation surface. Prolapse of the posterior leaflet may cause the anterior leaflet to prolapse because of the loss of this keystone function in the absence of any major pathologic change in the anterior leaflet or its chordae.

Myxomatous disease of the mitral valve may affect one or both leaflets and may affect many or only some of the chordae. Prolapse or flail of the posterior leaflet is the most common indication for surgical intervention. In one study of more than 1000 patients undergoing surgery for myxomatous MR, more than 50% had evidence of chordal rupture to the posterior leaflet.[24] The middle scallop (P2) is the segment most commonly affected, followed by the lateral and then the medial scallop.

Etiology and Pathology of Mitral Valve Prolapse

MVP is a degenerative condition of the mitral valve that usually becomes evident in adulthood and is associated with a number of connective tissue disorders. Each of these disorders is related to mutations in extracellular matrix genes, thus suggesting a role

in the anterior leaflet (A1, A2, and A3) and three in the posterior leaflet (P1, P2, and P3). The posterior leaflet segments consist of the naturally occurring scallops (P1, lateral; P2, middle; and P3, medial); the anterior segments constitute the areas adjoining each of the three posterior scallops (Figure 18-3).[21,22]

Normal chordae vary widely in number and appearance, and each papillary muscle provides chordae to both leaflets. Primary chordae are attached to the valve at the leaflet edge and serve to halt valve-edge prolapse. Secondary chordae attach the papillary muscle to the ventricular surface of the leaflets at the region of coaptation. Their role is to anchor the leaflets, and they are integral to optimal ventricular function (highlighting the idea of valvuloventricular synergy and providing a rationale for valve-sparing

for abnormalities of structural proteins in the pathogenesis of MVP.[19,25-29] MVP is seen in patients suffering with the Ehlers-Danlos syndrome and osteogenesis imperfecta, both of which are associated with mutations in collagen. Patients with the Marfan syndrome have a mutation in the *fbn1* gene encoding fibrillin, a major component of elastin, and also display MVP. In a related pathway, mutations in transforming growth factor-β (TGF-β) signaling may be responsible for the progression of Marfan syndrome and also result in the Loeys-Dietz syndrome, which is associated with a number of phenotypes, including MVP. Whether abrogation of the TGF-β pathway using angiotensin receptor blockade, as shown in Loeys-Dietz mice with aortic pathology, can slow the progression of MVP in humans is unknown but is an interesting concept. Ultimately, however, the majority of MVP cases are idiopathic in nature, and although characteristic abnormalities on both gross pathologic and histologic examinations are evident, the precise mechanism of disease remains to be determined.

Pathologically, myxoid degeneration of valve tissue is distinctive.[30] Grossly, there is enlargement and thickening of the leaflets and chords, interchordal hooding of the leaflets, and annular dilation with elongated and frequently ruptured chordae (Figure 18-4). The tissue has a spongy texture, and valve thickening is in large part due to the deposition of proteoglycans and collagen. The redundancy of leaflet tissue is often substantial, and fibrin deposits and even microthrombi may be evident in the folds at the base of the leaflets.[31-33] In addition to these microthrombi, platelet activation at the site of roughened endothelium in the valve has also been postulated as a source of emboli.[32] The increased motion of valves and chords often leads to fibrosis of both valve tissue and endocardium at points of contact in the atrium and ventricles. These fibrosed areas have been postulated by some to be a source of increased arrhythmogenicity.[34]

The mitral valve has three layers histologically: the atrialis, a layer of collagen and elastic tissue that forms the atrial aspect of the leaflet; the spongiosa, a middle layer that contains structural proteins and proteoglycans; and the fibrosa, or ventricularis, that consists predominantly of collagen and is on the ventricular side of the leaflet (Figure 18-5).[35] In myxomatous disease, the spongiosa shows an accumulation of proteoglycans and glycosaminoglycans that extends into the chords and the fibrosa and has

reduced collagen staining.[36] The increased extracellular matrix gives the tissue a blue color on hematoxylin and eosin staining and was the original basis for the "myxomatous" label. The increased proteoglycans in the fibrosa are postulated to interfere with tensile strength. An inflammatory infiltrate is not seen in

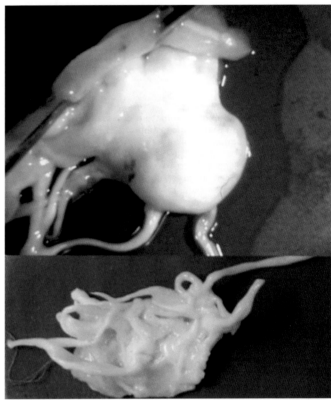

FIGURE 18-4 **Gross appearance of myxomatous valve and chordae illustrating the thickening and spongy appearance of the leaflets and chordae.**

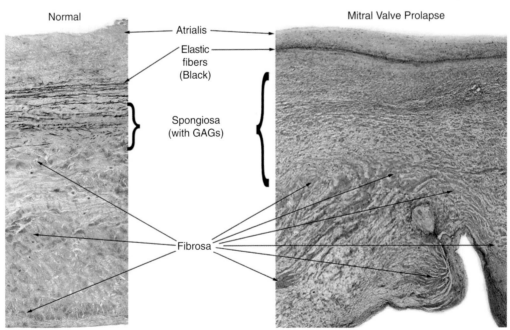

FIGURE 18-5 **Histologic appearance of a mitral valve leaflet.** The spongiosa is thicker in mitral valve prolapse than in the normal valve with a greater concentration of glycosaminoglycans (GAGs), some of which extend into the fibrosa. *(Courtesy Rene Rodriguez, MD, Department of Cardiovascular Pathology, Cleveland Clinic.)*

myxomatous tissue, but myofibroblasts are modulated to a more activated format.[37]

The myxomatous mitral valve has been classified into two types on the basis of its surgical appearance by Carpentier's group.[38] One type, called Barlow disease, is seen in younger patients with marked redundancy of the tissue and prolapse that may involve multiple segments and is more difficult to repair.[31,39] This type is also seen in connective tissue disorders such as Marfan syndrome. Fibroelastic deficiency, the other type, is seen in older patients in whom myxomatous changes are confined to a single segment, typically the posterior middle scallop (P2). The rest of the valve does not appear myxomatous. There is considerable overlap between these groups, and in our and others' experience it has proved difficult to differentiate the groups reproducibly on either the gross or histologic appearance of the valve.[38]

At a mechanical level, considerable abnormality is noted in myxomatous valve disease, which in part explains the pathophysiology. Fragmentation and irregularity of both collagen and elastin have been reported.[40-42] When myxomatous valve tissue obtained at the time of mitral valve surgery is subjected to formal stress/strain analysis, the leaflets are more extensible and less stiff than normal but have relatively minor reductions in tensile strength.[43] Tensile strength is seriously compromised in the chordae despite the increase in thickness and extensibility. Myxomatous chordae fail at 25% of the load that it takes to rupture a normal chord.[44] They exhibit areas of thickening due to glycosaminoglycans deposition and fibrous sheath formation.[45] The poor load-bearing qualities of these chordae suggest that the collagen in the fibrous sheath does not add any tensile strength.[46]

Biochemically, alterations in myxomatous tissue have also been noted. The major abnormalities relate not only to the increased amounts of glycosaminoglycans but also to the types produced. Glycosaminoglycans have multiple roles, including imparting specific qualities to connective tissue and modifying the structure of collagen. Glycosaminoglycans are incorporated with proteins as proteoglycans, which have also inherent specific properties.[47] These properties may in turn be further modified by combination with other proteoglycans. In myxomatous chordae, the amount of glycosaminoglycans is twice the normal amount, without any change in cellularity, suggesting that this increase occurs because of either greater production or reduced degradation or a combination. Thus far, mutations in proteoglycans have not been identified in association with MVP, but it is possible that improper processing of these proteins leads to degenerative valve disease (as shown in *Adamts*9 protease-deficient mice).[48]

As in the mechanical findings, the degree of biochemical abnormality in myxomatous tissue is more marked in chordal tissue than in the leaflets.[47] Although the individual glycosaminoglycans in valve and chordal tissue are similar, their proportions differ substantially. These proportions are further altered in myxomatous tissue, as is the chain length of the glycosaminoglycans themselves. In myxomatous chordae, there is an excess of hyaluronan and chondroitin-6-sulfate. Hyaluronan and chondroitin-6-sulfate are constituents of the proteoglycan versican. Versican is a large proteoglycan that in combination with hyaluronan is thought to increase hydration and sponginess of connective tissue. These properties are ideal to withstand compressive forces such as those that occur at the coaptation surface. In addition, myxomatous chordae have decreased amounts of 4-sulfated glycosaminoglycans commonly seen in the small proteoglycan decorin. Decorin is important in collagen fibrillogenesis, and its reduction may further explain the decrease in the tensile strength encountered in these chordae.[49]

Interestingly, the proportions of glycosaminoglycans seen in myxomatous chordae more closely resemble those in normal leaflets than those in normal chordae. It is unclear why this finding occurs, whether it is genetically determined or whether local environmental factors in the valve itself play a role. The finding that glycosaminoglycan production is modulated in a cell culture model of valve tissue by alterations in environmental factors such as tissue strain and location suggests that glycosaminoglycan synthesis or degradation is responsive to local environmental conditions.[50] A neural network that is impaired or damaged in the myxomatous process has also been described in valves.[51] This impairment too, could potentially be involved in aligning appropriate glycosaminoglycan production with a sensed physiologic stimulus such as tension or compression. In addition to changes in glycosaminoglycans, an increase in matrix metalloproteinases and other degradative enzymes is reported in myxomatous mitral valve disease.[37] These enzymes appear to be produced by cells within the valve tissue, are capable of structural protein degradation, and may play a role in the structural abnormalities in this disease or may occur in response to the alterations caused by the disease.

Genetic Factors

Myxoid degeneration of the mitral valve is often familial, although the severity of expression varies considerably within a given family, suggesting that environmental influences are also important.[52,53] The inheritance is considered to be autosomal dominant with variable penetrance that is influenced by both age and gender. It is uncommon in our experience at Cleveland Clinic to perform surgery for myxoid MR on more than one member of an affected family despite the familial nature of the disease. Work from Devereux's group suggested that although MVP occurs with frequency in the families of those affected, the severity of the lesion is very variable within the same kindred.[53,54] In one study, probands with thickened leaflets were more likely to have family members with MVP (53%) than those without significant leaflet thickening (27%). In multiple studies, heterogeneity of findings in relatives of probands is seen. Thus, leaflet thickening or involvement of one or both leaflets may vary in family members, suggesting that phenotypic expression is affected by many other factors rather than a specific genotype.[53]

At least three separate loci for the MVP trait have been identified in extended families with multiple affected members. These include a locus identified in 1999 in France (*MMVP1*), which was mapped to chromosome 16p11.2-p12.1.[55] A further locus, *MMVP2*, was identified in 2003 by Freed et al[56] on chromosome 11p15.4. A third locus (*MMVP3*) on chromosome 13 (13q31.3-q32.1) was reported by Nesta et al[57] in a family of 43 members, of whom 9 had conventional diagnostic criteria for MVP. Prolapse configuration was not uniform in those affected, and both thickened and nonthickened prolapsing leaflets were seen; prolapse involved the posterior leaflet in some and both leaflets in others. The proteins coded by the three reported MVP loci are unknown as yet because these studies were performed with linkage analysis.[58] However, the locus on chromosome 13 has genes of potential interest that involve cell growth and differentiation.

The occurrence of myxomatous MVP in association with other inherited connective tissue disorders raised the question whether proteins involved in these disorders might underlie idiopathic myxomatous degeneration. So far, however, the genes encoding the primary collagens in valve tissue have not been linked to autosomal dominant MVP.[59,60] Multiple single-nucleotide polymorphisms were detected at a higher frequency in people with idiopathic myxoid degeneration than in a control population, but their significance remains unclear.[61,62] In a rare related condition, X-linked myxomatous valvular dystrophy, in which all of the valves are thickened, mutations in filamin A, a gene that previously was identified only as a cause of neurologic and skeletal disorders, have been implicated.[63]

MVP is not confined to humans. Specific breeds of dog, including the Cavalier King Charles Spaniel and the dachshund, have a high prevalence of prolapse that may lead to severe MR and congestive heart failure later in life.[64,65] The disease is associated with dysmorphic leaflets and is inherited, suggesting a strong genetic linkage, although the specific genetic determinants remain to be elucidated. An experimental murine model of

Marfan syndrome–associated MVP has been described in which TGF-β signaling is increased as a result of fibrillin-1 deficiency.[66] Interestingly, the mitral valve changes progressed over time. Abnormal signaling involving the TGF-β system has also been postulated as a mechanism of abnormality in X-linked valve dystrophy.[67] Although these animal models provide very useful insights into mechanism of disease, the pathophysiologic mechanisms operating in human idiopathic MVP appear to differ from those in both Marfan syndrome and the X-linked disorder.[26,68]

Epidemiology and Natural History

The currently accepted prevalence of MVP in the community is based on the Framingham Heart Study.[69] In that population-based study, the echocardiograms of 3491 individuals (1845 men and 1646 women) were reviewed. The mean age of the population was 55 years. MVP was determined on long-axis views of the valve and was seen in 84 subjects or 2.4% of the population. Classic prolapse, in which leaflet thickness greater than 5 mm and leaflet prolapse are present, was seen in 1.3% of those studied; nonclassic prolapse, in which leaflet displacement alone was apparent, occurred in 1.1%. There was no significant gender difference in prevalence, unlike in earlier studies without a strict echocardiographic definition, in which women predominated. Prevalence was 2% to 3% in each decade of age from 30 to 80. The subjects with MVP had a greater likelihood of MR than those without prolapse, with more regurgitation being evident in the group with classic prolapse, who had, on average, mild regurgitation. Those with nonclassic prolapse had, on average, trace MR. Other complications, such as atrial fibrillation, congestive heart failure, cerebrovascular disease, and syncope, were no more common in the MVP group than in the rest of the population studied. MVP has been detected in many population groups of different ethnic and racial backgrounds.[70] In one Canadian study, the prevalences were similar in Caucasian, Indian, and Chinese populations.[71]

When MVP is suspected clinically and confirmed by echocardiography, long-term follow-up suggests a more complicated course than that experienced by subjects detected by community screening as in the Framingham study. A Mayo Clinic study identified 833 asymptomatic patients with MVP between 1989 and 1998 in Olmsted County, of whom about two thirds presented with a murmur, and in one third MVP was detected on an echocardiogram performed for another reason.[72] The mean age of this cohort was 47 years. Those presenting with a murmur tended to have more severe MR and a larger left atrium, and were less likely to have atrial fibrillation at the outset. Ten-year mortality for the total cohort was 19% but was not statistically greater than expected. Cardiovascular mortality at 10 years was 9%. Predictors of cardiovascular mortality were moderate or more severe MR and LV ejection fraction less than 50%. Site of prolapse, presence of flail, and LV size did not influence mortality. Cardiovascular morbid events in follow-up occurred in 171 patients. These included heart failure in 60, new-onset atrial fibrillation in 51, ischemic neurologic events in 38, peripheral thromboembolism in 11, endocarditis in 4, and mitral valve surgery in 65 patients. Ten-year cardiovascular morbidity was 30% and was predicted by age 50 or older, left atrial size 40 mm or greater, MR of any severity but higher odds ratio for more severe MR, flail leaflet, and baseline atrial fibrillation. Gender, location of prolapse, LV size, and valve thickening did not independently predict cardiovascular morbidity.

Prior studies of patients with MVP also suggested high-risk features detected clinically and on an echocardiogram. In a cohort of 237 asymptomatic or minimally symptomatic patients with MVP studied in the 1980s at the Mayo Clinic who were followed for an average of 6 years, the survival at 8 years was predicted to be 88%, no different from that of a control population. Factors indicative of worse outcome included an end-diastolic LV dimension greater than 6 cm, which was an indicator of a need for mitral valve surgery. Valve redundancy was another strong negative predictor, with sudden death, infective endocarditis, or a cerebral ischemic event occurring in 10% of the 97 patients with this finding, whereas only 1 of 140 patients without redundancy experienced such an event.[12] In another study of 456 patients reported in the late 1980s, the population was classified as having classic MVP on the basis of leaflet thickening and redundancy or nonclassic MVP on the basis of the absence of these features. Complications were more common in the classic group. These included endocarditis in 3.5% of the classic group versus 0% of the nonclassic group, significant MR in 12% and 0%, respectively, and the need for mitral valve surgery in 7% and 1%, respectively. The incidence of stroke was significant, being 6% to 7% in both groups.

The age of onset of MVP is variable. One study failed to detect MVP in neonates, even in offspring of affected parents.[73] It appears to be relatively uncommon in pediatric populations except in the setting of a primary disorder of connective tissue such as Marfan syndrome.[74] Symptomatic presentation is most common in midlife, and surgical intervention for severe MR is most likely in the sixth or seventh decade.[21,75] In one study, the average time from detection of a murmur to symptomatic presentation was 24 years.[76] Once symptoms occurred, surgical intervention was required within 1 year and the mean age at surgery was 60 years. Thus, by inference, it appears that the mean age at which the murmur was detected was 35 years.

Given the asymptomatic nature of MVP for many years, the earliest clinical abnormalities go undetected. Even in those who may be anticipated to have a likelihood of early detection, such as physicians or executives who have yearly physical examinations, detection of a murmur or click may occur only in middle age. This fact suggests that, at least in many people, the change in valve function sufficient to be clinically evident does occur relatively late and is not due solely to a failure in detection. Thus, in the Framingham study, a systolic murmur was heard in only 23% of patients with classic MVP, 10% of those with nonclassic prolapse, and 4% of those without prolapse, whereas a click was heard in 11%, 8%, and 1.5%, respectively, of these groups.

It was estimated, in the earlier era of echocardiographic diagnosis of MVP, that approximately 4% of men and 1.5% of women in Australia[77] with the condition would eventually require surgery, whereas the estimates for the United States were 5% and 1.5%, respectively.[78] Given the surfeit of diagnoses of MVP in this era, the likelihood is that with a stricter definition of prolapse a greater proportion of these patients will eventually need surgery. Thus, a later estimate of the need for mitral valve surgery by age 70 is 11% in men with mitral prolapse and 6% for women.[79]

Despite the risk of complications, MVP appears to have an excellent prognosis. When patients with severe MR from MVP undergo repair surgery at an appropriate time, there is considerable evidence that their survival is as good as, if not better than, that of a control population without MVP.[75,80,81] This is not necessarily true if a mitral valve replacement is performed or if MR has led to LV dysfunction.[82-84] The excellent prognosis in reported series of MVP may reflect a lower than expected rate of coronary artery disease in these series either by design (exclusion of patients with both coronary disease and mitral repair in surgical series) or by chance. In the Framingham study, subjects with MVP showed a trend toward a lower prevalence of coronary disease. In one surgical series in which patients who had coronary artery disease and myxomatous disease were compared with those who had ischemic heart disease alone, survival rates were impaired equally in both groups and depended on severity of ischemic heart disease and LV dysfunction.[85] Failure to appropriately intervene surgically in MVP with severe MR does lead to impairment of survival, however, illustrating the importance of careful follow-up of such patients at regular intervals.[86] Referral to surgery before the onset of symptoms or of LV dilation or dysfunction is now indicated by the most recent American College of Cardiology (ACC)/American Heart Association (AHA) guidelines if the likelihood of successful repair is greater than 90%.[87]

Diagnosis and Clinical Features

Symptoms

Most patients presenting with MVP for the first time are asymptomatic, and the diagnosis is made on the basis of the characteristic physical findings or because an echocardiogram is being performed for another reason. Nevertheless, patients with MVP may present with specific symptoms referable to the valve. These include shortness of breath and even heart failure when significant MR is already present. Sudden onset of shortness of breath and heart failure requiring immediate treatment may result from acute chordal rupture or from valve leaflet perforation or valve disruption in endocarditis.[88] Patients with MVP may experience chest pain that is atypical for angina.[89] The mechanism by which this pain occurs is unknown. Palpitations are common in patients with MVP, even in those with little or no MR.[90] Most frequently the palpitations consist of ventricular extrasystoles that may be multifocal or clustered. Atrial extrasystoles are also common.[91] However, in a blinded study of Holter monitor recordings from patients with MVP and from control subjects, no difference in frequency or complexity of rhythm disturbance was noted.[92] Nevertheless, once MR is present, arrhythmia is common and is more frequent in women and with advancing age.[91] Atrial fibrillation and atrial flutter are common later in the course of MVP, when significant MR has been established for some time and atrial enlargement has ensued.[93] Rarely, MVP manifests initially as ventricular tachycardia or sudden death.[34,94,95] MVP may also manifest as subacute bacterial endocarditis[96,97] with fever and systemic illness or with a stroke or transient ischemic attack.[98,99]

Cardiac Physical Findings

MVP is reliably diagnosed by both physical examination and 2D echocardiography. Classic physical findings for MVP include a dynamic midsystolic to late systolic click followed by a high-pitched systolic murmur heard at the cardiac apex. With more advanced MR, the murmur may extend throughout systole, and with severe MR or associated LV dysfunction, a third sound may be heard and the click may be inaudible, but the murmur is usually loud.[100,101] The click is thought to result from stretching of redundant valve and chordal tissue. A click may occur without any murmur when the leaflets are redundant but not regurgitant. In addition, systolic clicks may arise from other pathologic conditions, including bicuspid aortic valve, atrial myxoma, and pericarditis. A click, therefore, is sensitive but not very specific for the diagnosis of MVP, although a midsystolic click with late systolic murmur is highly likely to represent myxomatous degeneration of the mitral valve. Provocative maneuvers such as the Valsalva maneuver, squatting, and leg raises may improve the diagnostic likelihood of MVP by illustrating that the click moves within systole in response to volume and loading changes.[102] A reduction in end-diastolic volume, such as that occurring with the Valsalva maneuver or standing, causes the click to occur earlier, whereas an increase in end-diastolic volume such as that occurring with squatting or decreasing contractility or increasing afterload (hand-grip) moves the click later in systole. The murmur may radiate on the basis of the direction of the regurgitant leak and the leaflet that is prolapsing. Thus, with anterior leaflet prolapse and a posteriorly directed jet, the murmur may be appreciated very well at the back.

Noncardiac Physical Findings

Secondary causes of MVP such as Marfan syndrome have specific skeletal and morphologic findings that aid in their identification. These are not seen routinely in idiopathic MVP, which, in contrast, has no specific features other than the cardiac manifestations that render the diagnosis likely.[103] Patients with MVP in the Framingham study were significantly leaner, according to lower body mass index and waist-to-hip ratio, than those without prolapse.[69] Lower weight and lower blood pressure in patients with MVP have been described in other studies.[90] Older studies suggested a higher incidence of skeletal abnormalities associated with MVP, such as straight back and asthenic build.[90,104]

Echocardiographic Diagnosis

A 2D echocardiogram is required for precise diagnosis of MVP and to determine the presence of MR and other findings that affect prognosis and risk of complications (Figure 18-6). Prolapse was detected initially on echocardiography by M-mode echocardiography. The characteristic appearance of late systolic hammocking of the mitral leaflets was used to make the diagnosis. However, apart from demonstrative purposes, M-mode echocardiography has little role in the current diagnosis of prolapse. Usually a transthoracic echocardiogram is adequate for simple diagnostic purposes, although both transesophageal echocardiography (TEE) and three-dimensional (3D) echocardiography may provide specific information that is not available from the transthoracic window. In fact, 3D echocardiography has been most successfully applied to the evaluation of the mitral valve apparatus, providing greater insight into its pathologies as well as the likelihood of and operative plans for successful repair. Stress echocardiography provides powerful additional diagnostic and prognostic information in selected individuals.

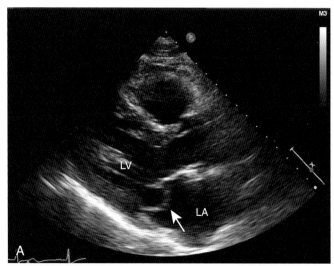

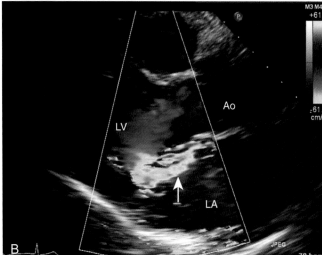

FIGURE 18-6 **A,** Parasternal long-axis view of prolapse of the posterior mitral leaflet into the left atrium (LA) (*arrow*). **B,** The anteriorly directed regurgitant jet of mitral regurgitation away from the prolapsing leaflet is demonstrated. *Ao,* aorta; *LV,* left ventricle.

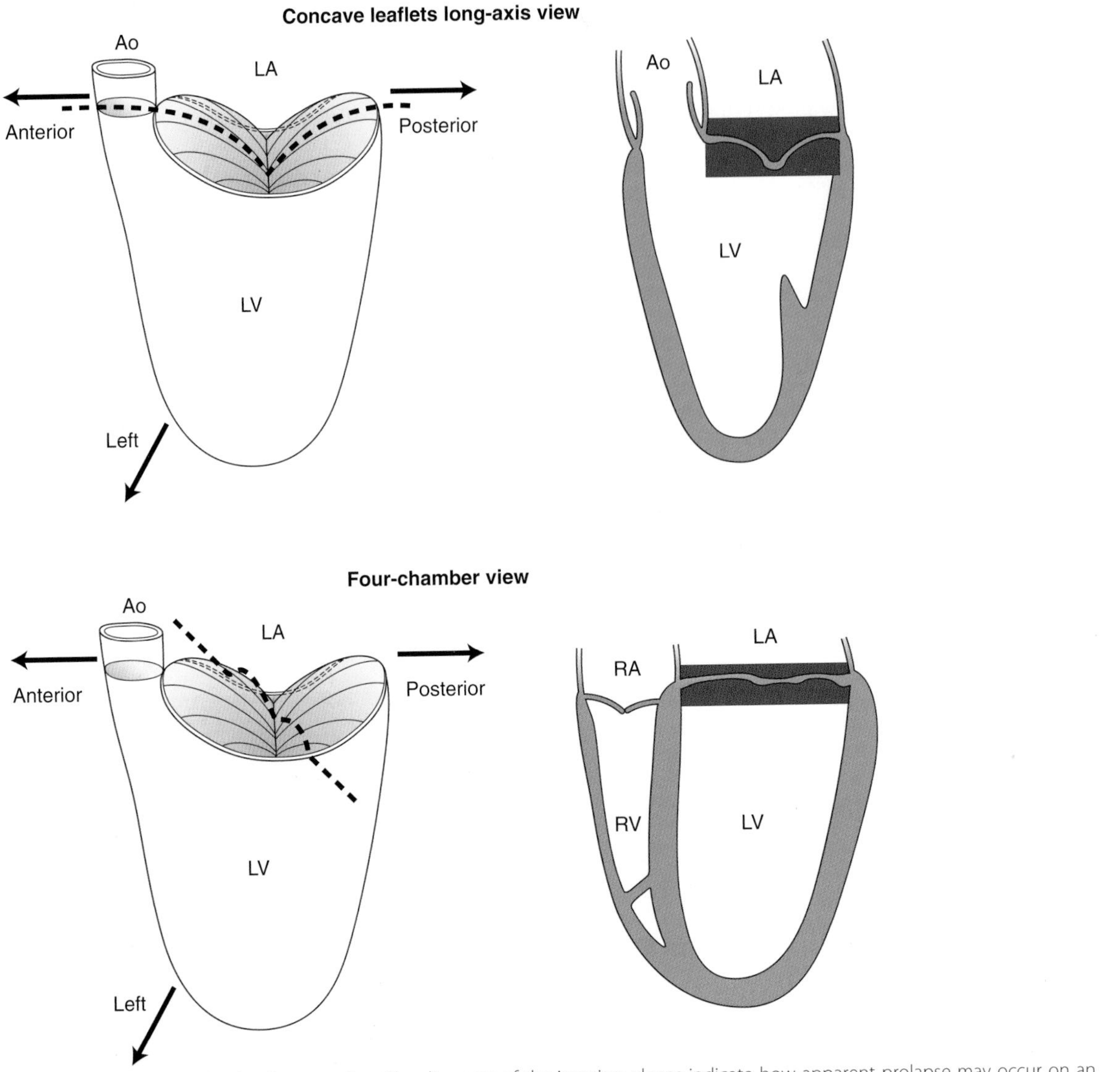

Concave leaflets long-axis view

Four-chamber view

FIGURE 18-7   Diagrams of saddle-shaped mitral valve annulus. The diagrams of the imaging planes indicate how apparent prolapse may occur on an apical cross-sectional image in the absence of any prolapse in a long-axis cross-section. *Ao,* Aorta; *LA,* left atrium; *LV,* left ventricle; *RA,* right atrium; *RV,* right ventricle. *(From Levine RA, Triulzi MO, Harrigan P, et al. The relationship of mitral annular shape to the diagnosis of mitral valve prolapse. Circulation 1987;75:756–67.)*

On 2D echocardiography, MVP is diagnosed when either or both of the leaflets are displaced 2 mm or more in systole above a line connecting the annular hinge points in the parasternal or apical long-axis view.[105-107] Displacement of the leaflets above this line in other imaging windows, specifically the apical four-chamber window, should not be considered abnormal. In an earlier era, however, prolapse identified on the apical four-chamber view was considered to be diagnostic of true MVP, leading to an epidemic of diagnosis in 38% of teenage girls.[13] Using 3D echocardiography, Levine et al[105-107] demonstrated in the late 1980s that the mitral annulus was not planar, but rather had a complex saddle-shaped structure in which the anterior and posterior portions of the annulus are higher than the lateral portions (Figure 18-7). Thus, in the anteroposterior axis, the annulus is concave upward, whereas in the mediolateral axis, the annulus is concave downward. The result is that in the apical four-chamber plane, even normal leaflets may appear to break the annular plane. Levine et al[105] went on to show that prolapse identified only on the apical four-chamber view did not exhibit the other features of pathologic MVP, such as chamber enlargement and leaflet thickening, and should not be considered abnormal.

Myxomatous changes in the mitral valve leaflets may lead to thickening of leaflets and chordae and to enlargement of the mitral valve annulus.[108] These are especially evident when MR is present. Thickening of the leaflets to 5 mm or more is considered "classic" for MVP and is predictive of subsequent complications (Figure 18-8).[109] Mitral valve thickening is measured in diastole from the leading edge to the trailing edge of the thickest area of the midportion of the leaflet and not as the dimension of maximal area of focal leaflet thickening.[69] In many instances, the leaflets and chordae are very thickened and redundant.[12,110] It is also common to identify tricuspid valve prolapse in patients with MVP.[111] Tricuspid valve prolapse may occur in up to 40% of all patients with MVP, whereas aortic valve prolapse is much less prevalent and occurs in 1% to 2% of patients with MVP.[87] The thickness of the leaflets changes much more than normally from systole to diastole in MVP on echocardiography.[112] This finding has been attributed to inherent increased thickening of the valve structures that has been demonstrated pathologically and also to increased redundancy of the leaflet tissue. Apical four-chamber views are not useful in detecting mild MVP, but once the diagnosis has been made, this imaging window is very helpful in defining the precise leaflet involvement and the severity of MR. In addition, prolapse of the lateral scallop of the posterior leaflet may be evident only on this view.

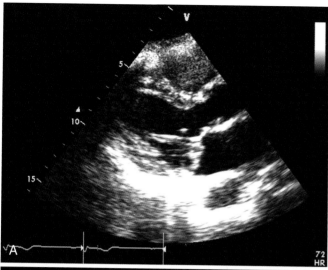

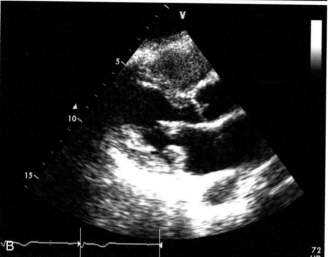

FIGURE 18-8   Parasternal long-axis echocardiogram of bileaflet prolapse in systole (A) and diastole (B). Significant thickening and redundancy of the leaflets in diastole can be seen, consistent with "classic" mitral valve prolapse.

In a substantial number of patients, there is echocardiographic evidence of chordal disruption.[113,114] In this instance, a portion of one or the other, or rarely both, leaflets may exhibit motion independent of normal leaflet tissue. Chordal rupture in this situation may either be partial or complete and usually leads to impaired coaptation over a substantial portion of the valve surface, giving rise to severe MR. This is not invariably the case, however. Coaptation may be maintained despite a flail segment if the other leaflet is large. Prolapsing and flail leaflets are usually reliably identified on transthoracic echocardiography, but TEE has been shown in multiple studies to improve the ability to detect a flail segment.[115-117]

CLASSIFICATION OF PROLAPSE ON ECHOCARDIOGRAPHY

MVP is classified on the basis of the leaflet involvement as involving the anterior leaflet, the posterior leaflet, or both. This classification has prognostic value in determining the likelihood of repair and may have some independent value in defining the nature of the disease itself. Unileaflet prolapse especially involving the posterior leaflet is more common than bileaflet prolapse and appears to be more likely to result in flail. Bileaflet prolapse tends to occur at a younger age, is more likely to be

associated with myxomatous changes in other valves, and tends to have more dynamic changes in severity of MR.[110] The leaflet involved in prolapse is determined not only by the apparent displacement of the leaflet but also by the direction of the jet or jets when regurgitation is present. Thus, anterior leaflet prolapse is associated with excess motion of the anterior leaflet and a posteriorly directed jet of MR. Posterior leaflet prolapse generally causes an anteriorly directed jet of MR. In bileaflet prolapse, two jets of regurgitation may be identified, or if the prolapse of the leaflets is symmetric, there may be one central jet. In the identification of bileaflet prolapse, jet direction is particularly important. As detailed in the section on anatomy, apparent prolapse of the anterior leaflet can occur with severe posterior leaflet prolapse owing to loss of the anchoring effect of the posterior leaflet. Unlike in true bileaflet prolapse, in which two jets or a central jet is evident, only an anteriorly directed jet is seen, and repair is as likely as with isolated posterior leaflet prolapse.[118]

LOCALIZATION OF PROLAPSE AND FLAIL BY ECHOCARDIOGRAPHY

In identifying the site of prolapse by echocardiography, first, the 2D appearance should be assessed and then the origin and direction of the accompanying jet of MR should be analyzed. In the 2D assessment, the long-axis views are paramount when the diagnosis is suspected rather than established. In more severe prolapse in the patient in whom the diagnosis is not in doubt but an assessment of the severity of the lesion is needed, additional views need to be taken into account, including the short-axis view of the valve on which the prolapsing or flail segment or segments may be apparent as a masslike lesion and may even simulate an infective vegetation.[119] Off-axis views and the four-chamber view may help determine which leaflet is prolapsing or whether both are. Lateral scallop involvement of the posterior leaflet may be particularly challenging to decipher. The regurgitant jet may appear to be directed anteriorly in some views but posteriorly in others, which is understandable because the lateral scallop is quite anteriorly located (see Figure 18-3). A short-axis view of the valve may be particularly helpful in identifying the excess motion of the lateral scallop in this situation and the origin of the regurgitant jet.

TEE is particularly useful in determining the precise site of prolapse and seems to be superior to transthoracic imaging in many instances.[120] Figure 18-3 demonstrates the portions of the MV that are interrogated at each imaging angle; it should be noted that at each angle, a number of parallel planes can be visualized, depending on the depth of the TEE probe in the esophagus and the extent of anteflexion or retroflexion of the probe. The key imaging planes on TEE are the midesophageal view at 40 to 60 degrees on multiplane imaging and the orthogonal view at 130 to 150 degrees. At 40 to 60 degrees, the imaging plane is parallel to a line between the commissures and is helpful in determining whether the prolapse involves the medial (to the left) or lateral (to the right) scallop. The orthogonal view at 130 to 150 degrees is most useful in identifying prolapse of the middle scallop or segment, because this imaging plane bisects that scallop. Short-axis views of the mitral valve may also be acquired by TEE in the short-axis transgastric view. 3D TEE is also quite helpful in defining the location of prolapse, as long as the image is of satisfactory quality (Figure 18-9).

When the mitral valve has been examined systematically in a segmental approach and the results are compared with the surgical findings, TEE is 96% accurate according to one study.[23] In another study of myxomatous mitral valve disease, localization of the abnormality to the posterior leaflet was 78% sensitive and 92% specific, with sensitivity being lowest when the medial scallop was affected.[121] Commissural prolapse is often difficult to detect because it may lead to prolapse of a portion of both leaflets with a large prolapsing mass that may simulate a vegetation.

Recognition is enhanced by a short-axis view of the valve on which the commissures are evident and by 3D echocardiography (discussed later).[122] In addition, the regurgitant jet is often very eccentric in origin in standard views and is seen to originate at the affected commissure in short-axis views.

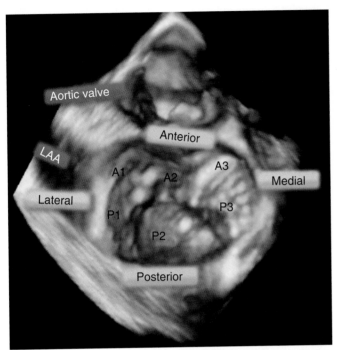

FIGURE 18-9   Three-dimensional echocardiogram of the mitral valve. Left atrial view demonstrates prolapse of the P2 scallop of the posterior leaflet. *A,* anterior leaflet; *LAA,* left atrial appendage; *P,* posterior scallop.

ASSESSMENT OF MITRAL REGURGITATION

MR is one of the major complications of MVP, and it is essential that an echocardiographic evaluation include a full assessment with quantification, when feasible, of the severity of the lesion. MR assessment is is discussed in detail elsewhere (see Chapter 6), so only important pitfalls in assessment specific to myxomatous mitral valve disease are summarized here.

1. MR from a prolapsing mitral valve is often eccentric in nature, and the color display may underestimate the true severity.[123] It is important to examine the left atrium in multiple views, including off-axis views, to fully define the jet. TEE is helpful to image the jet in this situation.

2. In quantifying MR with the proximal isovelocity surface area technique, care must be taken to account for the effects of wall constraint on the proximal isovelocity surface area, which is particularly common with a large flail segment (Figure 18-10).[124] Wall constraint of the proximal convergence area leads to the loss of a true hemispheric proximal convergence zone and measurement of a spuriously large radius. These factors lead to a gross overestimation of the regurgitant volume and the regurgitant orifice. Correction factors are available but are somewhat difficult to use because they involve calculating and allowing for the true angle made by the convergence area.[125] Fortunately, when constraint is present, the MR is usually already severe, and quantitation, although inaccurate, does not misrepresent the appropriate grading of MR as severe.

3. The duration of regurgitation is inconstant in myxomatous MR more so than in MR from other etiologies.[126] Thus, MR may be severe when it occurs but is confined to the latter half of systole rather than being holosystolic. In determination of the effects of MR on LV size and function (an important consideration in appropriately timing surgical intervention), not only the severity of the MR but also its duration is important.[127] Color M-mode echocardiography may be very helpful in determining the true duration of the regurgitation as may the continuous wave Doppler

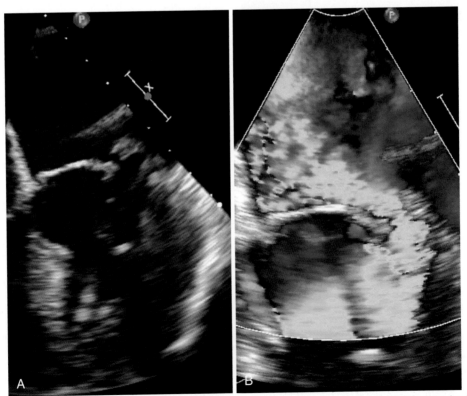

FIGURE 18-10   Flail posterior mitral valve leaflet on transesophageal echocardiography (A) and severe mitral regurgitation seen on color-flow Doppler imaging (B). The proximal convergence area is constrained by the wall and is no longer a true hemisphere. Proximal isovelocity surface area measurement of regurgitant orifice area from this image would overestimate the true area because of the change in the geometry of the convergence area.

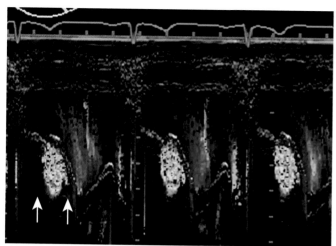

FIGURE 18-11   Color M-mode echocardiography of mitral regurgitation. This asymptomatic patient with bileaflet prolapse has a large regurgitant orifice area but normal left atrial and ventricular sizes. The regurgitant jet is confined to the second half of systole (between *arrows*) so that the total volume of regurgitation is much lower than would have been anticipated on the basis of the regurgitant orifice area.

echocardiography profile of the MR jet (Figure 18-11). Dynamic changes in the apparent severity of the lesion may involve the duration as well as the severity. The severity of MR is especially dynamic in prolapsing mitral valves, probably as a result of the effects of loading and geometry on the chordae and leaflets. Patients who are asymptomatic at rest and with apparently moderate MR may exhibit marked symptoms with exercise as a result of increases in both the severity and the duration of the regurgitation.[128,129] Stress echocardiography is very helpful in situations in which there is a discrepancy between the symptoms and apparent severity of MR at rest in myxomatous disease, and an increase in severity of MR with exercise may have predictive value in determining the need for earlier surgical intervention.[130]

ECHOCARDIOGRAPHY IN DEFINING LIKELIHOOD OF REPAIR

Myxomatous mitral valve disease is associated with excess tissue, which usually allows the possibility of repair in centers experienced in the necessary surgical techniques. The current ACC/AHA guidelines stipulate that surgical intervention should be predicated on the likelihood of repair as defined by the valve lesion and the center at which the surgery is to take place.[87] Surgical intervention is indicated earlier if repair appears likely because the short-term and long-term morbidity and mortality associated with repair are much more favorable than those associated with mitral valve replacement. It is increasingly possible to repair even complex myxomatous disease lesions that historically would have required valve replacement.[131-133] In experienced centers, it is now possible to repair a posterior leaflet prolapse or flail in more than 90% of instances.[21] Extensive calcification of the leaflet that precludes leaflet resection is the usual reason that a posterior leaflet lesion is not reparable. This situation too is usually evident echocardiographically, at least to an experienced reader. Currently, bileaflet prolapse lesions can usually be repaired in experienced centers.

Anterior leaflet prolapse, anterior leaflet flail, and flail of both leaflets have been the most difficult lesions to repair. It is difficult to resect diseased areas from the anterior leaflet because of its sail-like configuration and the absence of true segmentation. Anterior leaflet repair has therefore required chordal transfer techniques, and durability has not been as good as for repair of posterior leaflet lesions. With the advent of more physiologic and user-friendly artificial chordae, the likelihood of durable repair in this situation has also improved substantially.[134]

Given the importance of defining the likelihood of repair when one is helping a patient determine the optimal timing for surgical intervention, TEE should be used if the transthoracic images are suboptimal or fail to adequately define the mechanism of MR. Furthermore, because 3D TEE (see later) provides a better assessment of valvular pathology and may direct certain patients with complex disease to a referral center for surgical repair, 3D imaging should be performed in all patients if possible.

THREE-DIMENSIONAL ECHOCARDIOGRAPHY

Improvements in real-time 3D echocardiography, whether acquired from the transthoracic windows or by the transesophageal approach, have led to a rapid evolution of the ability to image complex structures and in particular the myxomatous mitral valve. In a number of institutions, including ours, 3D TEE is a standard part of the evaluation of MV pathology because it has been repeatedly shown to be more accurate in identifying pathologic changes than 2D imaging alone. In a study of 112 patients with myxomatous mitral valve disease who were undergoing mitral valve repair, Pepi et al[135] compared 3D TEE, 2D TEE, and both 3D and 2D transthoracic echocardiography in the localization of the site of prolapse, using the surgical findings as the "gold standard." 3D TEE was significantly more accurate, at 96%, than the other techniques. 3D transthoracic echocardiography and 2D TEE were similarly accurate, at 90% and 87%, respectively, with 2D transthoracic echocardiography being the least accurate, at 77%. Multiple areas of prolapse were more likely to be detected by the 3D approach, as were commissural lesions. Similarly, Grewal et al[136] demonstrated that, in comparison with surgical evaluation, 3D TEE was superior to 2D TEE in the diagnosis of disease involving the P1, A2, and A3 segments as well as of bileaflet disease. It is also possible to measure the regurgitant orifice directly in myxomatous mitral valves with 3D TEE. However, this measurement requires considerable off-line processing, which makes it of limited clinical feasibility.[137]

There is a significant discrepancy between the national rate of mitral valve repair (60% to 70%) and the rate in high-volume surgical centers (>90%). It is possible that much of this discrepancy is due to an incomplete diagnosis, and surgeons without significant mitral valve experience who encounter more complicated disease at the time of surgery than that suggested by 2D echocardiography forfeit the option of valve repair and simply replace the valve. Therefore, a thorough evaluation including 3D TEE may result in the more frequent referral of patients with complex prolapse to centers with adequate surgical experience to undertake a mitral valve repair successfully.

Other Diagnostic Techniques

ELECTROCARDIOGRAPHY

Electrocardiographic changes, particularly flattening or inversion of the T wave in the inferior leads, have been identified in patients with MVP.[10] QT prolongation is uncommon but has been reported in individual patients with prolapse. Patients with MVP may demonstrate abnormal electrocardiographic responses to exercise, and false-positive ST segment depression has been reported in 10% to 60% of patients studied.[10] An imaging study in addition to the electrocardiogram is likely to be more specific when coronary disease is being evaluated in these patients and is a useful screening tool in intermediate-risk patients.[138] An increase in ventricular ectopy with salvoes of ventricular premature beats may also occur with exercise, particularly in the cool-down phase.[10] Ventricular ectopy is usually worsened by concomitant MR and frequently improves but may not normalize after successful valve surgery. The cause and significance of the electrocardiographic changes and ectopy have been debated for years, with autonomic abnormalities being postulated as a cause by some.[139]

ANGIOGRAPHY

Although an LV angiogram is no longer used to make the diagnosis of MVP, certain characteristic findings are often evident. The right anterior oblique projection is best for posterior leaflet prolapse, whereas the left anterior oblique projection is optimal for anterior leaflet prolapse. The mitral leaflets are seen to be displaced beyond their point of attachment to the annulus. Other abnormalities may be evident, such as MR, annular calcification, and impaired motion of the basal portion of the left ventricle.[140]

Other Imaging Techniques

Nuclear scintigraphy may be of value in excluding coronary artery disease in those patients with chest pain. Echocardiography is usually adequate to assess LV function, but when another assessment of ejection fraction is required, a gated blood pool scan is usually the methodology of choice. Cardiac magnetic resonance and computed tomography at present have limited value in comparison with echocardiography in defining valve morphology and hemodynamics and are not routinely used in the evaluation of MVP.

Mitral Valve Prolapse Syndrome

MVP has been associated with numerous symptoms, such as atypical chest pain, fatigue, orthostatic hypotension, shortness of breath on exertion, palpitations, syncope, panic attack, and anxiety.[139] Asthenic build, low blood pressure, and electrocardiographic evidence of repolarization abnormalities have all been characterized as the MVP syndrome. In the era before the rationalization of the echocardiographic diagnosis of MVP, during which the apparent prevalence of MVP in the community was high, it is understandable that many of these manifestations appeared to be clustered with the diagnosis of MVP, which in turn gave a convenient and not too grave a diagnosis to account for them. Many studies indicated abnormalities in catecholamines, adrenergic activity, and autonomic function in the patient population.[141-143] Echocardiography was performed in many patients presenting with nonspecific symptoms as a screening tool to identify a possible cause of the symptoms. This selection bias amplified the association of MVP with many other disorders.

Newer studies have suggested that with a more appropriate diagnosis of MVP based on long-axis views there is little, if any, association between true MVP and this cluster of symptoms and clinical findings.[144] Thus, in the Framingham Heart Study, patients with MVP did not have a higher risk for development of psychiatric abnormalities or electrocardiographic changes or for experiencing atypical chest pain, panic disorder, or dyspnea than the general population.[145,146] Furthermore, studies that included asymptomatic patients with MVP failed to detect abnormal autonomic or neuroendocrine function at rest or with tilt testing.[147] Whether there are subgroups of patients with MVP who have true autonomic abnormalities remains to be determined. A polymorphism at the 1166 position of the angiotensin II receptor has been detected more commonly in patients with MVP than in control subjects and appears to be associated with postural hypotension and enhanced vasomotor response.[148]

Patients with MVP syndrome are managed symptomatically and with counseling on the benign nature of the condition. If there is concern about a true abnormality at the valve or if this issue is in doubt, echocardiography should be performed after an interval, usually of 1 year. Beta-blockade in small doses may be helpful in treating symptomatic palpitations or atypical chest pain. If anxiety disorder or panic disorder appears to be the underlying problem, referral to a specialist clinic is often beneficial.

Management of the Asymptomatic Patient

Patients with MVP, mild or no MR, and mild or no symptoms are managed expectantly with the assurance that their prognosis is excellent. Table 18-1 details the current ACC/AHA guidelines for echocardiography in these patients. Those who exhibit high-risk features on an echocardiogram, such as leaflet thickening, should be followed up more closely with a yearly echocardiogram. Those in whom no high-risk features are present may be followed up less frequently. Patients with mild prolapse and atypical chest pain should undergo a stress echocardiogram or stress nuclear study if the pretest probability of coronary artery disease is in the intermediate range. Stress electrocardiography in the setting of MVP is associated with a high incidence of false-positive ST depression and is best avoided when the diagnosis of ischemia is required. In patients with palpitations, Holter monitoring is useful to detect the precise cause of arrhythmia, although a serious rhythm disturbance is rare.

Good health measures, such as avoidance of caffeine and alcohol and an exercise program, along with reassurance often suffice in reducing or eliminating symptoms. In more refractory instances, symptomatic relief of atypical chest pain and palpitations may be afforded by the empiric use of small doses of beta-blockers. Exercise is encouraged in patients with MVP. Competitive exercise should be avoided by those with moderate LV enlargement, LV dysfunction, uncontrolled tachyarrhythmias, long QT interval, unexplained syncope, prior resuscitation from cardiac arrest, or aortic root enlargement.[149] Heavy weightlifting should also be avoided in those with MVP because it, theoretically at least, may lead to further chordal extension by increasing LV wall stress and thus worsening prolapse and MR. This prohibition generally remains in force even after successful surgical repair, given the residual abnormality of leaflet and chordal tissue. Pregnancy is not contraindicated in MVP on the basis of the diagnosis alone.[87]

Patients with severe MR and normal LV size and function but without clinical symptoms present a controversial scenario.

TABLE 18-1	American College of Cardiography/American Heart Association Guidelines for Echocardiography in Asymptomatic Mitral Valve Prolapse

Class I

Echocardiography is indicated for the diagnosis of MVP and assessment of MR, leaflet morphology, and ventricular compensation in asymptomatic patients with physical signs of MVP. (Level of Evidence: B)

Class IIa

1. Echocardiography can effectively exclude MVP in asymptomatic patients who have been diagnosed without clinical evidence to support the diagnosis. (Level of Evidence: C)
2. Echocardiography can be effective for risk stratification in asymptomatic patients with physical signs of MVP or known MVP. (Level of Evidence: C)

Class III

1. Echocardiography is not indicated to exclude MVP in asymptomatic patients with ill-defined symptoms in the absence of a constellation of clinical symptoms or physical findings suggestive of MVP or a positive family history. (Level of Evidence: B)
2. Routine repetition of echocardiography is not indicated for the asymptomatic patient who has MVP and no MR or MVP and mild MR with no changes in clinical signs or symptoms. (Level of Evidence: C)

MR, Mitral regurgitation; MVP, mitral valve prolapse.
From Bonow RO, Carabello B, Chatterjee K, et al. 2008 focused update incorporated into the ACC/AHA 2006 guidelines for the management of patients with valvular heart disease: a report of the American College of Cardiology/American Heart Association Task Force on Practice Guidelines. J am Coll Cardiol 2008;52:e1–142.

Although patients without symptoms were previously thought to have a benign prognosis, later studies have shown the opposite. Enriquez-Sarano et al[150] demonstrated a significantly lower rate of survival than expected (58% vs. 78% at 5 years, $P = 0.03$) for patients with severe MR without surgery. Similarly, Kang et al[151] studied 447 patients with severe MR, 161 of whom underwent surgery and the remainder of whom were followed up for development of symptoms or LV dysfunction (at which time they were referred for surgery). Those patients who underwent early surgery had a significantly better survival at 7 years than those in the "watchful waiting" group (99% vs. 85%, $P = 0.007$). It should be emphasized that operative mortality was 0% and that 94% of patients had successful mitral valve repair, important facts to consider when one is weighing the benefits of early surgery and those of conservative waiting. At our institution, given the level of surgical experience and likelihood of successful repair, we generally recommend early repair for patients with severe but asymptomatic MR who are reasonable candidates for open-heart surgery, with a high likelihood of repair.

Previously, the decision about endocarditis prophylaxis was complicated and somewhat obscure in patients with MVP and was predicated on the presence of MR on either clinical or echocardiographic grounds.[152,153] However, the latest AHA endocarditis prophylaxis guidelines have substantially clarified and simplified this decision. The AHA no longer recommends the use of antibiotic prophylaxis for patients with any form of MVP unless a prior episode of endocarditis has been documented or unless surgical repair or replacement of the valve has taken place.[154]

Complications of Mitral Valve Prolapse

Although in many respects a benign condition, MVP is associated with significant complications. These include endocarditis, sudden cardiac death, cerebrovascular events, and MR of a severity to necessitate surgery. Both clinical and echocardiographic parameters are useful in identifying patients at increased risk for these complications (Table 18-2). Although MVP is equally prevalent in men and women, men are much more likely to experience significant complications.[155] In most surgical series of patients

with myxomatous disease undergoing valve surgery, men outnumber women by a factor of $2:1$ or $3:1$.[21] Similarly, men are more prone to endocarditis. The reasons that men are more likely to present with a complicated course are unknown. It has been postulated that LV wall stress is higher in men and, thus, greater tension is exerted on valve tissue and chordae, thus leading to a higher risk of leaflet and chord rupture.[156] Other clinical factors associated with a higher risk of complications include higher blood pressure and higher body mass index.

The echocardiographic findings in multiple studies that have been associated with a complicated course include impaired LV function, more severe MR, and leaflet thickness greater than 5 mm (see Table 18-2). The last is associated with a greater than tenfold increase in risk of sudden death, infective endocarditis, or cerebrovascular event.

Infective Endocarditis

Patients with MVP have a threefold to eightfold higher risk for development of endocarditis, although the absolute risk, at approximately 0.2% per year, is relatively low.[155,157,158] Nevertheless, endocarditis is a cause of significant morbidity and mortality when it occurs and may bring forward the time at which surgical intervention is required because of an increase in severity of MR. Furthermore, the destruction of the valve tissue in severe cases of endocarditis may preclude successful repair. Risk factors for development of endocarditis include male gender, age more than 45 years, the presence of a systolic murmur, and thickening and redundancy of the leaflets.[12,97,109,155,158] Vortices produced by the turbulent jet of MR and the redundant thickened valve tissue are thought to increase the likelihood that a bacteremia of a suitable organism will infect the valve. Patients without MR do not appear to have an increased risk of endocarditis. The risk in those with prolapse and a systolic murmur has been estimated to be 0.05% per year.[159] The new guidelines suggest that the risk of bacteremia is as likely with everyday dental hygiene, such as flossing and cleaning, as with specific dental procedures and that specific prophylaxis therefore is probably not useful. When endocarditis occurs in MVP, it is treated as for other endocarditis of etiologies,

TABLE 18-2 Use of Echocardiography for Risk Stratification in MV Prolapse

STUDY (YEAR)	N	FEATURES EXAMINED	OUTCOME	P<
Chandraratna et al (1984)[189]	86	MV leaflets >5 mm	↑ Cardiovascular abnormalities (60% vs. 6%; Marfan syndrome, tricuspid valve prolapse, MR, dilated ascending aorta)	0.001
Nishimura et al (1985)[12]	237	MV leaflet ≥5 mm Left ventricular internal diameter ≥60 mm	↑ Sum of sudden death, endocarditis, and cerebral embolus ↑ MVR (26% vs. 3.1%)	0.02 0.001
Marks et al (1989)[109]	456	MV leaflet ≥5 mm	↑ Endocarditis (3.5% vs. 0%) ↑ Moderate-severe MR (11.9% vs. 0%) ↑ MVR (6.6% vs. 0.7%) ↑ Stroke (7.5% vs. 5.8%)	0.02 0.001 0.02 NS
Takamoto et al (1991)[190]	142	MV leaflet 3 mm or greater, redundant, low echo destiny	↑ Ruptured chordae (48% vs. 5%)	
Babuty et al (1994)[191]	58	Undefined MV thickening	No relation to complex ventricular arrhythmias	NS
Zuppiroli et al (1994)[91]	119	MV leaflet greater than 5 mm	↑ Complex ventricular arrhythmias	0.001
Avierinos et al (2002)[72]	833	Risk factors for: 　Moderate-severe MR 　Ejection fraction <50% Risk factors for: 　Left atrial size ≥40 mm 　Slight MR 　Moderate-severe MR 　Flail	↑ Cardiovascular mortality HR 3.0, CI 1.5-5.8 HR 3.8, CI 1.6-8.1 ↑ Cardiovascular morbidity (sum of heart failure, new atrial fibrillation, ischemic neurologic events, peripheral embolic events, endocarditis, MVR) HR 2.7, CI 1.9-3.8 HR 3.6, CI 2.0-7.0 HR 9.1, CI 4.9-18.3 HR 2.6, CI 1.5-2.6	 0.002 0.003 0.001 0.001 0.001 0.002

CI, 95% Confidence interval; *HR*, hazard ratio; *MR*, mitral regurgitation; *MV*, mitral valve; *MVR*, mitral valve surgery; *N*, number of patients *NS*, not significant; ↑, increase in.
Adapted and expanded from Bonow RO, Carabello B, Chatterjee K, et al. 2008 focused update incorporated into the ACC/AHA 2006 guidelines for the management of patients with valvular heart disease: a report of the American College of Cardiology/American Heart Association Task Force on Practice Guidelines. J Am Coll Cardiol 2008;52:e1-142.

on the basis of the susceptibility of the organism. Surgical repair, if feasible, is indicated when a hemodynamically severe regurgitant leak ensues, if bacteriologic cure proves impossible with antibiotics alone, or if embolization from a vegetation has occurred or appears to be likely. As discussed earlier, a flail portion of valve in MVP can simulate a vegetation and is a common source of a false-positive diagnosis of endocarditis. Awareness of this possibility and the use of more advanced imaging techniques such as TEE, in addition to repeated cultures and the involvement of an infectious disease specialist, usually help resolve the clinical problem. Because MR is frequently severe in patients with such findings anyway, surgical intervention is often warranted, and the final diagnosis is made on the basis of the pathologic findings.

Cerebrovascular Ischemic Events

An increased incidence of cerebrovascular events has been reported in MVP, especially in younger patients.[160-162] Multiple potential mechanisms for thromboembolism exist, including platelet and fibrin aggregates on the valve,[31] abnormal platelet aggregation,[163] other detritus such as calcium on the valve in older patients, onset of atrial arrhythmias especially in older patients with more severe MR, and left atrial enlargement. The earlier studies suggesting an increased risk of cerebral thromboembolism in young patients with MVP have been challenged. In a study of 213 consecutive patients 45 years or younger with ischemic stroke or a transient ischemic attack identified over a 10-year period, Gilon et al[164] found that only 1.9% had MVP, compared with 2.7% of control subjects. A study from the Mayo Clinic also indicated that the relative risk for stroke in younger patients with uncomplicated MVP was not increased, although the risk in patients with prolapse generally was increased by a factor of 2.[165] In a later study from the Mayo Clinic, of 777 patients with MVP followed up from 1989 to 1998, prolapse doubled the likelihood of a cerebral ischemic event. However, most of the events occurred in patients older than 50 and were predicted by advancing age, leaflet thickening, atrial fibrillation at follow-up, and cardiovascular surgery.[166] Thus, MVP, especially when complicated by other comorbidities, may increase the risk of cerebral embolism, but the risk is low in young people with uncomplicated MVP.

The greater risk imposed by altered platelet aggregation and fibrin or platelet aggregates has also been questioned. Platelet aggregates are uncommon in pathologic studies, and platelet activation studies have suggested that the severity of MR may be more important than myxomatous disease itself in causing activation.[163,167] Table 18-3 details the current ACC/AHA guidelines for the management of patients with MVP who have symptoms of transient ischemic attacks or stroke. Aspirin is usually considered the first line of therapy unless there is evidence for or substantial risk of thrombus generation within the heart, in which case full anticoagulation with warfarin is indicated.

Sudden Cardiac Death and Ventricular Arrhythmia

Sudden cardiac death occurs at a yearly rate of 40 per 10,000 in those with MVP, a rate that is low but still at least twice as high as that in the general population.[168] The presumed cause of this increased risk is ventricular arrhythmia,[7,34,169] although severe valve disruption due to acute chordal tear has been implicated in case reports.[170] Multiple electrical abnormalities have been reported in MVP, including increased QT dispersion and ventricular arrhythmia that may be accentuated by volume loading from MR.[171,172] In fact, MR may be more important in the genesis of ventricular arrhythmia than MVP itself.[172] The true significance of these findings and their relationship to sudden death are unknown.

TABLE 18-3	American College of Cardiology/American Heart Association Guidelines for Antithrombotic Therapy in Mitral Valve Prolapse

Class I

1. Aspirin therapy (75-325 mg/day) is recommended for symptomatic patients with MVP who experience cerebral transient ischemic attacks. (Level of Evidence: C)
2. In patients with MVP and atrial fibrillation, warfarin therapy is recommended for patients aged older than 65 or those with hypertension, MR murmur, or a history of heart failure. (Level of Evidence: C)
3. Aspirin therapy (75-325 mg/day) is recommended for patients with MVP and atrial fibrillation who are younger than 65 years old and have no history of MR, hypertension, or heart failure. (Level of Evidence: C)
4. In patients with MVP and a history of stroke, warfarin therapy is recommended for patients with MR, atrial fibrillation, or left atrial thrombus. (Level of Evidence: C)

Class IIa

1. In patients with MVP and a history of stroke, who do not have MR, atrial fibrillation, or left arterial thrombus, warfarin therapy is reasonable for patients with echocardiographic evidence of thickening (≥5 mm) and/or redundancy of the valve leaflets. (Level of Evidence: C)
2. In patients with MVP and a history of stroke, aspirin therapy is reasonable for patients who do not have MR, atrial fibrillation, left atrial thrombus, or echocardiographic evidence of thickening (≥5 mm) or redundancy of the valve leaflets. (Level of Evidence: C)
3. Warfarin therapy is reasonable for patients with MVP with transient ischemic attacks despite aspirin therapy. (Level of Evidence: C)
4. Aspirin therapy (75-325 mg/day) can be beneficial for patients with MVP and a history of stroke who have contraindications to anticoagulants. (Level of Evidence: B)

Class IIb

Aspirin therapy (75-325 mg/day) may be considered for patients in sinus rhythm with echocardiographic evidence of high-risk MVP. (Level of Evidence: C)

MR, Mitral regurgitation; *MVP,* mitral valve prolapse.
From Bonow RO, Carabello B, Chatterjee K, et al. 2008 focused update incorporated into the ACC/AHA 2006 guidelines for the management of patients with valvular heart disease: a report of the American College of Cardiology/American Heart Association Task Force on Practice Guidelines. J Am Coll Cardiol 2008;52:e1–142.

Risk factors for sudden death include significant MR,[168] redundant valve tissue,[12] and decreased LV systolic function.[173] Autopsy studies of sudden death victims in this population have indicated more severe myxomatous changes in the valve.[174] Other autopsy series suggest an excess of women, particularly in younger age groups.[34,94,175] MVP is a very rare cause of sudden death in competitive athletes.[176] The risk of sudden cardiac death is reported to be increased when the mitral valve is flail, with the mechanism presumably being the addition of severe MR to the increased susceptibility of myxomatous disease itself.[173,177] Sudden death rates of up to 2% per year were reported in this setting, which is five times higher than rates estimated in patients with uncomplicated MVP, but the group studied in the report tended to be older (mean age 67 years[173]). Predictors of risk include atrial fibrillation, worsening functional class, and lower ejection fraction. Early surgical intervention appears to offer protection from the risk of sudden death in this older patient population with severe MR.[86,178]

In patients with symptomatic ventricular arrhythmia and significant MR in whom the valve is likely to be repaired, surgical intervention will probably improve but not eradicate symptoms completely and is the best initial approach. Implantable cardiac defibrillators are indicated in survivors of a sudden death episode. Patients with impaired LV function, those with frequent episodes of nonsustained ventricular tachycardia, and those with sustained ventricular tachycardia are best referred to an electrophysiologist for assessment with electrophysiologic testing as needed. In those with normal LV function, symptomatic improvement may result from beta-blockade. In the rare patient with very frequent symptomatic unifocal ventricular arrhythmias, electrophysiologic mapping and ablation of the focus may allow improvement in symptoms.

Mitral Regurgitation

MR of a severity to cause severe volume loading of the left ventricle and to necessitate eventual surgical intervention is the most frequent complication of MVP. MR tends to progress over time for a number of reasons. Progressive lengthening of chordae predisposes to more MR. The ventricular and annular remodeling due to MR causes further chordal stretching and ever more MR. Eventually, chordal strength is sufficiently diminished or stress on the chordae exceeds its load-bearing capacity, and a chord ruptures, leading to a flail segment and even more severe MR.

Risk factors for development of progressively severe MR include male gender, hypertension, greater body mass index, and increasing age.[76,156] Severe MR is relatively uncommon in patients before the fifth decade.[77] Echocardiographic factors associated with increased risk of severe MR include redundant thickened leaflets, prolapse involving the posterior leaflet, and increased ventricular size.[12,109,179] Conversely, patients who have thin leaflets and little MR at the outset appear to have a relatively low risk for subsequent development of severe MR.[69,109] In a study of 285 patients with MVP and lesser degrees of MR over a 4- to 5-year follow-up, progression of a grade or more of MR developed in 38% and was predicted by age and initial grade of MR. Progression was associated with greater increases in left atrial and LV size.[180]

The indications for surgery in patients with severe MR and the management of these patients in the operating room by both the echocardiographer and surgeon are addressed in other chapters (see Chapters 20 and 21). Mitral valve repair is highly likely when MVP is the etiology of the MR. Therefore, the threshold to intervene surgically is lowered in these patients when severe MR is present and competent surgical expertise is available to the patient. Outcomes are better for mitral valve repair in this setting than in other etiologies of MR, such as ischemic and rheumatic diseases, in terms of the initial success of the repair, its durability over time, and the life expectancy of the patient. Excellent durability of mitral repair out to 20 years has now been reported.[181] In certain situations, percutaneous mitral valve repair using the MitraClip Mitral Valve Repair System (Abbott Laboratories, Abbott Park, Illinois) may be beneficial.[182] Indications and appropriate patient selection are discussed in other chapters (see Chapter 22).

FOLLOW-UP AFTER MITRAL VALVE REPAIR

Close follow-up is required in patients with MVP after successful valve surgery. Echocardiography is usually performed before discharge to redefine baseline data, including any residual MR, the valve gradient, presence of systolic anterior motion of the mitral valve and any resultant outflow obstruction, and LV size and function. Postoperative LV function has been shown to define the subsequent risk of heart failure and survival, so it is an important parameter in follow-up.[84] LV ejection fraction may decline with successful eradication of MR based on the changes in loading. An ejection fraction less than 50% is associated with worse outcomes postoperatively, and prophylactic use of angiotensin-converting enzyme inhibitors and beta-blockers is appropriate.[183] LV dysfunction may normalize subsequently as a result of successful remodeling of the ventricle.[184] Systolic anterior motion is less common with current surgical techniques such as sliding annuloplasty.[120,131] Older studies suggest that systolic anterior motion develops more frequently in the presence of an annuloplasty ring and in patients with relatively small ventricles preoperatively.[185] Mild systolic anterior motion and outflow obstruction or provocable outflow obstruction often improve with beta-blockade and may diminish or disappear over time as remodeling occurs.[186] Rarely, more severe outflow obstruction may require subsequent reoperation for correction. Repair with a sliding annuloplasty is often possible,

but when it is not feasible, a mechanical valve may need to be implanted to forestall obstruction from bioprosthetic struts.

Residual mitral stenosis is exceedingly rare after mitral valve repair performed in an experienced center, given the excess tissue present in myxomatous disease. Endocarditis is also rare after mitral valve repair, although endocarditis prophylaxis is indicated by the newest AHA guidelines.[154] When endocarditis occurs, medical management is usually successful if the leaflets alone are involved, whereas surgical débridement is required if the annuloplasty is involved.[187] In a study of 1072 patients, the risk of reoperation in myxomatous mitral valve disease was 7% in the first 10 years after initial surgery.[21] Risk factors for reoperation include more complex anatomy, chordal transfer procedures, and inadequate early results. In approximately 50% of patients requiring reoperation, progression of the degenerative or myxomatous process was the major factor, but these patients accounted for only 1.5% of the initial operative cohort. Occasionally such patients present abruptly with chordal rupture and a flail segment, which may manifest as severe heart failure or rarely as intravascular hemolysis.[188]

Conclusions and Future Perspectives

Myxomatous mitral valve disease with MVP has been recognized as a clinical entity since its first descriptions using phonocardiography and ventriculography in the mid 1960s. Theories about its prevalence, cause, and significance have varied widely over that time. During the last two decades there has been growing consensus based on considerable data regarding its prevalence, natural history, risk for complications, and effective treatment of MR by valve repair. We still have major knowledge gaps with regard to the pathogenesis of the condition and the molecular basis by which it occurs. We are still unable to detect true myxomatous mitral valve disease in its preclinical state, and affected patients are not identified until the onset of significant valve changes heralded by clinical manifestations or echocardiography. We hope that, as the understanding of the molecular and genetic nature of the condition increases, more precise diagnostic tools will become available that will allow early detection in those at risk and more precise stratification of those most likely to experience complications. Furthermore, with knowledge of the aberrant molecular pathways leading to disease, it may then be possible to intervene prophylactically to lessen the likelihood of complications or, in the most attractive scenario, to forestall complications and the need for surgical intervention.

REFERENCES

1. Barlow JB, Bosman CK. Aneurysmal protrusion of the posterior leaflet of the mitral valve: an auscultatory-electrocardiographic syndrome. Am Heart J 1966;71:166–78.
2. Criley JM, Lewis KB, Humphries JO, et al. Prolapse of the mitral valve: clinical and cine-angiocardiographic findings. Br Heart J 1966;28:488–96.
3. Olson LJ, Subramanian R, Ackermann DM, et al. Surgical pathology of the mitral valve: a study of 712 cases spanning 21 years. Mayo Clin Proc 1987;62:22–34.
4. Waller BF, Morrow AG, Maron BJ, et al. Etiology of clinically isolated, severe, chronic, pure mitral regurgitation: analysis of 97 patients over 30 years of age having mitral valve replacement. Am Heart J 1982;104:276–88.
5. Hayek E, Gring CN, Griffin BP. Mitral valve prolapse. Lancet 2005;365:507–18.
6. Nishimura RA, McGoon MD. Perspectives on mitral-valve prolapse. N Engl J Med 1999;341:48–50.
7. Davies MJ, Moore BP, Braimbridge MV. The floppy mitral valve: Study of incidence, pathology, and complications in surgical, necropsy, and forensic material. Br Heart J 1978;40:468–81.
8. Jeresaty RM, Edwards JE, Chawla SK. Mitral valve prolapse and ruptured chordae tendineae. Am J Cardiol 1985;55:138–42.
9. Barlow JB. Mitral valve billowing and prolapse—an overview. Aust N Z J Med 1992;22:541–9.
10. Devereux RB, Perloff JK, Reichek N, et al. Mitral valve prolapse. Circulation 1976;54:3–14.
11. Devereux RB, Kramer-Fox R, Kligfield P. Mitral valve prolapse: causes, clinical manifestations, and management. Ann Intern Med 1989;111:305–17.
12. Nishimura RA, McGoon MD, Shub C, et al. Echocardiographically documented mitral-valve prolapse: long-term follow-up of 237 patients. N Engl J Med 1985;313:1305–9.
13. Warth DC, King ME, Cohen JM, et al. Prevalence of mitral valve prolapse in normal children. J Am Coll Cardiol 1985;5:1173–7.

14. Lax D, Eicher M, Goldberg SJ. Mild dehydration induces echocardiographic signs of mitral valve prolapse in healthy females with prior normal cardiac findings. Am Heart J 1992;124:1533–40.
15. Aufderheide S, Lax D, Goldberg SJ. Gender differences in dehydration-induced mitral valve prolapse. Am Heart J 1995;129:83–6.
16. Lax D, Eicher M, Goldberg SJ. Effects of hydration on mitral valve prolapse. Am Heart J 1993;126:415–18.
17. Schreiber TL, Feigenbaum H, Weyman AE. Effect of atrial septal defect repair on left ventricular geometry and degree of mitral valve prolapse. Circulation 1980;61: 888–96.
18. Suchon E, Podolec P, Plazak W, et al. Mitral valve prolapse associated with ostium secundum atrial septal defect—a functional disorder. Acta Cardiol 2004;59:237–8.
19. Come PC, Fortuin NJ, White Jr RI, et al. Echocardiographic assessment of cardiovascular abnormalities in the Marfan syndrome: comparison with clinical findings and with roentgenographic estimation of aortic root size. Am J Med 1983;74:465–74.
20. Antunes MJ. Mitral Valve Repair. Starnberg, Germany: Verlag R.S. Schultz; 1989.
21. Carpentier A. Cardiac valve surgery—the "French correction." J Thorac Cardiovasc Surg 1983;86:323–37.
22. Foster GP, Isselbacher EM, Rose GA, et al. Accurate localization of mitral regurgitant defects using multiplane transesophageal echocardiography. Ann Thorac Surg 1998;65:1025–31.
23. Fann JI, Ingels Jr NB, Miller DC. Pathophysiology of mitral valve disease. In: Cohn L, editor. Cardiac Surgery in the Adult. New York: McGraw-Hill; 2008. p. 973–1012.
24. Gillinov AM, Cosgrove DM, Blackstone EH, et al. Durability of mitral valve repair for degenerative disease. J Thorac Cardiovasc Surg 1998;116:734–43.
25. Pyeritz RE, Wappel MA. Mitral valve dysfunction in the Marfan syndrome: clinical and echocardiographic study of prevalence and natural history. Am J Med 1983;74: 797–807.
26. Weyman AE, Scherrer-Crosbie M. Marfan syndrome and mitral valve prolapse. J Clin Invest 2004;114:1543–6.
27. Jaffe AS, Geltman EM, Rodey GE, et al. Mitral valve prolapse: a consistent manifestation of type IV Ehlers-Danlos syndrome. The pathogenetic role of the abnormal production of type III collagen. Circulation 1981;64:121–5.
28. Hortop J, Tsipouras P, Hanley JA, et al. Cardiovascular involvement in osteogenesis imperfecta. Circulation 1986;73:54–61.
29. Pyeritz RE, Weiss JL, Renie WA, et al. Pseudoxanthoma elasticum and mitral-valve prolapse. N Engl J Med 1982;307:1451–2.
30. van der Bel-Kahn J, Becker AE. The surgical pathology of rheumatic and floppy mitral valves: distinctive morphologic features upon gross examination. Am J Surg Pathol 1986;10:282–92.
31. Anyanwu AC, Adams DH. Etiologic classification of degenerative mitral valve disease: Barlow's disease and fibroelastic deficiency. Semin Thorac Cardiovasc Surg 2007;19: 90–6.
32. Fisher M, Weiner B, Ockene IS, et al. Platelet activation and mitral valve prolapse. Neurology 1983;33:384–6.
33. Virmani R, Atkinson JB, Forman MB. The pathology of mitral valve prolapse. Herz 1988;13:215–26.
34. Chesler E, King RA, Edwards JE. The myxomatous mitral valve and sudden death. Circulation 1983;67:632–9.
35. Olsen EG, Al-Rufaie HK. The floppy mitral valve: study on pathogenesis. Br Heart J 1980;44:674–83.
36. Baker PB, Bansal G, Boudoulas H, et al. Floppy mitral valve chordae tendineae: histopathologic alterations. Hum Pathol 1988;19:507–12.
37. Rabkin E, Aikawa M, Stone JR, et al. Activated interstitial myofibroblasts express catabolic enzymes and mediate matrix remodeling in myxomatous heart valves. Circulation 2001;104:2525–32.
38. Fornes P, Heudes D, Fuzellier JF, et al. Correlation between clinical and histologic patterns of degenerative mitral valve insufficiency: a histomorphometric study of 130 excised segments. Cardiovasc Pathol 1999;8:81–92.
39. Flameng W, Meuris B, Herijgers P, et al. Durability of mitral valve repair in Barlow disease versus fibroelastic deficiency. J Thorac Cardiovasc Surg 2008;135:274–82.
40. Tamura K, Fukuda Y, Ishizaki M, et al. Abnormalities in elastic fibers and other connective-tissue components of floppy mitral valve. Am Heart J 1995;129:1149–58.
41. King BD, Clark MA, Baba N, et al. "Myxomatous" mitral valves: collagen dissolution as the primary defect. Circulation 1982;66:288–96.
42. Akhtar S, Meek KM, James V. Immunolocalization of elastin, collagen type I and type III, fibronectin, and vitronectin in extracellular matrix components of normal and myxomatous mitral heart valve chordae tendineae. Cardiovasc Pathol 1999;8:203–11.
43. Barber JE, Kasper FK, Ratliff NB, et al. Mechanical properties of myxomatous mitral valves. J Thorac Cardiovasc Surg 2001;122:955–62.
44. Barber JE, Ratliff NB, Cosgrove 3rd DM, et al. Myxomatous mitral valve chordae. I: Mechanical properties. J Heart Valve Dis 2001;10:320–4.
45. Grande-Allen KJ, Ratliff NB, Griffin BP, et al. Case report: outer sheath rupture may precede complete chordal rupture in fibrotic mitral valve disease. J Heart Valve Dis 2001;10:90–3.
46. Lis Y, Burleigh MC, Parker DJ, et al. Biochemical characterization of individual normal, floppy and rheumatic human mitral valves. Biochem J 1987;244:597–603.
47. Grande-Allen KJ, Griffin BP, Ratliff NB, et al. Glycosaminoglycan profiles of myxomatous mitral leaflets and chordae parallel the severity of mechanical alterations. J Am Coll Cardiol 2003;42:271–7.
48. Kern CB; Wessels A, McGarity J, et al. Reduced versican cleavage due to Adamts9 haploinsufficiency is associated with cardiac and aortic anomalies. Matrix Biol 2010;29: 304–16.
49. Nasuti JF, Zhang PJ, Feldman MD, et al. Fibrillin and other matrix proteins in mitral valve prolapse syndrome. Ann Thorac Surg 2004;77:532–6.
50. Gupta V, Werdenberg JA, Mendez JS, et al. Influence of strain on proteoglycan synthesis by valvular interstitial cells in three-dimensional culture. Acta Biomat 2008;4: 88–96.
51. Oki T, Fukuda N, Kawano T, et al. Histopathologic studies of innervation of normal and prolapsed human mitral valves. J Heart Valve Dis 1995;4:496–502.
52. Devereux RB, Brown WT, Kramer-Fox R, et al. Inheritance of mitral valve prolapse: effect of age and sex on gene expression. Ann Intern Med 1982;97:826–32.
53. Zuppiroli A, Roman MJ, O'Grady M, et al. A family study of anterior mitral leaflet thickness and mitral valve prolapse. Am J Cardiol 1998;82:823–6.
54. Pini R, Greppi B, Kramer-Fox R, et al. Mitral valve dimensions and motion and familial transmission of mitral valve prolapse with and without mitral leaflet billowing. J Am Coll Cardiol 1988;12:1423–31.
55. Disse S, Abergel E, Berrebi A, et al. Mapping of a first locus for autosomal dominant myxomatous mitral-valve prolapse to chromosome 16p11.2–p12.1. Am J Hum Genet 1999;65:1242–51.
56. Freed LA, Acierno Jr JS, Dai D, et al. A locus for autosomal dominant mitral valve prolapse on chromosome 11p15.4. Am J Hum Genet 2003;72:1551–9.
57. Nesta F, Leyne M, Yosefy C, et al. New locus for autosomal dominant mitral valve prolapse on chromosome 13: clinical insights from genetic studies. Circulation 2005;112:2022–30.
58. Roberts R. Another chromosomal locus for mitral valve prolapse: close but no cigar. Circulation 2005;112:1924–6.
59. Henney AM, Tsipouras P, Schwartz RC, et al. Genetic evidence that mutations in the COL1A1, COL1A2, COL3A1, or COL5A2 collagen genes are not responsible for mitral valve prolapse. Br Heart J 1989;61:292–9.
60. Wordsworth P, Ogilvie D, Akhras F, et al. Genetic segregation analysis of familial mitral valve prolapse shows no linkage to fibrillar collagen genes. Br Heart J 1989;61:300–6.
61. Chou HT, Hung JS, Chen YT, et al. Association between angiotensinogen gene M235T polymorphism and mitral valve prolapse syndrome in Taiwan Chinese. J Heart Valve Dis 2002;11:830–6.
62. Chou HT, Chen YT, Shi YR, et al. Association between angiotensin I-converting enzyme gene insertion/deletion polymorphism and mitral valve prolapse syndrome. Am Heart J 2003;145:169–73.
63. Kyndt F, Schott JJ, Trochu JN, et al. Mapping of X-linked myxomatous valvular dystrophy to chromosome Xq28. Am J Hum Genet 1998;62:627–32.
64. Pedersen HD, Kristensen BO, Lorentzen KA, et al. Mitral valve prolapse in 3-year-old healthy Cavalier King Charles Spaniels: an echocardiographic study. Can J Vet Res 1995;59:294–8.
65. Olsen LH, Fredholm M, Pedersen HD. Epidemiology and inheritance of mitral valve prolapse in Dachshunds. J Vet Intern Med 1999;13:448–56.
66. Ng CM, Cheng A, Myers LA, et al. TGF-β-dependent pathogenesis of mitral valve prolapse in a mouse model of Marfan syndrome. J Clin Invest 2004;114:1586–92.
67. Charitakis K, Basson C. Degenerating heart valves; fill them up with filamin? Circulation 2007;115:2–4.
68. Levine R, Slaugenhaupt S. Molecular genetics of mitral valve prolapse. Curr Opin Cardiol 2007;22:171–5.
69. Freed LA, Levy D, Levine RA, et al. Prevalence and clinical outcome of mitral-valve prolapse. N Engl J Med 1999;341:1–7.
70. Oke DA, Ajuluchukwu JN, Mbakwem A, et al. Clinical and echocardiographic assessment of Nigerian patients seen at the Lagos University Teaching Hospital with features of mitral valve prolapse. West Afr J Med 2000;19:200–5.
71. Theal M, Sleik K, Anand S, et al. Prevalence of mitral valve prolapse in ethnic groups. Can J Cardiol 2004;20:511–15.
72. Avierinos JF, Gersh BJ, Melton 3rd LJ, et al. Natural history of asymptomatic mitral valve prolapse in the community. Circulation 2002;106:1355–61.
73. Nascimento R, Freitas A, Teixeira F, et al. Is mitral valve prolapse a congenital or acquired disease? Am J Cardiol 1997;79:226–7.
74. Tayel S, Kurczynski TW, Levine M, et al. Marfanoid children: etiologic heterogeneity and cardiac findings. Am J Dis Child 1991;145:90–3.
75. Mohty D, Orszulak TA, Schaff HV, et al. Very long-term survival and durability of mitral valve repair for mitral valve prolapse. Circulation 2001;104(Suppl I):I-1–I-7.
76. Kolibash Jr AJ, Kilman JW, Bush CA, et al. Evidence for progression from mild to severe mitral regurgitation in mitral valve prolapse. Am J Cardiol 1986;58:762–7.
77. Wilcken DE, Hickey AJ. Lifetime risk for patients with mitral valve prolapse of developing severe valve regurgitation requiring surgery. Circulation 1988;78:10–14.
78. Devereux RB. Mitral valve prolapse and severe mitral regurgitation. Circulation 1988;78:234–6.
79. St John Sutton M, Weyman AE. Mitral valve prolapse prevalence and complications: an ongoing dialogue. Circulation 2002;106:1305–7.
80. Rosenhek R, Rader F, Klaar U, et al. Outcome of watchful waiting in asymptomatic severe mitral regurgitation. Circulation 2006;113:2238–44.
81. Enriquez-Sarano M, Schaff HV, Orszulak TA, et al. Valve repair improves the outcome of surgery for mitral regurgitation: a multivariate analysis. Circulation 1995;91: 1022–8.
82. Ling LH, Enriquez-Sarano M, Seward JB, et al. Early surgery in patients with mitral regurgitation due to flail leaflets: a long-term outcome study. Circulation 1997;96: 1819–25.
83. Enriquez-Sarano M, Avierinos JF, Messika-Zeitoun D, et al. Quantitative determinants of the outcome of asymptomatic mitral regurgitation. N Engl J Med 2005;352: 875–83.
84. Enriquez-Sarano M, Schaff HV, Orszulak TA, et al. Congestive heart failure after surgical correction of mitral regurgitation: a long-term study. Circulation 1995;92: 2496–503.
85. Gillinov AM, Blackstone EH, Rajeswaran J, et al. Ischemic versus degenerative mitral regurgitation: does etiology affect survival? Ann Thorac Surg 2005;80:811–19.
86. Ling LH, Enriquez-Sarano M, Seward JB, et al. Clinical outcome of mitral regurgitation due to flail leaflet. N Engl J Med 1996;335:1417–23.
87. Bonow RO, Carabello B, Chatterjee K, et al. 2008 focused update incorporated into the ACC/AHA 2006 guidelines for the management of patients with valvular heart disease: a report of the American College of Cardiology/American Heart Association Task Force on Practice Guidelines (writing committee to revise the 1998 Guidelines for the

Management of Patients with Valvular Heart Disease). J Am Coll Cardiol 2008;52: e1–142.

88. Roberts WC, Braunwald E, Morrow AG. Acute severe mitral regurgitation secondary to ruptured chordae tendineae: clinical, hemodynamic, and pathologic considerations. Circulation 1966;33:58–70.

89. Alpert MA, Mukerji V, Sabeti M, et al. Mitral valve prolapse, panic disorder, and chest pain. Med Clin North Am 1991;75:1119–33.

90. Devereux RB. Recent developments in the diagnosis and management of mitral valve prolapse. Curr Opin Cardiol 1995;10:107–16.

91. Zuppiroli A, Mori F, Favilli S, et al. Arrhythmias in mitral valve prolapse: relation to anterior mitral leaflet thickening, clinical variables, and color Doppler echocardiographic parameters. Am Heart J 1994;128:919–27.

92. Kramer HM, Kligfield P, Devereux RB, et al. Arrhythmias in mitral valve prolapse: effect of selection bias. Arch Intern Med 1984;144:2360–4.

93. Kernis SJ, Nkomo VT, Messika-Zeitoun D, et al. Atrial fibrillation after surgical correction of mitral regurgitation in sinus rhythm: incidence, outcome, and determinants. Circulation 2004;110:2320–5.

94. Anders S, Said S, Schulz F, et al. Mitral valve prolapse syndrome as cause of sudden death in young adults. Forensic Sci Int 2007;171:127–30.

95. Dollar AL, Roberts WC. Morphologic comparison of patients with mitral valve prolapse who died suddenly with patients who died from severe valvular dysfunction or other conditions. J Am Coll Cardiol 1991;17:921–31.

96. Danchin N, Voiriot P, Briancon S, et al. Mitral valve prolapse as a risk factor for infective endocarditis. Lancet 1989;1:743–5.

97. MacMahon SW, Hickey AJ, Wilcken DE, et al. Risk of infective endocarditis in mitral valve prolapse with and without precordial systolic murmurs. Am J Cardiol 1987;59: 105–8.

98. Kelley RE, Pina I, Lee SC. Cerebral ischemia and mitral valve prolapse: case-control study of associated factors. Stroke 1988;19:443–6.

99. Watson RT. TIA, stroke, and mitral valve prolapse. Neurology 1979;29:886–9.

100. Desjardins VA, Enriquez-Sarano M, Tajik AJ, et al. Intensity of murmurs correlates with severity of valvular regurgitation. Am J Med 1996;100:149–56.

101. Tribouilloy CM, Enriquez-Sarano M, Mohty D, et al. Pathophysiologic determinants of third heart sounds: a prospective clinical and Doppler echocardiographic study. Am J Med 2001;111:96–102.

102. Weis AJ, Salcedo EE, Stewart WJ, et al. Anatomic explanation of mobile systolic clicks: implications for the clinical and echocardiographic diagnosis of mitral valve prolapse. Am Heart J 1995;129:314–20.

103. Roman MJ, Devereux RB, Kramer-Fox R, et al. Comparison of cardiovascular and skeletal features of primary mitral valve prolapse and Marfan syndrome. Am J Cardiol 1989;63:317–21.

104. Udoshi MB, Shah A, Fisher VJ, et al. Incidence of mitral valve prolapse in subjects with thoracic skeletal abnormalities—a prospective study. Am Heart J 1979;97:303–11.

105. Levine RA, Stathogiannis E, Newell JB, et al. Reconsideration of echocardiographic standards for mitral valve prolapse: lack of association between leaflet displacement isolated to the apical four chamber view and independent echocardiographic evidence of abnormality. J Am Coll Cardiol 1988;11:1010–19.

106. Levine RA, Triulzi MO, Harrigan P, et al. The relationship of mitral annular shape to the diagnosis of mitral valve prolapse. Circulation 1987;75:756–67.

107. Levine RA, Handschumacher MD, Sanfilippo AJ, et al. Three-dimensional echocardiographic reconstruction of the mitral valve, with implications for the diagnosis of mitral valve prolapse. Circulation 1989;80:589–98.

108. Weissman NJ, Pini R, Roman MJ, et al. In vivo mitral valve morphology and motion in mitral valve prolapse. Am J Cardiol 1994;73:1080–8.

109. Marks AR, Choong CY, Sanfilippo AJ, et al. Identification of high-risk and low-risk subgroups of patients with mitral-valve prolapse. N Engl J Med 1989;320:1031–6.

110. Mills WR, Barber JE, Skiles JA, et al. Clinical, echocardiographic, and biomechanical differences in mitral valve prolapse affecting one or both leaflets. Am J Cardiol 2002; 89:1394–9.

111. Brown AK, Anderson V. Two dimensional echocardiography and the tricuspid valve: leaflet definition and prolapse. Br Heart J 1983;49:495–500.

112. Louie EK, Langholz D, Mackin WJ, et al. Transesophageal echocardiographic assessment of the contribution of intrinsic tissue thickness to the appearance of a thick mitral valve in patients with mitral valve prolapse. J Am Coll Cardiol 1996;28:465–71.

113. Chandraratna PA, Aronow WS. Incidence of ruptured chordae tendineae in the mitral valvular prolapse syndrome: an echocardiographic study. Chest 1979;75:334–9.

114. Grenadier E, Alpan G, Keidar S, et al. The prevalence of ruptured chordae tendineae in the mitral valve prolapse syndrome. Am Heart J 1983;105:603–10.

115. Hozumi T, Yoshikawa J, Yoshida K, et al. Direct visualization of ruptured chordae tendineae by transesophageal two-dimensional echocardiography. J Am Coll Cardiol 1990;16:1315–19.

116. Enriquez-Sarano M, Freeman WK, Tribouilloy CM, et al. Functional anatomy of mitral regurgitation: accuracy and outcome implications of transesophageal echocardiography. J Am Coll Cardiol 1999;34:1129–36.

117. Sochowski RA, Chan KL, Ascah KJ, et al. Comparison of accuracy of transesophageal versus transthoracic echocardiography for the detection of mitral valve prolapse with ruptured chordae tendineae (flail mitral leaflet). Am J Cardiol 1991;67:1251–5.

118. Cho L, Gillinov AM, Cosgrove 3rd DM, et al. Echocardiographic assessment of the mechanisms of correction of bileaflet prolapse causing mitral regurgitation with only posterior leaflet repair surgery. Am J Cardiol 2000;86:1349–51.

119. Hickey AJ, Wolfers J. False positive diagnosis of vegetations on a myxomatous mitral valve using two-dimensional echocardiography. Aust N Z J Med 1982;12:540–2.

120. Stewart WJ, Griffin BP. Intraoperative echocardiography in mitral valve repair. In: Otto C, editor. The Practice of Clinical Echocardiography, 3rd ed. Philadelphia: WB Saunders; 2007. p. 459–80.

121. Grewal KS, Malkowski MJ, Kramer CM, et al. Multiplane transesophageal echocardiographic identification of the involved scallop in patients with flail mitral valve leaflet: intraoperative correlation. J Am Soc Echocardiogr 1998;11:966–71.

122. Muller S, Muller L, Laufer G, et al. Comparison of three-dimensional imaging to transesophageal echocardiography for preoperative evaluation in mitral valve prolapse. Am J Cardiol 2006;98:243–8.

123. Chen CG, Thomas JD, Anconina J, et al. Impact of impinging wall jet on color Doppler quantification of mitral regurgitation. Circulation 1991;84:712–20.

124. Pu M, Vandervoort PM, Greenberg NL, et al. Impact of wall constraint on velocity distribution in proximal flow convergence zone: implications for color Doppler quantification of mitral regurgitation. J Am Coll Cardiol 1996;27:706–13.

125. Pu MMDP, Vandervoort PMMD, Griffin BPMD, et al. Quantification of mitral regurgitation by the proximal convergence method using transesophageal echocardiography: clinical validation of a geometric correction for proximal flow constraint. Circulation 1995;92:2169–77.

126. Enriquez-Sarano M, Sinak LJ, Tajik AJ, et al. Changes in effective regurgitant orifice throughout systole in patients with mitral valve prolapse: a clinical study using the proximal isovelocity surface area method. Circulation 1995;92:2951–8.

127. Griffin BP. Timing of surgical intervention in chronic mitral regurgitation: is vigilance enough? Circulation 2006;113:2169–72.

128. Armstrong GP, Griffin BP. Exercise echocardiographic assessment in severe mitral regurgitation. Coron Artery Dis 2000;11:23–30.

129. Leung DY, Griffin BP, Snader CE, et al. Determinants of functional capacity in chronic mitral regurgitation unassociated with coronary artery disease or left ventricular dysfunction. Am J Cardiol 1997;79:914–20.

130. Tischler MD, Battle RW, Ashikaga T, et al. Effects of exercise on left ventricular performance determined by echocardiography in chronic, severe mitral regurgitation secondary to mitral valve prolapse. Am J Cardiol 1996;77:397–402.

131. Gillinov AM, Cosgrove DM. Mitral valve repair for degenerative disease. J Heart Valve Dis 2002;11(Suppl 1):S15–20.

132. Fedak PW, McCarthy PM, Bonow RO. Evolving concepts and technologies in mitral valve repair. Circulation 2008;117:963–74.

133. Lawrie GM. Mitral valve: toward complete repairability. Surg Technol Int 2006;15: 189–97.

134. Gillinov AM, Banbury MK. Pre-measured artificial chordae for mitral valve repair. Ann Thorac Surg 2007;84:2127–9.

135. Pepi M, Tamborini G, Maltagliati A, et al. Head-to-head comparison of two- and three-dimensional transthoracic and transesophageal echocardiography in the localization of mitral valve prolapse. J Am Coll Cardiol 2006;48:2524–30.

136. Grewal J, Mankad S, Freeman WK, et al. Real-time three dimensional transesophageal echocardiography in the intraoperative assessment of mitral valve disease. J Am Soc Echocardiogr 2009;22:34–41.

137. Breburda CS, Griffin BP, Pu M, et al. Three-dimensional echocardiographic planimetry of maximal regurgitant orifice area in myxomatous mitral regurgitation: intraoperative comparison with proximal flow convergence. J Am Coll Cardiol 1998;32:432–7.

138. Lin SS, Lauer MS, Asher CR, et al. Prediction of coronary artery disease in patients undergoing operations for mitral valve degeneration. J Thorac Cardiovasc Surg 2001;121:894–901.

139. Boudoulas H, Kolibash Jr AJ, Baker P, et al. Mitral valve prolapse and the mitral valve prolapse syndrome: a diagnostic classification and pathogenesis of symptoms. Am Heart J 1989;118:796–818.

140. Cohen MV, Shah PK, Spindola-Franco H. Angiographic-echocardiographic correlation in mitral valve prolapse. Am Heart J 1979;97:43–52.

141. Boudoulas H, Reynolds JC, Mazzaferri E, et al. Metabolic studies in mitral valve prolapse syndrome: a neuroendocrine-cardiovascular process. Circulation 1980;61:1200–5.

142. Boudoulas H, Wooley CF. Mitral valve prolapse syndrome: evidence of hyperadrenergic state. Postgrad Med 1988;Spec No:152–62.

143. Gaffney FA, Karlsson ES, Campbell W, et al. Autonomic dysfunction in women with mitral valve prolapse syndrome. Circulation 1979;59:894–901.

144. Devereux RB, Kramer-Fox R, Brown WT, et al. Relation between clinical features of the mitral prolapse syndrome and echocardiographically documented mitral valve prolapse. J Am Coll Cardiol 1986;8:763–72.

145. Savage DD, Devereux RB, Garrison RJ, et al. Mitral valve prolapse in the general population. 2. Clinical features: the Framingham Study. Am Heart J 1983;106:577–81.

146. Freed LA, Levy D, Levine RA, et al. Prevalence and clinical outcome of mitral-valve prolapse. N Engl J Med 1999;341:1–7.

147. Chesler E, Weir EK, Braatz GA, et al. Normal catecholamine and hemodynamic responses to orthostatic tilt in subjects with mitral valve prolapse: correlation with psychologic testing. Am J Med 1985;78:754–60.

148. Szombathy T, Janoskuti L, Szalai C, et al. Angiotensin II type 1 receptor gene polymorphism and mitral valve prolapse syndrome. Am Heart J 2000;139:101–5.

149. Fontana ME, Sparks EA, Boudoulas H, et al. Mitral valve prolapse and the mitral valve prolapse syndrome. Curr Probl Cardiol 1991;16:309–75.

150. Enriquez-Sarano M, Avierinos JF, Messika-Zeitoun D, et al. Quantitative determinants of the outcome of asymptomatic mitral regurgitation. N Engl J Med 2005;352: 875–83.

151. Kang DH, Kim JH, Rim JH, et al. Comparison of early surgery versus conventional treatment in asymptomatic severe mitral regurgitation. Circulation 2009;119:797–804.

152. Dajani AS, Taubert KA, Wilson W, et al. Prevention of bacterial endocarditis: recommendations by the American Heart Association. J Am Dent Assoc 1997;128:1142–51.

153. Devereux RB, Frary CJ, Kramer-Fox R, et al. Cost-effectiveness of infective endocarditis prophylaxis for mitral valve prolapse with or without a mitral regurgitant murmur. Am J Cardiol 1994;74:1024–9.

154. Wilson W, Taubert KA, Gewitz M, et al. Prevention of infective endocarditis: guidelines from the American Heart Association: a guideline from the American Heart Association Rheumatic Fever, Endocarditis, and Kawasaki Disease Committee, Council on Cardiovascular Disease in the Young, and the Council on Clinical Cardiology, Council on Cardiovascular Surgery and Anesthesia, and the Quality of Care and Outcomes Research Interdisciplinary Working Group. Circulation 2007;116:1736–54.

155. Devereux RB, Hawkins I, Kramer-Fox R, et al. Complications of mitral valve prolapse: disproportionate occurrence in men and older patients. Am J Med 1986;81:751–8.

156. Singh RG, Cappucci R, Kramer-Fox R, et al. Severe mitral regurgitation due to mitral valve prolapse: risk factors for development, progression, and need for mitral valve surgery. Am J Cardiol 2000;85:193–8.

157. Clemens JD, Horwitz RI, Jaffe CC, et al. A controlled evaluation of the risk of bacterial endocarditis in persons with mitral-valve prolapse. N Engl J Med 1982;307:776–81.

158. MacMahon SW, Roberts JK, Kramer-Fox R, et al. Mitral valve prolapse and infective endocarditis. Am Heart J 1987;113:1291–8.

159. Steckelberg JM, Wilson WR. Risk factors for infective endocarditis. Infect Dis Clin North Am 1993;7:9–19.

160. Barnett HJ, Boughner DR, Taylor DW, et al. Further evidence relating mitral-valve prolapse to cerebral ischemic events. N Engl J Med 1980;302:139–44.

161. Sandok BA, Giuliani ER. Cerebral ischemic events in patients with mitral valve prolapse. Stroke 1982;13:448–50.

162. Jackson AC, Boughner DR, Barnett HJ. Mitral valve prolapse and cerebral ischemic events in young patients. Neurology 1984;34:784–7.

163. Walsh PN, Kansu TA, Corbett JJ, et al. Platelets, thromboembolism and mitral valve prolapse. Circulation 1981;63:552–9.

164. Gilon D, Buonanno FS, Joffe MM, et al. Lack of evidence of an association between mitral-valve prolapse and stroke in young patients. N Engl J Med 1999;341:8–13.

165. Orencia AJ, Petty GW, Khandheria BK, et al. Risk of stroke with mitral valve prolapse in population-based cohort study. Stroke 1995;26:7–13.

166. Avierinos JF, Brown RD, Foley DA, et al. Cerebral ischemic events after diagnosis of mitral valve prolapse: a community-based study of incidence and predictive factors. Stroke 2003;34:1339–44.

167. Tse HF, Lau CP, Cheng G. Relation between mitral regurgitation and platelet activation. J Am Coll Cardiol 1997;30:1813–18.

168. Kligfield P, Levy D, Devereux RB, et al. Arrhythmias and sudden death in mitral valve prolapse. Am Heart J 1987;113:1298–307.

169. Pocock WA, Bosman CK, Chesler E, et al. Sudden death in primary mitral valve prolapse. Am Heart J 1984;107:378–82.

170. Ferguson DW, Kiefaber RW, Ziegelman DS, et al. Acute rupture of myxomatous mitral valve presenting as refractory cardiopulmonary arrest. J Am Coll Cardiol 1987;9:215–20.

171. Tieleman RG, Crijns HJ, Wiesfeld AC, et al. Increased dispersion of refractoriness in the absence of QT prolongation in patients with mitral valve prolapse and ventricular arrhythmias. Br Heart J 1995;73:37–40.

172. Kligfield P, Hochreiter C, Kramer H, et al. Complex arrhythmias in mitral regurgitation with and without mitral valve prolapse: contrast to arrhythmias in mitral valve prolapse without mitral regurgitation. Am J Cardiol 1985;55:1545–9.

173. Grigioni F, Enriquez-Sarano M, Ling LH, et al. Sudden death in mitral regurgitation due to flail leaflet. J Am Coll Cardiol 1999;34:2078–85.

174. Farb A, Tang AL, Atkinson JB, et al. Comparison of cardiac findings in patients with mitral valve prolapse who die suddenly to those who have congestive heart failure from mitral regurgitation and to those with fatal noncardiac conditions. Am J Cardiol 1992;70:234–9.

175. Corrado D, Basso C, Nava A, et al. Sudden death in young people with apparently isolated mitral valve prolapse. G Ital Cardiol 1997;27:1097–105.

176. Maron BJ, Epstein SE, Roberts WC. Causes of sudden death in competitive athletes. J Am Coll Cardiol 1986;7:204–14.

177. Ciancamerla F, Paglia I, Catuzzo B, et al. Sudden death in mitral valve prolapse and severe mitral regurgitation. Is chordal rupture an indication to early surgery? J Cardiovasc Surg (Torino) 2003;44:283–6.

178. Enriquez-Sarano M, Avierinos JF, Ling LH, et al. Surgical treatment of degenerative mitral regurgitation: should we approach differently patients with flail leaflets of simple mitral valve prolapse? Adv Cardiol 2004;41:95–107.

179. Fukuda N, Oki T, Iuchi A, et al. Predisposing factors for severe mitral regurgitation in idiopathic mitral valve prolapse. Am J Cardiol 1995;76:503–7.

180. Avierinos JF, Detaint D, Messika-Zeitoun D, et al. Risk, determinants, and outcome implications of progression of mitral regurgitation after diagnosis of mitral valve prolapse in a single community. Am J Cardiol 2008;101:662–7.

181. Braunberger E, Deloche A, Berrebi A, et al. Very long-term results (more than 20 years) of valve repair with Carpentier's techniques in nonrheumatic mitral valve insufficiency. Circulation 2001;104(Suppl I):I-8–I-11.

182. Feldman T, Foster E, Glower DG, et al. Percutaneous repair or surgery for mitral regurgitation. N Engl J Med 2011;364:1395–406

183. Enriquez-Sarano M, Tajik AJ, Schaff HV, et al. Echocardiographic prediction of left ventricular function after correction of mitral regurgitation: results and clinical implications. J Am Coll Cardiol 1994;24:1536–43.

184. Starling MR, Kirsh MM, Montgomery DG, et al. Impaired left ventricular contractile function in patients with long-term mitral regurgitation and normal ejection fraction. J Am Coll Cardiol 1993;22:239–50.

185. Freeman WK, Schaff HV, Khandheria BK, et al. Intraoperative evaluation of mitral valve regurgitation and repair by transesophageal echocardiography: incidence and significance of systolic anterior motion. J Am Coll Cardiol 1992;20:599–609.

186. Schiavone WA, Cosgrove DM, Lever HM, et al. Long-term follow-up of patients with left ventricular outflow tract obstruction after Carpentier ring mitral valvuloplasty. Circulation 1988;78(Suppl I):I-60–I-65.

187. Gillinov AM, Faber CN, Sabik JF, et al. Endocarditis after mitral valve repair. Ann Thorac Surg 2002;73:1813–16.

188. Garcia MJ, Vandervoort P, Stewart WJ, et al. Mechanisms of hemolysis with mitral prosthetic regurgitation: study using transesophageal echocardiography and fluid dynamic simulation. J Am Coll Cardiol 1996;27:399–406.

189. Chandraratna PA, Nimalasuriya A, Kawanishi D, et al. Identification of the increased frequency of cardiovascular abnormalities associated with mitral valve prolapse by two-dimensional echocardiography. Am J Cardiol 1984;54:1283–5.

190. Takamoto T, Nitta M, Tsujibayashi T, et al. The prevalence and clinical features of pathologically abnormal mitral valve leaflets (myxomatous mitral valve) in the mitral valve prolapse syndrome: an echocardiographic and pathological comparative study. J Cardiol Suppl 1991;25:75–86.

191. Babuty D, Cosnay P, Breuillac JC, et al. Ventricular arrhythmia factors in mitral valve prolapse. Pacing Clin Electrophysiol 1994;17:1090–9.

CHAPTER 19 Secondary Mitral Regurgitation

Elyse Foster and Rajni K. Rao

Key Points

- Secondary mitral regurgitation is the most common valve disease, with coronary artery disease accounting for approximately a third of cases.
- In contrast to primary mitral valve disease, secondary mitral regurgitation is best thought of as a ventricular process that alters the normal balance between the forces that close the valve and tethering forces that prevent the valve from prolapsing into the left atrium.
- Secondary MR is MR not due to primary valvular leaflet pathology. Secondary MR may be divided into MR due to ischemic heart disease (ischemic MR) and MR due to other causes (functional MR).
- Atrial enlargement with associated annular dilation may be responsible for mitral regurgitation in some patients with atrial fibrillation but is usually not severe.
- Criteria for grading the severity of secondary mitral regurgitation may differ from criteria for severity of primary mitral regurgitation.
- The primary treatment of secondary mitral regurgitation is targeted at treating the underlying ventricular dysfunction, including pharmacologic therapy, cardiac resynchronization therapy, and treatment of contributing ischemia.
- There are limited indications for surgery in the treatment of secondary mitral regurgitation.
- Percutaneous therapy for secondary mitral regurgitation is under investigation.

Epidemiology

Secondary mitral regurgitation (MR) is the most common valve disease. A population-based study combined the echocardiographic data from three separate studies funded by the National Institutes of Health (NIH) that examined young (Coronary Artery Revascularisation in Diabetes [CARDIA]), middle-aged (Atherosclerosis Risk in Communities [ARIC]) and older adults (Cardiovascular Health Study [CHS]) to determine the incidence of moderate to severe valvular disease. Their findings in approximately 12,000 adults demonstrated that valve disease was equally common among men and women and among blacks and whites, and that it increased in frequency with age. MR was the most common significant valve disease, with an incidence less than 1% before age 55 years but increasing each decade and reaching more than 9% after age 75 years.[1] The incidence of MR was similar among the residents of Olmsted County.[1] Patients with MR had larger ventricles without hypertrophy. This analysis did not differentiate between primary and secondary MR. However, a later meta-analysis attempted to examine the prevalence of MR in the U.S. population and categorize the type of MR according to Carpentier's classification (see Chapter 21). Although there were a number of limitations to the methodology, the analysis estimated that MR affected 2 to 2.5 million people in the United States in the year 2000. The largest group could be classified as having Carpentier type IIIb, with restricted motion due to left ventricular (LV) dysfunction, either ischemic or nonischemic.[2] The investigators of the meta-analysis estimated the prevalence of MR due to ischemic cardiomyopathy at 7500 to 9000 per million, and of MR due to LV dysfunction at 16,250 per million. The high number of individuals affected by secondary MR warrants an in-depth understanding of its pathophysiology, diagnosis, and management.

Pathophysiology

The mitral apparatus consists of the leaflets, annulus, chordae tendineae, papillary muscles, and supporting LV myocardium.[3] In contrast to organic mitral valve disease, most secondary MR is best thought of as a ventricular, rather than valvular, process. Mitral valve competency relies on a balance between the forces that close the valve and tethering forces that prevent the valve from prolapsing into the left atrium (Figure 19-1). The papillary muscles normally help counterbalance the force of LV contraction on the mitral valve by exerting force parallel to LV contraction and perpendicular to the mitral leaflets, thus preventing mitral valve prolapse. In secondary MR, altered geometry and reduced contractility, either global or regional, result in mitral valve incompetence.

Secondary Mitral Regurgitation in the Presence of Coronary Artery Disease

"Ischemic MR" may occur in the setting of acute myocardial infarction (MI) associated with a significant wall motion abnormality, acute MI with papillary muscle rupture, chronic ischemic heart disease with normal LV function, or end-stage ischemic heart disease with LV dilation and dysfunction. The mechanism of MR varies in each of these conditions. MR due to primary valvular pathology with coexisting coronary artery disease (CAD) is best considered separately from secondary MR in the setting of ischemic heart disease, the latter of which is the subject of this discussion.

The pathophysiology of ischemic MR varies with the distribution of CAD. In patients with disease of the right coronary artery and inferior infarction, the focal wall motion abnormality affecting the basal inferior wall leads to MR, often with preserved ejection fraction (EF). Papillary muscle infarction and rupture are most likely in patients with occlusion of the left circumflex or right coronary artery and affect the posteromedial papillary muscle. In anterior MI due to occlusion of the left anterior descending artery, MR is usually a result of spherical remodeling with overall reduced LV contractility.

Reduced contractility with dilation of the inferior wall in isolation or in association with global LV dilation results in lateral displacement of the papillary muscle and a longer distance from the papillary muscle tips to the mitral annulus. Consequently, altered tension on the chordae tendineae results in incomplete

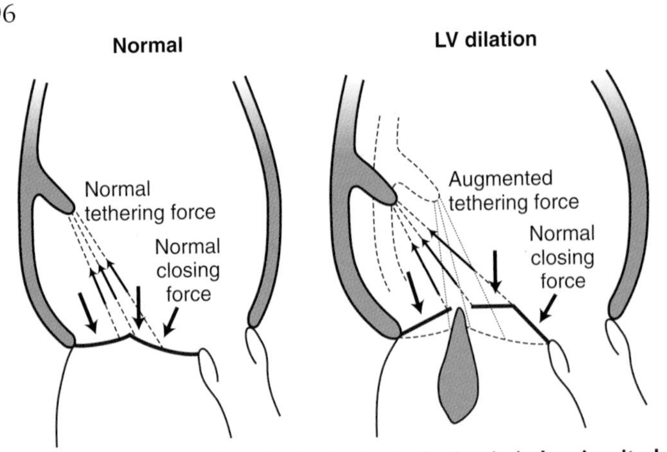

Normal **LV dilation**

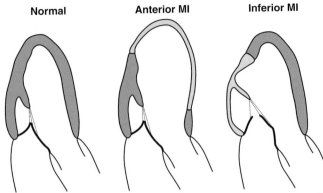

Normal **Anterior MI** **Inferior MI**

FIGURE 19-1 Principles of mitral valve tethering in ischemic mitral regurgitation. Basic principles of tethering mechanism for ischemic mitral regurgitation (MR) and balance of apposed closing and tethering forces acting on the leaflets. Augmented tethering force created by papillary muscle displacement apically displaces the leaflets and causes MR. *LV,* Left ventricular.

FIGURE 19-2 Ischemic mitral regurgitation in inferior versus anterior myocardial infarction. Potential mechanism for higher incidence of ischemic mitral regurgitation in inferior versus anterior myocardial infarction (MI), despite the lower level of global left ventricular (LV) remodeling in patients with inferior MI. LV remodeling in anterior MI may involve a broader region of the LV without causing major alterations in the mitral valve complex. In contrast, LV remodeling in response to inferior MI may involve less area but may cause major alterations in the mitral valve complex.

mitral leaflet closure. The term "papillary muscle dysfunction" may be misleading because it implies that an isolated reduction in the contractility of the papillary muscle is responsible for the MR. Rather than suffering from reduced contractility, the papillary muscle becomes *tethered* as a result of changes in the supporting LV wall and lateral displacement of the papillary muscle.[4] This process was elegantly shown by Kaul et al,[5] who demonstrated that hypoperfusion of the papillary muscle without an effect on other LV segments *did not* result in MR. However, global ischemia resulting in LV dilation and dysfunction with normal papillary muscle perfusion *did* cause incomplete mitral valve closure and MR.[5] Thus the papillary muscle is better thought of as a functional unit, composed of the papillary muscle and the subtending LV wall foundation.

Alterations in LV geometry, chiefly increased sphericity, change the position of the papillary muscle and the direction of tension exerted on the mitral leaflets. The normal papillary muscle position allows them to exert vertical tension on the chordae and leaflets, preventing prolapse. However, when the papillary muscles are laterally displaced due to LV dilation, the direction of force on the mitral leaflets is altered and inhibits proper closure. The leaflets become tethered and the zone of coaptation reduced. This is seen on echocardiography as tenting of the mitral valve. In the VALsartan In Acute myocardial iNfarcTion (VALIANT) study, tenting area, coaptation depth, annular dilation, and left atrial (LA) size were associated with the extent of baseline MR, but the degree of tenting after MI was the only variable that independently and significantly predicted progression of MR. A tenting area greater than 4 cm[2] was associated with the highest risk of MR progression after MI.[6]

In the setting of acute inferior MI, typically caused by right coronary artery or left circumflex CAD, a resultant inferior wall motion abnormality leads to tethering of the posteromedial papillary muscle and a loss of support for the medial aspects of the anterior and posterior mitral leaflets. On echocardiography the posterior leaflet appears to have restricted motion toward the annulus, and the anterior leaflet appears to override the posterior leaflet without rising above the annular plane. This appearance has been termed *pseudoprolapse.*[7] The altered leaflet coaptation leads to a posteriorly directed jet and may result in silent MR.

The extent of infarction may not necessarily correlate with the degree of MR. For the reasons described previously, patients with inferior MI may be more vulnerable to MR than those with anterior MI. Although anterior MI may affect a larger area of myocardium, the LV remodeling from inferior MI may involve a smaller area of myocardium with less global LV dilation but may cause

more dramatic alterations in the papillary muscle geometry (Figure 19-2).

Occasionally, active ischemia may cause "flash" pulmonary edema for which MR may be a contributing factor. However, ischemic MR need not imply the presence of active ischemia.[8] It usually reflects the consequences of chronic CAD, essentially postinfarction MR remodeling. In fact, many patients with ischemic MR are not found to have reversible ischemia, and conversely, persistent moderate or severe MR can occur in 77% of patients who have already undergone revascularization with coronary artery bypass grafting surgery (CABG), in whom presumably the ischemic substrate was addressed.[9]

Papillary muscle rupture is a different entity from other causes of ischemic MR. Infarction of the papillary muscle can occur in the setting of a relatively small MI, usually with infarction of the posteromedial papillary muscle because it receives blood from a single artery. The magnitude of MR depends on the site of papillary muscle rupture. Rupture of the head of the papillary muscle results in MR of a similar degree to that encountered with chordal rupture. Rupture of the body of the papillary muscle results in acute loss of support of half of the anterior leaflet and half of the posterior leaflet; the resultant MR is torrential and often immediately fatal.[10]

DYNAMIC CHANGES

MR severity is usually assessed by physical examination or echocardiography in the resting state. However, in the setting of coronary heart disease, exercise, labile hypertension, or other stressors may provoke dynamic changes in LV wall motion or otherwise result in further alterations of LV function and geometry. Dynamic changes in LV size and function may result in exercise-induced worsening of MR, thus contributing to heart failure symptoms. Addressing this question, Pierard and Lancellotti[8] looked at two groups of patients with LV dysfunction: one with and one without a history of acute pulmonary edema. The two groups were matched for resting MR severity, LV size, and EF. Despite similar heart rates and blood pressure responses to exercise, those patients with a history of acute pulmonary edema were more likely to have significant exercise-induced increases in MR volume, regurgitant orifice area (ROA), and pulmonary pressure.[8] The unmasking of significant MR with exercise may explain the clinical conundrum of patients who experience dyspnea on exertion that seems out of proportion to their resting LV function, resting MR grade, or degree of stress-induced ischemia.

Conversely, evaluation of MR during intraoperative transesophageal echocardiography (TEE) may underestimate true MR severity because sedation and inotropic agents can temporarily reduce LV size, improve LV function, and reduce papillary muscle tethering, thus complicating surgical decisions about procedures to reduce MR at the time of CABG. Thus, MR is best evaluated under normal loading conditions in the preoperative setting.[11]

Functional Mitral Regurgitation in the Absence of Coronary Artery Disease

MR is common in patients with all forms of nonischemic cardiomyopathy, including dilated cardiomyopathy, restrictive cardiomyopathy, and hypertrophic cardiomyopathy (HCM). The mechanism and the severity of MR vary widely as does the impact on the clinical status of the patient and prognostic significance.

The pathophysiology and mechanism for functional MR depend primarily on the geometry of the left ventricle and the left atrium as well as of the mitral annulus. Other contributing factors are the force of LV contraction and the degree of coordination of LV contraction.

DILATED CARDIOMYOPATHY

In patients with dilated cardiomyopathy, the mitral annulus is dilated and the papillary muscles are abnormally splayed. The papillary muscle architecture results from spherical remodeling of the ventricle. The chordae are stretched and the leaflets become tethered such that the point of coaptation lies within the LV chamber rather than in its normal position closer to the mitral annulus. There is a smaller total area of coaptation, which leads to valvular incompetence. In addition, the reduced closing force on the mitral leaflets due to diminished contractility contributes to the smaller area of coaptation. Thus, the extent of mitral closure depends on the balance between the tethering forces due to chordal stretch and the closing forces during systole.[12]

In 1972, on the basis of the work of early investigators,[13-15] Roberts and Perloff[10] formulated a postulate for the mechanism of MR in patients with dilated cardiomyopathy. The papillary muscles are located in the middle to apical third of the ventricle. In the normal elliptically shaped left ventricle, the contraction of the papillary muscles exerts a vertical force on the leaflets, which brings them together during isovolumic contraction and prevents them from prolapsing into the left atrium during ejection. As the ventricle becomes more spherical owing to remodeling, the papillary muscles migrate laterally and can no longer exert vertical force during systole, leading to reduced apposition of the leaflets with subsequent incompetence. As MR leads to further LV dilation, there was early recognition that "MR begets MR." In an experimental model of dilated cardiomyopathy created through sequential coronary microsphere embolization, progressive MR was observed.[16] The first parameter to change prior to the onset of MR was the sphericity of the left ventricle measured at end-systole. Increases in LV volume and mitral annular diameter ensued and were associated with worsening of the MR. The coaptation depth, measured as distance from the mitral annulus to the tips of the leaflets, was increased at the onset of MR and did not increase further over time. In additional experiments, the investigators observed that MR occurred only in dogs with increases in sphericity.[17] In clinical studies, the primary dependence of MR severity on LV sphericity is less certain. In a study of 128 patients with LV dysfunction (LVEF <50%), including patients with both ischemic and nonischemic etiologies, there was a correlation of ROA and sphericity. However, in multivariable analysis that included measures of mitral valve deformation, this index was no longer significant.[18] A later study confined to patients with nonischemic cardiomyopathy also showed that sphericity correlated with MR but was not an independent predictor of severity.[19]

Further observations on the depth of coaptation in functional MR were extended to include more robust measures based on two-dimensional (2D) and three-dimensional (3D) echocardiography, including tenting area and tenting volume, respectively. Yiu et al[18] examined patients with both ischemic and dilated cardiomyopathy and found that tenting area measured in the parasternal long-axis view on 2D echocardiography was related to posterior and apical displacement of the papillary muscles and correlated with ROA. The tenting area (cm^2) values were 6.66 ± 0.9, 7.46 ± 0.9, and 8.86 ± 1.5 in patients with ROA (mm^2) values of less than 10, 10 through 19, and more than 20.[18] In another study by Karaca et al,[19] tenting area was the best parameter to predict severe functional MR (ROA >20 mm^2) at a cutoff level of 3.4 cm^2 with 82% sensitivity and 77% specificity.[19] In a sheep model of pacing-induced dilated cardiomyopathy, the 3D tenting volume correlated best with the MR severity and was predicted by the severity of annular dilation rather than subvalvular remodeling.[20] A clinical study of 37 patients with functional MR used 3D echocardiography to measure maximal and minimal tenting volumes during systole as well as tenting areas on 2D apical long-axis, two-chamber, and four-chamber views. The best predictor of ROA was the tenting volume, measured at end-systole (minimum). These researchers defined the optimal cut-point for minimal tenting volume as 3.90 mL or larger, which identified significant functional MR (ROA >20 mm^2) with a sensitivity of 86% and a specificity of 100%.[21]

Annular dilation and shape also contribute to functional MR in patients with dilated cardiomyopathy. As the annulus dilates, the amount of leaflet tissue required to effectively occlude the annulus during systole increases occurring at the expense of coaptation zone area; in other words, the valve is closed but not sealed. Annular dilation exceeding a critical value eventually results in noncoaptation and MR. Using 2D echocardiography, Boltwood et al[22] demonstrated that mitral annular area was significantly larger in patients with dilated cardiomyopathy with MR than in those without MR and that the total leaflet area, derived mathematically, was significantly greater. LA size and mitral annular area were the major determinants of leaflet area and mitral regurgitant severity, whereas LV size was less important.[22] These findings suggest that the leaflet area relative to annular area in systole determines the extent of MR. This concept was supported by a study using 3D echocardiography in 44 patients with MR related to bilateral papillary muscle displacement. The investigators showed that the area of leaflet coaptation was significantly lower in patients with hemodynamically significant functional MR than in those without. They defined coaptation area as the difference between the leaflet area at the onset of systole and that in mid-systole. Coaptation length was measured at three sites: medial, middle, and lateral. The annular and the leaflet areas were greater in those with significant functional MR (cm/m^2) (annular: 6.8 ± 1.6 vs. 5.4 ± 0.9; leaflet: 9.2 ± 1.9 vs. 8.3 ± 1.6). The ratio of leaflet area to annular area and the coaptation length were also lower in the presence of significant MR.[23]

In addition to the specific anatomic properties in dilated cardiomyopathy, mechanical factors are important, specifically the force and coordination of LV contraction. The closing force on the leaflets, or transmitral pressure, is related to LV systolic pressure, which varies during systole. Schwammenthal et al[24] examined the instantaneous regurgitant orifice using M-mode echocardiography to measure the proximal flow convergence divided by instantaneous velocity. They demonstrated that in dilated cardiomyopathy there was a decrease in ROA throughout systole with an increase during LV relaxation, compared with a relatively constant ROA in rheumatic MR and an increase in ROA during systole in mitral valve prolapse.[24] Using an in vitro model, He et al[12] demonstrated the contributions of papillary muscle position, apical displacement of the papillary muscles, annular dilation, and the driving pressure.[12] Apical and posteromedial displacement of the papillary muscles increased both leaflet tethering and MR, as did annular dilation, whereas higher driving pressures reduced ROA and decreased MR. The severity of MR in their model varied during systole as in the clinical observation described earlier. Delayed closure of the mitral valve due to increased tethering caused early systolic MR. In mid-systole, the closing forces were maximal, and the regurgitant orifice size was at a minimum. As LV pressure fell, there was an increase in MR in late systole. An additional clinical study demonstrated that mitral annular area decreased during systole, but this change had a smaller contribution to the decrease in regurgitant orifice than the progressive rise in transmitral pressure.[25]

Intraventricular dyssynchrony due to conduction defects has become an important therapeutic target of the use of biventricular pacing for cardiac resynchronization therapy (CRT). CRT has been shown to reduce MR in clinical trials.[26] LV dyssynchrony may contribute to MR through a number of different mechanisms, including uncoordinated contraction of the papillary muscles with alteration in the timing of tethering forces exerted on the leaflets and reduced closing forces on the leaflets. However, the role of dyssynchrony is likely overridden by factors related to mitral deformation, as demonstrated in a clinical study using tissue Doppler imaging to derive the standard deviation of the time to peak systolic contraction as a measure of dyssynchrony. In this study, dyssynchrony contributed only weakly to MR severity after correction for tenting area and LV sphericity, and only in patients with nonischemic cardiomyopathy.[27] While dyssynchrony may only contribute a small part to the development of MR, improvement in synchrony with CRT may indeed relate to improved MR severity. For example, one study showed that reduction in MR with CRT was related to improved timing of coordinated contraction of the papillary muscles.[28] Another demonstrated that the improvements in total MR were related to reductions in LV end-systolic volumes and mitral valve tenting area. However, the reduction in early systolic MR was related to end-systolic volume and global dyssynchrony, whereas the reduction in late systolic MR was related to tenting area and dyssynchrony.[29]

In summary, altered geometry and reduced contractility contribute to MR in patients with nonischemic dilated cardiomyopathy. Therapeutic interventions can target one or more of the perturbations that lead to the incompetence of the mitral valve.

HYPERTROPHIC CARDIOMYOPATHY

In the obstructive form of HCM, late systolic MR is associated with the systolic anterior motion of the anterior mitral leaflet (SAM) and is coincident with the onset of LV outflow tract obstruction.[10] In 1969, Wigle et al[30] performed a clinical study that demonstrated that MR was reduced when the outflow tract obstruction was eliminated or reduced through the administration of angiotensin or through surgery as long as there were no primary abnormalities of the mitral valve. Conversely, MR worsened with pharmacologic interventions that increased the severity of obstruction, such as isoproterenol and amyl nitrite.

Jiang et al[31] further elucidated the mechanism of MR in HCM, demonstrating the following geometric contributions: anterior and inward displacement of the papillary muscles, anterior displacement of the anterior leaflet, and elongation of the anterior mitral leaflet. The displacement of the papillary muscles was believed to reduce the support of the central portions of the leaflets, causing them to slacken and to be subject to greater anterior drag. In a pathologic study of 43 mitral valve specimens from patients with HCM and basal outflow tract obstruction, 19 had enlarged, elongated mitral valves. The echocardiograms of these patients showed that their valves were situated more posteriorly and that they had greater systolic excursion of the anterior leaflet, which showed a more sharp-angled bend and localized contact of the tip with the septum. The echocardiograms of the patients with normal-sized leaflets showed more anteriorly situated valves with septal contact involving a greater portion of the valve. Those with normal-sized anterior leaflets were more likely to have diffuse thickening of the anterior leaflet that restricted the SAM, preventing the sharp right-angled bend.[32]

The geometric relationships of the papillary muscles to the LV outflow tract may be important in predicting outcomes after septal ablation. Delling et al[33] measured echocardiographic dimensions that reflected the malposition of the anterior leaflet (anterior-to-posterior leaflet coaptation position ratio) and the distance between the papillary muscle and anterior septum relative to the left ventricular internal diameter as well as the anterior position of coaptation relative to the septum (coaptation-to-septum distance). The patients who demonstrated persistent SAM after alcohol septal ablation had more severe anterior malposition at baseline and were more likely to have persistent obstruction.

There are numerous reported cases of ruptured chordae tendineae contributing to MR in patients with HCM. A surgical case series demonstrated that in the majority of patients with MR due to chordal rupture, the posterior leaflet was affected. At surgery, the leaflet tissue appeared normal, unlike in patients with degenerative mitral valve disease. The investigators in this series hypothesized that the cause was related to increased stress on the posterior leaflet, which is perpendicular to flow during systole.[34]

In summary, although the predominant cause of MR in patients with HCM is functional, being related to altered geometry and SAM of the anterior leaflet, anatomic abnormalities can include elongation and fibrosis of the leaflets as well as chordal rupture.

RESTRICTIVE CARDIOMYOPATHY

Restrictive cardiomyopathy is the least well-defined form of cardiomyopathy. The primary defect is the impairment in LV filling, which has a diverse set of etiologies. The ventricles are normal in size, and systolic function is generally preserved until late in the course of disease. The wall thickness may be increased in infiltrative disease (amyloid heart disease) or in storage diseases such as Fabry disease. However, in most genetic forms of restrictive cardiomyopathy, the wall thickness is normal. Endocardial processes, such as hypereosinophilic syndrome and endocmyocardial fibrosis, cause scarring that can impact the papillary muscles and chordae tendineae.

The mechanisms for MR in these patients are as diverse as the underlying etiologies. In amyloid heart disease, there may be primary valvular involvement due to amyloid deposition. However, functional MR may be associated with severe LA enlargement and annular dilation. In Fabry disease, mild MR is frequent but it is rarely hemodynamically significant.[35] In Loeffler endocarditis associated with hypereosinophilic syndrome, MR due to scarring and fibrosis of the chordae tendineae is common, occurring in almost 50% of patients. MR contributes to congestive heart failure, and valve surgery may be required.[36,37] However, because even bioprosthetic valve replacement may be complicated by thrombosis in this setting, long-term anticoagulation should be considered.[36]

Severe MR may mimic restrictive cardiomyopathy because there is often an increased mitral E velocity and severe LA enlargement. However, an abnormal mitral valve and LV dilation are consistent with primary MR, whereas an apparently normal valve with a small left ventricle would suggest restrictive cardiomyopathy with secondary MR.

ATRIAL FUNCTIONAL MITRAL REGURGITATION

It is well known that patients with hemodynamically significant primary MR are at risk for development of atrial fibrillation and that the occurrence of atrial fibrillation is associated with poor prognosis.[38] However, it has only been recently recognized that atrial fibrillation can lead to MR in patients with anatomically normal mitral valves.[39] In an observational cohort study of patients undergoing ablation for atrial fibrillation, the investigators studied 53 patients with normal mitral valves and normal LV function who had moderate to severe MR and compared them with a matched cohort of patients with grade mild or less MR. These patients represented approximately 7% of the cohort referred for ablation in whom preprocedural echocardiograms had been obtained. Patients with moderate or severe MR were older, more likely to be in persistent atrial fibrillation, and had a higher incidence of hypertension. They had greater LA volumes and larger annular dimensions. Mitral annular dimension was the strongest predictor of significant MR with an odds ratio of 8.4 per cm of annular size. The strongest evidence that atrial fibrillation caused MR was provided at follow-up. Only 18% of patients who maintained sinus rhythm still had moderate to severe MR, compared with 82% of those with recurrence of atrial fibrillation. Only the patients who maintained sinus rhythm had a significant reduction in annular dimension, suggesting that the primary cause of atrial functional MR is annular dilation.

This concept is not universally accepted. An earlier study compared patients with atrial fibrillation alone and patients with ischemic or dilated cardiomyopathy. Despite similar annular dimensions and annular areas in the two groups, the degree of MR, as measured by regurgitant fraction (RF), in those with atrial fibrillation was very modest (RF = 3%) compared to those with cardiomyopathy (RF = 36%). The investigators concluded that papillary muscle tethering due to LV dilation was the major cause of MR and that annular dilation did not have an important role.[40] One important difference in the studies is the method of measuring MR. In the study of patients undergoing ablation, MR severity was determined by the ratio of jet area to LA area, which is less rigorous that the measurements of RF used in the other study.

Although the observation that atrial fibrillation with secondary atrial enlargement and annular dilation can lead to MR is probably valid, it occurs in less than 10% of patients and the degree of MR is usually not severe. Hemodynamically significant tricuspid regurgitation is more common, probably because the fibrous skeleton of the tricuspid annulus is less developed than that of the mitral valve.[41]

Diagnosis

General

MR may be suspected from history and physical examination. Dyspnea is the predominant symptom associated with MR. However, in most patients with secondary MR, symptoms related to the underlying condition predominate; dyspnea and fatigue may result from ischemia or from nonischemic cardiomyopathy rather than from the MR per se. In addition, the typical holosystolic murmur of MR may be absent. In acute MR associated with ischemia or infarction, the murmur is often early systolic and may be high pitched or "cooing" in quality. In a small Thrombolysis In Myocardial Infarction (TIMI) substudy in the post-MI setting, a murmur was appreciated in only 50% of cases in which MR was clearly present on contrast-enhanced left ventriculography.[42] Even with moderate to severe MR, only two thirds of patients had appreciable murmurs.[43,44] When the MR is directed posteriorly, as occurs with an inferior wall motion abnormality and tethering of the posterior leaflet, the murmur may radiate to the back and may be missed on routine precordial examination.

Even the chronic MR associated with reduced LV function may be undetectable on physical examination. When LA pressures are severely elevated, the duration of MR is brief and the murmur ends in mid-systole, mimicking an ejection murmur.

Findings on chest radiographs are nonspecific and may include cardiomegaly with evidence of LV and LA enlargement as well as pulmonary vascular congestion.

Echocardiography

Echocardiography is the predominant modality for detection and evaluation of secondary MR (Table 19-1). The aims of the

TABLE 19-1	Comprehensive Echocardiographic Assessment of Secondary Mitral Regurgitation

Left Ventricular (LV) Size and Function

LV volume at end-systole and end-diastole
Sphericity index
LV ejection fraction
LV regional wall motion

Mitral Regurgitation Quantification

Regurgitant fraction and volume (volumetric method)
Regurgitant fraction and volume (proximal isovelocity surface area method—ideally using three-dimensional [3D] imaging to account for noncircular orifice)
Number of jets
Jet direction

Mitral Valve Morphology

Tenting area or volume:
  In parasternal long-axis or apical four-chamber view
  Use of 3D echocardiography to calculate tenting volume
Coaptation depth
Maximal annular diameter (measure in midsystole in apical four-chamber view)

Tethering

Presence/absence
Symmetric vs. asymmetric
Degree of tethering (measure posterior leaflet tethering angle > or < 45 degrees in apical four-chamber view)

Secondary Findings

Atrial volumes
Pulmonary artery pressure
Secondary tricuspid regurgitation
Associated right ventricular dilation and dysfunction

Dynamic Assessment

Reassessment under various loading conditions (sedation, blood pressure fluctuation)
Assessment of mitral regurgitation severity with exercise
Contractile reserve to identify hibernating or stunned myocardium
Reassessment after cardiac resynchronization therapy or cardiac resynchronization therapy optimization
Atrioventricular optimization
Ventriculoventricular optimization

Adapted from Ray S. The echocardiographic assessment of functional mitral regurgitation. Eur J Echocardiogr 2010;11;i11–7.

echocardiographic examination include: confirmation that the anatomy of the mitral valve is normal or near normal, evaluation of the mechanism for MR, and determination of the severity of MR. In the majority of cases, transthoracic echocardiography is adequate. However there are patients in whom TEE may be required to exclude the presence of specific valvular pathology. Although the valve may show evidence of nonspecific thickening and areas of calcification, especially in older patients, the valvular pathology is not the primary issue causing MR.

The Carpentier classification is the most widely adopted approach to the pathology of the mitral valve (see Chapter 21).[43] Atrial functional MR associated with atrial fibrillation is classified as type I, in which leaflet motion is normal and MR is due primarily to annular dilation. Type II MR involves excessive motion of the valve like that seen in degenerative MR. In type III, the leaflets are restricted. With use of this classification system, the majority of patients with secondary MR, either ischemic or nonischemic, are classified as having type IIIB, in which the leaflet motion is restricted predominantly in systole. In both ischemic and nonischemic MR, the mechanism is LV remodeling. Echocardiography demonstrates the apical displacement and/or splaying of the papillary muscles, their restricted systolic motion and the annular dilation to differing degrees.

The tethering may be asymmetric, affecting only one leaflet, or symmetric, affecting both leaflets.[45] In asymmetric tethering, the

TABLE 19-2	Echocardiographic Findings in Mitral Regurgitation due to Asymmetric versus Symmetric Tethering	
	ASYMMETRIC	SYMMETRIC
Etiology	Inferior myocardial infarction (MI)	Large anterior or multiple MIs Nonischemic cardiomyopathy
Tethering	Posterior leaflet	Both leaflets
Tenting	Increased	Markedly increased
Annulus	Mild to no dilation	Dilated, flattened
Left ventricular remodeling	Inferior wall alone	Global dilation with increased sphericity
Mitral regurgitation jet direction	Posterior	Usually central

Adapted from Ray S. The echocardiographic assessment of functional mitral regurgitation. Eur J Echocardiogr 2010;11:i11–7.

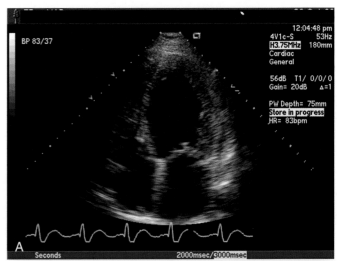

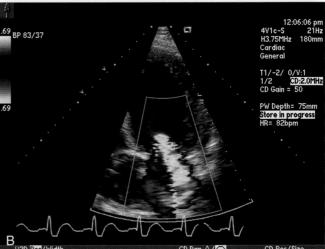

FIGURE 19-3   Restricted mitral valve motion in dilated cardiomyopathy. A, End-systolic frame from four-chamber view of patient with dilated cardiomyopathy demonstrating mitral valve tenting due to restricted systolic motion of both leaflets. **B,** The color-flow Doppler imaging jet of severe mitral regurgitation is predominantly central in association with bilateral leaflet restriction.

posterior leaflet is most commonly affected, usually in the setting of an inferior MI that caused focal remodeling. The annulus may or may not be significantly dilated but there is increased tenting. There is also pseudo-prolapse of the anterior leaflet.[7] The jet is directed posteriorly. When the tethering is symmetric, both leaflets are apically displaced and there is a markedly increased tenting area. The annulus is dilated and loses its normal saddle shape. The ventricle is dilated with global remodeling and greater sphericity. The jet direction is usually central when the tethering is symmetric (Table 19-2) (Figures 19-3 and 19-4).

In ischemic MR the extent of remodeling and its impact on the mitral apparatus can be evaluated by echocardiography in order to predict the likelihood of successful mitral valve surgery. The European Society of Echocardiography (ESE) has recommended the measurement of a number of anatomic parameters, which are illustrated in Figure 19-5.[46] The echocardiographic measurement values that predict an unfavorable result are listed in Table 19-3.[47]

One particular challenge with respect to grading secondary MR is its dynamic nature, which causes it to vary from one occasion to another. Factors influencing MR severity include loading conditions, rhythm, exercise, and ischemia. At the time of the echocardiogram, the blood pressure should be noted and, ideally, a patient's medications should be recorded. If the patient is in a paced rhythm, specific pacing parameters should be considered, including the use of biventricular pacing with specific atrioventricular and ventriculoventricular intervals. An excessively long atrioventricular delay may lead to presystolic MR. Exercise testing can be used to evaluate for the presence of ischemia and the impact of exercise on MR severity, although interpretation of color-flow Doppler imaging may be challenging.[48] An increase in the ROA with exercise in patients who have systolic heart failure has been associated with poor exercise tolerance in comparison with patients who have stable MR. During TEE, MR jets may have diminished area and penetration, leading to an underestimation of MR severity in comparison with findings on transthoracic echocardiography. This phenomenon can be particularly troublesome during intraoperative TEE, when a decision to repair the valve is at stake. Altering the loading conditions pharmacologically may be helpful to making a decision. In one study of 30 patients with ischemic MR referred for CABG, preload was adjusted with fluids to a pulmonary capillary wedge pressure of 15 mm Hg, and phenylephrine dose was titrated to achieve a systolic blood pressure of 160 mm Hg. The jet on color-flow on Doppler imaging, the ROA, and the regurgitant volume increased to levels observed on the preoperative echocardiogram.[11]

The American Society of Echocardiography (ASE) recommendations for grading severity of MR do not distinguish between functional and organic MR.[49] However, there is growing evidence of fundamental differences between these two categories of MR, suggesting that thresholds for MR severity should be specific to

the mechanism for MR.[50,51] The ESE has recommended different thresholds: An ROA ≥40 mm² or a regurgitant volume ≥60 mL indicates severe organic MR. In ischemic MR, an ROA ≥20 mm² or a regurgitant volume ≥30 mL identifies a subset of patients at increased risk of cardiovascular events.[46] The rationale for tailored thresholds is based on differences in the physiologic impact of a given mitral regurgitant volume depending on the function and total stroke volume of the left ventricle, as well as factors influencing the specific quantitative measures. Many factors affect the accuracy of quantitative measures of MR severity, including the jet direction, the timing of MR, the driving pressure, and the shape of the regurgitant orifices.

As previously mentioned, the color-flow Doppler imaging characteristics of the jet vary with the extent and pattern of tethering. Eccentric jets associated with asymmetric tethering entrain the LA wall (Coanda effect), tend to have smaller total area, and represent a smaller percentage of the total LA area.[52] When the MR is acute, such as that which occurs during active ischemia, the high LA pressure will result in rapid equilibration and the color-flow jet will be brief and of relatively low velocity. The corresponding continuous wave (CW) Doppler echocardiography signal will show rapid late systolic deceleration, so-called Doppler V wave or cutoff sign. Additionally the color-flow jet may

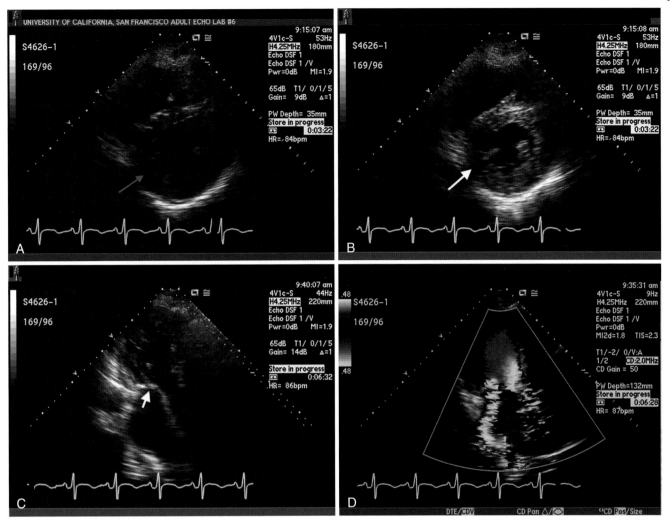

FIGURE 19-4 **Restricted posterior mitral leaflet motion with severe mitral regurgitation in a patient who has had an inferior myocardial infarction. A,** End-diastolic frame from parasternal short-axis (PSAX) view. There is thinning of the inferior wall *(arrow)*. **B,** End-systolic frame from PSAX view. There is no contraction of the inferior wall *(arrow)*. **C,** End-systolic frame from the apical long-axis view demonstrating bulging of the inferoposterior wall. The posterior leaflet is restricted, and there is overshoot of the anterior leaflet *(arrow)*. **D,** Posteriorly directed jet of mitral regurgitation.

TABLE 19-3	Unfavorable Echocardiographic Characteristics for Mitral Valve Repair in Ischemic and Functional Mitral Regurgitation

Mitral Valve Deformation

Coaptation distance ≥1 cm
Tenting area >2.5-3 cm²
Complex jets
Posterolateral angle >45 degrees

Local Left Ventricular Remodeling

Interpapillary muscle distance >20 mm
Posterior papillary–fibrosa distance >40 mm
Lateral wall motion abnormality

Global Left Ventricular Remodeling

End-diastolic dimension >65 mm; end-systolic dimension >51 mm
 (end-systolic volume >140 mL)
Systolic sphericity index >0.7

Adapted with permission from Lancellotti P, Marwick T, Pierard LA. How to manage ischaemic mitral regurgitation. Heart 2008;94:1497–502.

be relatively unimpressive in patients with chronic severe LV dysfunction associated with low systolic blood pressure and high LA pressure. The low driving pressure results in a lower-velocity color-flow jet, which is also reflected in the lower peak velocity of the CW signal, often less than 4 m/sec.

As previously mentioned, the MR is maximal in early systole, diminishes in mid-systole, when the regurgitant orifice is at its smallest, and then increases again in late systole. The corresponding CW signal may have a mid-systolic "dropout" that corresponds to the smaller volume of red blood cells available to reflect the ultrasound signal (Figures 19-6 and 19-7). The variation in regurgitant orifice was elegantly demonstrated in a study comparing the measurement of regurgitant volume on cardiac magnetic resonance imaging with proximal isovelocity surface area (PISA) measurements on echocardiography. In functional MR, the PISA measurement significantly underestimated mitral regurgitant volume, especially when a single-point measure at mid-systole was used. The regurgitant volume was more accurately represented when a method that integrated flow over the entire cardiac cycle was used because of the concave shape of the ROA curve over the course of the cardiac cycle (see Figure 19-6).[53] This complicated method has not been adapted for clinical use and could be superseded by 3D methods.

Further confounding the measurement of functional MR severity is the shape of the regurgitant orifice. In functional MR, the orifice is more likely to be elliptical rather than circular as is common in degenerative MR. The shape of the orifice affects the use of the vena contracta measurement to estimate MR severity as well as the application of the PISA formula for measurement of ROA. The elliptical shape of the orifice causes significant differences in the measurement of the vena contracta between the

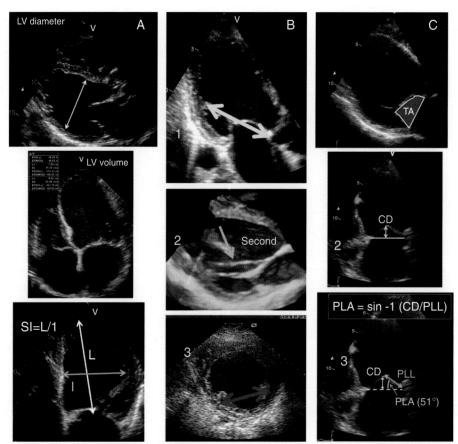

FIGURE 19-5 **Echocardiographic parameters in ischemic mitral regurgitation that predict the success of mitral valve repair. A,** Global left ventricular (LV) remodeling: *Top,* LV internal diameter in diastole *(arrow); middle,* LV volumes by method of disks; *bottom,* sphericity index *(SI = L/1; L,* major axis; *1,* minor axis). **B,** Local LV remodeling: *Top,* apical displacement of the posteromedial papillary muscle *(arrow); middle,* second-order chordae *(arrow); bottom,* interpapillary muscle distance *(arrow).* **C,** Mitral valve deformation: *Top,* systolic tenting area (TA); *middle,* coaptation distance (CD); *bottom,* posterolateral angle (PLA), posterolateral length (PLL). *(Reproduced with permission from Lancellotti P, Moura L, Pierard LA, et al. European Association of Echocardiography recommendations for the assessment of valvular regurgitation. Part 2: mitral and tricuspid regurgitation [native valve disease]. Eur J Echocardiogr 2010;11:307–32.)*

four-chamber and two-chamber views. The measurement in the parasternal long-axis view, which is considered standard, is closer to that of the four-chamber view, whereas the two-chamber view has a much larger vena contracta (Figure 19-8). Another factor influencing the accuracy of vena contracta measurements is the presence of multiple jets, which cannot be handled simply by adding multiple vena contracta widths. If the regurgitant orifice is not centrally located, off-axis views may be required. In functional MR, up to 35% of jets may be medial or lateral along the coaptation line.[54] Ideally, when measuring the vena contracta, the sonographer should use the zoom mode to maximize frame rate and minimize the measurement error. The Nyquist limit should be adjusted to visualize the color-flow Doppler imaging signal so the zone of proximal flow convergence is on the LV side of the valve, the narrowest portion of the jet at the valve (anatomic orifice), and the vena contracta just beyond the valve within the left atrium (physiologic orifice). The physiologic orifice is slightly smaller than the anatomic orifice and thus the vena contracta should be measured at this point.[55] The ESE guidelines recommend using the average of measurements in the two- and four-chamber views (biplane measurement) with a cut point of more than 8 mm for severe functional MR, whereas the ASE guidelines recommend the use of the parasternal long-axis view with a cut point of 7 mm for severe MR.

The PISA formula for estimation of the ROA is based on a circular orifice, rendering the shape of the proximal flow convergence zone a hemisphere. In most cases of primary degenerative MR, the MR flow can be calculated with use of the formula for a hemisphere, which is multiplied by the aliasing velocity. The

ROA is calculated by dividing by the peak velocity of the MR CW jet. However, as mentioned previously, this formula may be invalidated by the elliptical shape of the orifice with its correspondingly "sausage-shaped" flow convergence zone (Figure 19-9). In these cases, the PISA method may underestimate functional MR severity. In a study comparing ROA measured on 3D echocardiography and that measured on 2D echocardiography, this underestimation was most marked when the ratio of long-axis length to short-axis length of the orifice was greater than or equal to 1.5.[56] In functional MR, the use of emerging methods using 3D PISA for estimation of ROA should be considered.[57,58] An alternative PISA method has been proposed that corrects for the obtuse angle formed by the tented leaflets and appears to more accurate.[59]

There are three echocardiographic methods to estimate the regurgitant volume and to derive regurgitant fraction. Each method has advantages and disadvantages. If the ROA is underestimated by the PISA formula, the regurgitant volume derived by the product of the ROA and the velocity-time integral (VTI) of the mitral regurgitant jet on CW Doppler echocardiography will underestimate regurgitant volume.[57] When 3D measurements of ROA are used, the regurgitant volume is close to that derived with cardiac magnetic resonance imaging. The regurgitant volume can also be derived by subtracting the forward stroke volume from the total LV stroke volume. LV stroke volume is calculated through the use of the biplane method of disks or with 3D measurements of LV end-diastolic and end-systolic volumes. Forward stroke volume is calculated with use of the LV outflow tract area and the LV outflow tract VTI. High-quality 2D imaging is necessary for

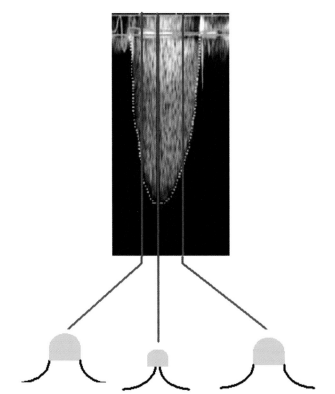

FIGURE 19-6 Variation in the proximal isovelocity surface area during systole in functional mitral regurgitation. Illustration demonstrating the variation of the proximal isovelocity surface area (PISA, represented by *yellow half-circles*)due to the variation of regurgitant orifice area (ROA) during systole. In early *(left)* and late *(right)* systole, closing forces are relatively low and so the ROA and PISA are relatively large. In mid-systole at the point of peak regurgitant velocity *(center)*, the closing forces are maximal, forcing the leaflet tips closer together and reducing the ROA and PISA. *(Reproduced with permission from Ray S. The echocardiographic assessment of functional mitral regurgitation. Eur J Echocardiogr 2010;11:i11–7.)*

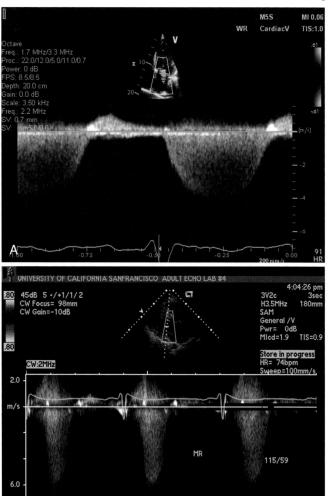

FIGURE 19-7 Mitral regurgitant jet contour in functional mitral regurgitation vs. hypertrophic obstructive cardiomyopathy. A, Continuous wave Doppler echocardiography tracing from a patient with functional mitral regurgitation (MR) in the setting of dilated cardiomyopathy. There is diminished signal in mid-systole, consistent with reduced regurgitation in mid-systole. There is a diminished rate of rise in velocity; the estimated dP/dt was 565 mm Hg/sec. **B,** Continuous wave Doppler echocardiography tracing from a patient with functional MR in the setting of hypertrophic obstructive cardiomyopathy. The MR peaks in late systole and the high peak transmitral gradient, 144 mm Hg, is consistent with dynamic outflow tract obstruction, given the patient's systolic blood pressure, which was 115 mm Hg.

accurate application of this method, and LV foreshortening often leads to underestimation of LV stroke volume. The third method is to calculate the difference between forward stroke volume and transmitral flow. An additional pitfall associated with this technique relates to inaccuracy in the measurement of the mitral annular area.[49] If this combined Doppler method is used, it may be most accurate to measure the annular area with 3D planimetry or to calculate an elliptical area based on the anterior-posterior (parasternal long-axis view) and commissure-commissure (parasternal short-axis view) diameters.[60] However, this method for measuring transmitral flow requires further study. A dimensionless index, consisting of the mitral VTI divided by the LV outflow tract VTI, has been studied in patients with primary MR but not in those with functional MR.[61]

Pulsed Doppler echocardiography patterns of pulmonary venous flow patterns can aid in grading MR severity. They are most helpful if there is systolic dominance consistent with normal filling pressures and mild MR or when there is systolic flow reversal suggesting severe MR. Blunted systolic flow in the pulmonary vein flow is a nonspecific finding that could be due to hemodynamically significant MR but could also represent elevated pressures in the absence of important MR and is often seen in patients with LV dysfunction. With eccentric jets of MR, there may be selective entrainment of one or more pulmonary veins lying in the path of flow. Because only the right upper pulmonary vein can be reliably sampled on transthoracic imaging, TEE may be needed to demonstrate this phenomenon.

The mitral inflow pattern is usually E dominant in the presence of significant MR with an increased peak E velocity up to

1.5 m/sec and may be helpful in patients with normal LV function.[62] In the patient with LV dysfunction, restrictive mitral inflow patterns may mimic severe MR. However, an A wave dominant mitral inflow pattern virtually excludes severe MR.

The left ventricle is usually dilated and EF usually reduced in patients with hemodynamically significant functional MR. One exception is the patient with isolated inferior wall remodeling and severe tethering of the posterior leaflet who may have near normal LV size and systolic function. The left atrium is enlarged unless the MR is acute, such as in a patient with acute inferior infarction or myocarditis. LV and LA volumes should be measured and recorded.

In summary, the echocardiographer faces many challenges in grading functional MR even when employing an integrative approach that incorporates both qualitative and quantitative parameters. There is a tendency to underestimate the severity of functional MR, which leads to potential minimization of its clinical impact.

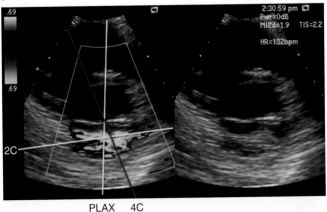

FIGURE 19-8 Vena contracta width dependency on imaging plane. Parasternal short-axis (PSAX) view at the mitral valve level with superimposed color-flow imaging demonstrating the variation in width of the vena contracta if measured from the four-chamber (4C) view *(red)*, the parasternal long-axis (PLAX) view *(yellow)*, and the two-chamber (2C) view *(light green)*. The vena contracta width would be smallest in the PLAX view and greatest in the two-chamber view.

Prognosis

In the Setting of Coronary Artery Disease

MR is often thought to be a bystander consequence of ischemic heart disease, and its clinical importance is overlooked. Evidence suggests that the MR itself may further compound the symptoms of ischemic heart disease and may contribute to the downward spiral of heart failure. Not only is MR in ischemic heart disease common (occurring in up to 20% of patients with acute MI and in 50% of patients with acute MI and heart failure), the presence of MR increases mortality twofold in the setting of MI, in chronic heart failure, and even after coronary revascularization, and even a mild degree of MR in the setting of ischemic heart disease affects survival negatively.[50,63-66] The prognostic significance is highlighted in Figure 19-10.[67] Finally, the degree of MR that is considered prognostically significant in ischemic heart disease is less than for primary MR; an ROA of just 0.2 cm² (unlike the value of 0.4 cm² in organic MR) predicted adverse outcomes.

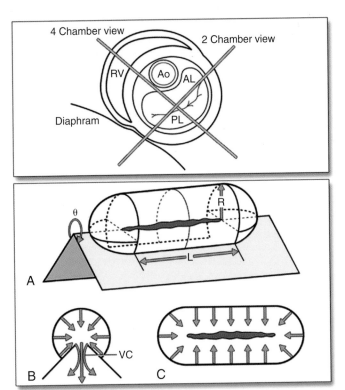

FIGURE 19-9 Proposed isovelocity surface area (ISVS) model in functional mitral regurgitation. *Top,* Short-axis left ventricular cross-section. Short-axis view demonstrating near parallel alignment of the two-chamber view with the long axis of the mitral commissures/orifice and perpendicular alignment of the four-chamber view across the commissures. *Bottom,* **A,** Schematic of ISVS. **B,** End-on view of model. **C,** Superior view of ISVS. Note that the true crescent orifice shape seen in the top is shown schematically as straight to simplify the illustration. *AL,* Anterior leaflet; *Ao,* aorta; *PL,* posterior leaflet; *RV,* right ventricle; *VC,* vena contracta. *(Reproduced with permission from Rifkin RD, Sharma S. An alternative isovelocity surface model for quantitation of effective regurgitant orifice area in mitral regurgitation with an elongated orifice application to functional mitral regurgitation. JACC Cardiovasc Imaging 2010;3: 1091–103.)*

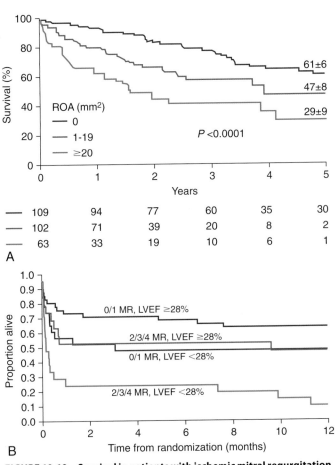

FIGURE 19-10 Survival in patients with ischemic mitral regurgitation (MR). A, Decreased survival after myocardial infarction (MI) with increasing MR. Regurgitant orifice area (ROA) of 20 mm² demarcates mild from moderate MR. Numbers below reflect the number of patients remaining in each group at various time points. **B,** Decreased survival after cardiogenic shock with increasing MR for comparable LV ejection fraction (LVEF). *(A reprinted with permission from Grigioni F, Enriquez-Sarano M, Zehr KJ, et al. Ischemic mitral regurgitation: long-term outcome and prognostic implications with quantitative Doppler assessment. Circulation 2001;103:1759–64. Copyright 2001, American Heart Association, Inc; B reprinted with permission from Picard MH, Davidoff R, Sleeper LA, et al. Echocardiographic predictors of survival and response to early revascularization in cardiogenic shock. Circulation 2003;107:279–84. Copyright 2003, American Heart Association, Inc.)*

In the Absence of Coronary Artery Disease

Several studies have analyzed the impact of functional MR on prognosis in patients with nonischemic cardiomyopathy. In a chart review of more than 1400 patients with severe LV systolic dysfunction defined as a LVEF less than 35%, predictors of poor outcome included increasing MR and tricuspid regurgitation grade, cancer, CAD, and absence of an implantable cardiac defibrillator. The relative risk of death was 1.84 in patients with severe MR. Survival was inversely related to MR grade (none to mild, 1004 days; moderate, 795 days; severe, 47 days; P <0.0001).[68] In the Beta-blocker Evaluation of Survival Trial (BEST), approximately 40% of patients had nonischemic cardiomyopathy. A substudy of 336 patients with complete echocardiograms showed that three variables predicted the combined end point of death, hospitalization for heart failure (HF), and transplant: LV end-diastolic volume index ≥120 mL/m², mitral deceleration time ≤150 milliseconds, and the MR vena contracta width ≥0.4 cm.[69] In another study of patients with severe MR and LV systolic dysfunction, the right ventricular systolic function as measured by tricuspid annular plane systolic excursion (TAPSE) was a strong predictor of prognosis.[70] In a European study of 1256 patients with HF due to dilated cardiomyopathy, 27% had no functional MR, 49% had mild to moderate functional MR, and 24% had severe functional MR. There was a strong independent association between severe functional MR and prognosis (hazard ratio [HR] 2.0) after adjustment for LVEF and restrictive filling pattern. The independent association of severe functional MR with prognosis was seen in both ischemic and nonischemic cardiomyopathy.[71]

Treatment

Medical

Medical therapy can be aimed at reducing MR in the short term and inducing LV reverse remodeling over the long term. Patients with dynamic outflow tract obstruction/HCM aside, acute treatment with inotropic agents or inodilators (e.g., dobutamine, milrinone) can improve contractility, raise LV systolic pressure, and reduce LV volume, thus increasing the closing forces and reducing the tethering forces, resulting in reduced MR severity. Agents to reduce afterload, preload, or a combination of the two (e.g., diuretics, nitrates, vasodilators) work to reduce LV size, improve papillary muscle geometry, and reduce tethering forces, thus improving MR. Hydralazine, nitroprusside, and angiotensin-converting enzyme (ACE) inhibitors have been shown to improve forward cardiac output in patients with severe MR.[72,73] For long-term therapy, diuretics, ACE inhibitors, aldosterone blockers, and beta-blockers along with other afterload-reducing agents lead to a complex process of reverse remodeling in which fibrosis, dilation, and LV dysfunction are stabilized or improved. Vasodilators such as ACE inhibitors are indicated for chronic MR in the setting of LV dysfunction. In the absence of heart failure, LV dysfunction, or symptoms, there is no evidence that vasodilators are useful for treatment of the MR.

Intra-aortic Balloon Pump

Intra-aortic balloon pump treatment may be useful in acute severe MR because it reduces afterload, preload, and ischemia. Because of the complications that can result from its prolonged use, however, there are few data for its use in the treatment of MR in the absence of papillary muscle rupture or other post-MI complications such as ventricular septal defect and cardiogenic shock.

Cardiac Resynchronization Therapy

CRT has been shown to reduce MR in a substantial number of patients with ischemic and nonischemic functional MR.[26]

Biventricular pacing can induce reverse remodeling and reduced LV volumes, thereby reducing tethering. CRT has been shown to reduce early systolic and mid-systolic MR. (Different determinants of the improvement of early and late systolic MR contributed after CRT.[29]) CRT can increase the closing force of contraction, as can be evidenced by higher dP/dt and more prolonged duration of peak transmitral closing pressures in systole.[74] Because delayed posterolateral wall contraction is characteristic of left bundle branch block, CRT may also reduce discoordinate papillary muscle contraction, thereby reducing MR. Finally, improvement in atrioventricular electrical and mechanical delay may reduce presystolic MR.

In the InSync trial, implantation of the cardiac resynchronization therapy defibrillator (CRT-D) (InSync ICD, Medtronic Inc., Minneapolis, Minnesota) in patients with ischemic and nonischemic HF, those with clinically significant MR at baseline had the following 12-month results with respect to MR grade: 67% had an improvement of MR grade; 28% had no change; and 5% had a worsening in MR grade. For patients with no significant MR at baseline, development of new or worsened MR was also very infrequent (5%).[75] The Multicenter Automatic Defibrillator Implantation with Cardiac Resynchronization Therapy (MADIT-CRT) trial also demonstrated that CRT improved MR, but the effect was more modest owing to the smaller number of patients with significant MR in the trial (only 15% had more than mild MR).[76]

As a corollary, the very presence of significant MR *at baseline* does not necessarily portend a worse response to CRT. In the InSync trial, event-free survival in patients with clinically significant MR was similar to that in patients without significant MR.[75] In fact, patients with severe MR at baseline may actually exhibit more reverse remodeling in response to CRT.[77] However, other studies have shown that patients with severe MR at baseline have less reverse remodeling after CRT—the latter CRT nonresponse may be more common in patients with an ischemic etiology of HF in whom leads may be placed in areas of nonviable or scarred myocardium.[78]

However, persistence or worsening of significant MR *after CRT* does portend a worse prognosis. Patients with this finding exhibit less reverse remodeling and have higher clinical event rates.[79,80]

Importantly, the frequency of response to CRT in terms of both reverse remodeling and MR reduction is two to three times higher in nonischemic than in ischemic etiologies of heart failure. Akinesis with scarring of the inferior wall is a common problem in ischemic MR, and CRT has been shown to be less beneficial in patients with scarring.[81,82] Even among patients with early CRT response, at 6 months, those with an ischemic etiology are less likely to sustain an initial favorable response to CRT at 12 months, likely as a result of progression of ischemic disease.[83]

Reperfusion and Percutaneous Revascularization

In the setting of acute inferior or posterior MI, reperfusion with thrombolytic therapy dramatically reduces MR immediately and at 30 days. The patients with the most advanced posterobasal wall motion abnormalities are more likely to have significant MR, and it has been found that reperfusion with thrombolysis likely reduces MR by improving posterobasal wall motion.[84,85] In the SHould we emergently revascularize Occluded Coronaries for cardiogenic shocK (SHOCK) trial, moderate or severe MR was seen in 39% of the patients. The presence of 2+ to 4+ grade MR increased the odds of death more than sixfold. Degree of MR was the only echocardiographic variable other than LVEF that independently predicted death. Despite their much higher mortality, patients with moderate to severe MR still demonstrated a survival benefit with early revascularization. This effect may have been due to early revascularization itself and also in part to the aggressive use of intra-aortic balloon counterpulsation in 86% of the patients.[86,87]

In contrast, delayed reperfusion or revascularization is less beneficial in chronic ischemic MR. Studies have shown persistence of MR after revascularization in up to 77% of patients with chronic CAD.[9]

Surgical Techniques

Surgical techniques include procedures on the valve itself, such as restrictive annuloplasty, mitral valve repair, mitral valve replacement, and procedures that primarily address LV dilation or dysfunction and may thus improve MR. Mitral annuloplasty with undersized rings is best suited for patients in whom remodeling has led to annular dilation as the primary mechanism of MR. Although an immediate salutary effect may be apparent, recurrent MR is a significant problem, affecting at least 30% of patients.[88] Lack of efficacy and durable response may be due to the nature of the MR itself. If the primary problem is papillary muscle tethering, annuloplasty will not be corrective. Annuloplasty may even exacerbate posteromedial papillary muscle tethering because the posterior annulus is pushed further anteriorly by the ring but the position of the posteromedial papillary muscle itself is unchanged (Figure 19-11). The posterior mitral valve leaflet becomes further restricted and fixed in some cases. Unless reverse remodeling also occurs in response to improved perfusion with concomitant CABG, thus allowing the papillary muscle to become less tethered, recurrent MR will remain a challenging problem.[89-93]

The data from examination of the role of mitral valve repair at the time of CABG have been conflicting.[94] If the role of mitral valve repair with CABG is unclear, the indication for mitral valve repair along with CABG in patients with severely reduced EF (<30%) is even murkier. A desire to address the problem of LV remodeling at the time of CABG in patients with EF values of 35% or less formed the basis of the Surgical Treatment for Ischemic Heart Failure (STICH) trial.[95,96] The first hypothesis of the trial tested whether CABG is superior to medical therapy alone; ultimately no difference was found in the primary end point of death or hospitalization. In STICH Hypothesis 1, patients were randomly assigned to surgery, and the decision to repair the mitral valve at the time of CABG was left to the discretion of the surgeon. Adjusted for baseline prognostic variables, observational data from the STICH Hypothesis I group showed a 59% lower hazard (HR 0.41, 95% confidence interval [CI] 0.22-0.77; P = 0.006) of death among the patients who received CABG plus mitral valve repair than in those who underwent CABG alone. A reduced hazard of death was also found in patients who received CABG plus mitral valve repair than in those undergoing medical therapy alone, but only after adjustment for baseline prognostic variables.[97] Because the decision for mitral valve repair was not randomized, these findings leave room for doubt.[97] A randomized trial to address the question of adding mitral valve repair to CABG for moderate MR is now under way, though this trial is not limited to patients with low EF (ClinicalTrials.gov; identifier: NCT00806988).

The second hypothesis of the STICH trial tested whether adding surgical ventricular reconstruction (SVR), a procedure that reduces LV volume, to CABG would have better outcomes than CABG alone. Although LV volume was reduced by 19% in the CABG plus SVR arm, compared with 6% in the CABG alone arm, there was no difference in the primary end point of death or hospitalization.[96] It is not yet known what effect the CABG plus SVR approach has on papillary muscle tethering or MR.

Other authorities have advocated resection of akinetic segments at the time of CABG to better restore LV geometry, external compression to prevent outward expansion of akinetic segments, and LV wrapping among other techniques to address the problem of papillary muscle tethering and altered LV geometry. However, data from robust randomized controlled trials for these procedures are lacking. All of these ancillary surgical procedures add

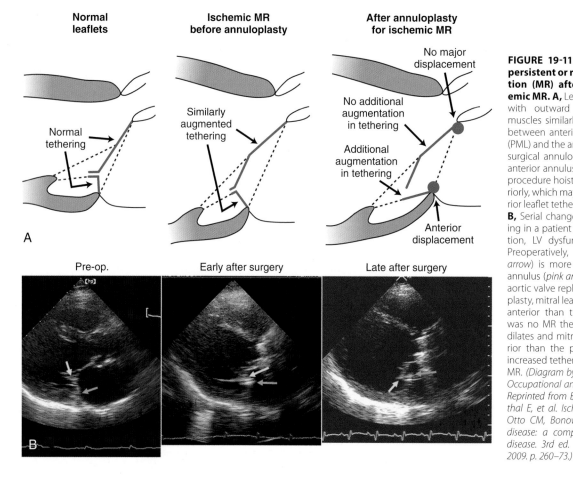

FIGURE 19-11 Potential mechanism of persistent or recurrent mitral regurgitation (MR) after annuloplasty for ischemic MR. A, Left ventricular (LV) remodeling with outward displacement of papillary muscles similarly increases tethering angles between anterior leaflet or posterior leaflet (PML) and the annular line (*middle*). Although surgical annuloplasty may not displace the anterior annulus fixed at the aortic root, this procedure hoists the posterior annulus anteriorly, which may specifically augment posterior leaflet tethering with recurrent MR (*right*). **B,** Serial changes in posterior leaflet tethering in a patient with severe aortic regurgitation, LV dysfunction, and functional MR. Preoperatively, leaflet coaptation (*yellow arrow*) is more anterior than the posterior annulus (*pink arrow*). Early after surgery with aortic valve replacemem and mitral annuloplasty, mitral leaflet coaptation is barely more anterior than the posterior annulus; there was no MR then. Late after surgery, the LV dilates and mitral coaptation is more posterior than the posterior annulus, indicating increased tethering as the basis for recurrent MR. (*Diagram by Yutaka Otsuji of University of Occupational and Environment Health, Japan. Reprinted from Beeri R, Otsuji Y, Schwammenthal E, et al. Ischemic mitral regurgitation. In: Otto CM, Bonow RO, editors. Valvular heart disease: a companion to Braunwald's heart disease. 3rd ed. Philadelphia: Elsevier Science; 2009. p. 260–73.*)

to operative and ischemic time. The choice of procedure also depends on a very clear understanding of the mechanism of MR. Given the neutral outcome of the STICH trial, recommending extensive ancillary SVR procedures at the time of CABG without more data is difficult.

Percutaneous Edge-to-Edge Repair

The MitraClip (Medtronic, Inc.) is an investigational device currently in clinical trials for MR. This percutaneously placed device clips the central portion of the anterior and posterior leaflets together, creating a double-orifice valve (see Chapter 22). Its role in secondary MR is still under active investigation. In the pivotal trial comparing percutaneous mitral repair with surgery, approximately 30% of the patients enrolled had functional MR.[98] Therefore the numbers of patients were too small for conclusions to be drawn regarding efficacy of the device in this subset of patients. Because the technique requires adequate leaflet approximation to enable the clip to appose the anterior and posterior leaflets, it may be best studied in selected patients with ischemic MR, a narrow coaptation depth, and less leaflet tethering. In a feasibility study that involved 69 patients with functional MR in whom surgery was deemed to be high risk because of critical illness and advanced age, device success could be achieved in 92% and improvement in MR grade to 2+ or lower achieved in 83%. Median follow-up was almost 1 year.[99] In another feasibility study, 51 patients thought to be "nonresponders" to CRT with moderate to severe secondary MR underwent MitraClip treatment. Clip placement was feasible in all patients, and 73% of patients had an acute improvement in New York Heart Association functional class at discharge that was judged to be durable at follow-up. For the secondary MR population, longer follow-up and randomized trials using MitraClip therapy are needed.[100]

Treatment Guidelines for Secondary Mitral Regurgitation

The 2006 American College of Cardiology (ACC)/American Heart Association (AHA) guidelines for the management of valvular heart disease are scant with regard to the management of secondary MR.[101] There is one specific recommendation (Class IIb) that mitral valve repair may be considered for patients with chronic severe secondary MR due to severe LV dysfunction (EF <0.30) who have persistent New York Heart Association functional class III to IV symptoms despite optimal therapy for heart failure, including biventricular pacing (level of evidence: C).[101] The 2012 guidelines from the European Society of Cardiology (ESC) contain specific guidelines for surgical indications in patients with ischemic cardiomyopathy (Table 19-4).[102] In patients without CAD, the ESC guidelines recommend medical therapy as the first line of therapy as well as CRT when indicated.

TABLE 19-4	European Society of Cardiology Guidelines for Surgery in Chronic Ischemic Mitral Regurgitation

Class IC

Patients with severe MR and LVEF >30% undergoing CABG

Class IIaC

Patients with moderate MR undergoing CABG if repair is feasible
Symptomatic patients with severe MR, LVEF <30%, option for CABG, and evidence of viability

Class IIbC

Patients with severe MR, LVEF >30%, no option for CABG, MR refractory to medical therapy, and low comorbidity

From Vahanian A, Alfieri O, Andreotti F, et al. Guidelines on the management of valvular heart disease (version 2012). Joint Task Force on the Management of Valvular Heart Disease of the European Society of Cardiology and the European Association for Cardio-Thoracic Surgery. Eur Heart J 2012;33:2451–96.
CABG, Coronary artery bypass grafting surgery; *LVEF,* left ventricular ejection fraction; *MR,* mitral regurgitation.

REFERENCES

1. Nkomo VT, Gardin JM, Skelton TN, et al. Burden of valvular heart diseases: a population-based study. Lancet 2006;368:1005–11.
2. de Marchena E, Badiye A, Robalino G, et al. Respective prevalence of the different carpentier classes of mitral regurgitation: a stepping stone for future therapeutic research and development. J Cardiac Surg 2011;26:385–92.
3. Perloff JK, Roberts WC. The mitral apparatus: Functional anatomy of mitral regurgitation. Circulation 1972;46:227–39.
4. Otsuji Y, Levine RA, Takeuchi M, et al. Mechanism of ischemic mitral regurgitation. J Cardiol 2008;51:145–56.
5. Kaul S, Spotnitz WD, Glasheen WP, et al. Mechanism of ischemic mitral regurgitation: an experimental evaluation. Circulation 1991;84:2167–80.
6. Meris A, Amigoni M, Verma A, et al. Mechanisms and predictors of mitral regurgitation after high-risk myocardial infarction. J Am Soc Echocardiogr 2012;25:535–42.
7. Hashim SW, Youssef SJ, Ayyash B, et al. Pseudoprolapse of the anterior leaflet in chronic ischemic mitral regurgitation: identification and repair. J Thorac Cardiovasc Surg 2012;143:S33–7.
8. Pierard LA, Lancellotti P. The role of ischemic mitral regurgitation in the pathogenesis of acute pulmonary edema. N Engl J Med 2004;351:1627–34.
9. Aklog L, Filsoufi F, Flores KQ, et al. Does coronary artery bypass grafting alone correct moderate ischemic mitral regurgitation? Circulation 2001;104:I68-I75.
10. Roberts WC, Perloff JK. Mitral valvular disease: a clinicopathologic survey of the conditions causing the mitral valve to function abnormally. Ann Intern Med 1972;77:939–75.
11. Shiran A, Merdler A, Ismir E, et al. Intraoperative transesophageal echocardiography using a quantitative dynamic loading test for the evaluation of ischemic mitral regurgitation. J Am Soc Echocardiogr 2007;20:690–7.
12. He S, Fontaine AA, Schwammenthal E, et al. Integrated mechanism for functional mitral regurgitation: leaflet restriction versus coapting force: in vitro studies. Circulation 1997;96:1826–34.
13. Levy MJ, Edwards JE. Anatomy of mitral insufficiency. Prog Cardiovasc Dis 1962;5:119–44.
14. Brolin I. The mitral orifice. Acta Radiol Diagn (Stockh) 1967;6:273–95.
15. Moller JH, Lucas Jr RV, Adams Jr P, et al. Endocardial fibroelastosis: a clinical and anatomic study of 47 patients with emphasis on its relationship to mitral insufficiency. Circulation 1964;30:759–82.
16. Kono T, Sabbah HN, Rosman H, et al. Left ventricular shape is the primary determinant of functional mitral regurgitation in heart failure. J Am Coll Cardiol 1992;20:1594–8.
17. Sabbah HN, Kono T, Rosman H, et al. Left ventricular shape: a factor in the etiology of functional mitral regurgitation in heart failure. Am Heart J 1992;123:961–6.
18. Yiu SF, Enriquez-Sarano M, Tribouilloy C, et al. Determinants of the degree of functional mitral regurgitation in patients with systolic left ventricular dysfunction: a quantitative clinical study. Circulation 2000;102:1400–6.
19. Karaca O, Avci A, Guler GB, et al. Tenting area reflects disease severity and prognosis in patients with non-ischaemic dilated cardiomyopathy and functional mitral regurgitation. Eur J Heart Fail 2011;13:284–91.
20. Tibayan FA, Wilson A, Lai DT, et al. Tenting volume: three-dimensional assessment of geometric perturbations in functional mitral regurgitation and implications for surgical repair. J Heart Valve Dis 2007;16:1–7.
21. Song JM, Fukuda S, Kihara T, et al. Value of mitral valve tenting volume determined by real-time three-dimensional echocardiography in patients with functional mitral regurgitation. Am J Cardiol 2006;98:1088–93.
22. Boltwood CM, Tei C, Wong M, et al. Quantitative echocardiography of the mitral complex in dilated cardiomyopathy: the mechanism of functional mitral regurgitation. Circulation 1983;68:498–508.
23. Saito K, Okura H, Watanabe N, et al. Influence of chronic tethering of the mitral valve on mitral leaflet size and coaptation in functional mitral regurgitation. JACC Cardiovasc Imaging 2012;5:337–45.
24. Schwammenthal E, Chen C, Benning F, et al. Dynamics of mitral regurgitant flow and orifice area: physiologic application of the proximal flow convergence method: clinical data and experimental testing. Circulation 1994;90:307–22.
25. Hung J, Otsuji Y, Handschumacher MD, et al. Mechanism of dynamic regurgitant orifice area variation in functional mitral regurgitation: physiologic insights from the proximal flow convergence technique. J Am Coll Cardiol 1999;33:538–45.
26. St John Sutton MG, Plappert T, Abraham WT, et al. Effect of cardiac resynchronization therapy on left ventricular size and function in chronic heart failure. Circulation 2003;107:1985–90.
27. Agricola E, Oppizzi M, Galderisi M, et al. Role of regional mechanical dyssynchrony as a determinant of functional mitral regurgitation in patients with left ventricular systolic dysfunction. Heart 2006;92:1390–5.
28. Kanzaki H, Bazaz R, Schwartzman D, et al. A mechanism for immediate reduction in mitral regurgitation after cardiac resynchronization therapy: insights from mechanical activation strain mapping. J Am Coll Cardiol 2004;44:1619–25.
29. Liang YJ, Zhang Q, Fung JW, et al. Different determinants of improvement of early and late systolic mitral regurgitation contributed after cardiac resynchronization therapy. J Am Soc Echocardiogr 2010;23:1160–7.
30. Wigle ED, Adelman AG, Auger P, et al. Mitral regurgitation in muscular subaortic stenosis. Am J Cardiol 1969;24:698–706.
31. Jiang L, Levine RA, King ME, et al. An integrated mechanism for systolic anterior motion of the mitral valve in hypertrophic cardiomyopathy based on echocardiographic observations. Am Heart J 1987;113:633–44.

32. Klues HG, Roberts WC, Maron BJ. Morphological determinants of echocardiographic patterns of mitral valve systolic anterior motion in obstructive hypertrophic cardiomyopathy. Circulation 1993;87:1570–9.

33. Delling FN, Sanborn DY, Levine RA, et al. Frequency and mechanism of persistent systolic anterior motion and mitral regurgitation after septal ablation in obstructive hypertrophic cardiomyopathy. Am J Cardiol 2007;100:1691–5.

34. Zhu WX, Oh JK, Kopecky SL, et al. Mitral regurgitation due to ruptured chordae tendineae in patients with hypertrophic obstructive cardiomyopathy. J Am Coll Cardiol 1992;20:242–7.

35. Weidemann F, Strotmann JM, Niemann M, et al. Heart valve involvement in Fabry cardiomyopathy. Ultrasound Med Biol 2009;35:730–5.

36. Ogbogu PU, Rosing DR, Horne 3rd MK. Cardiovascular manifestations of hypereosinophilic syndromes. Immunol Allergy Clin North Am 2007;27:457–75.

37. Ommen SR, Seward JB, Tajik AJ. Clinical and echocardiographic features of hypereosinophilic syndromes. Am J Cardiol 2000;86:110–3.

38. Grigioni F, Avierinos JF, Ling LH, et al. Atrial fibrillation complicating the course of degenerative mitral regurgitation: determinants and long-term outcome. J Am Coll Cardiol 2002;40:84–92.

39. Gertz ZM, Raina A, Saghy L, et al. Evidence of atrial functional mitral regurgitation due to atrial fibrillation: reversal with arrhythmia control. J Am Coll Cardiol 2011;58:1474–81.

40. Otsuji Y, Kumanohoso T, Yoshifuku S, et al. Isolated annular dilation does not usually cause important functional mitral regurgitation: comparison between patients with lone atrial fibrillation and those with idiopathic or ischemic cardiomyopathy. J Am Coll Cardiol 2002;39:1651–6.

41. Zhou X, Otsuji Y, Yoshifuku S, et al. Impact of atrial fibrillation on tricuspid and mitral annular dilatation and valvular regurgitation. Circ J 2002;66:913–6.

42. Lehmann KG, Francis CK, Dodge HT. Mitral regurgitation in early myocardial infarction: incidence, clinical detection, and prognostic implications. TIMI Study Group. Ann Intern Med 1992;117:10–7.

43. Carpentier A. Cardiac valve surgery—the "French correction". J Thorac Cardiovasc Surg 1983;86:323–37.

44. Hashim SW, Youssef SJ, Ayyash B, et al. Pseudoprolapse of the anterior leaflet in chronic ischemic mitral regurgitation: identification and repair. J Thorac Cardiovasc Surg 2012;143:S33–7.

45. Ray S. The echocardiographic assessment of functional mitral regurgitation. Eur J Echocardiogr 2010;11:i11–7.

46. Lancellotti P, Moura L, Pierard LA, et al. European Association of Echocardiography recommendations for the assessment of valvular regurgitation: part 2: mitral and tricuspid regurgitation (native valve disease). Eur J Echocardiogr 2010;11:307332.

47. Lancellotti P, Marwick T, Pierard LA. How to manage ischaemic mitral regurgitation. Heart 2008;94:1497–502.

48. Izumo M, Suzuki K, Moonen M, et al. Changes in mitral regurgitation and left ventricular geometry during exercise affect exercise capacity in patients with systolic heart failure. Eur J Echocardiogr 2011;12:54–60.

49. Zoghbi WA, Enriquez-Sarano M, Foster E, et al. Recommendations for evaluation of the severity of native valvular regurgitation with two-dimensional and Doppler echocardiography. J Am Soc Echocardiogr 2003;16:777–802.

50. Grigioni F, Enriquez-Sarano M, Zehr KJ, et al. Ischemic mitral regurgitation: long-term outcome and prognostic implications with quantitative Doppler assessment. Circulation 2001;103:1759–64.

51. Enriquez-Sarano M, Avierinos JF, Messika-Zeitoun D, et al. Quantitative determinants of the outcome of asymptomatic mitral regurgitation. N Engl J Med 2005;352:875–83.

52. McCully RB, Enriquez-Sarano M, Tajik AJ, et al. Overestimation of severity of ischemic/functional mitral regurgitation by color Doppler jet area. Am J Cardiol 1994;74:790–3.

53. Buck T, Plicht B, Kahlert P, et al. Effect of dynamic flow rate and orifice area on mitral regurgitant stroke volume quantification using the proximal isovelocity surface area method. J Am Coll Cardiol 2008;52:767–78.

54. Song JM, Kim MJ, Kim YJ, et al. Three-dimensional characteristics of functional mitral regurgitation in patients with severe left ventricular dysfunction: a real-time three-dimensional colour Doppler echocardiography study. Heart 2008;94:590–6.

55. Roberts BJ, Grayburn PA. Color flow imaging of the vena contracta in mitral regurgitation: technical considerations. J Am Soc Echocardiogr 2003;16:1002–6.

56. Iwakura K, Ito H, Kawano S, et al. Comparison of orifice area by transthoracic three-dimensional Doppler echocardiography versus proximal isovelocity surface area (PISA) method for assessment of mitral regurgitation. Am J Cardiol 2006;97:1630–7.

57. Shanks M, Siebelink HM, Delgado V, et al. Quantitative assessment of mitral regurgitation: comparison between three-dimensional transesophageal echocardiography and magnetic resonance imaging. Circ Cardiovasc Imaging 2010;3:694–700.

58. Marsan NA, Westenberg JJ, Ypenburg C, et al. Quantification of functional mitral regurgitation by real-time 3D echocardiography: comparison with 3D velocity-encoded cardiac magnetic resonance. JACC Cardiovascular imaging 2009;2:1245–52.

59. Rifkin RD, Sharma S. An alternative isovelocity surface model for quantitation of effective regurgitant orifice area in mitral regurgitation with an elongated orifice application to functional mitral regurgitation. JACC Cardiovasc Imaging 2010;3:1091–103.

60. Hyodo E, Iwata S, Tugcu A, et al. Accurate measurement of mitral annular area by using single and biplane linear measurements: comparison of conventional methods with the three-dimensional planimetric method. Eur Heart J Cardiovasc Imaging 2012;13:605–11.

61. Tribouilloy C, Shen WF, Rey JL, et al. Mitral to aortic velocity-time integral ratio: a non-geometric pulsed-Doppler regurgitant index in isolated pure mitral regurgitation. Eur Heart J 1994;15:1335–9.

62. Thomas L, Foster E, Schiller NB. Peak mitral inflow velocity predicts mitral regurgitation severity. J Am Coll Cardiol 1998;31:174–9.

63. Ellis SG, Whitlow PL, Raymond RE, et al. Impact of mitral regurgitation on long-term survival after percutaneous coronary intervention. Am J Cardiol 2002;89:315–18.

64. Pellizzon GG, Grines CL, Cox DA, et al. Importance of mitral regurgitation in patients undergoing percutaneous coronary intervention for acute myocardial infarction: the Controlled Abciximab and Device Investigation to Lower Late Angioplasty Complications (CADILLAC) trial. J Am Coll Cardiol 2004;43:1368–74.

65. Feinberg MS, Schwammenthal E, Shlizerman L, et al. Prognostic significance of mild mitral regurgitation by color Doppler echocardiography in acute myocardial infarction. Am J Cardiol 2000;86:903–7.

66. Barra S, Providencia R, Paiva L, et al. Mitral regurgitation during a myocardial infarction—new predictors and prognostic significance at two years of follow-up. Acute Card Care 2012;14:27–33.

67. Levine RA, Schwammenthal E. Ischemic mitral regurgitation on the threshold of a solution: from paradoxes to unifying concepts. Circulation 2005;112:745–58.

68. Koelling TM, Aaronson KD, Cody RJ, et al. Prognostic significance of mitral regurgitation and tricuspid regurgitation in patients with left ventricular systolic dysfunction. Am Heart J 2002;144:524–9.

69. Grayburn PA, Appleton CP, DeMaria AN, et al. Echocardiographic predictors of morbidity and mortality in patients with advanced heart failure: the Beta-blocker Evaluation of Survival Trial (BEST). J Am Coll Cardiol 2005;45:1064–71.

70. Dini FL, Conti U, Fontanive P, et al. Right ventricular dysfunction is a major predictor of outcome in patients with moderate to severe mitral regurgitation and left ventricular dysfunction. Am Heart J 2007;154:172–9.

71. Rossi A, Dini FL, Faggiano P, et al. Independent prognostic value of functional mitral regurgitation in patients with heart failure: a quantitative analysis of 1256 patients with ischaemic and non-ischaemic dilated cardiomyopathy. Heart 2011;97:1675–80.

72. Harshaw CW, Grossman W, Munro AB, et al. Reduced systemic vascular resistance as therapy for severe mitral regurgitation of valvular origin. Ann Intern Med 1975;83:312–16.

73. Greenberg BH, Massie BM, Brundage BH, et al. Beneficial effects of hydralazine in severe mitral regurgitation. Circulation 1978;58:273–9.

74. Breithardt OA, Sinha AM, Schwammenthal E, et al. Acute effects of cardiac resynchronization therapy on functional mitral regurgitation in advanced systolic heart failure. J Am Coll Cardiol 2003;41:765–70.

75. Boriani G, Gasparini M, Landolina M, et al. Impact of mitral regurgitation on the outcome of patients treated with CRT-D: data from the InSync ICD Italian Registry. Pacing Clin Electrophysiol 2012;35:146–54.

76. Solomon SD, Foster E, Bourgoun M, et al. Effect of cardiac resynchronization therapy on reverse remodeling and relation to outcome: multicenter automatic defibrillator implantation trial: cardiac resynchronization therapy. Circulation 2010;122:985–92.

77. Verhaert D, Popovic ZB, De S, et al. Impact of mitral regurgitation on reverse remodeling and outcome in patients undergoing cardiac resynchronization therapy. Circ Cardiovasc Imaging 2012;5:21–6.

78. Senechal M, Lancellotti P, Magne J, et al. Impact of mitral regurgitation and myocardial viability on left ventricular reverse remodeling after cardiac resynchronization therapy in patients with ischemic cardiomyopathy. Am J Cardiol 2010;106:31–7.

79. Cabrera-Bueno F, Molina-Mora MJ, Alzueta J, et al. Persistence of secondary mitral regurgitation and response to cardiac resynchronization therapy. Eur J Echocardiogr 2010;11:131–7.

80. Uretsky BF, Thygesen K, Daubert JC, et al. Predictors of mortality from pump failure and sudden cardiac death in patients with systolic heart failure and left ventricular dyssynchrony: results of the CARE-HF trial. J Card Fail 2008;14:670–5.

81. Petryka J, Misko J, Przybylski A, et al. Magnetic resonance imaging assessment of intraventricular dyssynchrony and delayed enhancement as predictors of response to cardiac resynchronization therapy in patients with heart failure of ischaemic and non-ischaemic etiologies. Eur J Radiol 2012;81:2639–47.

82. Xu YZ, Cha YM, Feng D, et al. Impact of myocardial scarring on outcomes of cardiac resynchronization therapy: extent or location? J Nucl Med 2012;53:47–54.

83. Sutton MG, Plappert T, Hilpisch KE, et al. Sustained reverse left ventricular structural remodeling with cardiac resynchronization at one year is a function of etiology: quantitative Doppler echocardiographic evidence from the Multicenter InSync Randomized Clinical Evaluation (MIRACLE). Circulation 2006;113:266–72.

84. Leor J, Feinberg MS, Vered Z, et al. Effect of thrombolytic therapy on the evolution of significant mitral regurgitation in patients with a first inferior myocardial infarction. J Am Coll Cardiol 1993;21:1661–6.

85. Tenenbaum A, Leor J, Motro M, et al. Improved posterobasal segment function after thrombolysis is associated with decreased incidence of significant mitral regurgitation in a first inferior myocardial infarction. J Am Coll Cardiol 1995;25:1558–63.

86. Hochman JS, Sleeper LA, Webb JG, et al. Early revascularization in acute myocardial infarction complicated by cardiogenic shock: SHOCK Investigators: Should We Emergently Revascularize Occluded Coronaries for Cardiogenic Shock. N Engl J Med 1999;341:625–34.

87. Picard MH, Davidoff R, Sleeper LA, et al. Echocardiographic predictors of survival and response to early revascularization in cardiogenic shock. Circulation 2003;107:279–84.

88. Hung J, Papakostas L, Tahta SA, et al. Mechanism of recurrent ischemic mitral regurgitation after annuloplasty: continued LV remodeling as a moving target. Circulation 2004;110:II85–II90.

89. Kongsaerepong V, Shiota M, Gillinov AM, et al. Echocardiographic predictors of successful versus unsuccessful mitral valve repair in ischemic mitral regurgitation. Am J Cardiol 2006;98:504–8.

90. Digiammarco G, Liberi R, Giancane M, et al. Recurrence of functional mitral regurgitation in patients with dilated cardiomyopathy undergoing mitral valve repair: how to predict it. Interact Cardiovasc Thorac Surg 2007;6:340–4.

91. Magne J, Pibarot P, Dagenais F, et al. Preoperative posterior leaflet angle accurately predicts outcome after restrictive mitral valve annuloplasty for ischemic mitral regurgitation. Circulation 2007;115:782–91.

92. Roshanali F, Mandegar MH, Yousefnia MA, et al. A prospective study of predicting factors in ischemic mitral regurgitation recurrence after ring annuloplasty. Ann Thorac Surg 2007;84:745–9.

93. Agricola E, Oppizzi M, Pisani M, et al. Ischemic mitral regurgitation: mechanisms and echocardiographic classification. Eur J Echocardiogr 2008;9:207–21.

94. Trichon BH, Glower DD, Shaw LK, et al. Survival after coronary revascularization, with and without mitral valve surgery, in patients with ischemic mitral regurgitation. Circulation 2003;108(Suppl 1):II103–II10.

95. Jones RH, Velazquez EJ, Michler RE, et al. Coronary bypass surgery with or without surgical ventricular reconstruction. N Engl J Med 2009;360:1705–17.

96. Velazquez EJ, Lee KL, Deja MA, et al. Coronary-artery bypass surgery in patients with left ventricular dysfunction. N Engl J Med 2011;364:1607–16.

97. Deja MA, Grayburn PA, Sun B, et al. Influence of mitral regurgitation repair on survival in the surgical treatment for ischemic heart failure trial. Circulation 2012;125: 2639–48.

98. Feldman T, Foster E, Glower DD, et al. Percutaneous repair or surgery for mitral regurgitation. N Engl J Med 2011;364:1395–406.

99. Rudolph V, Knap M, Franzen O, et al. Echocardiographic and clinical outcomes of MitraClip therapy in patients not amenable to surgery. J Am Coll Cardiol 2011;58: 2190–5.

100. Auricchio A, Schillinger W, Meyer S, et al. Correction of mitral regurgitation in nonresponders to cardiac resynchronization therapy by MitraClip improves symptoms and promotes reverse remodeling. J Am Coll Cardiol 2011;58:2183–9.

101. Bonow RO, Carabello BA, Kanu C, et al. ACC/AHA 2006 guidelines for the management of patients with valvular heart disease: a report of the American College of Cardiology/ American Heart Association Task Force on Practice Guidelines (writing committee to revise the 1998 Guidelines for the Management of Patients With Valvular Heart Disease): developed in collaboration with the Society of Cardiovascular Anesthesiologists: endorsed by the Society for Cardiovascular Angiography and Interventions and the Society of Thoracic Surgeons. Circulation 2006;114:e84–231.

102. Vahanian A, Alfieri O, Andreotti F, et al. Guidelines on the management of valvular heart disease (version 2012). Joint Task Force on the Management of Valvular Heart Disease of the European Society of Cardiology and the European Association for Cardio-Thoracic Surgery. Eur Heart J 2012;33:2451–96.

SECONDARY MITRAL REGURGITATION

CHAPTER 20

Mitral Regurgitation: Timing of Surgery

Rick A. Nishimura and Hartzell V. Schaff

Key Points

- Irreversible left ventricular (LV) dysfunction may occur with the long-standing volume overload of mitral regurgitation (MR) and leads to a poor prognosis.
- Predictors of outcome in patients with MR include symptoms, LV function, and severity of MR. Left atrial size and natriuretic peptide levels may also predict outcome in patients with MR.
- Mitral valve repair is preferred over mitral valve replacement because of a lower operative mortality and better long-term outcome.
- The important clinical predictors of late mortality and heart failure following operation are older age, elevated serum creatinine, elevated systolic blood pressure, presence of coronary artery disease, and advanced functional class.
- The important echocardiographic predictors of late mortality following operation are LV ejection fraction (EF) and end-systolic dimension. Mitral valve operation is indicated for patients with severe MR due to a primary valvular abnormality when LV dysfunction is present on echocardiography (EF ≤60% or end-systolic dimension ≥40 mm).
- Operation for severe MR should ideally be performed before the onset of LV dysfunction, because residual LV dysfunction may occur even with "normal" preoperative systolic function.
- Patients with severe MR in whom severe symptoms have already developed (New York Heart Association functional class III or IV) despite normal LV function will benefit from mitral valve operation.
- In institutions with surgical expertise in mitral valve repair, it is reasonable to proceed with operation in the asymptomatic patient with severe MR and normal LV systolic function
- Patients with severe acute MR should undergo early operation, despite hemodynamic stabilization.

The optimal timing for surgery for severe mitral regurgitation (MR) has been controversial.[1-6] In the symptomatic patient with severe MR, relief of volume overload by mitral valve repair or replacement improves symptoms and functional status.[7] Thus, the primary indication for operation in a patient with severe MR has been the presence of severe symptoms. However, the natural history of severe MR is not benign, and surgical correction of MR in asymptomatic patients may improve survival and reduce risk of complications such as heart failure and atrial fibrillation. In the past, clinicians have been reluctant to subject asymptomatic patients with MR to operation owing to an in-hospital operative mortality and morbidity as well as potential long-term complications of a valve prosthesis. In current practice, however, severe MR due to degenerative disease can be repaired in more than 90% of patients with very low operative risk (<1% to 2%).

It is well known that chronic volume overload may lead to irreversible left ventricular (LV) systolic dysfunction, and this systolic dysfunction can develop before the onset of symptoms.[8-10]

Once systolic dysfunction occurs, the outcome becomes poorer, whether or not operation is performed. Conventional measurements of LV function do not reliably predict the onset of LV dysfunction, owing to changes in load on the ventricle imposed by the MR.[8,9,11,12] It is important, therefore, to identify and correct severe MR before irreversible LV dysfunction occurs.[1,2]

There have been advances in our knowledge, diagnosis, and treatment of MR. The pathophysiology of the volume overload on the left ventricle and its eventual outcome on LV function is now better understood.[6,13] The natural history of severe MR has been clarified and elucidated by multiple centers.[14-16] Echocardiography can now accurately assess the valve morphology and severity of the regurgitation noninvasively in most patients as well as determine the effect of the volume overload on the left ventricle. Current operative interventions have resulted in a much lower operative mortality and better long-term outcome than was possible several decades ago, with clear benefits of mitral valve repair over valve replacement.[2,3,5,17,18] All of these advances have provided an incentive to change the indication for timing of operation in patients with MR, setting the paradigm of early operation before the onset LV dysfunction. This chapter outlines these advances and provide recommendations regarding optimal timing of surgery for MR.

Recent Advances

Pathophysiology

The diagnosis of severe MR is made when 50% of the total stroke volume is diverted to regurgitant flow.[13] Several general stages describe the hemodynamic response to the excessive volume overload of MR in terms of intrinsic LV myocardial as well as circulatory responses (Table 20-1). These stages are (1) an acute volume overload stage, (2) a chronic compensated volume overloaded stage, and (3) the decompensated stage of MR with irreversible LV dysfunction.[1,6,8,13,19,20]

ACUTE VOLUME OVERLOAD STAGE

In patients with acute MR, an acute volume load is placed on the left atrium and an unconditioned left ventricle, resulting in an immediate increase in left atrial (LA) pressure that is reflected back to the pulmonary circulation. This process causes symptoms of severe shortness of breath and many times leads to pulmonary congestion. As blood is directed back into the left atrium, there is less forward stroke volume, and thus, systemic cardiac output falls.

The short-term LV response to volume overload is an increase in LV volume from a lengthening of sarcomeres along their normal length tension curve so that total stroke volume increases via the

TABLE 20-1	Stages of Mitral Regurgitation		
		Chronic	
	ACUTE	COMPENSATED	DECOMPENSATED
Symptoms	↑↑	–	↑↑↑
Left ventricular size	↑	↑↑	↑↑↑
Ejection fraction (%)	>70	>60	≤60
End-systolic dimension (mm)	<40	<40	≥40
Wall stress	?	N	↑↑
Preload (myofiber)	↑	N	↑↑↑

Starling mechanism.[8] Fractional shortening of the left ventricle increases and end-systolic volume decreases as the result of the low resistance runoff into the low-pressure left atrium. There is thus a decrease in the integrated systolic wall tension. If forward cardiac output can be maintained by these compensatory mechanisms, and if LA pressure is lowered by therapy, an evolution from the acute to the chronic compensated stage of MR occurs.[6,8,13,19,20]

CHRONIC COMPENSATED STAGE

The major compensatory mechanism that occurs in this chronic steady state of MR is LV enlargement. LV dilation occurs from rearrangement of sarcomeres, added in series and parallel.[19] The individual sarcomeres are not extended beyond their optimal contractile length and, thus, the stretch (or preload) on the individual sarcomere is normalized. The increase in LV cavity size allows a greater LV volume as a result of the MR while maintaining normal diastolic pressures.

Wall stress on the left ventricle depends on LV pressure, volume, and wall thickness. The initial unloading of the left ventricle by the low-resistance runoff into the left atrium is countered by an increase in LV size during this compensatory stage, returning systolic wall stress to normal levels.[6,13] In this chronic compensated stage of MR, appropriate LV adaptation occurs by dilation with adequate forward cardiac output and maintenance of normal filling pressures. Patients remain asymptomatic during this state, and the normalized preload and wall stress help the left ventricle maintain normal contractility. Patients may remain in this chronic compensated stage for years to decades following the onset of MR.[6,8,11,13,19]

DECOMPENSATED STAGE WITH IRREVERSIBLE LEFT VENTRICULAR DYSFUNCTION

In patients with severe MR, there will eventually be progressive LV enlargement beyond that of a compensated stage.[6,8,13,19-22] This progressive LV enlargement is due to increasing severity of MR, continued compensatory chamber enlargement, or a combination of both. Mitral valve competence is highly dependent on the integrated function of the entire mitral valve apparatus—the mitral annulus, papillary muscle orientation, chordae, and leaflets. Progressive LV enlargement itself can cause increasing degrees of MR from altered LV geometry and annular dilation; thus the saying "MR begets MR." In degenerative MR, disruption of supporting structures such as rupture of chordae tendineae may occur, further increasing the severity of MR. As disease progresses, systolic wall stress on the left ventricle is increased as a result of increased circumferential stress from a larger LV minor axis as the left ventricle assumes a more spherical shape.[8,11,12,20,22] An increase in end-diastolic stress occurs from further stretching of the myocytes beyond their normal contractile length, leading to an increase in end-diastolic pressure as the ventricle overfills. The effect of the continued abnormally elevated wall stresses on

the ventricle is a decreased contractile state, with reduced myofiber content and interstitial fibrosis. The cumulative effects of prolonged oxidative stress with secondary lipofuscin accumulation and cardiomyocyte myofibrillar degeneration further account for LV contractile dysfunction.[23] As this process continues, irreversible LV dysfunction occurs, leading to the decompensated stage of MR. Once irreversible LV dysfunction is present, the prognosis is poor.

TRANSITION STAGE (FROM COMPENSATED TO DECOMPENSATED STAGE)

Development of symptoms is an unreliable guide to the transition from the compensated to the uncompensated stage. By the time significant symptoms of dyspnea occur, there may already be significant irreversible dysfunction. The usual ejection phase indices of LV contractility may not reflect deterioration of LV systolic function, owing to the dependence of these indices on the load imposed on the left ventricle. Preload, afterload, and wall stress are abnormal and variable in patients with MR, and indices such as ejection fraction (EF) and fractional shortening may remain normal despite progressive decrease in contractile function of the left ventricle. Therefore, other parameters, such as preload-corrected EF, end-systolic wall stress normalized for end-systolic volume index, mass normalization of LV elastance, and end-systolic wall stress normalization of EF, have all been proposed as possible indices of a deterioration in intrinsic LV function.[9,12,20,22,24,25] However, although studies of these indices have been able to identify patients who are already in the decompensated stage, none has been shown to determine when the transition stage begins. Indeed, as discussed later, the outcome of patients with MR depends largely on the severity of valve leakage, and in current practice, criteria for optimal timing of intervention rely mainly on quantitative measurements of the severity of mitral valve leakage rather than indices of LV function, size, or wall stress. The goal of optimal timing is to intervene *before* the decompensated stage of irreversible LV dysfunction occurs.

Natural History

Prior reports on the natural history of MR have been highly variable, for a multitude of reasons, including the small populations of patients studied, selection bias and multiple etiologies of valve disease, presence of other concomitant cardiovascular disease, as well as incomplete hemodynamic data. Also, many of these studies did not compare outcome in patients with MR with expected survival in patients without heart disease.

The natural history of severe MR in the modern era is now well documented,[2,14,18,26,27] on the basis of studies of patients followed up with flail posterior leaflet (a surrogate for severe MR) (Figure 20-1). In an initial study by Ling et al,[14] of patients who were followed up for more than 10 years, mortality rate was higher (6.3% yearly) than the expected survival rate (see Figure ON20-1 on website). Twenty percent of patients receiving medical management died; 69% of the deaths were from cardiac causes. High morbidity was also noted, with 10-year incidences of atrial fibrillation of 30% and of heart failure 63%. Once heart failure developed, the prognosis was worse, with a 5-year survival of less than 20%. At 10 years, 90% of patients with a flail posterior leaflet had either died or undergone surgical repair because of the development of symptoms.[14] These high event rates were confirmed in a multicenter study, linearized event rates/year for those receiving nonsurgical management being 5.4% for atrial fibrillation, 8.0% for heart failure, and 2.6% for death[27] (Figure 20-2). Sudden death is a frequent catastrophic event, responsible for approximately one fourth of deaths in patients receiving medical treatment.[28]

The natural history of predominantly asymptomatic patients with moderately severe MR and normal LV function has been controversial. Rosen et al[15] in 1994 reported a benign prognosis, with no deaths and no progression to subnormal LV function,

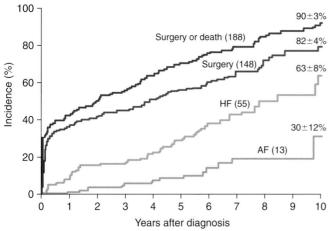

FIGURE 20-1   Incidence of atrial fibrillation (AF), heart failure (HF), mitral valve surgery, and surgery or death. In 229 patients with isolated mitral regurgitation due to flail mitral valve leaflet between 1980 and 1989, there was a high event rate at 10-year follow-up. *(From Ling LH, Enriquez-Sarano M, Seward JB, et al. Clinical outcome of mitral regurgitation due to flail leaflet. N Engl J Med 1996;335:1417–23.)*

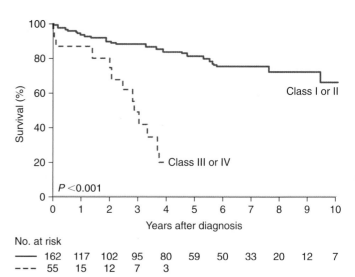

FIGURE 20-3   Overall long-term survival with medical treatment in patients with flail mitral valve leaflet. Patients are subdivided according to New York Heart Association functional class. *(From Ling LH, Enriquez-Sarano M, Seward JB, et al. Clinical outcome of mitral regurgitation due to flail leaflet. N Engl J Med 1996;335:1417–23.)*

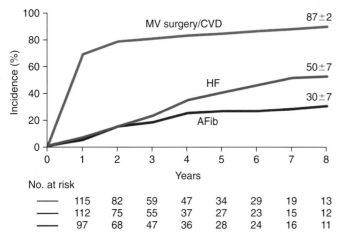

FIGURE 20-2   Long-term outcomes for patients with mitral regurgitation due to a flail mitral valve receiving medical treatment in a multicenter study. Note the high 8-year event rate, similar to the outcome seen in Figure 20-1. *AFib,* Atrial fibrillation; *CVD,* cardiovascular death; *HF,* heart failure; *MV,* mitral valve. *(From Grigioni F, Tribouilloy C, Avierinos JF, et al. Outcomes in mitral regurgitation due to flail leaflets a multicenter European study. JACC Cardiovasc Imaging 2008:1:133–41.)*

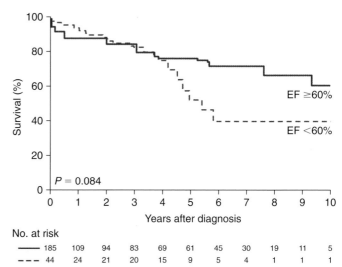

FIGURE 20-4   Long-term survival with medical treatment in 229 patients with flail mitral valve leaflet. Patients are subdivided according to ejection fraction (EF) value. *(From Ling LH, Enriquez-Sarano M, Seward JB, et al. Clinical outcome of mitral regurgitation due to flail leaflet. N Engl J Med 1996; 335:1417–23.)*

after 5 years of follow-up. However, in this report, there was a 10% average annual risk for development of symptoms leading to surgery. In addition, the patients in this study most likely had less severe MR than those in other studies, given the smaller LV size and lack of quantitative measurements.[5] In a subset of patients from a multicenter study who were completely asymptomatic with normal LV function, the 5-year combined incidence of atrial fibrillation, heart failure, or cardiovascular death was 42% ± 8%.[27]

Predictors of Outcome

The outcome of patients with severe MR is highly dependent on initial symptoms and LV function. In the study reported by Ling et al,[14] patients with New York Heart Association (NYHA) functional class III or IV symptoms who did not undergo an operation had considerable mortality (34% yearly) (Figure 20-3). Even those patients with NYHA functional class I or II symptoms had a mortality of 4.1% per year. Those patients with an EF of less than 60% also had a substantial mortality in comparison with those whose

EF was 60% or greater. Ten-year survival was 61% in patients with an EF greater than 60%, compared with 40% for patients with an EF less than 60% (Figure 20-4).[14]

More data on the natural history of asymptomatic patients with MR has been accumulated on the basis of the ability not only to measure LV function but also to quantify the degree of MR.[29] After stratification by quantitative Doppler echocardiography, 456 patients with asymptomatic primary MR were prospectively followed. Five years after the diagnosis, 22% of patients had died (14% from cardiac causes) and one third of patients suffered a cardiac event, defined as death from cardiac cause, heart failure, or new atrial fibrillation. Independent determinants of survival were age, presence of diabetes, but also the regurgitant orifice area (ROA), which provides a quantitative measure of severity of MR. Those patients with an ROA of at least 40 mm² had a 5-year survival rate lower than expected on the basis of U.S. census data (58% versus 78%). In comparison with patients with an ROA of less than 20 mm², those with an ROA of at least 40 mm² had a

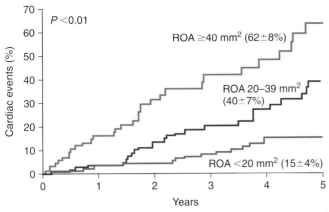

FIGURE 20-5 **Kaplan-Meier estimates of the mean (± SE) rates of cardiac events among patients with asymptomatic mitral regurgitation receiving medical management.** Patients are subdivided according to the regurgitant orifice area (ROA). Cardiac events were defined as death from cardiac causes, heart failure, or new atrial fibrillation. Values in *parentheses* are survival rates at 5 years. *(From Enriquez-Sarano M, Avierinos J-F, Messika-Zeitoun D, et al. Quantitative determinants of the outcome of asymptomatic mitral regurgitation. N Engl J Med 2005;352:875–83.)*

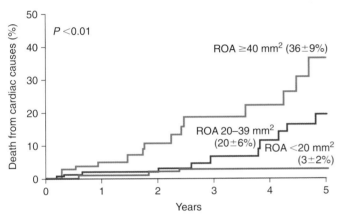

FIGURE 20-6 **Kaplan-Meier estimates of the mean (± SE) rates of death from cardiac causes among patients with asymptomatic mitral regurgitation receiving medical management.** Patients are subdivided according to the regurgitant orifice area (ROA). Values in *parentheses* are survival rates at 5 years. *(From Enriquez-Sarano M, Avierinos J-F, Messika-Zeitoun D, et al. Quantitative determinants of the outcome of asymptomatic mitral regurgitation. N Engl J Med 2005;352:875–83.)*

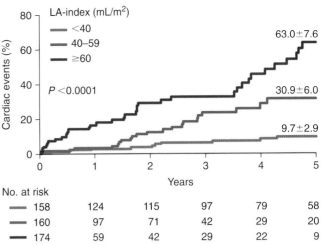

FIGURE 20-7 **Cardiac events after diagnosis of severe mitral regurgitation.** Patients are subdivided according to left atrial (LA) volume. *(From Le Tourneau T, Messika-Zeitoun D, Russo A, et al. Impact of left atrial volume on clinical outcome in organic mitral regurgitation. J Am Coll Cardiol 2010;56:570–8.)*

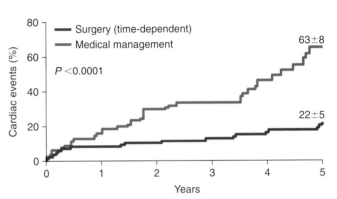

FIGURE 20-8 **Cardiac events after diagnosis of mitral regurgitation in patients with markedly enlarged left atrium.** Patients receiving medical management are compared to those treated surgically. *(From Le Tourneau T, Messika-Zeitoun D, Russo A, et al. Impact of left atrial volume on clinical outcome in organic mitral regurgitation. J Am Coll Cardiol 2010;56:570–8.)*

higher risk of death from any cause, of death from cardiac causes, and of cardiac deaths (Figures 20-5 and 20-6). This finding has been confirmed in a study of 286 patients with asymptomatic severe MR who were monitored medically. The ROA as well as the baseline grade of pulmonary hypertension were independent predictors of heart failure or need for surgery.[30]

Overall, the presence of severe MR portends a poor prognosis, even in the asymptomatic patient with preserved EF. This insight into the natural history of patients with MR has important implications regarding timing of operation. Data show very clearly that patients with a regurgitant volume of at least 60 mL/beat or an ROA of at least 40 mm[2] have a poor outcome with medical management alone. In addition, close follow-up of patients with intermediate grades of MR (ROA 20 to 39 mm[2]) is essential. Although these patients with less severe MR have low risk of death and cardiac events during the first 12 to 18 months after diagnosis, the rates of death and other complications increase substantially thereafter.[29]

LA enlargement is the end result of the pathophysiologic response to MR. LA enlargement strongly predicts survival and other cardiac events (heart failure, atrial fibrillation) in patients with MR managed medically (Figure 20-7; see also Figure ON20-2). Compared with patients with LA volume less than 40 mL/m[2], those with LA volume greater than 60 mL/m[2] have increased mortality and rate of cardiac events[31,32] Among patients with marked LA dilation, mortality and cardiac event rates are lower in those treated surgically compared to those maintained on medical management (Figure 20-8; see also Figure ON20-3).

There has been interest in the use of measurements of natriuretic peptides for predicting outcome in patients with MR.[33-35] Brain natriuretic peptide (BNP) activation in MR increases with the severity of MR.[35] BNP Levels of brain natriuretic peptide are independently predictive of heart failure and mortality in patients with MR[33-35] (Figure 20-9; see also Figures ON20-4 and ON20-5).

Advances in Surgical Intervention

Determination of optimal timing of valve operation requires knowledge of the risks and benefits of the operation itself. There have been significant changes in the surgical treatment of MR, with substantial effect on the operative mortality and long-term outcome (Figure 20-10). In North America, the most common cause of MR is primary degenerative valve disease, and the most common pathophysiologic mechanism is leaflet prolapse. More than 95% of patients with leaflet prolapse can undergo surgery

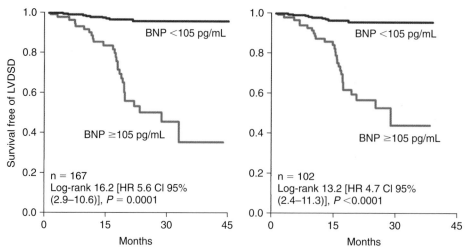

FIGURE 20-9 **Survival free of heart failure or left ventricular systolic dysfunction (LVDSD) according to initial brain natriuretic peptide (BNP) levels.** *Left,* derivation set of patients; *Right,* validation set of patients. *CI,* confidence interval; *HR,* hazard ratio. *(From Pizarro R, Bazzino OO, Oberti PF, et al. Prospective validation of the prognostic usefulness of brain natriuretic peptide in asymptomatic patients with chronic severe mitral regurgitation. J Am Coll Cardiol 2009;54:1099–106.)*

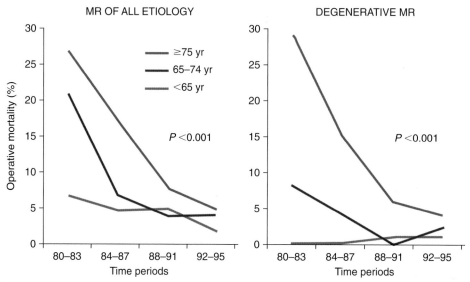

FIGURE 20-10 **Trends in operative mortality for surgery for mitral regurgitation (MR) throughout four time periods (1980-1983, 1984-1987, 1988-1991, and 1992-1995).** The operative mortality is shown for patients in three age ranges. *Left,* Trends in operative mortality for all causes of MR. *Right,* Trends in operative mortality for primary degenerative MR. The probability *(P)* values apply to the time trends for all patients irrespective of age. *(From Detaint D, Sundt TM, Nkomo VT, et al. Surgical correction of mitral regurgitation in the elderly: outcomes and recent improvements. Circulation 2006;114:265–72.)*

with low operative risk and high feasibility of repair (see Figure ON20-6), with a durability that approaches that of prosthetic replacement. In our clinic, operative risk for valve repair in patients 75 years or younger is less than 1%. Linearized risk of reoperation after repair of posterior leaflet prolapse is approximately 0.5% per year, and rates of reintervention after repair of anterior or bileaflet prolapse are similarly low (1.6% and 0.9% per year, respectively). Indeed, the durability of mitral repair for all subsets of patients with leaflet prolapse in the current era (0.74% per year overall) is similar to that following mitral valve replacement.[36]

Mitral valve repair is preferred over prosthetic replacement because of low operative mortality and elimination of device-related complications such as ventricular rupture, thrombus formation, or mechanical malfunction.[5,18] With valve repair, the chordal apparatus is preserved, and studies in patients undergoing valve replacement show that the preservation of mitral valve attachments preserves LV geometry and systolic function.[37] Also, valve repair has a much lower rate of late complications than prosthetic replacement. The survival advantage of repair over replacement extends to patients who undergo reoperation for late failure of initial repair.[36]

There have also been improvements in outcome for patients who cannot undergo mitral valve repair but require mitral valve replacement. Studies have shown that preservation of the chordal apparatus at the time of valve insertion results in a smaller postoperative chamber size, prevents the postoperative increase in systolic stress, and maintains normal ejection performance.[38-41] Thus, the preservation of the chordal apparatus has a lower risk of LV dysfunction following mitral valve operation than the resection of supporting mitral valve structures.[38-41]

Predictors of Surgical Outcome

EARLY MORTALITY

The factors that have been shown to influence early mortality following mitral valve operation are the patient's age and NYHA functional class.[42] Operative mortality continues to improve each decade and is related to surgical expertise.[5,6,27]

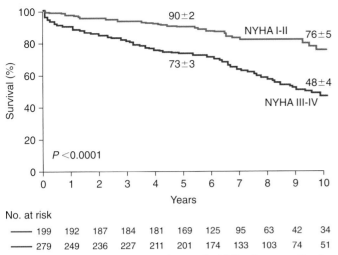

FIGURE 20-11 Overall postoperative survival following operation for severe mitral regurgitation. Patients in New York Heart Association *(NYHA)* functional classes I and II are compared to patients in NYHA functional class III and IV. *(From Tribouilloy CM, Enriquez-Sarano M, Schaff HV, et al. Impact of preoperative symptoms on survival after surgical correction of organic mitral regurgitation: rationale for optimizing surgical indications. Circulation 1999;99:400–5.)*

LATE OUTCOME

The major cause of death after surgical correction of MR is continued heart failure.[2,11,19,42-44] The important clinical predictors of late mortality and heart failure following operation are older age, elevated serum creatinine, elevated systolic blood pressure, presence of coronary artery disease, and advanced functional class[42,43] (Figure 20-11). Echocardiographic parameters that predict late mortality after operation are EF and end-systolic dimension.[5,16]

As would be expected, postoperative LV dysfunction, as assessed by EF, remains a major predictor of poor outcome.[2,11,19,42-44] A decreased EF postoperatively is highly associated with future mortality and the onset of heart failure. Thus, it is essential to attempt to determine factors associated with postoperative LV dysfunction.

PREDICTION OF POSTOPERATIVE LEFT VENTRICULAR DYSFUNCTION

A multitude of studies have attempted to predict residual postoperative LV systolic dysfunction.[9,12,20,22,24,25] The ejection phase indices of LV function (EF and fractional shortening) were not thought to be of benefit in evaluating intrinsic contractility of the left ventricle or patient outcome because of the changes in load on the ventricle from the severe MR (see Figure ON20-7). Thus, other parameters had been identified, such as preload-corrected EF, end-systolic volume index normalized to wall stress, and diastolic volume mass normalization of LV elastance. Despite the elegant pathophysiologic theoretical models underlying these parameters, these studies showed only that all these parameters demonstrated when it was "too late" for operation (see Figure ON20-8).[9,12,20,22,24,25] The "cutoff" values from each study predicted when patients had a high risk of severe heart failure or death following operation but did not predict the optimal timing of operation. It must be noted that these prior studies might not be applicable to surgical outcomes today, because they included small number of patients, mixed valve disease, conservative selection bias, as well as the use of valve replacement with or without chordal sparing.[9,12,20,22,24,25]

Later studies have looked at the determinants of residual postoperative LV dysfunction in the era of mitral valve repair.[2,3,18,42-46] Overall, EF drops by approximately 10% in patients with degenerative MR, on average from 58% to 50%.[42,43] Several theories have been put forward to explain this observation, including acute increase in LV afterload and myocardial injury during operation as a result of global ischemia and reperfusion.

An echocardiographic and hemodynamic study of LV function immediately after mitral valve repair demonstrated that indexes of global systolic function decreased significantly from preoperative values (*P* <0.001), primarily because of an increase in LV end-systolic size.[47,48] At the same time, hemodynamic parameters, including cardiac output and forward stroke volume, were maintained after surgery, suggesting preservation of cardiac pump function. Indeed, control patients in the investigation, who were undergoing coronary artery bypass grafting and had cardioplegic arrest for intervals similar to or longer than those in patients undergoing MV repair, exhibited no change in postoperative LV systolic function and hemodynamic parameters except for increased heart rate. The best explanation for these data is that immediately after correction of MR, the LV undergoes volumetric adjustments to ensure constant forward stroke volume at the expense of decreased EF. With time, there is reverse remodeling with decrease in LV end-diastolic dimension and appropriate increase in EF to maintain stroke volume.

An important issue for clinicians and their patients is the extent to which LV function and reverse remodeling occurs late after correction of MR. In a retrospective study from our clinic, Enriquez-Sarano et al[43] reported that in 217 patients with organic mitral valve disease, average EF 1 year after correction of MR was 52%, compared with 62% preoperatively (*P* < 0.001), and this decline was due to decreased LV end-diastolic dimension and minimal change in LV end-systolic dimension. Suri et al[48] extended these studies and reported that after an early decrease, the EF in patients undergoing mitral valve repair or replacement improved steadily throughout the follow-up period, which extended to 10 years. Predictors of recovery of EF included larger preoperative EF, smaller LV chamber size, mitral valve repair rather than replacement, and surgery during the 1990s versus operation in an earlier era. Taken together, these findings further support the advantage of early repair of severe MR, before there is an important drop in EF. Indeed, in this study the most important thresholds predicting recovery of normal LV EF were preoperative EF 65% or larger and LV systolic dimension less than 36 mm.

Despite the limitations of the EF, this measurement has emerged as the best predictor for determining postoperative LV systolic dysfunction as well as the onset of heart failure and/or mortality (Figure 20-12).[2,3,18,42-46] Patients with a preoperative EF of less than 60% have a higher incidence of postoperative LV dysfunction as well as an increased incidence of poor outcome.[2,42,43] Even those with EF between 50% and 60% had a poorer outcome than patients with EF greater than 60%.

LV end-systolic volume (or dimension) has been another useful parameter that has emerged in the predicting of adverse outcome following mitral valve operation.[9,11,12] The end-systolic dimension incorporates both the increased preload of the heart and the intrinsic contractility, because ejection will cease when the ventricle can no longer contract against its afterload. The end-systolic dimension is also a direct single measurement rather than a calculated value and therefore has excellent reproducibility if properly obtained by echocardiography. A LV end-systolic dimension greater than 40 mm independently predicts overall mortality and cardiac mortality in patients with MR undergoing conservative management (Figure 20-13). After adjustment for age, sex, comorbidity, and EF, each 1 mm increment in LV end-systolic dimension is associated with a 7% increase in overall mortality and a 13% increase in cardiac mortality (Figure 20-14; see also Figure ON20-9). There is also an excess mortality in patients with end-systolic dimension greater than 40 mm after surgery[16] (see Figure ON20-10).

In patients with severe MR, women have a higher mortality than men, perhaps in relation to the smaller body size of women.[49] Normalization of the LV end-systolic dimension to body surface area may be indicated in those patients with a small body size,

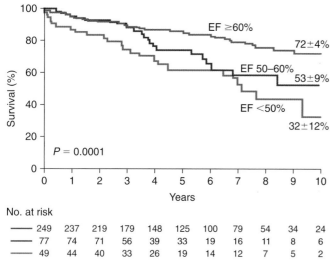

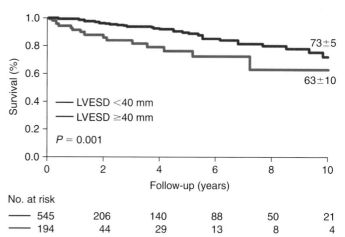

No. at risk

— 249	237	219	179	148	125	100	79	54	34	24
— 77	74	71	56	39	33	19	16	11	8	6
— 49	44	40	33	26	19	14	12	7	5	2

FIGURE 20-12   Late survival of patients undergoing operation for severe mitral regurgitation. Patients are subdivided according to the preoperative echocardiographic ejection fraction (EF) value. Numbers of patients at risk for each EF and time interval are shown indicated under the graph. *(From Enriquez-Sarano M, Tajik AJ, Schaff HV, et al. Echocardiographic prediction of survival after surgical correction of organic mitral regurgitation. Circulation 1994;90: 830–7.)*

No. at risk

— 545	206	140	88	50	21
— 194	44	29	13	8	4

FIGURE 20-14   Survival of patients with primary mitral regurgitation undergoing conservative nonsurgical management. Patients are subdivided according to left ventricular end-systolic diameter (LVESD). *Pt*, number of patients. *(From Tribouilloy C, Grigioni F, Aviernos JF, et al. Survival implication of left ventricular end-systolic diameter in mitral regurgitation due to flail leaflets: a long-term follow-up multicenter study. J Am Coll Cardiol 2009;54:1961–8.)*

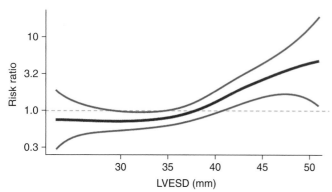

FIGURE 20-13   The association between the left ventricular end-systolic dimension (LVESD) and risk of death with conservative management for patients with primary mitral regurgitation. The hazard line *(solid line)* and 95% confidence limits *(blue lines)* were estimated in a Cox multivariate model with left ventricular end-systolic dimension represented as a spline function. *(From Tribouilloy C, Grigioni F, Aviernos JF, et al. Survival implication of left ventricular end-systolic diameter in mitral regurgitation due to flail leaflets: a long-term follow-up multicenter study. J Am Coll Cardiol 2009;21:1961–8.)*

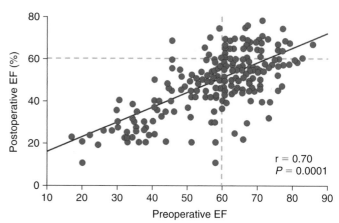

FIGURE 20-15   Correlation between postoperative and preoperative ejection fraction (EF). Although a linear correlation can be seen between the preoperative and postoperative EF values, there remain a number of patients in whom the postoperative EF is less than 60% despite a preoperative EF greater than 60%. This group represents the patients with "unexpected left ventricular dysfunction" following operation. *(From Enriquez-Sarano M, Tajik AJ, Schaff HV, et al. Echocardiographic prediction of left ventricular function after correction of mitral regurgitation: results and clinical implications. J Am Coll Cardiol 1994;24:1536–43.)*

and an LV end-systolic dimension greater than 22 mm/m^2 is associated with excess mortality.[16]

Thus, the combination of end-systolic dimension and EF has been valuable in identifying patients who have already reached the irreversible stage of LV dysfunction.[11,21,43] In those patients with an EF value less than 60% or an end-systolic dimension greater than 40 mm, irreversible LV dysfunction is assumed to be present.[1]

"UNEXPECTED LEFT VENTRICULAR DYSFUNCTION"

The criteria of EF less than 60% and end-systolic dimension greater than 40 mm determine when the patient has reached the stage of irreversible LV dysfunction.[1,43] However, it does not determine when the transition to LV dysfunction begins to occur. Thus, "unexpected LV dysfunction," which is defined as a depressed EF after the correction of MR, may occur even before these parameters are reached (Figure 20-15). It is important to recognize that the "cutoff criteria" are measurements of when the decompensated stage of LV dysfunction is reached. Ideally, operation should be performed before this end stage occurs.[5,6,13]

Effect of Surgical Correction on Outcome

From the foregoing discussion, it is clear that hemodynamically severe MR does not have a benign course. A strategy of initial medical treatment and delayed surgical intervention for symptomatic patients is accompanied by excess morbidity and mortality (Figure 20-16).[5,18,27,30] Several lines of investigation indicate that earlier referral for correction of severe MR improves the outlook for these patients.

In a further analysis of 221 patients with flail mitral valve leaflets, patients were stratified according to the timing of surgery.[18] Sixty-three patients who had mitral valve surgery within 1 month of diagnosis were categorized as having early surgery. Among the remaining 158 patients designated as the "conservatively" managed group, 80 had later surgery. Because this was an observational, nonrandomized study, some patient characteristics other than timing of surgery were different in the two groups. Patients having early surgery were younger and more likely to have symptoms and atrial fibrillation, but there was no difference

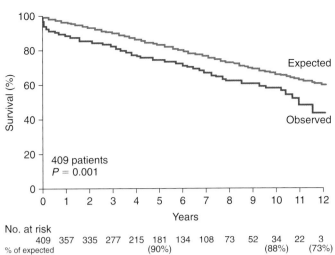

FIGURE 20-16 Postoperative survival compared with expected survival in 409 patients undergoing mitral valve operation. Survival was 75% at 5 years, 58% at 10 years, and 44% at 12 years. Numbers across the bottom represent the numbers of patients at risk for each time interval and the percentage of the expected survival for specific intervals. *(From Enriquez-Sarano M, Tajik AJ, Schaff HV, et al. Echocardiographic prediction of survival after surgical correction of organic mitral regurgitation. Circulation 1994;90:830–7.)*

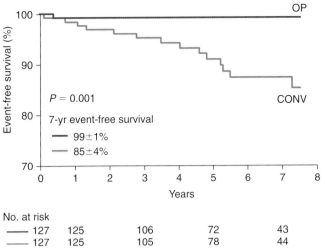

FIGURE 20-18 Comparison of event-free survival rates between the operated (OP) and conventional treatment (CONV) groups in propensity-matched pairs. *(From Kang D-H, Kim JH, Rim JH, et al. Comparison of early surgery versus conventional treatment in asymptomatic severe mitral regurgitation. Circulation 2009;119:797–804.)*

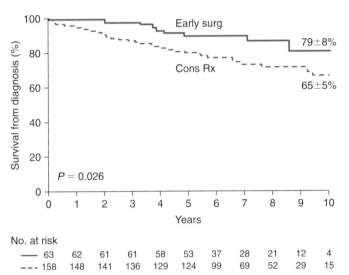

FIGURE 20-17 The outcomes for 221 patients with flail leaflets undergoing operation. The group undergoing early surgery (Early surg), defined as mitral valve surgery within 1 month after diagnosis, comprised 63 patients. The conservative therapy group (Cons Rx) contained 158 patients initially treated conservatively (80 of whom who underwent operation later). Overall 10-year survival is shown, with long-term survival being better in patients who underwent the strategy of early surgery. *(From Ling LH, Enriquez-Sarano M, Seward JB, et al. Early surgery in patients with mitral regurgitation due to flail leaflets: a long-term outcome study. Circulation 1997;96:1819–25.)*

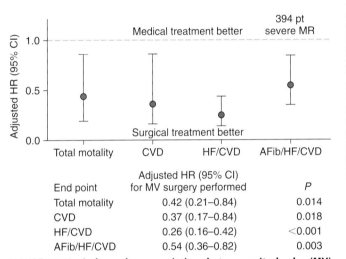

FIGURE 20-19 Independent associations between mitral valve (MV) surgical treatment and outcome in 394 patients with flail leaflets. Time-dependent analysis shows favorable associations between MV surgery and outcome in patients with degenerative mitral regurgitation due to flail leaflet (after adjustment for age, New York Heart Association functional class, and left ventricular ejection fraction). The results support the rationale for considering MV surgery early in the course of the disease. Cases of perioperative (i.e., within 30 days) atrial fibrillation (AFib) (n = 24) were excluded from the analysis. Point estimates of hazard ratios (HRs) are graphically depicted as *circles*, with their 95% confidence intervals shown as *lines. CVD,* Cardiovascular death; *HF,* heart failure. *(From Grigioni F, Tribouilloy C, Avierinos JF, et al. Outcomes in mitral regurgitation due to flail leaflets a multicenter European study. JACC Cardiovasc Imaging 2008;1:133–41.)*

in EF between the groups. Patients in the early surgery group had better overall survival rate than those managed conservatively (10-year survival 79% vs. 65%; P = 0.028) (Figure 20-17). The beneficial effect of early surgery was observed in asymptomatic and minimally symptomatic patients as well as those with more serious heart failure. Other investigators have confirmed the advantage of early surgery over conventional therapy in patients with severe asymptomatic MR (Figure 20-18; see also Figure ON20-11).[30]

A clear weakness among observational studies comparing the outcomes of early surgery and conservative management is the potential for selection bias. The improved outcome of patients undergoing early surgery might theoretically be attributable to the more favorable risk profile. However, multivariate analysis as well as a propensity-matched analysis in these studies suggested that early surgery is an independent predictor of better survival, along with greater freedom from heart failure and new-onset atrial fibrillation (Figure 20-19; see also Figure ON20-12).[27]

An analysis of the causes of death also strongly indicated that the beneficial effect of correction of the MR was due to improved postoperative cardiovascular physiology and not simply patient selection.[27] In the study of patients with flail mitral valve leaflets, a high percentage of all deaths was attributable to cardiovascular causes. However, there were only 6 cardiovascular deaths during follow-up among patients having early surgery compared with 35 in the conservatively managed group. The mortality rate was 11%

± 2% at 5 years and 21% ± 5% at 10 years for patients having early correction of MR compared to 14% ± 4% at 5 years for conservatively managed patients ($P = 0.025$), and in multivariate analysis, early surgery was associated with decreased cardiovascular mortality (adjusted risk ratio, 0.18; $P = 0.002$). Similar data in patients with flail leaflets were reported by Ling et al18: the mortality rate was 11% ± 4% at 5 years and 21% ± 8% at 10 years for patients having early correction of MR compared to 22% ± 3% at five years and 35% ± 5% at 10 years for conservatively managed patients ($P = 0.028$).

Acute Mitral Regurgitation

Etiology and Presentation

Acute MR is usually due to an acute structural problem of the mitral valve apparatus—infection causing destruction of the mitral valve leaflets or chordae, spontaneous chordal rupture, or papillary muscle rupture from a myocardial infarction. In acute severe MR, a sudden volume overload is imposed on an unprepared left atrium and left ventricle, with a severe increase in LA pressure and a reduction in forward stroke volume and cardiac output.[8,11] Pulmonary edema usually occurs, sometimes even accompanied by cardiogenic shock. If the volume overload is not tolerated, urgent operation must be performed.

Clinical Evaluation

Acute severe MR must be considered in any patient presenting with hemodynamic compromise. In patients with acute severe MR, the physical examination itself may be misleading. The systolic murmur of MR may be soft, early in systole, and may even be absent because there is rapid equilibration of LA and LV pressures. Transthoracic echocardiography is useful to demonstrate a hyperdynamic left ventricle, which rules out a myocardial or pericardial etiology for the hemodynamic compromise. However, owing to problems with obtaining high-resolution imaging in a critically ill patient, transthoracic echocardiography may not be able to demonstrate a structural abnormality of the mitral valve. Transesophageal echocardiography should be performed to accurately assess the etiology and severity of MR. The structural abnormality causing the MR should be visualized, such as leaflet perforation, chordal rupture, or rupture of the papillary muscle. The presence of other abnormalities, such as vegetations and regional wall motion abnormalities, is useful to determine the etiology of the MR.

Visualization of an unsupported segment of the mitral apparatus coupled with an eccentric jet of MR on color-flow imaging in this clinical setting is all that is required to confirm acute severe MR. Cardiac catheterization is no longer required for diagnosis, and left ventriculography can be potentially harmful. A limited coronary angiogram should be performed prior to operation if the patient is hemodynamically stable.

Treatment

Medical therapy has a limited role in patients with acute severe MR causing hemodynamic compromise, mainly to stabilize the patient in preparation for operation. Intravenous diuretics are used to decrease pulmonary congestion, and afterload reduction with drugs such as nitroprusside will improve forward cardiac output and reduce filling pressures.[50] Antibiotics should be given if infective endocarditis is suspected. An intraaortic balloon pump can stabilize hemodynamics to a greater degree than medical therapy. The intra-aortic balloon should be placed if the patient is stable enough to go to the catheterization laboratory for preoperative coronary angiography. However, the ultimate goal is to proceed to operation as soon as possible for mitral valve repair or replacement.[51] The operative mortality for severe MR due to papillary muscle rupture is less than 10%, and the 5-year survival for patients surviving more than 30 days after surgery is 79% ± 4%.[52]

There may be a subset of patients who present with lesser degrees of acute MR. They have mild pulmonary congestion that responds initially to medical therapy. These patients may be the subset who have either a rupture of secondary chordae or a partial papillary muscle rupture associated with myocardial infarction. In these patients, early operation is still warranted because they have a high likelihood of acute deterioration during medical observation.[51,52]

Chronic Mitral Regurgitation

Etiology of Mitral Regurgitation

It is important to determine the etiology of chronic MR when one is considering timing of operation (Figure 20-20). Different surgical techniques are performed on the basis of valve morphology and underlying etiologies, and the performance of these different surgical techniques has important implications such as when a particular operation should be performed (see Chapter 21). The competent mitral valve depends on the coordinated function of all the components of the mitral valve apparatus: valve leaflets, annulus, papillary muscles, chordae tendineae, and the LV myocardium (see Chapter 2). The maintenance of the chordal-annular-subvalvular continuity and the mitral geometric relationships are important in the preservation of overall LV function. Under normal conditions, mitral valve competence is maintained during systole by both passive and active function of the mitral annulus and cusps, subvalvular apparatus, and ventricular wall. The posterior annulus is a muscular structure that shortens at end-systole with a sphincter-like contraction, thus narrowing the annulus and promoting leaflet coaptation. The papillary muscle–to-annular distance during normal posterolateral LV segmental contraction facilitates the closing motion of normal mitral valve leaflets, permitting their free edges to move centrally. Prolapse into the left atrium is prevented early in systole by papillary muscle contraction and shortening, which produce tension along the chordae and subsequently draw the free edges apically.

MR occurs when there is either an abnormality of the mitral valve leaflets, chordal apparatus, and papillary muscle structures or a functional and structural abnormality of the underlying supporting LV myocardium. A clinically relevant categorization for the etiology of chronic MR is to divide it into two categories: primary valvular abnormality and secondary MR caused by abnormality of supporting structures (Table 20-2).

In the United States, the most common cause of primary valvular abnormality causing severe MR is degenerative mitral valve disease. In degenerative mitral valve disease there is myxomatous degeneration of the mitral valve leaflets and elongated and redundant chordal apparatus (see Chapter 18). The thickened redundant leaflets prolapse into the left atrium, causing malcoaptation of leaflet edges and subsequent MR. Rupture of the chordae structures is not uncommon in degenerative mitral valve disease, especially in older men, which causes abrupt increases in severity of MR due to unsupported segments of the mitral leaflets. Other etiologies for primary valvular MR include rheumatic disease, senile calcific disease, and rare causes such as drug-induced mitral valve disease, healed infective endocarditis, and MR associated with systemic disease. It is important to be able to differentiate among these etiologies, because there is a higher chance of successful repair with degenerative MR, than with other etiologies of primary MR.

MR can also result from abnormalities of the underlying supporting structures (see Chapter 19). Ischemic MR occurs when myocardial ischemia or infarction interrupts the normal mechanics of contraction of the annulus, posterolateral myocardium, and shortening of the papillary muscle.[53-58] This disruption of the normal contraction sequence results in loss of cusp coaptation. Hypokinesia of the myocardial segments adjacent to the posterior annulus may disrupt annular contraction and early leaflet coaptation, and may even result in acute dilation during systole. Although

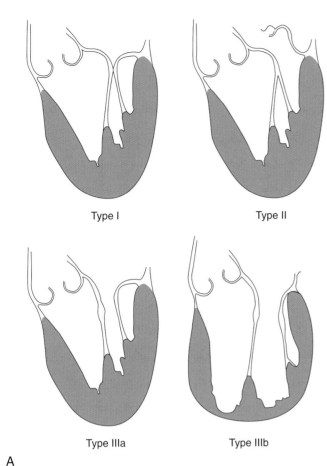

TABLE 20-2	Categorization of Etiology of Mitral Regurgitation
Primary Valvular Causes	
Degenerative	
Rheumatic	
Infective	
Other:	
Systemic disease	
Drug-induced	
Senile calcific	
Abnormal Supporting Structures	
Ischemic mitral regurgitation	
Functional mitral regurgitation	

Functional MR is due to progressive dilation of the left ventricle in the presence of a normal mitral valve apparatus.[59,60] The LV dilation leads to a circle of volume overload within an already dilated left ventricle, progression of annular dilation, increased LV wall tension, and loss of coaptation of mitral leaflets. Myocardial thinning and dilation, blunting of the aortomitral angle, widening of the intrapapillary muscle distance, increased leaflet tethering, and decreased leaflet closing forces all lead to altered forces generated by the papillary muscles. These morphologic changes combine to cause loss of the zone of coaptation and the central jet of MR.

Clinical Evaluation

The clinical evaluation of a patient with chronic MR requires a comprehensive history and physical examination as well as properly selected noninvasive and invasive testing. Two-dimensional and Doppler echocardiography are used to determine the etiology of MR and the LV response to MR as well as to evaluate the severity of MR. Direct visualization of mitral valve leaflets, chordal structure, and papillary muscle can help differentiate primary valvular abnormality (e.g., degenerative mitral valve disease or rheumatic mitral valve disease) from abnormalities of the supporting structures. A critical feature that must be assessed by echocardiography is feasibility of valve repair, which depends on the etiology of the MR.[61] The determination whether a valve can be repaired or replaced has significant implications for timing of operation. It is the degenerative mitral valve that has the highest chance of mitral repair. In diseases that produce calcification, fibrosis, and chordal shortening, such as rheumatic disease and calcific senile disease, and in MR associated with systemic diseases, there is a very low likelihood of valve repair. For patients with degenerative mitral valve disease, the overall morphology of the mitral valve leaflets, the primary abnormality causing the regurgitation, as well as surrounding structures such as the mitral annulus determine whether or not a valve can be successfully repaired.

In ischemic MR, there is tethering of the posterior leaflet and an akinetic posterolateral segment of the myocardium. This results in "tenting" of the mitral coaptation point and a posteriorly directed jet. The degree of tenting of the posterior leaflet on echocardiography may predict the outcome of a restrictive annuloplasty alone.[62] In functional MR related to LV dilation, there is usually a central jet of MR due to asymmetric loss of coaptation of the anterior and posterior leaflet.

It is important to take into consideration LV and LA size in the assessment of patients with MR, both of which can be accurately assessed by two-dimensional echocardiography. Measurement of LV systolic and diastolic dimensions on two-dimensional directed M-mode echocardiography is the most reproducible measurement of LV size in the absence of regional wall motion abnormalities.[1] LA dimension or volume is also an important part of the assessment of the patient with MR. Despite any quantitative

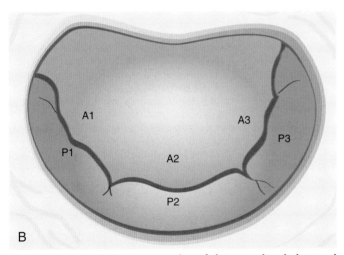

FIGURE 20-20 **Artist's representation of the normal and abnormal mitral valve. A,** Different etiologies of mitral regurgitation compared to the normal valve. *Type I,* normal; *Type II,* degenerative mitral regurgitation; *Type IIIa,* ischemic mitral regurgitation; *Type III b,* functional mitral regurgitation due to left ventricular dilation. **B,** *A1* to *A3,* segments of anterior mitral valve leaflet; *P1* to *P3,* segments of posterior mitral valve leaflet.

rupture of the head of the papillary muscle produces severe regurgitation in the acute setting, ischemic MR requires a chronically infarcted fibrotic and shortened papillary muscle in conjunction with an akinetic adjacent scar of the LV wall.[53-58] Overall, there is a restricted cusp motion due to leaflet tethering and tenting. The tenting may also occur in combination with annular dilation from dysfunction of the base of the heart. Because of the influence of cardiac loading conditions on LV geometry, the degree of MR depends on changes in load imposed on the left ventricle.

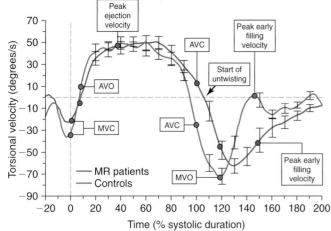

FIGURE 20-21 Evaluation of left ventricular torsion in patients with mitral regurgitation (MR). The average plots of all subjects for torsional velocity versus time are shown. The *blue line* refers to MR patients and the *red line* refers to control patients. *Error bars* are shown at 10% time point intervals and each represents one standard error. *Arrow* indicates the start of untwisting—that is, the point where the curve crosses the x-axis. Note that in patients with MR, there is delayed onset of the untwisting beyond aortic valve closure (AVC), peaking of untwisting after mitral valve opening (MVO), such that rapid untwisting persists during early filling, and ongoing untwisting during peak early filling velocities. *AVO,* aortic valve opening. *(From Borg AN, Harrison JL, Argyle RA, Ray SG. Left ventricular torsion in primary chronic mitral regurgitation. Heart 2008;94:597–603.)*

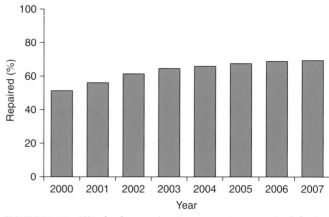

FIGURE 20-22 Mitral valve repair rates, percentage repaired, for isolated mitral regurgitation for the years 2000 to 2007. *(From Gammie JS, Sheng S, Griffith BP, et al. Trends in mitral valve surgery in the United States: results from the Society of Thoracic Surgeons Adult Cardiac Database. Ann Thorac Surg 2009;87:1431–9.)*

assessment of MR severity, a normal LV size precludes the possibility of surgically significant chronic MR. More sophisticated analyses of wall stress, preload-corrected EF, and LV elastance have been studied but do not add to the simple measurements of LV dimensions and EF. Noninvasive measurements of myocardial strain or LV torsion have promise for detection of early LV dysfunction[23,63] (Figure 20-21).

The comprehensive two-dimensional and Doppler echocardiographic examinations must also include a systematic approach to determining severity of MR. A comprehensive evaluation using multiple parameters is needed to fully assess the severity of MR. Because decisions for timing of operation for MR are based on the severity of MR, especially in the asymptomatic patient, it is of value to be able to quantitate the degree of MR. Measurement of regurgitant volume and ROA can now be obtained using proximal isovelocity surface area measurements, and these parameters should be a part of all echocardiographic examinations in which MR is a key element. Pulmonary pressure is an important parameter to obtain in all patients.

There may be situations in which a discrepancy is found between the severity of MR on history and physical examination and that on echocardiography. Right heart catheterization may be helpful in these instances by determining the pulmonary pressure, LA pressure, and the absence or presence of a large v wave on the pulmonary artery wedge pressure. Although a ventriculogram is not necessary in most patients with MR, left ventriculography can be useful in further aiding the decision whether the severity of MR is enough to warrant intervention when the physical findings do not correlate with the echocardiographic findings.

Exercise testing may be of benefit to evaluate a select subset of patients with MR. It is particularly useful in patients in whom the presence or absence of symptoms is unclear. Oxygen consumption testing may be performed, which can determine not only whether a limited exercise tolerance is present but whether or not the limitation is due to deconditioning or a cardiac etiology. With a cardiac etiology, there should be a plateau of the myocardial oxygen consumption at peak exercise concomitant with symptoms. The LV response or pulmonary response to exercise as

assessed by exercise echocardiography or radionuclide angiography may be of further benefit in determining timing of operation. Exercise-induced pulmonary hypertension (pulmonary artery systolic pressure >60 mm Hg) has been found to be an independent predictor of symptoms in patients with asymptomatic MR.[64]

Primary Valvular Mitral Regurgitation: Indications for Operation

The optimal timing for surgery in the patient with primary valvular MR depends on multiple factors.[1,6,13] These include the patient's symptoms, the severity of MR, and the response of the left ventricle to the volume overload. In addition, a major determinant for timing of operation is the available surgical expertise. The ability to repair rather than replace the valve may have a substantial influence on whether or not early surgery should be considered.[1] Although the number of patients undergoing mitral valve repair for MR has been rising over the past two decades in the United States and Canada, this technique is still underutilized. Of 47,000 patients undergoing isolated primary mitral valve operations in the United States in a 7-year period, the rate of repair increased from 51% in 2000 to only 69% in 2007[65] (Figure 20-22). In contrast, data from surgical centers that are experienced in mitral valve repair show that the frequency of repair is 95% or higher in patients with severe isolated MR due to degenerative disease.[5] There is a high variation in the number of mitral valve operations among all surgical centers, which also correlates with the rate of successful repair (see Figure ON20-13).[65] Because MV repair results in a lower operative mortality (1% to 2% vs. 6%), better preservation of LV function, and overall better survival than replacement, cardiologists are encouraged to refer candidates for mitral valve repair to these experienced surgical centers.[1]

The following indications for operation are based on the American College of Cardiology (ACC)/American Heart Association (AHA) guidelines for management of patients with valvular heart disease (Figure 20-23).[1]

SYMPTOMATIC PATIENTS: NORMAL LEFT VENTRICULAR FUNCTION

It is well documented that patients with severe MR who already have severe symptoms (NYHA class III or IV) despite normal LV function will benefit from mitral valve operation.[66] Normal LV function is defined as an EF greater than 60% and end-systolic dimension less than 40 mm on echocardiography.[1] In patients

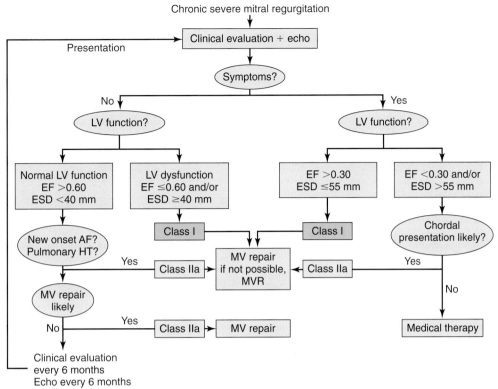

FIGURE 20-23 Management strategy for patients with chronic severe mitral regurgitation. Mitral valve repair may be performed in asymptomatic patients with normal left ventricular (LV) function if performed by an experienced surgical team and the likelihood of successful mitral valve repair is higher than 90%. New York Heart Association functional classes are shown. *AF,* Atrial fibrillation; *echo,* echocardiography; *EF,* ejection fraction; *ESD,* end-systolic dimension; *HT,* hypertension; *MV,* mitral valve; *MVR,* mitral valve replacement. *(From Bonow RO, Carabello B, Chatterjee K, et al. ACC/AHA 2006 guidelines for the management of patients with valvular heart disease: a report of the American College of Cardiology/American Heart Association Task Force on Practice Guidelines [writing committee to revise the 1998 Guidelines for the Management of Patients With Valvular Heart Disease]. Circulation 2006;114:e84–231.)*

with small body size, an end-systolic dimension greater than 22 mm/m^2 may be used.[16,33] The benefit in terms of relief of symptoms and prolongation of life occurs irrespective of whether the valve can be repaired or replaced. The occurrence of severe symptoms indicates an inadequate ability of the left ventricle to respond to the volume overload, and once symptoms occur, there is a progressive downhill course with medical treatment alone.

Even patients with mild symptoms (NYHA class II) should be considered for operation. These patients with mild symptoms may be having a gradual insidious onset of symptoms but will note a decrease in exercise tolerance with time. The mildly symptomatic patients are most likely entering the transition phase to LV decompensation, because even mild symptoms indicate that the LV compensatory mechanisms are becoming overwhelmed by the volume overload. Therefore, patients with any symptoms (NYHA classes II, III, and IV), preserved LV function, and severe MR due to a primary valvular abnormality should be considered for operation.[1]

SYMPTOMATIC OR ASYMPTOMATIC PATIENTS: LEFT VENTRICULAR DYSFUNCTION

Mitral valve operation is indicated for patients with severe MR due to a primary valvular abnormality when LV dysfunction is demonstrated on echocardiography (EF ≤60% or end-systolic dimension ≥40 mm).[1] This applies to patients who are symptomatic but also to those who are asymptomatic. The latter patients have already progressed to the stage of irreversible LV dysfunction from the long-standing volume overload. Although it would have been ideal to have operated on such patients before they reached this stage, operation will likely prevent further deterioration in LV function and improve long-term outlook. Operation should be considered irrespective of whether the valve can be repaired or

replaced, although valve repair is preferable, given the better effect on LV function.

SYMPTOMATIC PATIENTS: SEVERE LEFT VENTRICULAR DYSFUNCTION

There is a subset of patients presenting with severe MR that is "end stage," in whom LV function has significantly deteriorated (EF <30%, end-systolic dimension >55 mm). If a primary valvular abnormality is causing the MR, a concomitant myocardial process is almost always contributing to the severe LV dysfunction. Nonetheless, a careful assessment of valve morphology and quantitation of the severity of MR are important in this distinction, because surgery may still be contemplated. Even though the operative risk is increased and persistent LV dysfunction will be present postoperatively, operation may be performed to improve symptoms and prevent progressive LV deterioration. In this subset of patients, it is of great importance to ensure that the chordal apparatus can be preserved to prevent acute LV dilation; thus, these highest-risk patients are best treated with mitral valve repair.

ASYMPTOMATIC PATIENTS: NORMAL LEFT VENTRICULAR FUNCTION

It is the management of asymptomatic patients with severe MR due to a primary valvular abnormality who maintain normal systolic function that has been most controversial.[1,2,4,11,19,67] If such patients are followed up until they reach the "cutoff" values already described (EF <60%, end-systolic dimension >40 mm), the patient has already entered into the decompensation stage of LV dysfunction.[11,19,67] Their postoperative survival is already reduced, and they have a high incidence of postoperative LV systolic dysfunction and eventual recurrent heart failure.[42,43] Thus,

322

there has been impetus to operate before the onset of LV dysfunction to prevent the sequelae of chronic severe MR.

There are no randomized data on which to base a recommendation of this approach to all patients. However, in experienced centers, there is a move to operate on patients who maintain normal systolic function if the likelihood of successful valve repair is high. This change in paradigm for early operation is based on multiple advances in our understanding of these patients with MR, as has been discussed previously. If severe MR is truly present, the natural history studies have uniformly indicated a high likelihood of development of symptoms and/or LV dysfunction over the course of 6 to 10 years.[14,27,30,68] The greater utilization of artificial chordae for repair of the anterior or severe bileaflet prolapse has resulted in a higher success rate for mitral valve repair.[69,70] Early repair can now be performed with a mortality less than 1% in experienced centers[65] and a chance of successful repair higher than 90%. The long-term outcome for the asymptomatic patient who undergoes early operation is excellent, with an overall survival comparable to that of an age-matched, control-matched population (see Figure ON20-14).[2,3]

For operation to be recommended in these patients, they must have several features. First, it is important to document severe MR. Thus, correlation of the physical examination and the diagnostic modalities is essential, and quantitative Doppler echocardiographic assessment is helpful. It is also important to correlate the severity of MR with the effect on the left ventricle and left atrium. Patients with severe MR by necessity have LV and LA enlargement. Finally, the feasibility of mitral valve repair is determined by the morphology of the mitral valve and the surgical expertise available.

Thus, in institutions with a surgical expertise in mitral valve repair, it is reasonable to proceed with operation in the asymptomatic patient with severe MR and normal systolic function.[1] This decision must be individualized for each patient, however, and the operative risk, patient lifestyle, and patient preference must be taken into consideration. These "early operations" should be performed only in experienced centers in which the the mortality is less than 1% and the likelihood of repair exceeds 90%.[5,70]

There is still controversy in regard to the optimal approach in this patient population. Not all institutions have surgical expertise in mitral valve repair. If a mitral repair cannot be done with a high likelihood of success, early operation in the asymptomatic patient with preserved LV function may not be warranted. Several series have shown a good outcome for patients with "watchful waiting," in which patients with MR were monitored medically until they reached the criterion of LV dysfunction (EF <60%).[4,15] When these guidelines were followed, no patients experienced residual LV dysfunction following operation, but a substantial proportion eventually required operation. Nearly 50% of all patients had symptoms of either LV dysfunction or atrial fibrillation by 8 years (Figure 20-24). Adherence to this more conservative approach does require meticulous and continuous follow-up of the patient, which may not be possible for every patient and care facility. In addition, there is always "unexpected LV dysfunction" which continues to occur even when patients undergo operation with a normal EF and a small end-systolic dimension. Thus, if this conservative approach is undertaken, the patient and physician must be willing to continue with frequent follow-up visits, with the understanding that the development of irreversible LV dysfunction cannot be predicted.

Other factors that may influence the decision to proceed with earlier operation include marked enlargement of the left atrium (>60 mL/m²),[32] elevated BNP level,[33,34] and pulmonary hypertension (pulmonary artery systolic pressure >50 mm Hg).[16,30,64]

ATRIAL FIBRILLATION

In patients with MR due to degenerative disease, there is a high risk for development of atrial fibrillation, which is independently associated with high risk of cardiac death or heart failure.[71]

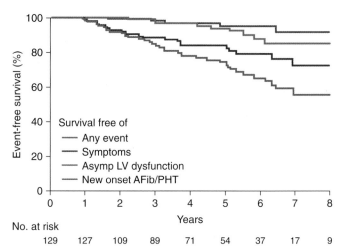

FIGURE 20-24 Kaplan-Meier event-free survival for patients with asymptomatic severe degenerative mitral regurgitation managed according to a watchful waiting strategy. *AFib,* atrial fibrillation; *LV,* left ventricular; *PHT,* pulmonary hypertension. *(From Rosenheck R, Rader F, Klaar U, et al. Outcome of watchful waiting in asymptomatic severe mitral regurgitation. Circulation 2006;113:2238–44.)*

Preoperative atrial fibrillation is an independent predictor of reduced long-term survival after mitral valve surgery for chronic severe MR.[72-74] Predictors of postoperative atrial fibrillation are an enlarged left atrium and a prolonged duration of preoperative atrial fibrillation; in one study, persistent atrial fibrillation after surgery occurred in 80% of patients who had preoperative atrial fibrillation for 3 months or longer but in no patient who had preoperative atrial fibrillation for less than 3 months.[72]

To prevent the adverse long-term sequelae of atrial fibrillation, the onset of this condition is an indication for operation in the patient with severe MR and a valve suitable for repair.[1] In patients presenting for mitral valve operation with chronic atrial fibrillation, a concomitant maze procedure or pulmonary vein isolation should be considered.[75-77]

GUIDELINE ADHERENCE FOR OPERATION

Despite the poor natural history of untreated severe MR and the excellent results of operation, it is not uncommon that eligible patients do not undergo surgery. In one study using the American College of Cardiology/American Heart Association guidelines,[1] one or more accepted indications for operation were present in nearly three of every four patients from a large tertiary referral center who did not undergo surgery.[78] Those unoperated patients had a high mortality rate, even though their perioperative mortality risk was no greater than that of a concomitant group of patients who were sent for surgery. This study highlights the necessity of a comprehensive and knowledgeable team for evaluation of patients with severe valve disease. Although there has been a trend toward earlier operation, before the onset of severe symptoms, almost 50% of mitral valve procedures are still being performed in patients with NYHA class III or IV symptoms (Figure 20-25).[65]

Ischemic Mitral Regurgitation: Indications for Operation

Many patients with ischemic heart disease have ischemic MR, and the presence of ischemic MR has subsequently been shown to have a significant impact on prognosis (see Figure ON20-15).[79-81] Some degree of ischemic MR is detected in as many as 40% of individuals suffering from acute myocardial infarction.[79,80] Those who have even mild degrees of ischemic MR after infarction have a cardiovascular risk two to four times higher than those without

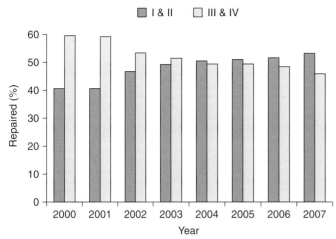

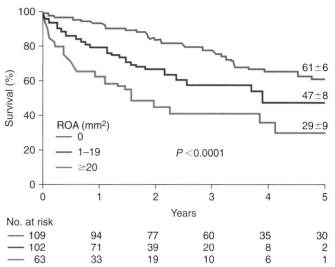

FIGURE 20-25   New York Heart Association functional class in patients undergoing mitral valve surgery for the years 2000 to 2007. *(From Gammie JS, Sheng S, Griffith BP, et al. Trends in mitral valve surgery in the United States: results from the Society of Thoracic Surgeons Adult Cardiac Database. Ann Thorac Surg 2009;87:1431–9.)*

FIGURE 20-26   Survival of patients after the diagnosis of ischemic mitral regurgitation. Patients are subdivided according to the degree of mitral regurgitation as graded by the regurgitant orifice area (ROA). *(From Grigioni F, Enriquez-Sarano M, Zehr KJ, et al. Ischemic mitral regurgitation: long-term outcome and prognostic implications with quantitative Doppler assessment. Circulation 2001;103:1759–64.)*

ischemic MR, both within the first 2 weeks and over the long term after myocardial infarction. Those patients with ischemic MR have greater degrees of heart failure and more likely to experience recurrent myocardial infarction than those without ischemic MR.[79,80] The more severe the MR, the poorer the survival (Figure 20-26).[79] In patients coming to coronary artery bypass grafting, one out of 10 have some degree of ischemic MR, and these patients have a higher operative mortality and lower long-term survival than patients without MR.

Revascularization alone can result in improvement of the ischemic MR in selected patients, because MR arises when ischemia or infarction interrupts the normal interaction between the mitral annulus, subvalvular apparatus, and LV wall.[82,83] It is difficult to determine whether revascularization alone will influence the severity of MR in an individual patient. The presence of viable myocardium and absence of dyssynchrony may help identify which patients will experience improvement with revascularization alone.[84,85] In addition, changes in load will significantly influence the severity of MR with ischemic MR, particularly when the patient is undergoing cardiopulmonary bypass. The late survival after bypass alone in the patient with ischemic MR has been reported to be between 60% and 94% at 3 years and 52% and 81% at 5 years.[83,86-88] In patients with only mild ischemic MR, 3-year survival is reported to be between 84% and 94%. In patients with moderate MR, the 3-year survival varies from 61% to 84% following bypass alone, with only a modest improvement in NYHA functional status and angina severity score.[83,86-88]

In the past, it was believed that the addition of mitral valve repair or replacement to bypass operation doubled the operative risk. However, later series have shown a lower operative mortality when mitral valve operation is added to coronary bypass grafting. It is still unclear whether mitral valve repair has become the preferred method to treat MR with concomitant coronary artery bypass grafting.[37,86,89-91] Residual regurgitation of moderate or even mild degree appears to affect late survival negatively.[92] Newer surgical techniques, such as posterior leaflet extension[93] and chordal cutting,[94] may enhance the long-term outcome of valve repair.[95] A survival advantage for combined procedures over isolated bypass operation in selected patient, has been reported by some investigators.[90,96,97] Others have not found a survival benefit when mitral repair was added to bypass operation (see Figures ON20-16 and ON20-17).[37,98] Overall survival after combined coronary bypass grafting and mitral valve surgery in patients with EF less than 45% is mostly influenced by factors related to patient condition at the time of surgery rather than to whether repair or replacement was performed.[91]

The surgical approach to ischemic MR remains controversial.[86,95,98,99] Most would agree that the finding of severe MR on echocardiography or angiography constitutes the need for mitral intervention at the time of bypass operation. Patients in whom there is only mild ischemic MR would probably not benefit from any operative intervention. However, there is debate regarding the management of patients with moderate degrees of ischemic MR, not only in the optimal treatment but when "mild" becomes "moderate." Prior studies that have evaluated the outcomes of the different approaches to ischemic MR have all been retrospective, with significant selection bias. Prospective randomized trials are under way that we hope will provide guidance for treatment of this subset of patients in the future.

Functional Mitral Regurgitation: Indications for Operation

Functional MR is due to progressive dilation of the annular-ventricular apparatus with altered LV geometry and a resultant loss of leaflet coaptation. The severity of MR in patients with severe LV dysfunction is highly dependent on the load on the heart. Thus, with aggressive medical therapy to decrease LV volume and annular dilation, a significant decrease in dynamic MR can occur. However, some patients continue to have severe MR despite optimal medical therapy.

In these patients with severe functional MR, there is a significant decrease in the efficiency of LV contraction and work expended by the left ventricle because the work used to generate regurgitant flow does not contribute to effective forward cardiac output. Some authorities believe that eliminating reversal of flow alleviates the excess of work placed on the left ventricle. With mitral valve repair to change the detrimental alterations in the annular-ventricular unit, both valve competency and LV function may be restored.[59,60,100]

Valve repair appears to be relatively safe in this patient population at high risk for operation, which consists of patients with severe functional MR, NYHA class II to IV symptoms, EF less than 35%, and a dilated left ventricle.[59,100] Several studies have shown an overall operative mortality of 1.5% to 5%, along with improvement in NYHA class for each patient. There were also improvements in EF, cardiac output, and end-diastolic volumes with a reduction in sphericity index and regurgitant fraction, all changes consistent with reverse remodeling.

However, these data have not been replicated in other centers.[101] Thus, the optimal indication and therapy for patients with functional MR remains unknown. Until more data are available, aggressive medical therapy, including the use of biventricular pacing, should be considered the first line of care for patients with severe LV dysfunction and functional MR. We reserve operation for patients with significant functional MR who remain symptomatic despite optimal medical treatment.

REFERENCES

1. Bonow RO, Carabello B, Chatterjee K, et al. ACC/AHA 2006 guidelines for the management of patients with valvular heart disease: a report of the American College of Cardiology/American Heart Association Task Force on Practice Guidelines (writing committee to revise the 1998 Guidelines for the Management of Patients With Valvular Heart Disease): developed in collaboration with the Society of Cardiovascular Anesthesiologists: endorsed by the Society for Cardiovascular Angiography and Interventions and the Society of Thoracic Surgeons. Circulation 2006;114:e84–231.
2. Enriquez-Sarano M, Orszulak TA, Schaff HV, et al. Mitral regurgitation: a new clinical perspective. Mayo Clin Proc 1997;72:1034–43.
3. Enriquez-Sarano M, Schaff HV, Frye RL. Early surgery for mitral regurgitation: the advantages of youth. Circulation 1997;96:4121–3.
4. Rosenhek R, Rader F, Klaar U, et al. Outcome of watchful waiting in asymptomatic severe mitral regurgitation. Circulation 2006;113:2238–44.
5. Schaff HV. Asymptomatic severe mitral valve regurgitation. Circulation 2009;119:768–9.
6. Carabello BA. The current therapy for mitral regurgitation. J Am Coll Cardiol 2008;52:319–26.
7. Crawford MH, Souchek J, Oprian CA, et al. Determinants of survival and left ventricular performance after mitral valve replacement. Department of Veterans Affairs Cooperative Study on Valvular Heart Disease. Circulation 1990;81:1173–81.
8. Carabello BA. Mitral regurgitation: basic pathophysiologic principles. Mod Concept Cardiovasc Dis 1988;57:53–8.
9. Carabello BA, Nolan SP, McGuire LB. Assessment of preoperative left ventricular function in patients with mitral regurgitation: value of the end-systolic wall stress-end-systolic volume ratio. Circulation 1981;64:1212–7.
10. Schuler G, Peterson KL, Johnson A, et al. Temporal response of left ventricular performance to mitral valve surgery. Circulation 1979;59:1218–31.
11. Carabello BA, Crawford Jr FA. Valvular heart disease.[erratum appears in N Engl J Med 1997 Aug 14;337(7):507]. N Engl J Med 1997;337:32–41.
12. Carabello BA, Williams H, Gash AK, et al. Hemodynamic predictors of outcome in patients undergoing valve replacement.[erratum appears in Circulation 1987;75:650]. Circulation 1986;74:1309–16.
13. Gaasch WH, Meyer TE. Left ventricular response to mitral regurgitation. Circulation 2008;118:2298–303.
14. Ling LH, Enriquez-Sarano M, Seward JB, et al. Clinical outcome of mitral regurgitation due to flail leaflet. N Engl J Med 1996;335:1417–23.
15. Rosen SE, Borer JS, Hochreiter C, et al. Natural history of the asymptomatic/minimally symptomatic patient with severe mitral regurgitation secondary to mitral valve prolapse and normal right and left ventricular performance. Am J Cardiol 1994;74:374–80.
16. Tribouilloy C, Grigioni F, Aviernos JF, et al. Survival implication of left ventricular end-systolic diameter in mitral regurgitation due to flail leaflets: a long-term follow-up multicenter study. J Am Coll Cardiol 2009;54:1961–8.
17. Enriquez-Sarano M, Schaff HV, Orszulak TA, et al. Valve repair improves the outcome of surgery for mitral regurgitation: a multivariate analysis. Circulation 1995;91:1022–8.
18. Ling LH, Enriquez-Sarano M, Seward JB, et al. Early surgery in patients with mitral regurgitation due to flail leaflets: a long-term outcome study. Circulation 1997;96:1819–25.
19. Gaasch WH, John RM, Aurigemma GP. Managing asymptomatic patients with chronic mitral regurgitation. Chest 1995;108:842–7.
20. Gaasch WH, Zile MR. Left ventricular function after surgical correction of chronic mitral regurgitation. Eur Heart J 1991;12(Suppl B):48–51.
21. Wisenbaugh T, Skudicky D, Sareli P. Prediction of outcome after valve replacement for rheumatic mitral regurgitation in the era of chordal preservation. Circulation 1994;89:191–7.
22. Zile MR, Gaasch WH, Carroll JD, et al. Chronic mitral regurgitation: predictive value of preoperative echocardiographic indexes of left ventricular function and wall stress. J Am Coll Cardiol 1984;3(2 Pt 1):235–42.
23. Ahmed MI, Gladden JD, Litovsky SH, et al. Increased oxidative stress and cardiomyocyte myofibrillar degeneration in patients with chronic isolated mitral regurgitation and ejection fraction >60%. J Am Coll Cardiol 2010;55:671–9.
24. Mirsky I, Corin WJ, Murakami T, et al. Correction for preload in assessment of myocardial contractility in aortic and mitral valve disease: application of the concept of systolic myocardial stiffness. Circulation 1988;78:68–80.
25. Wisenbaugh T. Does normal pump function belie muscle dysfunction in patients with chronic severe mitral regurgitation? Circulation 1988;77:515–25.
26. Enriquez-Sarano M, Basmadjian AJ, Rossi A, et al. Progression of mitral regurgitation: a prospective Doppler echocardiographic study. J Am Coll Cardiol 1999;34:1137–44.
27. Grigioni F, Tribouilloy C, Avierinos JF, et al. Outcomes in mitral regurgitation due to flail leaflets a multicenter European study. JACC Cardiovasc Imaging 2008;1:133–41.
28. Grigioni F, Enriquez-Sarano M, Ling LH, et al. Sudden death in mitral regurgitation due to flail leaflet. J Am Coll Cardiol 1999;34:2078–85.
29. Enriquez-Sarano M, Avierinos J-F, Messika-Zeitoun D, et al. Quantitative determinants of the outcome of asymptomatic mitral regurgitation. N Engl J Med 2005;352:875–83.
30. Kang D-H, Kim JH, Rim JH, et al. Comparison of early surgery versus conventional treatment in asymptomatic severe mitral regurgitation. Circulation 2009;119:797–804.
31. Rusinaru D, Tribouilloy C, Grigioni F, et al. Left atrial size is a potent predictor of mortality in mitral regurgitation due to flail leaflets: results from a large international multicenter study. Circ Cardiovasc Imaging 2011;4:473–81.
32. Le Tourneau T, Messika-Zeitoun D, Russo A, et al. Impact of left atrial volume on clinical outcome in organic mitral regurgitation. J Am Coll Cardiol 2010;56:570–8.
33. Pizarro R, Bazzino OO, Oberti PF, et al. Prospective validation of the prognostic usefulness of brain natriuretic peptide in asymptomatic patients with chronic severe mitral regurgitation. J Am Coll Cardiol 2009;54:1099–106.
34. Detaint D, Messika-Zeitoun D, Avierinos J-F, et al. B-type natriuretic peptide in organic mitral regurgitation: determinants and impact on outcome. Circulation 2005;111:2391–7.
35. Sutton TM, Stewart RAH, Gerber IL, et al. Plasma natriuretic peptide levels increase with symptoms and severity of mitral regurgitation. J Am Coll Cardiol 2003;41:2280–7.
36. Suri RM, Schaff HV, Dearani JA, et al. Recurrent mitral regurgitation after repair: should the mitral valve be re-repaired? J Thorac Cardiovasc Surg 2006;132:1390–7.
37. Magne J, Girerd N, Sénéchal M, et al. Mitral repair versus replacement for ischemic mitral regurgitation. Circulation 2009;120(11 suppl 1):S104–11.
38. David TE, Burns RJ, Bacchus CM, et al. Mitral valve replacement for mitral regurgitation with and without preservation of chordae tendineae. J Thorac Cardiovasc Surg 1984;88:718–25.
39. Hennein HA, Swain JA, McIntosh CL, et al. Comparative assessment of chordal preservation versus chordal resection during mitral valve replacement. J Thorac Cardiovasc Surg 1990;99:828–36; discussion 836–7.
40. Horskotte D, Schulte HD, Bircks W, et al. The effect of chordal preservation on late outcome after mitral valve replacement: a randomized study. J Heart Valve Dis 1993;2:150–8.
41. Rozich JD, Carabello BA, Usher BW, et al. Mitral valve replacement with and without chordal preservation in patients with chronic mitral regurgitation: mechanisms for differences in postoperative ejection performance. Circulation 1992;86:1718–26.
42. Enriquez-Sarano M, Tajik AJ, Schaff HV, et al. Echocardiographic prediction of survival after surgical correction of organic mitral regurgitation. Circulation 1994;90:830–7.
43. Enriquez-Sarano M, Tajik AJ, Schaff HV, et al. Echocardiographic prediction of left ventricular function after correction of mitral regurgitation: results and clinical implications. J Am Coll Cardiol 1994;24:1536–43.
44. Essop MR. Predictors of left ventricular dysfunction following mitral valve repair for mitral regurgitation. J Am Coll Cardiol 2004;43:1925.
45. Dujardin KS, Seward JB, Orszulak TA, et al. Outcome after surgery for mitral regurgitation: determinants of postoperative morbidity and mortality. J Heart Valve Dis 1997;6:17–21.
46. Mohty D, Enriquez-Sarano M. The long-term outcome of mitral valve repair for mitral valve prolapse. Curr Cardiol Rep 2002;4:104–10.
47. Ashikhmina EA, Schaff HV, Ommen SR, et al. Intraoperative direct measurement of left ventricular outflow tract gradients to guide surgical myectomy for hypertrophic cardiomyopathy. J Thorac Cardiovasc Surg 2011;142:53–9.
48. Suri RM, Schaff HV, Dearani JA, et al. Determinants of early decline in ejection fraction after surgical correction of mitral regurgitation. J Thorac Cardiovasc Surg 2008;136:442–7.
49. Avierinos J-F, Inamo J, Grigioni F, et al. Sex differences in morphology and outcomes of mitral valve prolapse. Ann Intern Med 2008;149:787–95.
50. Yoran C, Yellin EL, Becker RM, et al. Mechanism of reduction of mitral regurgitation with vasodilator therapy. Am J Cardiol 1979;43:773–7.
51. Nishimura RA, Schaff HV, Gersh BJ, et al. Early repair of mechanical complications after acute myocardial infarction. JAMA 1986;256:47–50.
52. Russo A, Suri RM, Grigioni F, et al. Clinical outcome after surgical correction of mitral regurgitation due to papillary muscle rupture. Circulation 2008;118:1528–34.
53. Kumanohoso T, Otsuji Y, Yoshifuku S, et al. Mechanism of higher incidence of ischemic mitral regurgitation in patients with inferior myocardial infarction: quantitative analysis of left ventricular and mitral valve geometry in 103 patients with prior myocardial infarction. J Thorac Cardiovasc Surg 2003;125:135–43.
54. Levine RA. Dynamic mitral regurgitation—more than meets the eye. N Engl J Med 2004;351:1681–4.
55. Levine RA, Schwammenthal E. Ischemic mitral regurgitation on the threshold of a solution: from paradoxes to unifying concepts. Circulation 2005;112:745–58.
56. Otsuji Y, Gilon D, Jiang L, et al. Restricted diastolic opening of the mitral leaflets in patients with left ventricular dysfunction: evidence for increased valve tethering. J Am Coll Cardiol 1998;32:398–404.
57. Otsuji Y, Handschumacher MD, Schwammenthal E, et al. Insights from three-dimensional echocardiography into the mechanism of functional mitral regurgitation: direct in vivo demonstration of altered leaflet tethering geometry. Circulation 1997;96:1999–2008.
58. Yiu SF, Enriquez-Sarano M, Tribouilloy C, et al. Determinants of the degree of functional mitral regurgitation in patients with systolic left ventricular dysfunction: a quantitative clinical study. Circulation 2000;102:1400–6.
59. Bolling SF. Mitral reconstruction in cardiomyopathy. J Heart Valve Dis 2002;11(Suppl 1):S26–31.
60. Bolling SF, Pagani FD, Deeb GM, et al. Intermediate-term outcome of mitral reconstruction in cardiomyopathy. J Thorac Cardiovasc Surg 1998;115:381–6; discussion 387–8.

61. Enriquez-Sarano M, Schaff HV, Frye RL. Mitral regurgitation: what causes the leakage is fundamental to the outcome of valve repair. Circulation 2003;108:253–6.
62. Magne J, Lancellotti P, Pierard LA. Exercise pulmonary hypertension in asymptomatic degenerative mitral regurgitation. Circulation 2007;122:33–41.
63. Borg AN, Harrison JL, Argyle RA, et al. Left ventricular torsion in primary chronic mitral regurgitation. Heart 2008;94:597–603.
64. Magne J, Lancellotti P, Piérard LA. Exercise pulmonary hypertension in asymptomatic degenerative mitral regurgitation. Circulation 2010;122(1):33–41.
65. Gammie JS, Sheng S, Griffith BP, et al. Trends in mitral valve surgery in the United States: results from the Society of Thoracic Surgeons Adult Cardiac Database. Ann Thorac Surg 2009;87:1431–9.
66. Tribouilloy CM, Enriquez-Sarano M, Schaff HV, et al. Impact of preoperative symptoms on survival after surgical correction of organic mitral regurgitation: rationale for optimizing surgical indications. Circulation 1999;99:400–5.
67. Ross Jr J. The timing of surgery for severe mitral regurgitation. N Engl J Med 1996;335:1456–8.
68. St John Sutton MG, Plappert T, Abraham WT, et al. Effect of cardiac resynchronization therapy on left ventricular size and function in chronic heart failure. Circulation 2003;107:1985–90.
69. Salvador L, Mirone S, Bianchini R, et al. A 20-year experience with mitral valve repair with artificial chordae in 608 patients. J Thorac Cardiovasc Surg 2008;135:1280–7.
70. Fedak PWM, McCarthy PM, Bonow RO. Evolving concepts and technologies in mitral valve repair. Circulation 2008;117:963–74.
71. Grigioni F, Avierinos JF, Ling LH, et al. Atrial fibrillation complicating the course of degenerative mitral regurgitation: determinants and long-term outcome. J Am Coll Cardiol 2002;40:84–92.
72. Chua YL, Schaff HV, Orszulak TA, et al. Outcome of mitral valve repair in patients with preoperative atrial fibrillation: should the maze procedure be combined with mitral valvuloplasty? J Thorac Cardiovasc Surg 1994;107:408–15.
73. Eguchi K, Ohtaki E, Matsumura T, et al. Pre-operative atrial fibrillation as the key determinant of outcome of mitral valve repair for degenerative mitral regurgitation. Eur Heart J 2005;26:1866–72.
74. Lim E, Barlow CW, Hosseinpour AR, et al. Influence of atrial fibrillation on outcome following mitral valve repair. Circulation 2001;104(12 Suppl 1):I59–63.
75. Bando K, Kasegawa H, Okada Y, et al. Impact of preoperative and postoperative atrial fibrillation on outcome after mitral valvuloplasty for nonischemic mitral regurgitation. J Thorac Cardiovasc Surg 2005;129:1032–40.
76. Handa N, Schaff HV, Morris JJ, et al. Outcome of valve repair and the Cox maze procedure for mitral regurgitation and associated atrial fibrillation. J Thorac Cardiovasc Surg 1999;118:628–35.
77. Kobayashi J, Sasako Y, Bando K, et al. Eight-year experience of combined valve repair for mitral regurgitation and maze procedure. J Heart Valve Dis 2002;11:165–71; discussion 171–2.
78. Bach DS, Awais M, Gurm HS, et al. Failure of guideline adherence for intervention in patients with severe mitral regurgitation. J Am Coll Cardiol 2009;54:860–5.
79. Grigioni F, Enriquez-Sarano M, Zehr KJ, et al. Ischemic mitral regurgitation: long-term outcome and prognostic implications with quantitative Doppler assessment. Circulation 2001;103:1759–64.
80. Lamas GA, Mitchell GF, Flaker GC, et al. Clinical significance of mitral regurgitation after acute myocardial infarction. Survival and Ventricular Enlargement Investigators. Circulation 1997;96:827–33.
81. Schroder JN, Williams ML, Hata JA, et al. Impact of mitral valve regurgitation evaluated by intraoperative transesophageal echocardiography on long-term outcomes after coronary artery bypass grafting. Circulation 2005;112(9 Suppl):I293–8.
82. Bursi F, Enriquez-Sarano M, Nkomo VT, et al. Heart failure and death after myocardial infarction in the community: the emerging role of mitral regurgitation. Circulation 2005;111:295–301.
83. Duarte IG, Shen Y, MacDonald MJ, et al. Treatment of moderate mitral regurgitation and coronary disease by coronary bypass alone: late results. Ann Thorac Surg 1999;68:426–30.
84. Penicka M, Linkova H, Lang O, et al. Predictors of improvement of unrepaired moderate ischemic mitral regurgitation in patients undergoing elective isolated coronary artery bypass graft surgery. Circulation 2009;120:1474–81.
85. Mihaljevic T, Gillinov AM, Sabik JF. Functional ischemic mitral regurgitation. Circulation 2009;120:1459–61.
86. Hamner CE, Sundt 3rd TM. Trends in the surgical management of ischemic mitral regurgitation. Curr Cardiol Rep 2003;5:116–24.
87. Prifti E, Bonacchi M, Frati G, et al. Ischemic mitral valve regurgitation grade II-III: correction in patients with impaired left ventricular function undergoing simultaneous coronary revascularization. J Heart Valve Dis 2001;10:754–62.
88. Prifti E, Bonacchi M, Frati G, et al. Should mild-to-moderate and moderate ischemic mitral regurgitation be corrected in patients with impaired left ventricular function undergoing simultaneous coronary revascularization? J Cardiac Surg 2001;16:473–83.
89. Gillinov AM, Wierup PN, Blackstone EH, et al. Is repair preferable to replacement for ischemic mitral regurgitation? J Thorac Cardiovasc Surg 2001;122:1125–41.
90. Grossi EA, Goldberg JD, LaPietra A, et al. Ischemic mitral valve reconstruction and replacement: comparison of long-term survival and complications. J Thorac Cardiovasc Surg 2001;122:1107–24.
91. Maltais S, Schaff HV, Daly RC, et al. Mitral regurgitation surgery in patients with ischemic cardiomyopathy and ischemic mitral regurgitation: factors that influence survival. J Thorac Cardiovasc Surg 2011;142:995–1001.
92. Aklog L, Filsoufi F, Flores KQ, et al. Does coronary artery bypass grafting alone correct moderate ischemic mitral regurgitation? Circulation 2001;104(12 Suppl 1):I68–75.
93. de Varennes B, Chaturvedi R, Sidhu S, et al. Initial results of posterior leaflet extension for severe type IIIb ischemic mitral regurgitation. Circulation 2009;119:2837–43.
94. Messas E, Pouzet B, Touchot B, et al. Efficacy of chordal cutting to relieve chronic persistent ischemic mitral regurgitation. Circulation 2003;108 (Suppl 1):II111–5.
95. Bolman RM. Have we found the surgical solution for ischemic mitral regurgitation? Circulation 2009;119:2755–7.
96. Adams DH, Filsoufi F, Aklog L. Surgical treatment of the ischemic mitral valve. J Heart Valve Dis 2002;11 (Suppl 1):S21–5.
97. Harris KM, Sundt 3rd TM, Aeppli D, et al. Can late survival of patients with moderate ischemic mitral regurgitation be impacted by intervention on the valve? Ann Thorac Surg 2002;74:1468–75.
98. Mihaljevic T, Lam BK, Rajeswaran J, et al. Impact of mitral valve annuloplasty combined with revascularization in patients with functional ischemic mitral regurgitation. J Am Coll Cardiol 2007;49:2191–201.
99. Badiwala MV, Verma S, Rao V. Surgical management of ischemic mitral regurgitation. Circulation 2009;120:1287–93.
100. Grossi EA, Crooke GA. Mitral valve surgery in heart failure: insights from the ACORN clinical trial. J Thorac Cardiovasc Surg 2006;132:455–6.
101. Wu AH, Aaronson KD, Bolling SF, et al. Impact of mitral valve annuloplasty on mortality risk in patients with mitral regurgitation and left ventricular systolic dysfunction. J Am Coll Cardiol 2005;45:381–7.

CHAPTER 21

Mitral Valve Repair and Replacement

Javier G. Castillo and David H. Adams

Key Points

- The mitral valve is a complex three-dimensional assembly of independent anatomic components including the annulus, the leaflets and commissures, the chordae tendineae, the papillary muscles, and the left ventricle. The presence of abnormalities (etiologic implications) in any of these components (lesions) may cause the alteration in closure (dysfunction) against left ventricular (LV) pressure and, consequently, mitral regurgitation (MR) or stenosis.

- Degenerative disease is the most prevalent cause of MR in Western countries. In the setting of severe MR, surgery is the only definitive treatment and mitral valve repair is currently the "gold standard." However, mitral valve repair is underutilized in patients with complex lesions.

- During the last decade, several variables have been identified as significantly affecting the natural history of MR caused by mitral valve prolapse, including the presence of LV dysfunction with an ejection fraction less than 60%, New York Heart Association functional class III or IV, regurgitant orifice area 40 mm^2 or larger, LV end-systolic dimension greater than 40 mm, left atrial index 60 mL/m^2 or less, left atrial dimension greater than 55 mm, the presence of pulmonary hypertension at rest or during exercise, and the presence of atrial fibrillation.

- Recent data have demonstrated that it is possible to repair practically all prolapsing degenerative mitral valves with a low operative risk (mortality risk <1%) and the absence of residual MR with procedures performed in high-volume reference centers. This finding is crucial because of the increasing number of asymptomatic patients referred for surgery.

- Although mitral valve replacement should be rare in patients with degenerative disease, it is fairly prevalent in patients with rheumatic disease and might be considered as a viable option in selected patients with ischemic MR. In this last scenario, mitral valve replacement might provide a good alternative because prosthetic valve function is not affected by degree of LV dysfunction, although there is the risk of complications related to the prosthesis.

- If the decision to proceed with mitral valve replacement is made, a chordal sparing approach should be employed to preserve chordal-ventricular-annular continuity, which is important to preserve long-term LV shape and performance.

- Currently, there is a significant trend toward the use of bioprostheses. In middle-aged patients, a mechanical prosthesis is reasonable according to the desire of the informed patient if there are no contraindications to anticoagulation and if there is a clear risk of accelerated structural valve deterioration. On the other hand, bioprostheses should be recommended when good-quality anticoagulation is unlikely (compliance problems or contraindication), for reoperation for mechanical thrombosis despite excellent anticoagulant control, in women contemplating pregnancy, and in patients wishing to avoid anticoagulation.

The normal mitral valve is located in the left atrioventricular groove and allows unidirectional flow of oxygenated blood from the left atrium into the left ventricle in a near frictionless fashion during diastole.[1] The valve is a complex three-dimensional assembly of independent anatomical components: the annulus, the leaflets and commissures, the chordae tendineae, the papillary muscles, and the left ventricle (see Chapter 2). During systole, a coordinated interaction of these anatomic components seals the valve against left ventricular (LV) pressure. Although even a normal competent valve may present a physiologically trivial amount of reversed flow into the left atrium, more than a trace of mitral regurgitation (MR) is considered pathologic.[2] According to the natural history of the disease, although mild to moderate MR might be well tolerated indefinitely, severe MR eventually leads to LV remodeling, heart failure, and ultimately death (see Chapter 20).[3] In this context, the natural history of MR depends intimately on its etiology, the severity of LV volume overload as well as its contractile performance, and the appearance of overlapping clinical conditions secondary to reversal of flow, such as atrial fibrillation and pulmonary hypertension.[4]

Primary degenerative mitral valve disease is the most prevalent cause of isolated severe MR in the United States.[5] Distinct pathologic features of the disease include mitral valve billowing (intact valve coaptation) and prolapse (deficient valve coaptation) due to myxomatous degeneration of the mitral leaflets, chordal elongation or rupture, or papillary muscle elongation or rupture.[6] In the setting of severe MR, even in the absence of symptoms, mitral valve repair is currently the gold standard procedure for patients who require surgery for degenerative MR.[7] In this particular subset of patients, mitral valve repair has become feasible and safe, and repair techniques have been proven to have an excellent durability, especially when performed in high-volume institutions.[8] In this regard, the latest guidelines for the management of patients with valvular heart disease suggest targeted referral to "reference centers" with experienced surgeons to ensure a repair rate greater than 90% and a mortality rate equal to or less than 1%.[9] Although these new standards have triggered a more liberal referral of asymptomatic patients, mitral valve repair is still underutilized in the United States.[10] Simple lesions such as posterior leaflet prolapse are associated with very high mitral valve repair rates in many centers,[11,12] but the overall repair rate for more complex scenarios, as defined by leaflet involvement (e.g., isolated anterior leaflet or bileaflet prolapse), lesion complexity (e.g., significant annular calcification, significant excess tissue), or patient comorbidities (e.g., older age, reoperations), remains uncertain and seems to be well below guidelines' recommendations.[13,14] A data analysis from the Society of Thoracic Surgeons (STS) observed an average mitral valve repair rate of only 70%.[15] The following section is a review of the surgical anatomy of the mitral valve as well as an updated summary of causes, consequences, and surgical treatment of mitral valve disease. We focus on mitral valve repair for primary forms of MR such as annular dilation and mitral valve prolapse, controversies on mitral valve repair versus mitral valve replacement for patients with secondary MR (see next section), and, finally, on mitral valve replacement for those etiologies of MR not as amenable to mitral valve repair, such as rheumatic mitral valve disease.

Surgical Anatomy of the Mitral Valve

As previously noted, the normal mitral valve is a dynamic complex of independent anatomic structures. The presence of abnormalities in any of these components (lesions) may cause the alteration in closure (dysfunction) against LV pressure and, consequently, MR. Structural abnormalities of the mitral valve are referred to as primary mitral valve disease, whereas valve dysfunction secondary to perturbations in LV geometry is termed ischemic MR in ischemic cardiomyopathy and functional MR in dilated cardiomyopathy (see Chapter 19).

Mitral Annulus

The mitral annulus is a discontinuous fibromuscular D-shaped ring located in the left atrioventricular groove (between the left ventricle and the left atrium) that serves as an anchor and hinge point for the mitral valve leaflets. The mitral annulus might be subjectively divided into anterior and posterior segments according to the attachments of the anterior and posterior mitral leaflets. In addition, it can also be segmented by location into septal and lateral components. The anterior part of the mitral annulus is in continuity with the fibrous skeleton of the heart, and is limited by the right and left fibrous trigones and the aortic mitral curtain (continuity at the level of the left and noncoronary aortic valve cusps). In contrast, the posterior part of the mitral annulus lacks a fibrous skeleton and is more prone to dilation and calcification.[16] The resultant changes in annular dimensions lead to a more circular annulus, compared with its normal "kidney bean" shape, which in turn compromises the coaptation of the mitral leaflets. The normal mitral annulus also has a three-dimensional saddle shape with two lower points at the level of both trigones and one peak at the midpoint of the anterior leaflet. This peak point is always above the midpoint of the posterior leaflet, allowing bulging during systole to accommodate the aortic root and optimize stress distribution over both leaflets. The overall circumference of the annulus may decrease by as much as 20% during systole (less eccentricity), promoting central leaflet coaptation.[17] Reduction in annular size begins with atrial contraction and reaches its maximum halfway through the systolic cycle.

Mitral Leaflets and Commissures

The mitral valve has two leaflets (anterior and posterior) with similar surface areas and thicknesses ($\approx$1 mm) but significantly different shapes. The anterior leaflet is taller and has a shorter base than the posterior leaflet, extends vertically, and is anchored to one third of the annular circumference between the right and left fibrous trigones.[18] The posterior leaflet is broader based, has a shorter height than the anterior leaflet, lies transverse to the mitral valve orifice, and, together with the commissures, is fixed to the remaining two thirds of the annulus. The posterior leaflet is closely related to the LV wall base, the point of greatest systolic stress. It is important to emphasize that the different orientation of the two leaflets ensures a competent closure line of the mitral valve during systole, located in the posterior one third of the valve orifice, which naturally prevents systolic anterior motion.[19] Additionally, both leaflets present two zones from its base to the free border or margin: *the atrial or membranous zone* (smooth and translucent) and *the coaptation zone* (rough, nodular, and thicker due to the attachment and fusion of chordae tendineae). As a surgical reference, the leaflets of the mitral valve can be "segmented" by location of the clefts or indentations in the posterior leaflet. If one counts both commissures as individual segments, a total of eight segments can be identified. Unlike the anterior leaflet, the posterior leaflet has two clefts in its free margin that allow full opening during LV filling and that, in turn, demarcate three segments or scallops. The middle scallop of the posterior leaflet is designated *P2* and adjacent medial and lateral scallops are designated as *P1* and *P3*, respectively. The corresponding areas of the anterior leaflet are designated by opposition to the segments in the posterior leaflet as *A1, A2,* and *A3* (Figure 21-1).

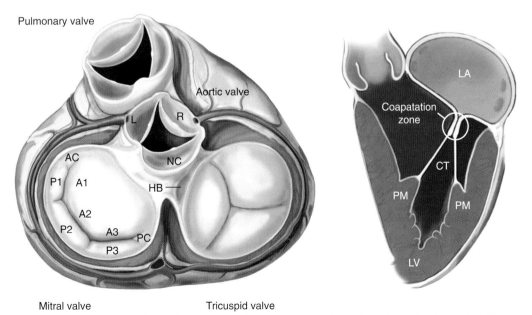

FIGURE 21-1 **Anatomy of the mitral valve and mitral apparatus.** *Left,* Anatomic view of the cardiac valves in systole with the left and right atrium cropped away and the great vessels transected. The mitral valve apparatus consists of the mitral leaflets, mitral annulus, chordae tendineae, the papillary muscles, and the left ventricle. *Right,* Normal function of the mitral apparatus brings both leaflets together in systole and creates the coaptation zone. *AC,* Anterior commissure; *A1, A2, A3,* segments of the anterior leaflet; *CT,* chordae tendineae; *HB,* His bundle; *L,* left coronary cusp; *LA,* left atrium; *NC,* noncoronary cusp; *P1, P2, P3,* segments of the posterior leaflet; *PC,* posterior commissure; *PM,* papillary muscle; *LV,* left ventricle; *R,* right coronary cusp.

In addition to the anterior and posterior leaflet scallops or segments, the mitral valve has two triangular segments that establish continuity between the two leaflets, also known as commissures. These distinct areas of leaflet tissue are supported by chordal fans and are critical to achieving a good surface of coaptation at the junctions of the two leaflets. For their identification, the vertical axis of the papillary muscles and their corresponding chordae tendineae is used as a reference point, thus obtaining an anterior commissure and a posterior commissure.

The Chordae Tendineae

The chordate tendineae are filament-like structures of connective fibrous tissue that join the LV surface and free border of the mitral leaflets to the papillary muscles and, by default, the posterior wall of the left ventricle. They create a suspension system that allows full opening of the leaflets during diastole and prevents the excursion of the leaflets above the annular plane during systole.[20] A total of about 25 primary chordae begin in the papillary muscles and progressively subdivide to insert into the leaflets. Chordae tendineae are classified according to their insertion point between the free border and the base of the mitral leaflets. Primary or marginal chordae attach along the margin (every 3 to 5 mm) of the leaflets and are critical to prevent leaflet prolapse and to align the rough zone of the anterior and posterior leaflets during systole. Secondary or intermediate chordae, which are inserted in the ventricular side of the body of the leaflets, relieve excess tension during systole.[21] Tertiary or basal chordae are only found on the posterior leaflet and connect its base and the posterior annulus to the papillary muscles, providing additional linkage to the ventricle.

Papillary Muscles and the Left Ventricle

The mitral valve leaflets are attached by the chordae tendineae to the papillary muscles, which are considered an extension of the left ventricle. The papillary muscles vary in the number of heads and exact position in the ventricle, but generally two organized groups can be identified. Each papillary muscle is designated according to the relationship to the valve commissures, and each provides a fan chord to its corresponding commissure as well as to both the anterior and posterior leaflets. The anterior papillary muscle has a single body, is larger, and is irrigated by the first obtuse marginal branch of the circumflex artery and the first diagonal branch of the anterior descending artery. The posterior papillary muscle has two bodies, is smaller, and is irrigated only by the posterior descending artery, a branch of the right coronary artery, in 90% of cases and by the circumflex artery in the other 10%. This arrangement explains the relative vulnerability of the posterior papillary muscle to ischemia, and subsequent involvement in localized remodeling in the setting of ischemic MR.[22] The left ventricle supports the entire mitral apparatus, owing to its continuation with the papillary muscles, and thus LV dimensional changes in the setting of volume overload and remodeling, whether ischemic or not, can lead to leaflet tethering and MR.[23]

The Pathophysiologic Triad of Mitral Valve Regurgitation

MR is defined as the existence of blood flow in systole from the left ventricle into the left atrium. The presence of minimal structural lesions might cause MR by reducing mitral leaflet coaptation. Therefore, the exhaustive interrogation (identification, localization, and magnitude) for mitral lesions is essential to determining the chances of successful valve repair and proceeding with a tailored therapeutic plan for each patient. Three decades ago, Carpentier described a systematic analytic approach to patients with MR known as the "pathophysiologic triad of MR."[24]

The triad emphasizes the importance of distinguishing between the medical conditions causing MR (etiology), identifying the resulting lesions, and finally how these lesions affect leaflet motion (dysfunction). Nowadays, besides promoting mutual understanding among surgeons and specialists in cardiac imaging, the triad also represents an organized and very consistent way to elucidate the most appropriate techniques to achieve a successful repair.

Dysfunction

The differentiation of valve dysfunctions (I, II, and III) is based on the position of the leaflet margins with respect to the mitral annular plane (Figure 21-2). Type I dysfunction implies normal leaflet motion, and the most common cause of significant MR is the perforation of one of the leaflets (e.g., endocarditis) or severe annular dilation with a central regurgitant jet (e.g., primary atrial fibrillation) (Figure 21-3A). Type II dysfunction denotes excess leaflet motion generally secondary to chordal elongation or rupture or to myxomatous degeneration of the leaflets (regurgitant jet directed to the opposite site of the prolapsing leaflet). Type III dysfunction designates restricted leaflet motion and results typically from retraction of the subvalvular apparatus (IIIA, rheumatic valve disease or other inflammatory scenarios that lead to scarring and calcification) or from papillary muscle displacement (leaflet tethering) due to LV remodeling or dilation (IIIB, ischemic or dilated cardiomyopathy).

Etiology and Lesions

Worldwide, rheumatic disease remains the most common cause of MR, but it has ceased to be the leading cause in developed countries.[25] Ischemic disease, currently responsible for 20% of cases of MR, may lose importance as a result of the ever more aggressive percutaneous treatment of coronary artery disease. Thus, degenerative disease is today the most frequent cause of MR in western countries.[26]

Degenerative mitral valve disease is characterized by a wide spectrum of lesions,[27] varying from a simple chordal rupture leading to prolapse of an isolated segment (frequently P2) in an otherwise normal valve, to multiple segment prolapse of both leaflets in a valve with significant excess tissue (Figure 21-3A and B).[28] This range of lesions gives rise to two opposing entities: fibroelastic deficiency and Barlow disease.[29] Fibroelastic deficiency occurs in older patients (generally more than 60-years-old) with a short history of severe holosystolic murmur. As the term *fibroelastic* implies, this disease is a condition associated with a deficit of the protein fibrillin that often leads to weakening, elongation, and ultimately rupture of chordae tendineae.[30] Chordal rupture of P2 is considered the most common lesion in patients with fibroelastic deficiency. The mitral leaflets are usually thin and translucent, although the prolapsing scallop might have a myxomatous aspect if the disease has been present for a long time. Distinguishing fibroelastic deficiency from other entities within the spectrum of degenerative mitral valve disease requires an exhaustive analysis of those segments immediately contiguous to the prolapsing one, which are generally normal in size, height, and tissue properties. Finally, the annular size in patients with this condition is often less than 32 mm. In contrast, at the opposite end of the spectrum of degenerative disease is Barlow disease.[31] Affected patients are younger, usually less than 60 years old, and present with a long history of holosystolic murmur that has been monitored by the referring cardiologist for many years. In this context, patients with Barlow disease have a more diffuse and complex redundancy of the leaflets. The most common lesions are excess leaflet tissue, leaflet thickening and distension, with diffuse chordal elongation, thickening, and/or rupture.[32] In these patients, the annular size exceeds 36 mm, and it is not uncommon to find varying degrees of annular calcification (often involving the anterior papillary

Dysfunction	Ventricular View	Atrial View	Etiology
Type I Normal leaflet motion	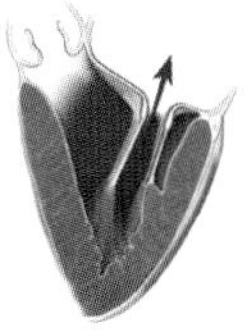	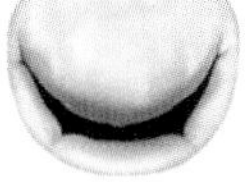	Ischemic cardiomyopathy Dilated cardiomyopathy Endocarditis Congenital

Type II
Increased leaflet motion
(leaflet prolapse)
	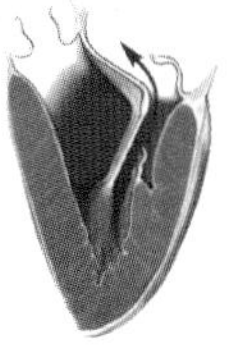	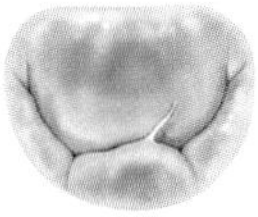	Degenerative disease
			    Fibroelastic deficiency
			    Marfan syndrome
			    Forme fruste Barlow
			    Barlow disease
			
			Endocarditis
			Rheumatic disease
			Trauma
			Ischemic cardiomyopathy
			Ehler-Danlos syndrome

Type IIIA Restricted leaflet motion (restricted opening)	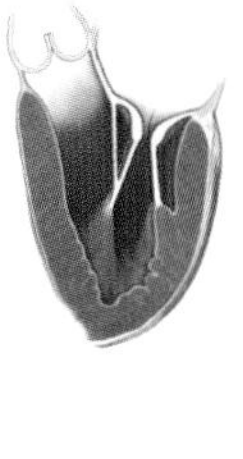	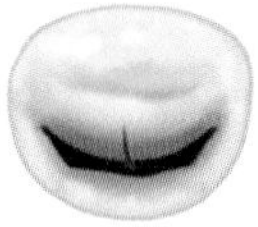	Rheumatic disease Carcinoid disease Radiation Lupus eythematosus Ergotamine use Hypereosinophilic syndrome Mucoploysaccharidosis
Type IIIB Restricted leaflet motion (restricted closure)	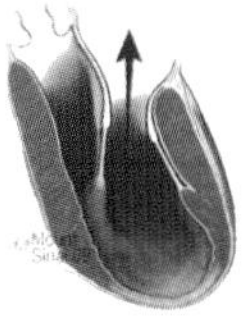	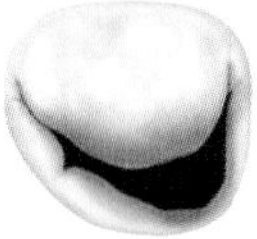	Ischemic cardiomyopathy Dilated cardiomyopathy

FIGURE 21-2 Pathophysiologic triad approach to mitral valve regurgitation, composed of leaflet dysfunction, ventricular and atrial views, and etiology.

muscle) as well as fibrosis of the subvalvular apparatus[33] (Figure 21-4).

Rheumatic disease is still the main cause of mitral disease in underdeveloped or developing countries (see Chapter 17). A systemic exudative inflammatory reaction involves the connective tissue of skin, joints, and heart.[25] Cardiac involvement has been described as a pancarditis with characteristic implication of the left-sided valves. Severe edema and cellular infiltration (severe leaflet thickening extending toward the commissures) is followed by the formation of rheumatic nodules along the free borders of the leaflets. In addition, all the components of the subvalvular apparatus are also affected, leading to chordal thickening and retraction and chordal and commissural fusion. The annulus then dilates in a very asymmetric fashion predominantly along the P3 segment (see Figure 21-3C). It is important to highlight that the anterior leaflet is generally less affected than the posterior leaflet, which is often retracted. Owing to the complexity of lesions, rheumatic mitral disease is not as amenable to valve repair.[34]

Ischemic MR is a consequence of myocardial ischemia and remodeling. In this context, ischemic MR can manifest acutely after papillary muscle rupture (primary) or secondary to LV remodeling and apical and inferior displacement of the papillary

muscles.[35] In the presence of ischemic MR, the mitral leaflets are tethered, and their coaptation point is below the mitral annulus (see Figure 21-3D). When restricted leaflet movement occurs principally in systole, the pattern is asymmetric and is mainly observed in patients with posterior infarction and posterior leaflet restriction (eccentric regurgitant jet)[36] (Figure 21-5). In contrast, in patients with dilated cardiomyopathy or anterior and posterior infarctions, both leaflets have a restrictive deficit, giving rise to a symmetric pattern (central jet).[37] In order to understand ischemic MR and its surgical approach, it is critical to understand the mechanism (secondary classification) and the dynamics of the disease (possible progression).[38] The analysis of the mechanism of MR, which is even more critical, answers prognostic questions such as How tethered and angulated are the leaflets? Is there a pseudoprolapse? Is the regurgitation jet eccentric or central? What are the ventricular dimensions? How reversible is the ischemic insult?[39]

Mitral Valve Surgery

MR predisposes the left ventricle to a volume overload in order to compensate for the volume lost to regurgitation. Although mild to

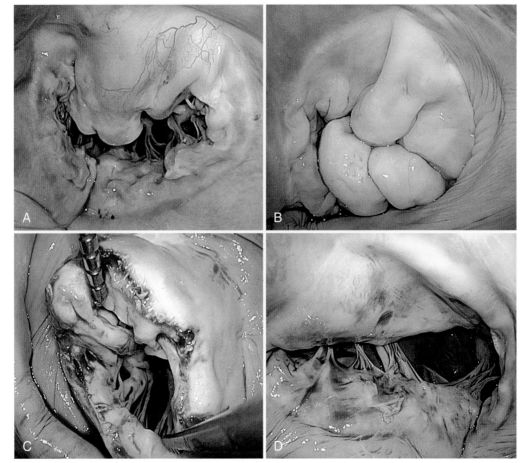

FIGURE 21-3 **Valve lesions in mitral valve regurgitation. A,** Severe annular dilation leading to type I dysfunction. **B,** Severe myxomatous changes with redundant, thick, and bulky segments in a patient with Barlow disease and type II dysfunction. **C,** Rheumatic mitral valve disease with classic "fish-mouth" appearance and type IIIA dysfunction. **D,** Ischemic mitral valve disease due to severe tethering of P3 leading to type IIIB dysfunction.

moderate MR might be well tolerated for long periods, severe MR is fatal at a determined stage. Severe MR can be mainly divided into three clinical stages—acute, chronic compensated, and chronic decompensated—each of which requires different management and has different surgical triggers. In this regard, severe MR is a mechanical problem with surgery as the only definitive solution, either mitral valve repair or mitral valve replacement. Although the lack of randomized trials comparing mitral valve repair with replacement has led to controversy, particularly in the setting of secondary MR, repair is favored over replacement for multiple reasons, especially in patients with degenerative mitral valve disease[40] (Figure 21-6). The reasons include a likely lower perioperative risk and improved event-free survival in the majority of operated patients, freedom from the various complications of prosthetic heart valves (Figure 21-7), and better postoperative LV function.[41]

Surgical Approach

Several surgical approaches for access to the mitral valve have been described. Although the earliest mitral valve procedures were performed through a right thoracotomy, the mitral valve has traditionally been exposed through a median sternotomy. Nowadays, median sternotomy remains as the gold standard and it is still the most popular approach.[42] Central cannulation and direct aortic clamping enable mitral surgery with generous exposure and excellent results. Some groups have significantly transformed the incision to a lower hemisternotomy, thus limiting the length of the incision to 7 to 9 cm. However, in an effort to reduce invasiveness and the potential operative morbidity, cardiac surgeons

have adopted nonsternotomy, also known as video-assisted approaches, including right thoracotomy and robotic surgery[43-45] (Table 21-1). Although the safety and efficacy of minimally invasive cardiac surgery have been established in several high-volume specialized centers, potential issues have been raised, including a higher incidence of certain complications, such as postoperative stroke.[46] Moreover, one of the issues implies the compromise of repair rates because minimally invasive cardiac surgery has been shown to be most predictably effective when utilized in simple pathology rather than in complex valve surgery. Finally, it is important to emphasize that to date there have been no clearly demonstrable clinical benefits of minimally invasive access other than cosmetic advantages.

The most important goal for patients with MR as well as for the physicians involved in their perioperative care is to achieve, when possible, not only a repair of the mitral valve but a good and durable one, as emphasized in the newest guidelines from the European Society of Cardiology and the European Association for Cardio-Thoracic Surgery.[47] In this regard, achieving a competent and symmetric line of closure, a good surface of coaptation, and an effective preservation of leaflet mobility is key to providing the patient with a competent and durable repair. In ideal conditions, these axioms could be met in the presence of either simple or complex lesions regardless of the preferred surgical approach. However, in the real world, complex mitral valve repair still remains challenging in patients undergoing median sternotomy in most centers and certainly is unpredictable when attempted with minimally invasive strategies. This issue is crucial when referring young asymptomatic patients, in whom durability of repair is critical and the occurrence of stroke is particularly

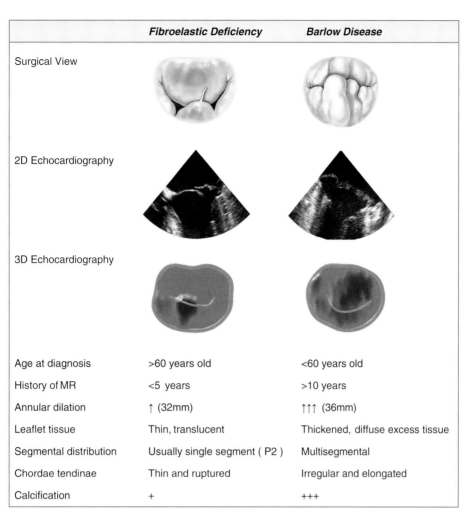

	Fibroelastic Deficiency	Barlow Disease
Surgical View		
2D Echocardiography		
3D Echocardiography		
Age at diagnosis	>60 years old	<60 years old
History of MR	<5 years	>10 years
Annular dilation	↑ (32mm)	↑↑↑ (36mm)
Leaflet tissue	Thin, translucent	Thickened, diffuse excess tissue
Segmental distribution	Usually single segment (P2)	Multisegmental
Chordae tendinae	Thin and ruptured	Irregular and elongated
Calcification	+	+++

FIGURE 21-4 **Most typical clinical and surgical differences between fibroelastic deficiency and Barlow disease.** *2D,* two-dimensional; *3D,* three-dimensional; *MR,* mitral regurgitation; *P2,* middle segment of posterior leaflet.

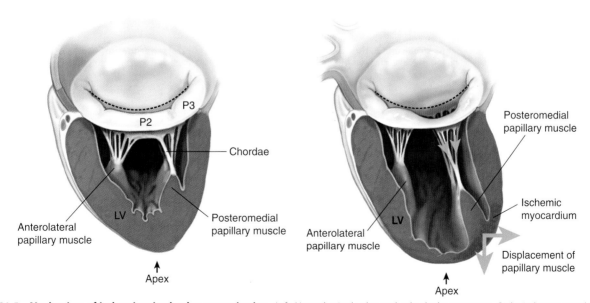

FIGURE 21-5 **Mechanism of ischemic mitral valve regurgitation.** *Left,* Normal mitral valve and subvalvular apparatus. *Right,* Ischemic mitral valve with pronounced posterior restriction in P3 after an episode of ventricular ischemia. *LV,* Left ventricle; *P2, P3,* segments of posterior leaflet.

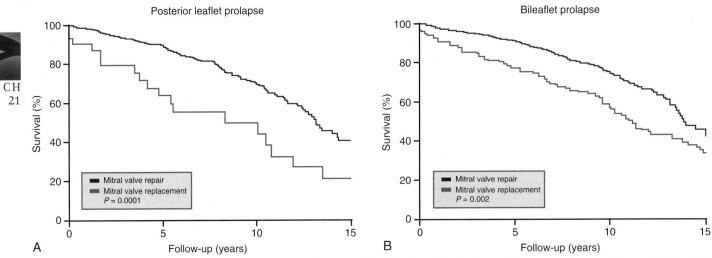

FIGURE 21-6   Probability of survival (death from any cause) among patients having mitral valve repair versus replacement for posterior leaflet prolapse (A) and bileaflet prolapse (B). *(From Suri RM, Schaff HV, Dearani JA, et al: Survival advantage and improved durability of mitral repair for leaflet prolapse subsets in the current era. Ann Thorac Surg 2006;82:819-826.)*

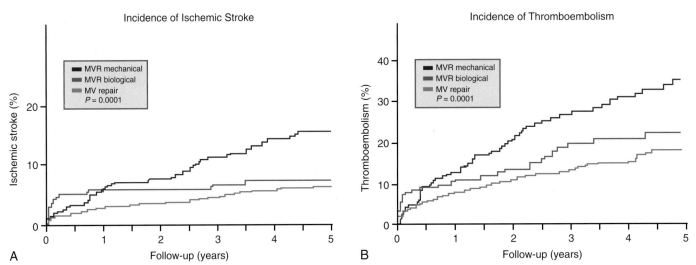

FIGURE 21-7   A, Incidence of first ischemic stroke and B, thromboembolism after surgery for mitral regurgitation. *(From Russo A, Grigioni F, Avierinos JF, et al: Thromboembolic complications after surgical correction of mitral regurgitation incidence, predictors, and clinical implications. J Am Coll Cardiol 2008;51:1203-1211.)*

TABLE 21-1	Technical Variations and Limitations According to Surgical Approach	
SURGICAL APPROACH	**STERNOTOMY**	**VIDEO-ASSISTED APPROACHES**
Incisions	Median sternotomy or lower hemisternotomy (7 to 9 cm)	Several 2- to 3-cm intercostal ports and an additional 4- to 6-cm working port for nonrobotic approaches
Arterial perfusion	Antegrade (aorta)	Retrograde (right femoral artery)
Venous drainage	Central	Peripheral
Aortic clamping	Clamp, site detected by direct palpation and verified by epi-aortic ultrasound	Endoscopic clamp or balloon
Myocardial protection	Direct	Indirect by rapid injection
Visualization of field	Direct and wide for all members of the team	Limited to the endoscopic device
Annuloplasty devices	As desired	Flexible posterior bands
Annuloplasty sutures	Braided polyester	Braided polyester, running polypropylene, nitinol clips
Repair techniques	As desired	Predilection for nonresectional techniques
Ventilation	Two-lung ventilation	Single-lung ventilation, potential rib spreading

devastating. As technology advances and training for surgical subspecialties develops, minimally invasive techniques may be applied to a wider spectrum of lesions. However, at this time, the use of these strategies to attempt mitral valve repair seems restricted to selected, high-volume, specialized centers and reserved for selected patients without complex pathology.

Mitral Valve Repair

As mentioned previously, degenerative mitral valve disease is defined by a wide spectrum of lesions and therefore requires a wide variety of surgical techniques to be repaired.[48] After a systematic valve analysis and identification of the lesions, mitral valve repair should be performed following a sequential approach as follows: (1) repair of the posterior leaflet, (2) ring annuloplasty using preferably a complete semirigid remodeling ring, and (3) repair of any residual prolapse of the anterior leaflet or commissures after inspection of the line of closure during saline testing.[49]

If posterior leaflet prolapse is due to fibroelastic disease, it is most commonly treated by a triangular (Figure 21-8A) or limited resection of the segment affected. The prolapsing segment is subsequently removed, and direct suturing of the leaflet remnants and edges restores leaflet continuity. Occasionally, to relieve leaflet tension, annular plication techniques might be applied. In the setting of very limited or normal leaflet tissue, it may be preferable to avoid leaflet resection and proceed with a chordal transfer or surgical techniques using polytetrafluoroethylene (PTFE) (loop technique, loop-in-loop technique, or single neochordoplasty) (Figure 21-8C). If a more extensive leaflet resection is needed, it is usually performed where the prolapse is greatest or the leaflet is tallest. This resection is typically 1 cm or less wide (additional excess tissue can be removed later). If the height is more than 15 mm in any residual leaflet segment, a sliding leaflet-plasty (including secondary chordal cutting) to reduce the residual leaflet height to 12 to 15 mm across the posterior leaflet may be performed (Figure 21-8B). Reattachment of the leaflet to the annulus will reduce the leaflet height several millimeters, depending on the depth of suture bites. Therefore, the leaflet height before suturing should ideally be about 15 mm in all segments. If the leaflet is taller than 2 cm, a horizontal wedge excision is made at the base of the appropriate segment to further reduce its height before reattachment. The margins of the reconstructed posterior leaflet are then examined to ensure all segments are adequately supported. Any gaps in support, or any areas supported by thinned-out chordae (even in the absence of prolapse), are reinforced by transposition of previously detached secondary chordae, or artificial PTFE neochords.

After posterior leaflet repair, annular remodeling needs to be addressed, because annular dilation is the most commonly associated lesion in the setting of leaflet prolapse. Annuloplasty sutures are generally placed around the annulus prior to leaflet height/prolapse correction. Annular sizing is performed by measuring the intercommissural distance and the surface area of the anterior leaflet. Sutures are passed through the annuloplasty ring, and the ring is tied down securely.

Correction of anterior leaflet dysfunction is usually addressed after a remodeling ring is placed. The anatomic disposition of the anterior leaflet does not allow aggressive resection of the leaflet margins. Therefore, surgical strategy to fix opposing anterior leaflet prolapse includes minimal (limited to the rough area of the leaflet) or no resection. After saline testing with moderate pressurization of the left ventricle, correction of the anterior leaflet prolapse using one or a combination of the following techniques might be performed: (1) chordal transfer of basal chords, secondary chords, or small segment of posterior leaflet with attached chords (flip technique;) (2) neochordoplasty with PTFE sutures; (3) PTFE loop or loop-in-loop technique to correct multiple prolapsing segments; or (4)) limited triangular resection of a prolapsing segment. Finally, commissural prolapse (often seen in patients with Barlow disease) might be achieved by placing

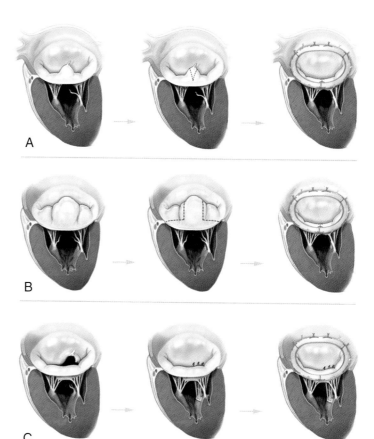

FIGURE 21-8 Currently most commonly applied surgical approaches to posterior leaflet prolapse. A, Triangular resection; **B,** quadrangular resection and sliding leaflet plasty; **C,** neochordoplasty with polytetrafluoroethylene sutures. *Dashed lines* represent the area of leaflet to be excised.

one or two vertical mattress sutures (Carpentier's "magic" suture) to fix opposing segments of A1/P1 or A3/P3, advancing the commissures. As a useful alternative, PTFE neochords may be placed to support opposing segments at the commissures, with one arm of the suture passed through opposing anterior and posterior leaflet segments.[50]

An optimal mitral valve repair should meet the following criteria:

• The valve is competent on saline testing
• There is a good surface of coaptation
• The line of closure where the anterior leaflet occupies 80% or more of the valve area is symmetric
• There is no residual billowing
• There is no tendency to systolic anterior motion

Evaluation for all these points may require two different intraoperative tests, the saline test and the ink test. The saline test is performed by filling the ventricle with saline. Examination of the valve confirms the absence of prolapse, billowing and incompetence, a symmetric closure line, and an anterior leaflet that occupies most of the valve orifice. The ink test is performed by drawing a line on the valve closure line during maximum saline insufflations. The coaptation zone beyond the ink is examined and should be at least 6 mm in length (this will transform to approximately 10 mm on echocardiography because part of the ink is within the coaptation zone). Also, there should be no more than 1 cm of anterior leaflet beyond the ink line, as presence of more would signify a risk for systolic anterior motion.[51]

Current practice guidelines separate recommendations for surgery not according to the etiology of MR but rather according to the severity of MR and the severity of symptoms. Most patients with severe ischemic MR have symptoms of heart failure. Thus, according to current guidelines, patients with severe, symptomatic MR have a class I indication for mitral valve surgery if the LV ejection fraction is more than 30% and or the end-systolic LV dimension is 55 mm or smaller. In these patients, the valvular apparatus is examined systematically to assess tissue pliability and identify leaflet restriction, with P1 as a reference point. The mitral annulus is also examined to assess the severity of annular dilation, which is very common. If mitral valve repair is the procedure of choice, restrictive remodeling annuloplasty should be the technique[52] (Figure 21-9). Because leaflet restriction in ischemic MR results in less leaflet tissue available for coaptation, it is necessary to downsize a complete remodeling ring by one or two sizes or to use a true-sized Carpentier-McCarthy-Adams IMR Etlogix ring[53] (Edwards Lifesciences Corporation, Irvine, California) to ensure an adequate surface of coaptation after

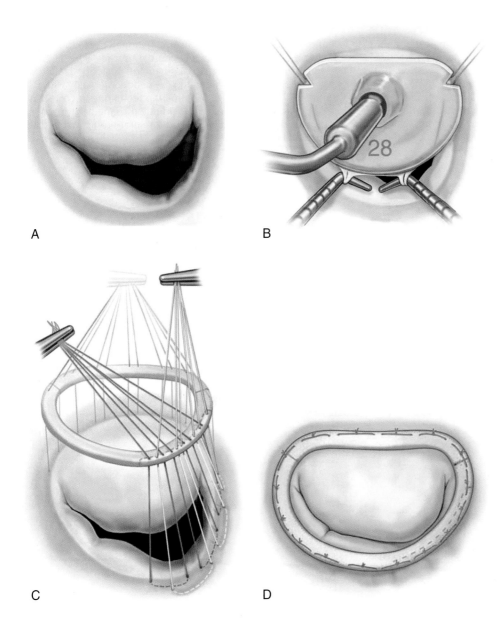

A

B

C

D

FIGURE 21-9 Surgical approach to ischemic mitral regurgitation. A, Typical findings with leaflet restriction predominantly in the P2-P3 region. **B,** Sizing of the annulus with a Carpentier-Edwards sizer is based primarily on the surface area and height of the anterior leaflet. One places 2-0 braided sutures into the mitral annulus, taking advantage of the full curve of the needle, with the angle directed toward the ventricle to ensure passage through the annulus. **C,** The sutures in the annulus at the position of the anterior commissure and trigone are placed last, taking advantage of previously placed sutures to expose this area. **D,** After placement of a full-remodeling Carpentier-McCarthy-Adams IMR Etlogix ring (Edwards Lifesciences Corporation, Irvine, California), the surface of coaptation is restored (below the plane of the annulus). *(Modified with permission from Carpentier A, Adams A, Filsoufi F: Carpentier's reconstructive valve surgery. Philadelphia: Saunders Elsevier; 2010.)*

annuloplasty.[54] This ring combines the principles of undersizing with the specific asymmetric deformation (severe tethering along P3) observed in type IIIb ischemic MR. In cases of severe leaflet tethering and moderate to severe LV dilation, restrictive annuloplasty and combined coronary artery bypass graft (CABG) surgery alone may not provide durable results. Hence, several adjunctive techniques as well as alternative procedures have been advocated, including division of secondary chords,[55] posterior leaflet extension with a pericardial patch, repositioning of the papillary muscles, and mitral valve replacement with chordal sparing.[56]

Rheumatic mitral valve disease is characterized mainly by mitral stenosis secondary to fibrotic restrictions of the subvalvular apparatus. Nonetheless, there are still some patients who present with MR due to varying degrees of restriction, chordal thickening, and commissural fusion. On many occasions, if the valve is severely calcified and there is freezing of the chordal structures, mitral valve repair is extremely complex and often fruitless. If there is mitral stenosis due to isolated commissural fusion or a more preserved subvalvular apparatus, as occurs in younger patients, mitral valve repair becomes feasible.[57] Techniques for rheumatic repair include commissurotomy and commissural reconstruction, calcium débridement, chordal fenestration and cutting, and patch extension of both leaflets with glutaraldehyde-fixed pericardium (this technique usually requires leaflet resuspension with PTFE neochords).

Mitral Valve Replacement

Although mitral valve replacement should be uncommon in patients with degenerative mitral disease if patients are appropriately referred to experienced surgeons, it still remains fairly prevalent in patients with complex lesions. This situation is inversely proportional in patients with rheumatic disease, in whom replacement rates are as high as 50% in reference centers. In patients with chronic ischemic MR, the best approach, mitral valve replacement or mitral valve repair with annuloplasty, remains debatable. This is in part due to the fact that prosthetic valve function is not affected by worsening LV function if there is further negative remodeling.[58] Recent studies have suggested better echocardiographic outcomes in patients undergoing mitral valve replacement, with no significant difference in mortality at 2.5 years.[59] Obviously, these data need longer follow-up to analyze the occurrence of classic complications of valve replacement, such as structural valve degeneration, nonstructural dysfunction, valve thrombosis, embolism, bleeding events, and endocarditis. If the decision to proceed with mitral valve replacement is made, a chordal sparing approach should be employed. The posterior leaflet with chords, and often all or portions of the anterior leaflet with chords are incorporated into the sutures used to secure the replacement valve prosthesis. This technique preserves chordal-ventricular-annular continuity, which is important to preserving long-term LV shape and performance.

Guidelines recommend that patient preference be considered in the decision to use a mechanical valve or a bioprosthetic valve in patients younger than 65 years,[9] and in real practice, more and more patients are selecting bioprostheses regardless of age because of their desire not to commit to a lifetime of warfarin therapy. Currently there is an important trend toward favoring the use of bioprostheses in the United States, where between 1999 and 2008, the implantation of mechanical valves among Medicare beneficiaries declined from 53% to 21%, and the implantation of bioprostheses increased from 22% to 34%.[60] This phenomenon has occurred despite the lack of data suggesting a significant difference in long-term survival associated with a specific type of prosthesis. However, two tenets may play an important role in decision making when it comes to choosing the type of prosthesis. First, patients older than 65 years, who gain most benefit from biologic prostheses, represent a growing proportion of patients undergoing valve surgery. Second, cardiologists and physicians

in general have potentiated a greater awareness of the lifetime risk of using anticoagulation. Furthermore, historical variables once considered strong reasons to implant a mechanical valve, including the presence of atrial fibrillation (availability of more advanced intraoperative antiarrhythmic procedures) and dialysis-dependent renal failure (poor long-term survival with either choice may favor the use of bioprostheses), are no longer valid.[9]

Although the choice of prosthesis in elderly patients or young patients seem to be clear-cut, it is important to emphasize that there are no current data suggesting any significant difference in survival benefit between mechanical and bioprosthetic valves in middle-aged patients. Indeed, after a thorough discussion about the potential risks of reoperation in comparison with lifelong risks of thromboembolic and hemorrhagic complications, either choice seems reasonable for patients in this age range.[9,61] According to the latest update of the guidelines on the management of valvular heart disease, mechanical prostheses are reasonable according to the desire of the informed patient if there are no contraindications to anticoagulation. Additionally, mechanical valves are preferred if there is risk of accelerated structural valve deterioration, or if the patient is already undergoing anticoagulation because he or she has a mechanical prosthesis in another position. On the other hand, bioprostheses should be recommended when good-quality anticoagulation is unlikely (compliance problems or contraindication), for reoperation for mechanical thrombosis despite excellent anticoagulant control, in women contemplating pregnancy, and in patients wishing to avoid anticoagulation.

Outcomes of Mitral Valve Repair

Contemporary data show low mortality rates after mitral valve repair regardless of the etiology.[60] In patients with degenerative mitral valve disease, the rate of long-term freedom from reoperation is very low,[62] although a return of moderate to severe MR has been reported in later series to occur at a rate of 1% to 4% per year[48,63-65] (Figure 21-10). The failure to use an annuloplasty ring, chordal shortening techniques (which are now uncommon), the presence of anterior leaflet pathology, and, of course, the unavailability of pliable leaflet tissue are all associated with higher repair failure rates[13,66] (Table 21-2). In the following section we analyze the outcomes of mitral valve repair according to the etiology encountered.

Degenerative Mitral Valve Disease

As mentioned previously, contemporary series of mitral valve procedures in many high-volume valve surgery centers for degenerative disease have reported valve replacement rates of 5% to 15% in higher-risk groups, such as elderly patients,[67] and for more complex pathology, including anterior leaflet involvement.[68] However, the latest reports have demonstrated that it is possible to repair practically all prolapsing degenerative mitral valves with a low operative risk (mortality less than 1%) and the absence of residual MR in high-volume reference centers (Table 21-3). As a growing number of asymptomatic patients with degenerative mitral valve disease are referred for surgery,[69] it seems mandatory that surgeons can reasonably ensure a repair at minimal risk with good long-term results. This goal has been proved to be feasible by specialized valve teams that include cardiologists, anesthesiologists, intensivists, and surgeons.[48]

The use of a systematic surgical strategy (same surgical approach and strategies) and a wide spectrum of surgical technique to attempt repair in all valves should lead to achieve very high repair rates in experienced hands. Subscribing to a technique[70,71] (for instance the use of PTFE) or philosophy (resect or respect) might endanger repair rates because specific techniques and philosophies are not applicable to the full spectrum of lesions potentially encountered. In addition, repairing certain valves (calcified annulus, advanced Barlow disease, re-repairs) might

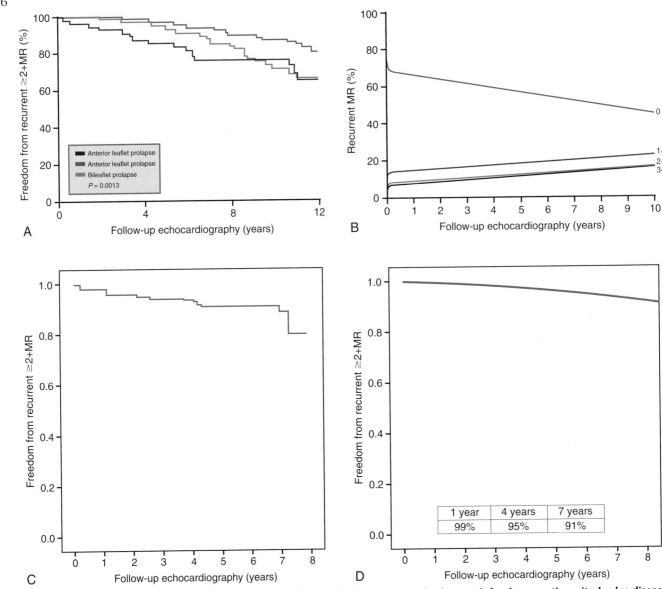

FIGURE 21-10 **Freedom from moderate to more severe mitral regurgitation after mitral valve repair for degenerative mitral valve disease.** (*A from David TE, Ivanov J, Armstrong S, et al: A comparison of outcomes of mitral valve repair for degenerative disease with posterior, anterior, and bileaflet prolapse. J Thorac Cardiovasc Surg 2005;130:1242-1249; **B** from Gillinov AM, Mihaljevic T, Blackstone EH, et al: Should patients with severe degenerative mitral regurgitation delay surgery until symptoms develop? Ann Thorac Surg 2010;90:481-488; **C** from Flameng W, Herijgers P, Bogaerts K: Recurrence of mitral valve regurgitation after mitral valve repair in degenerative valve disease. Circulation 2003;107:1609-1613; **D** from Castillo JG, Anyanwu AC, Fuster V, Adams DH: A near 100% repair rate for mitral valve prolapse is achievable in a reference center: implications for future guidelines. J Thorac Cardiovasc Surg 2012;144:308-312.)*

require long cross-clamp times, and one must be willing to take as long as necessary to repair achieve a successful repair. Moreover, no patient should leave the operating room with more than trivial MR as shown by post-bypass transesophageal echocardiography. If there is still even mild MR, surgeons should resume bypass and perfect the repair, as such a repair usually requires chordal adjustments or closure of clefts, which will take limited time.[72]

Postoperative mortality has been shown to be affected by age, with an averaged risk of about 1% for patients younger than 65 years, 2% for those aged 65 to 80 years, and 4% to 5% for those older than 80 years.[73] Preoperative factors that significantly affect survival in patients with MR include the presence of LV dysfunction (ejection fraction <60%), New York Heart Association functional class III or IV, regurgitant orifice area of 40 mm² or more, a LV end-systolic dimension greater than 40 mm, a left atrial index of 60 mL/m² or higher, a left atrial dimension greater than 55 mm, pulmonary hypertension at rest or with exercise, and

atrial fibrillation.[74-78] After surgery, patients who had severe symptoms before surgery continue to have increased mortality despite symptom relief (especially those with an LV ejection fraction <50%), whereas in those who had no or few preoperative symptoms, restoration of life expectancy can be achieved.[79,80]

Durability of mitral valve repair, defined as freedom from moderate or greater degree of MR, has been reported to be between 90% and 95% at 5 years in high-volume centers, with a recurrent MR rate of 1% to 1.5% a year (see Figure 21-10). If durability rates are stratified by leaflet involvement, those patients with isolated anterior leaflet prolapse have lower durability, ranging between 75% and 85% at 5 years.[40,81] This fact might have a potential etiologic explanation. Patients with isolated anterior leaflet prolapse usually present with fibroelastic disease and have thin leaflets with limited tissue availability. After repair, the coaptation height is not as robust as it is in patients with a minimal degree of myxomatous degeneration, potentially affecting the durability of the repair.

TABLE 21-2 Probability of Mitral Valve Repair According to Echocardiographic Findings and Medical Center

ETIOLOGY	DYSFUNCTION LEVEL	CALCIFICATION	LESIONS	Probability of Repair	
				<50 CASES/YEAR	≥50 CASES/YEAR
Fibroelastic deficiency	II	None/annular	Posterior localized prolapse	Certain	Certain
		None/annular	Anterior prolapse	Possible	Certain
Barlow's disease	II	None/annular	Posterior localized prolapse	Certain	Certain
		None/annular	Multisegmental prolapse	Possible	Certain
		Leaflets	Multisegmental prolapse	Unlikely	Possible
		None/annular	Anterior prolapse	Unlikely	Possible
Endocarditis	I	None	Perforation	Possible	Certain
	II	None	Prolapse	Possible	Certain
		None	Destructive lesions	Unlikely	Possible
Rheumatic	IIIA	Annular	Pliable anterior leaflet	Possible	Certain
		Leaflets	Stiff anterior leaflet	Unlikely	Unlikely
Secondary	I	None	Annular dilation	Certain	Certain
	IIIB	None	Tethering	Unlikely	Possible
		None	Predictors of failed repair	Unlikely	Unlikely

TABLE 21-3 Contemporary Results of Mitral Valve Repair for Degenerative Mitral Valve Prolapse in a Reference Center

Study period	2002 to 2010
Number of patients	744
Exclusions	None
Age (range, years)	58 ± 13 (12-90)
Isolated posterior prolapse	556 (75%)
Isolated anterior prolapse	42 (6%)
Bileaflet	146 (19%)
Previous sternotomy	44 (5.9%)
Previous mitral surgery	18 (2.4%)
Median sternotomy	724 (97%)
Mitral valve repair	743 (99.9%)
Mitral valve replacement	1 (0.1%)
Adjuvant tricuspid repair	465 (62.5%)
In-hospital mortality	6 (0.8%)
No major complications	690 (92.7%)
Major stroke	4 (0.5%)
Minor stroke	8 (1.1%)
Respiratory failure	38 (5.1%)
Length of stay (interquartile range, days)	6 (5-8)
Predischarge TTE: No MR	697 (94.5%)
Predischarge TTE: 1+ MR	41 (4.5%)

MR, Mitral regurgitation; TTE, Transthoracic echocardiogram.

Ischemic Mitral Regurgitation

The increasing life expectancy of the general population, together with the improved survival rates after myocardial infarction, is expected to contribute to even a higher prevalence of ischemic MR in a near future. Although mitral valve repair is generally considered more beneficial than valve replacement,[82] especially in patients with degenerative disease, the best approach for chronic ischemic MR remains debatable,[83] and as a consequence only a small number of patients are referred for surgery. Postoperative improvement in functional class and LV dimensions have been demonstrated in patients who undergo restrictive annuloplasty,[84] but the lack of a firm evidence of survival benefit still precludes surgical referral in many cardiology practices.[85] In addition, significant rates (between 15% and 25%) of recurrent MR as early as 6 months after surgery have triggered a search for alternative therapies, including mitral valve replacement and percutaneous approaches.[86] This search has been further supported by later studies that reported a possible induction of mitral stenosis after restrictive annuloplasty.[87]

The presence of immediate residual MR in the early postoperative period after restrictive annuloplasty is likely related to a progressive leaflet tethering in both symmetric and asymmetric patterns.[88] On the other hand, the recurrence of MR is likely secondary to negative LV remodeling and worsening sphericity. In this scenario, mitral valve replacement might provide a good alternative since prosthetic valve function is not affected by changes in severity of LV dysfunction but with an increased risk of complications (see section on mitral valve replacement).[89] It is important to highlight that in the setting of ischemic MR, even the presence of mild MR after surgery must be taken into consideration (mild MR is associated with reduced postoperative survival), as opposed to what occurs in other etiologies such as degenerative mitral valve disease, in which this can be obviated by valve replacement instead of repair.[84]

Current evidence demonstrates that CABG surgery alone does not correct ischemic MR.[90] One of the initial publications on ischemic MR found that 40% of patients with moderate MR who underwent CABG surgery alone were left with moderate or severe (3+ to 4+) residual ischemic MR.[91] The results of the Randomized Ischemic Mitral Evaluation (RIME) trial, published in 2012, demonstrated a significantly better outcome if annuloplasty was added to CABG in patients with moderate MR and an ejection fraction higher than 30%.[92] Consequently, a ring-remodeling annuloplasty with complete, rigid, or semirigid rings should be strongly recommended in patients with ischemic MR, because the use of flexible rings or annuloplasty bands has been associated with recurrent moderate or greater MR rates of 29% and 30%, respectively, as early as 18 months after surgery.[58] These failure rates in mitral valve repair, potentially related to the asymmetric tethering

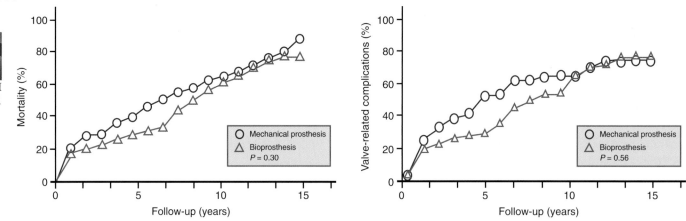

FIGURE 21-11 **Outcomes after mechanical versus bioprosthetic mitral valve replacment. A,** Mortality after mitral valve replacement. **B,** Valve related complications after mitral valve replacement. (*A adapted from Hammermeister K, Sethi GK, Henderson WG, et al: Outcomes 15 years after valve replacement with a mechanical versus a bioprosthetic valve: final report of the Veterans Affairs randomized trial. J Am Coll Cardiol 2000;36:1152-1158; B adapted from Grunkemeier GL, Li HH, Naftel DC, et al: Long-term performance of heart valve prostheses. Curr Probl Cardiol 2000;25:73-154.)*

of the mitral valve towards P2 and P3, have been improved with restrictive asymmetric rings, the rate of freedom from recurrent MR of 2+ severity or greater being 95% at 15 months and 89% at 25 months.[53,54,93] Echocardiographic factors associated with repair failure are listed in Table 21-2.

Later publications have demonstrated better midterm (2.5 years) echocardiographic outcomes with mitral valve replacement in terms of freedom from mild to moderate MR and similar results when the variable analyzed was freedom from moderate to severe MR, supporting the use of mitral valve replacement as a viable option.[59] In terms of survival benefit, unadjusted survival is generally lower in patients undergoing mitral valve replacement.[94] However, in high-risk patients with multiple comorbidities, survival has been observed to be similar regardless the type of procedure.[95]

Outcomes of Mitral Valve Replacement

Disparities in reporting morbidity and mortality after cardiac valve interventions led to the publication of consensus guidelines by the American Association for Thoracic Surgery and the STS in order to provide clear definitions of perioperative mortality, survival, structural and nonstructural valve dysfunction, valve thrombosis, embolism, hemorrhagic events, endocarditis, and freedom from reoperation.[96] In this section we analyze the most relevant and updated series on mitral valve replacement according to the most frequent complications after valve replacement. Among these, despite the generous number of observational studies comparing clinical outcomes of mechanical valves and bioprostheses, only a very limited number of studies have been randomized.

The latest executive summary from the STS national database reported an unadjusted in-hospital mortality between 4% and 6% in patients undergoing isolated mitral valve replacement. If concomitant CABG was performed, in-hospital mortality increased up to 13%.[97] Of course these are not absolute numbers, and several experiences from high-volume centers have observed operative mortalities lower than 1%. Currently, there are no data suggesting that the choice of mechanical or bioprosthetic valve has a significant impact on operative mortality. Mortality and long-term survival after valve replacement have been significantly linked to demographic variables such as age or to comorbidities, including the presence of coronary artery disease and LV dysfunction.[98] Randomized trials failed to show any difference in long-term survival (Figure 21-11) between bioprosthetic and mechanical valves.[99] The Edinburgh Heart Valve Trial reported 20-year

survival rates of 28% and 31% (*P* = 0.57) for patients with mechanical and bioprosthetic valves, respectively.[100]

Valve dysfunction is often divided into structural (inevitable degeneration inherent to the valve, mostly seen in biological prostheses) and nonstructural (any abnormality not inherent to the valve, such as pannus formation, paravalvular leaks, or a technical error, but excluding endocarditis and thromboembolic complications). Structural valve degeneration is considered the most common nonfatal complication in patients having bioprosthetic valves. Although there has been a clear improvement in durability with each "generation" of valves, freedom from structural degeneration remains 70% to 80% at 10 years, although it decreases rapidly after, with ranges between 40% and 50% at 15 years.[98] As mentioned before, even though renal failure might predispose to an accelerated calcification of bioprosthetic valves, the lower life expectancy of patients in renal failure with either type of valve have probably biased observational studies, and no difference has been observed. Although structural degeneration is barely seen in mechanical valves, nonstructural dysfunction is almost exclusively seen in mechanical valves. In this regard, rotating the valve (sewing the ring to a position where the leaflet opening is not impinged) is believed to reduce the risk of this complication.

Valve thrombosis is believed to be more common in mechanical valves, especially in the mitral position (<0.2% per year for mechanical valves versus <0.1% per year for biological valves). Large randomized trials have observed a probability of valve thrombosis between 1% and 2% up to 15 years after surgery regardless the type of valve.[99] Patients with mechanical valves are obviously at a higher risk of presenting with embolic events. Major embolism occurs in approximately 9% of patients with prosthetic valves. If stratified by type of prosthesis, the incidence of systemic embolism at 15 years has been reported to be 18% and 22% (*P* = 0.96) for mechanical valves and bioprostheses, respectively.[99] Further long-term results have demonstrated an incidence of all embolism at 20 years of 53% for mechanical valves versus and incidence of 32% for bioprostheses (*P* = 0.13). Moreover, it also seems reasonable that hemorrhagic events are more likely to occur in patients who receive mechanical valves and consequent anticoagulation. However, as with thromboembolic complications, this likelihood is highly dependent on adherence to anticoagulation and patient comorbidities.

Prosthetic valve endocarditis (see Chapter 25) may occur years after surgery or early during the perioperative course (field contamination, wound infection, or indwelling catheters and cannulas). In the latter case, the most frequent causative agents are *Staphylococcus aureus*, *Staphylococcus epidermidis*, and gram-negative bacteria. This complication is slightly more frequent in patients receiving mechanical valves, with an overall incidence of 1%.[100] Late endocarditis has an incidence of 0.2% to 0.4% per patient-year, and there is no difference in incidence between types of prostheses.

REFERENCES

1. Quill JL, Hill AJ, Laske TG, et al. Mitral leaflet anatomy revisited. J Thorac Cardiovasc Surg 2009;137:1077–81.
2. Freed LA, Benjamin EJ, Levy D, et al. Mitral valve prolapse in the general population: the benign nature of echocardiographic features in the framingham heart study. J Am Coll Cardiol 2002;40:1298–304.
3. Anders S, Said S, Schulz F, et al. Mitral valve prolapse syndrome as cause of sudden death in young adults. Forensic Sci Int 2007;171:127–30.
4. Carabello BA. The current therapy for mitral regurgitation. J Am Coll Cardiol 2008;52:319–26.
5. Nkomo VT, Gardin JM, Skelton TN, et al. Burden of valvular heart diseases: a population-based study. Lancet 2006;368:1005–11.
6. Carpentier A. Cardiac valve surgery—the "french correction". J Thorac Cardiovasc Surg 1983;86:323–37.
7. Enriquez-Sarano M, Akins CW, Vahanian A. Mitral regurgitation. Lancet 2009; 373:1382–94.
8. David TE, Armstrong S, Ivanov J. Chordal replacement with polytetrafluoroethylene sutures for mitral valve repair: a 25-year experience. J Thorac Cardiovasc Surg 2012. Epub ahead of print Jun 17. doi:10.1016/j.jtcvs.2012.05.030.
9. Bonow RO, Carabello BA, Chatterjee K, et al. 2008 focused update incorporated into the ACC/AHA 2006 guidelines for the management of patients with valvular heart disease: a report of the American College of Cardiology/American Heart Association task force on practice guidelines (writing committee to revise the 1998 guidelines for the management of patients with valvular heart disease). Endorsed by the Society of Cardiovascular Anesthesiologists, Society for Cardiovascular Angiography and Interventions, and Society of Thoracic Surgeons. J Am Coll Cardiol 2008;52:e1–142.
10. Gammie JS, O'Brien SM, Griffith BP, et al. Influence of hospital procedural volume on care process and mortality for patients undergoing elective surgery for mitral regurgitation. Circulation 2007;115:881–7.
11. Johnston DR, Gillinov AM, Blackstone EH, et al. Surgical repair of posterior mitral valve prolapse: implications for guidelines and percutaneous repair. Ann Thorac Surg 2010;89:1385–94.
12. Mihaljevic T, Jarrett CM, Gillinov AM, et al. Robotic repair of posterior mitral valve prolapse versus conventional approaches: potential realized. J Thorac Cardiovasc Surg 2011;141:72–80 e71–4.
13. Gillinov AM, Blackstone EH, Alaulaqi A, et al. Outcomes after repair of the anterior mitral leaflet for degenerative disease. Ann Thorac Surg 2008;86:708–17; discussion 708–17.
14. Umakanthan R, Leacche M, Petracek MR, et al. Safety of minimally invasive mitral valve surgery without aortic cross-clamp. Ann Thorac Surg 2008;85:1544–9; discussion 1549–50.
15. Gammie JS, Sheng S, Griffith BP, et al. Trends in mitral valve surgery in the united states: results from the Society of Thoracic Surgeons Adult Cardiac Surgery database. Ann Thorac Surg 2009;87:1431–7; discussion 1437–9.
16. Levine RA. Dynamic mitral regurgitation—more than meets the eye. N Engl J Med 2004;351:1681–4.
17. Levine RA, Handschumacher MD, Sanfilippo AJ, et al. Three-dimensional echocardiographic reconstruction of the mitral valve, with implications for the diagnosis of mitral valve prolapse. Circulation 1989;80:589–98.
18. Ranganathan N, Lam JH, Wigle ED, et al. Morphology of the human mitral valve. II. The value leaflets. Circulation 1970;41:459–67.
19. Dent JM, Spotnitz WD, Nolan SP, et al. Mechanism of mitral leaflet excursion. Am J Physiol 1995;269:H2100–2108.
20. Lam JH, Ranganathan N, Wigle ED, et al. Morphology of the human mitral valve. I. Chordae tendineae: a new classification. Circulation 1970;41:449–58.
21. Rodriguez F, Langer F, Harrington KB, et al. Importance of mitral valve second-order chordae for left ventricular geometry, wall thickening mechanics, and global systolic function. Circulation 2004;110:II115–122.
22. Kron IL, Green GR, Cope JT. Surgical relocation of the posterior papillary muscle in chronic ischemic mitral regurgitation. Ann Thorac Surg 2002;74:600–1.
23. Kono T, Sabbah HN, Rosman H, et al. Left ventricular shape is the primary determinant of functional mitral regurgitation in heart failure. J Am Coll Cardiol 1992;20:1594–8.
24. Carpentier A, Chauvaud S, Fabiani JN, et al. Reconstructive surgery of mitral valve incompetence: ten-year appraisal. J Thorac Cardiovasc Surg 1980;79:338–48.
25. Essop MR, Nkomo VT. Rheumatic and nonrheumatic valvular heart disease: Epidemiology, management, and prevention in Africa. Circulation 2005;112:3584–91.
26. Iung B, Baron G, Butchart EG, et al. A prospective survey of patients with valvular heart disease in Europe: the Euro Heart Survey on Valvular Heart Disease. Eur Heart J 2003;24:1231–43.
27. Fornes P, Heudes D, Fuzellier JF, et al. Correlation between clinical and histologic patterns of degenerative mitral valve insufficiency: a histomorphometric study of 130 excised segments. Cardiovasc Pathol 1999;8:81–92.
28. Adams DH, Anyanwu AC. Seeking a higher standard for degenerative mitral valve repair: Begin with etiology. J Thorac Cardiovasc Surg 2008;136:551–6.
29. Anyanwu AC, Adams DH. Etiologic classification of degenerative mitral valve disease: Barlow's disease and fibroelastic deficiency. Semin Thorac Cardiovasc Surg 2007;19: 90–6.
30. Carpentier A, Lacour-Gayet F, Camilleri J. Fibroelastic dysplasia of the mitral valve: an anatomical and clinical entity. Circulation 1982;3:307.
31. Barlow JB, Bosman CK. Aneurysmal protrusion of the posterior leaflet of the mitral valve. an auscultatory-electrocardiographic syndrome. Am Heart J 1966;71:166–78.
32. Barlow JB, Pocock WA. Billowing, floppy, prolapsed or flail mitral valves? Am J Cardiol 1985;55:501–2.
33. Adams DH, Anyanwu AC, Rahmanian PB, et al. Large annuloplasty rings facilitate mitral valve repair in barlow's disease. Ann Thorac Surg 2006;82:2096–100; discussion 2101.
34. Lee R, Li S, Rankin JS, et al. Fifteen-year outcome trends for valve surgery in North America. Ann Thorac Surg 2011;91:677–84; discussion p 684.
35. Agricola E, Oppizzi M, Pisani M, et al. Ischemic mitral regurgitation: mechanisms and echocardiographic classification. Eur J Echocardiogr 2008;9:207–21.
36. Bax JJ, Braun J, Somer ST, et al. Restrictive annuloplasty and coronary revascularization in ischemic mitral regurgitation results in reverse left ventricular remodeling. Circulation 2004;110:II103–08.
37. Levine RA, Hung J. Ischemic mitral regurgitation, the dynamic lesion: clues to the cure. J Am Coll Cardiol 2003;42:1929–32.
38. Unger P, Magne J, Dedobbeleer C, et al. Ischemic mitral regurgitation: not only a bystander. Curr Cardiol Rep 2012;14:180–9.
39. Mesana T. Ischemic mitral regurgitation: the challenge goes on. Curr Opin Cardiol 2012;27:108–10.
40. Suri RM, Schaff HV, Dearani JA, et al. Survival advantage and improved durability of mitral repair for leaflet prolapse subsets in the current era. Ann Thorac Surg 2006;82:819–26.
41. Russo A, Grigioni F, Avierinos JF, et al. Thromboembolic complications after surgical correction of mitral regurgitation: incidence, predictors, and clinical implications. J Am Coll Cardiol 2008;51:1203–11.
42. Gammie JS, Zhao Y, Peterson ED, et al. Maxwell chamberlain memorial paper for adult cardiac surgery. Less-invasive mitral valve operations: Trends and outcomes from the Society of Thoracic Surgeons adult cardiac surgery database. Ann Thorac Surg 2010;90:1401–8, 1410 e1401; discussion 1408–10.
43. Casselman FP, Van Slycke S, Dom H, et al. Endoscopic mitral valve repair: feasible, reproducible, and durable. J Thorac Cardiovasc Surg 2003;125:273–82.
44. Chitwood Jr WR, Rodriguez E, Chu MW, et al. Robotic mitral valve repairs in 300 patients: a single-center experience. J Thorac Cardiovasc Surg 2008;136:436–41.
45. Seeburger J, Borger MA, Falk V, et al. Minimal invasive mitral valve repair for mitral regurgitation: results of 1339 consecutive patients. Eur J Cardiothorac Surg 2008;34: 760–5.
46. Casselman FP, Van Slycke S, Wellens F, et al. Mitral valve surgery can now routinely be performed endoscopically. Circulation 2003;108(Suppl 1):II48–54.
47. Vahanian A, Alfieri O, Andreotti F, et al. Guidelines on the management of valvular heart disease (version 2012). Joint Task Force on the Management of Valvular Heart Disease of the European Society of Cardiology and the European Association for Cardiothoracic Surgery. Eur Heart J 2012;33:2451–96.
48. Castillo JG, Anyanwu AC, Fuster V, et al. A near 100% repair rate for mitral valve prolapse is achievable in a reference center: implications for future guidelines. J Thorac Cardiovasc Surg 2012;144:308–12.
49. Adams DH, Anyanwu AC, Rahmanian PB, et al. Current concepts in mitral valve repair for degenerative disease. Heart Fail Rev 2006;11:241–57.
50. Carpentier AC, Adams DH, Filsoufi F. Carpentier's reconstructive valve surgery. Maryland Heights: Saunders Elsevier; 2010.
51. Anyanwu AC, Adams DH. The intraoperative "ink test": a novel assessment tool in mitral valve repair. J Thorac Cardiovasc Surg 2007;133:1635–6.
52. Braun J, van de Veire NR, Klautz RJ, et al. Restrictive mitral annuloplasty cures ischemic mitral regurgitation and heart failure. Ann Thorac Surg 2008;85:430–6; discussion 436–7.
53. Filsoufi F, Castillo JG, Rahmanian PB, et al. Remodeling annuloplasty using a prosthetic ring designed for correcting type-iiib ischemic mitral regurgitation. Rev Esp Cardiol 2007;60:1151–8.
54. Daimon M, Fukuda S, Adams DH, et al. Mitral valve repair with Carpentier-Mccarthy-Adams IMR Etlogix annuloplasty ring for ischemic mitral regurgitation: early echocardiographic results from a multi-center study. Circulation 2006;114(Suppl 1):I588–93.
55. Borger MA, Murphy PM, Alam A, et al. Initial results of the chordal-cutting operation for ischemic mitral regurgitation. J Thorac Cardiovasc Surg 2007;133:1483–92.
56. Borger MA. Chronic ischemic mitral regurgitation: insights into pandora's box. Circulation 2012;126:2674–6.
57. Chauvaud S, Fuzellier JF, Berrebi A, et al. Long-term (29 years) results of reconstructive surgery in rheumatic mitral valve insufficiency. Circulation 2001;104(Suppl 1):I12–15.
58. Magne J, Senechal M, Dumesnil JG, et al. Ischemic mitral regurgitation: a complex multifaceted disease. Cardiology 2009;112:244–59.
59. Chan V, Ruel M, Mesana TG. Mitral valve replacement is a viable alternative to mitral valve repair for ischemic mitral regurgitation: a case-matched study. Ann Thorac Surg 2011;92:1358–65; discussion 1365–56.
60. Dodson JA, Wang Y, Desai MM, et al. Outcomes for mitral valve surgery among medicare fee-for-service beneficiaries, 1999 to 2008. Circ Cardiovasc Qual Outcomes 2012;5:298–307.
61. Rahimtoola SH. Choice of prosthetic heart valve in adults an update. J Am Coll Cardiol 2010;55:2413–26.
62. Seeburger J, Borger MA, Doll N, et al. Comparison of outcomes of minimally invasive mitral valve surgery for posterior, anterior and bileaflet prolapse. Eur J Cardiothorac Surg 2009;36:532–8.
63. David TE. Outcomes of mitral valve repair for mitral regurgitation due to degenerative disease. Semin Thorac Cardiovasc Surg 2007;19:116–20.
64. Flameng W, Meuris B, Herijgers P, et al. Durability of mitral valve repair in Barlow disease versus fibroelastic deficiency. J Thorac Cardiovasc Surg 2008;135:274–82.
65. Gillinov AM, Mihaljevic T, Blackstone EH, et al. Should patients with severe degenerative mitral regurgitation delay surgery until symptoms develop? Ann Thorac Surg 2010;90:481–8.

66. Flameng W, Herijgers P, Bogaerts K. Recurrence of mitral valve regurgitation after mitral valve repair in degenerative valve disease. Circulation 2003;107:1609–13.

67. Badhwar V, Peterson ED, Jacobs JP, et al. Longitudinal outcome of isolated mitral repair in older patients: results from 14,604 procedures performed from 1991 to 2007. Ann Thorac Surg 2012;94:1870–9.

68. Pfannmuller B, Seeburger J, Misfeld M, et al. Minimally invasive mitral valve repair for anterior leaflet prolapse. J Thorac Cardiovasc Surg 2012 Epub ahead of print. July 14. doi.org/10.1016/j.jtcvs.2012.06.044.

69. Tietge WJ, de Heer LM, van Hessen MW, et al. Early mitral valve repair versus watchful waiting in patients with severe asymptomatic organic mitral regurgitation; rationale and design of the Dutch AMR trial, a multicenter, randomised trial. Neth Heart J 2012;20:94–101.

70. Lawrie GM, Earle EA, Earle NR. Nonresectional repair of the barlow mitral valve: importance of dynamic annular evaluation. Ann Thorac Surg 2009;88:1191–6.

71. Perier P, Hohenberger W, Lakew F, et al. Toward a new paradigm for the reconstruction of posterior leaflet prolapse: midterm results of the "respect rather than resect" approach. Ann Thorac Surg 2008;86:718–25; discussion 718–25.

72. Bolling SF, Li S, O'Brien SM, et al. Predictors of mitral valve repair: clinical and surgeon factors. Ann Thorac Surg 2010;90:1904–11; discussion 1912.

73. Kilic A, Shah AS, Conte JV, et al. Operative outcomes in mitral valve surgery: combined effect of surgeon and hospital volume in a population-based analysis. J Thorac Cardiovasc Surg 2012 Epub ahead of print. Aug 20. doi.org/10.1016/j.jtcvs.2012.07.070.

74. Le Tourneau T, Messika-Zeitoun D, Russo A, et al. Impact of left atrial volume on clinical outcome in organic mitral regurgitation. J Am Coll Cardiol 2010;56:570–8.

75. Ling LH, Enriquez-Sarano M, Seward JB, et al. Clinical outcome of mitral regurgitation due to flail leaflet. N Engl J Med 1996;335:1417–23.

76. Magne J, Lancellotti P, O'Connor K, et al. Prediction of exercise pulmonary hypertension in asymptomatic degenerative mitral regurgitation. J Am Soc Echocardiogr 2011;24:1004–12.

77. Rusinaru D, Tribouilloy C, Grigioni F, et al. Left atrial size is a potent predictor of mortality in mitral regurgitation due to flail leaflets: results from a large international multicenter study. Circ Cardiovasc Imaging 2011;4:473–81.

78. Tribouilloy C, Grigioni F, Avierinos JF, et al. Survival implication of left ventricular end-systolic diameter in mitral regurgitation due to flail leaflets: a long-term follow-up multicenter study. J Am Coll Cardiol 2009;54:1961–8.

79. Enriquez-Sarano M, Avierinos JF, Messika-Zeitoun D, et al. Quantitative determinants of the outcome of asymptomatic mitral regurgitation. N Engl J Med 2005;352:875–83.

80. Enriquez-Sarano M, Nkomo V, Mohty D, et al. Mitral regurgitation: predictors of outcome and natural history. Adv Cardiol 2002;39:133–43.

81. David TE, Ivanov J, Armstrong S, et al. A comparison of outcomes of mitral valve repair for degenerative disease with posterior, anterior, and bileaflet prolapse. J Thorac Cardiovasc Surg 2005;130:1242–9.

82. Reece TB, Tribble CG, Ellman PI, et al. Mitral repair is superior to replacement when associated with coronary artery disease. Ann Surg 2004;239:671–5; discussion 675–7.

83. Gillinov AM, Wierup PN, Blackstone EH, et al. Is repair preferable to replacement for ischemic mitral regurgitation? J Thorac Cardiovasc Surg 2001;122:1125–41.

84. Deja MA, Grayburn PA, Sun B, et al. Influence of mitral regurgitation repair on survival in the Surgical Treatment For Ischemic Heart Failure trial. Circulation 2012;125:2639–48.

85. Vassileva CM, Boley T, Markwell S, et al. Meta-analysis of short-term and long-term survival following repair versus replacement for ischemic mitral regurgitation. Eur J Cardiothorac Surg 2011;39:295–303.

86. Penicka M, Linkova H, Lang O, et al. Predictors of improvement of unrepaired moderate ischemic mitral regurgitation in patients undergoing elective isolated coronary artery bypass graft surgery. Circulation 2009;120:1474–81.

87. Magne J, Senechal M, Mathieu P, et al. Restrictive annuloplasty for ischemic mitral regurgitation may induce functional mitral stenosis. J Am Coll Cardiol 2008;51:1692–701.

88. Anyanwu AC, Adams DH. Ischemic mitral regurgitation: recent advances. Curr Treat Options Cardiovasc Med 2008;10:529–37.

89. Glower DD, Tuttle RH, Shaw LK, et al. Patient survival characteristics after routine mitral valve repair for ischemic mitral regurgitation. J Thorac Cardiovasc Surg 2005;129:860–8.

90. Mihaljevic T, Lam BK, Rajeswaran J, et al. Impact of mitral valve annuloplasty combined with revascularization in patients with functional ischemic mitral regurgitation. J Am Coll Cardiol 2007;49:2191–201.

91. Aklog L, Filsoufi F, Flores KQ, et al. Does coronary artery bypass grafting alone correct moderate ischemic mitral regurgitation? Circulation 2001;104:I68–75.

92. Chan KM, Punjabi PP, Flather M, et al. Coronary artery bypass surgery with or without mitral valve annuloplasty in moderate functional ischemic mitral regurgitation: final results of the Randomized Ischemic Mitral Evaluation (RIME) trial. Circulation 2012;126:2502–10.

93. de Varennes B, Chaturvedi R, Sidhu S, et al. Initial results of posterior leaflet extension for severe type IIIb ischemic mitral regurgitation. Circulation 2009;119:2837–43.

94. Lorusso R, Gelsomino S, Vizzardi E, et al. Mitral valve repair or replacement for ischemic mitral regurgitation? The Italian Study on the Treatment of Ischemic Mitral Regurgitation (ISTIMIR). J Thorac Cardiovasc Surg 2013;145:128–39.

95. Diodato MD, Moon MR, Pasque MK, et al. Repair of ischemic mitral regurgitation does not increase mortality or improve long-term survival in patients undergoing coronary artery revascularization: a propensity analysis. Ann Thorac Surg 2004;78:794–9; discussion 794–9.

96. Edmunds Jr LH, Clark RE, Cohn LH, et al. Guidelines for reporting morbidity and mortality after cardiac valvular operations. J Thorac Cardiovasc Surg 1996;112:708–11.

97. Society of Thoracic Surgery adult cardiac database executive summary, 2012. Available at <http://www.sts.org/sts-national-database/database-managers/executive-summaries>

98. Grunkemeier GL, Li HH, Naftel DC, et al. Long-term performance of heart valve prostheses. Curr Probl Cardiol 2000;25:73–154.

99. Hammermeister K, Sethi GK, Henderson WG, et al. Outcomes 15 years after valve replacement with a mechanical versus a bioprosthetic valve: final report of the Veterans Affairs randomized trial. J Am Coll Cardiol 2000;36:1152–8.

100. Oxenham H, Bloomfield P, Wheatley DJ, et al. Twenty year comparison of a Bjork-Shiley mechanical heart valve with porcine bioprostheses. Heart 2003;89:715–21.

CHAPTER 22

Transcatheter Mitral Valve Repair and Replacement

Howard C. Herrmann

Key Points

- The risks of surgery in patients with severe mitral regurgitation, particularly with consideration of morbidity and patient preference, have stimulated attempts to develop less invasive solutions. The risks of surgery are particularly high in patients who are elderly and have left ventricular dysfunction and/or medical comorbidities.
- Unlike the extensive toolbox available to the mitral surgeon, transcatheter approaches are much more limited and often able to address only a single major element of the dysfunctional valve that contributes to mitral regurgitation (MR).
- The MitraClip is a device that clips the middle scallops of the anterior and posterior leaflets, analogous to the surgical Alfieri procedure. It is an approved device in Europe and remains investigational in the United States. A series of trials with this device confirmed feasibility (EVEREST I), and a randomized trial provided safety and efficacy data in comparison with surgical repair in (EVEREST II).
- The MitraClip is undergoing further investigation in patients for whom surgery poses a high risk in a new randomized trial (COAPT) that will compare outcomes of the use of the device and outcomes of medical therapy.
- Other investigations are under way to test efficacy of other nonsurgical devices, including mitral annuloplasty devices, left ventricular remodeling devices (to reduce severity of MR in patients with dilated left ventricles), and transcatheter mitral valve replacements.

Rationale for Transcatheter Therapy

Surgery to repair or replace the mitral valve in patients with severe MR appears to improve survival in observational studies.[8] However, the risks of surgery, particularly in consideration of morbidity and patient preference, have stimulated attempts to develop less invasive solutions.[9] Surgery is associated with mortality rates of 1% to 5% and additional morbidity rates of 10% to 20%, the morbidity including stroke, reoperation, renal failure, and prolonged ventilation.[10] Furthermore, in one study of Medicare-age patients, more than 20% required rehospitalization in the first 30 days after surgery.[11]

The risks of surgery are particularly high in patients who are elderly or have LV dysfunction.[10,12] In one study of more than 30,000 patients undergoing mitral valve replacement, the mortality increased from 4.1% in those younger than 50 years to 17.0% in octogenarians (Figure 22-1). Similarly, significant morbidity (stroke, prolonged ventilation, renal failure, reoperation, sternal infection) occurred in more than a third of octogenarians. Predictors of risk in addition to age in this study included hemodynamic instability, severe symptoms, renal failure, and prior coronary artery bypass grafting surgery (CABG).[12]

In patients with LV dysfunction and secondary MR, whether ischemic or functional, survival with or without surgery is not as good as in patients with preserved LV function and primary MR etiology.[4] Whether the increased mortality is a consequence of the preexisting LV dysfunction and whether the MR contributes to the reduced survival remain a controversial issues. In vitro studies have demonstrated progressive adverse LV remodeling in sheep even after successful MR repair.[13] Other studies have not shown benefit with annuloplasty repair of MR in dilated cardiomyopathy[14] or at the time of revascularization with CABG.[15] In both ischemic and nonischemic functional MR, age and comorbidities are the most important predictors of survival.[16]

Thus, the major reason for surgery in most patients with ischemic MR is to provide symptomatic improvement and in those with primary MR to forestall the development of LV dysfunction. For this reason, it is essential to also discuss the efficacy of surgery in terms of MR reduction. In relatively young patients (mean age 55 to 60 years) with primary MR, long-term freedom from repeat surgery is well documented.[17,18] However, recurrent 3+ and 4+ MR may occur in up to 30% of patients within 15 years.[17,18] Recurrent MR is even more frequent in patients with ischemic MR, providing a potential target for the development of transcatheter therapies.[19]

Classification of Percutaneous Repair Therapies

In keeping with the earlier discussion of the complexity of the mitral valve apparatus, it is useful to consider the percutaneous approaches according to the major structural abnormality that they address.[20] Unlike the extensive toolbox available to the mitral

Mitral regurgitation (MR) is a diverse disease that results from dysfunction of any of the portions of the complex mitral valve apparatus, including the leaflets, chords, annulus, and left ventricle. It is convenient to classify MR on the basis of two broad categories of dysfunction, namely primary (organic or degenerative) disease, which primarily affects the leaflets (e.g., fibromuscular dysplasia, mitral valve prolapse, rheumatic disease), and secondary (ischemic or functional) diseases, which spare the leaflets (e.g., diseases of the atrium and ventricle, including ischemic dysfunction and dilated cardiomyopathy) (see Chapters 18 and 19). More recently, it has been appreciated that even in secondary functional or ischemic MR, there may be changes that affect the leaflets.[1] Finally, some diseases such as ischemic MR may affect more than one portion of the valve apparatus. For example, both leaflet tethering and annular dilation may be present and may contribute to MR.[2]

Patients with severe MR have decreased survival,[3] whether symptomatic[4] or not,[5] and surgery is often recommended. However, some studies have demonstrated that asymptomatic patients with severe MR and preserved left ventricular (LV) function can be safely monitored with a "watchful waiting" approach until the development of symptoms, LV dysfunction, pulmonary hypertension, or atrial fibrillation without a morbidity penalty at the time of surgery.[6] For these reasons, current guidelines recommend surgery for symptomatic patients and asymptomatic patients with abnormal LV function.[7] Surgery may also be considered for asymptomatic patients with normal LV function when there is a high likelihood of successful repair.

surgeon, transcatheter approaches are much more limited and often able to address only a single major element of the dysfunctional valve that contributes to MR. The remainder of this chapter addresses these transcatheter approaches with an emphasis on devices that have been approved in some part of the world, those that have entered first-in-human or phase 1 clinical investigation, and those with published data (either clinical or preclinical). Some devices that have been evaluated in vivo without success or are no longer under development are discussed only as they relate to other current approaches. Table 22-1 lists the devices along with their manufacturers, state of development, and any available published reports.

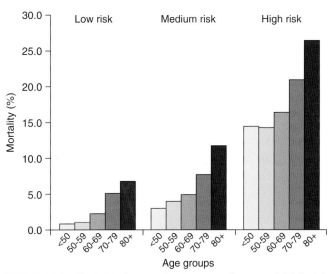

FIGURE 22-1 Mortality by age for low-, medium-, and high-risk categories of patients undergoing mitral valve replacement. *(From Mehta RH, Eagle KA, Coombs LP, et al: Influence of age on outcomes in patients undergoing mitral valve replacement. Ann Thorac Surg 2002;74:1459-1467.)*

Leaflet and Chordal Technology

MITRACLIP

The major technology in this category, MitraClip (Abbott Vascular), was also the first transcatheter mitral valve repair technology to receive CE Mark approval (Figure 22-2). This system has its roots in the Alfieri stitch operation, in which the middle scallops of the posterior and anterior leaflets (P2 and A2, respectively) are sutured together to create a double-orifice mitral valve. This operation, though usually performed with adjunctive ring annuloplasty, has proved effective and durable in a wide variety of pathologies and even in selected patients without annuloplasty.[21,22]

The concept of a percutaneous replicate of an Alfieri stitch was initially conceived by St. Goar and subsequently developed as MitraClip by Evalve, Inc. (which was later acquired by Abbott Vascular).[23] A series of trials with this device confirmed its feasibility (Endovascular Valve Edge-to-Edge Repair Study [EVEREST] I), and its safety and efficacy were compared with those of surgical repair in a randomized trial (EVEREST II), providing a wealth of data on this technology as described later.[24,25]

The procedure is performed with standard catheterization techniques utilizing a transseptal approach from the right femoral vein.[26] The clip delivery system is introduced through a 24F sheath into the left atrium, where it can be guided using a series of turning knobs under transesophageal (both two- and three-dimensional) echocardiography guidance through the mitral valve into the left ventricle. A properly aligned and oriented clip can be placed on the P2 and A2 segments of leaflets, grasping them from the ventricular side to create leaflet opposition. Once leaflet insertion is confirmed by echocardiography, the clip can be released. If a suboptimal grasp occurs, the leaflet can be released, allowing repositioning prior to a second grasp attempt. Additionally, a second or more clips can be placed as needed for optimal MR reduction (Figure 22-3).[26]

In the 2:1 randomized EVEREST II trial, 184 patients were designated to receive MitraClip therapy and 95 to undergo surgical repair or replacement. These patients were almost a decade older (mean age 67 years) than in usual surgical series and had more comorbidities. Major adverse events at 30 days were significantly less frequent with MitraClip therapy (9.6% versus 57% with surgery;

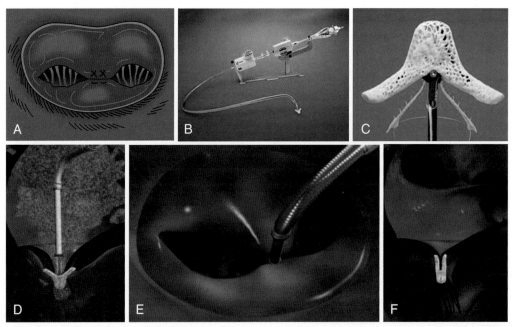

FIGURE 22-2 The MitraClip leaflet coaptation system. This device (Abbott Vascular, Inc.) creates a bridge between the P2 and A2 segments of the mitral valve similar to the Alfieri stitch operation **(A)** utilizing a clip delivery system **(B)** and the MitraClip **(C)**. **D** and **E,** Side view and left atrial view of the clip delivery system as it is advanced through the mitral valve in the open position prior to grasping of the leaflets. **F,** The final result is illustrated after the clip has been released and the delivery system removed.

TABLE 22-1   Devices for Transcatheter Mitral Valve Therapy

ANATOMIC TARGET	DEVICE NAME	MANUFACTURER	DEVELOPMENT STATUS	REFERENCE(S)
Leaflet/Chordal				
	MitraClip	Abbott Vascular, Abbott Park, Illinois	CE Mark Phase III (US)	24-32
	NeoChord DS1000 System	Neochord, Inc., Eden Prairie, Minnesota	Phase 1 (outside US)	33
	Mitra-Spacer	Cardiosolutions, Inc., West Bridgewater, Massachusetts	Phase 1 (outside US)	34
	MitraFlex	TransCardiac Therapeutics, LLC, Atlanta, Georgia	Preclinical	—
Indirect Annuloplasty				
	CARILLON XE2 Mitral Contour System	Cardiac Dimensions, Inc., Kirkland, Wisconsin	CE Mark	37,38
	Kardium MR	Kardium, Inc., Richmond, British Columbia, Canada	Preclinical	—
	Cerclage annuloplasty	National Heart, Lung, and Blood Institute, Bethesda, Maryland	Preclinical	42
Direct or Left Ventricular Annuloplasty				
	Mitralign Percutaneous Annuloplasty System	Mitralign, Inc., Tewksbury, Massachusetts	Phase 1 (outside US)	44
	GDS Accucinch System	Guided Delivery Systems, Santa Clara, California	Phase 1 (outside US)	47
	Boa RF Catheter	QuantumCor, Inc., Laguna Niguel, California	Preclinical	—
	Cardioband	Valtech Cardio, Or Yehuda, Israel	Preclinical	—
	Millipede system	Millipede LLC, Ann Arbor, Michigan	Preclinical	—
Hybrid Surgical				
	Adjustable Annuloplasty Ring	Mitral Solutions, Fort Lauderdale, Florida	Phase 1	—
	Dynaplasty ring	MiCardia Corporation, Irvine, California	Phase 1	—
LV Remodeling				
	The Basal Annuloplasty of the Cardia Externally (BACE)	Mardil Medical, Minneapolis, Minnesota	Phase 1	—
	Tendyne Repair	Tendyne Holdings, Inc., Baltimore	Preclinical	—
Replacement				
	Endovalve	Micro Interventional Devices, Inc., Langhorne, Pennsylvania	Preclinical	48
	CardiAQ	CardiAQ Valve Technologies, Inc., Irvine, California	Preclinical	—
	Lutter	Universitatsklinikum, Kiel, Germany	Preclinical	62,63
	Tiara	Neovasc, Inc., Richmond, British Columbia, Canada	Preclinical	—
	Ventor Embracer	Medtronic, Inc., Minneapolis, Minnesota	Preclinical	—
	PCS Mitral Valve	Percutaneous Cardiovascular Solutions, Pty, Ltd, Newcastle, New South Wales, Australia	Preclinical	—

$P < 0.0001$), although much of the difference could be attributed to the greater need for blood transfusions with surgery[27] (Figure 22-4). The freedom from the combined outcome of death, mitral valve surgery, and MR severity greater than 2+ at 12 months was higher with surgery (73%) than with MitraClip therapy (55%; $P = 0.0007$). Importantly, in patients with acute MitraClip therapy success, the result appears durable with a very low rate of later mitral valve surgery (Figure 22-5).

Subsequent analyses of this rich database have demonstrated persistent reductions in MR grade, improvement in New York Heart Association (NYHA) functional class, and reduction in LV dimensions[27] with MitraClip therapy. Other studies have demonstrated a lack of mitral stenosis, no effect of initial rhythm on results, and benefit in higher-risk subjects.[28-30]

In the EVEREST II High-Risk Study, 78 patients with an estimated surgical mortality rate of 12% or higher (mean 14%) were treated with MitraClip, with an actual 30-day mortality of 8%. Survival at 12 months was 76% and significantly better than that of a concurrently screened comparison group, the majority of whom (86%) were treated medically. Patients treated with Mitra-Clip had improved MR grade at 12 months (78% ≤2+), LV dimensions, New York Heart Association functional class, and quality of life, and a reduced need for hospitalization.[30] Similar benefit was demonstrated in another series of extreme-risk patients.[31] In addition, a group of European investigators have demonstrated the feasibility of MitraClip therapy in a group of 51 severely symptomatic patients with secondary ischemic or functional MR that failed to respond to cardiac resynchronization therapy.[32]

The future of MitraClip therapy and its role in the management of patients with MR remains unclear in the United States because of its investigational status. The EVEREST II trial failed to demonstrate efficacy equivalent to that of surgery for a diverse group of patients with varied risk and etiology. The EVEREST High-Risk Registry and experience outside the United States point to a more appropriate role in high-risk patients with secondary functional and ischemic MR. A new randomized trial (Clinical Outcomes Assessment of the MitraClip Percutaneous Therapy for High Surgical Risk Patients [COAPT]) is under way to compare the device with medical therapy in these patients.

OTHER DEVICES

Other devices discussed in this category are NeoChord, Mitra-Spacer, and MitraFlex (Figure 22-6). The NeoChord DS1000 system is a transapically inserted tool that can capture a flail leaflet segment and pierce it with a semidull needle to attach a standard polytetrafluoroethylene (PTFE) artificial chord, which is then anchored to the apical entry site with a pledgeted suture. A

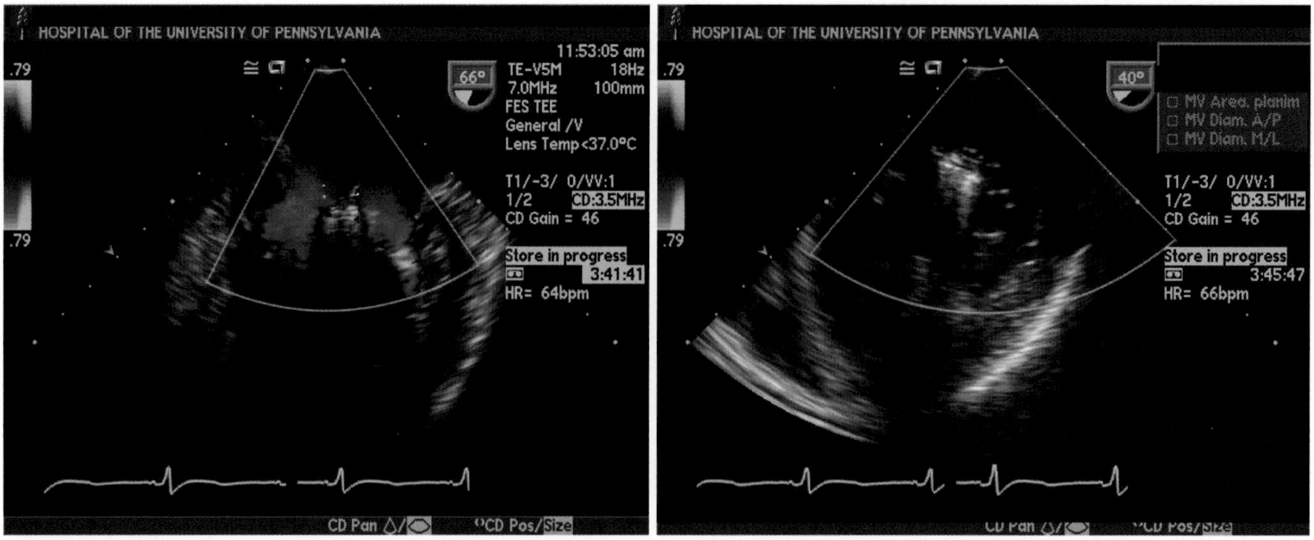

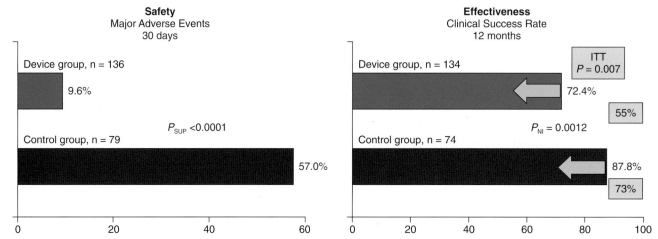

FIGURE 22-3 Echocardiograms after deployment of two MitraClip devices. *Left panel,* Mitral inflow view demonstrating flow around the MitraClips (Abbott Vascular) into the ventricle through both orifices. *Right panel,* Dual orifices in the transgastric view.

FIGURE 22-4 Primary safety and efficacy endpoints for EVEREST II. Rates of major adverse events at 30 days were reduced by MitraClip (Abbott Vascular) from 57.0% to 9.6% (*P* <0.0001). The rates of clinical success at 12 months for patients with immediate procedural success were similar, although by intent-to-treat (ITT) analysis of all patients *(yellow arrows),* effectiveness was better with surgery (73%) than with MitraClip (55%; p = 0.007). *EVEREST,* Endovascular Valve Edge-to-Edge Repair Study; *NI,* non-inferiority; *SUP,* superiority. *(From Feldman T, Foster E, Glower D, et al. Percutaneous repair or surgery for mitral regurgitation. N Engl J Med. 2011;364:1395-1406.)*

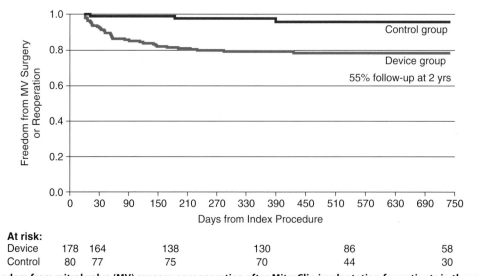

FIGURE 22-5 The freedom from mitral valve (MV) surgery or reoperation after MitraClip implantation for patients in the randomized EVEREST II. Note that patients with good results at 90 days after MitraClip (Abbott Vascular) appear to have a durable outcome to 2 years. EVEREST, Endovascular Valve Edge-to-Edge Repair Study. *(From Feldman T, Foster E, Glower D, et al: Percutaneous repair or surgery for mitral regurgitation. N Engl J Med 2011;364:1395-1406.)*

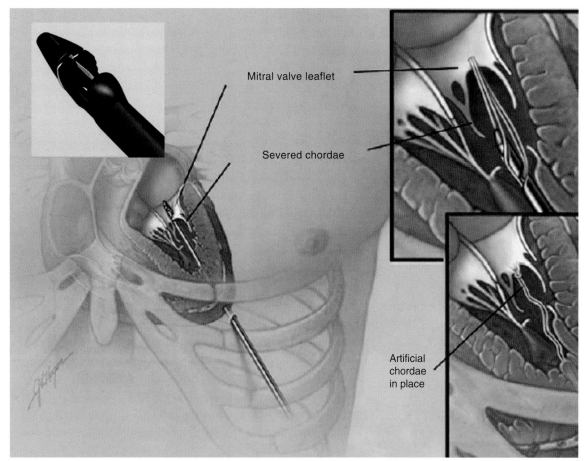

Mitral valve leaflet

Severed chordae

Artificial
chordae
in place

FIGURE 22-6   Additional leaflet repair technology. Neochord insertion of a transapically-anchored PTFE chord (NeoChord, Inc., Eden Praire, MN).

first-in-human case has been reported,[33] and the device is currently undergoing a phase 1 evaluation in Europe in the Transapical Artificial Chordae Tendineae (TACT) trial.

Mitra-Spacer (Cardiosolutions, Inc.) is an occluder device that is anchored in the LV apex via transseptal or transapical insertion with an anchor fixed outside the heart. The tethered "balloon-like" spacer floats in the mitral inflow pathway, providing a space occluder around which the mitral leaflets coalesce. This device has entered outside US first-in-human evaluation and has been deployed in four patients, with a reported reduction of one to two MR grades.[34] The MitraFlex device (Transcardiac Therapeutics) is designed as a transapically inserted thorascopic device to implant artificial chordae tendineae and is in preclinical development.

Indirect Annuloplasty

The venous anatomy of the heart is of particular interest for treating MR because of the ease of access (from the right internal jugular vein) and the location of the great cardiac vein in proximity to the posterior mitral annulus. Some of the first attempts to treat MR without surgery did so by mimicking surgical ring annuloplasty through placement of devices in the coronary sinus, so-called indirect or percutaneous coronary sinus annuloplasty. The goal of this approach is to remodel the posterior annulus cinching the great cardiac vein or pushing in on the posterior annulus from the vein in order to improve leaflet coaptation.

Two early attempts to do this highlight some of the difficulties encountered with this approach. The MONARC annuloplasty system (Edward Lifesciences, Irvine, California) consisted of two stent anchors with a shortening bridge between them that pulled the anchors together over several weeks with the intent to cinch the vein and shorten the circumference of the mitral valve in its posterior portion (Figure 22-7). The device was initially implanted in 59 of 72 patients, with a modest reduction in MR grade at 12 months: among 22 patients with matched echocardiograms at baseline and 12 months, 50% achieved ≥1 grade reduction in MR severity. More concerning, however, was a high incidence of major adverse cardiovascular events, which included tamponade, early and late myocardial infarction, and nine deaths (at least one of which appeared to be device-related).[35] The combination of modest efficacy and safety concerns caused the manufacturer to abandon subsequent development.

In another approach, the Viacor Percutaneous Transvenous Mitral Annuloplasty (Viacor, Inc., Wilmington, Massachusetts) involved a nitinol rod placed in the coronary sinus to push on the P2 segment of the annulus to reduce the septal-lateral dimension and improve leaflet coaptation (see Figure 22-7). This device had the advantage of not requiring permanent implantation until efficacy could be determined in vivo, but it suffered from the same limitations as the MONARC: only mild efficacy, the potential risk for myocardial infarction, and the additional risk for rupture of the great cardiac vein.[36] This approach was also abandoned.

One coronary sinus approach has met with sufficient success and promise to obtain CE Mark, and a U.S. investigational device exemption (IDE) trial is planned. The CARILLON XE2 Mitral Contour System (Cardiac Dimensions, Inc.) uses novel anchors placed permanently in the coronary sinus that are pulled toward each other with a cinching device to reduce the mitral annular dimension by traction (see Figure 22-7). Early evaluation in the

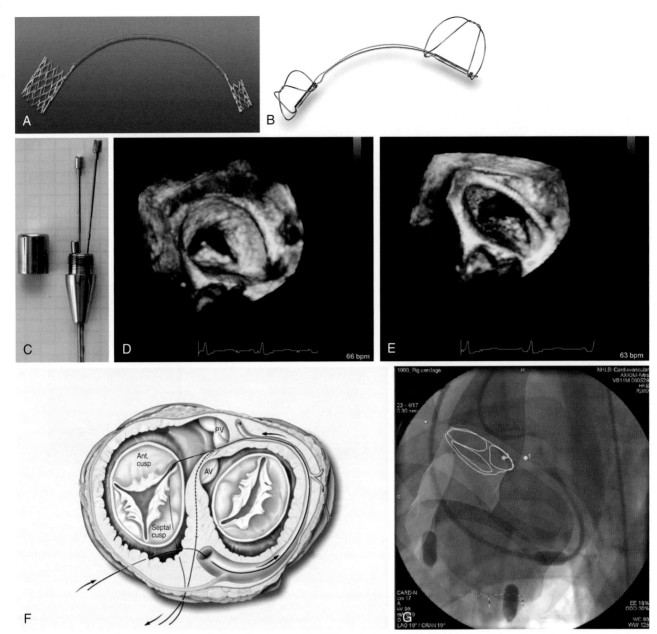

FIGURE 22-7   Several indirect annuloplasty devices. A, Edwards MONARC annuloplasty system (Edwards Lifesciences LLC, Irvine, California; Edwards and Edwards Lifesciences are trademarks of Edwards Lifesciences Corporation.). **B,** CARILLON XE2 Mitral Contour System (Cardiac Dimension, Inc., Kirkland, WA) coronary sinus cinching device. **C,** Viacor, Inc. (Wilmington, Massachusetts) coronary sinus device. Three-dimensional transesophageal echocardiograms before **(D)** and **(E)** after use of the Viacor device in a patient, in whom the device has pushed on the P2 segment to remodel the annulus and improve leaflet coaptation. Cerclage technique, shown in a schematic **(F)** and an angiogram with superimposed magnetic resonance images **(G)**. *AV,* aortic valve; *PV,* pulmonary valve. *(F and G from Kim JH, Kocaturk O, Ozturk C, et al. Mitral Cerclage annuloplasty, a novel transcatheter treatment for secondary mitral valve regurgitation: initial results in swine. J Am Coll Cardiol 2009;54:638–51.)*

Amadeus study demonstrated feasibility, with implantation in 30 of 48 patients and modest improvement in quantitative measures of MR with a small risk of coronary compromise (15%) and death (1 patient).[37] More recently, a redesigned device was tested in the Transcatheter Implantation of Carillon Mitral Annuloplasty Device (TITAN) trial.[38] Among 65 enrolled subjects with secondary MR (62% ischemic), the device was implanted successfully in 36 patients with a mean age of 62 years, mean ejection fraction 29%, with predominantly New York Heart Association functional class III symptoms, and with 2+ (30%), 3+ (55%), or 4+ (15%) grade MR. Quantitative measures of MR were better at 6 and 12 months than in 17 patients who were enrolled in the trial and did not receive implants.

In general, indirect annuloplasty devices may be able to provide modest MR reduction in selected patients, but likely less than is achievable with surgery. Whether this level of efficacy will result in sufficient symptomatic improvement and LV remodeling to justify the procedure requires further study. The limited efficacy is related to the location of the coronary sinus relative to the annulus (up to 10 mm more cranial), great individual anatomic variability, and the limited benefit of partial annular remodeling.[39,40] Possibly, some "super-responders" may be able to be identified on the basis of anatomic considerations before the procedure.

The risks of this approach must also be considered. In addition to the risk for damage to the cardiac venous system, devices in this location can compress the left circumflex or diagonal coronary arteries, which traverse between the coronary sinus and the mitral annulus in most patients.[41]

In this regard, one novel indirect approach to reduce the septal-lateral dimension that deserves further consideration is the

Cerclage annuloplasty technique. This approach attempts to create a more complete circumferential annuloplasty by placing a suture from the coronary sinus through a septal perforator vein into the right atrium or ventricle, where it is snared and tensioned with the proximal end from the right atrium to create a closed pursestring.[42] The procedure is guided by cardiac magnetic resonance and also uses a novel rigid protection device to avoid coronary compression.

Direct Annuloplasty and Hybrid Techniques

In part because of the limitations of the coronary sinus devices just described, other attempts to more directly remodel the mitral annulus have been developed (Figure 22-8). These include both transcatheter devices and hybrid devices that require surgical implantation with subsequent transcatheter adjustment.

The Mitralign Percutaneous Annuloplasty System (Mitralign, Inc.) was originally based on the surgical techniques of Paneth's posterior suture plicaton.[43] In this procedure, a transaortic catheter is advanced to the left ventricle and used to deliver pledgeted anchors through the posterior annulus that can be pulled together to shorten (plicate) the annulus up to 17 mm (with two implants) (see Figure 22-8). In 16 patients treated in a phase 1 trial, septal-lateral dimension could be reduced up to 8 mm.[44] A CE Mark trial is planned.

The Accucinch (Guided Delivery Systems) device utilizes a similar catheter approach to place up to 12 anchors along the ventricular surface of the posterior mitral annulus. A cable running through the anchors is tensioned to create posterior plication. In a later development, the anchors have been placed in the ventricular myocardium just below the valve plane (percutaneous ventriculoplasty). This device has been characterized as more of a ventricular remodeling approach rather than one that is truly annular.

In addition to these devices that have entered clinical investigation, a preclinical device that deserves mention is the QuantumCor Device (QuantumCor Inc.). This technology uses low-radiofrequency energy delivered via a transseptal catheter (Boa RF Catheter) to shrink the collagen within the mitral annulus.

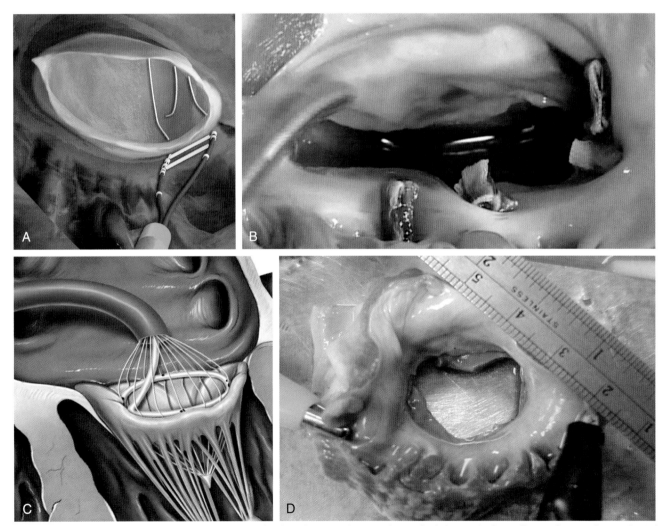

FIGURE 22-8 **Devices that directly remodel a portion of either the posterior annulus or the left ventricular wall near the annulus. A,** The Bident (Mitralign Inc., Tewksbury, MA) direct annuloplasty system and the result in an animal annulus **(B)**; **C,** the Boa radiofrequency collagen remodeling catheter is illustrated based on the QuantumCor device; **D,** the results of heat remodeling of an animal's annulus in vitro.

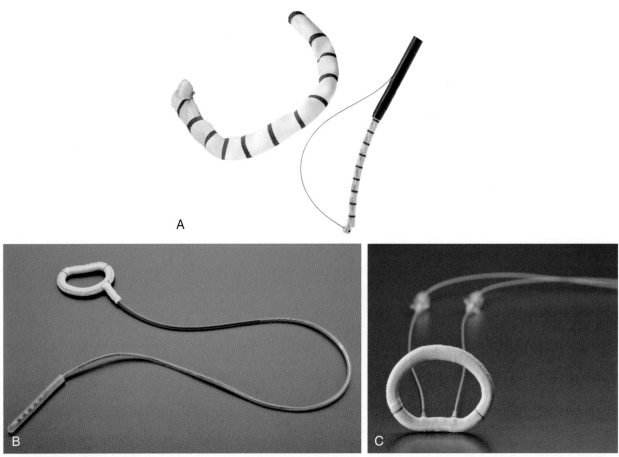

FIGURE 22-9 **Additional annuloplasty devices.** Several systems more directly mimic surgical ring annuloplasty either by direct insertion *(top)* or by requiring initial surgical implantation with subsequent size modification *(bottom).* **A,** Cardioband (Valtech Cardio, Or Yehuda, Israel); **B** and **C,** Dynaplasty ring (MiCardia Corp., Irvine, CA).

In animals, a 20% to 25% reduction in anterior-posterior dimension was achieved with a durability to 6 months (see Figure 22-8). A first-in-human validation study during open-heart surgery is planned.

Two devices that are under development represent a hybrid of surgical and transcatheter approaches. Both the Adjustable Annuloplasty Ring (Mitral Solutions) and the enCor Dynaplasty ring (MiCardia Corporation) are surgically implanted annuloplasty rings (Figure 22-9). The former can be adjusted (circumferentially reduced) with a mechanical catheter attachment. Similarly, the enCor ring is placed surgically and can be reshaped with radiofrequency energy supplied via removable leads passed externally from the left atrium through the incision for connection to an activation generator. This latter device has CE Mark and a U.S. investigational device exemption trial is under way. A subcutaneous version that may allow late activation and shape changing on an outpatient basis as well as a transcatheter version are under development (see Figure 22-9). These devices may improve surgical annuloplasty outcomes by allowing for fine tuning of the ring size and shape under more physiologic conditions (e.g., not during cardiopulmonary bypass) or at a future time if further MR or ventricular enlargement develops.

Finally, two devices are under development that attempt to further mimic surgical ring annuloplasty with a transcatheter approach. The Millipede nitinol ring (MC3, Inc.) is envisioned as a self-expanding, catheter-delivered device. The Cardioband (Valtech Cardio) is an adjustable, catheter-delivered, sutureless device that is inserted transseptally or transatrially and anchored on the atrial side of the annulus with the potential for subsequent adjustment (see Figure 22-9). Both are undergoing preclinical development.

Left Ventricular Remodeling Techniques

The basis for devices to treat MR by affecting the shape of the left ventricle arises from the pathophysiology of secondary ischemic or functional MR. Changes in the inferior and lateral left ventricle due to infarction can lead to tethering or tenting of the posterior leaflet, allowing anterior leaflet override as the mechanism of MR.[1,2] Similarly, failure of leaflet coaptation due to global LV enlargement causing annular distension is the major mechanism for MR in dilated cardiomyopathy.[45] Although ring annuloplasty can often ameliorate MR caused by LV distortion, procedures that specifically address the underlying LV pathology may also be beneficial.

The Coapsys annuloplasty system (Myocor Inc., Maple Grove, Minnesota) was originally developed as an adjunct to surgical revascularization (Figure 22-10). This device has two extracardiac epicardial pads connected by a flexible, transventricular subvalvular chord that can be shortened intraoperatively. In the Randomized Evaluation of a Surgical Treatment for Off-Pump Repair of the Mitral Valve (RESTORE-MV) Trial, 165 patients were randomly assigned to undergo CABG with or without Coapsys ventricular reshaping.[46] Patients treated with the device had greater reductions in LV end-diastolic dimension, lower MR grades, and better survival at 2 years. Despite the benefit and proof of concept demonstrated in this trial as well as early success with a percutaneous prototype (iCoapsys), the company ran out of funding and ceased operations.

Other companies are continuing to develop approaches to LV remodeling. The VenTouch System (Mardil Medical, Inc., Plymouth, MN) is a surgically implanted targeted ventricular reshaping therapy placed externally around the heart to treat functional MR

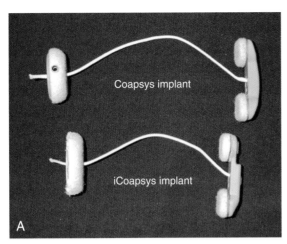

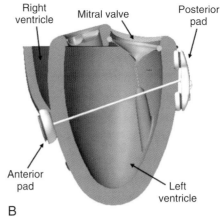

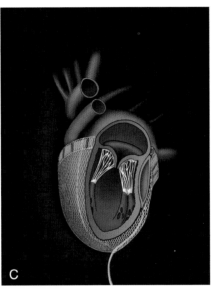

FIGURE 22-10 **Two devices that directly alter left ventricular shape. A** and **B,** Coapsys (Myocor Inc, Maple Glen, Minnesota), which is no longer in development, achieved the shape change with an external band and internal connection, delivered surgically (Coapsys) or percutaneously (iCoapsys). **A** also shows the iCoapsys, a percutaneous version. **C,** The VenTouch System (Mardil Medical, Inc, Plymouth, MN).

(see Figure 22-10). In a preliminary report of 11 patients treated in India, MR grade was reduced acutely from grade 3.3 to 0.6.[47] Preclinical work with a transcatheter approach to approximate the papillary muscles is also in development (Tendyne Repair, Tendyne Holdings, Inc.).

Transcatheter Mitral Valve Replacement

The rationale for transcatheter mitral valve replacement has as its basis several lessons learned from surgical valve replacement.[48] Surgical valve replacement is the most effective method to reliably reduce MR. This is particularly apparent in comparisons with transcatheter repairs, which do not appear to reduce MR to the same extent as surgical repairs. Despite its proven efficacy, the risks of surgery may include significant morbidity and mortality related to the incision and the need for cardiopulmonary bypass.[10-12]

One of the most touted advantages of surgical repair over replacement is the improved survival related to better LV remodeling.[8] However, this and other observational comparisons may be confounded by differences in patient baseline characteristics and comorbid conditions. In one study utilizing propensity scoring, 322 patients undergoing mitral valve repair were matched with an equal number of patients undergoing valve replacement.[49] During a median follow-up of 3.4 years, a modest survival benefit was associated with repair, but the rate of freedom from reoperation was twofold higher with replacement. Importantly, only 15% of these patients had MR with an ischemic etiology. In a comparison of 397 patients with ischemic MR undergoing repair and 85 patients undergoing replacement, Gillinov et al[50] did not find a survival benefit for repair in patients with the most complex and severe conditions.

In the absence of a randomized comparison of repair and replacement, historical comparisons are limited by the use of older prostheses and the lack of chordal sparing techniques.[51,52] For this reason, a randomized trial comparing repair and replacement with complete subvalvular preservation in severe ischemic MR, sponsored by the National Heart, Lung, and Blood Institute, is now under way (clinicaltrials.gov, NCT00807040). Finally, both surgical[15,18,19] and transcatheter[24,25,27,32] valve repairs are characterized by higher rates of MR recurrence than are seen after valve replacement.

For these reasons, several companies are working to develop percutaneous or minimally invasive transcatheter methods to replace the mitral valve with a prosthesis (Figure 22-11). These devices will likely first be used in elderly and other patients at high surgical risk for whom the benefits of repair are unproven and the risks of surgery are high. In this regard, early experience utilizing transcatheter aortic valve implantation (TAVI) devices in previously implanted and now degenerating surgical bioprostheses

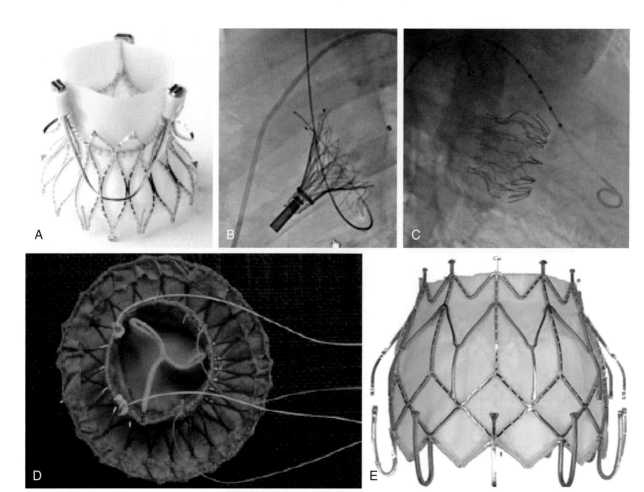

FIGURE 22-11 Transcatheter mitral valve replacement. Transcatheter mitral valve replacement remains mostly in pre-clinical development. Prototypes are: **A,** Ventor Embracer (Medtronic, Inc., Minneapolis, MN); **B** and **C,** Tiara transcatheter mitral valve (Neovasc, Richmond BC, Canada); **D,** Lutter valve (Courtesy of Georg Lutter, MD); **E,** CardiAQ valve (Irvine, CA).

and rings has confirmed the feasibility of this approach (Table 22-2). Balloon-expandable prostheses have been implanted in degenerating bioprostheses[53-58] and previous surgical annuloplasty rings,[59-61] predominantly via a transapical approach. However, the feasibility of transseptal delivery[54,60,61] and transatrial[54,56] delivery has also been demonstrated. Complications, including valve embolization, bleeding, and death, have been reported, but the early results have been generally favorable with excellent reduction in MR grade and low residual transmitral gradients (see Table 22-2).

Despite these early demonstrations of the feasibility of transcatheter mitral valve-in-valve implantation, it is likely that de novo placement of such devices in native valves will be more challenging. The devices will need to be larger than most aortic devices, and fixation to the diseased mitral apparatus will be hampered by the greater valve complexity, the lack of calcium, the potential need for orientation, and the noncircular annular shape. Paravalvular leaks, already demonstrated to reduce survival after TAVI, will likely be even less well tolerated in the mitral valve, with the higher driving pressures and more common development of hemolysis. Finally, all such devices will need to preserve the subvalvular apparatus and not create LV outflow tract obstruction. Most current designs utilize a stent-based bioprosthesis that is self-expanding and inserted transseptally (CardiAQ) or transapically (Ventor, Tiara) (see Figure 22-11). Devices that do not rely on radial force for fixation in the annulus may be advantageous to reduce the risk for outflow tract obstruction (Endovalve, Lutter).

The Lutter group published their initial experience with a transapical, off-pump, porcine self-expanding stent prosthesis in pigs.

Seven of the 8 animals died because of paravalvular leaks, suboptimal positioning, or failure of fixation.[62] A subsequent bovine pericardial design with a ventricular tethering fixation system reduced embolization, but malpositioning and failure of ventricular fixation resulted in death in 6 of 8 animals.[63]

CardiAQ Valve Technologies, Inc., is developing a transseptally inserted stent device with a foreshortening frame and anchor barbs. The device sits in the left atrium to a significant degree above the annulus, a characteristic that has hampered the experimental evaluation. Nonetheless, investigators reported on its use in 82 pigs with acute and subchronic MR, with delivery system failure in 36% and unsuccessful implant positions in 21% of the remaining completed procedures.[64]

Micro Interventional Devices, Inc., is developing the Endovalve prosthesis. This foldable (nonstent) nitinol prosthesis with proprietary gripper technology was initially developed for insertion via a minimally invasive right minithoracotomy. Novel features of this device included cabling to contract, reposition, and release the prosthesis as well as a sewn fabric skirt to provide perivalvular sealing. Initial in vivo sheep implants demonstrated fixation, valve function, and lack of LV outflow tract obstruction and MR. However, fixation was judged to be suboptimal, and the Endovalve prosthesis has now been redesigned for transapical insertion utilizing active annular fixation with proprietary Permaseal anchoring technology.

Finally, several self-expanding bovine pericardial prostheses for transapical delivery are also under development: Tiara, (Neovasc Inc.) and Ventor Embracer (Medtronic, Inc.). Both these devices and the Endovalve transapical prosthesis will benefit from the growing experience with transapical TAVI[65] and

TABLE 22-2 Transcatheter Mitral Valve-in-Valve Implantation

FIRST AUTHOR (YEAR)	N	ACCESS ROUTE (n)	PROCEDURE SUCCESS (n/total)	POSTPROCEDURE MR GRADE	RESIDUAL MEAN GRADIENT (mm Hg)	30-DAY MORTALITY (%)	COMMENT
Seiffert (2010)[53]	1	TA	1/1	0-1+	2	100	
Webb (2010)[54]	7	Transseptal (1), transaortic (1), transapical (5)	6/7	0-1+	8	29	
Cerillo (2011)[55]	3	Transapical	2/3	1+	5	33	
Cheung (2011)[56]	11	Transaortic (1), transapical (10)	9/10	0-1+	7	10	Includes some patients in reference 54
Van Garsse (2011)[57]	1	Transapical	1/1	0	3	0	
de Weger (2011)[59]	1	Transapical	1/1	1+	4	0	Status after ring annuloplasty
Himbert (2011)[60]	1	Transseptal	1/1	1+	8	0	Status after ring annuloplasty
Gaia (2012)[58]	1	Transatrial	1/1	0	5	0	
Vahanian (2012)[61]	8	Transseptal					Status after ring annuloplasty (n = 6)

paravalvular leak closure.[66] Furthermore, several companies are developing transapical closure devices to simplify insertion of both aortic and mitral prostheses via catheters.

Both transseptal and transapical insertion of mitral valve replacement prostheses may be an attractive future option for patients for whom surgery poses a high risk. The potential advantages of this approach include the avoidance of both the surgical incision and the effects of cardiopulmonary bypass. Such devices could be fully sparing of the subvalvular apparatus and provide MR reduction that is equivalent to that achieved with surgical valve replacement.

Conclusions

The complexity of the mitral valve apparatus and the myriad causes of MR have caused the field of transcatheter mitral valve repair and replacement to develop more slowly than treatments for other valve diseases. The release of devices to treat MR in Europe and aortic stenosis throughout the world has reenergized the development of new transcatheter valve therapies. Fueled by the ever-growing prevalence of heart failure in the aging U.S. population[67]—most of these older patients with heart failure have significant MR—and aided by the ingenuity of physicians and engineers, transcatheter mitral valve therapies will probably also become an available option for such patients.

REFERENCES

1. Chaput M, Handschumacher MD, Tournoux F, et al. Mitral leaflet adaptation to ventricular remodeling: occurrence and adequacy in patients with functional mitral regurgitation. Circulation 2008;118:845–52.
2. Silbinger JJ. Mechanistic Insights into Ischemic Mitral regurgitation: echocardiographic and surgical implications. J Am Soc Echocardiogr 2011;24:707–19.
3. Bursi F, Enriquez-Sarano M, Nkomo VT, et al. Heart failure and death after myocardial infarction in the community: the emerging role of mitral regurgitation. Circulation 2005;111:295–301.
4. Trichon BH, Felker GM, Shaw LK, et al. Relation of frequency and severity of mitral regurgitation to survival among patients with left ventricular systolic dysfunction and heart failure. Am J Cardiol 2003;91:538–43.
5. Enriquez-Sarano M, Avierinos JF, Messika-Zeitoun D, et al. Quantitative determinants of the outcome of asymptomatic mitral regurgitation. N Engl J Med 2005;352:875–83.
6. Rosenhek R, Rader F, Klaar U, et al. Outcome of watchful waiting in asymptomatic severe mitral regurgitation. Circulation 2006;113:2238–44.
7. Bonow RO, Carabello BA, Chatterjee K, et al. 2008 focused update incorporated into the ACC/AHA 2006 guidelines for the management of patients with valvular heart disease: a report of the American College of Cardiology/American Heart Association Task Force on Practice Guidelines (Writing Committee to revise the 1998 guidelines for the management of patients with valvular heart disease). Endorsed by the Society of Cardiovascular Anesthesiologists, Society for Cardiovascular Angiography and Interventions, and Society of Thoracic Surgeons. J Am Coll Cardiol 2008;52:e1–142.
8. Enriquez-Sarano M, Schaff HV, Orszulak TA, et al. Valve repair improves the outcome of surgery for mitral regurgitation: a multivariate analysis. Circulation 1995;91:1022–8.
9. Masson JB, Webb JG. Percutaneous treatment of mitral regurgitation. Circ Cardiovasc Interv 2009;2:140–6.
10. Gammie JS, O'Brien SM, Griffith BP, et al. Influence of hospital procedural volume on care process and mortality for patients undergoing elective surgery for mitral regurgitation. Circulation 2007;115:881–7.
11. Goodney PP, Stuke TA, Lucas FL, et al. Hospital volume, length of stay, and readmission rates in high-risk surgery. Ann Surg 2003;238:161–7.
12. Mehta RH, Eagle KA, Coombs LP, et al. Influence of age on outcomes in patients undergoing mitral valve replacement. Ann Thorac Surg 2002;74:1459–67.
13. Guy TS, Moainie SL, Gorman JH, et al. Prevention of ischemic mitral regurgitation does not influence the outcome of remodeling after posterolateral myocardial infarction. J Am Coll Cardiol 2004;43:377–83.
14. Wu AH, Aaronson KD, Bolling SF, et al. Impact of mitral valve annuloplasty on mortality risk in patients with mitral regurgitation and left ventricular systolic dysfunction. J Am Coll Cardiol 2005;45:381–7.
15. Mihaljevic T, Lam BK, Rajeswaran J, et al. Impact of mitral valve annuloplasty combined with revascularization in patients with functional ischemic mitral regurgitation. J Am Coll Cardiol 2007;49:2191–201.
16. Glower DD, Tuttle RH, Shah LK, et al. Patient survival characteristics after routine mitral valve repair for ischemic mitral regurgitation. J Thorac Cardiovasc Surg 2005;129:860–8.
17. David TE. Outcomes of mitral valve repair for mitral regurgitation due to degenerative disease. Semin Thorac Cardiovasc Surg 2007;19:116–20.
18. Flameng W, Herijgers P, Bogaerts K. Recurrence of mitral valve regurgitation after mitral valve repair in degenerative valve disease. Circulation 2003;107:1609–13.
19. McGee EC, Gillino AM, Blackstone EH, et al. Recurrent mitral regurgitation after annuloplasty for functional ischemic mitral regurgitation. J Thorac Cardiovasc Surg 2004;128:916–24.
20. Chaim PTL, Ruiz CE. Percutaneous mitral valve repair: a classification of the technology. J Am Coll Cardiol Interv 2011;4:1–13.
21. Alfieri O, Maisano F, DeBonis M, et al. The double-orifice technique in mitral valve repair: a simple solution for complex problems. J Thorac Cardiovasc Surg 2001;122:674–81.
22. Maisono F, Caldarola A, Blasio A, et al. Midterm results of edge-to-edge mitral valve repair without annuloplasty. J Thorac Cardiovasc Surg 2003;126:1987–97.
23. St. Goar FG, James FI, Komtebedde J, et al. Endovascular edge-to-edge mitral valve repair: short-term results in a porcine model. Circulation, 2003;108:1990–3.
24. Feldman T, Wasserman HS, Herrmann HC, et al. Percutaneous mitral valve repair using the edge-to-edge technique: six-month results of the EVEREST Phase 1 Clinical Trial. J Am Coll Cardiol 2005;46:2134–40.
25. Herrmann HC, Feldman T. Percutaneous mitral valve edge-to-edge repair with the Evalve MitraClip System: rationale and phase 1 results. EuroIntervention 2006;1(supplement A):A36–9.
26. Silvestry FE, Rodriguez LL, Herrmann HC, et al. Echocardiographic guidance and assessment of percutaneous repair for mitral regurgitation with the Evalve MitraClip: lessons learned from EVEREST 1. J Am Soc Echocardiogr 2007;20:1131–40.
27. Feldman T, Foster E, Glower D, et al. Percutaneous repair or surgery for mitral regurgitation. N Engl J Med 2011;364:1395–406.
28. Herrmann HC, Kar S, Siegel R, et al. Effect of percutaneous mitral repair with the Mitra-Clip device on mitral valve area and gradient. EuroIntervention 2009;4:437–42.
29. Herrmann HC, Gertz ZM, Silvestry FE, et al. Effects of atrial fibrillation on treatment of mitral regurgitation in the EVEREST II Randomized Trial. J Am Coll Cardiol 2012;59:A17–20.

30. Whitlow PL, Feldman T, Pedersen WR, et al. Acute and 12-month results with catheter-based mitral valve leaflet repair. J Am Coll Cardiol 2012;59:130–9.

31. Rudolph V, Knap M, Frnazen O, et al. Echocardiographic and clinical outcomes of MitraClip therapy in patients not amenable to surgery. J Am Coll Cardiol 2011;58:2190–5.

32. Auricchio A, Schillinger W, Meyer S, et al. Correction of mitral regurgitation in nonresponders to cardiac resynchronization therapy by MitraClip improves symptoms and promotes reverse remodeling. J Am Coll Cardiol 2011;58:2183–9.

33. Seeburger J, Borger MA, Tschernich H, et al. Transapical beating heart mitral valve repair. Circ Cardiovasc Interv 2010;3:611–12.

34. Svensson L. Presentation at TransCatheter Therapeutics 23rd Annual Scientific Symposium, November 7-11, 2011, San Francisco.

35. Harnek J, Webb JG, Kuck KH, et al. Transcatheter implantation of the MONARC coronary sinus device for mitral regurgitation. J Am Coll Cardiol Intv 2011;4:115–22.

36. Sack S, Kahlert P, Bilodeau L, et al. Percutaneous transvenous mitral annuloplasty: initial human experience with a novel coronary sinus implant device. Circ Cardiovasc Interv 2009;2:277–84.

37. Schofer J, Siminiak T, Haude M, et al. Percutaneous mitral annuloplasty for functional mitral regurgitation: results of the Carillon Mitral Annuloplasty Device European Union Study. Circulation 2009;120:326–33.

38. Goldberg S. Presentation at TransCatheter Therapeutics 23rd Annual Scientific Symposium, November 7-11, 2011, San Francisco.

39. Choure AJ, Barcia MJ, Hesse B, et al. In vivo analysis of the anatomical relationship of coronary sinus to mitral annulus and left circumflex coronary artery using cardiac multidetector computed tomography. J Am Coll Cardiol 2006;48:1938–45.

40. Maselli D, Guarracino F, Chiaramonti F, et al. Percutaneous mitral annuloplasty: an anatomic study of human coronary sinus and its relation with mitral valve annulus and coronary arteries. Circulation 2006;114:377–80.

41. Spongo S, Bertrand OF, Philippon F, et al. Reversible circumflex coronary artery occlusion during percutaneous transvenous mitral annuloplasty with the Viacor system. J Am Coll Cardiol 2012;59:288.

42. Kim JH, Kocaturk O, Ozturk C, et al. Mitral Cerclage annuloplasty, a novel transcatheter treatment for secondary mitral valve regurgitation: initial results in swine. J Am Coll Cardiol 2009;54:638–51.

43. Tibayan FA, Rodriguez F, Liang D, et al. Paneth suture annuloplasty abolishes acute ischemic mitral regurgitation but preserves annular and leaflet dynamics. Circulation 2003;108(suppl II):II-128–II-133.

44. Grube E. Presentation at TransCatheter Therapeutics 23rd Annual Scientific Symposium, November 7-11, 2011, San Francisco.

45. Komeda M, Glasson JR, Bolger AF, et al. Geometric determinants of ischemic mitral regurgitation. Circulation 1997;96(Suppl):II-128–II-33.

46. Grossi EA, Patel N, Woo YJ, et al. Outcomes of the RESTOR-MV Trial (Randomized Evaluation of a Surgical Treatment for Off-Pump Repair of the Mitral Valve). J Am Coll Cardiol 2010;56:1984–93.

47. Presentation at TransCatheter Therapeutics 23rd Annual Scientific Symposium, November 7-11, 2011, San Francisco.

48. Herrmann HC. Transcatheter mitral valve implantation. Cardiac Interventions Today, August/September 2009:82–5.

49. Moss RR, Humphries KH, Gao M, et al. Outcome of mitral valve repair or replacement: a comparison by propensity score analysis. Circulation 2003;108(suppl II):II90–II97.

50. Gillinov AM, Wierup PN, Blackstone EH, et al. Is repair preferable to replacement for ischemic mitral regurgitation? J Thorac Cardiovasc Surg 2001;122:1125–41.

51. Rozich JD, Carabello BA, Usher BW, et al. Mitral valve replacement with and without chordal preservation in patients with chronic mitral regurgitation: mechanisms for differences in postoperative ejection performance. Circulation 1992;86:1718–26.

52. Yun KL, Sinteck CF, Miller DC, et al. Randomized trial comparing partial versus complete chordal-sparing mitral valve replacement: effects on left ventricular volume and function. J Thorac Cardiovasc Surg 2002;123:707–14.

53. Seiffert M, Franzen O, Conradi L, et al. Series of transcatheter valve-in-valve implantations in high-risk patients with degenerated bioprostheses in aortic and mitral position. Cath Cardiovasc Interv 2010;76:608–15.

54. Webb JG, Wood DA, Ye J, et al. Transcatheter valve-in-valve implantation for failed bioprosthetic heart valves. Circulation 2010;121:1848–57.

55. Cerillo AG, Chiaramonti F, Murzi M, et al. Transcatheter valve in valve implantation for failed mitral and tricuspid bioprostheses. Cath Cardiovasc Interv 2011;78:987–95.

56. Cheung AW, Gurvitch R, Ye J, et al. Transcatheter transapical mitral valve-in-valve implantations for a failed bioprosthesis: a case series. J Thorac Cardiovasc Surg 2011;141:711–15.

57. Van Garsse LAFM, Gelsomino S, Van Ommen V, et al. Emergency transthoracic transapical mitral valve-in-valve implantation. J Interv Cardiol 2011;24:474–6.

58. Gaia DF, Palma JH, de Souza JAM, et al. Transapical mitral valve-in-valve implant: an alternative for high risk and multiple reoperative rheumatic patients. Int J Cardiol 2012;154:e6–e7.

59. de Weger A, Ewe SH, Delagado V, et al. First in man implantation of a transcatheter aortic valve in a mitral annuloplasty ring: novel treatment modality for failed mitral valve repair. Eur J Cardiothorac Surg 2011;39:1054–6.

60. Himbert D, Brochet E, Radu C, et al. Transseptal implantation of a transcatheter heart valve in a mitral annuloplasty ring to treat mitral repair failure. Circ Cardiovasc Interv 2011;4:396–8.

61. Himbert D, Descoutures F, Brochet E, et al. Transvenous mitral valve replacement after failure of surgical ring annuloplasty. J Am Coll Cardiol 2012;60:1205–6.

62. Lozonschi L, Quaden R, Edwards NM, et al. Transapical mitral valved stent implantation. Ann Thorac Surg 2008;86:745–8.

63. Lozonschi L, Bombien R, Osaki S, et al. Transapical mitral valved stent implantation: a survival series in swine. J Thorac Cardiovasc Surg 2010;140:4220–6.

64. Mack M. Presentation at TransCatheter Therapeutics 23rd Annual Scientific Symposium, November 7-11, 2011, San Francisco.

65. Dewey TM, Thourani V, Bavaria JE, et al. Transapical aortic-valve replacement for critical aortic stenosis: results from the nonrandomized continued-access cohort of the PARTNER trial. Presented to Society of Thoracic Surgeons 48th Annual Meeting, January 30, 2012, Fort Lauderdale, Florida.

66. Sorajja P, Cabalks AK, Hagler DJ, et al. Percutaneous repair of paravalvular prosthetic regurgitation: acute and 30-day outcomes in 115 patients. Circ Cardiovasc Interv 2011;4:314–21.

67. Roger VL, Go AS, Lloyd-Jones DM, et al. Heart disease and stroke statistics-2011 update. A report from the American Heart Association. Circulation 2011;123:e18–e209.

CHAPTER 23

Intraoperative Echocardiography for Mitral Valve Surgery

Donald C. Oxorn

Key Points

- Mitral regurgitation (MR) and mitral stenosis (MS) may be the result of abnormalities of the mitral valvular complex; leaflets, annulus, chordae, papillary muscles, as well as the left atrium and ventricle.
- Intraoperative echocardiography is a vital diagnostic technique for mitral valve (MV) surgery and is recommended for all valve repair procedures.
- The alterations in loading conditions from general anesthesia and positive pressure ventilation have dramatic effects on indices of MR and MS severity. The high-flow state after the use of cardiopulmonary bypass may falsely raise pressure gradients across prosthetic mitral valves.
- There are numerous options for MV repair, which have different effects on the appearance on post-bypass transesophageal echocardiography (TEE). Each prosthetic valve type (mechanical, biological) has unique echocardiographic patterns.
- Epicardial echocardiography may be employed by the surgeon to evaluate the MV in its dynamic state if questions still exist about the mechanism of MV dysfunction after sternotomy.
- Residual MR after MV repair portends a poor prognosis. Location (central, eccentric) and mechanism of MR (undercorrection of annulus, residual leaflet abnormalities, repair breakdown, ring dehiscence, and systolic anterior motion [SAM]) are just as important as the degree of regurgitation.
- Common prosthetic valves abnormalities are impairment of leaflet opening and closing (thrombus, pannus, calcification, entrapment by subvalvular tissue) and paravalvular regurgitation. Native mitral tissue left after valve replacement has the potential to create SAM. Small paravalvular leaks after valve replacement usually resolve after heparin reversal.

Mitral Valve Disease in the Twenty-First Century

Although the prevalence of rheumatic mitral valve (MV) disease remains high worldwide,[1] early treatment of rheumatic fever has altered etiologic patterns in industrialized countries, resulting in a higher prevalence of degenerative and ischemic etiologies (see Chapter 1). As patients age, the prevalence of valve disease increases, with a disproportionate representation of those with mitral valve involvement;[3] this change is in part due to the prolonged survival of patients with severe heart failure and ischemic MR. Therefore the population of patients who present for mitral valve surgery has altered considerably over the past few decades.

A tremendous body of literature has evolved, describing more and more complex techniques of MV repair and replacement. Knowledge of these techniques, the preoperative and postoperative echocardiographic assessment, and the ability to effectively communicate findings to the surgeon are essential in ensuring successful surgical planning.

This chapter describes the intraoperative milieu, the major objectives of the echocardiographic examinations performed before and after cardiopulmonary bypass, the published guidelines for intraoperative MV assessment, and the impact of intraoperative transesophageal echocardiography (TEE) on the success of MV surgery.

Anatomic Background

The Mitral Valve Complex

Understanding the components and function of the MV complex is essential to the proper interpretation of preoperative and postoperative echocardiographic anatomy.

The MV complex consists primarily of the anterior and posterior leaflets but also includes a number of anatomic entities that are in close proximity to the valve, and all components of the valve must act in a coordinated fashion to ensure proper valve function[4] (see Chapter 2).

The mitral annulus effectively separates the left atrium (LA) and left ventricle (LV) and provides support for the anterior and posterior leaflets[5] (Figure 23-1). Anteriorly, the annulus is interrupted by the aortic-mitral fibrous continuity, with thickened tissue at the right and left fibrous trigones. From the trigones emanates the fibrous tissue of the annulus that encircles the orifice of the valve, but it is rarely continuous; it is deficient in some areas and curtain-like in others. The annulus is not a static structure; it changes size during the cardiac cycle to facilitate filling and minimize regurgitation.[6] The annulus is saddle-shaped, with the low points at the commissures and the high points at the mid-portions of the leaflets. This shape facilitates valve closure and may minimize leaflet stress.[7]

Whereas the echocardiographer readily identifies the annulus as the hinge point at the base of the leaflets, the surgical identification is the level of the visible transition between the LA myocardium and the denser white leaflet (Figure 23-2).

The mitral leaflets are in fact a single structure that becomes confluent at the lateral and medial commissures. The anterior leaflet, though longer, covers approximately one third of the annular circumference, and the posterior leaflet covers the remaining two thirds. The posterior leaflet has three scallops: P1, or lateral; P2, or central; and P3, or medial, with the central scallop usually the largest.[8] Although the anterior leaflet lacks distinctive scallops, the nomenclature is such that the portions opposite the corresponding posterior segments are named A1, A2, and A3 (Figure 23-3).[9]

Each leaflet consists of a smooth zone and a rough zone. The rough zone is involved in coaptation and is subtended by primary (marginal, first-order) chordae that insert into the leaflet edges, and secondary (basal, second-order) chordae that insert into the ventricular surface of the rough zone (Figure 23-4). During systole, the rough zones are in contact over a distance of approximately 1 cm. The excess valvular tissue relative to orifice size offers some functional reserve, thus ensuring proper coaptation and preventing regurgitation.

Some especially large second-order chordae, known as strut chords, attach to the rough zone of the anterior leaflet and maintain direct continuity among the valve, the papillary muscles, and the ventricular myocardium. Cutting these strut chords during surgical procedures may lead to LV dysfunction.[10,11] Tertiary chordae insert into the basal portion of the posterior leaflet only and are of uncertain significance. The remainder of each leaflet is made up of a smooth zone that is devoid of chordae.

The lateral and medial papillary muscles provide a continuum between the ventricular myocardium and the valve and are critical in supporting proper valve closure. Each papillary muscle supplies chordae to both leaflets.

Finally, LV shape and myocardial function are also key components in normal MV function. Disturbances in LV function or shape, such as chronic myocardial ischemia, may lead to valvular tethering and mitral regurgitation.[12]

Nomenclature

One of the keys to successful communication between the echocardiographer and the surgeon is make sure they speak the same "language." The same structure may be named differently depending on the anatomical terms of reference used.[13] For example, the lateral and medial commissures are sometimes referred to as anterior or left and posterior or right commissures, respectively.

The anterior leaflet is intimately associated with the aortic mitral curtain and thus is sometimes referred to as the aortic leaflet. The posterior leaflet may be referred to as the mural leaflet, owing to its proximity to the LV wall. The classification

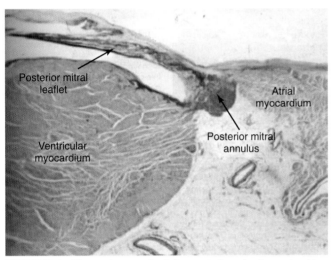

FIGURE 23-1 Photomicrograph of the posterior mitral annulus. Note that the posterior mitral annulus separates the musculature of the left ventricle from that of the left atrium, where it forms a hinge point with base of the posterior mitral leaflet. *(Wilcox, BR, Cook AC, Anderson RH, Surgical anatomy of the valves of the heart. New York: Cambridge University Press; 2004. p. 55, with permission)*

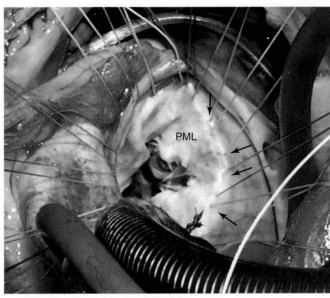

FIGURE 23-2 Surgical exposure of the mitral valve. The surgeon has placed sutures in the posterior annulus, which is identified as the transition between the pink atrial myocardium and the white leaflet *(arrows)*. *PML,* Posterior mitral leaflet.

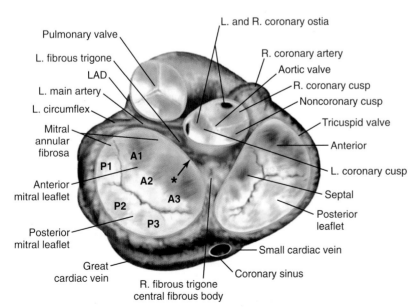

FIGURE 23-3 Anatomic view of the cardiac valves from the perspective of the base of the heart with the left and right atria "cut away" and the great vessels transected. Note the close anatomic relationships of all four cardiac valves. In particular the aortic valve is adjacent to the mitral valve along the midsegment of the anterior mitral valve leaflet. The pulmonic valve is slightly superior to the aortic valve, and the aortic and pulmonic valve planes are nearly perpendicular to each other. The three scallops of the posterior mitral leaflet are lateral *(P1),* central *(P2),* and medial *(P3)* with the corresponding segments for the anterior leaflet *(A1, A2, A3)* shown. *Asterisk* indicates the mitral-aortic curtain. *L,* Left; *LAD,* left anterior descending artery; *R,* right.

endorsed by the American Society of Echocardiography and Society of Cardiovascular Anesthesiologists is illustrated in Figure 23-5. From left to right (or lateral to medial), the posterior leaflet is divided into scallops P1, P2, P3, and corresponding segments of the non-scalloped anterior leaflet into A1, A2, A3. Deviant clefts may be found in up to 30% of posterior leaflet specimens.[14]

The Intraoperative Milieu

The intraoperative setting can be daunting, even to experienced practitioners who do not spend the bulk of their clinical time in the operating room. Numerous factors constrain optimal image acquisition, including bright lights and noise. Time may be limited because several different physicians and nurses have responsibilities in surgical preparation and the surgical procedure. If feasible, the echocardiographer should request that room lighting be dimmed, or at a minimum should request that any overhead surgical lighting be directed away from the echocardiographic system screen.

Most general anesthetic medications diminish vascular tone and decrease contractility. In addition patients are often taking preoperative vasodilator medications such as angiotensin-converting enzyme (ACE) inhibitors. The echocardiographer must take effects of decreased afterload into account when quantifying the degree of mitral regurgitation. As well, positive pressure ventilation and cardiopulmonary bypass have numerous hemodynamic effects with the potential to alter echocardiographic findings.

Once the surgical procedure commences, electrocautery is used, which causes interference with quality of two-dimensional (2D) echocardiography, spectral Doppler echocardiography, and especially color-flow Doppler imaging data. Electrocautery also creates stitching artifacts during multiple beat acquisitions on three-dimensional (3D) transesophageal echocardiography (TEE).

The electrocardiogram is distorted, preventing appropriate triggering of cine loop recording from the QRS complex; instead, the echocardiography instrument should be set to store data for a set length of time, such as 2 seconds, rather than a set number of beats.

Pre-Bypass Assessment

Presurgical Preparation

The variety and acuity of diagnoses seen in patients coming to the operating room for treatment of valve disease has increased considerably as surgical options have expanded over the past few decades.[15] In addition to regurgitant or stenotic lesions, mixed stenosis and regurgitation and "repeat" surgery for prosthetic valve dysfunction or after a prior valve repair procedure are increasingly common. Ideally the echocardiographer and surgeon should discuss the nature of the mitral disease and the planned operative approach, including any ancillary procedures, such as a maze procedure for atrial fibrillation. Remaining uncertainties after preoperative evaluation should be defined, with a plan for their resolution. Knowledge of preoperative data is crucial. Along with clinical data, the preoperative transthoracic echocardiography (TTE) data should be reviewed, and if possible, the actual images should be examined to assess data quality. Cardiac catheterization findings, computed tomography images, and cardiac magnetic resonance imaging data also should be reviewed when available. The preoperative evaluation helps define the information needed from the intraoperative examination. If, as often occurs, previously undiagnosed pathology is discovered on echocardiography, this information should be promptly shared with the surgeon. In some cases, the referring cardiologist may be consulted if findings are substantially

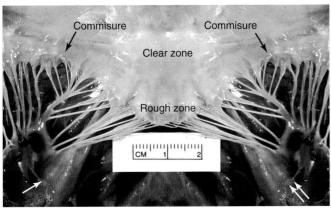

FIGURE 23-4   Mitral valve anatomy. The posterior leaflet has been sectioned at its midpoint. The commissures and the clear and rough zones of the anterior mitral leaflet are shown. The anterolateral *(single white arrow)* and the posteromedial *(double arrow)* papillary muscles both give cords to both leaflets. *(Image courtesy Dr. Dennis Reichenbach.)*

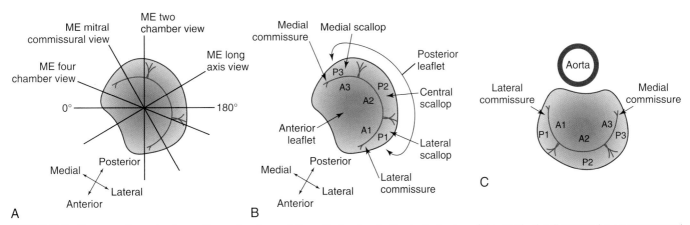

FIGURE 23-5   Transesophageal echocardiography views of the mitral valve. A, Short-axis drawing of the mitral valve illustrating how it is transected by midesophageal views. Rotating through multiplane angles from 0 degrees to 180 degrees moves the imaging plane axially through the entire mitral valve. **B,** Anatomy of mitral valve. **C,** The surgeon's view of the mitral valve. *A1,* Lateral third of the anterior leaflet; *A2,* central third of the anterior leaflet; *A3,* medial third of the anterior leaflet; *ME,* midesophageal; *P1,* lateral scallop of the posterior leaflet; *P2,* central scallop of the posterior leaflet; *P3,* medial scallop of the posterior leaflet. *(From Shanewise JS, Cheung AT, Aronson S, et al. ASE/SCA guidelines for performing a comprehensive intraoperative multiplane transesophageal echocardiography examination: recommendations of the American Society of Echocardiography Council for Intraoperative Echocardiography and the Society of Cardiovascular Anesthesiologists Task Force for Certification in Perioperative Transesophageal Echocardiography. J Am Soc Echocardiogr 1999;12:884–900.)*

TABLE 23-1 Perioperative Implications of Lesions Associated with Mitral Valve Disease

SECONDARY CONDITION	PREOPERATIVE SIGNIFICANCE	POSTOPERATIVE SIGNIFICANCE
Pulmonary hypertension	May indicate left ventricular failure, left ventricular outflow tract obstruction, aortic valve disease, severe mitral regurgitation	Aortic valve surgery may be needed Pharmacologic therapy may be needed
Right heart failure	Often secondary to elevated left-sided filing pressures	Aggressive pharmacologic support may be needed
Tricuspid regurgitation	Often secondary to elevated left-sided filling pressures, consideration for reparative procedure at time of mitral surgery	Must be differentiated from primary tricuspid valve disease
Mitral leaflet systolic anterior motion	Consideration for reparative procedure; i.e., myomectomy	Aggressive pharmacologic manipulation may be needed; may necessitate valve replacement
Rheumatic valvular disease	May have aortic stenosis, aortic regurgitation, tricuspid stenosis/regurgitation necessitating intervention Aortic regurgitation may confound mitral valve area calculation by pressure half time method	Reassessment of native valves, or of repaired/replaced valves after mitral valve surgery, required

different from expected or a major alteration in surgical approach is needed.

Systematic Examination

A comprehensive baseline intraoperative TEE examination is recommended to confirm or refute the mechanism and severity of the MV abnormality, assess valve reparability, and provide comparison images for the postoperative evaluation.

The baseline TEE examination includes 2D, spectral, and color-flow Doppler with quantitation of mitral stenosis and regurgitation using standard approaches (see Chapter 6). 3D imaging if available, enhances the understanding of abnormal mitral function.,[16]

Secondary effects on other structures, specifically the left-sided chambers and the tricuspid valve, may help determine the chronicity of the process. A number of lesions are often associated with MV disease, both primarily and secondarily (Table 23-1), that may require correction at the time of mitral surgery.

TWO-DIMENSIONAL IMAGING

On 2D imaging, the general condition of the leaflets is assessed, with the degree of thickness, mobility, and calcification, and subvalvular disease noted.[17] The LA is assessed for the presence of thrombus and ruptured chordae. The presence of masses should alert the echocardiographer to the likelihood of endocarditis, with the possibility of para-annular extension, leaflet perforation, and the involvement of other valves (see Chapter 25). Although uncommon, involvement of the mitral-aortic intravalvular fibrosa (MAIVF) with pseudoaneurysm formation may result from primary mitral rather than aortic endocarditis.[18]

Next, a systematic examination of the MV is performed using schemata such as described by Shanewise et al[19] and Foster et al[9] (Figures 23-5 and 23-6, Table 23-2), which provide a "roadmap" for recognizing where the pathologic aspects of the valve lie. Basic views of the MV leaflets are obtained from a high TEE position (Figure 23-7). Once each view is obtained, slight movements of the probe—withdrawal and advancement, rotation left and right, and flexion and extension—are used to completely examine each leaflet segment. At this stage of the examination, color-flow Doppler imaging may be used, but more to help clarify the mechanism of MR (Figures 23-8 and 23-9). The subvalvular apparatus is best seen with transgastric views, which allow visualization of cordal thickening, redundancy, or frank rupture along with the orientation of the papillary muscles. On the basis of these images, the Carpentier classification can be used to define the mechanism and etiology of MR, which may be helpful in the planning of the surgical approach[2] (Table 23-3; Figure 23-10).

Measurement of annular diameter may help define the etiology of MR and guide the surgeon in selection of a prosthesis or annuloplasty ring. The saddle shape of the annulus is demonstrated with 3D reconstructions (see Figure 2-3). The low points of the "saddle" are at the commissures, seen in the bicommissural view, and the high points in the anterior-posterior axis, seen in the midesophageal long-axis view.

On the basis of comparison with cardiac computed tomography, the best approach for annular measurement is the commissure-to-commissure peak systolic diameter in the TEE bicommissural view the and anterior-to-posterior diameter in the long-axis view.[19a] The annulus is also assessed for the degree of calcification, which may be predictive of paravalvular leaks[20] and perioperative vascular events.[21]

Examination of global and segmental LV function is also needed in evaluation of the mechanism of MR. Secondary MR is due to either global or regional LV systolic dysfunction or to altered LV geometry. However, chronic primary MR also leads to LV dilation with the potential for progressive LV dysfunction[22] (see Chapter 5), which may complicate the perioperative management of MV surgery.

EPICARDIAL ECHOCARDIOGRAPHY

If TEE images are suboptimal, the surgeon can employ the technique of epicardial echocardiography both before and after cardiopulmonary bypass.[23] A transthoracic probe is placed inside a sterile sheath, which is then placed directly on the heart. Most standard transthoracic views can be obtained, with excellent resolution.

DOPPLER ECHOCARDIOGRAPHY QUANTIFICATION

Ideally, any method for intraoperative assessment of MR severity should be easy to perform, reliable, and independent of the etiology of the MR and loading conditions. The time for intraoperative assessment is limited, thereby making more complex calculations, such as the proximal isovelocity surface area (PISA) approach and its derivatives, prohibitive. The presence of rhythm disturbances and the ubiquitous use of electrocautery confound any quantitative measurements.

No single tool is optimal for the intraoperative assessment of MR. Variations in etiology (ischemic versus nonischemic) and chronicity, secondary effect on chamber size and compliance, and acute changes in loading conditions influence the size and direction of the jet. Thus before any attempt at quantification is made, supportive information such as the history, physical findings, preoperative hemodynamics, and the secondary effects on chamber size and function must be reviewed. Intraoperative findings must be interpreted in conjunction with the preoperative echocardiographic data and with consideration of the clinical conditions during the intraoperative study. For example, a patient

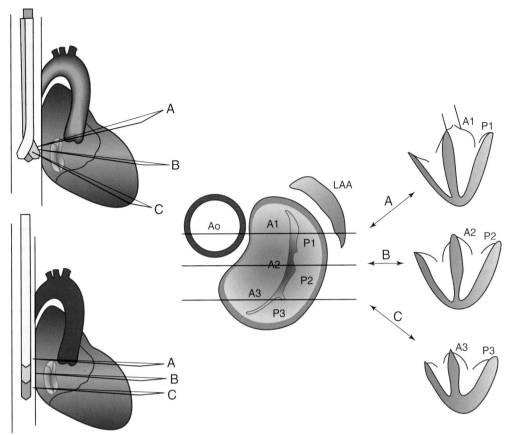

FIGURE 23-6 **Effect of changes in transesophageal echocardiography probe position.** Effect of flexion or withdrawal and retroflexion or advancement of the transesophageal probe tip on the imaging plane in relation to the mitral valve at a transducer rotational angle of 0 degrees. *A1, A2, A3,* Anterior leaflet sections; *Ao,* aorta; *LAA,* left atrial appendage; *P1, P2, P3,* posterior leaflet sections. *(From Foster GP, Isselbacher EM, Rose GA, et al. Accurate localization of mitral regurgitant defects using multiplane transesophageal echocardiography. Ann Thorac Surg 1998;65:1025–31.)*

TABLE 23-2   Recommended Intraoperative Transesophageal Echocardiography (TEE) Examination

Two-Dimensional TEE							
WINDOW	**VIEW**	**APPROXIMATE MULTIPLANE ANGLE (DEGREES)**	**STRUCTURES**	**IMAGING SPECIFICS**	**COMMENTS**	**SPECTRAL DOPPLER**	**COLOR DOPPLER**
Mid-esophageal	Four-chamber	0-20	A2, P2	Flexion and slight withdrawal to image A1 and P1; retroflexion and slight advancement to image A3 and P3	Good for initial assessment of leaflet structure, mobility	Mitral inflow with pulsed or continuous wave as appropriate, for calculation of mean gradient, aortic valve area	Initial assessment of MR; flexion and retroflexion of probe may pick up jet not initially seen
	Mitral commissural	50-80	P3, A2, P1	Low points of annulus, make annular measurement at peak systole In P2 flail/prolapse, P2 seen coming up "behind" A2	Ultrasound plane intersects coaptation zone twice; don't mistake for leaflet perforation or cleft		If MR present, two jets often seen
	Two-chamber	80-100	A1, A2, A3, P3	Left atrial appendage usually seen lateral to mitral annulus	Anterior mitral leaflet seen in its entirety		Posterior jets of MR seen
	Long-axis	110-140	A2, P2 High points of annulus, make annular measurement at peak systole Measure leaflet length	Aortic valve and LVOT seen		May measure mitral inflow here	Optimal view for vena contracta measurement Check for AR following repair, replacement of MV

Continued

TABLE 23-2   Recommended Intraoperative Transesophageal Echocardiography (TEE) Examination—cont'd

Two-Dimensional TEE

WINDOW	VIEW	APPROXIMATE MULTIPLANE ANGLE (DEGREES)	STRUCTURES	IMAGING SPECIFICS	COMMENTS	SPECTRAL DOPPLER	COLOR DOPPLER
Transgastric	Basal short-axis	0-20	The zone of coaptation from posterior (A3, P3) through middle (A2, P2) to anterior (A1, P1)	From midpapillary view of LV, flex and slightly withdraw probe	Difficult to avoid oblique cut	NA	May help in localizing jet
	Two-chamber	80-100	Long axis of papillary muscles, chordae, leaflet attachments	Papillary muscles often not in same plane, may have to rotate probe to see both	Useful in rheumatic disease to assess subvalvular involvement Leaflet tethering appreciated	NA	Not as good as esophageal views
	Long axis	90-120°	Images subvalvular apparatus, LVOT, AoV	Important to align LVOT and AV with cursor when looking for LVOT gradient Probe flexion may be required	SAM may be seen	Gradient across LVOT, useful with SAM	In LVOT obstruction by SAM, acceleration of CD seen
	Deep transgastric	0-20°	Images LVOT, AV	Advance and flex probe Important to align LVOT and AoV with cursor when looking for LVOT gradient	SAM may be seen	Gradient across LVOT, useful with SAM	In LVOT obstruction by SAM, acceleration of CD seen

Three-Dimensional TEE

VIEW	MODE	STRUCTURES	IMAGING SPECIFICS	COMMENTS	SPECTRAL DOPPLER	COLOR DOPPLER
"En face"	3D zoom mode based on the midesophageal four-chamber view	Anterior and posterior mitral leaflets, commissures	Use 3D rotate so that aortic valve is en face and at 12 o'clock Using rotation may view atrial and ventricular aspects of the MV	Replicates surgeon's view of the MV Improved localizing of flail/prolapse/cleft of specific segments* May see ruptured chordae from atrial aspect	NA	NA
Full-volume 3D data set		Mitral valvular complex	Multiple beat acquisition Use of various cropping modes to view structures of interest	Interrelationship between the MV, the papillary muscles, the myocardial walls, and the LVOT	NA	NA
3D color	Full-volume 3D or live 3D		Multiple beat acquisition Size and location of jet accurately measured	Size and location of jet accurately measured	NA	Shape, size, and complexity of MR jet Vena contracta shape

2D, Two-dimensional; *3D,* three-dimensional; *A1, A2, A3,* segments of anterior leaflet; *AR,* aortic regurgitation; *AoV,* aortic valve; *CD,* color Doppler; *LV,* left ventricular; *OT,* outflow tract; *MR,* mitral regurgitation; *MV,* mitral valve; *NA,* not applicable; *P1, P2, P3,* segments of posterior leaflet; *SAM,* mitral systolic anterior motion of the mitral valve.
*Mahmood F, Hess PE, Matyal R, et al. Echocardiographic anatomy of the mitral valve—a critical appraisal of two-dimensional imaging protocols with a three-dimensional perspective. J Cardiothorac Vasc Anesth 2012;26:777–84.

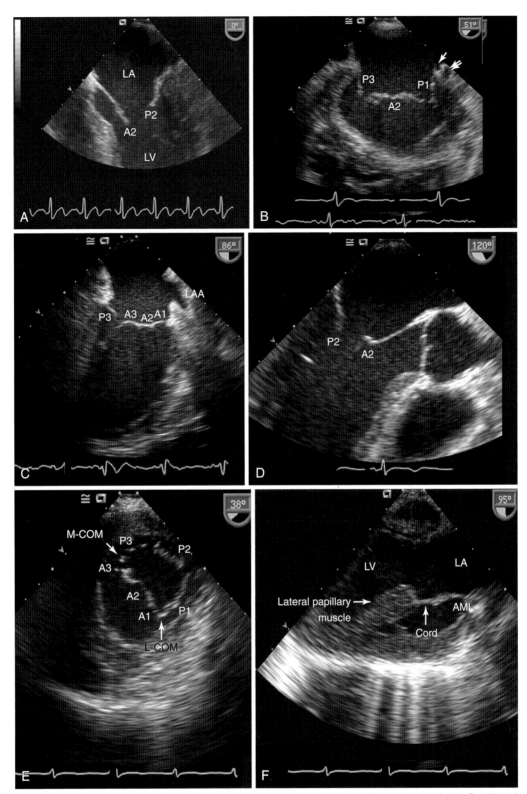

FIGURE 23-7 **Basic transesophageal echocardiography views of the MV. A,** Four-chamber view; **B,** bicommissural view; **C,** midesophageal two-chamber view; **D,** midesophageal long-axis view; **E,** transgastric short-axis view; **F,** transgastric two-chamber view. *A1, A2, A3,* Anterior leaflet sections; *AML,* anterior mitral leaflet; *LA,* left atrium; *L-COM,* anterior commissure; *LV,* left ventricle; *M-COM,* posterior commissure, *P1, P2, P3,* posterior leaflet sections.

who is acutely ischemic during the preoperative examination may have significantly less MR after anesthesia induction.

LOADING CONDITIONS

The most important confounding variables in the intraoperative assessment of MR are the loading conditions, which are affected to a great degree by (1) the depressive effects of general anesthetic on myocardial contractility and vascular tone and (2) the effects of positive pressure ventilation on systemic venous return in both open heart and closed chest procedures.[24] For these reasons, the degree of intraoperative MR is often significantly less than seen on preoperative transthoracic studies.[25] Sometimes this finding creates uncertainty as to the proper surgical course of action.

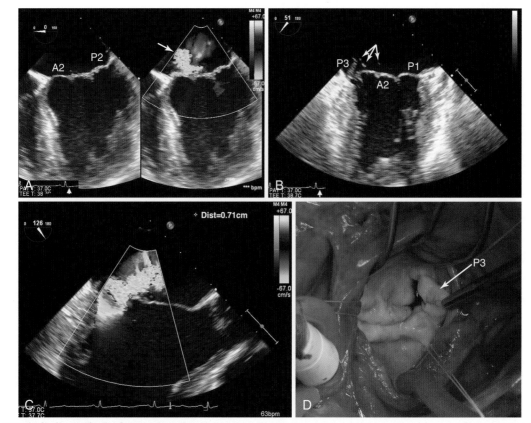

FIGURE 23-8 Anteriorly directed mitral regurgitant jet. The 46-year-old patient presented with increasing shortness of breath over several years and an acute increase in dyspnea over the last week. **A,** A four-chamber view *(left)* demonstrates normal coaptation, but a color-flow Doppler image *(right)* shows an anteriorly directed jet of mitral regurgitation (MR) *(arrow)*, indicative of either posterior leaflet prolapse or anterior leaflet restriction. **B,** The bicommissural view shows a flail P3 scallop with numerous ruptured chordae *(arrows)*. **C,** A vena contracta of 0.71 cm, indicative of severe MR. **D,** Surgical exposure revealed involvement of the P3 scallop. *A2,* Anterior section; *P1, P2,* posterior leaflet sections.

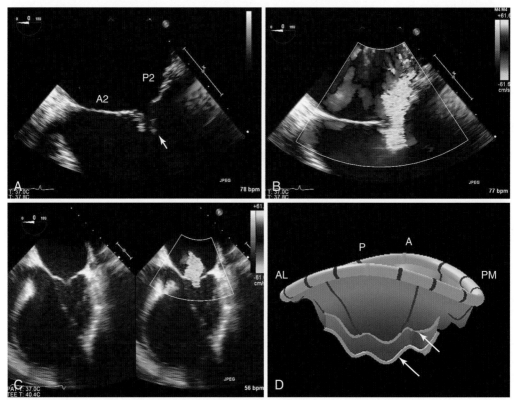

FIGURE 23-9 Ischemic mitral regurgitation (MR). In this patient with previous inferior wall infarction, **A** demonstrates tethering of the posterior mitral leaflet *(arrow)* in the four-chamber view. **B,** Color-flow Doppler image shows a posterior directed jet of MR. **C,** In another patient with a dilated cardiomyopathy and symmetric tethering, a central jet of MR is shown. **D,** MVQ (mitral valve quantification) illustrates the bileaflet tethering *(arrows). (With permission, Stefan Lombaard)* *A,* anterior; *AL,* antero-lateral; *P,* posterior; *PM,* postero-medial.

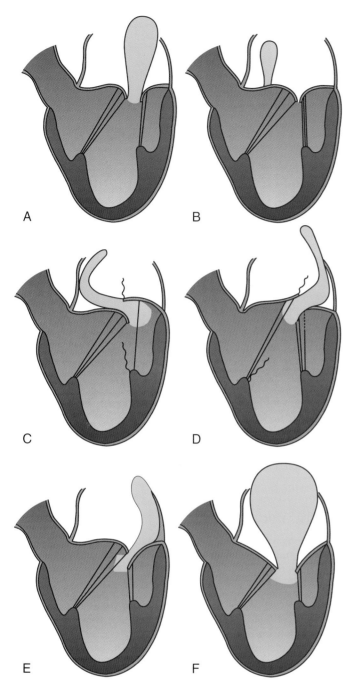

TABLE 23-3	Common Causes of Mitral Regurgitation (MR) Seen in the Operating Room
Structural MR	Mitral valve prolapse Rheumatic disease Congenital valve disease Mitral valve endocarditis
Secondary MR	Ischemic heart disease Nonischemic dilated cardiomyopathy
MR associated with obstruction of left ventricular outflow tract	Hypertrophic cardiomyopathy (HCM) Underfilled/hyperdynamic left ventricle (rare without HCM) After mitral valve repair (usually in the setting of underfilling/hyperdynamic states)

FIGURE 23-10 Carpentier's classification of mitral regurgitation (MR) based on leaflet motion. Leaflet motion is classified as normal (Type I), excessive (Type II) or restricted (Type III). In type I (**A** and **B**) the leaflet motion is normal and the jet tends to be central. The cause of MR is usually annular dilatation (**A**) or leaflet perforation (**B**). In type II (**C** and **D**) there is excessive leaflet motion and the jet is directed away from the diseased leaflet. In type III lesions (**E** and **F**) the leaflet motion is restricted. Type III lesions are further subdivided into IIIA and IIIB. The jet can be directed towards the affected leaflet, or it can be central if both leaflets are equally affected. (*Modified from Perrino AC, Reeves ST. The practice of perioperative transesophageal echocardiography. Philadelphia: Lippincott William & Wilkins; 2003.*)

A number of strategies have been proposed to replicate findings in the preoperative state. In a prospective study of patients with at least moderate MR from a variety of etiologies, TEE was performed at three stages: with conscious sedation prior to induction of anesthesia, after induction, and after use of phenylephrine to bring the blood pressure back to pre-induction levels.[25a] Blood pressure dropped significantly after induction and was driven

over baseline with phenylephrine. Compared with pre-induction findings, there were decreases in measurements of vena contracta, regurgitant orifice area (ROA), and regurgitant volume (RV), although the decreases were not statistically significant. Phenylephrine resulted in the return of regurgitant parameters to baseline, with a significant increase in MR severity compared to post-induction values, regardless of the underlying etiology, likely as a result of the combination of increased blood pressure, changes in preload, and possible myocardial ischemia.

In another study of patients with ischemic MR, both phenylephrine and fluids were used to restore pre-induction hemodynamics. Again, parameters of MR severity dropped after anesthesia induction, though not significantly. With loading, blood pressure, ROA, and regurgitant volume superseded baseline measurements.[25b]

However, these effects are not seen uniformly in all patients. In a diverse group of patients with MR, MR severity remained less than baseline values in 20% of patients despite the use of vasoactive agents to bring blood pressure back to baseline.[25c]

These studies, in combination with clinical experience, emphasize that intraoperative Doppler estimation of MR is complex. Measures of MR severity are affected by the degree of blood pressure drop, changes in preload and afterload, LV contractility, LV dyssynchrony,[26] mitral closing force,[12] the etiology of mitral disease, other concurrent valve lesions, and the possible induction of myocardial ischemia. The use of pharmacologic manipulation to reestablish baseline conditions is to some extent artificial, and the significance of increased MR severity with "overdriving" of loading parameters is uncertain. It is axiomatic that a high-quality preoperative echocardiogram performed without general anesthesia should be readily available for review in the operating room. Decisions based on the patient's clinical course and symptoms, degree of LV dilation and systolic dysfunction, and quantitation of MR on the preoperative study should rarely be overruled simply on the basis of differences in the quantitative parameters of MR severity on intraoperative TEE.

COLOR DOPPLER IMAGING

The MR jet as defined by color Doppler imaging is complex.[27] The size of the jet as it fans out into the LA is of limited quantitative value because of numerous technical and physiologic factors.[28] The direction of the jet gives useful information about the mechanism of the MR (Figure 23-11), and the presence of multiple jets may be indicative of leaflet perforation (Figure 23-12). However, eccentric jets appear smaller than central jets because they flatten out against the wall of the receiving chamber. Physiologic factors affect the size of the jet in the LA, for example, the driving pressure across the valve or changes in LA compliance related to chronicity of regurgitation. In addition, instrument settings, such as color gain and pulse repetition frequency, affect jet size independently of ROA.

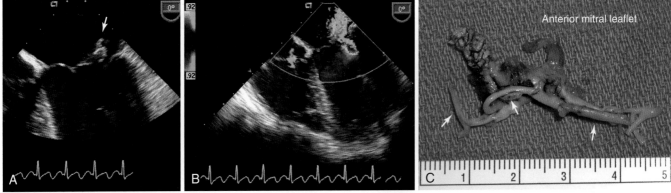

FIGURE 23-11   Mitral valve endocarditis. A, The anterior mitral leaflet has a large vegetation *(arrow)* and is flail. **B,** A posteriorly directed jet of MR can be seen. **C,** The resected valve has numerous torn chordae.

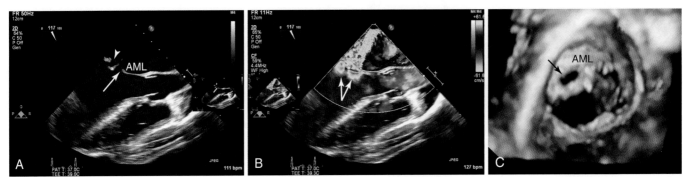

FIGURE 23-12   Anterior mitral leaflet perforation. A, In a midesophageal long-axis view, the *arrowhead* indicates the normal point of coaptation, whereas the *arrow* indicates another regurgitant orifice. **B,** Color Doppler applied to **A.** Two jets of mitral regurgitation *(double arrow)* can be seen—a normal central jet and another jet that appears to be through a leaflet perforation. **C,** Three-dimensional transesophageal echocardiography confirms the presence of a perforation *(arrow)* in the anterior mitral leaflet (AML).

VENA CONTRACTA

The *vena contracta* (see Figure 6-15) is defined as the narrowest central flow region of a jet that occurs at, or just downstream to, the orifice of a regurgitant valve.[29] The vena contracta is characterized by high-velocity, laminar flow and is slightly smaller than the *anatomic* regurgitant orifice because of boundary effects. The vena contracta measurement is easily obtained in the operating room and can be used to assess regurgitation severity. The vena contracta is measured as the narrow neck between the proximal flow convergence area and expansion of the jet in the receiving chamber. Vena contracta measurements correlate with invasive measures of MR regardless of etiology of regurgitation and compare favorably with more complex measures such as regurgitant volume and ROA.[30,31] However, the following caveats apply:

1. The technical aspects of image acquisition must be adhered to, with the Nyquist limit set at 50-60 cm/sec, the use of zoom mode, and a narrow color sector width.
2. Measurements are made in the midesophageal long-axis plane to avoid overestimation.
3. The method can be applied to central and eccentric jets but is not validated for multiple jets.
4. Vena contracta measurement is predicated on the assumption that the regurgitant orifice is circular, which may not be the case in secondary MR, leading to erroneous measurements.[32]

Current guidelines recommend that vena contracta widths between 3 and 7 mm need confirmation by more quantitative methods when feasible.[33] These include other Doppler imaging–based techniques, such as proximal isovelocity surface area and volumetric methods based on calculations of stroke volume through the mitral and aortic annuli.[27,33] However, these methods can be challenging with intraoperative TEE.

SPECTRAL DOPPLER IMAGING

Continuous wave Doppler echocardiography is used to examine the temporal characteristics of the MR jet, and jet density; dense, early peaking and triangular jets are more indicative of significant MR (Figure 23-13).

Pulsed wave Doppler echocardiography interrogation of the pulmonary veins is easy to perform. The presence of systolic reversal has high specificity but low sensitivity for severe MR; systolic blunting may indicate moderate MR but is often present with other causes of elevated LA pressure.

Mitral inflow velocities are measured with either pulsed wave or continuous wave Doppler echocardiography to assess for mitral stenosis (see Chapter 6).

THREE-DIMENSIONAL TRANSESOPHAGEAL ECHOCARDIOGRAPHY

With the availability of real-time methods of imaging that make 3D TEE use in the operating room practical,[16,34,35] it is not surprising that there has been a surge in interest in using 3D TEE in that setting. Because the number and complexity of mitral procedures is high, it is fortuitous that the MV is the easiest valve to image by 3D TEE (see Fig 2-1 and 2-2). Potential benefits include better assessment of the pathologic components of the valve that need to be addressed surgically, evaluation of MV repair and replacement, and localization of postprocedural leaks.[36] Some of the basic tenets of MR quantification have been challenged with the use of 3D TEE by color Doppler imaging.[32,37]

Grewal et al[38] compared 2D TEE and 3D TEE in the setting of MV surgery and found that the two methods were equally reliable in diagnosing the etiology, but that 3D TEE had greater sensitivity and specificity for disease involving the P1 segment of the

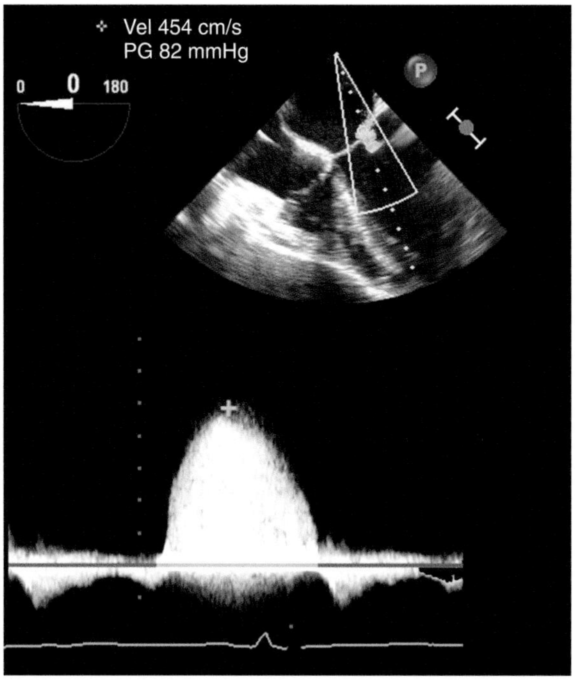

Vel 454 cm/s
PG 82 mmHg

0   0   180

FIGURE 23-13   Continuous wave Doppler echocardiography of mitral regurgitation. The velocity profile is very dense, indicative of significant mitral regurgitation.

TABLE 23-4	Transthoracic Echocardiographic Characteristics Unfavorable for Mitral Valve Repair in Secondary Mitral Regurgitation
Mitral valve deformation	
Coaptation distance ≥1 cm	
Tenting area >2.5-3 cm^2	
Complex jets	
Posterolateral angle >45 degrees	
Local left ventricular (LV) remodelling	
Interpapillary muscle distance >20 mm	
Posterior papillary-fibrosa distance >40 mm	
Lateral wall motion abnormality	
Global LV remodelling	
End-diastolic diameter >65 mm, end-systolic diameter >51 mm (end-systolic volume >140 mL)	
Systolic sphericity index >0.7	

From Lancellotti, P, Moura, L, Pierard, LA, et al. European Association of Echocardiography recommendations for the assessment of valvular regurgitation. Part 2: mitral and tricuspid regurgitation (native valve disease). Eur J Echocardiogr 2010;11:307–32.

posterior leaflet or the A3 segment of the anterior leaflet and for bileaflet disease. Similarly, Ben Zekry et al[39] reported that both 2D and 3D methods of TEE were highly accurate in diagnosing mitral disease, but that 3D TEE could localize the lesion more predictably. Both studies acknowledge the limitations inherent in such comparisons. Importantly, surgical observation is considered the "gold standard" although it is performed with the heart in a flaccid state.

In an elegant study, Maffessanti et al[40] evaluated a large group of patients with Carpentier type II disease and found not only improved localization of leaflet abnormalities with 3D TEE, but greater ability to define annular shape before and after surgical repair.

Numerous other studies report high accuracy with 3D TEE in the evaluation of mitral pathology[41-45] and mitral annular dimensions before and after surgery.[46] Mukherjee et al,[47] however, found no statistically significant difference between 2D TEE and 3D TEE for imaging complex mitral disease involving multiple segments.

3D TEE has enhanced both our understanding of mitral leaflet and annular mechanics and our ability to define complex lesions both before and after bypass (see Figure 6-6). The valve can be imaged from the LA and LV sides. MV quantification software may improve our ability to fully define MV lesions and may help the surgeon better plan the procedure—what to resect, the shape of annular ring to choose, and prediction of the effect of remodeling procedures such as papillary muscle repositioning.[48] Optimal use of 3D imaging requires considerable expertise; however, as practitioners become more experienced, its use in the operating room will undoubtedly increase.

Reparability

Numerous techniques of MV repair exist and are in constant evolution (see Chapter 21). The reparability of a given valve depends on both the lesion (Tables 23-4 and 23-5) and the skill of the surgeon. The echocardiographer must present the information needed to make the appropriate surgical decision.

CARPENTIER TYPE I (NORMAL LEAFLET MOTION)

Mitral regurgitation with normal leaflet motion (see Figure 23-10) often is repaired with a patch in the presence of leaflet perforation, or ring annuloplasty with or without coronary artery bypass grafting (CABG) in patients with dilated cardiomyopathy.

CARPENTIER TYPE II (EXCESSIVE LEAFLET MOTION)

Excessive leaflet motion, as in mitral valve prolapse, is often repairable, most frequently with resection of redundant posterior leaflet segment(s) and the placement of an annuloplasty ring (Figure 23-14). Altering leaflet lengths and annular diameter may change the distance between the coaptation point and the interventricular septum and therefore has the potential to produce postoperative systolic anterior motion (SAM) of the mitral valve. The pathophysiology of SAM is complex, but is believed to involve both drag (ejected blood pushing the redundant anterior leaflet into the LV outflow tract) and push (the anterior leaflet causing turbulence in the LV outflow tract, creating a Venturi effect and pulling the leaflet towards the septum).[49] LV outflow obstruction and the refractory MR that ensue portend a poor long-term outcome.[50] Systolic anterior motion is associated with factors that either (1) push the coaptation point closer to the septum, such as a small LV outflow tract dimension, excessive posterior leaflet length, a bulging septum,[51] or overcorrection of the annulus or (2) pull the coaptation point into the LV outflow tract, such as a large anterior leaflet.[52] Maslow et al[53] stress the importance of the pre-bypass examination and emphasize the significance of small anterior-to-posterior leaflet ratio and coaptation point-to-septal distance. There are surgical modifications that may be used to decrease the likelihood of SAM; these include posterior leaflet reduction with a sliding annuloplasty,[54] anterior leaflet shortening,[55,56] sizing of the annuloplasty ring to the anterior leaflet,[57] and LV outflow tract myomectomy[51] (see Chapter 21). Patients presenting with Barlow disease and bileaflet prolapse (see Fig 2-1) are usually not candidates for repair.

Correction of anterior leaflet prolapse is more complex because of its association with the rigid mitral-aortic curtain (see Figure 23-3). Options include placing synthetic chordae and edge-to-edge plication of both anterior and posterior leaflets.[58]

If excessive leaflet motion is the result of endocarditis, valve replacement is usually indicated (see Figure 23-12).

TABLE 23-5	Probability of Successful Mitral Valve Repair in Primary Mitral Regurgitation Based on Echocardiography Findings				
ETIOLOGY	**DYSFUNCTION (CARPENTIER CLASS)**	**CALCIFICATION**	**MITRAL ANNULUS DILATION**	**PROBABILITY OF REPAIR**
Degenerative	II: Localized prolapse (leaflet P2 and/or A2)	No/localized	Mild/moderate	Feasible
Ischemic/secondary	I or IIIb	No	Moderate	Feasible
Barlow disease	II: Extensive prolapse (≥3 scallops, posterior commissure)	Localized (annulus)	Moderate	Difficult
Rheumatic	IIIa but pliable anterior leaflet	Localized	Moderate	Difficult
Severe Barlow disease	II: Extensive prolapse (>3 scallops, anterior commissure)	Extensive (annulus + leaflets)	Severe	Unlikely
Endocarditis	II: Prolapse but destructive lesions	No	No/mild	Unlikely
Rheumatic	IIIa but stiff anterior leaflet	Extensive (annulus + leaflets)	Moderate/severe	Unlikely
Ischemic/secondary	IIIb but severe valvular deformation	No	No or severe	Unlikely

From Lancellotti, P, Moura, L, Pierard, LA, et al. European Association of Echocardiography recommendations for the assessment of valvular regurgitation. Part 2: mitral and tricuspid regurgitation (native valve disease). Eur J Echocardiogr 2010;11:307–32.

TABLE 23-6	Characteristics of Mitral Regurgitation Due to Symmetric and Asymmetric Tethering	
	ASYMMETRIC	**SYMMETRIC**
Etiology	Inferoposterior myocardial infarction	Multiple myocardial infarctions or nonischemic cardiomyopathy
Tethering	Marked posterior tethering of the posterior leaflet	Both leaflets are tethered and displaced apically
Tenting	Increased	Markedly increased
Annulus	May be dilated	Dilated, flattened, and decreased systolic contraction
Remodeling	Localized to inferoposterior wall	Global dilation with increased sphericity
Mitral regurgitation jet	Posteriorly directed, eccentric	Usually central

From Ray S. The echocardiographic assessment of secondary mitral regurgitation. Eur J Echocardiogr 2010;11:i11–7.

Rarely, papillary muscle rupture complicates myocardial infarction, usually involving the inferoposterior wall. The flail segment may or may not be visualized in the LA. Surgical treatment is usually valve replacement.

CARPENTIER TYPE IIIB (RESTRICTED SYSTOLIC LEAFLET MOTION)

Leaflet tethering (symmetric or asymmetric) often occurs in the setting of ischemic heart disease (Table 23-6). The greater the degree of leaflet restriction, the less likely a surgical repair will be successful.[12] Magne et al[59] found that the most robust predictor of residual MR after ring annuloplasty for ischemic MR was a posterior leaflet angle greater than 45 degrees. Because the abnormality is not in the valve leaflets but in the LV and subvalvular apparatus, novel restorative approaches are being slowly introduced into the therapeutic realm.[48,60] In the presence of leaflet restriction and concavity toward the left atrium, some investigators have advocated cutting specific second-order chordae in order to improve coaptation and move the coaptation point away from the ventricular apex.[61,62] However, adverse effects on LV systolic function may result from interruption of the valvular-ventricular continuity.[63]

CARPENTIER TYPE IIIA (RESTRICTED SYSTOLIC AND DIASTOLIC LEAFLET MOTION)

Adults with rheumatic MV disease usually present for valve replacement, especially if there is coexistent mitral stenosis.[64,65] These are commonly individuals who have extensive distortion of the valve apparatus, often with extensive chordal involvement, and for whom balloon valvuloplasty has been rejected as likely unsuccessful.[17] However, when valve thickening and chordal fusion are not as prominent but valvuloplasty is judged as

inappropriate because of excessive regurgitation, ring annuloplasty may be feasible.

The probability of successful MV repair in secondary and primary mitral regurgitation based on echocardiography findings is presented in Tables 23-4 and 23-5.

Prosthetic Valves

Problems with prosthetic valves may be detected prior to chest closure (perivalvular regurgitation from valve dehiscence, "stuck" leaflets), and such problems should be rectified before the patient leaves the operating room (as discussed later).

Patients with prosthetic mitral valves may return later for replacement of these valves (see Table 23-7). The pattern of presentation depends on the type of prosthesis. Tissue valves become fibrotic and calcified over time. Leaflet degeneration may lead to regurgitation, whereas calcification often results in stenosis. Abnormalities of leaflet motion in mechanical valves may be due to pannus or thrombus formation and may lead to varying degrees of stenosis and regurgitation. Endocarditis is a concern for both kinds of valves and may lead to emboli, leaflet dysfunction, and paravalvular infectious complications resulting in valve dehiscence and fistula formation.

On echocardiographic imaging, the issue of distal shadowing is more of a concern for mechanical than for tissue prosthetic valves. With TTE, the LA and the MR jet may be obscured, whereas with TEE, the LV and LV outflow tract are not well visualized. For this reason, the two techniques are complementary, and both typically are needed in patient evaluation.

A complete intraoperative evaluation requires careful scanning of the prosthetic mitral valve from both the stomach and esophagus, and from different angles of interrogation (see Table 23-8). The appearance of the valve leaflets and whether tissue leaflet

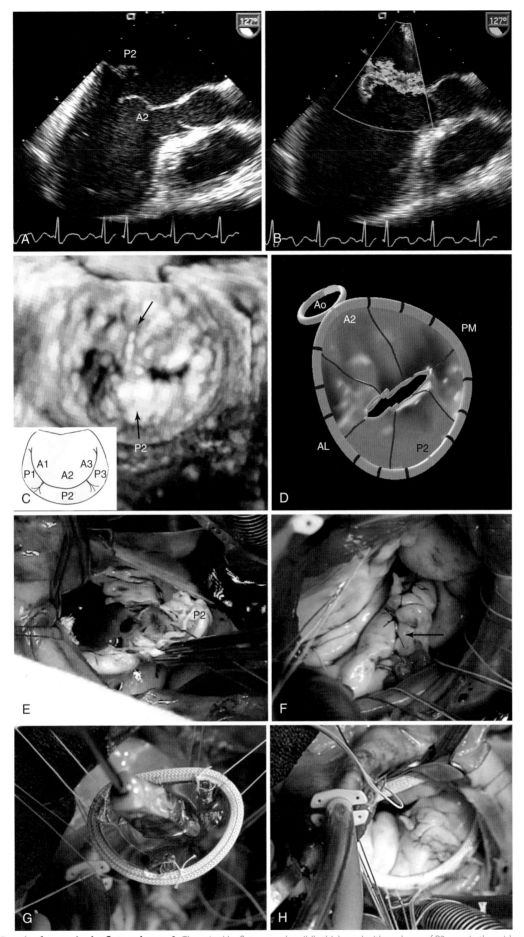

FIGURE 23-14   Repair of posterior leaflet prolapse. A, The mitral leaflets are only mildly thickened with prolapse of P2 seen in the midesophageal long-axis view. **B,** Color-flow Doppler imaging shows an anteriorly directed jet of mitral regurgitation. **C,** Real-time three-dimensional (3D) echocardiography of the mitral valve from the surgeons' view *(inset)* shows the P2 prolapse with a torn cord *(arrows).* **D,** A 3D reconstruction of the mitral valve shows P2 prolapse *(red)* and the coaptation defect. **E,** At surgery, the affected P2 segment is grasped by the surgeon. **F,** After its excision, P1 and P3 are sutured together *(arrows).* The annuloplasty ring has been sized to the anterior leaflet **(G),** and subsequently sutured in place **(H).** *AL,* lateral commissure; *Ao,* aortic valve; *PM,* medial commissure; *MVQ,* mitral valve quantification *(Courtesy Kris Natrajan, MD.)*

motion is excessive or restricted are noted. Spectral Doppler imaging is used to obtain the mean pressure gradient and pressure half-time, and color-flow Doppler echocardiography to determine the severity of MR and the relationship of the jet to the sewing ring (Figures 23-15 and 23-16). 3D TEE may be helpful in the evaluation and percutaneous closure of mitral paravalvular leaks[66] (see Chapter 16).

Tricuspid Regurgitation

Tricuspid regurgitation is commonly seen secondary to the right ventricular and tricuspid annular dilation that often accompany MV disease. The pathophysiology of secondary TR is complex (Figure 23-17), and in some instances, lesser degrees of TR in relatively healthy patients might regress after mitral surgery alone. However, with TR of moderate or greater severity, consideration should be given to annular reduction. This approach is justified by the reduced rate of TR progression, the reverse remodeling of

TABLE 23-7	Early and Late Complications of Prosthetic Valves
Patient prosthesis mismatch	
Geometric mismatch	
Dehiscence	
Primary failure	
Thrombosis and thromboembolism	
Pannus formation	
Pseudoaneurysm formation	
Endocarditis	
Hemolysis	

Reproduced from Zoghbi, WA, Chambers, JB, Dumesnil, JG, et al. Recommendations for evaluation of prosthetic valves with echocardiography and Doppler ultrasound: a report From the American Society of Echocardiography's Guidelines and Standards Committee and the Task Force on Prosthetic Valves. J Am Soc Echocardiogr 2009;22:975–1014.

TABLE 23-8	Echocardiographic and Doppler Parameters in the Evaluation of Prosthetic Mitral Valve Function (Stenosis or Regurgitation)
Doppler echocardiography of the valve	Peak early velocity Mean gradient Heart rate at the time of examination Pressure half-time Doppler valve index*: VTI_{PrMV}/VTI_{LVOT} Regurgitant orifice area* Presence, location, and severity of regurgitation†
Other pertinent echocardiographic and Doppler imaging parameters	Left ventricular size and function Left atrial size‡ Right ventricular size and function Estimation of pulmonary artery pressure

LVOT, Left ventricular outflow tract; *PrMV*, prosthetic mitral valve; *VTI*, velocity time integral.
Reproduced from Zoghbi, WA, Chambers, JB, Dumesnil, JG, et al. Recommendations for evaluation of prosthetic valves with echocardiography and Doppler ultrasound: a report From the American Society of Echocardiography's Guidelines and Standards Committee and the Task Force on Prosthetic Valves. J Am Soc Echocardiogr 2009; 22:975–1014.
*These indices are used when further information is needed about valve function. Regurgitant orifice area is calculated by means of the continuity equation.
†Often needs transesophageal echocardiographic evaluation because of acoustic shadowing.
‡May be difficult in the presence of shadowing or reverberation from the valve.

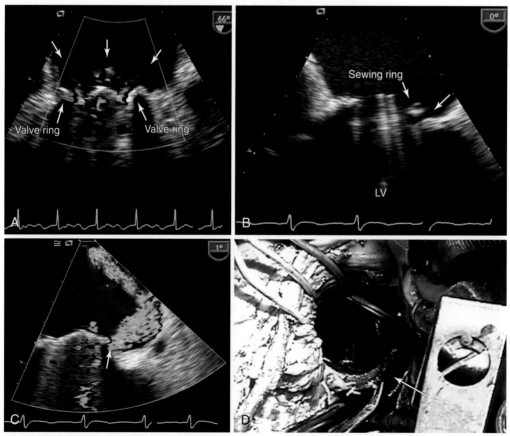

FIGURE 23-15 Dehiscence of a mechanical mitral valve. A, The normal appearance of a bileaflet mechanical prosthesis is demonstrated, with several "cleaning" jets, which are designed to keep the edges of the leaflets clean. **B,** In a patient with valve dehiscence *(arrow)*, rocking motion is seen with **(C)** a large jet of paravalvular mitral regurgitation. **D,** At surgery, the dehisced portion of the mitral sewing ring can be seen *(arrow)*.

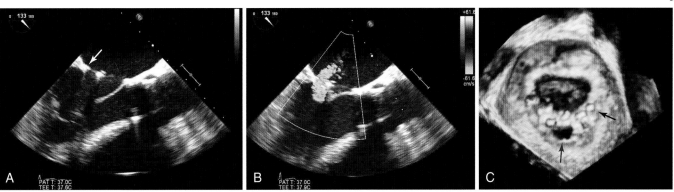

FIGURE 23-16 Annular ring dehiscence. The patient presented with worsening symptoms after mitral valve annuloplasty. **A,** In a midesophageal long-axis view, dehiscence of the annuloplasty ring *(red arrows)* from the posterior native annulus *(white arrow)* is shown. **B,** Color-flow Doppler imaging shows severe mitral regurgitation. **C,** The posterior defect is demonstrated *(red arrow)* with three-dimensional transesophageal echocardiography with the *black arrow* indicting the annuloplasty ring.

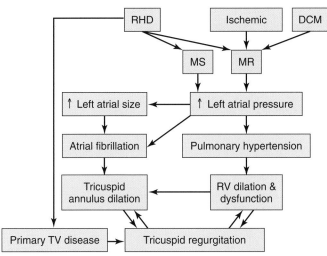

FIGURE 23-17 Pathogenesis of tricuspid regurgitation in mitral valve disease. *DCM,* dilated cardiomyopathy; *MR,* mitral regurgitation; *MS,* mitral stenosis; *RHD,* rheumatic heart disease; *RV,* right ventricular; *TV,* tricuspid valve. *(From Shiran A, Sagie A. Tricuspid regurgitation in mitral valve disease: incidence, prognostic implications, mechanism, and management. J Am Coll Cardiol 2009;53: 401–8.)*

remodeling. The echocardiographer must recognize both conditions requiring immediate attention in the operating room as well as situations in which late failure is predictable.

Following MV repair and prior to removal of the cross-clamps, the surgeon distends the ventricle with saline to address gross inadequacies of the repair.

The postprocedural evaluation begins in earnest after separation from cardiopulmonary bypass is complete. At this point the echocardiographer should have a complete understanding of what the surgeon did and what problems can be anticipated. This is a time of rapid hemodynamic change, so the final opinion on the result should await restoration of baseline conditions. The components of the post–cardiopulmonary bypass examination are outlined in Table 23-9.

Left and right ventricular function should be carefully assessed, especially if coronary bypass with or without a ventricular remodeling procedure has been performed. Right ventricular dysfunction may be the result of persistent severe MR, intracoronary air emboli, or inadequate ventricular protection during the period of aortic cross-clamping. Any ancillary procedures, such as tricuspid annuloplasty, must be carefully evaluated.

The detection of residual MR is the most important component of the postoperative examination. As with the pre-bypass evaluation, multiple views of the MV, including off-axis views, must be examined to determine the presence or absence of residual MR. Severity is assessed with use of the same criteria as for native valves on the baseline study. Normal loading conditions must be established prior to the final determination.

Residual MR may be secondary to several factors. If the annulus has not been downsized appropriately, residual central MR may occur. If the MR is eccentric, the valve must be reexamined to determine whether there are persistent coaptation abnormalities. If the residual jet occurs outside the zone of coaptation, the suture used to close the post excision leaflet defect may have broken down. If the MR jet lies outside the annuloplasty ring, the ring may have become detached from the native annulus. It is important to realize that the direction of the postoperative jet is often different from that seen preoperatively.[76]

If the postoperative regurgitation is graded as greater than mild or if it results from a significant technical breakdown, the patient should be returned to cardiopulmonary bypass and the valve repaired again or an MV replacement performed.[77] Only in exceptional circumstances, such as patient instability, should a second session of bypass be denied.

The presence of an adequate length of coaptation is essential for MV repair success. The concept of adequate coaptation length index has been proposed as a predictor of repair failure even in the presence of minimal post-bypass MR.[78] However, cutoff values have not yet been proposed.

the dysfunctional right ventricle, and better outcomes.[67-70] Severe tethering, increased age, and severe TR preoperatively are predictive of a high likelihood of residual TR after annuloplasty[71] (Figure 23-18). The risk of underestimating TR in the anesthetized patient, which is theoretically an issue because of a change in right ventricular loading conditions, must be considered in clinical decision making.

In patients whose tricuspid valve disease is due to disease of the leaflets, there is a higher likelihood of valve replacement.

Post-Bypass Evaluation

Native Valve Assessment

MV repair in properly selected patients has excellent long-term durability. However, residual regurgitation after MV repair portends a poor long-term prognosis.[59,72]

In a 2009 editorial, Anyanwu and Adams[73] broadly categorized the causes of MV repair failure as resulting either from technical inadequacies such as inappropriate annular ring selection or from progression of underlying disease with global[74] or localized[75] LV

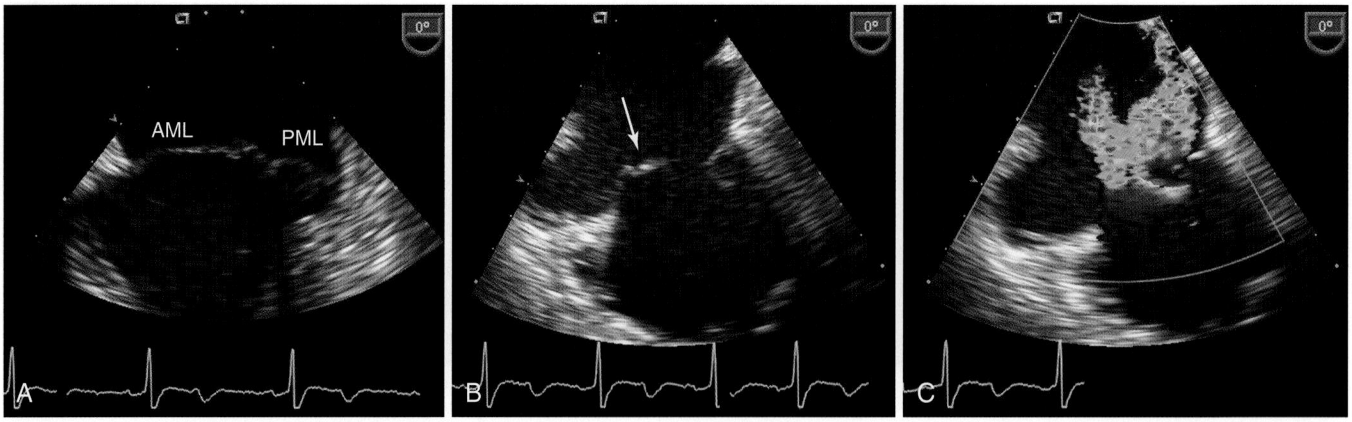

FIGURE 23-18 Combined mitral and tricuspid disease. A, Bileaflet mitral valve prolapse is present. **B,** Examination of the tricuspid valve revealed a flail anterior leaflet *(arrow),* with severe tricuspid regurgitation. **(C)**. Both valves were replaced. *AML,* Anterior mitral leaflet; *PML,* posterior mitral leaflet.

TABLE 23-9   Post–Cardiopulmonary Bypass Examination of the Mitral Valve

STRUCTURE/SUBJECT OF INTEREST	PARTICULARS OF EXAMINATION	VIEWS	FOCUS
Mitral Valve Repair			
LV	Regional and global function, volume status	Midesophageal two- and four-chamber, midesophageal long-axis, transgastric long- and short-axis	Adequate contractility important for valve closure; hypovolemia/hypercontractility predispose to SAM Examine LV restraint, papillary repositioning if performed
Right ventricle	Regional and global function	Midesophageal four-chamber, transgastric long- and short-axis	New dysfunction may indicate right coronary artery air, significant residual MR
MV competence	Define residual jets for severity, direction Assess coaptation length, residual prolapse, flail, tethering	Views as outlined in Figure 23-7 Color-flow Doppler with appropriate technical settings PW Doppler of pulmonary veins	Small central jets usually acceptable Eccentric jets may indicate breakdown of valve repair
MV gradients	Excessive gradients may indicate undersized annuloplasty ring	PW and CW Doppler of mitral inflow	Gradients may be present due to high flow state of after cardiopulmonary bypass[81,82]
Annulus	Assess for seating, MR outside the annuloplasty ring	Views as outlined in Figure 23-7	Regurgitation outside the ring always abnormal, may indicate separation from native annulus, poor valve seating
LVOT	LVOT obstruction	Midesophageal four-chamber and long-axis, deep transgastric, transgastric long-axis with color-flow and CW Doppler	Abnormal flow acceleration may be indicative of LVOT obstruction Look for SAM
Surrounding structures	Aortic valve, circumflex artery, AV nodal artery*	Check aortic valve competence, circumflex territory, heart block	
Prosthetic Valve Replacement			
Mechanical valve	Evaluate proper bileaflet motion Color-flow Doppler, PW and CW Doppler gradients	Scan valve from midesophageal position Leaflet best viewed at about 0-20 degrees if valve placement anatomic, 50-70 degrees if anti-anatomic	Small "washing jets" acceptable Paravalvular MR, if small, often disappears after heparin reversed
	LVOT obstruction	Midesophageal four-chamber and long axis, deep transgastric, transgastric long axis with color and CW Doppler	Preserved anterior leaflet may result in SAM
Tissue valve	Evaluate leaflet motion Color-flow Doppler gradients		Small central MR often present
	LVOT obstruction	Midesophageal 4 chamber and long axis, deep transgastric, transgastric long axis with color and CW Doppler	Preserved anterior leaflet may result in SAM Prosthetic struts may protrude into LVOT, infrequently a cause of LVOT obstruction

AV, atrioventricular; *CW,* Continuous wave; *Doppler,* Doppler echocardiography/imaging; *LV,* left ventricle/ventricular; *MR,* mitral regurgitation; *MV,* mitral valve; *OT,* outflow tract; *PW,* pulsed-wave; *SAM,* systolic anterior motion of the mitral valve.
*Berdajs D, Schurr UP, Wagner A, et al. Incidence and pathophysiology of atrioventricular block following mitral valve replacement and ring annuloplasty. Eur J Cardio-Thorac Surg 2008;34:55–61.

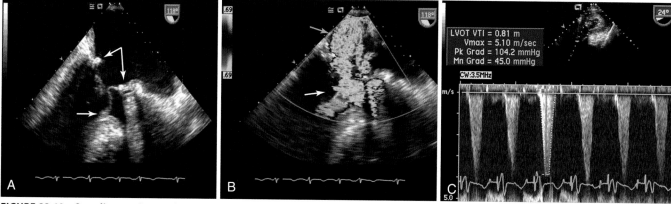

FIGURE 23-19 Systolic anterior motion (SAM) after mitral valve repair. A, Following P2 excision and ring annuloplasty *(double arrow)*, SAM developed secondary to hypovolemia *(single arrow)*. **B,** Color-flow Doppler imaging showed mitral regurgitation (MR) *(purple arrow)* and left ventricular outflow tract obstruction manifest as color Doppler aliasing *(white arrow)*. **C,** Deep transgastric imaging allowed parallel alignment of continuous wave Doppler echocardiography beam with the outflow tract, showing evidence of obstruction. Both MR and outflow obstruction resolved with measures to increase blood volume and a decrease in inotropic support.

Mitral Valve Systolic Anterior Motion

SAM after MV repair is often first suspected from the presence of color-flow Doppler aliasing in the LV outflow tract with residual MR, evident on both four-chamber and long-axis views (Figure 23-19). The late-peaking high-velocity ("dagger") appearance on continuous wave Doppler echocardiography can often be demonstrated in the transgastric long-axis and deep transgastric views and may allow calculation of gradient across the outflow tract, although one must keep in mind that the gradient may be underestimated because of a nonparallel angle between the Doppler beam and the high-velocity jet. SAM is less of a problem in ischemic MR because the outflow tract is usually large.

The presence of decreased preload and afterload along with increased heart rate and contractility is known to predispose to SAM and should be addressed through manipulations of vascular tone, volume, and inotropy. If MR cannot be ameliorated, cardiopulmonary bypass should be reinitiated and the valve repaired again or replaced. Patients who have intraoperative SAM that resolves with medical management in the operating room should be closely monitored for late recurrence.[50,79]

It is crucial that assessment be made in a timely fashion so that problems can be rectified before systemic heparin anticoagulation is reversed and the bypass cannulae are removed.

Prosthetic Valve Assessment

Following replacement, the prosthetic valve should be imaged by 2D, spectral, and color-flow Doppler echocardiography. This process is more straightforward for tissue prostheses. For mechanical valves, scanning from 0 to 180 degrees in the midesophageal position enables the optimal angle for leaflet assessment to be found. Both leaflets should move in an unrestricted fashion (Figure 23-20).

Pressure gradients across a newly placed prosthetic valve are often higher than expected. Assessing pressure gradients after cardiopulmonary bypass may be confounded by several factors: increased post-bypass cardiac output and anemia, pressure recovery, complex flow patterns of prosthetic valves, and use of the simplified Bernoulli equation (Pressure gradient = $4v^2$), which does not take into account high velocities through the LV outflow tract.[80] Any increased gradient takes on significance if there is obvious valvular dysfunction. The posts of a tissue prosthesis have the potential to obstruct the LV outflow tract, especially if it is small and the valve has a high profile.

Later in follow-up, the presence of high gradients as defined in the literature[81,82] should prompt examination for pathologic valve obstruction or patient prosthesis mismatch (see Chapter 26).

Color-flow Doppler evidence of MR is seen with most prosthetic valves. With a tissue prosthesis there is often a small jet of central MR, and a bileaflet mechanical prosthesis has small intravalvular "cleaning" jets (see Figure 23-15A). Echocardiographic interrogation at multiple angles will help determine whether the jets are "physiologic" or pathologic.

Abnormally large intravalvular jets may result if valve closure is impeded by retained mitral tissue.[83] Return to cardiopulmonary bypass is usually needed, so that rotation of the valve within the sewing ring or excision of the redundant tissue may be performed. Paravalvular jets are always abnormal (see Figure 23-15B-D) and are due to inadequate seating to the native annulus, especially in the presence of mitral annular calcification. Small paravalvular leaks often disappear after heparin reversal, but larger leaks should be addressed in the operating room prior to decannulation. 3D TEE may help pinpoint their location (Figure 23-21).

SAM can compound mitral valve replacement if native anterior leaflet preservation is undertaken and can occur after both bioprosthetic and mechanical valve replacement (Figure 23-22).

Assessment of Proximate Structures

There are a number of vulnerable anatomic structures proximate to the mitral annulus. Sutures placed in the MV sewing ring may entrap the left and noncoronary leaflets of the aortic valve. In an elegant study, Veronesi et al[84] demonstrated that even in the absence of injury, ring annuloplasty of the MV can alter the dynamics of flow through the aortic valve.

The circumflex artery is also vulnerable as it passes posterior to the MV annulus (Figure 23-23).[85,86] Appropriate 2D TEE and Doppler echocardiography examinations should be performed to rule out injury to these structures.[87]

Guidelines and Outcome

The American Heart Association (AHA)/American College of Cardiology (ACC)/American Society of Echocardiography (ASE) guidelines recommend the use of intraoperative TEE (class I recommendation) for all surgical valve repair and complex valve replacement procedures.[88] The latest updates from the American Society of Anesthesiologists/Society of Cardiovascular Anesthesia[89] and European Association of Echocardiography/European Association of Cardiothoracic Anesthesiologists[90] strongly recommend the use of intraoperative TEE in all adult patients undergoing cardiac surgery.

The impact of intraoperative TEE on surgical outcomes in valvular heart disease has never been studied in prospective, randomized fashion, nor is it likely ever to be. Several questions arise.

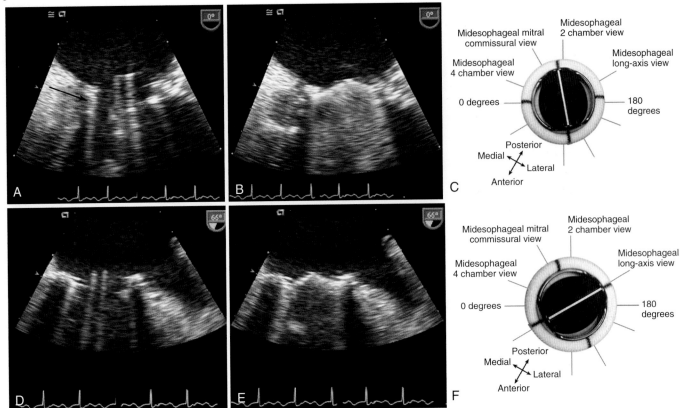

FIGURE 23-20 Prosthetic mitral valve orientation. A to **C,** When the bileaflet prosthetic valve occluders are aligned parallel to the position of the native valve leaflets, midesophageal images at 0 degrees and in a long axis plane show both leaflets opening normally in diastole **(A)** and closing in systole **(B). D** to **F,** When the prosthetic occluders are aligned perpendicular to the normal leaflet alignment ("anti-anatomic"), the transesophageal echocardiography image plane must be rotated to about 65 degrees to show normal occluder motion in diastole **(D)** and systole **(E)**. The *arrow* in **A** indicates a reverberation or "comet tail" artifact originating from the sewing ring.

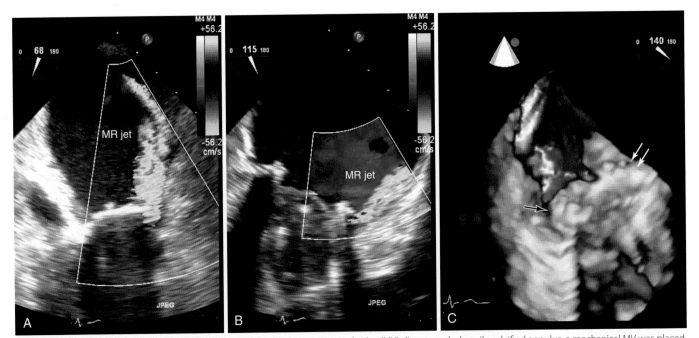

FIGURE 23-21 Paravalvular regurgitation. In a patient with rheumatic mitral valve (MV) disease and a heavily calcified annulus, a mechanical MV was placed. **A** and **B,** Following separation from cardiopulmonary bypass, two-dimensional transesophageal echocardiography revealed a paravalvular leak in what appeared to be the vicinity of the native anterior commissure. **C,** Three-dimensional color-flow Doppler imaging confirmed a large jet at the lateral commissure *(black arrow)*, and extending around to the native A1-A2 region. Cardiopulmonary bypass was reinstituted, the position of the leak was confirmed, and reinforcement sutures were successfully placed. *Double arrow* indicates the medial commissure.

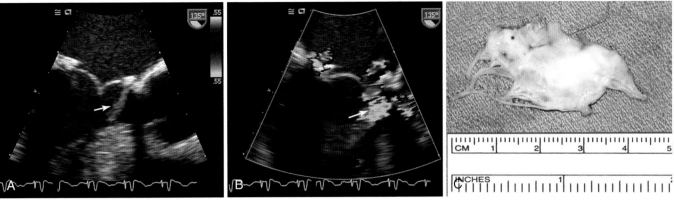

FIGURE 23-22   Subaortic obstruction. Following prosthetic tissue mitral valve replacement and subvalvular preservation, native anterior leaflet tissue can be seen obstructing the left ventricular outflow tract (**A**; *arrow*) with color-flow Doppler aliasing in the left ventricular outflow tract indicative of flow acceleration. **(B). C,** Cardiopulmonary bypass was reinstituted and when the native anterior leaflet was excised (shown here), the left ventricular outflow gradient resolved.

TABLE 23-10		Studies Addressing the Specific Impact of Intraoperative Transesophageal Echocardiography in Surgery for Valvular Heart Disease					
STUDY	**DESIGN**	**YEAR**	**NO. OF PATIENTS**	**VALVE SURGERY (%)**	**PRE-CPB IMPACT* (%)**	**POST-CPB FINDINGS**	**SECOND CPB SESSION (%)**
Sheikh et al[92]	Prospective Nonconsecutive	1985-1988	154	MV surgery (60) (repair [26]) Aortic surgery (40) (repair [11])	9	Residual regurgitation	6.0 All mitral surgery
Grimm & Stewart[93]	Retrospective Nonconsecutive	1984-1996	4066	Mitral repair (75) Aortic repair (12) Tricuspid repair (13)	NS	Inadequate repair Residual regurgitation	7.0 Total 5.0 Mitral 1.8 Aortic[†] 0.2 Tricuspid
Mishra et al[94]	Prospective Nonconsecutive	1993-1997	1356	Mitral (62) (repair or MVR) AVR (38)	13	Inadequate repair	2.0 All mitral repair
Click et al[95]	Prospective Nonconsecutive	1993-1997	2369	Mitral repair (36) MVR (18) AVR (30) Aortic repair (5) Other (11)	14	Inadequate repair Perivalvular leak LVOT obstruction	2.0 All mitral repair
Nowrangi et al[96]	Retrospective Nonconsecutive	1993-1996	383	AVR for aortic stenosis (100)	7	New RWMA	0.0
Shapira et al[97]	Retrospective Nonconsecutive	1999-2003	352	MVR (47) AVR (43) TVR (10)	29	Perivalvular leak Immobilized leaflet Coronary obstruction	4.0 Total 2.0 MVR 1.7 AVR 0.3 TVR
Bajzer et al[98]	Prospective Nonconsecutive	1990s	335	Tricuspid surgery (100) (repair or replacement)	6	Failed repair	4.0
Eltzschig et al[99]	Retrospective Nonconsecutive	1990-2005	6525	MVR or repair (28) AVR or repair (25) Both (6) CABG + aortic (21) CABG + mitral (20)	9	Inadequate mitral or aortic repair/ replacement New RWMA	3.0 Total 1.2 MVR or repair 0.6 AVR or repair 0.2 Both 0.3 CABG + aortic 0.7 CABG + mitral
Summary		1984-2005	15,540	Mitral surgery (56) Aortic surgery (36) Tricuspid surgery (8)	11 (n = 11,474)	Abnormal valve result most common	4.0

From Michelena HI, Abel MD, Suri RM, et al. Intraoperative echocardiography in valvular heart disease: an evidence-based appraisal. Mayo Clin Proc 2010;85:646–55. *AVR,* Aortic valve replacement; *CABG,* coronary artery bypass graft; *CPB,* cardiopulmonary bypass; *IOTEE,* intraoperative transesophageal echocardiography; *LVOT,* left ventricular outflow tract; *MVR,* mitral valve replacement; *NS,* not specified; *RWMA,* regional wall motion abnormality; *TVR,* tricuspid valve replacement.
*Pre-CPB findings that altered the planned surgery.
[†]This represented 14% of all aortic repairs, compared with 7% of all mitral repairs requiring a second pump run.

What is the additive value of pre-bypass TEE in clarifying MV pathology? What is the impact of post-bypass TEE on the rates of immediate and late reoperation, and does it result in improved outcomes?

In an extensive meta-analysis, Michelena et al[91] examined whether the use of intraoperative TEE in valvular heart disease had beneficial effects on patient outcome (Table 23-10). The availability of images obtained before surgery, before and after cardiopulmonary bypass, and during follow-up was a prerequisite for inclusion in the study. In 11% of patients, pre-bypass findings altered management. The most common finding was an undiagnosed patent foramen ovale; the actual number of patients with MV disease in whom intraoperative TEE findings refuted preoperative TTE findings was not stated. Post-bypass TEE resulted in a second bypass session in only 4% of patients, in the majority of whom there were residual valvular problems.

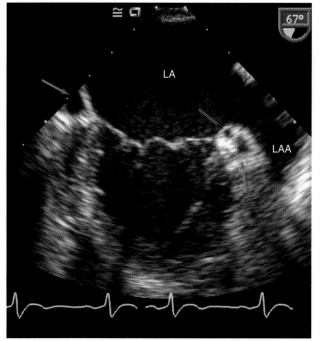

FIGURE 23-23 Para-annular anatomy. In this bicommissural view, the circumflex artery can be seen adjacent to the mitral annulus *(red arrow)*. The *blue arrow* indicates the coronary sinus. *LA*, Left atrium; *LAA*, left atrial appendage.

Two questions remain. First, if pre-bypass findings contradict preoperative TTE findings, should the surgical plan be changed? The answer is yes, but only if it can be demonstrated that the new finding was not the result of changes in loading conditions, but something that could reasonably have been missed on preoperative TTE, such as leaflet perforation. Second, if post-bypass imaging identifies abnormalities, should the finding prompt a second bypass session to allow correction? Clearly a gross technical failure of repair or an obvious abnormality of a prosthetic valve (i.e., stuck leaflet, large paravalvular leak, persistent SAM after medical optimization) should be addressed in the operating room, but more subtle degrees of MR in the adequately loaded patient present a greater challenge. Evidence seems to support an aggressive strategy to correct anything more serious than trivial MR, but this approach is not uniformly accepted.[77]

Outcomes following the use of 3D TEE in MV surgery have not been studied, and it is unlikely that a head-to-head comparison of outcomes with 3D TEE and 2D TEE will be forthcoming.

Conclusion

Decision making in MV surgery is a complex task that must incorporate precise imaging with knowledge of current surgical techniques and outcomes. Recognizing what constitutes an acceptable result or a surgical failure is the most important aspect of intraoperative echocardiography. Ongoing developments in 3D technology as well as a better understanding of the pathophysiology of MV disease make this an exciting area of clinical practice and research.

REFERENCES

1. Marijon E, Ou P, Celermajer DS, et al. Prevalence of rheumatic heart disease detected by echocardiographic screening. N Engl J Med 2007;357:470–6.
2. Carpentier A. Cardiac valve surgery—the "French correction." J Thorac Cardiovasc Surg 1983;86:323–37.
3. Nkomo VT, Gardin JM, Skelton TN, et al. Burden of valvular heart diseases: a population-based study. Lancet 2006;368:1005–11.
4. Muresian H. The clinical anatomy of the mitral valve. Clin Anat 2009;22:85–98.
5. Angelini A, Ho SY, Anderson RH, et al. A histological study of the atrioventricular junction in hearts with normal and prolapsed leaflets of the mitral valve. Br Heart J 1988;59:712–16.
6. Khoo NS Smallhorn JF. Mechanism of valvular regurgitation. Curr Opin Pediatr 2011;23:512–17.
7. Nii M, Roman KS, Macgowan CK, et al. Insight into normal mitral and tricuspid annular dynamics in pediatrics: a real-time three-dimensional echocardiographic study. J Am Soc Echocardiogr 2005;18:805–14.
8. Ranganathan N, Lam JH, Wigle ED, et al. Morphology of the human mitral valve. II: the value leaflets. Circulation 1970;41:459–67.
9. Foster GP, Isselbacher EM, Rose GA, et al. Accurate localization of mitral regurgitant defects using multiplane transesophageal echocardiography. Ann Thorac Surg 1998;65:1025–31.
10. Nielsen SL, Timek TA, Green GR, et al. Influence of anterior mitral leaflet second-order chordae tendineae on left ventricular systolic function. Circulation 2003;108:486–91.
11. Timek TA, Nielsen SL, Green GR, et al. Influence of anterior mitral leaflet second-order chordae on leaflet dynamics and valve competence. Ann Thorac Surg 2001;72:535–40; discussion 541.
12. Levine RA Schwammenthal E. Ischemic mitral regurgitation on the threshold of a solution: from paradoxes to unifying concepts. Circulation 2005;112:745–58.
13. Anderson RH Loukas M. The importance of attitudinally appropriate description of cardiac anatomy. Clin Anat 2009;22:47–51.
14. Quill JL, Hill AJ, Laske TG, et al. Mitral leaflet anatomy revisited. J Thorac Cardiovasc Surg 2009;137:1077–81.
15. Jamieson WR, Cartier PC, Allard M, et al. Surgical management of valvular heart disease 2004. Can J Cardiol 2004;20(Suppl E):7E–120E.
16. Lang RM, Badano LP, Tsang W, et al. EAE/ASE Recommendations for image acquisition and display using three-dimensional echocardiography. J Am Soc Echocardiogr 2012;25:3–46.
17. Wilkins GT, Weyman AE, Abascal VM, et al. Percutaneous balloon dilatation of the mitral valve: an analysis of echocardiographic variables related to outcome and the mechanism of dilatation. Br Heart J 1988;60:299–308.
18. Kunavarapu C, Olkovsky Y, Lafferty JC, et al. Unusual Cardiac complications of Staphylococcus aureus endocarditis. J Am Soc Echocardiogr 2008;21:187.e183–187.e185.
19. Shanewise JS, Cheung AT, Aronson S, et al. ASE/SCA guidelines for performing a comprehensive intraoperative multiplane transesophageal echocardiography examination: recommendations of the American Society of Echocardiography Council for Intraoperative Echocardiography and the Society of Cardiovascular Anesthesiologists Task Force for Certification in Perioperative Transesophageal Echocardiography. J Am Soc Echocardiogr 1999;12:884–900.
19a. Foster GP, Dunn AK, Abraham S, et al. Accurate measurement of mitral annular dimensions by echocardiography: importance of correctly aligned imaging planes and anatomic landmarks. J Am Soc Echocardiogr 2009;22:458–63.
20. Wasowicz M, Meineri M, Djaiani G, et al. Early complications and immediate postoperative outcomes of paravalvular leaks after valve replacement surgery. J Cardiothorac Vasc Anesth 2011;25:610–14.
21. Kohsaka S, Jin Z, Rundek T, et al. Impact of mitral annular calcification on cardiovascular events in a multiethnic community: the Northern Manhattan Study. JACC Cardiovasc Imaging 2008;1:617–23.
22. Gaasch WH Meyer TE. Left ventricular response to mitral regurgitation. Circulation 2008;118:2298–303.
23. Reeves ST, Glas KE, Eltzschig H, et al. Guidelines for performing a comprehensive epicardial echocardiography examination: recommendations of the American Society of Echocardiography and the Society of Cardiovascular Anesthesiologists. J Am Soc Echocardiogr 2007;20:427–37.
24. Kubitz JC, Annecke T, Kemming GI, et al. The influence of positive end-expiratory pressure on stroke volume variation and central blood volume during open and closed chest conditions. Eur J Cardio-Thorac Surg 2006;30:90–5.
25. Grewal KS, Malkowski MJ, Piracha AR, et al. Effect of general anesthesia on the severity of mitral regurgitation by transesophageal echocardiography. Am J Cardiol 2000;85:199–203.
25a. Gisbert A, Souliere V, Denault AY, et al. Dynamic quantitative echocardiographic evaluation of mitral regurgitation in the operating department. J Am Soc Echocardiogr 2006;19:140–6.
25b. Shiran A, Merdler A, Ismir E, et al. Intraoperative transesophageal echocardiography using a quantitative dynamic loading test for the evaluation of ischemic mitral regurgitation. J Am Soc Echocardiogr 2007;20:690–7.
25c. Mihalatos DG, Gopal AS, Kates R, et al. Intraoperative assessment of mitral regurgitation: role of phenylephrine challenge. J Am Soc Echocardiogr 2006;19:1158–64.
26. Agricola E, Oppizzi M, Galderisi M, et al. Role of regional mechanical dyssynchrony as a determinant of functional mitral regurgitation in patients with left ventricular systolic dysfunction. Heart 2006;92:1390–5.
27. Roberts BJ Grayburn PA. Color flow imaging of the vena contracta in mitral regurgitation: technical considerations. J Am Soc Echocardiogr 2003;16:1002–6.
28. Zoghbi WA, Enriquez-Sarano M, Foster E, et al. Recommendations for evaluation of the severity of native valvular regurgitation with two-dimensional and Doppler echocardiography. J Am Soc Echocardiogr 2003;16:777–802.
29. Tribouilloy C, Shen WF, Quere JP, et al. Assessment of severity of mitral regurgitation by measuring regurgitant jet width at its origin with transesophageal Doppler color flow imaging. Circulation 1992;85:1248–53.
30. Lesniak-Sobelga A, Kostkiewicz M, Olszowska M, et al. Chronic mitral regurgitation—significance of the echocardiographic determinants in predicting severity. Acta Cardiol 2009;64:187–93.
31. Lesniak-Sobelga A, Olszowska M, Pienazek P, et al. Vena contracta width as a simple method of assessing mitral valve regurgitation. Comparison with Doppler quantitative methods. J Heart Valve Dis 2004;13:608–14.

32. Kahlert P, Plicht B, Schenk IM, et al. Direct assessment of size and shape of noncircular vena contracta area in functional versus organic mitral regurgitation using real-time three-dimensional echocardiography. J Am Soc Echocardiogr 2008;21:912–21.
33. Lancellotti P, Moura L, Pierard LA, et al. European Association of Echocardiography recommendations for the assessment of valvular regurgitation. Part 2: mitral and tricuspid regurgitation (native valve disease). Eur J Echocardiogr 2010;11:307–32.
34. Biaggi P, Gruner C, Jedrzkiewicz S, et al. Assessment of mitral valve prolapse by 3D TEE angled views are key. JACC Cardiovasc Imaging 2011;4:94–7.
35. Lang RM, Tsang W, Weinert L, et al. Valvular heart disease: the value of 3-dimensional echocardiography. J Am Coll Cardiol 2011;58:1933–44.
36. Kronzon I, Sugeng L, Perk G, et al. Real-time 3-dimensional transesophageal echocardiography in the evaluation of post-operative mitral annuloplasty ring and prosthetic valve dehiscence. J Am Coll Cardiol 2009;53:1543–7.
37. Yosefy C, Hung J, Chua S, et al. Direct measurement of vena contracta area by real-time 3-dimensional echocardiography for assessing severity of mitral regurgitation. Am J Cardiol 2009;104:978–83.
38. Grewal J, Mankad S, Freeman WK, et al. Real-time three-dimensional transesophageal echocardiography in the intraoperative assessment of mitral valve disease. J Am Soc Echocardiogr 2009;22:34–41.
39. Ben Zekry S, Nagueh SF, Little SH, et al. Comparative accuracy of two- and three-dimensional transthoracic and transesophageal echocardiography in identifying mitral valve pathology in patients undergoing mitral valve repair: initial observations. J Am Soc Echocardiogr 2011;24:1079–85.
40. Maffessanti F, Marsan NA, Tamborini G, et al. Quantitative analysis of mitral valve apparatus in mitral valve prolapse before and after annuloplasty: a three-dimensional intraoperative transesophageal study. J Am Soc Echocardiogr 2011;24:405–13.
41. Müller S, Müller L, Laufer G, et al. Comparison of three-dimensional imaging to transesophageal echocardiography for preoperative evaluation in mitral valve prolapse. Am J Cardiol 2006;98:243–8.
42. Pepi M, Tamborini G, Maltagliati A, et al. Head-to-head comparison of two- and three-dimensional transthoracic and transesophageal echocardiography in the localization of mitral valve prolapse. J Am Coll Cardiol 2006;48:2524–30.
43. Sugeng L, Shernan SK, Weinert L, et al. Real-Time Three-Dimensional Transesophageal Echocardiography in Valve Disease: comparison With Surgical Findings and Evaluation of Prosthetic Valves. J Am Soc Echocardiogr 2008;21:1347–54.
44. La Canna G, Arendar I, Maisano F, et al. Real-time three-dimensional transesophageal echocardiography for assessment of mitral valve functional anatomy in patients with prolapse-related regurgitation. Am J Cardiol 2011;107:1365–74.
45. Chen X, Sun D, Yang J, et al. Preoperative assessment of mitral valve prolapse and chordae rupture using real time three-dimensional transesophageal echocardiography. Echocardiography 2011;28:1003–10.
46. Mahmood F, Subramaniam B, Gorman 3rd JH, et al. Three-dimensional echocardiographic assessment of changes in mitral valve geometry after valve repair. Ann Thorac Surg 2009;88:1838–44.
47. Mukherjee C, Tschernich H, Kaisers UX, et al. Real-time three-dimensional echocardiographic assessment of mitral valve: is it really superior to 2D transesophageal echocardiography? Ann Card Anaesth 2011;14:91–6.
48. Fattouch K, Murana G, Castrovinci S, et al. Mitral valve annuloplasty and papillary muscle relocation oriented by 3-dimensional transesophageal echocardiography for severe functional mitral regurgitation. J Thorac Cardiovasc Surg 2012;143:S38–42.
49. Sherrid MV, Chaudhry FA Swistel DG. Obstructive hypertrophic cardiomyopathy: echocardiography, pathophysiology, and the continuing evolution of surgery for obstruction. Ann Thorac Surg 2003;75:620–32.
50. Sorrell VL, Habibzadeh MR, Kalra N, et al. Transient severe mitral regurgitation after mitral valve repair is associated with a poor clinical outcome: a small case series. Echocardiography 2008;25:835–9.
51. Said SM, Schaff HV, Suri RM, et al. Bulging subaortic septum: an important risk factor for systolic anterior motion after mitral valve repair. Ann Thorac Surg 2011;91:1427–32.
52. Shah PM Raney AA. Echocardiography in mitral regurgitation with relevance to valve surgery. J Am Soc Echocardiogr 2011;24:1086–91.
53. Maslow AD, Regan MM, Haering JM, et al. Echocardiographic predictors of left ventricular outflow tract obstruction and systolic anterior motion of the mitral valve after mitral valve reconstruction for myxomatous valve disease. J Am Coll Cardiol 1999;34: 2096–104.
54. George KM Gillinov AM. Posterior leaflet shortening to correct systolic anterior motion after mitral valve repair. Ann Thorac Surg 2008;86:1699–700.
55. Quigley RL, Garcia FC Badawi RA. Prevention of systolic anterior motion after mitral valve repair with an anterior leaflet valvuloplasty. J Heart Valve Dis 2004;13: 927–30.
56. Saunders PC, Grossi EA, Schwartz CF, et al. Anterior leaflet resection of the mitral valve. Semin Thorac Cardiovasc Surg 2004;16:188–93.
57. Kahn RA, Mittnacht AJ Anyanwu AC. Systolic anterior motion as a result of relative "undersizing" of a mitral valve annulus in a patient with Barlow's disease. Anesth Analg 2009;108:1102–4.
58. De Bonis M, Lorusso R, Lapenna E, et al. Similar long-term results of mitral valve repair for anterior compared with posterior leaflet prolapse. J Thorac Cardiovasc Surg 2006;131: 364–70.
59. Magne J, Pibarot P, Dagenais F, et al. Preoperative posterior leaflet angle accurately predicts outcome after restrictive mitral valve annuloplasty for ischemic mitral regurgitation. Circulation 2007;115:782–91.
60. Timek TA Miller DC. Another multidisciplinary look at ischemic mitral regurgitation. Semin Thorac Cardiovasc Surg 2011;23:220–31.
61. Messas E, Bel A, Szymanski C, et al. Relief of mitral leaflet tethering following chronic myocardial infarction by chordal cutting diminishes left ventricular remodeling. Circ Cardiovasc Imaging 2010;3:679–86.
62. Da Col U, Di Bella I, Bardelli G, et al. Echocardiographic evaluation of mitral tethering for 'chordal cutting' procedure. Eur J Echocardiogr 2008;9:54–5.
63. Rodriguez F, Langer F, Harrington KB, et al. Importance of mitral valve second-order chordae for left ventricular geometry, wall thickening mechanics, and global systolic function. Circulation 2004;110:II115–22.
64. Yankah CA, Siniawski H, Detschades C, et al. Rheumatic mitral valve repair: 22-year clinical results. J Heart Valve Dis 2011;20:257–64.
65. Zakkar M, Amirak E, Chan KM, et al. Rheumatic mitral valve disease: current surgical status. Prog Cardiovasc Dis 2009;51:478–81.
66. Garccía-Ferníndez MA, Cortés M, García-Robles JA, et al. Utility of real-time three-dimensional transesophageal echocardiography in evaluating the success of percutaneous transcatheter closure of mitral paravalvular leaks. J Am Soc Echocardiogr 2010;23:26–32.
67. Benedetto U, Melina G, Angeloni E, et al. Prophylactic tricuspid annuloplasty in patients with dilated tricuspid annulus undergoing mitral valve surgery. J Thorac Cardiovasc Surg 2012;143:632–8.
68. De Bonis M, Lapenna E, Sorrentino F, et al. Evolution of tricuspid regurgitation after mitral valve repair for functional mitral regurgitation in dilated cardiomyopathy. Eur J Cardiothorac Surg 2008;33:600–6.
69. Kim JB, Yoo DG, Kim GS, et al. Mild-to-moderate functional tricuspid regurgitation in patients undergoing valve replacement for rheumatic mitral disease: the influence of tricuspid valve repair on clinical and echocardiographic outcomes. Heart 2012;98: 24–30.
70. Navia JL, Brozzi NA, Klein AL, et al. Moderate tricuspid regurgitation with left-sided degenerative heart valve disease: to repair or not to repair? Ann Thorac Surg 2012;93:59–67; discussion 68–59.
71. Fukuda S, Song J-M, Gillinov AM, et al. Tricuspid valve tethering predicts residual tricuspid regurgitation after tricuspid annuloplasty. Circulation 2005;111:975–9.
72. David TE, Ivanov J, Armstrong S, et al. A comparison of outcomes of mitral valve repair for degenerative disease with posterior, anterior, and bileaflet prolapse. J Thorac and Cardiovasc Surg 2005;130:1242–9.
73. Anyanwu AC Adams DH. Why do mitral valve repairs fail? J Am Soc Echocardiogr 2009;22:1265–8.
74. Hung J, Papakostas L, Tahta SA, et al. Mechanism of recurrent ischemic mitral regurgitation after annuloplasty: continued LV remodeling as a moving target. Circulation 2004;110:II85–90.
75. Magne J, Pibarot P, Dumesnil JG, et al. Continued global left ventricular remodeling is not the sole mechanism responsible for the late recurrence of ischemic mitral regurgitation after restrictive annuloplasty. J Am Soc Echocardiogr 2009;22:1256–64.
76. Senechal M, Magne J, Pibarot P, et al. Direction of persistent ischemic mitral jet after restrictive valve annuloplasty: implications for interpretation of perioperative echocardiography. Can J Cardiol 2007;23(Suppl B):48B–52B.
77. Adams DH Anyanwu AC. Pitfalls and limitations in measuring and interpreting the outcomes of mitral valve repair. J Thorac Cardiovasc Surg 2006;131:523–9.
78. Yamauchi T, Taniguchi K, Kuki S, et al. Evaluation of the mitral valve leaflet morphology after mitral valve reconstruction with a concept "coaptation length index". J Cardiac Surg 2005;20:432–5.
79. Varghese R, Anyanwu AC, Itagaki S, et al. Management of systolic anterior motion after mitral valve repair: an algorithm. J Thorac Cardiovasc Surg 2012;143:S2–7.
80. Schroeder RA Mark JB. Is the valve OK or not? Immediate evaluation of a replaced aortic valve. Anesth Analg 2005;101:1288–91.
81. Pibarot P Dumesnil JG. Doppler echocardiographic evaluation of prosthetic valve function. Heart 2012;98:69–78.
82. Zoghbi WA, Chambers JB, Dumesnil JG, et al. Recommendations for evaluation of prosthetic valves with echocardiography and doppler ultrasound: a report From the American Society of Echocardiography's Guidelines and Standards Committee and the Task Force on Prosthetic Valves, developed in conjunction with the American College of Cardiology Cardiovascular Imaging Committee, Cardiac Imaging Committee of the American Heart Association, the European Association of Echocardiography, a registered branch of the European Society of Cardiology, the Japanese Society of Echocardiography and the Canadian Society of Echocardiography, endorsed by the American College of Cardiology Foundation, American Heart Association, European Association of Echocardiography, a registered branch of the European Society of Cardiology, the Japanese Society of Echocardiography, and Canadian Society of Echocardiography. J Am Soc Echocardiogr 2009;22:975–1014; quiz 1082–14.
83. Oxorn D Verrier ED. Echocardiographic diagnosis of incomplete St. Jude's bileaflet valvular closure after mitral valve replacement with subvalvular preservation. Eur J Cardiothorac Surg 2003;24:298.
84. Veronesi F, Caiani EG, Sugeng L, et al. Effect of Mitral Valve Repair on Mitral-Aortic Coupling: a Real-Time Three-Dimensional Transesophageal Echocardiography Study. J Am Soc Echocardiogr 2012;25:524–31.
85. Tavilla G Pacini D. Damage to the circumflex coronary artery during mitral valve repair with sliding leaflet technique. Ann Thorac Surg 1998;66:2091–3.
86. Ender J, Singh R, Nakahira J, et al. Echo didactic: visualization of the circumflex artery in the perioperative setting with transesophageal echocardiography. Anesth Analg 2012;115:22–6.
87. Ender J, Selbach M, Borger MA, et al. Echocardiographic identification of iatrogenic injury of the circumflex artery during minimally invasive mitral valve repair. Ann Thorac Surg 2010;89:1866–72.
88. Shanewise JS, Cheung AT, Aronson S, et al. ASE/SCA guidelines for performing a comprehensive intraoperative multiplane transesophageal echocardiography examination: recommendations of the American Society of Echocardiography Council for Intraoperative Echocardiography and the Society of Cardiovascular Anesthesiologists Task Force for Certification in Perioperative Transesophageal Echocardiography. Anesth Analg 1999;89:870–84.
89. Practice guidelines for perioperative transesophageal echocardiography: an updated report by the American Society of Anesthesiologists and the Society of Cardiovascular Anesthesiologists Task Force on Transesophageal Echocardiography. Anesthesiology 2010;112:1084–96.

374

CH
23

90. Flachskampf FA, Badano L, Daniel WG, et al. Recommendations for transoesophageal echocardiography: update 2010. Eur J Echocardiogr 2010;11:557–76.

91. Michelena HI, Abel MD, Suri RM, et al. Intraoperative echocardiography in valvular heart disease: an evidence-based appraisal. Mayo Clin Proc 2010;85:646–55.

92. Sheikh KH, de Bruijn NP, Rankin JS, et al. The utility of transesophageal echocardiography and Doppler color flow imaging in patients undergoing cardiac valve surgery. J Am Coll Cardiol 1990;15:363–72.

93. Grimm RA Stewart WJ. The role of intraoperative echocardiography in valve surgery. Cardiol Clin 1998;16:477–89, ix.

94. Mishra M, Chauhan R, Sharma KK, et al. Real-time intraoperative transesophageal echocardiography—how useful? Experience of 5,016 cases. J Cardiothorac Vasc Anesth 1998;12:625–32.

95. Click RL, Abel MD Schaff HV. Intraoperative transesophageal echocardiography: 5-year prospective review of impact on surgical management. Mayo Clin Proc 2000;75:241–7.

96. Nowrangi SK, Connolly HM, Freeman WK, et al. Impact of intraoperative transesophageal echocardiography among patients undergoing aortic valve replacement for aortic stenosis. J Am Soc Echocardiogr 2001;14:863–6.

97. Shapira Y, Vaturi M, Weisenberg DE, et al. Impact of intraoperative transesophageal echocardiography in patients undergoing valve replacement. Ann Thorac Surg 2004;78:579–83; discussion 583–74.

98. Bajzer CT, Stewart WJ, Cosgrove DM, et al. Tricuspid valve surgery and intraoperative echocardiography: factors affecting survival, clinical outcome, and echocardiographic success. J Am Coll Cardiol 1998;32:1023–31.

99. Eltzschig HK, Rosenberger P, Loffler M, et al. Impact of intraoperative transesophageal echocardiography on surgical decisions in 12,566 patients undergoing cardiac surgery. Ann Thorac Surg 2008;85:845–52.

CHAPTER 24

Diseases of the Tricuspid and Pulmonic Valves

Grace Lin, Charles J. Bruce, and Heidi M. Connolly

Key Points

- Tricuspid regurgitation is most frequently "functional," not related to primary tricuspid leaflet pathology but rather secondary to another disease process causing right ventricular dilation, distortion of the subvalvular apparatus, tricuspid annular dilation or a combination of these.
- Severe tricuspid regurgitation due to a flail leaflet is associated with adverse outcomes favoring early surgical repair.
- Tricuspid regurgitation negatively impacts clinical outcome and survival regardless of left ventricular ejection fraction and severity of pulmonary hypertension.
- Tricuspid valve repair is the preferred treatment for tricuspid regurgitation in the absence of severely dysplastic or damaged leaflets.
- Tricuspid stenosis occurs infrequently and is essentially never seen in isolation.
- Pulmonic stenosis is related to a congenital or genetic disorder in 95% of cases; 80% of cases of valvular pulmonic stenosis occur in isolation.
- Balloon valvotomy is the procedure of choice for children and adults with severe or symptomatic pulmonic stenosis.
- Pulmonic stenosis with hypoplastic pulmonic annulus or dysplastic leaflets may require pulmonic valve replacement.
- Pathologic pulmonic regurgitation in adults is most often the consequence of prior interventions for congenital heart disease, including tetralogy of Fallot repair and surgical or balloon valvotomy for relief of pulmonic stenosis.
- Chronic severe pulmonic regurgitation results in progressive right ventricular dilation and dysfunction and right heart failure as well as an increased risk of arrhythmias.

Pathophysiology of Right-Sided Valve Disease

Primary versus Secondary Right-Sided Valve Disease

Differentiation of primary valve abnormalities from valve dysfunction secondary to pulmonary hypertension or primary right heart disease is an important first step in the evaluation of patients with tricuspid or pulmonic valve disease. Primary anatomic abnormalities of the tricuspid and pulmonic valves are often congenital and are usually diagnosed in childhood. In adults, right-sided valve disease is more commonly secondary to pulmonary hypertension, which in turn is often due to left-sided heart disease.

Response of the Right Heart to Pressure and/or Volume Overload

In the setting of chronic tricuspid or pulmonic regurgitation, the right ventricle dilates in response to chronic volume overload, which is visualized on echocardiography predominantly as enlargement in the short axis rather than in the longitudinal axis dimension.[1,2] Right ventricular volume overload is also associated with abnormal or "paradoxic" ventricular septal motion, because the septum moves toward the center of the right ventricle in systole and moves rapidly posteriorly in diastole—a pattern opposite of normal.[3-5] The reversed curvature of the septum is most marked in end-diastole, in contrast to pressure overload in which the maximum reversed curvature is more evident and occurs early in diastole.[6]

In chronic right ventricular volume overload, right ventricular systolic dysfunction occurs earlier in the disease course than is typical for left-sided volume overload conditions.[7,8] As with left-sided valve disease, right ventricular volume and systolic function typically improve after intervention for valvular regurgitation unless an irreversible decline in contractility has occurred.

The response of the right ventricle to chronic pressure overload, such as pulmonary hypertension or pulmonic stenosis, also differs from that of the left ventricle. Although the initial response is an increase in wall thickness, ventricular dilation may occur and depends on the acuteness and severity of the pressure overload state. With a gradual increase in right ventricular pressure, right ventricular size and systolic function may remain normal with a compensatory increase in right ventricular wall thickness.[9] After intervention, such as relief of pulmonic stenosis, an improvement in right ventricular hypertrophy and systolic function is expected because of the decreased right ventricular afterload. Although few studies have analyzed the extent of improvement in right ventricular function after relief of pulmonic stenosis, the improvement in right ventricular dimensions and systolic function in most patients after lung transplantation supports the concept that systolic function improves with decreased afterload.[10,11]

In contrast, with an acute increase in right ventricular pressure, for example with acute pulmonary embolism, decreased right ventricular systolic function and clinical right heart failure may be seen with mean pulmonary pressures of only 20 to 40 mm Hg.[12] Acute or subacute right ventricular pressure overload often results in right ventricular dilation with secondary annular dilation and tricuspid regurgitation. This combination superimposes a volume overload state, engendering a vicious circle of right ventricular dilation and worsening tricuspid regurgitation.

Principles of Diagnosis

VALVE STENOSIS AND REGURGITATION

After a thorough history and physical examination, echocardiography remains the cornerstone of diagnosis of right-sided valve disease and follows the same principles as those of evaluation for left-sided disease (see Chapter 6), confirming the presence and severity of valvular stenosis and regurgitation and providing important information about etiology. Assessment of the consequences of the valve abnormality for right ventricular size and function is also important.

Specific echocardiographic assessment of each right-sided valve lesion is outlined in detail later in this chapter.

RIGHT VENTRICULAR SIZE AND FUNCTION

Although echocardiography can provide morphologic assessment of right ventricular dimensions and function, accurate measurements are difficult because of the complex three-dimensional (3D) anatomy of the right ventricle.[13] Three-dimensional echocardiographic imaging improves estimation of right ventricular volumes over two-dimensional (2D) imaging, but cardiac magnetic resonance (CMR) imaging is more accurate.[14-16] For routine clinical assessment, tricuspid annular plane systolic excursion is a simple and reproducible measurement of right ventricular longitudinal function that correlates well with right ventricular ejection fraction by CMR.[14,15] Other measures of right ventricular function, including the right-sided index of myocardial performance (Tei index)[17], measurements of the peak systolic velocity, and displacement of the tricuspid annulus using tissue Doppler imaging[18-20] are feasible and have prognostic value in patients with pulmonary hypertension and other pathologies.[14] Right ventricular strain is a promising method of evaluating regional right ventricular contractility, and reduced strain predicts disease progression in pulmonary arterial hypertension.[14,21]

The extent of right ventricular hypertrophy can be assessed qualitatively from the thickness of the right ventricular free wall.[13,14] The timing of ventricular septal motion also provides insight into right ventricular function. Although patterns of abnormal septal motion may be appreciated on 2D imaging, the timing and extent of septal motion are best evaluated using M-mode echocardiography. When right ventricular enlargement is present, careful assessment of the atrial septum and pulmonary veins is critical to exclude left-to-right shunt, and transesophageal echocardiography should be performed if uncertainty remains after transthoracic imaging.

CMR methods for the assessment of right ventricular size and function are discussed in greater detail in Chapter 8.

PULMONARY ARTERY PRESSURES

Estimation of pulmonary pressures is an essential component of the examination in patients with right-sided valve disease. Right ventricular pressures can be estimated noninvasively from the velocity of the tricuspid regurgitant jet (V_{TR}) and the appearance of the inferior vena cava. Most patients have some degree of tricuspid regurgitation that permits estimation of the right ventricular-to-right atrial pressure gradient (ΔP_{RV-RA}), as described in the simplified Bernoulli equation:

$$\Delta P_{RV-RA} = 4(V_{TR})^2$$

This Doppler imaging–derived pressure gradient is added to an estimate of right atrial pressure, which is based on the size and respiratory variation of the inferior vena cava caliber (see Chapter 6).

Tricuspid Valve Anatomy

The normal tricuspid valve is characterized by three sail-like leaflets: anterior, posterior, and septal (Figure 24-1). The anterior leaflet is the most anatomically constant of the three, the other leaflets varying more often in size and position. The leaflets are attached to the tricuspid valve annulus and are restrained by chordae tendineae attached to the papillary muscles, which in turn insert into the right ventricular wall. However, tricuspid valve chordae may also insert directly into the right ventricular free wall, a feature distinguishing the right and left ventricles.

Tricuspid Regurgitation

Etiology

Tricuspid regurgitation that is at least moderate or greater in severity is most frequently "functional" or secondary in nature. Secondary tricuspid regurgitation by definition is not due to primary tricuspid leaflet pathology but is secondary to another disease process causing right ventricular dilation, distortion of the subvalvular apparatus, tricuspid annular dilation, or a combination of these problems. Causes of clinically significant tricuspid regurgitation are listed in Table 24-1. Furthermore, a moderate or greater degree of tricuspid regurgitation, regardless of etiology, usually engenders worsening tricuspid regurgitation owing to adverse hemodynamic consequences of right ventricular volume

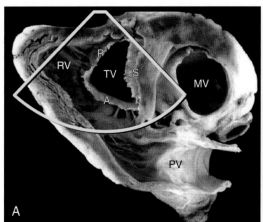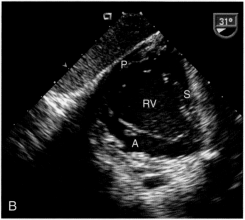

FIGURE 24-1   Tricuspid Valve Anatomy. A, Pathology image demonstrating the right ventricle (RV) with tricuspid valve (TV) in short axis. The pathologic section is oriented to replicate the transesophageal transgastric view obtained at a transducer angle of 31 degrees. Note septal (S), anterior (A), and posterior (P) leaflets. *MV,* Mitral valve; *PV,* pulmonic valve; **B,** Transesophageal transgastric echocardiographic image using same imaging plane (defined by the border in **A**) demonstrating the right ventricle with tricuspid valve septal, anterior, and posterior leaflets. *(Pathologic image courtesy Dr. William D. Edwards, Department of Laboratory Medicine and Pathology, Mayo Clinic College of Medicine).*

overload, resulting in a slow and inexorable clinical and hemodynamic deterioration.

Tricuspid regurgitation secondary to pulmonary hypertension is seen in patients with significant left-sided heart disease, those with primary pulmonary hypertension, and those with pulmonary disease leading to cor pulmonale.[22] As a general rule, when systolic pulmonary artery pressures increase beyond 55 mm Hg, tricuspid regurgitation can occur despite anatomically normal tricuspid leaflets, whereas more than mild tricuspid regurgitation occurring in the setting of lower systolic pulmonary pressures (<55 mm Hg) likely reflects a structural abnormality of the valve leaflets or the subvalvular apparatus.[23,24] Secondary tricuspid regurgitation also results from tricuspid annular dilation in patients with right ventricular enlargement resulting from right ventricular infarction, dilated cardiomyopathy, or chronic left-to-right shunt due to an atrial septal defect or anomalous pulmonary venous drainage.[25-27]

TABLE 24-1   Causes of Tricuspid Valve Regurgitation

Congenital Tricuspid Valve Disease

Ebstein anomaly
Tricuspid valve dysplasia
Tricuspid valve hypoplasia
Tricuspid valve cleft
Double-orifice tricuspid valve
Unguarded tricuspid valve orifice

Right Ventricular Disease

Right ventricular dysplasia
Endomyocardial fibrosis

Acquired Tricuspid Valve Disease

Annular dilation
Left-sided valvular heart disease
Endocarditis
Trauma
Carcinoid heart disease
Rheumatic heart disease
Tricuspid valve prolapse
Iatrogenic (irradiation, drugs, biopsy, pacemaker, implantable cardioverter-defibrillator)

Right Ventricular Dilation

Pulmonary hypertension:
  Primary
  Secondary to left-sided heart disease (valvular heart disease, cardiomyopathy, etc.)
Right ventricular volume overload
Atrial septal defect
Anomalous pulmonary venous drainage

Primary tricuspid valve pathology leading to tricuspid regurgitation may result from blunt trauma, iatrogenic injury, or specific diseases. When it is caused by permanent pacemaker or internal cardiac defibrillator leads, the mechanism of valve injury is variable, related to lead entrapment in the tricuspid apparatus, direct leaflet perforation, fibrotic adhesion of the lead to the leaflet, or avulsion or laceration of the tricuspid valve leaflets upon lead removal.[28] Because leaflet injury may be underappreciated, a high clinical index of suspicion is warranted, particularly when the patient with such an injury later presents with worsening right heart failure. Echocardiography, including 3D imaging, may be useful in localizing the leads relative to the tricuspid valve leaflets (Figure 24-2). The device leads can be visualized on computed tomography,[29] but because of artifact from the leads, their position relative to the tricuspid valve leaflets can be difficult to determine. Tricuspid valve repair or replacement may be required in symptomatic patients;[28] the role of pacemaker or defibrillator extraction to improve tricuspid regurgitation in patients without infection is less clear.

Direct tricuspid valve leaflet or chordal trauma may occur from transvenous endomyocardial biopsy, particularly in patients who have undergone cardiac transplantation who have repeated biopsies for rejection surveillance[30] (Figure 24-3). Echocardiographic guidance using real-time three-dimensional imaging during the biopsy may prevent damage to the tricuspid valve or subvalvular apparatus.[31]

The tricuspid leaflets and supporting structures may be damaged by blunt chest trauma, most often after a motor vehicle accident resulting in papillary muscle, valve, or chordal rupture. Affected patients may be asymptomatic and remain so for years following the trauma, and the murmur of tricuspid regurgitation is often not initially recognized.[32] Conduction abnormalities, including right and left bundle branch block and left anterior hemiblock, occur in more than 90% of patients with traumatic tricuspid regurgitation. Severe tricuspid regurgitation due to a flail leaflet is associated with adverse outcomes favoring early surgical repair (see natural history discussion).[30]

Damage to the tricuspid valve may also occur as a result of infective and marantic endocarditis.[30,33] Right-sided infective endocarditis is usually a manifestation of intravenous drug abuse, indwelling dialysis or chemotherapy venous catheters, or infected pacemakers or implantable cardioverter defibrillators[24,34-38] (Figure 24-4). *Staphylococcus aureus* accounts for 80% of these tricuspid valve infections, although in pacemaker- or defibrillator-associated endocarditis, coagulase-negative staphylococcus may be more common.[24,35,36] In cases of implantable cardiac device or indwelling catheter infections, early device extraction reduces mortality, and in most cases, the pacemaker or defibrillator can be explanted safely even with large vegetations.[36,39] Infrequently, marantic or

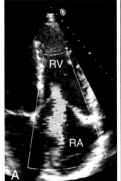
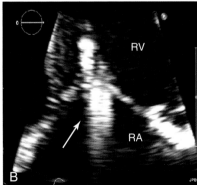
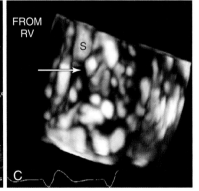

FIGURE 24-2   Device Lead Related Tricuspid Regurgitation. A, Color-flow Doppler image demonstrates tricuspid regurgitation related to multiple device leads. **B,** Zoomed view of tricuspid valve in apical four-chamber view with multiple leads *(arrow)* crossing the valve. **C,** Three-dimensional echocardiographic image of the tricuspid valve. Full volume 3D image of the heart was obtained, and image was cropped to obtain a short-axis view of the tricuspid valve, shown here from the right ventricular aspect of the valve. The device leads *(arrow)* are seen impinging on the motion of the septal leaflet. *RA,* Right atrium; *RV,* right ventricle; *S,* septal leaflet.

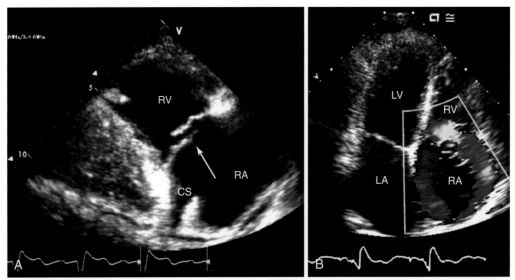

FIGURE 24-3   Flail tricuspid valve leaflet that occurred as a complication of an endomyocardial biopsy. A, Parasternal right ventricular inflow view; the posterior leaflet is flail *(arrow)*. *CS,* Coronary sinus; *RA,* right atrium; *RV,* right ventricle. **B,** Apical four-chamber view with color-flow Doppler imaging. Eccentric, laterally directed jet of tricuspid regurgitation. *LA,* left atrium; *LV,* left ventricle.

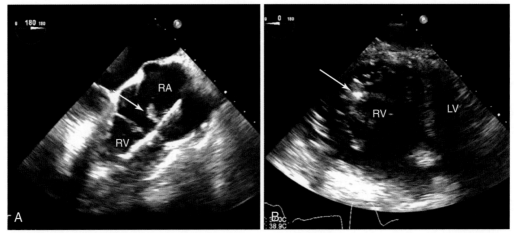

FIGURE 24-4   Endocarditis associated with a device lead. A, Transesophageal echocardiography shows vegetation *(arrow)* attached to the right atrial (RA) portion of the right ventricular (RV) defibrillator lead and to the posterior leaflet of the tricuspid valve. **B,** On transgastric short-axis image, the tricuspid valve and the defibrillator lead and vegetation *(arrow)* are visualized moving together with the posterior leaflet. Following device extraction, the vegetation was still attached to the posterior leaflet. *LV,* Left ventricle.

noninfective endocarditis occurs in the setting of systemic lupus erythematosus, rheumatoid arthritis, or antiphospholipid antibody syndrome.[40] The tricuspid valve may also be affected in up to 30% to 50% of patients with rheumatic valve disease.[41]

Serotonin-active drugs can induce fibroproliferative changes to the tricuspid valve leaflets, which are mediated by the 5-HT$_{2B}$ receptor.[42] These changes result in pathologic and echocardiographic features similar to those seen in carcinoid heart disease, with thickened tethered leaflets leading to tricuspid regurgitation. This association was first described with the ergot alkaloids, ergotamine and methysergide, used for migraine therapy.[43] The anorectic agents fenfluramine and dexfenfluramine were subsequently implicated and have since been withdrawn from the market.[44] Pergolide and cabergoline, dopamine agonists used in the treatment of Parkinson disease and restless leg syndrome, induce valve thickening and regurgitation by a similar mechanism and have also been withdrawn.[45-47]

Carcinoid heart disease is a rare but distinctive form of valve disease affecting primarily the right-sided cardiac valves. Carcinoid tumors arise from argentaffin cells; the primary tumor is usually located in the small bowel and metastasizes to the liver.

Serotonin produced by the primary tumor and metastases is recognized to be an agent involved in the development and progression of valve disease in patients with carcinoid syndrome.[48] Carcinoid heart disease involves a combination of tricuspid regurgitation (Figure 24-5) with rare stenosis as well as pulmonic stenosis and regurgitation. Left-sided valvular involvement occurs in approximately 10% of patients with carcinoid, generally in relation to right-to-left shunting of serotonin-rich blood through a patent foramen ovale or primary lung metastases.[49] Rarely, carcinoid valve disease occurs in patients without hepatic metastases; an ovarian carcinoid tumor should be sought in this setting.[50]

Mediastinal irradiation can directly damage the tricuspid leaflets (Figure 24-6). The associated post-inflammatory fibrosis and calcification, which usually manifest 5 years or longer after the radiation insult, result in distortion of the leaflets, causing tricuspid regurgitation.[24,51,52] Assessment and treatment of tricuspid regurgitation in this setting may be complicated by concomitant dysfunction of other cardiac valves as well as pericardial, myocardial, and coronary artery involvement.

Endomyocardial fibrosis, which is prevalent in tropical Africa, causes fibrosis of the papillary muscle tip and thickening and

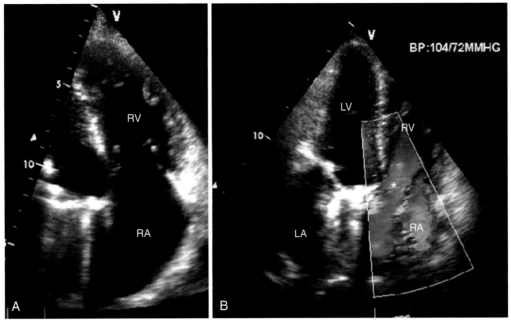

FIGURE 24-5   Tricuspid Regurgitation due to Carcinoid Heart Disease. A, Apical four-chamber view demonstrates thickened septal and anterior tricuspid valve leaflets with right ventricular (RV) enlargement and dysfunction in carcinoid heart disease. The patient previously had mitral valve replacement. **B,** Color-flow Doppler image shows severe tricuspid regurgitation in the same patient. Note the laminar color flow *(asterisk)* filling an enlarged right atrium (RA). *LA,* Left atrium, *LV,* left ventricle.

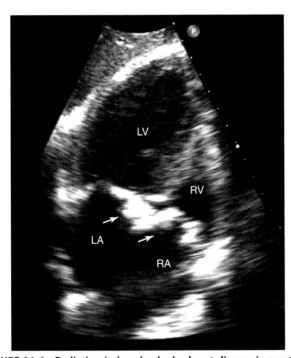

FIGURE 24-6   Radiation-induced valvular heart disease in a patient treated for lymphoma. Extensive thickening and calcification of both the mitral and tricuspid annuli *(arrows)* and leaflets., *LA,* Left atrium; *LV,* left ventricle; *RA,* right atrium; *RV,* right ventricle.

shortening of the leaflets and chordae, leading to regurgitation. This process may affect both mitral and tricuspid valves.

Congenital causes of tricuspid regurgitation are rare and include congenital tricuspid valve prolapse, which may occur as an isolated abnormality or may be associated with mitral valve prolapse and other connective tissue disorders.[53,54] The most common congenital cause of tricuspid regurgitation is Ebstein anomaly[55] (Figure 24-7). In this entity there is apical displacement of the septal and posterior tricuspid valve leaflets into the right

ventricle and variable tethering of the anterior leaflet as well as variability in the severity of tricuspid regurgitation. A patent foramen ovale or atrial septal defect occurs in more than 50% of patients. Other associated defects include accessory conduction pathways, pulmonic stenosis, and ventricular septal defect.[56]

Diagnosis

The course and presentation of tricuspid regurgitation are variable; moderate to severe tricuspid regurgitation is often well tolerated, and patients can remain asymptomatic for years. Symptoms depend on the acuity and chronicity of valve dysfunction and resultant right chamber dilation, and they are usually related to hemodynamic changes that occur as a result of elevated right atrial pressure due to tricuspid regurgitation. Chronic, severe tricuspid regurgitation leads to right heart failure and low cardiac output, resulting in fatigue and decreased exercise tolerance. Peripheral edema and hepatic congestion with associated anorexia and abdominal fullness can occur, and eventually, ascites and anasarca may develop.

Physical examination findings are characterized by jugular venous distention with a visible systolic v wave in 35% to 75% of patients.[25-27] Hepatomegaly is present in 90% of patients, but palpable systolic pulsation of the liver is less common. Classically the holosystolic murmur of tricuspid regurgitation is heard along the left sternal border with radiation to the hepatic region and increases in intensity with inspiration because of increased systemic venous return.[26] However, the murmur is often inaudible and can be auscultated in fewer than 20% of patients with documented tricuspid valve regurgitation.[25-27] In addition, many patients have atrial fibrillation, which further confounds interpretation of the characteristic respiratory variation in murmur intensity.[25-27,57]

As many as 80% to 90% of patients referred for echocardiography have some degree of tricuspid regurgitation.[58] Tricuspid regurgitation can be qualitatively graded with use of color-flow Doppler imaging according to the extent of the systolic color-flow disturbance in the right atrium and semiquantitatively from the density of the continuous wave Doppler echocardiography signal (Figure 24-8A). Severe tricuspid regurgitation is characterized by a dense and dagger-shaped continuous wave Doppler signal appearance

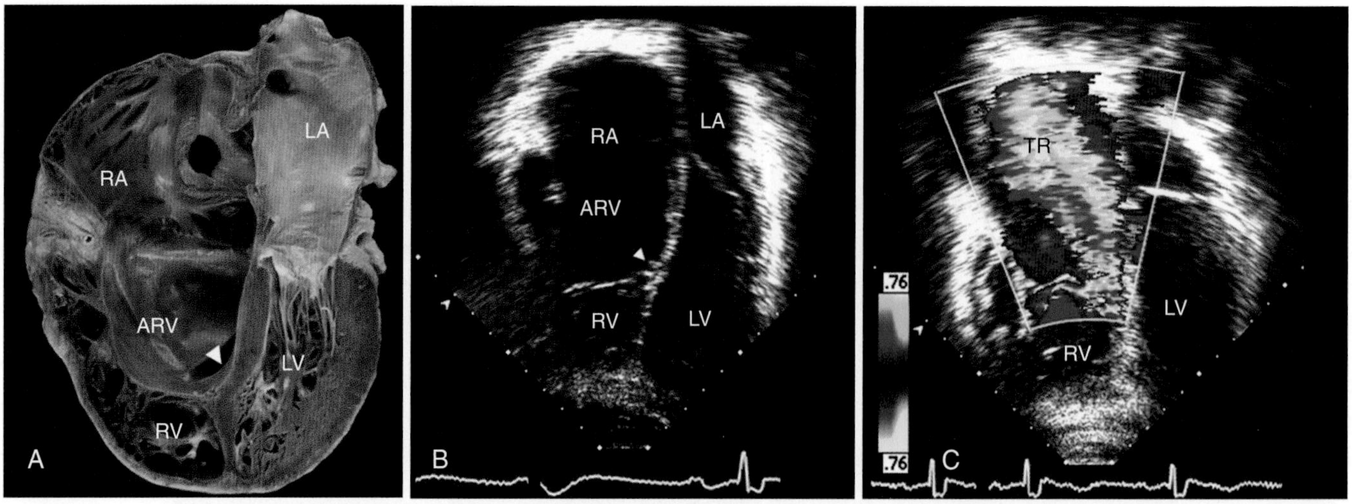

FIGURE 24-7 Ebstein anomaly. Characteristic findings are apical displacement of the septal leaflet of the tricuspid valve (arrowhead) and variable tethering of the anterior leaflet. The segment of right ventricular (RV) myocardium between the leaflet insertion and the anatomic annulus is "atrialized" (ARV), as seen in the pathology specimen demonstrated in the apical four-chamber "apex down" imaging format **(A)** and the two-dimensional echocardiographic image demonstrated in the same format **(B)**. **C,** Because of associated valve disease, severe tricuspid regurgitation (TR) was noted on color-flow imaging, resulting in severely enlarged right heart chambers. *LA,* left atrium; *LV,* Left ventricle; *RA,* right atrium. *(Pathology image courtesy Dr. William D. Edwards, Department of Laboratory Medicine and Pathology, Mayo Clinic College of Medicine.)*

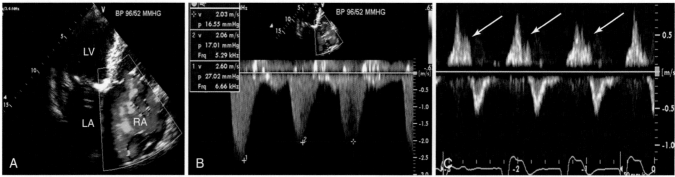

FIGURE 24-8 Severe tricuspid regurgitation. A, Apical four-chamber view. With color-flow Doppler imaging, the tricuspid regurgitant jet fills >10 cm², or ≥30% of the right atrium (RA). **B,** Continuous wave Doppler signal across the tricuspid valve demonstrates a dagger-shaped signal consistent with rapid equalization of right ventricular and right atrial pressures. **C,** Hepatic vein pulsed wave Doppler signal with accompanying electrocardiogram tracing demonstrating systolic flow reversals *(arrows),* reflecting retrograde flow in the hepatic veins that can be appreciated clinically as a pulsatile liver and a v wave on the jugular venous examination. Hepatic vein systolic reversal may not be specific for severe tricuspid regurgitation when atrial fibrillation is present. *LA,* Left atrium; *LV,* left ventricle.

due to rapid equalization of pressures between the right atrium and right ventricle (Figure 24-8B). Ancillary echocardiographic findings in patients with severe tricuspid regurgitation include inferior vena cava dilation of more than 2 cm and systolic flow reversals in the hepatic veins[59-62] (Figure 24-8C).

The effective regurgitant orifice area can be estimated by measuring the vena contracta on color-flow Doppler imaging; a vena contracta larger than 0.7 cm indicates severe tricuspid regurgitation.[24,61-63] Quantitative Doppler assessment is also feasible with use of the proximal isovelocity surface area (PISA) method, although this requires angle correction.[61] As with auscultation of the tricuspid regurgitant murmur, respiratory changes occur that may impact Doppler quantification of tricuspid regurgitation. Both the effective regurgitant orifice and the regurgitant volume significantly increase with inspiration, independent of both the severity and pathophysiology of tricuspid regurgitation and the degree of pulmonary hypertension.[64]

Natural History

The natural history of severe tricuspid regurgitation is often one of a prolonged latent period with eventual progressive right ventricular and later right atrial volume overload. Atrial arrhythmias are common secondary to right atrial enlargement and may be difficult to treat in the presence of persistent tricuspid regurgitation. Initially symptoms of right heart failure and volume overload can be palliated with diuretics, but as hepatic congestion and resultant anorexia develop, patients may become nutritionally depleted.

Tricuspid valve regurgitation has an important impact on clinical outcome and survival in patients with cardiovascular disease. Mortality is higher in patients with tricuspid regurgitation regardless of ejection fraction or severity of pulmonary hypertension.[65] Severe tricuspid regurgitation following percutaneous mitral balloon valvotomy has a negative effect on survival,[66] and as in patients who have undergone mitral valve replacement, subsequent severe tricuspid regurgitation is associated with a significant reduction in exercise capacity.[67]

Tricuspid regurgitation from flail leaflets is associated with an increased risk of atrial fibrillation, heart failure, need for surgery, or death.[30] The natural history of tricuspid regurgitation due to flail tricuspid valve leaflets was demonstrated in a cohort of 60 patients at Mayo Clinic, half of whom underwent operative intervention (27 tricuspid valve repair, 6 tricuspid valve replacement). In this series, operative risk was low, and symptomatic improvement was noted in 88% of operated patients. Unoperated patients experienced higher than expected mortality (4.5% yearly; P <0.01) than a matched U.S. population. Right-sided chamber enlargement, even in asymptomatic patients, was associated with a marked increase in morbidity. Unfortunately, risk of atrial arrhythmia may persist even after successful repair.

Medical and Surgical Treatment

GENERAL

The patient's clinical status and the etiology of the tricuspid valve regurgitation determine the appropriate therapeutic strategy (Tables 24-2 and 24-3).[24] Correctable causes should be identified and addressed. Medical management of symptomatic tricuspid regurgitation centers on treatment of right heart failure and primarily involves the use of diuretics combined with fluid and sodium restriction to manage volume status. In patients with left ventricular dysfunction, additional medical therapy may be required for management of left heart failure, but care should be taken to avoid exacerbating fatigue and hypotension related to a low cardiac output.

Tricuspid valve surgery is the only treatment demonstrated to be effective for symptomatic tricuspid valve regurgitation. At our institution, tricuspid valve repair or replacement is recommended for patients with severe tricuspid valve regurgitation without important comorbidities and (1) symptomatic right heart failure (reduced cardiac output, fatigue, exertional dyspnea, diminished exercise capacity), (2) mitral valve disease or other cardiac disease that requires operative intervention, (3) progressive right ventricular enlargement or dysfunction, and (4) select asymptomatic patients, such as patients with traumatic tricuspid valve flail with severe tricuspid valve regurgitation. Tricuspid valve operation is also recommended in patients with moderate or more tricuspid valve regurgitation undergoing other cardiac surgery. The American Heart Association (AHA)/American College of Cardiology (ACC) and European Society of Cardiology (ESC) guidelines for indications for tricuspid valve repair and replacement are summarized in Tables 24-2 and 24-3; both guidelines specify the presence of symptoms or need for additional cardiac surgery as important indications.[24,62]

TIMING OF SURGERY

Timing of surgery for tricuspid regurgitation remains controversial, in part because of limited and heterogenous data on postoperative outcomes.[24] Reported short- and long-term mortality rates following tricuspid valve surgery are high, with up to 20% operative mortality and 50% mortality at 10 years.[68-71] These rates may reflect the latent course of tricuspid regurgitation, operation for which often occurs in patients with advanced disease and heart failure. Advanced age, emergency status, associated atrial fibrillation, and pulmonary hypertension are preoperative predictors of poor outcome,[69] but heart failure and elevated right-sided filling pressures (defined by short tricuspid regurgitation duration) are among the most important determinants.[71] In a cohort of patients at Mayo Clinic who underwent tricuspid valve surgery and were stratified according to according to severity of preoperative heart failure, operative mortality was higher (18%) in patients with New York Heart Association class IV symptoms than in those with less advanced heart failure (0% for class II, 9% for class III; $P = 0.02$). Similarly, long-term outcomes, regardless of whether concomitant left-sided valve replacement was performed, were better in patients without advanced heart failure symptoms preoperatively.[71] These findings argue for earlier intervention, before the onset of severe right ventricular dysfunction and heart failure.

TABLE 24-2	Management of Patients with Severe Tricuspid Regurgitation (American College of Cardiology/American Heart Association Guidelines)*[24]

Class I

Tricuspid valve repair is beneficial for severe TR in patients with MV disease requiring MV surgery. (*Level of Evidence: B*)

Class IIa

1. Tricuspid valve replacement or annuloplasty is reasonable for severe primary TR when symptomatic. (*Level of Evidence: C*)
2. Tricuspid valve replacement is reasonable for severe TR secondary to diseased/abnormal tricuspid valve leaflets not amenable to annuloplasty or repair. (*Level of Evidence: C*)

Class IIb

Tricuspid annuloplasty may be considered for less than severe TR in patients undergoing MV surgery when there is pulmonary hypertension or tricuspid annular dilation. (*Level of Evidence: C*)

Class III

1. Tricuspid valve replacement of annuloplasty is not indicated in asymptomatic patients with TR whose pulmonary artery systolic pressure is less than 60 mm Hg in the presence of a normal MV. (*Level of Evidence: C*)
2. Tricuspid valve replacement or annuloplasty is not indicated in patients with mild primary TR (*Level of Evidence: C*)

MV, Mitral valve; *TR,* tricuspid regurgitation.
*Classification of recommendations and level of evidence are expressed in the ACC/AHA format are as follows:
Class I: Conditions for which there is evidence for and/or general agreement that the procedure or treatment is beneficial, useful, and effective.
Class II: Conditions for which there is conflicting evidence and/or a divergence of opinion about the usefulness/efficacy of a procedure or treatment:
  Class IIa: Weight of evidence/opinion is in favor of usefulness/efficacy.
  Class IIb: Usefulness/efficacy is less well established by evidence/opinion.
Class III: Conditions for which there is evidence and/or general agreement that the procedure/treatment is not useful/effective and in some cases may be harmful.
Level of Evidence B: Data derived from a single randomized trial or nonrandomized studies.
Level of Evidence C: Only consensus opinion of experts, case studies, or standard-of-care.

TABLE 24-3	Indications for Intervention in Tricuspid Valve Disease (European Society of Cardiology Guidelines)*[62]	
INDICATION		**CLASS**
Symptomatic severe TS		IC
Severe TS in patients undergoing left-sided valve intervention		IC
Severe primary or secondary TR in patients undergoing left-sided valve surgery[†]		IC
Symptomatic severe isolated primary TR without severe RV dysfunction[†]		IC
Moderate primary TR in a patient undergoing left-sided valve surgery		IIaC
Moderate secondary TR with dilated annulus (>40 mm or >21 mm/m²) in a patient undergoing left-sided valve surgery		IIaC
Severe TR and symptoms, after left-sided valve surgery, in the absence of left-sided myocardial, valve, or right ventricular dysfunction and without severe pulmonary vascular disease		IIaC
Severe isolated primary TR with mild or no symptoms and progressive dilation or deterioration of RV function		IIbC

TR, Tricuspid regurgitation; *TS,* tricuspid stenosis.
*Recommendation classes and levels of evidence:
Class I: Evidence and/or general agreement that a given treatment or procedure is beneficial, useful, and effective.
Class II: Conflicting evidence and/or a divergence of opinion about the usefulness/efficacy of a given treatment or procedure:
  Class IIa: Weight of evidence/opinion is in favor of usefulness/efficacy.
  Class IIb: Usefulness/efficacy is less well established by evidence/opinion.
Level of evidence A: Data derived from multiple randomized clinical trials or meta-analyses.
Level of evidence B: Data derived from a single randomized clinical trial or large nonrandomized studies.
Level of evidence C: Consensus of opinion of the experts and/or small studies, retrospective studies, registries.
[†]Percutaneous technique can be attempted as a first approach if TS is isolated.

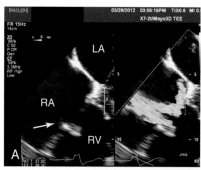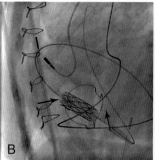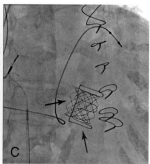

FIGURE 24-9 **Dysfunctional tricuspid valve prosthesis treated with Melody stented valve (valve-in-valve procedure). A,** Transesophageal echocardiography demonstrating a transverse view of the right atrium (RA), left atrium (LA), right ventricle (RV), and tricuspid valve bioprosthesis *(arrow; left panel).* Severe prosthetic tricuspid regurgitation is noted on color-flow Doppler imaging *(right panel).* **B,** Fluoroscopy image, left lateral view. A catheter with the Melody valve *(black arrow)* is placed through the tricuspid valve bioprosthesis *(red arrow).* Note the dual-chamber pacemaker with a coronary sinus lead as the primary ventricular pacing lead; no right ventricular lead was placed through the tricuspid valve bioprosthesis. **C,** Right anterior oblique view following completed placement of the Melody valve *(black arrow)* with the stent fully deployed through the tricuspid valve bioprosthetic valve *(red arrow).*

TRICUSPID VALVE REPAIR VERSUS REPLACEMENT

Accurate imaging of the tricuspid valve anatomy prior to surgery is paramount. Although intraoperative transesophageal echocardiography may allow refinement of annuloplasty techniques to optimize outcome,[72-74] assessment of the tricuspid valve with intraoperative transesophageal echocardiography is difficult owing to limited Doppler echocardiography angles of interrogation and periprocedural hemodynamic alterations that may reduce the severity of tricuspid regurgitation. A comprehensive assessment of the severity of tricuspid regurgitation is best undertaken by careful preoperative transthoracic echocardiography.[24]

In the setting of tricuspid annular dilation in the absence of significant abnormalities of the tricuspid valve leaflets, tricuspid valve repair is generally the preferred approach. Singh et al,[75] comparing tricuspid valve replacement with repair in "primary" tricuspid valve disease, demonstrated that tricuspid valve repair was associated with better perioperative and mid-term event-free survival than tricuspid valve replacement, and despite increased severity of recurrent tricuspid regurgitation in patients undergoing repair, there was no difference in reoperation rates or New York Heart Association functional class during follow-up.[75]

Options for tricuspid valve repair include ringed or flexible band annuloplasty, DeVega (purse-string) annuloplasty, edge-to-edge (Alfieri-type) repairs, and posterior annular bicuspidalization.[76,77] Robotically assisted, minimally invasive tricuspid valve repair techniques have also been employed and may be a potential alternative.[78] Compared with a purse-string annuloplasty, ringed annuloplasty is associated with better long-term event-free survival and greater freedom from recurrent tricuspid regurgitation.[79] The degree of tricuspid valve tethering and the severity of early postoperative left ventricular dysfunction and recurrent tricuspid regurgitation are important determinants of residual and persistent tricuspid regurgitation following tricuspid valve repair.[80,81] Although preoperative and postoperative pulmonary hypertension was not predictive of recurrent tricuspid regurgitation, postoperative increase in pulmonary artery pressures was a risk factor.[81]

Tricuspid valve replacement is indicated for patients who have abnormal tricuspid valves not amenable to repair, including those with carcinoid heart disease, rheumatic heart disease, some patients with Ebstein anomaly, and those with recurrent tricuspid valve regurgitation after prior repair. Most commonly, tricuspid valve replacement is undertaken with a bioprosthesis, which avoids the need for long-term anticoagulation, and the durability of right-sided bioprostheses is superior to that of left-sided prostheses, likely related to lower transvalvular pressure gradients.[82] Pericardial bioprostheses are generally avoided in the tricuspid position owing to leaflet stiffness and the associated risk of obstruction. Mechanical tricuspid valve prostheses can be considered in

the patient with an established indication for long-term anticoagulation, for example, concomitant mechanical left-sided prosthesis or atrial fibrillation. Although there is a risk of thrombosis or bleeding due to long-term anticoagulation with mechanical valves, several large series have reported no differences in mortality between bioprosthetic and mechanical tricuspid valves.[68,70,83,84]

Percutaneous native tricuspid valve replacement has been performed in animal studies. Off-label use of the Melody bioprosthetic percutaneous pulmonic valve placed in a dysfunctional tricuspid bioprosthesis has been reported in a small number of patients and has yielded promising results with reduction in tricuspid regurgitation or transvalvular gradient and clinical improvement[85,86] (Figure 24-9). Video-assisted minimal-access procedures to replace the tricuspid valve may be another alternative treatment option.[87]

TRICUSPID REGURGITATION WITH MITRAL VALVE DISEASE

In the setting of left-sided valvular heart disease, both the latest ACC/AHA and ESC valvular heart disease guidelines suggest that tricuspid valve annuloplasty should be considered at the time of left-sided valve surgery even when less than severe or even mild tricuspid regurgitation is present, if there is associated annular dilation.[24,62] The outlook is poor for patients who have previously undergone left-sided valvular heart disease surgery and subsequently present with symptomatic severe tricuspid regurgitation. Although "repeat" surgery to specifically address the tricuspid valve regurgitation in these patients can be performed with acceptable early mortality (9%) and symptomatic improvement, late mortality remains high (event-free survival 42% ± 9%), especially in those with advanced age and multiple previous cardiac operations.[88]

Despite the recommendation from the ACC/AHA and the ESC, tricuspid valve procedures represent only one tenth the number of mitral valve procedures performed in the United States yearly, suggesting that tricuspid valve repair is still underutilized in this setting.[77] Some observational studies have documented improvement in tricuspid regurgitation severity when percutaneous balloon mitral valvotomy is performed in patients with mitral stenosis, severe pulmonary hypertension, and significant secondary tricuspid regurgitation, as a result of relief of pulmonic stenosis and resultant drop in pulmonary artery pressures.[89,90] Nevertheless, tricuspid valve repair combined with mitral valve replacement has been shown to be better than percutaneous balloon mitral valvotomy alone in patients with mitral stenosis and severe secondary tricuspid regurgitation, especially if they also have atrial fibrillation or right ventricular enlargement.[91]

Yilmaz et al,[92] reporting on 699 patients undergoing mitral valve repair for degenerative mitral valve prolapse with

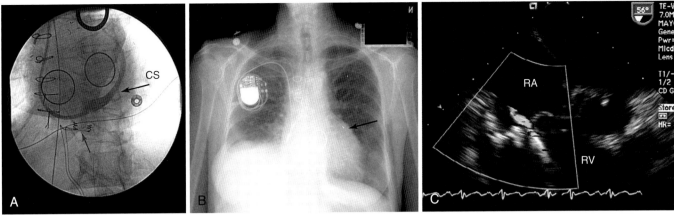

FIGURE 24-10 Pacemaker lead placement options in patients with tricuspid valve prostheses. A, Coronary sinus (CS) venogram *(arrow)* in a patient with radiation-induced valvular heart disease, and mitral and tricuspid mechanical prostheses. Note the abandoned epicardial pacing leads *(red arrow)*. **B,** CS lead *(arrow)* placed for ventricular pacing in the same patient. **C,** Transesophageal echocardiography depicting a transverse view of the right atrium (RA) and right ventricle (RV) with trivial tricuspid regurgitation on color-flow Doppler imaging after a pacemaker lead was placed through the tricuspid valve bioprosthesis. Two years later, only trivial tricuspid regurgitation was still present.

associated less-than-severe tricuspid regurgitation, observed that tricuspid regurgitation improved following surgery and remained clinically insignificant at 5 years of follow-up, arguing for a selective approach to tricuspid valve repair in this patient population. However, the likelihood of developing or worsening secondary tricuspid regurgitation is affected by the etiology of mitral valve disease, and because the etiology of mitral valve disease is not homogenous, these results cannot be generalized.[77,92]

SPECIFIC CONSIDERATIONS BASED ON ETIOLOGY

FLAIL TRICUSPID VALVE LEAFLETS. Early surgery should be considered for patients with severe tricuspid regurgitation resulting from blunt chest trauma, because the long-term prognosis of flail tricuspid leaflets is poor[30] and the likelihood of repair is high.

EBSTEIN ANOMALY. Although tricuspid valve replacement may be required, tricuspid valve repair options are possible for patients with Ebstein anomaly.[55] Appropriate patient selection is critical, and these procedures should be performed at tertiary care centers by congenital cardiac surgeons. A series from Mayo Clinic of 539 patients with Ebstein anomaly suggests that 20-year survival may be higher in patients who undergo tricuspid valve repair, but residual tricuspid regurgitation persisted in 33% of patients undergoing repair compared with none in those who underwent replacement. Considerations for valve replacement rather than repair include older age (>12 years) and more-than-moderate residual tricuspid regurgitation at the end of the operation.[93]

CARCINOID HEART DISEASE. Carcinoid heart disease is best treated surgically with valve replacement, and operative intervention has a beneficial impact on patient survival and functional class.[48,94,95] Indications for operative intervention in patients with controlled carcinoid disease include progressive fatigue, dyspnea or right heart failure, and progressive right heart enlargement or dysfunction. Asymptomatic patients with severe carcinoid heart disease may be candidates for valve replacement, which might permit partial hepatic resection or liver transplantation.

SECONDARY TRICUSPID REGURGITATION DUE TO PULMONARY HYPERTENSION. In patients with pulmonary hypertension secondary to pulmonary thromboembolic disease, pulmonary thromboendarterectomy alone has been shown to reduce not only pulmonary hypertension but also tricuspid regurgitation without the need for concomitant tricuspid annuloplasty even if the tricuspid valve annulus is dilated.[96] Tricuspid regurgitation secondary to severe primary pulmonary hypertension is usually treated with pulmonary vasodilator and diuretic therapy alone because of the risk of cardiac surgical intervention and the poor overall prognosis.

PACEMAKER- OR DEFIBRILLATOR-INDUCED TRICUSPID REGURGITATION. Patients with severe tricuspid regurgitation due to pacemaker or implantable cardioverter defibrillator lead impingement or perforation demonstrate symptomatic improvement following tricuspid valve repair or replacement.[28] Repair involves suture repair of a defect in the leaflet and positioning of the device lead by suture fixation in the recess of either the posteroseptal or anteroposterior commissure. With tricuspid valve replacement, the device lead is placed outside the sewing ring. When pacing is required in the setting of an existing tricuspid mechanical prosthetic valve, a ventricular lead cannot be placed across the valve, and an epicardial lead or endovascular coronary sinus pacing lead may be required (Figure 24-10A and B). In selected patients, device leads can be placed across a bioprosthetic valve without causing significant tricuspid valve prosthesis dysfunction (Figure 24-10C).[97]

TRICUSPID REGURGITATION IN PATIENTS UNDERGOING LEFT VENTRICULAR ASSIST DEVICE PLACEMENT. Left ventricular assist devices are increasingly utilized to treat advanced heart failure, and severe right ventricular dysfunction is a predictor of high postoperative mortality.[98] Concomitant tricuspid valve repair for severe tricuspid regurgitation promotes right ventricular reverse remodeling and improved clinical outcomes.[99] In one study, outcomes with tricuspid valve repair at the time of surgery for left ventricular assist device placement were comparable to those with biventricular assist device or total artificial heart implantation in patients with severe right ventricular dysfunction and tricuspid regurgitation.[100]

ATRIAL FIBRILLATION. Patients with severe tricuspid valve regurgitation and atrial arrhythmias referred for surgical intervention should be considered for concomitant partial or full maze procedure. Although this latter procedure may not alleviate atrial fibrillation, it may decrease the clinical impact.[101]

PREGNANCY. The patient with isolated severe tricuspid regurgitation generally tolerates pregnancy well in the absence of right heart failure, unless an arrhythmia occurs.

ATRIAL SEPTAL DEFECT. Adult patients with an atrial septal defect or other shunt lesion causing tricuspid annular dilation and more-than-moderate tricuspid regurgitation should be considered for operative atrial septal defect closure and tricuspid valve repair to decrease the extent of right heart enlargement, given the unpredictable reduction in regurgitation following atrial septal defect closure alone.

TABLE 24-4   Causes of Tricuspid Stenosis

Rheumatic heart disease
Congenital tricuspid stenosis
Right atrial tumors
Carcinoid heart disease
Endomyocardial fibrosis
Valvular vegetations
Extracardiac tumors

Tricuspid Stenosis

Etiology

In developed countries, tricuspid valve stenosis is an exceptionally rare clinical condition. Although rheumatic heart disease accounts for about 90% of all cases, concurrent tricuspid stenosis occurs in only 3% to 5% of patients with rheumatic mitral valve disease.[102,103] Other, more unusual causes of tricuspid stenosis include carcinoid heart disease,[104] congenital anomalies, infective endocarditis due to large (often fungal) vegetations and Whipple disease.[105] Bioprosthetic tricuspid valves can degenerate and become stenotic. A right atrial myxoma might manifest as signs and symptoms mimicking those of obstruction at the tricuspid valve level (Table 24-4).

Diagnosis

Because patients with rheumatic tricuspid stenosis invariably have coexisting mitral valve disease, it is difficult to separate symptoms specific to tricuspid valve obstruction from those of mitral valve stenosis and/or regurgitation, which include fatigue, dyspnea, and peripheral edema.[103,106,107]

On physical examination, venous pressure is elevated with a prominent a wave and characteristically an opening snap, followed by a diastolic rumbling murmur at the right sternal border that varies with respiration.[108] As with tricuspid regurgitation, the murmur is often inaudible.

Atrial fibrillation is present in 50% of cases, but right atrial enlargement may be evident on electrocardiography in patients in sinus rhythm.[103,106-108] An enlarged right atrium is often present on chest radiography with normal pulmonary artery size and clear lung fields. The transvalvular pressure gradient and valve area of the stenotic tricuspid valve can be measured by hemodynamic catheterization, but evaluation by Doppler echocardiography has replaced the need for routine catheterization.[109-111]

Echocardiography enables a definitive diagnosis of the etiology and severity of tricuspid stenosis. Rheumatic involvement parallels the changes seen with rheumatic mitral valve disease, including commissural fusion and diastolic doming with thickened and shortened chordae. Even on echocardiography, findings can be subtle, so tricuspid valve involvement may be overlooked unless specific attention is directed to the tricuspid valve in patients with rheumatic mitral valve disease. Unlike in mitral stenosis, short-axis 2D imaging of the valve orifice is rarely feasible in tricuspid stenosis; 3D imaging may be useful to better define the valve anatomy and orifice size.[112]

Evaluation of the degree of tricuspid stenosis includes calculation of the mean pressure gradient and valve area. Tricuspid stenosis is considered hemodynamically significant when the mean gradient is 5 mm Hg or greater, valve area is 1.0 cm^2 or less, and the pressure half-time is 190 milliseconds or longer.[112] During assessment of the mean gradient, measurements should be averaged throughout the respiratory cycle. If atrial fibrillation is present, a minimum of five cardiac cycles should be recorded, and the measurements averaged. The valve area can be calculated by the pressure half-time method as in mitral stenosis, using a constant of 190, or, in the absence of significant tricuspid regurgitation, with the continuity equation.[112]

Natural History

Few data are available on the natural history of isolated tricuspid stenosis because it typically accompanies rheumatic mitral valve disease. In a retrospective study of 13 patients with severe rheumatic tricuspid stenosis, 12 underwent surgery for mitral and/or aortic valve involvement, and 6 of these had concurrent tricuspid valve surgery.[113] Like mitral stenosis, tricuspid valve obstruction is the result of a chronic, slowly progressive disease process correlating with a gradual increase in stenosis severity and gradual symptom onset.

Medical and Surgical Treatment

Medical therapy for hemodynamically significant tricuspid stenosis consists of diuresis to improve systemic venous congestion and heart rate control to promote effective diastolic filling. However, these methods are only temporizing, and tricuspid valve replacement is usually required[24,62] (see Tables 24-2 and 24-3).

Tricuspid balloon valvotomy has been advocated for tricuspid stenosis of various causes. However, severe tricuspid regurgitation is a common consequence of this procedure, and results are poor when severe tricuspid regurgitation develops.[24,114,115] Percutaneous valve replacement (valve-in-valve) may be an option in selected patients with previous valve replacement and bioprosthetic valve stenosis.[86]

Pulmonic Stenosis

Etiology

Pulmonic valve stenosis is related to a congenital or genetic disorder in 95% of cases. Although pulmonic stenosis may be a feature of complex congenital cardiac lesions, such as tetralogy of Fallot, 80% of cases occur in isolation. Rarely, carcinoid syndrome and rheumatic valve disease may cause pulmonic valve stenosis but these lesions essentially always occur in conjunction with other valve disease.[105]

The abnormal pulmonic valve may be classified as *acommissural,* with prominent systolic doming of the valve cusps and an eccentric orifice; *unicommissural,* with a single asymmetric commissure; *bicuspid,* with fused commissures; or *dysplastic,* with severely thickened and deformed valve cusps (Figure 24-11). Evaluation of valve morphology is important because dysplastic valves respond poorly to balloon dilation. The pulmonic annulus and outflow tract may also be narrowed; this type of valve morphology is common in patients with Noonan syndrome.

Pulmonic stenosis may be associated with pulmonary artery aneurysms. Most patients with pulmonary artery enlargement and congenital pulmonic stenosis do not require operative intervention unless they have either symptomatic compression of adjacent structures or pulmonic regurgitation with associated right heart enlargement. However, rupture or dissection may occur when severe pulmonary artery dilation occurs in the setting of severe pulmonary hypertension.[116,117]

The patient with repaired congenital heart disease involving placement of an extracardiac conduit from the right ventricle to pulmonary arteries requires long-term monitoring. Such a conduit is prone to degeneration, resulting in pulmonic stenosis or regurgitation.

Diagnosis

Most patients with mild or moderate pulmonic stenosis are asymptomatic, and even those with severe obstruction can be asymptomatic. Typical symptoms include fatigue and dyspnea due to reduced cardiac output. Patients can delay symptom onset by adjusting their lifestyle and level of exertion. Exertional lightheadedness or syncope may occur in adults with pulmonic stenosis associated with systemic or suprasystemic right ventricular

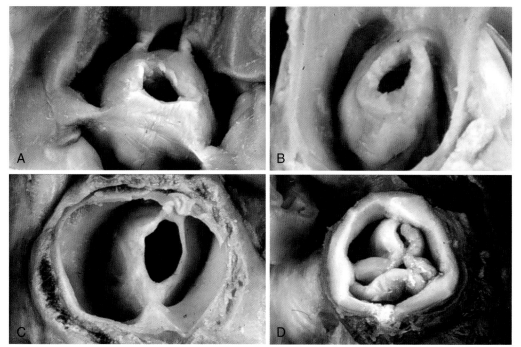

FIGURE 24-11 **Classification of the abnormal pulmonic valve.** The abnormal pulmonic valve may be classified as **(A)** *acommisural* with prominent systolic doming of the valve cusps and an eccentric orifice, **(B)** *unicommissural*, **(C)** *bicuspid* with fused commissures, or **(D)** *dysplastic* with severely thickened and deformed valve cusps. *(Pathology image courtesy Dr. William D. Edwards, Department of Laboratory Medicine and Pathology, Mayo Clinic College of Medicine.)*

pressures. With long-standing severe pulmonic stenosis, right heart failure may occur.

Most adults with pulmonic stenosis have a normal appearance. In the Noonan syndrome, characteristic features include short stature, webbed neck, hypertelorism, low-set ears and hairline, chest wall deformities and lymphedema. This autosomal dominant disorder is important to recognize because of the high frequency of associated cardiac anomalies (≈85%), most commonly pulmonic stenosis (60%).[118] The dysplastic pulmonic valve in Noonan syndrome is less amenable to balloon intervention, and surgical treatment should be considered.

Clinical findings depend on the severity of pulmonic stenosis, valve pathology, and other associated cardiac lesions. In mild pulmonic stenosis, the physical findings are characterized by a normal jugular venous pulse, no right ventricular lift, and a pulmonic ejection sound that tends to decrease with inspiration. A pulmonic ejection murmur ending in mid-systole is usually heard; this murmur increases in intensity with inspiration.

In severe pulmonic stenosis, the jugular venous pressure demonstrates a prominent a wave, and a right ventricular lift is common. A palpable systolic murmur may be noted at the upper left sternal border. A loud and long crescendo-decrescendo pulmonic ejection systolic murmur is present, loudest at the upper left sternal border and radiating to the suprasternal notch and left side of the neck. Although an ejection click is common in mild pulmonic stenosis, the click moves closer to the first heart sound with increasing stenosis severity and may be absent in severe stenosis. As the severity of pulmonic stenosis progresses, the second heart sound becomes widely split. Delayed pulmonic valve closure is secondary to prolongation of the right ventricular ejection time, and eventually pulmonic valve closure is no longer audible. As a consequence of right ventricular hypertrophy, a right-sided fourth heart sound may also be heard.

The electrocardiogram is usually normal in patients with pulmonic stenosis. With severe pulmonic stenosis, features of right atrial enlargement, right axis deviation, and right ventricular hypertrophy may be present (Figure 24-12A). In Noonan syndrome, however, left axis deviation is more common.[119]

The chest radiograph findings may be normal or may demonstrate features of right heart enlargement and dilation of the pulmonary artery (Figure 24-12B). In severe pulmonic stenosis, the vascular lung markings may be diminished.

Transthoracic Doppler echocardiography is recommended for initial and serial follow-up evaluations of pulmonic stenosis.[24,120] Two-dimensional echocardiography demonstrates the thickened pulmonic valve cusps with characteristic doming in systole as the cusps reach their limit of excursion. The severity of pulmonic stenosis is determined by the peak transpulmonic velocity with the use of continuous wave Doppler echocardiography to calculate the transvalvular pressure gradient (Figure 24-13). Severe pulmonic stenosis is defined as a peak gradient greater than 60 mm Hg, moderate as a peak gradient 36 to 60 mm Hg, and mild as a peak gradient less than 36 mm Hg.[24,120] The degree of coexisting pulmonic regurgitation should be evaluated with color-flow Doppler imaging and continuous wave Doppler recordings of signal intensity and Doppler profile (see discussion of pulmonic regurgitation). It is particularly important to evaluate for subvalvular or supravalvular obstruction, in addition to valvular stenosis, because right ventricular outflow obstruction may take any one of these forms, which have similar clinical manifestations. Rarely, echocardiography is nondiagnostic, and CMR, computed tomography, or cardiac catheterization is needed to define the exact level of obstruction (Figure 24-14).

In uncomplicated pulmonic stenosis, the use of CMR or computed tomography is simply confirmatory. These studies provide excellent imaging of the pulmonary arteries and are useful when associated lesions are suspected (see Chapter 7).

Exercise testing is not routinely performed for evaluation of pulmonic stenosis but may be useful to unmask symptoms in the "asymptomatic" patient. Patients are able to maintain normal oxygen consumption, cardiac output, and right ventricular diastolic pressure when pulmonic stenosis is mild or moderate. However, a marked increase in right ventricular end-diastolic pressure is seen as the pulmonic valve area falls below 0.5 cm^2/m^2.[121]

The role of cardiac catheterization in pulmonic stenosis is discussed in Chapter 7. Catheterization should be considered when

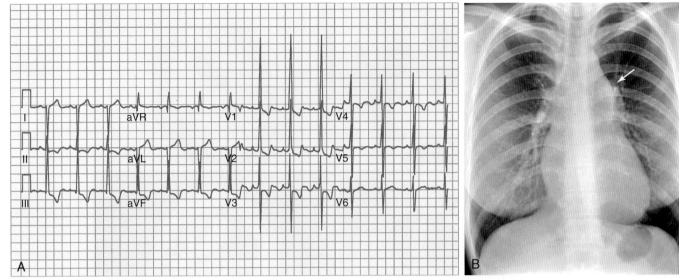

FIGURE 24-12 Electrocardiographic and chest radiographic findings with pulmonic valve stenosis. A, The electrocardiogram from a patient with critical pulmonic stenosis demonstrates right-axis deviation and right ventricular hypertrophy with a strain pattern. **B,** The chest radiograph from the same patient with critical pulmonic valve stenosis demonstrates features of right atrial and ventricular enlargement, dilation of the pulmonary artery *(arrow)*, and diminished vascular markings.

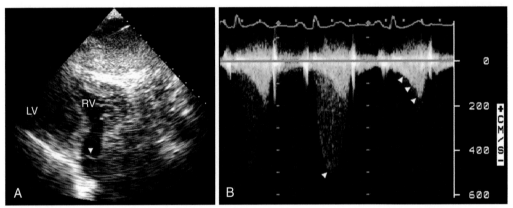

FIGURE 24-13 Echocardiographic findings with pulmonic valve stenosis. A, Two-dimensional echocardiogram from a patient with severe pulmonic valve stenosis. The best alignment between the Doppler beam and the pulmonic flow signal was from a subcostal long-axis window with the transducer angled anteriorly. Marked right ventricular (RV) hypertrophy was noted and there was systolic doming of the pulmonic valve *(arrowhead)*. *LV,* Left ventricle. **B,** In the same patient, the peak velocity recorded with continuous wave Doppler ultrasound for calculation of the transvalvular pressure gradient *(single arrowhead)* suggests a peak gradient of more than 100 mm Hg. Note the late-peaking infundibular gradient *(three arrowheads)* from dynamic right ventricular outflow tract obstruction.

the clinical assessment of pulmonic stenosis severity and imaging data are discordant or to facilitate intervention.

Natural History

In the Second Natural History Study of Congenital Heart Defects (conducted 1958-1969), event-free survival of patients with pulmonic stenosis was closely related to the pressure gradient, with survival of 31% for those with a gradient of 50 to 79 mm Hg, 77% for those with a gradient between 25 and 49 mm Hg, and 96% for those with a gradient less than 25 mm Hg[122] (Figure 24-15). These data suggest that relief of pulmonic stenosis should be strongly considered for all patients with a peak gradient greater than 50 mm Hg. Intervention during the Second Natural History Study was surgical valvotomy, but in the current era, owing to the option of percutaneous balloon valvotomy, intervention is undertaken at a lower peak gradient.

Mild pulmonic stenosis (peak gradient <36 mm Hg) in adults has a benign course with little progression of disease and excellent clinical outcomes.[122-124] The ACC/AHA guidelines for management of congenital heart disease recommend serial follow-up

evaluations every 5 years for asymptomatic patients in whom the peak gradient is less than 30 mm Hg.[120]

Patients with moderate pulmonic stenosis (peak gradient 36 to 60 mm Hg) may be symptomatic with exertional dyspnea or fatigue. Approximately 24% of initially asymptomatic patients with moderate pulmonic stenosis who were followed in the Second Natural History Study eventually required intervention. Independent predictors of the need for intervention included higher peak systolic gradient and reduced cardiac output. There were few clinical differences between medically and surgically treated patients with moderate pulmonic stenosis; both groups have excellent clinical status and low likelihood of requiring medications.[122] In symptomatic patients with peak gradients higher than 30 mm Hg, the ACC/AHA guidelines recommend follow-up evaluation every 2 years.[120]

In contrast, patients with severe stenosis (peak gradient ≥60 mm Hg) are usually symptomatic, and those with a peak gradient of 80 mm Hg or higher often have evidence of right heart failure.[122,125] Outcomes following intervention are excellent. In the Second Natural History Study, only 4% of patients required reoperation during 10-year follow-up.[122] In a cohort of 90 patients with

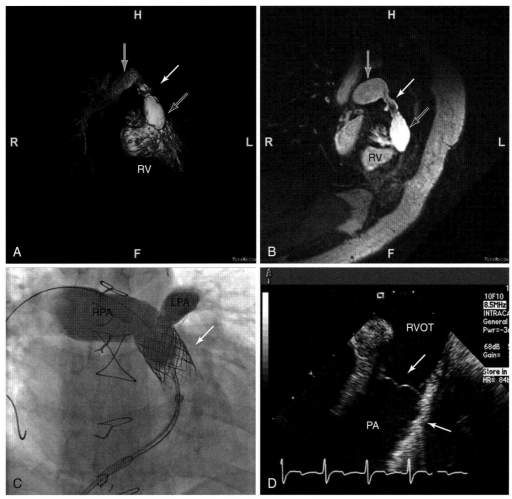

FIGURE 24-14   Dysfunctional right ventricle-to-pulmonary artery conduit in a patient with double-outlet right ventricle and D-transposition of the great vessels. Surface-rendered three-dimensional reformatted magnetic resonance imaging **(A)** and cardiac magnetic resonance imaging **(B)** of the dysfunctional right ventricular outflow tract (RVOT) conduit. The conduit and valve and the level of obstruction were adequately delineated by echocardiography, although a mean gradient of 38 mmHg was noted. Both **A** and **B** demonstrate oblique views through the RVOT conduit *(red arrow)* with stenosis *(white arrow)* proximal to the conduit valve. The *green arrow* indicates the right pulmonary artery (RPA). **C,** Subsequent cardiac catheterization demonstrated a peak-to-peak gradient of 51 mmHg, and a Melody stented valve was placed *(white arrow)*. In this right anterior oblique fluoroscopy image, a catheter remains across the Melody valve extending into the right pulmonary artery. The left pulmonary artery (LPA) had been previously stented. **D,** Post-procedure transthoracic echocardiography demonstrating the Melody stented valve *(white arrows)*. *PA,* Pulmonary artery; *RV,* right ventricle.

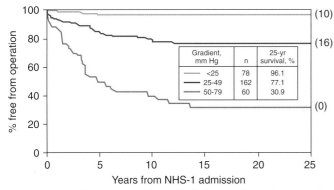

FIGURE 24-15   Outcomes with medical therapy for pulmonic valve stenosis. Kaplan-Meier curves of the percentage free from surgery for 300 patients with pulmonic stenosis managed medically, grouped by gradient at admission to the First Natural History Study (NHS-1). Numbers in *parentheses* indicate the numbers of patients remaining under observation 25 years after admission. *(From Hayes C, Gersony WM, Driscoll DJ, et al: Second natural history study of congenital heart defects: results of treatment of patients with pulmonic valve stenosis. Circulation 1993;87[Suppl]:I28-I37.)*

pulmonic stenosis treated with surgery from the Netherlands, survival at 25 years was 93%, and at last follow-up, 67% still had New York Heart Association class I symptoms. However, re-intervention was required in 15%, primarily for pulmonic regurgitation (9%). At last follow-up, moderate to severe pulmonic regurgitation was present in 37%; supraventricular arrhythmias occurred in patients with severe pulmonic regurgitation and resolved after valve replacement.[126]

Medical, Interventional, and Surgical Treatment

Balloon valvotomy was initially described in 1982 and has become the procedure of choice for children and adults with uncomplicated severe or symptomatic pulmonic stenosis. The ACC/AHA and ESC congenital heart disease guidelines concerning the management of pulmonic stenosis are summarized in Tables 24-5 and 24-6.[24,120,127] The ACC/AHA valvular heart disease guidelines rely on right ventricular-to-pulmonary artery peak-to-peak catheter-derived gradients across the pulmonic valve (>30 mmHg in symptomatic patients or >40 mmHg in asymptomatic patients) to determine appropriate timing of intervention; the ACC/AHA and

TABLE 24-5	American College of Cardiology/American Heart Association Congenital Heart Disease Guidelines for Management of Pulmonic Valve Stenosis (PS)*[120]

Class I

1. Balloon valvotomy is recommended for asymptomatic patients with a domed pulmonic valve and a peak instantaneous Doppler gradient greater than 60 mm Hg or a mean Doppler gradient greater than 40 mm Hg (in association with less than moderate pulmonic valve regurgitation). *(Level of Evidence: B)*
2. Balloon valvotomy is recommended for symptomatic patients with a domed pulmonic valve and a peak instantaneous Doppler gradient greater than 50 mm Hg or a mean Doppler gradient greater than 30 mm Hg (in association with less than moderate pulmonic regurgitation). *(Level of Evidence: C)*
3. Surgical therapy is recommended for patients with severe PS and an associated hypoplastic pulmonary annulus, severe pulmonary regurgitation, subvalvular PS, or supravalvular PS. Surgery is also preferred for most dysplastic pulmonic valves and when there is associated severe tricuspid regurgitation or the need for a surgical maze procedure. *(Level of Evidence: C)*
4. Surgeons with training and expertise in congenital heart disease should perform operations for the RVOT and pulmonic valve. *(Level of Evidence: B)*

Class IIb

1. Balloon valvotomy may be reasonable in asymptomatic patients with a dysplastic pulmonic valve and a peak instantaneous gradient by Doppler greater than 60 mm Hg or a mean Doppler gradient greater than 40 mm Hg. *(Level of Evidence: C)*
2. Balloon valvotomy may be reasonable in selected symptomatic patients with a dysplastic pulmonic valve and peak instantaneous gradient by Doppler greater than 50 mm Hg or a mean Doppler gradient greater than 30 mm Hg. *(Level of Evidence: C)*

Class III

1. Balloon valvotomy is not recommended for asymptomatic patients with a peak instantaneous gradient by Doppler less than 50 mm Hg in the presence of normal cardiac output. *(Level of Evidence: C)*
2. Balloon valvotomy is not recommended for symptomatic patients with PS and severe pulmonic regurgitation. *(Level of Evidence: C)*
3. Balloon valvotomy is not recommended for symptomatic patients with a peak instantaneous gradient by Doppler less than 30 mm Hg. *(Level of Evidence: C)*

*Classification of recommendations and level of evidence are expressed in the ACC/AHA format as described in the footnote for Table 24-2.

TABLE 24-6	Indications for Intervention in Right Ventricular Outflow Tract Obstruction (ESC Grown-up Congenital Heart Disease Guidelines)[127]	
		CLASS*
RVOT obstruction at any level should be repaired regardless of symptoms when Doppler peak gradient is >64 mmHg (peak velocity >4.0 m/s) provided that RV function is normal and no valve substitute is required		IC
In valvular PS, balloon valvotomy should be the intervention of choice		IC
In asymptomatic patients in whom balloon valvotomy is ineffective and surgical valve replacement is the only option, surgery should be performed in the presence of a systolic RV pressure >80 mmHg		IC
Intervention in patients with gradient <64 mmHg should be considered in the presence of any of the following: • Symptoms related to PS • Decreased RV function (which is usually progressive) • Important arrhythmias • Right to left shunting via ASD or VSD		IIaC
Peripheral PS regardless of symptoms should be considered for repair if >50% diameter narrowing and RV systolic pressure >50 mmHg and/or lung perfusion abnormalities are present		IIaC

ASD, Atrial septal defect; *PS,* pulmonic stenosis; *RV,* right ventricle; *RVOT,* right ventricular outflow tract; *VSD,* ventricular septal defect.
*Recommendation classes and levels of evidence are as described in Table 24-3.

ESC guidelines for management of congenital heart disease, however, utilize Doppler-derived gradients measured by echocardiography. Some data suggest that the Doppler-derived maximum instantaneous gradient may overestimate peak-to-peak gradient by up to 20 mm Hg and that the mean Doppler gradient may have better correlation with the peak-to-peak gradient measured at the time of catheterization prior to balloon valvotomy.[128] The ACC/AHA guidelines for the management of congenital heart disease recommend balloon valvotomy for asymptomatic patients with maximum instantaneous gradient greater than 60 mm Hg or mean gradient greater than 40 mm Hg, and for symptomatic patients with maximum instantaneous gradient greater than 50 mm Hg and mean gradient greater than 30 mm Hg.[120]

No significant risk of restenosis has been reported after pulmonic balloon valvotomy, although there is risk for subsequent pulmonic regurgitation.[117,129-133] Garty et al[133] from Toronto reported on outcomes in 150 children after pulmonic balloon valvotomy (mean follow-up of 12 ± 3 years, range 3.7 to 19.3); 57% of the children had moderate or severe pulmonic regurgitation at last follow-up. The rate of freedom from reintervention at 15 years was 77%, emphasizing the need for lifelong follow-up in these patients.

Pulmonic balloon valvotomy is most often performed with a circular balloon, which is oversized by about 20% to 40% relative to the pulmonic annulus, although both double-balloon and Inoue balloon approaches have been described.[117,134-136] The mechanism of successful dilation is thought to be separation of congenitally fused commissures, to achieve a decrease in transpulmonic gradient by two thirds of its baseline value (Table 24-7).[117, 129, 132, 137-142] Results are likely to be suboptimal when the valve is dysplastic, the valve cusps are excessively thickened, or the annulus is hypoplastic.[142,143] Excessive dilation or unfavorable valve morphology may lead to tearing or avulsion of the cusps, with consequent severe pulmonic regurgitation, or to rupture of the pulmonary artery. Although balloon valvotomy can be performed in patients with acquired pulmonic stenosis due to carcinoid or rheumatic disease, it is generally not recommended because of the nature of valve involvement, associated pulmonic regurgitation, and concomitant involvement of other valves.[142,144]

Outcomes of balloon valvotomy are excellent, with low mortality (0 to 1% risk of death) and morbidity.[136,142,145] Potential complications include transient hypotension, bradycardia, ventricular tachycardia, right bundle branch block, complete heart block, cardiac arrest, pulmonary artery tear, right ventricular outflow tract perforation, tricuspid valve injury, pulmonic valve tear causing pulmonic regurgitation, cardiac perforation, and endocarditis. Tricuspid insufficiency occurs in 0.2% of patients after balloon valvotomy, as a result of inadvertent disruption of the right ventricular papillary muscle.

A potentially serious complication following balloon valvotomy is acute severe infundibular obstruction due to the subvalvular muscular hypertrophy that is often associated with pulmonic valvular stenosis, as a result of chronic pressure overload of the right ventricle (Figure 24-16). After relief of pulmonic stenosis, infundibular obstruction may transiently worsen, but then the hypertrophy tends to regress over months with eventual resolution.[132,138,141,146] Acute severe obstruction can cause "suicide" right ventricle, resulting in suprasystemic right ventricular pressure with cyanosis and hemodynamic instability. Beta-blocker therapy is recommended before pulmonic balloon valvotomy to prevent or reduce the severity of this complication; therapy is continued for 3 to 6 months after the procedure.

In patients who have a poor result with percutaneous valvotomy or have unfavorable valve morphology, coexisting

TABLE 24-7   Percutaneous Pulmonic Valvotomy in Adults

SERIES	N	MEAN AGE, YEARS (RANGE)	BASELINE PEAK GRADIENT, mm Hg	POST-PROCEDURE PEAK GRADIENT, mm Hg	LONG-TERM OUTCOME
Sievert et al (1989)[141]	24	39 (17-72)	92 ± 36	43 ± 19	Subvalvular hypertrophy decreased over 3-12 months
Fawzy et al (1990)[138]	22	25 (16-45)	111 ± 33	38 ± 26	Infundibular stenosis decreased from 35 ± 26 to 15 ± 9 mm Hg after 1 year
David et al (1993)[137]	38	14 (1-63)	97 ± 43	26 ± 17	Median transpulmonic gradient at 8 months decreased from 84 mm Hg to 27 mm Hg
Lau and Hung (1993)[140]	14	27 (17-47)	102 ± 41	52 ± 19	No restenosis at repeat catheterization in 8 patients (12-30 months post-procedure)
Kaul et al (1993)[139]	40	28 (18-56)	107 ± 29	37 ± 25	No restenosis at follow-up of 25 ± 12 months
Chen et al (1996)[117]	53	26 (13-55)	9 1± 46	38 ± 32	No restenosis at follow-up of 6.9 ± 3.1 years
Teupe et al (1997)[132]	14	31 (19-65)	82 ± 19	37 ± 14	No restenosis at 5- to 9-year follow-up with a residual gradient of 25 ± 12 mm Hg
Fawzy et al (2001)[129]	87	23 (15-54)	105 ± 39	34 ± 26	No restenosis at 14-month follow-up

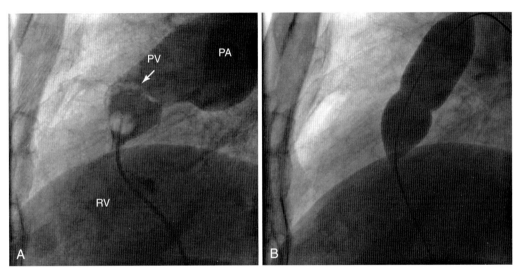

FIGURE 24-16   **Cardiac catheterization images from pulmonic balloon valvotomy. A,** Right ventricular anteroposterior angiogram demonstrates systolic doming *(arrow)* of a stenotic pulmonic valve (PV) due to severe valve stenosis. Dynamic subvalvular obstruction can also be seen below the valve. Post-stenotic dilation of the pulmonary artery (PA) is present. *RV,* Right ventricle. **B,** Pulmonic balloon valvotomy resulted in marked reduction in the transpulmonic gradient.

hypoplastic pulmonic annulus, fixed subvalvar pulmonic stenosis, supravalvular pulmonic stenosis, or associated severe pulmonic regurgitation, surgical valvotomy or valve replacement may be preferred. Operations on the pulmonic valve or right ventricular outflow tract should be performed by experienced congenital heart surgeons.

The decision regarding type of pulmonic valve prosthesis must be individualized, although bioprostheses, which are nonthrombogenic, are preferred. These valves are subject to degradation, but durability of biological pulmonic prostheses is generally favorable compared with that of left-sided valves because of the lower-pressure environment of the right heart, especially in adults.[147] Homograft valve replacements are not thrombogenic, and the length of the graft can be used to reconstruct the annulus and outflow tract, but they have unpredictable durability and may degenerate prematurely, with obstruction, regurgitation, or both, especially in the setting of pulmonary hypertension.[148,149]

Mechanical valves are more durable but thrombogenic and generally are not favored in the low-pressure right side of the heart, unless the patient has other mechanical valves or requires anticoagulation for another reason.[150] Data now suggest that with adequate anticoagulation, the risk of thromboembolic events with mechanical pulmonic prosthetic valves is low. Among 54 patients with mechanical pulmonic valve prostheses in one series, only 1 experienced an embolic event during long-term follow-up, in the setting of subtherapeutic anticoagulation. Previously reported high rates of thrombosis in other series also occurred with subtherapeutic levels or lack of anticoagulation. However, the rate of freedom from bleeding complications was higher with bioprosthetic than mechanical valves, although this difference was not statistically significant (96% vs. 88%, $P = 0.08$).[151]

Another alternative is the valved bovine jugular vein (Contegra, Medtronic, Inc., Minneapolis, Minnesota) conduit for right ventricular outflow tract reconstruction in children.[152,153]

Percutaneous pulmonic valve replacement can be performed in patients with mixed pulmonic valve disease.[154] The Melody transcatheter pulmonic valve (Medtronic, Inc.) is now approved in the United States for treatment of dysfunctional right ventricular outflow tract valve conduits (see Figure 24-14). McElhinney et al,[155] reporting on 124 patients implanted with the Melody transcatheter pulmonic valve, demonstrated a decreased mean right ventricular outflow tract gradient, from 28 mm Hg to 19 mm Hg, immediately after implantation, and a decrease in pulmonic regurgitation. The rate of freedom from valve dysfunction was 93.5% ± 2.4% at 1 year and 85.7% ± 4.7% at 2 years.[155]

SPECIFIC CONSIDERATIONS

PREGNANCY. Severe pulmonic stenosis may be associated with an increased risk. If indicated, percutaneous balloon valvotomy can be performed with low risk during pregnancy.[156] Patients with pulmonic stenosis are at an increased risk of having an infant with congenital heart disease.[157] Pulmonic stenosis occurs primarily in offspring of patients with Noonan syndrome but may also occur in patients with sporadic pulmonic stenosis.

ATHLETES. Physical activity recommendations should follow the guidelines summarized in an article by Task Force 2 on Congenital Heart Disease.[158]

Athletes with pulmonic stenosis with a peak systolic gradient lower than 40 mm Hg and normal right ventricular function can participate in all competitive sports if they have no symptoms. Annual reevaluation is recommended.

Athletes with a peak systolic gradient higher than 40 mm Hg can participate in low-intensity competitive sports. Patients in this category usually are referred for balloon valvotomy or operative valvotomy before sports participation. Following intervention, athletes with no or only mild residual pulmonic stenosis and normal ventricular function without symptoms can participate in all competitive sports within 2 to 4 weeks after balloon valvotomy but after a suggested interval of approximately 3 months after surgery. Athletes with a persistent peak systolic gradient higher than 40 mm Hg can participate in low-intensity competitive sports.

Pulmonic Regurgitation

Etiology

A trivial or mild degree of pulmonic regurgitation is detectable by Doppler echocardiography in most normal individuals.[58] In adults, pathologic pulmonic regurgitation is most often the consequence of prior interventions for congenital heart disease. Severe pulmonic regurgitation is the most common postoperative complication in patients with prior tetralogy of Fallot repair, because of the valvotomy and outflow tract patch placement used for relief of pulmonic stenosis.[159-162] Patients who have undergone surgical or balloon valvotomy for isolated congenital pulmonic valvular stenosis are also at risk for late pulmonic regurgitation, as are those with extracardiac conduits from the right ventricle to the pulmonary arteries, which are prone to degeneration, resulting in either stenosis or regurgitation.[122,163]

Other causes of pulmonic regurgitation include rheumatic or carcinoid heart disease, trauma, endocarditis, pulmonary artery and annular dilation, and pulmonary hypertension.[105] In patients undergoing dialysis, a transient murmur of pulmonic regurgitation is common, most likely reflecting transient pulmonary hypertension associated with intravascular volume overload; the murmur typically diminishes during dialysis with volume removal.[164]

Diagnosis

Physical examination findings may be unimpressive, even in the patient with severe pulmonic regurgitation. Typically the murmur is a soft, diastolic, decrescendo murmur best heard in the left upper sternal region, beginning after the pulmonic closure sound, and it may be accompanied by a systolic ejection murmur. During inspiration, the murmur increases in intensity. The murmur is easily audible in patients with pulmonary hypertension but may be difficult to appreciate when pulmonary pressures are normal, even if pulmonic regurgitation is severe. A right ventricular lift may be palpable when the right ventricle is enlarged.

Electrocardiogram findings are generally nonspecific in pulmonic regurgitation, although in patients with tetralogy of Fallot, QRS widening and the rate of increase in QRS duration reflect the severity of pulmonic regurgitation and consequent right ventricular dilation.[165,166] Chest radiography may demonstrate cardiomegaly, particularly involving the right-sided chambers, and in some cases pulmonary artery dilation.

The diagnosis of pulmonic regurgitation is often initially made on echocardiography. In contrast to the narrow jet of mild regurgitation, severe pulmonic regurgitation is characterized by a wide, diastolic jet in the right ventricular outflow tract on color-flow imaging (Figure 24-17). The duration of the jet increases with the severity of pulmonic regurgitation; however, severe pulmonic regurgitation often terminates in early or mid-diastole owing to rapid equalization of diastolic pulmonary artery and right ventricular pressures, and color imaging may be misleading. A large vena contracta width can distinguish severe pulmonic regurgitation in this setting.[61] Quantification of vena contracta by 3D echocardiography may be an adjunct to further define the severity of pulmonic regurgitation.[167] Planimetered color-flow jet areas correlate well with pulmonic regurgitation severity on angiography; however, there is a high degree of variability and overlap among different grades of regurgitation.[168] Importantly, the characteristics of the color-flow jet are also affected by the right ventricular pressures, so pulmonic regurgitation may appear laminar and brief when pulmonary pressures are normal.

The density of the continuous wave Doppler echocardiography signal is a qualitative method of assessing pulmonic regurgitation severity. Severe pulmonic regurgitation is characterized by equal intensities of antegrade and retrograde "to-and-fro" flows across the pulmonic valve, with the signal rapidly reaching baseline (Figure 24-17D). The deceleration pressure half-time corresponds to the degree of regurgitation; a pressure half-time less than 100 milliseconds is suggestive of severe pulmonic regurgitation, with a sensitivity of 76% and specificity of 94%.[169] As on color-flow imaging, the pulmonic regurgitant signals on continuous wave Doppler echocardiography are subject to right-sided pressures; early and rapid equilibration of diastolic pressures also occurs in patients with low pulmonary artery end-diastolic pressure and/or increased right ventricular diastolic pressure.

The value of cardiac catheterization and CMR are discussed in Chapters 7 and 8.

Natural History

Most patients with mild degrees of pulmonic regurgitation have a benign clinical course and do not go on to have progressive disease. Chronic severe pulmonic regurgitation is often well tolerated for many years, but eventually, chronic volume overload of the right ventricle leads to progressive dilation, systolic dysfunction, and heart failure.[170-172] Patients experience functional limitation owing to inability to augment cardiac output with exercise. In tetralogy of Fallot, progressive right ventricular dilation and dysfunction are associated with increased risk of ventricular arrhythmias and sudden cardiac death.[165,166,173,174] The clinical course of pulmonic regurgitation is related to the underlying etiology, and in the evaluation of patients with severe pulmonic regurgitation in the setting of prior congenital cardiac surgery, the surgical records must be obtained.

Medical and Surgical Treatment

No specific therapy is needed for most adults with pulmonic regurgitation because disease severity is usually mild. With severe regurgitation and evidence of progressive right ventricular enlargement or the onset of right ventricular systolic dysfunction, surgical intervention should be considered. Medical therapy has not been demonstrated to be effective in reducing the degree of pulmonic regurgitation or affecting the impact of severe pulmonic regurgitation on the right ventricle.

The most common indication for intervention for pulmonic regurgitation in adults is seen in patients with previous surgery for tetralogy of Fallot or pulmonic valvular stenosis.[175-178] As the intervention options improve and the morbidity related to long-standing pulmonic regurgitation is increasingly recognized,

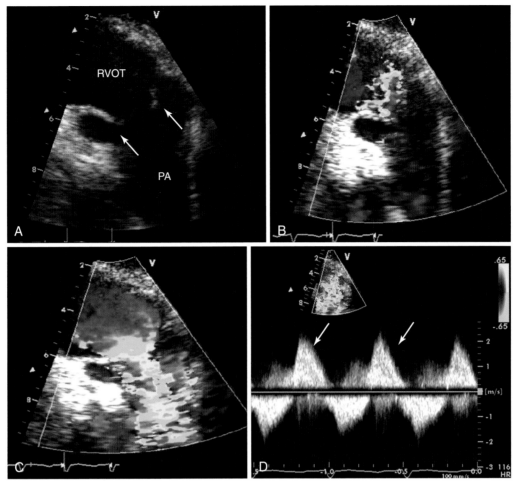

FIGURE 24-17 **Carcinoid involvement of the pulmonic valve. A,** Two-dimensional imaging shows thickened, retracted pulmonic valve cusps *(arrows)* with limited mobility and incomplete coaptation. **B,** Color-flow Doppler imaging during diastole features a broad pulmonic regurgitant jet into the right ventricular outflow tract (RVOT). **C,** Color-flow imaging during systole into the pulmonary artery (PA). **D,** Continuous wave Doppler echocardiography shows an intense diastolic flow signal *(arrows)* that decelerates rapidly to baseline. There is no pulmonic stenosis (antegrade velocity of 1.0 m/s).

indications for intervention are being refined. Data suggest that pulmonic valve replacement for severe pulmonic regurgitation should be strongly considered if there is evidence of any of the following:[165,166,173,174,179-181]

1. Symptoms related to pulmonic regurgitation, including arrhythmias, which indicate a New York Heart Association functional class higher than II.
2. Decreased right ventricular systolic function (ejection fraction <40% as assessed on CMR).
3. Progressive right ventricular dilation (right ventricular end-diastolic volume ≥160 mL/m^2 or end-systolic volume ≥82 mL/m^2 on CMR).
4. Decline in functional aerobic capacity related to pulmonic regurgitation.
5. Moderate or more tricuspid valve regurgitation related to progressive annular dilation.
6. Severe pulmonic regurgitation in a patient with another cardiac lesion that requires operative intervention.
7. Concern about risk of arrhythmia in patients with prolonged or increasing QRS duration (total QRS duration ≥180 msec, or QRS duration increase >3.5 msec per year).

The timing of surgical intervention is important because, according to some studies, right ventricular function may not fully recover after pulmonic valve replacement once right ventricular enlargement and systolic dysfunction are evident (Figure 24-18);[179,180,182,183] other investigations, however, have reported improvement with pulmonic homograft insertion late after surgery

to repair tetralogy of Fallot. Possible reasons for these different results might relate to older mean age at initial repair or older age at time of surgery for pulmonic regurgitation. In a series of patients with repaired tetralogy of Fallot who underwent pulmonic valve replacement, right ventricular volumes decreased by a mean of 28%, but right ventricular ejection fraction did not change significantly. A preoperative right ventricular end-diastolic volume of 160 mL/m^2 or higher or right ventricular end-systolic volume of 82 mL/m^2 or higher have been reported to be associated with low likelihood for recovery of right ventricular function.[181]

The type of pulmonic valve prosthesis should be individualized, and the operation should be performed by a cardiac surgeon experienced in the management of congenital cardiac disease. Percutaneous placement of a transcatheter pulmonic valve prosthesis may be an option in some patients with pulmonic conduits (see earlier discussion of pulmonic stenosis). Annual echocardiography is appropriate for patient monitoring, ideally beginning soon after the initial operation so that residual right ventricular dilation can be distinguished from progressive disease.

Summary

Tricuspid and pulmonic valve diseases have been historically underappreciated, but improved diagnostic testing and increasing awareness have led to substantial advances in both earlier diagnosis and treatment of right-sided valvular heart disease.[184] Development and application of cardiac magnetic resonance

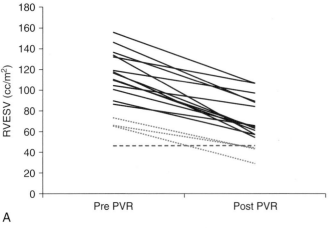

A

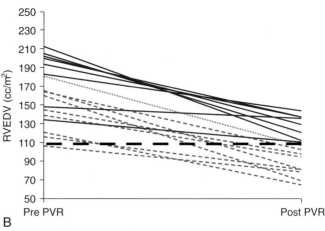

B

FIGURE 24-18 **Impact of pulmonic valve replacement on right ventricular size.** Normalization of RV volumes occurred only in patients with pre-operative right ventricular end-systolic volume (RVESV) <85 ml/m² or right ventricular end-diastolic volume (RVEDV) <70 ml/m². **A,** Normalization of RVESV (<47 ml/m² *black hatched line*) is noted in 3 of 17 patients. *Dotted lines,* patients whose RVESV normalized. *Solid lines,* patients whose RVESV did not normalize. **B,** Normalization of RVEDV (<108 ml/m² black hatched line) in 9 of 17 patients. *Hatched lines,* patients in whom the RVEDV normalized. *Solid lines,* patients whose RVEDV did not normalize. One patient (*dotted line*) with a preoperative RVEDV >170 ml/m² normalized to 108 ml/m² after surgical resection of a RV outflow tract aneurysm. One patient (59-years-old) (*hatched line*) with a preoperative RVEDV of <170 ml/m² did not normalize to 108 ml/m² after the operation. (*Therrien J, et al. Optimal timing for pulmonary valve replacement in adults after tetralogy of Fallot repair. Am J Cardiol 2005;95:779–782.*)

imaging has facilitated more accurate characterization of right ventricular size and function and of the impact of tricuspid and pulmonic valvular heart disease. Newer techniques for valve intervention allow for tricuspid and pulmonic valve repair and replacement with improved outcomes in increasingly complex situations. Appropriate application of these new technologies and vigilance in recognition of the consequences of right-sided valvular heart disease will continue to lead to better patient outcomes.

REFERENCES

1. Bommer W, Weinert L, Neumann A, et al. Determination of right atrial and right ventricular size by two dimensional echocardiography. Circulation 1979;60:91–100.
2. Watanabe T, Katsume H, Matsukubo H, et al. Estimation of right ventricular volume with two dimensional echocardiography. Am J Cardiol 1982;49(8):1946–53.
3. Dell'Italia L, Walsh R. Right ventricular diastolic pressure-volume relations and regional dimensions during acute alterations in loading conditions. Circulation 1988;77(6):1276–82.
4. Feneley M, Gavaghan T. Paradoxical and pseudoparadoxical interventricular septal motion in patients with right ventricular volume overload. Circulation 1986;74(2):230–8.
5. Pearlman A, Clark C, Henry W, et al. Determinants of ventricular septal motion: influence of relative right and left ventricular size. Circulation 1976;54(1):83–91.
6. Louie E, Rich S, Levitsky S, et al. Doppler echocardiographic demonstration of the differential effects of right ventricular pressure and volume overload on left ventricular geometry and filling. J Am Coll Cardiol 1992;19(1):84–90.
7. Dell'Italia L. The right ventricle: anatomy, physiology, and clinical importance. Curr Probl Cardiol 1991;16(10):653–720.
8. Lee F. Hemodynamics of the right ventricle in normal and disease states. Cardiol Clin 1992;10(1):59–67.
9. Spann J, Buccino R, Sonnenblick E, et al. Contractile state of cardiac muscle obtained from cats with experimentally produced ventricular hypertrophy and heart failure. Circ Res 1967;21(3):341–54.
10. Kramer M, Valantine H, Marshall S, et al. Recovery of the right ventricle after single-lung transplantation in pulmonary hypertension. Am J Cardiol 1994;73(7):494–500.
11. Scuderi L, Bailey S, Calhoon J, et al. Echocardiographic assessment of right and left ventricular function after single-lung transplantation. Am Heart J 1994;127(3):636–42.
12. Jardin F, Dubourg O, Gueret P, et al. Quantitative two-dimensional echocardiography in massive pulmonary embolism: emphasis on ventricular interdependence and leftward septal displacement. J Am Coll Cardiol 1987;10(6):1201–6.
13. Lang RM, Bierig M, Devereux RB, et al. Recommendations for chamber quantification: a report from the American Society of Echocardiography's Guidelines and Standards Committee and the Chamber Quantification Writing Group, developed in conjunction with the European Association of Echocardiography, a branch of the European Society of Cardiology. J Am Soc Echocardiogr 2005;18(12):1440–63.
14. Rudski LG, Lai WW, Afilalo J, et al. Guidelines for the echocardiographic assessment of the right heart in adults: a report from the American Society of Echocardiography: Endorsed by the European Association of Echocardiography, a registered branch of the European Society of Cardiology, and the Canadian Society of Echocardiography. J Am Soc EchocardiogrJ 2010;23(7):685–713.
15. Kjaergaard J, Petersen CL, Kjaer A, et al. Evaluation of right ventricular volume and function by 2D and 3D echocardiography compared to MRI. Eur J Echocardiogr 2006;7(6):430–8.
16. van der Zwaan HB, Geleijnse ML, McGhie JS, et al. Right ventricular quantification in clinical practice: two-dimensional vs. three-dimensional echocardiography compared with cardiac magnetic resonance imaging. Eur J Echocardiogr 2011;12(9):656–64.
17. Tei C, Dujardin KS, Hodge DO, et al. Doppler echocardiographic index for assessment of global right ventricular function. J Am Soc Echocardiogr 1996;9(6):838–47.
18. LaCorte JC, Cabreriza SE, Rabkin DG, et al. Correlation of the Tei index with invasive measurements of ventricular function in a porcine model. J Am Soc Echocardiogr 2003;16(5):442–7.
19. Meluzin J, Spinarova L, Bakala J, et al. Pulsed Doppler tissue imaging of the velocity of tricuspid annular systolic motion; a new, rapid, and non-invasive method of evaluating right ventricular systolic function. Eur Heart J 2001;22(4):340–8.
20. Miller D, Farah MG, Liner A, et al. The relation between quantitative right ventricular ejection fraction and indices of tricuspid annular motion and myocardial performance. J Am Soc Echocardiogr 2004;17(5):443–7.
21. Sachdev A, Villarraga HR, Frantz RP, et al. Right Ventricular Strain for Prediction of Survival in Patients With Pulmonary Arterial Hypertension. Chest 2011;139(6):1299–309.
22. Cohen S, Sell J, McIntosh C, et al. Tricuspid regurgitation in patients with acquired, chronic, pure mitral regurgitation. II: nonoperative management, tricuspid valve annuloplasty, and tricuspid valve replacement. J Thorac Cardiovasc Surg 1987;94(4):488–97.
23. Waller BF, Moriarty AT, Eble JN, et al. Etiology of pure tricuspid regurgitation based on anular circumference and leaflet area: analysis of 45 necropsy patients with clinical and morphologic evidence of pure tricuspid regurgitation. J Am Coll Cardiol 1986;7(5):1063–74.
24. Bonow RO, Carabello BA, Chatterjee K, et al. 2008 focused update incorporated into the ACC/AHA 2006 guidelines for the management of patients with valvular heart disease: a report of the American College of Cardiology/American Heart Association Task Force on Practice Guidelines (Writing Committee to Revise the 1998 Guidelines for the Management of Patients With Valvular Heart Disease) Endorsed by the Society of Cardiovascular Anesthesiologists, Society for Cardiovascular Angiography and Interventions, and Society of Thoracic Surgeons. J Am Coll Cardiol 2008;52(13):e1–e142.
25. Muller O, Shillingford J. Tricuspid incompetence. Br Heart J 1954;16:195.
26. Salazar E, Levine H. Rheumatic tricuspid regurgitation. Am J Med 1962;33:111.
27. Sepulveda G, Lukas D. The diagnosis of tricuspid insufficiency – clinical features in 60 cases with associated mitral valve disease. Circulation 1955;11:552.
28. Lin G, Nishimura RA, Connolly HM, et al. Severe symptomatic tricuspid valve regurgitation due to permanent pacemaker or implantable cardioverter-defibrillator leads. J Am Coll Cardiol 2005;45(10):1672–5.
29. Piekarz J, Lelakowski J, Rydlewska A, et al. Heart perforation in patients with permanent cardiac pacing—pilot personal observations. Arch Med Sci 2012;8(1):70–4.
30. Messika-Zeitoun D, Thomson H, Bellamy M, et al. Medical and surgical outcome of tricuspid regurgitation caused by flail leaflets. J Thorac Cardiovasc Surg 2004;128:296–302.
31. Sloan KP, Bruce CJ, Oh JK, et al. Complications of echocardiography-guided endomyocardial biopsy. J Am Soc Echocardiogr 2009;22(3):324.
32. Marvin R, Schrank J, Nolan S. Traumatic tricuspid insufficiency. Am J Cardiol 1973;32(5):723–6.

33. van Son JA, Danielson GK, Schaff HV, et al. Traumatic tricuspid valve insufficiency. Experience in thirteen patients. J Thorac Cardiovasc Surg 1994;108(5):893–8.
34. Chan P, Ogilby JD, Segal B. Tricuspid valve endocarditis. Am Heart J 1989;117(5): 1140–6.
35. Sohail MR, Uslan DZ, Khan AH, et al. Management and outcome of permanent pacemaker and implantable cardioverter-defibrillator infections. J Am Coll Cardiol 2007; 49(18):1851–9.
36. Sohail MR, Uslan DZ, Khan AH, et al. Infective endocarditis complicating permanent pacemaker and implantable cardioverter-defibrillator infection. Mayo Clinic Proceedings 2008;83(1):46–53.
37. Greenspon AJ, Prutkin JM, Sohail MR, et al. Timing of the most recent device procedure influences the clinical outcome of lead-associated endocarditis: Results of the MEDIC (Multicenter Electrophysiologic Device Infection Cohort). J Am Coll Cardiol 2012;59(7): 681–7.
38. FitzGerald SF, O'Gorman J, Morris-Downes MM, et al. A 12-year review of *Staphylococcus aureus* bloodstream infections in haemodialysis patients: more work to be done. J Hospital Infection 2011;79(3):218–21.
39. Le KY, Sohail MR, Friedman PA, et al. Impact of timing of device removal on mortality in patients with cardiovascular implantable electronic device infections. Heart Rhythm 2011;8(11):1678–85.
40. Waller BF, Knapp WS, Edwards JE. Marantic valvular vegetations. Circulation 1973;48(3):644–50.
41. Duran C. Tricuspid valve surgery revisited. J Card Surg 1994;9(2 Suppl):242–7.
42. Rothman RB, Baumann MH, Savage JE, et al. Evidence for possible involvement of 5-HT(2B) receptors in the cardiac valvulopathy associated with fenfluramine and other serotonergic medications. Circulation 2000;102(23):2836–41.
43. Redfield MM, Nicholson WJ, Edwards WD, et al. Valve disease associated with ergot alkaloid use: echocardiographic and pathologic correlations. Ann Intern Med 1992; 117(1):50–2.
44. Connolly HM, Crary JL, McGoon MD, et al. Valvular heart disease associated with fenfluramine-phentermine. N Engl J Med 1997;337(9):581–8.
45. Pritchett AM, Morrison JF, Edwards WD, et al. Valvular heart disease in patients taking pergolide. Mayo Clin Proc 2002;77(12):1280–6.
46. Schade R, Andersohn F, Suissa S, et al. Dopamine agonists and the risk of cardiac-valve regurgitation. N Engl J Med 2007;356(1):29–38.
47. Zanettini R, Antonini A, Gatto G, et al. Valvular heart disease and the use of dopamine agonists for Parkinson's disease. N Engl J Med 2007;356(1):39–46.
48. Moller JE, Pellikka PA, Bernheim AM, et al. Prognosis of carcinoid heart disease: analysis of 200 cases over two decades. Circulation 2005;112(21):3320–7.
49. Connolly HM, Schaff HV, Mullany CJ, et al. Surgical management of left-sided carcinoid heart disease. Circulation 2001;104(12 Suppl 1):I36–40.
50. Chaowalit N, Connolly HM, Schaff HV, et al. Carcinoid heart disease associated with primary ovarian carcinoid tumor. Am J Cardiol 2004;93(10):1314–5.
51. Adams MJ, Hardenbergh PH, Constine LS, et al. Radiation-associated cardiovascular disease. Crit Rev Oncol Hematol 2003;45(1):55–75.
52. Crestanello JA, McGregor CG, Danielson GK, et al. Mitral and tricuspid valve repair in patients with previous mediastinal radiation therapy. Ann Thorac Surg 2004;78(3):826–31; discussion 826-31.
53. Chandraratna P, Lopez J, Fernandez J, et al. Echocardiographic detection of tricuspid valve prolapse Circulation 1975;51(5):823–6.
54. Weinreich D, Burke J, Bharati S, et al. Isolated prolapse of the tricuspid valve. J Am Coll Cardiol 1985;6(2):475–81.
55. Attenhofer Jost CH, Connolly HM, Dearani JA, et al. Ebstein's anomaly. Circulation 2007;115(2):277–85.
56. Celermajer D, Bull C, Till J, et al. Ebstein's anomaly: presentation and outcome from fetus to adult. J Am Coll Cardiol 1994;23(1):170–6.
57. Hansing C, Rowe G. Tricuspid insufficiency. A study of hemodynamics and pathogenesis. Circulation 1972;45(4):793–9.
58. Klein A, Burstow D, Tajik A, et al. Age-related prevalence of valvular regurgitation in normal subjects: a comprehensive color flow examination of 118 volunteers. J Am Soc Echocardiogr 1990;3(1):54–63.
59. Pennestri F, Loperfido F, Salvatori MP, et al. Assessment of tricuspid regurgitation by pulsed Doppler ultrasonography of the hepatic veins. Am J Cardiol 1984;54(3):363–8.
60. Sakai K, Nakamura K, Satomi G, et al. Evaluation of tricuspid regurgitation by blood flow pattern in the hepatic vein using pulsed Doppler technique. Am Heart J 1984;108 (3 Pt 1):516–23.
61. Zoghbi WA, Enriquez-Sarano M, Foster E, et al. Recommendations for evaluation of the severity of native valvular regurgitation with two-dimensional and Doppler echocardiography. J Am Soc Echocardiogr 2003;16(7):777–802.
62. Vahanian A, Alfieri O, Andreotti F, et al. Guidelines on the management of valvular heart disease (version 2012): the Joint Task Force on the Management of Valvular Heart Disease of the European Society of Cardiology (ESC) and the European Association for Cardio-Thoracic Surgery (EACTS). Eur Heart J 2012;33(19):2451–96.
63. Baumgartner FJ, Milliken JC, Robertson JM, et al. Clinical patterns of surgical endocarditis. J Card Surg 2007;22(1):32–8.
64. Topilsky Y, Tribouilloy C, Michelena HI, et al. Pathophysiology of tricuspid regurgitation— clinical perspective. Circulation 2010;122(15):1505–13.
65. Nath J, Foster E, Heidenreich PA. Impact of tricuspid regurgitation on long-term survival. J Am Coll Cardiol 2004;43(3):405–9.
66. Sagie A, Schwammenthal E, Newell J, et al. Significant tricuspid regurgitation is a marker for adverse outcome in patients undergoing percutaneous balloon mitral valvuloplasty. J Am Coll Cardiol 1994;24:696–702.
67. Groves P, Lewis N, Ikram S, et al. Reduced exercise capacity in patients with tricuspid regurgitation after successful mitral valve replacement for rheumatic mitral valve disease. Br Heart J 1991;66:295–301.
68. Garatti A, Nano G, Bruschi G, et al. Twenty-five year outcomes of tricuspid valve replacement comparing mechanical and biologic prostheses. Ann Thorac Surg 2012;93(4):1146–53.
69. Filsoufi F, Anyanwu AC, Salzberg SP, et al. Long-term outcomes of tricuspid valve replacement in the current era. Ann Thorac Surg 2005;80(3):845–50.
70. Chang B-C, Lim S-H, Yi G, et al. Long-Term Clinical results of tricuspid valve replacement. Ann Thorac Surg 2006;81(4):1317–24.
71. Topilsky Y, Khanna AD, Oh JK, et al. Preoperative factors associated with adverse outcome after tricuspid valve replacement—clinical perspective. Circulation 2011; 123(18):1929–39.
72. De Simone R, Lange R, Tanzeem A, et al. Adjustable tricuspid valve annuloplasty assisted by intraoperative transesophageal color Doppler echocardiography. Am J Cardiol 1993;71(11):926–31.
73. Pellegrini A, Colombo T, Donatelli F, et al. Evaluation and treatment of secondary tricuspid insufficiency. Eur J Cardiothorac Surg 1992;6(6):288–96.
74. Yada I, Tani K, Shimono T, et al. Preoperative evaluation and surgical treatment for tricuspid regurgitation associated with acquired valvular heart disease. The Kay-Boyd method vs the Carpentier-Edwards ring method. J Cardiovasc Surg (Torino) 1990;31(6): 771–7.
75. Singh SK, Tang GH, Maganti MD, et al. Midterm outcomes of tricuspid valve repair versus replacement for organic tricuspid disease. Ann Thorac Surg 2006;82(5):1735–41; discussion 1741.
76. Thapa R, Dawn B, Nath J. Tricuspid regurgitation: pathophysiology and management. Current Cardiol Rep 2012;14:190–9.
77. Rogers JH, Bolling SF. The Tricuspid Valve. Circulation 2009;119(20):2718–25.
78. Panos A, Myers P, Kalangos A. Thorascopic and robotic tricuspid valve annuloplasty with a biodegradeable ring: an initial experience. J Heart Valve Dis 2010;19(2): 201–5.
79. Tang GH, David TE, Singh SK, et al. Tricuspid valve repair with an annuloplasty ring results in improved long-term outcomes. Circulation 2006;114(Suppl):I577–I581.
80. Fukuda S, Song JM, Gillinov AM, et al. Tricuspid valve tethering predicts residual tricuspid regurgitation after tricuspid annuloplasty. Circulation 2005;111(8):975–9.
81. Fukuda S, Gillinov AM, McCarthy PM, et al. Determinants of recurrent or residual functional tricuspid regurgitation after tricuspid annuloplasty. Circulation 2006;114(1 suppl):I-582–I-587.
82. Ohata T, Kigawa I, Tohda E, et al. Comparison of durability of bioprostheses in tricuspid and mitral positions. Ann Thorac Surg 2001;71(Suppl):S240–3.
83. Ratnatunga C, Edwards M, Dore C, et al. Tricuspid valve replacement: UK Heart Valve Registry mid-term results comparing mechanical and biological prostheses. Ann Thorac Surg 1998;1998:1940–7.
84. Rizzoli G, Vendramin I, Nesseris G, et al. Biological or mechanical prostheses in tricuspid position? A meta-analysis of intra-institutional results. Ann Thorac Surg 2004;77(5): 1607–14.
85. Boudjemline Y, Agnoletti G, Bonnet D, et al. Steps toward the percutaneous replacement of atrioventricular valves: an experimental study. J Am Coll Cardiol 2005;46(2): 360–5.
86. Roberts PA, Boudjemline Y, Cheatham JP, et al. Percutaneous tricuspid valve replacement in congenital and acquired heart disease. J Am Coll Cardiol 2011;58(2):117–22.
87. Casselman FP, La Meir M, Jeanmart H, et al. Endoscopic mitral and tricuspid valve surgery after previous cardiac surgery. Circulation 2007;116(Suppl):I270–5.
88. Staab ME, Nishimura RA, Dearani JA. Isolated tricuspid valve surgery for severe tricuspid regurgitation following prior left heart valve surgery: analysis of outcome in 34 patients. J Heart Valve Dis 1999;8(5):567–74.
89. Hannoush H, Fawzy ME, Stefadouros M, et al. Regression of significant tricuspid regurgitation after mitral balloon valvotomy for severe mitral stenosis. Am Heart J 2004;148(5):865–70.
90. Song JM, Kang DH, Song JK, et al. Outcome of significant functional tricuspid regurgitation after percutaneous mitral valvuloplasty. Am Heart J 2003;145(2):371–6.
91. Song H, Kang DH, Kim JH, et al. Percutaneous mitral valvuloplasty versus surgical treatment in mitral stenosis with severe tricuspid regurgitation. Circulation 2007; 116(Suppl):I246–50.
92. Yilmaz O, Suri RM, Dearani JA, et al. Functional tricuspid regurgitation at the time of mitral valve repair for degenerative leaflet prolapse: the case for a selective approach. J Thorac Cardiovasc Surg 2011;142(3):608–13.
93. Brown ML, Dearani JA, Danielson GK, et al. The outcomes of operations for 539 patients with Ebstein anomaly. J Thorac Cardiovasc Surg 2008;135(5):1120–36.
94. Bhattacharyya S, Raja SG, Toumpanakis C, et al. Outcomes, risks and complications of cardiac surgery for carcinoid heart disease. Eur J Cardio-Thorac Surg 2011;40(1): 168–72.
95. Mokhles P, van Herwerden LA, de Jong PL, et al. Carcinoid heart disease: outcomes after surgical valve replacement. Eur J Cardio-Thorac Surg J 2012;41:1278–1283.
96. Sadeghi HM, Kimura BJ, Raisinghani A, et al. Does lowering pulmonary arterial pressure eliminate severe functional tricuspid regurgitation? Insights from pulmonary thromboendarterectomy. J Am Coll Cardiol 2004;44(1):126–32.
97. Eleid MF, Blauwet LA, Cha Y-M, et al. Bioprosthetic tricuspid valve regurgitation associated with pacemaker or defibrillator lead implantation. J Am Coll Cardiol 2012;59(9): 813–18.
98. Topilsky Y, Oh JK, Shah DK, et al. Echocardiographic predictors of adverse outcomes after continuous left ventricular assist device implantation. JACC: Cardiovasc Imaging 2011;4(3):211–22.
99. Maltais S, Topilsky Y, Tchantchaleishvili V, et al. Surgical treatment of tricuspid valve insufficiency promotes early reverse remodeling in patients with axial-flow left ventricular assist devices. J Thorac Cardiovasc Surg 2012;143:1370–6.
100. Potapov EV, Scweiger M, Stepanenko A, et al. Tricuspid valve repair in patients supported with left ventricular assist devices. ASAIO 2011;57(5):363–7.
101. Stulak JM, Dearani JA, Puga FJ, et al. Right-sided maze procedure for atrial tachyarrhythmias in congenital heart disease. Ann Thorac Surg 2006;81(5):1780–4; discussion 1784-5.
102. Bousvaros G, Stubington D. Some auscultatory and phonocardiographic features of tricuspid stenosis Circulation 1964;29:26.
103. Kitchin A, Turner R. Diagnosis and treatment of tricuspid stenosis. Br Heart J 1964;16:354.

104. Pellikka PA, Tajik AJ, Khandheria BK, et al. Carcinoid heart disease: clinical and echocardiographic spectrum in 74 patients. Circulation 1993;87(4):1188–96.
105. Waller B, Howard J, Fess S. Pathology of tricuspid valve stenosis and pure tricuspid regurgitation—Part III. Clin Cardiol 1995;18(4):225–30.
106. Gibson R, Wood P. The diagnosis of tricuspid stenosis. Br Heart J 1955;17:552.
107. Killip T, Lukas D. Tricuspid stenosis—clinical features in twelve cases. Am J Med 1958;24:836.
108. el-Sherif N. Rheumatic tricuspid stenosis: a haemodynamic correlation. Br Heart J 1971;33(1):16–31.
109. Guyer D, Gillam L, Foale R, et al. Comparison of the echocardiographic and hemodynamic diagnosis of rheumatic tricuspid stenosis. J Am Coll Cardiol 1984;3(5):1135–44.
110. Perez J, Ludbrook PJ, Ahumada G. Usefulness of Doppler echocardiography in detecting tricuspid valve stenosis. Am J Cardiol 1985;55(5):601–3.
111. Shimada R, Takeshita A, Nakamura M, et al. Diagnosis of tricuspid stenosis by M-mode and two-dimensional echocardiography. Am J Cardiol 1984;53(1):164–8.
112. Baumgartner H, Hung J, Bermejo J, et al. Echocardiographic assessment of valve stenosis: EAE/ASE recommendations for clinical practice. J Am Soc Echocardiogr 2009;22(1):1–23.
113. Roguin A, Rinkevich D, Milo S, et al. Long-term follow-up of patients with severe rheumatic tricuspid stenosis. Am Heart J 1998;136(1):103–8.
114. Onate A, Alcibar J, Inguanzo R, et al. Balloon dilation of tricuspid and pulmonary valves in carcinoid heart disease. Tex Heart Inst J 1993;20(2):115–9.
115. Orbe LC, Sobrino N, Arcas R, et al. Initial outcome of percutaneous balloon valvuloplasty in rheumatic tricuspid valve stenosis. Am J Cardiol 1993;71(4):353–4.
116. Lopez Candales A, Kleiger R, Aleman Gomez J, et al. Pulmonary artery aneurysm: review and case report. Clin Cardiol 1995;18(12):738–40.
117. Chen C, Cheng T, Huang T, et al. Percutaneous balloon valvuloplasty for pulmonic stenosis in adolescents and adults. N Engl J Med 1996;335(1):21–5.
118. Sznajer Y, Keren B, Baumann C, et al. The spectrum of cardiac anomalies in Noonan syndrome as a result of mutations in the PTPN11 gene. Pediatrics 2007;119(6): e1325–31.
119. Raaijmakers R, Noordam C, Noonan J, et al. Are ECG abnormalities in Noonan syndrome characteristic for the syndrome? Eur J Pediatrics 2008;167(12):1363–7.
120. Warnes CA, Williams RG, Bashore TM, et al. ACC/AHA 2008 guidelines for the management of adults with congenital heart disease: a report of the American College of Cardiology/American Heart Association Task Force on Practice Guidelines (Writing Committee to Develop Guidelines on the Management of Adults With Congenital Heart Disease) Developed in collaboration with the American Society of Echocardiography, Heart Rhythm Society, International Society for Adult Congenital Heart Disease, Society for Cardiovascular Angiography and Interventions, and Society of Thoracic Surgeons. J Am Coll Cardiol 2008;52(23):e143–263.
121. Krabill K, Wang Y, Einzig S, et al. Rest and exercise hemodynamics in pulmonary stenosis: comparison of children and adults. Am J Cardiol 1985;56(4):360–5.
122. Hayes C, Gersony W, Driscoll D, et al. Second natural history study of congenital heart defects: results of treatment of patients with pulmonary valvar stenosis. Circulation 1993;87(Suppl):I28–I37.
123. Johnson L, Grossman W, Dalen J, et al. Pulmonic stenosis in the adult. Long-term follow-up results. N Engl J Med 1972;287(23):1159–63.
124. Nugent E, Freedom R, Nora J, et al. Clinical course in pulmonary stenosis. Circulation 1977;56(Suppl):I138–I147.
125. Nadas A. Report from the Joint Study on the Natural History of Congenital Heart Defects. IV: clinical course: introduction. Circulation 1977;56(2 Suppl):I136–I138.
126. Roos-Hesselink J, Meijboom F, Spitaels SV, et al. Long-term outcome after surgery for pulmonary stenosis (a longitudinal study of 22-33 years). Eur Heart J 2006;27(4): 482–8.
127. Baumgartner H, Bonhoeffer P, De Groot NMS, et al. ESC guidelines for the management of grown-up congenital heart disease (new version 2010). European Heart Journal 2010;31(23):2915–57.
128. Silvilairat S, Cabalka AK, Cetta F, et al. Outpatient echocardiographic assessment of complex pulmonary outflow stenosis: Doppler mean gradient is superior to the maximum instantaneous gradient. J Am Soc Echocardiogr 2005;18(11):1143–8.
129. Fawzy M, Awad M, Galal O, et al. Long-term results of pulmonary balloon valvulotomy in adult patients. J Heart Valve Dis 2001;10(6):812–18.
130. Masura J, Burch M, Deanfield J, et al. Five-year follow-up after balloon pulmonary valvuloplasty. J Am Coll Cardiol 1993;21(1):132–6.
131. McCrindle B, Kan J. Long-term results after balloon pulmonary valvuloplasty. Circulation 1991;83(6):1915–22.
132. Teupe C, Burger W, Schrader R, et al. Late (five to nine years) follow-up after balloon dilation of valvular pulmonary stenosis in adults. Am J Cardiol 1997;80(2):240–2.
133. Garty Y, Veldtman G, Lee K, et al. Late outcomes after pulmonary valve balloon dilatation in neonates, infants and children. J Invasive Cardiol 2005;17(6):18–22.
134. Herrmann H, Hill J, Krol J, et al. Effectiveness of percutaneous balloon valvuloplasty in adults with pulmonic valve stenosis [see comments]. Am J Cardiol 1991;68(10):1111–3.
135. Lau K, Hung J, Wu J, et al. Pulmonary valvuloplasty in adults using the Inoue balloon catheter. Cathet Cardiovasc Diagn 1994;29:99.
136. Ports T, Grossman W. Balloon Valvuloplasty. In: Baim D, Grossman W, editors. Cardiac catheterization, angiography, and intervention. Baltimore: Williams and Wilkins; 2000. p. 667–84.
137. David S, Goussous Y, Harbi N, et al. Management of typical and dysplastic pulmonic stenosis, uncomplicated or associated with complex intracardiac defects, in juveniles and adults: use of percutaneous balloon pulmonary valvuloplasty with eight-month hemodynamic follow-up. Cathet Cardiovasc Diagn 1993;29(2):105–12.
138. Fawzy M, Galal O, Dunn B, et al. Regression of infundibular pulmonary stenosis after successful balloon pulmonary valvuloplasty in adults. Cathet Cardiovasc Diagn 1990;21(2):77–81.
139. Kaul U, Singh B, Tyagi S, et al. Long-term results after balloon pulmonary valvuloplasty in adults. Am Heart J 1993;126(5):1152–5.
140. Lau K, Hung J. Controversies in percutaneous balloon pulmonary valvuloplasty: timing, patient selection and technique. J Heart Valve Dis 1993;2(3):321–5.
141. Sievert H, Kober G, Bussman W, et al. Long-term results of percutaneous pulmonary valvuloplasty in adults. Eur Heart J 1989;10(8):712–17.
142. Stanger P, Cassidy S, Girod D, et al. Balloon pulmonary valvuloplasty: results of the Valvuloplasty and Angioplasty of Congenital Anomalies Registry. Am J Cardiol 1990;65(11):775–83.
143. McCrindle B. Independent predictors of immediate results of percutaneous balloon aortic valvotomy in children: Valvuloplasty and Angioplasty of Congenital Anomalies (VACA) Registry Investigators. Am J Cardiol 1996;77(4):286–93.
144. McCrindle B. Independent predictors of long-term results after balloon pulmonary valvuloplasty: Valvuloplasty and Angioplasty of Congenital Anomalies (VACA) Registry Investigators. Circulation 1994;89(4):1751–9.
145. Pepine C, Gessner I, Feldman R. Percutaneous balloon valvuloplasty for pulmonic valve stenosis in the adult. Am J Cardiol 1982;50(6):1442–5.
146. Ben-Shachar G, Cohen M, Sivakoff M, et al. Development of infundibular obstruction after percutaneous pulmonary balloon valvuloplasty. J Am Coll Cardiol 1985;5:754–6.
147. Fukada J, Morishita K, Komatsu K, et al. Influence of pulmonic position on durability of bioprosthetic heart valves Ann Thorac Surg 1997;64(6):1678–80.
148. Brown J, Ruzmetov M, Rodefeld M, et al. Right ventricular outflow tract reconstruction with an allograft conduit in non-ross patients: risk factors for allograft dysfunction and failure. Ann Thorac Surg 2005;80(2):655–63.
149. Dearani J, Danielson G, Puga F, et al. Late follow-up of 1095 patients undergoing operation for complex congenital heart disease utilizing pulmonary ventricle to pulmonary artery conduits. Ann Thorac Surg 2003;75(2):399–410.
150. Waterbolk T, Hoendermis E, den Hamer I, et al. Pulmonary valve replacement with a mechanical prosthesis. Promising results of 28 procedures in patients with congenital heart disease. Eur J Cardiothorac Surg 2006;30(1):28–32.
151. Stulak JM, Dearani JA, Burkhart HM, et al. The increasing use of mechanical pulmonary valve replacement over a 40-year period. Ann Thorac Surg 2010;90(6):2009–15.
152. Brown J, Ruzmetov M, Rodefeld M, et al. Valved bovine jugular vein conduits for right ventricular outflow tract reconstruction in children: an attractive alternative to pulmonary homograft. Ann Thorac Surg 2006;82(3):909–16.
153. Corno A, Qanadli S, Sekarski N, et al. Bovine valved xenograft in pulmonary position: medium-term follow-up with excellent hemodynamics and freedom from calcification. Ann Thorac Surg 2004;78(4):1382–8.
154. Coats L, Khambadkone S, Derrick G, et al. Physiological and clinical consequences of relief of right ventricular outflow tract obstruction late after repair of congenital heart defects. Circulation 2006;113(17):2037–44.
155. McElhinney DB, Hellenbrand WE, Zahn EM, et al. Short- and medium-term outcomes after transcatheter pulmonary valve placement in the expanded multicenter US Melody Valve trial. Circulation 2010;122(5):507–16.
156. Presbitero P, Prever S, Brusca A. Interventional cardiology in pregnancy. Eur Heart J 1996;17(2):182–8.
157. Drenthen W, Pieper P, Roos-Hesselink J, et al. ZAHARA Investigators. Outcome of pregnancy in women with congenital heart disease: a literature review. J Am Coll Cardiol 2007;49(24):2303–11.
158. Graham Jr T, Driscoll D, Gersony W, et al. Task Force 2: congenital heart disease. J Am Coll Cardiol 2005;45:1326–33.
159. Friedli B, Bolens M, Taktak M. Conduction disturbances after correction of tetralogy of Fallot: are electrophysiologic studies of prognostic value? J Am Coll Cardiol 1988; 11(1):162–5.
160. Murphy J, Gersh B, Mair D, et al. Long-term outcome in patients undergoing surgical repair of tetralogy of Fallot. N Engl J Med 1993;329:593–9.
161. Rosenthal A, Behrendt D, Sloan H, et al. Long-term prognosis (15 to 26 years) after repair of tetralogy of Fallot: I: survival and symptomatic status. Ann Thorac Surg 1984;38(2):151–6.
162. Oechslin E, Harrison D, Harris L, et al. Reoperation in adults with repair of tetralogy of Fallot: indications and outcomes. J Thorac Cardiovasc Surg 1999;118(2):245–51.
163. Earing M, Connolly H, Dearani J, et al. Long-term follow-up of patients after surgical treatment for isolated pulmonary valve stenosis. Mayo Clin Proc 2005;80(7): 871–6.
164. P'eres J, Smith C, Meltzer V. Pulmonic valve insufficiency: a common cause of transient diastolic murmurs in renal failure. Ann Intern Med 1985;103(4):497–502.
165. Gatzoulis M, Balaji S, Webber S, et al. Risk factors for arrhythmia and sudden cardiac death late after repair of tetralogy of Fallot: a multicentre study. Lancet 2000;356: 975–81.
166. Gatzoulis M, Till J, Somerville J, et al. Mechanoelectrical interaction in tetralogy of Fallot: QRS prolongation relates to right ventricular size and predicts malignant ventricular arrhythmias and sudden death. Circulation 1995;92(2):231–7.
167. Pothineni KR, Wells BJ, Hsiung MC, et al. Live/real time three-dimensional transthoracic echocardiographic assessment of pulmonary regurgitation. Echocardiography 2008; 25(8):911–7.
168. Kobayashi J, Nakano S, Matsuda H, et al. Quantitative evaluation of pulmonary regurgitation after repair of tetralogy of Fallot using real-time flow imaging system. Jpn Circ J 1989;53(7):721–7.
169. Silversides C, Veldtman G, Crossin J, et al. Pressure half-time predicts hemodynamically significant pulmonary regurgitation in adult patients with repaired tetralogy of Fallot. J Am Soc Echocardiogr 2003;16:1057–62.
170. Ebert P. Second operations for pulmonary stenosis or insufficiency after repair of tetralogy of Fallot. Am J Cardiol 1982;50(3):637–40.
171. Shimazaki Y, Blackstone E, Kirklin J. The natural history of isolated congenital pulmonary valve incompetence: surgical implications. Thorac Cardiovasc Surg 1984;32(4): 257–9.
172. Zahka K, Horneffer P, Rowe S, et al. Long-term valvular function after total repair of tetralogy of Fallot: relation to ventricular arrhythmias Circulation 1988;78(5 Pt 2): III14–III19.

173. Harrison D, Harris L, Siu S, et al. Sustained ventricular tachycardia in adult patients late after repair of tetralogy of Fallot. J Am Coll Cardiol 1997; 30:1368–73.
174. Therrien J, Siu S, Harris L, et al. Impact of pulmonary valve replacement on arrhythmia propensity late after repair of tetralogy of Fallot. Circulation 2001;103(20): 2489–94.
175. Bove E, Kavey R, Byrum C, et al. Improved right ventricular function following late pulmonary valve replacement for residual pulmonary insufficiency or stenosis. J Thorac Cardiovasc Surg 1985;90(1):50–5.
176. d'Udekem Y, Rubay J, Shango-Lody P, et al. Late homograft valve insertion after transannular patch repair of tetralogy of Fallot. J Heart Valve Dis 1998;7(4):450–4.
177. Waien S, Liu P, Ross B, et al. Serial follow-up of adults with repaired tetralogy of Fallot. J Am Coll Cardiol 1992;20(2):295–300.
178. Warner K, Anderson J, Fulton D, et al. Restoration of the pulmonary valve reduces right ventricular volume overload after previous repair of tetralogy of Fallot. Circulation 1993;88(5 Pt 2):II189–II197.
179. Buechel E, Dave H, Kellenberger C, et al. Remodelling of the right ventricle after early pulmonary valve replacement in children with repaired tetralogy of Fallot: assessment by cardiovascular magnetic resonance. Eur Heart J 2005;26:2721–7.
180. Therrien J, Provost Y, Merchant N, et al. Optimal timing for pulmonary valve replacement in adults after tetralogy of Fallot repair. Am J Cardiol 2005;95:779–82.
181. Oosterhof T, van Straten A, Vliegen H, et al. Preoperative thresholds for pulmonary valve replacement in patients with corrected tetralogy of Fallot using cardiovascular magnetic resonance. Circulation 2007;116(5):545–51.
182. Therrien J, Siu S, McLaughlin P, et al. Pulmonary valve replacement in adults late after repair of tetralogy of Fallot: are we operating too late? J Am Coll Cardiol 2000;36(5): 1670–5.
183. Hazekamp M, Kurvers M, Schoof P, et al. Pulmonary valve insertion late after repair of Fallot's tetralogy. Eur J Cardiothorac Surg 2001;19(5):667–70.
184. Bruce CJ, Connolly HM. Right-sided valve disease deserves a little more respect. Circulation 2009;119(20):2726–34.

CH
24

DISEASES OF THE TRICUSPID AND PULMONIC VALVES

Thomas M. Bashore

Key Points

- Infective endocarditis (IE) remains a rare but deadly disease, causing death in one of every four patients affected despite advances in antimicrobial and surgical therapy.
- In the past, IE was a disease that most commonly involved Streptococcus viridans species in younger patients who had rheumatic valvular disease. Now endocarditis is caused mainly by staphylococcal infections, and most patients are elderly, are injection drug users, or have an implanted medical device (prosthetic valve, pacemaker, or defibrillator). Only three fourths of patients with IE have known underlying heart disease.
- Endocarditis begins with platelet and fibrin deposition in an area of endothelial damage, with formation of a nonbacterial thrombotic lesion. Transient bacteremias can result in bacterial adherence to this lesion, particularly with organisms such as staphylococcal species that have adhesion molecules on their surfaces. Bacterial growth leads to recruitment of inflammatory cells, and valvular damage ensues. Certain host factors play a role as well.
- Many of the classic features of IE are less often manifest because of earlier diagnosis today. The modified Duke criteria are important in establishing the diagnosis. The criteria rely on the determination of a likely organism and on imaging evidence for valvular vegetations or leaflet destruction. Epiphenomena, such as fever, evidence of inflammatory markers, and signs of peripheral emboli, contribute to the criteria. Biomarkers (brain natriuretic protein, troponin, procalcitonin, C-reactive protein) may provide important supplemental information for both diagnosis and prognosis.
- Echocardiography is the key diagnostic tool and provides major diagnostic Duke criteria. In many patients transesophageal echocardiography offers important additional information for diagnosis and evaluation of vegetation size, abscess formation, fistula formation, leaflet perforation, or prosthetic valve dehiscence.
- The prognosis of IE is poorest in patients with heart failure, altered mental state, general debility, poor left ventricular function, and/or diabetes. Patients undergoing hemodialysis also are at higher risk for morbidity and death, as are those with significant emboli. Injection drug users tend to do better than others because of their younger age and higher likelihood of tricuspid endocarditis (right-sided rather than left-sided disease). Concurrent human immunodeficiency virus infection in injection drug users does not contribute added risk unless the CD4+ counts are low.
- Prosthetic valve endocarditis early (<60 days) after surgery tends to be nosocomial, whereas late infections are more similar to native valve IE. The presence of a prosthetic valve identifies the highest risk for development of endocarditis.
- Cardiac device infections are a major source of new cases of IE, and the use of intracardiac devices is growing. In addition to antibiotic therapy, device removal is generally necessary for cure of the infection.

- Patients undergoing surgery often do better than those receiving medical treatment, although medical cure rates continue to improve. Heart failure remains the primary reason for surgical intervention. Other indications for surgery are extensive valvular destruction and large vegetations, a paravalvular abscess, ineffective antimicrobial therapy, recurrent emboli, and the presence of a highly resistant organism. A scoring system has been developed to better define the advantage of early surgery.
- Surgical options have expanded, and valve repair is preferred whenever feasible.
- Results of blood culture are negative in about 5% to 10% of patients with IE. An aggressive approach to uncovering the infective source may be necessary and involves novel culture methods, antibody titers, and molecular and immunologic methods. Newer guidelines outline the use of such methods to confirm the infecting organism, leading causes being Coxiella burnetii and Bartonella spp.
- The type of organism determines the type and duration of antimicrobial therapy. For most cases of native valve endocarditis, 4 weeks of therapy are warranted, whereas prosthetic valve endocarditis generally requires 6 weeks. In select situations with right heart involvement, 2 weeks of therapy may be adequate. More resistant organisms require 8 weeks of treatment, and some unusual organisms may require months or years. New guidelines published in 2012 outline currently recommended regimens.

Historical Background

The earliest description of the vegetative lesions of infective endocarditis (IE) has been attributed to Lazarus Riverius (1589-1655).[1] Later, Giovanni Lancisi (1654-1720) provided a more complete description of these pathologic lesions of the heart in De Subitaneis Mortibus written in 1709.[2] Throughout the eighteenth and early nineteenth centuries there were many descriptions of endocarditis by investigators such as Morgagni and Corvisart, yet it was not until the middle to late 19th century that a link was made among the lesions, the associated inflammation, and the sequelae of the disease. In 1841, Bouillard (1796-1881) made the important connection between the inflamed endocardium, a "typhoid" state, and "gangrenous endocarditis." This event was followed by the observations of Virchow (1821-1902), in 1847, and Kirkes (1823-1864), in 1852, connecting the dots between the presence of vegetative lesions and embolic events.[1]

In his famous 1885 Gulstonian lectures Sir William Osler summarized the knowledge at that time and in addition made several important observations. First he described the acute and fulminating forms of the disease and was able to articulate specific characteristics of a more chronic and insidious form. He then improved the nomenclature of the disease and suggested calling the clinical course of the disease either "simple" or "malignant."[3,4] In addition, he described the classic presentation of a typical case and noted the diagnostic uncertainty in many cases. Finally, Osler believed that endocarditis would turn out to be a "mycotic" process, describing it as, "in all its forms, an essentially mycotic process; the local and constitutional effects being produced by the growth on valves, and the transference to distant parts of microbes, which vary in character with the disease in which it develops."

Since the days of Osler there have been many advances in our understanding of IE from pathophysiology to diagnosis, prognosis, and treatment; yet our knowledge remains remarkably incomplete. What is clear is that IE was, and remains, a serious and dynamic disease process. Over the past 30 years the incidence has remained relatively unchanged, and the associated mortality remains between 10% and 30% (depending on the organism, noncardiac conditions of the patient, and whether a native or prosthetic valve is involved).[5] Guidelines regarding endocarditis prophylaxis and therapeutic approaches to treatment have been now published and are the focus of this review.

Epidemiology

Overall Incidence

The true incidence of IE is difficult to ascertain. In a Swedish urban setting, Hogevik et al[6] found an incidence of 5.9 episodes per 100,000 person-years from 1984 to 1988. During a similar period in a Philadelphia metropolitan study, the total incidence was calculated to be 9.29 episodes per 100,000 person-years.[7] When intravenous drug users were excluded, this incidence fell to 5.02 episodes per 100,000 person-years. In both urban and rural settings in France, the incidence was estimated to be around 2.43 episodes per 100,000 person-years in 1991[8] and increased to 3.1 episodes per 100,000 person-years in 1999[9] with a peak incidence of 14.5 episodes per 100,000 person-years in the elderly. The growing incidence in elderly individuals has been confirmed in the Medicare population in the United States, in which it was 20.4 episodes per 100,000 person-years in 1998 (a 13.7% increase from 1986).[10] In fact, more than half of all cases of IE in the United States and Europe now occur in patients older than 60 years, and the median age of patients has increased steadily during the past 40 years.[11] Health care–associated IE results from health care–associated bacteremias. They include both nosocomial and nonnosocomial infections, have a high mortality rate, and are frequent in patients who are undergoing hemodialysis and/or who have other debilitating diseases. The typical patient nowadays is therefore less likely to be one with poor dentition and rheumatic disease[12] and more likely to be elderly and to have undergone a procedure to implant a device such as a prosthetic valve, pacemaker, and/or defibrillator[5] or to have a major comorbid condition.

Incidence of Infective Endocarditis and Associated Mortality

Table 25-1 summarizes cardiac conditions and the subsequent estimated incidence of IE per 100,000 patient-years.[13] Sex and age also influence the incidence of IE, with males predominating. Male:female ratios have been noted to range from 3.2:1 to 9:1.[11,14] Of interest, 50% to 70% of children younger than 2 years in whom IE develops have no apparent underlying heart disease, whereas older children usually have a congenital heart condition.[15] Endocarditis in patients with injection drug use (IDU)—defined as the intravenous injection of recreational drugs such as heroin, cocaine, and amphetamines—also may occur when there is no

TABLE 25-1	Estimated Incidence of Endocarditis
	PER 100,000 PATIENT-YEARS
General population	5-7
In patients with the following underlying cardiac conditions:	
Mitral valve prolapse with no murmur	4.6
Mitral valve prolapse with mitral regurgitation	52
Ventricular septal defect	145 (½ risk if closed)
Aortic stenosis	271
Rheumatic heart disease	380-440
Prosthetic heart valve	308-383
Cardiac surgery for native infective endocarditis	630
Prior native endocarditis	740
Surgery for prosthetic infective endocarditis	2160

Modified from Pallasch TJ. Antibiotic prophylaxis: problems in paradise. Dent Clin North Am 2003;47:665-679.

TABLE 25-2	Estimated Predisposing Valvular Lesions in Patients with Endocarditis
	PERCENTAGE OF ENDOCARDITIS CASES AFFECTED
Native Valve Disease	
Left-sided:	70
Mitral regurgitation	21-33
Aortic regurgitation	17-30
Aortic stenosis	10-18
Congenital heart disease:	4-18
Cyanotic heart disease	8
Tetralogy of Fallot	2
Ventricular septal defect	1.5
Patent ductus arteriosus	1.5
Eisenmenger syndrome	1.2
Atrial septal defect, coarctation of aorta	<1
Right-sided (including device infection)	5-10
Prosthetic Valve	20

apparent underlying valvular pathologic lesions.[16] Despite these exceptions, most patients do have identifiable underlying structural heart disease at the time of their endocarditis diagnosis.[17,18] Earlier reports, before 1967, showed that rheumatic heart disease was the most common cardiac abnormality, being present in 39% of patients,[19] whereas later series suggest its presence in only about 6%.[18] Estimates of specific valvular lesion involvement is summarized in Table 25-2.

Despite advances in the diagnosis and management of IE, it remains a disease with unacceptably high morbidity and mortality. More than 50% of patients with IE have some type of serious complication, including HF, stroke, and paravalvular extension, whereas the in-hospital mortality rates (15% to 20%) and 1-year mortality rates (30% to 40%) have changed little over the past 20 years.[5,9,20-22] Death is still disturbingly frequent and usually relates to cardiogenic shock, multiorgan failure, or stroke. Surgery is necessary and important for survival in around half the cases.[23]

When valvular disease is considered as a whole, endocarditis still is an uncommon disease process. In the Euro Heart Survey[24] of the incidence of valvular disease in a general population, endocarditis was the major diagnosis in less than 1% of patients who were found to have aortic or mitral stenosis, in only 7.5% of those with aortic regurgitation, and in 3.5% of those who had mitral regurgitation.

Left-sided native valve endocarditis (NVE) remains the most common presentation, accounting for 70% of all cases of IE. Mortality depends on comorbidities but still is at least 15% as a whole.[25] Degenerative mitral valve disease (mitral valve prolapse) is the leading predisposing valve lesion, with the risk particularly high in children and in patients older than 50 years. Patients with degenerative aortic valve disease are also at risk, helping explain the rising age of patients presenting with IE. One review estimated a slightly greater incidence of mitral than aortic involvement, 8% involving both, 4% involving the tricuspid valve, and 3.5% occurring in patients with congenital heart disease.[26] Endocarditis is unusual in patients with isolated pulmonary stenosis, atrial septal defect, mitral stenosis, or hypertrophic cardiomyopathy.

Prosthetic valve endocarditis (PVE) accounts for up to 20% of the patients with endocarditis reported in a recent series from the International Collaboration on Endocarditis-Prospective Cohort Study.[27] *Staphylococcus aureus* was the most common organism. Having a prosthetic heart valve is the greatest risk for development of IE in every series. It is estimated that IE will develop in 1.4% to 3.1% of all patients with prosthetic valve at 1 year and 3% to 5.7% at 5 years.[28] There are two disparate risk periods for the development of PVE, an early period and a late period, although some writers believe it is more useful to consider early (2 months), middle (2 to 12 months), and late (>12 months) periods as the organisms involved shift gradually rather than abruptly.[28] The early period is generally defined as the first 60 days after heart surgery, and most of the implicated organisms are considered nosocomial. The late period involves organisms more like those involved in NVE. Although there has always been a suggestion that the mechanical valves are more susceptible to IE, by 5 years there appears to be no real difference, and most series do not suggest a difference in the risk by model, position, or type of valve (mechanical or bioprosthetic).[29] Some patient factors have been associated with PVE, including renal dysfunction, young age, prior endocarditis, and perioperative wound infections.[30] Health care–associated prosthetic valve endocarditis is identified in 36.5% of all cases, and most infections (71%) occur in the first year after the valve was implanted. The rate of in-hospital death remains high, at 23%, and its occurrence is associated with older age and the complications related to the surgical intervention. The higher risk of "redo" aortic valve replacement (AVR) for endocarditis is emphasized in a report of 313 patients by Leontyev et al.[31] Perioperative mortality was 24.3% in "redo" AVR for IE compared with 6.8% for redo AVR for reasons other than endocarditis.

Right-sided endocarditis is seen in about 5% to 10% of IE surveys[16,25] and has a better prognosis than left-sided disease, though the mortality remains high in patients with human immunodeficiency virus (HIV).[32] Right-sided endocarditis typically occurs in patients with illicit IDU (including patients with HIV) and those with structural abnormalities of the right heart due to congenital heart disease, pacemaker or defibrillator implantation, or central venous catheters. The most significant risk factor for right-sided IE is certainly IDU; however, left-sided disease may be more common in some groups of addicts. In one series, left-sided involvement occurred in 57% of patients with IDU compared with 40% with right-sided disease.[33] The most common infecting organism in patients with IDU is *S. aureus*, where it has been reported as the offending organism in up to 82%.[34]

Prognosis in patients with IDU and IE is generally better than that in overall patients with IE who do not have a history of IDU, because of the lower risk of IE on the right side.[32] The patients with IDU and IE generally are also much younger than other IE populations. Of importance, the presence of HIV infection does not appear to alter the diagnostic use of the Duke criteria or the course of the disease,[35] although patients with a very low CD4[+] count (<200 cells/mm[3]) are at greater risk.[9]

The expanded use of cardiovascular electronic devices has resulted in infections not only on the device leads themselves but also on the tricuspid leaflet. A pocket infection appears to predispose to this form of IE.[36] A study from the Medicare database indicates that although the device implantation rate rose 42% in the 1990s, the IE infection rate rose 124%.[36] One estimate of the rate of these device-related infections suggests it is about 0.55 cases per 1,000 implants.[37] Removal of the device is almost always required for cure.[38,39]

Groups at High Risk for Development of Infective Endocarditis, and the Determination of Prognosis

A summary of a variety of noncardiac clinical conditions predisposing to IE and the organisms frequently associated with these conditions is given in Table 25-3.

IDU is clearly a risk factor for IE, and those who use cocaine may have the greatest risk.[40] A prior history of endocarditis is an important predisposing factor in recurrent IE in patients with IDU. Recurrent endocarditis occurred in 4.5% of one large cohort of nonaddicts who survived their initial episode.[41]

Pacemaker-associated infections have increased with the increased use of electrophysiologic (EP) devices. A report from the Multicenter Electrophysiologic Device Infection Cohort (MEDIC) registry[42] from 2009 through 2011 found that early (<6 months after implantation) device infections were generally related to pocket infections and that later IE was the result of other bacteremias. Staphylococci (coagulase-negative, methicillin-resistant, and methicillin-sensitive) were the most common organisms involved. As mentioned, effective treatment almost always requires removal of leads.

Patients undergoing hemodialysis are the largest subgroup with health care–related IE.[43,44] Predisposing factors in this population include intravascular access, calcific valvular disease, and impairment of the immune system. Of patients with health care–associated IE who are not undergoing dialysis, most have underlying predisposing conditions, including diabetes, cancer, and immunosuppressive therapy use. Identifiable underlying cardiac predisposition to IE occurs in less than 50% of this group.[5] Most invasive organisms originate from the skin or urinary tract, and the presence of intravenous lines or other invasive procedures is frequently evident.[45] *Staphylococcus* is the predominant offender.

Other noncardiac conditions also can predispose to IE and are often associated with specific infecting organisms. For instance, in the International Collaboration on Endocarditis-Prospective Cohort Study, patients with IE due to *S. aureus* were significantly more likely to be hemodialysis dependent, to have diabetes, to have a presumed intravascular device source, to receive vancomycin, to be infected with methicillin-resistant *S. aureus* (MRSA), and/or to have persistent bacteremia.[46]

Nosocomial endocarditis infections are also becoming more common. They are defined as a diagnosis of IE made more than 72 hours after admission in patients with no evidence of IE on admission or as development of IE within 60 days of a prior hospital admission during which there was risk for bacteremia or IE.[47] Nosocomial IE is usually a complication of bacteremia caused by an invasive intravascular procedure or an intravenous catheter–related device infection.[47,48] It accounts for almost 10% of cases of IE in some series.

A number of cases of IE have been reported in patients with HIV infection.[49,50] Some valves have been infected with unusual organisms such as *Salmonella* and *Listeria*.[50] It has been reported that HIV infection is an independent risk factor for IE in injection drug users,[51] although this finding has not been confirmed in other studies.[50]

The clinical examination, the organism involved and its response to therapy, and the echocardiographic information can establish the prognosis and guide decision making in the treatment of IE. A number of studies have examined other factors in an effort to understand prognosis in patients with IE. Chu et al[52]

TABLE 25-3 Epidemiologic Factors Associated with the Development of Infective Endocarditis and the Commonly Associated Organisms

EPIDEMIOLOGIC FEATURE	COMMON MICROORGANISM(S)
Injection drug usage	*Staphylococcus aureus*, coagulase-negative staphylococci, β-hemolytic streptococci, fungi, aerobic gram-negative bacilli (including *Pseudomonas*), polymicrobial
Indwelling medical devices	*S. aureus*, coagulase-negative staphylococci, β-hemolytic streptococci, fungi, aerobic gram-negative bacilli, *Corynebacterium* spp.
Poor dental health	Viridans group streptococci, HACEK group (*Haemophilus, Actinobacillus, Cardiobacterium, Eikenella*, and *Kingella*), nutritionally deficient streptococci, *Abiotrophia defectiva, Granulicatella* spp., *Gemella* spp.
Diabetes mellitus	*S. aureus*, β-hemolytic streptococci, *Streptococcus pneumoniae*
Acquired immunodeficiency syndrome	*Salmonella* spp., *S. pneumoniae, S. aureus*
Chronic skin infections, burns	*S. aureus*, β-hemolytic streptococci, aerobic gram-negative bacilli, fungi
Genitourinary infections or manipulation, including pregnancy, abortion, and delivery	*Enterococcus* spp., group B streptococci, *Listeria monocytogenes*, aerobic gram-negative bacilli, *Neisseria gonorrhoeae*
Alcoholic cirrhosis	*Bartonella* spp., *Aeromonas* spp., *Listeria* spp., *S. pneumoniae*, β-hemolytic streptococci
Gastrointestinal lesions	*Streptococcus bovis, Enterococcus* spp., *Clostridium septicum*
Solid organ transplantation	*S. aureus, Aspergillus fumigatus, Candida* spp., *Enterococcus* spp.
Homelessness, body lice	*Bartonella* spp.
Pneumonia, meningitis	*S. pneumoniae*
Contact with containerized milk or infected farm animals	*Brucella* spp., *Pasteurella* spp., *Coxiella burnetii, Erysipelothrix* spp.
Dog/cat exposure	*Bartonella* spp., *Pasteurella* spp., *C. septicum*

Modified from Baddour LM, Wilson WR, Bayer AS, et al. Infective endocarditis: diagnosis, antimicrobial therapy, and management of complications. Circulation 2005;111:e394-e434.

examined 267 consecutive patients with acute IE to determine factors early in the course of the disease that were independently associated with mortality. After controlling data for severity of illness with Acute Physiology and Chronic Health Evaluation (APACHE) II scoring, they found that the independent predictors of early mortality were the presence of diabetes mellitus (odds ratio [OR], 2.48; 95% confidence interval [CI], 1.24-4.96), *S. aureus* infection (OR, 2.06; 95% CI, 1.01-4.20), and an embolic event (OR, 2.79; 95% CI, 1.15-6.80). In a similar fashion, Hasbun et al[53] found that five baseline features were independently associated with mortality and developed a scoring system that included the following: mental status, lethargy or disorientation (4 points); Charlson comorbidity scale, 2 or greater (3 points); HF, moderate to severe (3 points); microbiology, *S. aureus* (6 points), other non-viridans infection (8 points); and therapy, medical therapy only (5 points). On the basis of this point system, patients with a score of 6 points or less only had 6% mortality at 6 months, whereas patients with a score of more than 15 points had 63% mortality. In other studies, the need for hemodialysis has also been found to portend a poor outcome,[43,54] as has the presence of poor ventricular function.[55] Another study identified patients with an altered mental state, those with mobile vegetations, and those undergoing hemodialysis as the cohort with the highest risk.[56]

Prophylaxis

Newer guidelines for endocarditis prophylaxis have created a great deal of controversy. In a population-based case-control study from Philadelphia, pulmonary, cardiac, gastrointestinal, and genitourinary procedures or surgery did not emerge as risk factors for the development of community-acquired endocarditis, and dental flossing reduced the risk only modestly.[57] One review emphasized that despite the known association of endocarditis with poor dental hygiene and a visit to the dentist's office, the actual risk of endocarditis from a dental procedure (such as a tooth extraction) is exceedingly low[13] (Table 25-4). In fact the

TABLE 25-4 Absolute Risks for Development of Infective Endocarditis from a Dental Procedure

	RISK
General population	1 per 14 million procedures
Patients with:	
Mitral valve prolapse	1 per 1.1 million
Congenital heart disease	1 per 475,000
Rheumatic heart disease	1 per 142,000
Prosthetic valve	1 per 114,000
Prior endocarditis	1 per 95,000

Modified from Pallasch TJ. Antibiotic prophylaxis: problems in paradise. Dent Clin North Am 2003;47:665-679.

event rate is so low, even in supposedly high-risk patients, that a trial designed to demonstrate an increased risk of IE from a dental procedure would require a prohibitively large number of patients and is likely not feasible.

As part of the rationale eliminating most scenarios requiring endocarditis prophylaxis, both the American Heart Association (AHA)[58] and the British Cardiac Society[59] have now published guidelines suggesting its use only in patients who not only have the greatest risk for endocarditis but who also would suffer the most from the consequences of the disease. The two lists of such patients differ slightly. The AHA/American College of Cardiology (ACC) Adult Congenital Heart Disease guidelines also weighed in by suggesting that endocarditis prophylaxis be extended to coverage of the high-risk group during vaginal delivery.[60]

The United Kingdom National Institute for Health and Clinical Excellence (NICE) working group has now taken the final step in this evolving process and suggests eliminating all prophylaxis before any procedure.[61] The NICE guidelines acknowledge that certain conditions predisposing to endocarditis—acquired valvular heart disease, valve replacement, structural congenital disease (including surgically corrected or palliated structural conditions,

TABLE 25-5	**Conditions That Pose Greatest Risk for Infective Endocarditis: Comparison of the American Heart Association and the British Cardiac Society Recommendations for Endocarditis Prophylaxis Therapy Following Dental Procedures***

American Heart Association	Prosthetic heart valve or prosthetic material used for valve repair
	Prior endocarditis
	Cyanotic heart disease
	Congenital heart disease:
	  Unrepaired cyanotic heart disease (including palliative shunts and conduits)
	  For 6 months after complete repair with prosthetic material or percutaneous device
	  Repaired with residual defect (jet lesion) at site of or adjacent to prosthetic material
	Cardiac transplant valvulopathy with regurgitation

British Cardiac Society	Prosthetic heart valve Prior endocarditis Cyanotic heart disease Transposition of the great vessels Tetralogy of Fallot Surgical systemic-to-pulmonary conduits Left ventricle-to-right atrium fistula Mitral valve prolapse with regurgitation or thickened valve leaflet

*Note that the American College of Cardiology (ACC)/American Heart Association (AHA) Guidelines for the Management of Adults With Congenital Heart Disease also suggest coverage of the high-risk patient during vaginal delivery[60] and that the National Institute for Health and Care Excellence (NICE) guidelines recommend no antibiotic coverage in any situation.[61]

fully repaired ventricular septal defect or patent ductus arteriosus, and closure devices), previous endocarditis, and hypertrophic cardiomyopathy—may increase the risk of IE should bacteremia occur. On the basis of their review of all available data, the NICE guidelines working group recommends eliminating antibiotic prophylaxis for all dental or nondental procedures. They also note no preventive advantage of chlorhexidine mouthwash. Although there remain questions as to the value of eliminating endocarditis prophylaxis entirely,[62] most physicians have gradually accepted the current endocarditis prophylaxis guidelines with some trepidation.[63-66] A comparison of the various recommendations from these guideline committees is summarized in Table 25-5.

Pathophysiology and Pathogenesis

The normal heart valve is a three-layer histologic structure of endothelium, spongiosa, and ventricularis. Its endothelium is in continuity with the endothelium over the arterial, atrial, and ventricular walls. The endothelial lining is resistant to infection by bacteria and fungi except for a few highly virulent organisms. Events that result in endocarditis constitute a complex interaction between the host and the invading microorganisms and involve the vascular endothelium, the host immune system, hemostatic mechanisms, cardiac anatomic characteristics, surface properties, enzyme and toxin production by the microorganisms, and peripheral events that have caused the bacteremia.[28] Endothelial damage is the inciting event, followed by a platelet-fibrin deposition that provides a milieu for bacterial colonization. The role of

endothelial damage as the inciting event is supported by the observation that the most likely areas of vegetation formation are similar to those where blood flow injury is most likely to occur: on the ventricular side of the semilunar valves and the atrial side of atrioventricular valves.[67] Jet lesions from insufficient valves may also damage endothelium, and vegetations may form on such sites of injury, for example, the mitral chordae in aortic regurgitation, the atrial wall (McCallum patch) in mitral regurgitation, and the septal leaflet of the tricuspid valve in a ventricular septal defect. Figure 25-1 illustrates the classic locations of endocardial and valvular lesions as well as the vegetation formation.

Interaction of damaged endothelium or microorganisms with intact endothelium results in exposure of the thrombogenic subendothelial valve collagen. This exposure is believed to result in platelet and fibrin deposition and the development of a nonbacterial thrombotic endocarditis (NBTE) lesion in most cases. If transient bacteremia is present, and the organisms can adhere to the NBTE lesion, an infective vegetation may be formed.

The vegetation is an amorphous platelet and fibrin mass. For it to evolve into an infective vegetation, microorganisms must adhere. In untreated infected vegetations, neutrophils and bacteria are present, and elastin and collagen become disrupted, quickly leading to valvular destruction. Extremely high concentrations of bacteria (e.g., 10^9 to 10^{11} bacteria per gram of tissue) may accumulate within the endocarditis vegetation. This process can become fulminant, extending into surrounding tissue and at times forming large friable vegetations that embolize. As the process continues, abscess formation may occur.

A critical component in the formation of the infected vegetation is adherence of organisms to the endothelium or to the NBTE lesion. This adherence is facilitated by adhesive surface matrix molecules on the microorganism. Certain organisms appear to possess these surface molecules more than others, a difference that may explain their particular affinity for the NBTE lesion. For instance, streptococci that produce surface glucans and dextran appear to be more likely to cause endocarditis than those that do not.[68] It is undoubtedly no accident that the most common pathogens are gram-positive bacteria and enterococci, because these organisms not only have the greatest ability to adhere and colonize these initial lesions but also have multiple identifiable surface adhesins, sometimes referred to collectively as MSCRAMMS (microbial surface components reacting with adhesive matrix molecules).[69]

For example *S. aureus* possesses clumping factor A (or fibrinogen-binding protein A) and fibronectin-binding protein A, both of which are known to be involved in valve colonization and invasion. The clumping factor appears to mediate the primary attachment of the bacteria to the NBTE lesion, and this step is followed by internalization of the organism, which is promoted by fibronectin-binding protein. Eventually proinflammatory and procoagulant responses occur.[70] Once safely inside the cells, the bacteria can survive, protected from antibiotics and host defense.[71] This process may explain why certain organisms, such as staphylococcal species and streptococci, which have the ability to bind to platelets and incite the clotting mechanism, may be more virulent than those organisms that are more readily shed into the bloodstream. The fact that *S. aureus* may also induce endothelial cells to produce a clotting tissue factor could, at least partially, explain why *S. aureus* adheres to relatively normal valve tissue. Particulate material that may be injected by intravenous drug users may also promote *S. aureus* adherence by stimulating adhesive binding molecules on normal heart valves.[72] This concept has been postulated to explain the distinct predilection for tricuspid valve involvement in intravenous drug users.[73] A potential therapeutic approach to prevent this binding was attempted by use of the St. Jude Silzon prosthetic valve ring, a silver-coated polyester ring (St. Jude Medical, Inc., St. Paul, Minnesota). Unfortunately, concerns regarding increased paravalvular regurgitation and emboli led to the product's early withdrawal from clinical trials.[74]

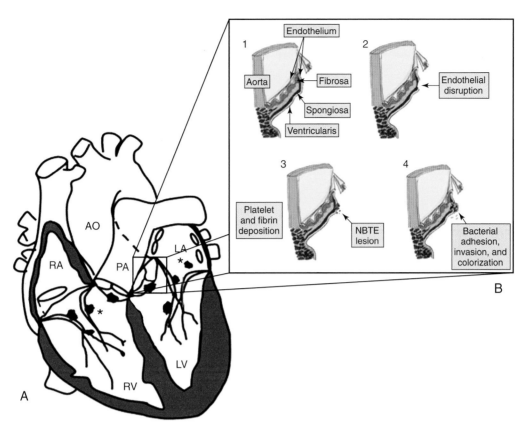

FIGURE 25-1　Pathogenesis of infective endocarditis. A, Sites of high-velocity jets where endocarditis vegetations occur. Note that these are on the atrial side of an atrioventricular valve and on the ventricular side of a semilunar valve. In addition, jet lesions from semilunar valves can result in lesions on chordae. *Asterisk* marks areas of jet lesions (McCallum patches) on endocardium from lesions such as a ventricular septal defect (on tricuspid septal leaflet) or on the left atrium from a mitral regurgitation jet. **B,** The steps in the development of the endocarditis lesion on the aortic valve. (1) The normal aortic valve leaflet. A thickened portion below the commissural line is the area where the leaflets coapt and trauma is most likely to occur. Endothelium covers the valve and is an extension of aortic and ventricular endothelium. The fibrosa provides major support for the leaflet. The ventricularis underlies the free edge, and the spongiosa lies between the two in the central portion. (2) The initial insult with endothelial injury and exposure of valve collagen. (3) Platelet and fibrin deposition with the formation of the nonbacterial thrombotic endocardial (NBTE) lesion. (4) Adhesion of microorganisms and then invasion into the NBTE lesion followed by colonization. Inflammatory cells become evident, elastin and collagen disruption occurs, and the valve destruction begins. *AO,* Aorta; *LA,* left atrium; *LV,* left ventricle; *PA,* pulmonary artery; *RA,* right atrium; *RV,* right ventricle. *(Adapted from Bashore TM, Cabell C, Fowler V Jr. Update on infective endocarditis. Curr Probl Cardiol 2006;31:274-352.)*

Enterococcus faecalis and other enterococcal species are also equipped with collagen adhesions[75] and aggregation substances[75] and are capable of biofilm production.[76] The clinical importance of biofilm production by these organisms has been strongly implicated in their antibiotic resistance and provides a potential therapeutic target for attacking the infections.[76]

Some writers have postulated that local inflammation from degenerative lesions might have a direct role in endothelial infection.[5] Inflammatory mechanisms could potentially play a role in the pathogenesis of certain fastidious infections involving pathogens, such as *Coxiella burnetii* (Q fever), *Chlamydia* spp., *Legionella* spp., and *Bartonella* spp.[77]

In up to 30% of patients, a preexisting cardiac abnormality may not be evident.[68] Several organisms appear capable of infecting apparently normal valves, including *S. aureus*, some streptococci, *Salmonella, Rickettsia, Borrelia,* and *Candida* spp. In addition to the mechanisms already described, it has even been postulated that some endothelial cells may contain metabolically latent organisms that eventually damage the endothelium.[78]

The role of transient bacteremia in vegetation formation is indisputable.[79] Transient bacteremia is unavoidable, however, and occurs even during such mundane activities as chewing food and toothbrushing. Toothbrushing twice a day for a year has been found to result in a 154,000 times greater risk of bacteremia than would result from a single tooth extraction, the dental procedure associated with the highest bacteremia.[80] Taken overall, the cumulative exposure from such routine activities may be as high

as 5.6 million times greater than that derived from a single tooth extraction.[80] Data such as these have led to the skepticism regarding the value of endocarditis prophylaxis during dental procedures.

Host defenses against infection likely also play an important but poorly defined role. Perhaps surprisingly, IE is not more prevalent in immunocompromised patients, with the possible exception of those with HIV disease.[81] Endocarditis involving gram-positive organisms is much more common than gram-negative, in part because of differences in the organism itself, but possibly also related to host defenses. For instance, the C5b-C9 membrane-attack complex of complement has a much greater killing effect on the membranes of gram-negative than of gram-positive organisms.[5] Platelet microbicidal proteins may also play some role,[82] especially because platelet deposition is so important in in vegetation formation.

The role of viruses as causative agents in IE remains unproven. A 2011 report revealing coxsackievirus cultured from an infected intracardiac patch raises the issue anew.[83] Burch et al[84] have suggested the possibility for many years, though later reviews of culture-negative endocarditis have not provided much evidence for viral etiologies.[85]

All of these interacting processes eventually lead to proliferation of the infecting organism within the vegetation. The cycle of adherence, organism growth, and platelet-fibrin deposition is then repeated again and again as the vegetation grows and develops. After treatment, capillaries and fibroblasts may appear in the lesion, but untreated lesions tend to be avascular. Necrosis with various stages of healing may occur along with vasculitic components in the healed lesion. Even after successful antimicrobial therapy, many sterile vegetation masses persist indefinitely.[86]

Diagnosis

Clinical Manifestations

The prevalences of the clinical features observed in patients with IE are summarized in Table 25-6. Many of these features were espoused by Osler in the Gulstonian lectures[4,87] but are rarely

seen in an era when diagnostic testing is better and there is antimicrobial therapy. Most patients continue to have an initial indolent course from 2 weeks to many months with vague symptoms. Symptoms include fever, chills, anorexia, weight loss, night sweats, and malaise.

Fever is the most common symptom, occurring in from 64% to 93% of patients with NVE, 85% with PVE, and 75% to 88% of patients with IDU and IE. It is less common in elderly patients and in patients with HF, renal failure, severe debility, or previous antibiotic therapy.[88] Persistent fever more than 1 week after therapy requires further investigation into its cause (e.g., an abscess somewhere), a nosocomial infection, drug fever, or inadequate IE therapy.

A murmur is apparent in 80% to 85% of patients,[28] although auscultation is a dying art in cardiology and a murmur may not always be recognized by health care providers even when present. The murmur of acute and fulminant aortic regurgitation may be particularly difficult to hear because there is little diastolic gradient. Whereas tricuspid regurgitation should be evident from examination of the jugular venous pulse, the murmur is often quite soft when right ventricular systolic pressure is normal.

A variety of peripheral cutaneous manifestations highlight the classic endocarditis examination (Figure 25-2). Unfortunately many of these peripheral stigmata are rare today. Emboli can be observed in many areas, such as mouth and conjunctival petechiae, nail bed splinters, skin Janeway lesions, Osler nodes, and Roth spots. Splinter hemorrhages tend to occur in the proximal half of the nail bed, as opposed to splinters due to trauma, which occur in the outer half. Janeway lesions are painless, erythematous skin lesions that often appear in crops on the hands or feet. They represent embolic events similar to those in splinters. Biopsies reveal that they are microabscesses without arteritis, and organisms can often be cultured from them.

Osler nodes are painful lesions that manifest as nodules on the pads of the toes or the fingertips and may persist for days. The cause for Osler nodes is unclear, but the fact that they may be seen in other settings, such as systemic lupus erythematosus (and there is histologic evidence for perivasculitis on biopsy), has led many to regard them as immunologic phenomena. Rarely,

TABLE 25-6	Clinical Manifestations of Infective Endocarditis
SYMPTOM OR PHYSICAL FINDING	**PREVALENCE (%)**
Fever	58-90
Weight loss	25-35
Headache	15-40
Musculoskeletal pain	15-40
Altered mentation	10-20
Murmur	80-85
Peripheral stigmata:	
Petechiae	10-40
Janeway lesions	6-10
Osler nodes	7-23
Splinter hemorrhages	5-15
Clubbing	10-15
Neurologic manifestations	30-40
Roth spots	4-10
Splenomegaly or infarct	15-50

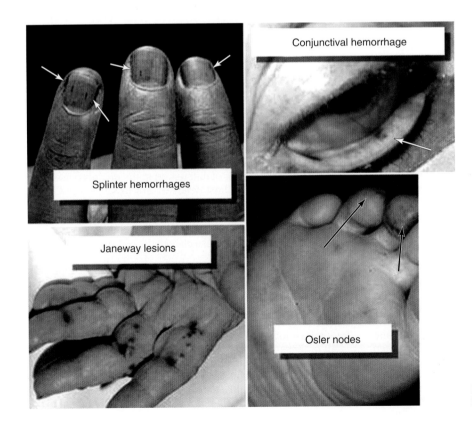

FIGURE 25-2 Peripheral manifestations of infective endocarditis. See text for discussion.

organisms have been cultured from Osler nodes, suggesting that emboli may at least be the inciting mechanism.[89]

Roth spots are retinal hemorrhages with a white center. They most likely represent septic emboli, but like Osler nodes, they have been described in other clinical settings and especially as a manifestation of systemic lupus erythematosus, anemia, diabetes, multiple myeloma, and HIV infection.[90] Frank retinal artery occlusion may also occur.

Musculoskeletal aches and pains are common in IE and often occur early in the course.[91] Any joint can be involved, but back and shoulder pains are most frequently cited.[92] Septic emboli may result in osteomyelitis or bone abscess formation (especially in the spine). Musculoskeletal pain must be taken seriously if it persists during the course of therapy.

Neurologic symptoms are common, being seen in as many as 30% to 50% of patients with IE. Symptoms appear to be more common in patients with IDU and those with staphylococcal IE.[93] Embolic stroke is the most common and serious manifestation. Intracranial hemorrhage may occur from a ruptured arterial vessel, a ruptured mycotic aneurysm, or bleeding into a thrombotic stroke distribution.[94] In addition, neurologic symptoms may be related to cerebritis or meningitis or to toxic or immune-mediated injury. Brain abscess is rare, but microabscesses from virulent organisms, such as *S. aureus*, occur with some frequency.[95] Meningitis may be a major feature in IE due to *Streptococcus pneumoniae*.

Splenic emboli are probably underreported. In the preantibiotic era, splenomegaly was common. Now about 25% to 50% of patients may have evidence of enlarged spleen. Autopsy series suggest that splenic infarcts are often present without clinical symptoms.[96]

The Evolution of the Duke Criteria

IE has traditionally been defined as an infection of the valves and chordae within the cardiac chambers. This definition has now been expanded to include infection on any structure within the heart, including normal endothelial surfaces (e.g., myocardium and valvular structures), prosthetic heart valves (e.g., mechanical or bioprosthetic valves, homografts, and autografts), and implanted devices (e.g., pacemakers, implantable defibrillators, and ventricular assist devices). Much of the increase in the incidence of IE described over the last couple of decades has come from infections on intracardiac devices, and the number of devices being implanted has grown dramatically.

The diagnosis of IE hinges on clinical suspicion and the demonstration of continuous bacteremia. It was not until the late 1970s that Pelletier and Petersdorf[97] developed a case definition based on a 30-year experience of caring for patients with IE in Seattle. Although this definition was highly specific, it lacked sufficient sensitivity. In 1981, von Reyn et al[98] published an analysis that provided four diagnostic categories for cases of suspected IE (rejected, possible, probable, and definite), and the effort improved both the sensitivity and the specificity of the previous case definition. The definition did not incorporate imaging information, however.

In 1994, Durack et al[99] from Duke University Medical Center incorporated echocardiography into the criteria for the first time, giving rise to what have come to be known as the Duke criteria. These criteria have been validated subsequently by many other studies,[100-102] including the latest modifications (Table 25-7).[103,104] There are now three diagnostic categories. *Definite* endocarditis is considered to be present if there is *pathologic* evidence (surgical pathologic histology or culture or vegetation histology or culture) *or* if there is *clinical* evidence as demonstrated by the presence of two major criteria *or* one major criterion and three minor criteria *or* five minor criteria. *Possible* endocarditis is defined as having one major criterion and one minor criterion *or* three minor criteria. *Rejected* diagnosis is defined as having a firm alternative diagnosis *or* sustained resolution of the evidence for

TABLE 25-7	The Modified Duke Criteria for Diagnosis of Infective Endocarditis*

I. Major Criteria

A. Microbiologic:
  Typical microorganisms isolated or identified from a pathologic specimen *or* found in positive blood cultures (all 3 or 3 of 4 specimens drawn over 1 hour or 2 positive cultures separated by >12 hours), *or* a single positive blood culture for *Coxiella burnetii* (or phase I immunoglobulin G antibody titer to *C. burnetii* >1:800)
B. Evidence of endocardial involvement:
  New valvular regurgitation murmur *or* positive echocardiogram results (intracardiac or device mass, *or* para-annular abscess, *or* new dehiscence of prosthetic valve)

II. Minor Criteria

A. Predisposition to infective endocarditis:
  1. Previous infective endocarditis
  2. Injection drug use
  3. Prosthetic heart valve
  4. Mitral valve prolapse
  5. Cyanotic congenital heart disease
  6. Other cardiac lesions creating turbulent flow within the intracardiac chambers
B. Fever >38°C (100.4°F)
C. Vascular phenomenon (e.g., embolic event, mycotic aneurysm, Janeway lesion)
D. Immunologic phenomenon (e.g., presence of serologic markers, glomerulonephritis, Osler nodes, or Roth spots); polymerase chain reaction assay for 16S ribosomal RNA has been added by Working Party of the British Society for Antimicrobial Therapy[22]
E. Microbiologic findings not meeting major criteria *or* serologic evidence for an active infection with typical organism

*Definite infective endocarditis = 2 major criteria *or* 1 major criterion and 3 minor *or* 5 minor criteria. Possible infective endocarditis = 1 major criterion and 1 minor criterion *or* 3 minor criteria.

endocarditis after 4 or fewer days of antibiotic therapy *or* no pathologic evidence of endocarditis at surgery or autopsy after 4 or fewer days of therapy.

Major criteria focus on identifying an organism and providing evidence that there is valvular, cardiac, or device infection from that organism. Positive blood culture results play an important role, and the occurrence of two separate blood cultures showing a typical organism, such as *S. aureus*, *Streptococcus viridans* species, *Streptococcus bovis*, HACEK group (*Haemophilus*, *Actinobacillus*, *Cardiobacterium*, *Eikenella*, and *Kingella*), or enterococci in the absence of a primary focus *or* persistently positive blood culture results (in ≥2 cultures of specimens collected >12 hours apart *or* in all 3 blood specimens or 3 of 4 blood specimens drawn within an hour period) qualifies as a major criterion for the diagnosis. Because of the difficulty in diagnosing Q fever, a single blood culture result or an immunoglobulin (Ig) G antibody titer greater than 1:800 for *C. burnetii* also qualifies. The other major criteria include clear-cut evidence for cardiac or device vegetation or valve destruction as demonstrated by echocardiographic evidence of a vegetation, abscess, and dehiscence of a prosthetic valve *or* the clinical presence of a new (not changing) regurgitant valve lesion on examination.

Minor criteria focus on the epiphenomena that are part of the endocarditis complex of clinical findings. These include having a predisposition (known heart condition or IDU), fever, vascular phenomena (major arterial emboli, septic pulmonary infarction, mycotic aneurysm, intracranial hemorrhage, conjunctival hemorrhage, Janeway lesions), immunologic phenomena (glomerulonephritis, Osler nodes, Roth spots, rheumatoid factor, C-reactive protein [CRP] level), and soft microbiologic evidence (positive blood culture results that do not qualify as major criteria) or serologic evidence of an active infection with an organism consistent with IE. A scheme to facilitate the diagnosis of IE in those patients who prove culture-negative is discussed later.

Emerging Roles for Biomarkers and Polymerase Chain Reaction Analysis

There is growing interest in the evaluation of certain biomarkers that are present in patients with endocarditis, but their use has focused on predicting outcomes rather than diagnosis. A CRP value that is elevated at baseline and normalizes with therapy has been associated with good outcomes,[105] whereas a persistently elevated CRP value despite therapy has been associated with a higher rate of cardiovascular events.[106] Procalcitonin, a marker of systemic bacterial infection, has also been shown to be elevated in IE and may be an early marker of the disease.[107,108] Troponin T has been found in 93% of patients with endocarditis, and its maximal level has also been correlated with a poor outcome.[109] In addition, the brain natriuretic peptide (BNP) value has been associated with poor outcomes, both alone and in association with the troponin level.[110]

There is also now growing evidence that molecular diagnostic techniques may eventually help refine the Duke criteria, especially regarding culture-negative endocarditis. Molecular and immunologic diagnostic techniques may have a role in discovering infection from fastidious agents such as *C. burnetii*, *Legionella pneumophila*, *Tropheryma whippelii*, *Bartonella* species, HACEK group organisms, and fungi. The most readily applicable techniques amplify trace amounts of a given nucleic acid target of microbial DNA in host tissues. In the form of the broad range or the universal 16S RNA gene polymerase chain reaction (PCR) test, most etiologic agents involved in IE have been identified. The bacterial 16S ribosomal RNA gene has both highly conserved and variable regions, and PCR is able to detect all known bacteria at the genus level and provide identification.[111] Fungal organisms can also be identified. PCR, however, is costly and requires meticulous technique to avoid contaminants and false-positive results. The technique has improved the sensitivity and specificity of diagnosis in excised heart valves,[112,113] but the advantage will come when real-time, effective PCR can readily be performed on blood samples. Newer reports of the use of PCR are encouraging.[114-117]

The 2012 Endocarditis Guidelines from the Working Party of the British Society for Antimicrobial Therapy added a broad-range PCR of 16S ribosomal RNA as a minor criterion to the Modified Duke Criteria.[22] To date this addition has yet to be confirmed as appropriate. Unfortunately, serologic tests for the specific strain of *Staphylococcus* do not seem to be useful in distinguishing IE in patients with staphylococcal sepsis.[118]

Transthoracic and Transesophageal Echocardiography

The modified Duke criteria depend on identification of the infected lesion, and echocardiography is the key imaging tool. With the use of echocardiography, several findings provide evidence consistent with IE, including vegetations, evidence of annular tissue destruction (abscess), aneurysm, fistula, leaflet perforation, and valvular dehiscence. Echocardiography also provides data regarding ventricular function, evidence of pulmonary hypertension, and an assessment of the hemodynamic consequences of the infection.

Both transthoracic echocardiography (TTE) and transesophageal echocardiography (TEE) play significant roles in the diagnosis and management of patients with suspected IE. TTE is widely available and can provide important diagnostic information rapidly. Under ideal conditions, TTE can reliably identify structures as small as 5 mm in diameter, although TEE can depict structures as small as 1 mm. It is widely accepted that the sensitivity and specificity of TEE are superior to those of TTE (93% and 96% versus 46% and 95%). As a generality, TEE should be performed whenever TTE is likely to have a low yield, such as in the definition of a paravalvular abscess or in the patient with a prosthetic valve or suspected infection of a lead or dwelling catheter. TEE may be particularly helpful in culture-negative IE. However, TEE may not detect the presence of a paravalvular abscess.[119]

Figure 25-3 outlines the current guidelines for appropriate use of TTE and TEE in the diagnosis and follow-up of patients with IE.[120] This algorithm reflects studies showing that an initial

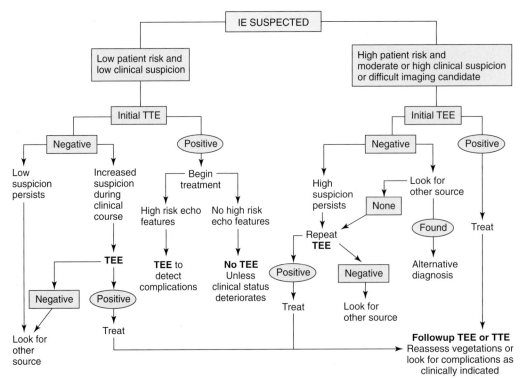

FIGURE 25-3 Algorithm for the effective use of transthoracic echocardiography (TTE) and transesophageal echocardiography (TEE) with suspicion of infective endocarditis (IE). *Echo*, echocardiographic. *(Modified from Bayer AS, Bolger AF, Taubert KA, et al. Diagnosis and management of infective endocarditis and its complications. Circulation 1998;98:2936-2948.)*

strategy of TEE imaging is the most cost-effective in many clinical situations. For instance, Heidenreich et al[121] have shown that in suspected endocarditis, a diagnostic strategy that focuses on TEE as the initial imaging modality may actually be more cost-effective than a staged procedure with TTE as the initial procedure, and that initial TEE is a better strategy for diagnosis than empiric antimicrobial therapy alone. In a similar study, Rosen et al[122] determined the cost-effectiveness of TEE in establishing the duration of therapy for catheter-associated bacteremia. The following three management strategies were compared: (1) empirical treatment with 4 weeks of antibiotics (long course), (2) empirical treatment with 2 weeks of antibiotic therapy (short course), and (3) TEE-guided therapy. In the case of the TEE strategy, positive TEE results dictated long-course therapy, and negative TEE results dictated short-course therapy. The empiric long-course strategy and the TEE-guided strategy were both superior in effectiveness to empirical short-course therapy. When costs were accounted for, the TEE-guided strategy was better than the empirical long-course strategy; an estimated cost saving of more than $1,500,000 per quality-adjusted life year was calculated.

The algorithm allows that multiple echocardiographic evaluations may be useful in determining the prognosis of patients with IE. For instance, whether a vegetation stays static or enlarges may affect prognosis.

Serial examinations can be taken to extreme, however. In a review of 262 patients with 266 episodes of suspected IE, TTE was repeated at least once in 192 (72.2%) patients, whereas TEE was repeated in 49 (18.4%) of patients. The average number of TTE examinations was 2.4, but 6 patients had at least 6. In a similar fashion, the mean number of TEE examinations was 1.7, although 4 patients had at least 4, and 1 patient had 5. The investigators found that repeated echocardiograms were not always helpful, and no additional diagnostic information was provided after the second or third echocardiogram (TTE or TEE).[123] This finding is important to keep in mind in an era in which cost containment is vital.

Echocardiographic Features in Infective Endocarditis

VEGETATIONS

On echocardiography, a vegetation appears as an irregularly shaped, discrete echogenic mass that is adherent to yet distinct from the endothelial cardiac surface. Oscillation of the mass with high-frequency movement independent of that of intrinsic structures is supportive but not mandatory for the echocardiographic diagnosis. Vegetations have the consistency of mid-myocardium (Figure 25-4) but may also have areas of both echolucency and echodensity. Their expected locations were described earlier (see Figure 25-1). Vegetations may also appear on nonvalvular intravascular structures, such as pacemaker leads (Figure 25-5), or on the windsock deformity associated with a ventricular septal defect. Vegetations on prosthetic material may be a particular challenge, and TEE is usually required for confirmation. Over time vegetations tend to decrease in size with therapy, although they may persist indefinitely as less mobile and more echogenic masses.

Not all intracardiac mass lesions are vegetations from IE. For instance, in systemic lupus erythematosus, inflammatory mass lesions (Libman-Sacks) related to the disease usually have broad bases and are small. Other sterile vegetations, such as in marantic endocarditis, may also occur in patients with advanced malignancies. A mass effect may be seen in patients with myxomatous valves, ruptured chordae unrelated to infection, cardiac tumors, and degenerative valvular changes, especially when there is considerable calcium. Moreover, normal variants, such as prominent Lambl excrescences[124] (small filiform processes on the medial tips of the aortic valve), a Chiari network, and a eustachian valve in the right atrium, may mimic IE vegetations on an

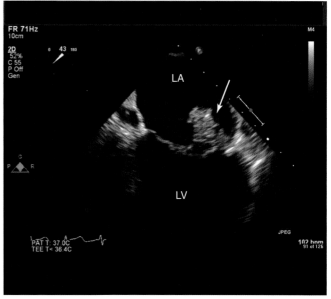

FIGURE 25-4 Typical endocarditis vegetative lesion on the native mitral valve *(arrow)* **as seen on a transesophageal echocardiogram.** Echocardiographic consistency of vegetation is similar to that of the myocardium. *LA,* Left atrium; *LV,* left ventricle. *(From Bashore TM, Cabell C, Fowler V Jr. Update on infective endocarditis. Curr Probl Cardiol 2006;31:274-352.)*

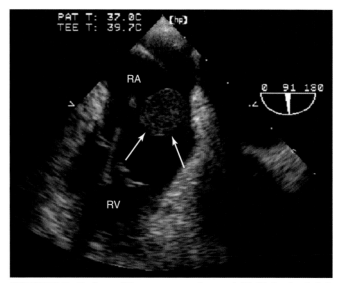

FIGURE 25-5 Endocarditis on a pacemaker or defibrillator lead. Ball-like vegetation *(arrows)* on a pacemaker lead (vertical echoes seen in right atrium [RA]). Horizontal echoes between RA and right ventricle (RV) represent the tricuspid valve. *(From Bashore TM, Cabell C, Fowler V Jr. Update on infective endocarditis. Curr Probl Cardiol 2006;31:274-352.)*

echocardiogram. To complicate matters, each of these structures has been reported as a site for infection.

Since the early 1990s multiple studies have shown an association between vegetation size and subsequent thromboembolic risk. Some have found that the risk of embolization was directly related to vegetation size.[125] Tischler and Vaitkus[126] conducted a meta-analysis that incorporated 10 studies involving 738 patients with IE. They found that the pooled OR for risk of embolization was three times higher in patients with large vegetations (>10 mm) than in patients with no detectable or small vegetations (OR, 2.90; 95% CI, 1.95-4.02). Di Salvo et al[127] also found that both size and mobility were predictive of embolic events. Unfortunately, there is a relatively high degree of interobserver variability in recording

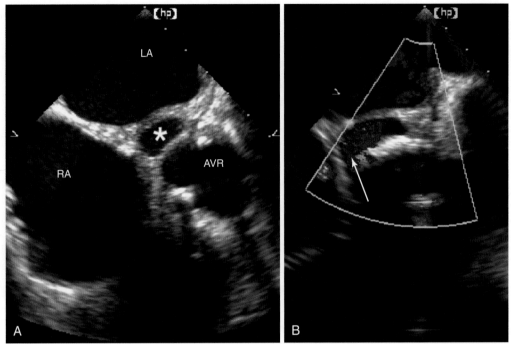

FIGURE 25-6 **Annular abscess formation in endocarditis. A,** *Asterisk* denotes the area of the paravalvular abscess between the aortic valve replacement (AVR) and the left atrium (LA). **B,** The color-flow Doppler imaging shows the presence of flow in and out of the abscess. *RA,* Right atrium. *(From Bashore TM, Cabell C, Fowler V Jr. Update on infective endocarditis. Curr Probl Cardiol 2006;31:274-352.)*

the specific characteristics of vegetations,[128] which has led some investigators to be skeptical of using a definitive cutoff size measurement to define risk. Large vegetations have now been incorporated into the criteria for surgical intervention, with large being defined as more than 10 mm and very large as more than 15 mm.

PARAVALVULAR EXTENSION OF INFECTION (MYOCARDIAL ABSCESS FORMATION)

Paravalvular extension of infection, or abscess formation, is one of the most serious complications of IE, being an indication for surgical therapy. A myocardial abscess can be defined as a thickened area or mass in the myocardium or annular region with an appearance that is generally nonhomogeneous. There is usually evidence of flow within the cavity, but flow is not mandatory for the diagnosis. An echo-free space suggests that complete liquefaction of the myocardium or aortic wall has occurred. A rupture with formation of a fistula or pseudoaneurysm may result. An example of an annular abscess is shown in Figure 25-6.

Abscess formation is associated with substantial morbidity and mortality. Extension into the septum may affect the conduction system, leading to heart block. Abscess formation is more commonly associated with IE of aortic valves—particularly prosthetic valves—the presence of new atrioventricular heart block, and coagulase-negative staphylococcus infection.[129] The mortality rate for patients with untreated abscess formation is 1.5 to 2.0 times higher than that for similar patients without abscess formation, although surgical mortality rates for the two groups are similar.[129] At times TTE can establish the diagnosis of abscess formation, but overall the resolution associated with typical TTE in adults is insufficient for the full characterization of most intracardiac abscess cavities, and TEE is preferred.

FISTULA FORMATION

Spread of infection from valvular structures to the surrounding paravalvular tissue may increase the patient's risk of adverse outcomes, including HF and death. This risk is particularly seen with aortic valve IE, in which aortic abscesses and mycotic pseudoaneurysms involving the sinuses of Valsalva may rupture, leading to the development of aortocavitary or aortopericardial fistulas. Aortocavitary communications, especially to right heart structures, create intracardiac shunts, which may result in further clinical deterioration and hemodynamic instability (Figure 25-7).

PERFORATION AND VALVULAR REGURGITATION

Little information is available about the implications of valvular perforation, but it is generally accepted that this event either is associated with a virulent microorganism, such as *S. aureus*, or occurs when the infection process continues for an extended time without detection. Once a perforation occurs, a significant amount of valvular regurgitation may develop.

PROSTHETIC VALVE DEHISCENCE

Dehiscence of a prosthetic valve due to IE is a serious complication. Dehiscence is generally defined fluoroscopically as a rocking motion of the prosthetic valve more than 15 degrees in any one plane. This complication may lead to a gross separation of the prosthetic annulus from the native tissue. Prosthetic valve dehiscence is invariably associated with significant paravalvular regurgitation and is usually associated with hemodynamic compromise. An example of prosthetic valve dehiscence demonstrated by echocardiography is shown in Figure 25-8. Dehiscence in acute IE represents an urgent indication for surgical therapy.

Other Imaging Modalities in the Diagnosis of Infective Endocarditis

Other imaging modalities may support the diagnosis of IE and/or may be used to evaluate the possibility of complications. Chest radiography can be used to provide supporting evidence of IE,

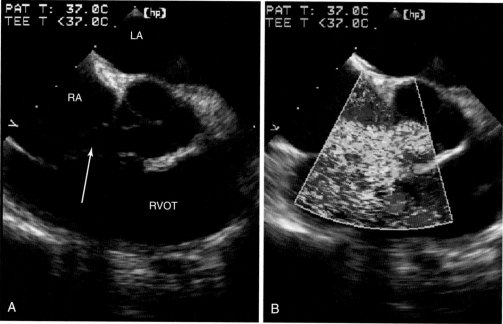

FIGURE 25-7 **Fistula formation during infective endocarditis. A,** An infected sinus of Valsalva aneurysm that has ruptured into the right ventricular outflow tract (RVOT) and right atrium (RA). **B,** Color-flow Doppler imaging shows a pattern of high-velocity flow from the high-pressure aorta into the lower-pressure right atrium and ventricle. *LA,* left atrium. *(From Bashore TM, Cabell C, Fowler V Jr: Update on infective endocarditis. Curr Probl Cardiol 2006;31:274-352.)*

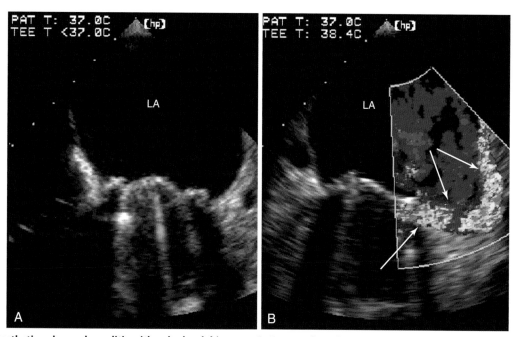

FIGURE 25-8 **Prosthetic valve endocarditis with valvular dehiscence. A,** Transesophageal two-dimensional echocardiogram of a St. Jude mitral valve. **B,** Color-flow Doppler image shows severe paravalvular mitral regurgitation *(arrows)* into the left atrium (LA) due to dehiscence of the mitral valve replacement. *(From Bashore TM, Cabell C, Fowler V Jr. Update on infective endocarditis. Curr Probl Cardiol 2006;31:274-352.)*

such as nodular pulmonary infiltrates in a febrile IDU, suggesting right-sided IE with septic pulmonary emboli, or evidence of pulmonary congestion from a left-sided lesion.

Computed tomography (CT), positron emission tomography, and cardiac magnetic resonance (CMR) imaging have all been reported to help assess the evidence for complications such as stroke and visceral embolic events, but these imaging modalities have little role in identifying the cardiac pathologic lesions themselves. Coronary CT angiography is useful for excluding coronary artery disease and avoiding cardiac catheterization in middle-aged or younger patients.

Specific Complications

Endocarditis vegetations on native valves may interfere mechanically with valve motion and lead to valvular regurgitation. Vegetation growth can also result in leaflet perforation and may cause chordal rupture. Endocarditis on a prosthetic valve usually begins on the valvular cuff and often extends outside the valvular apparatus, resulting in valvular dehiscence, abscess formation, and myocardial involvement. Vegetations can be large enough to interfere directly with mechanical prosthetic leaflet function and cause both regurgitation and obstruction. Mechanical prosthetic

TABLE 25-8	Complications from Infective Endocarditis: Estimates of the Incidence of Complications in the Modern Era
COMPLICATION	**INCIDENCE (%)**
Death	12-45 (24% average)
Heart failure (aortic regurgitation > mitral regurgitation > tricuspid regurgitation)	50-60
Embolization (mitral > aortic valve):	20-25
Cardiovascular accident	15
Other major emboli:	
Limb	2-3
Mesenteric	2
Splenic	2-3
Glomerulonephritis	15-25
Annular abscess	10-15
Mycotic aneurysm	10-15
Conduction system involvement	5-10
Central nervous system abscess	3-4
Other, less common complications (pericarditis, myocarditis, myocardial infarction, intracardiac fistula, metastatic abscess)	1-2

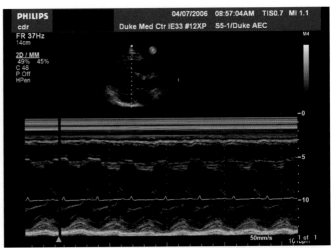

FIGURE 25-9   Pre-closure of mitral valve in acute aortic regurgitation. In this M-mode echocardiogram, the closure point of the anterior and posterior mitral valves can be identified to occur prior to the superimposed initiation of the electrocardiographic QRS. This early closure is due to the rapid rise in the left ventricular diastolic pressures as a result of acute aortic regurgitation into a noncompliant left ventricle.

valves appear to have a greater risk for endocarditis in the early period after surgery, and bioprosthetic valves later on.[130] By 5 years, though, there is no real difference in incidence of endocarditis between mechanical and bioprosthetic valves.[27,131] Implantable rings (inserted as part of valve repair) have the least risk for endocarditis,[132] but valve repair is still considered a higher risk for recurrent endocarditis.[63] Despite improvements in diagnostic tests and antibiotics, the incidence of complications in patients with endocarditis has not changed much over the last few decades.[133] Table 25-8 provides estimates of the incidence of clinical complication from IE in the modern era.[130]

Cardiac Complications

The most frequent complication of IE is HF, which is usually the result of acute or semiacute valvular regurgitation and not myocardial failure. It is most common with aortic valve involvement, followed by mitral and then tricuspid valve infections.[134] The ability of the heart to withstand the volume overload–related valvular regurgitation depends on several factors: the severity of the regurgitation, the valve involved, the rapidity of the volume overload, and both the size and function of the chamber receiving the volume overload. Mitral regurgitation, for instance, presents both a volume overload and an afterload decrease to the left ventricle, perhaps explaining why it is better tolerated than acute aortic regurgitation, in which the lesion results in both a volume overload and an afterload increase. The rapid rise in left ventricular diastolic pressures in acute aortic regurgitation may even close the mitral valve prematurely, before ventricular systole is initiated. This pre-closure is readily observed on M-mode echocardiography and has been used as an indication that surgical correction is urgently warranted[135] (Figure 25-9).

Abscess formation has already been discussed. At times the only clue to abscess formation may be the development of first-degree or more severe atrioventricular block. Abscess formation is much more common in aortic than in mitral valve endocarditis. Aortic root involvement may result not only in abscess formation but also in a true rupture, leading to fistula formation or a pseudoaneurysm.

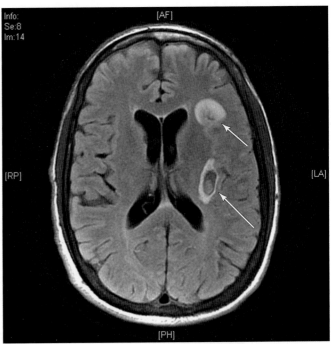

FIGURE 25-10   Magnetic resonance imaging of central nervous system bleed in endocarditis. Brain magnetic resonance imaging showing intracranial hemorrhage (arrows) from a ruptured mycotic aneurysm.

Embolization

The second most common cardiac complication of IE is embolization. Stroke is the most commonly observed major clinical consequence of embolization, and the risk of such embolization appears much greater for mitral than for aortic valve endocarditis.[136] Indeed, cerebral infarction due to either emboli or mycotic aneurysm may be the presenting sign of endocarditis in up to 14% of patients.[137] CMR is useful in detecting stroke and deciphering an embolic event from a bleed (Figure 25-10). The rate of embolic events declines rapidly after the initiation of effective antibiotics, dropping from an initial 13 events per 1000 patient-days in the first week to less than 1.2 events per 1000 patient-days after 2 weeks

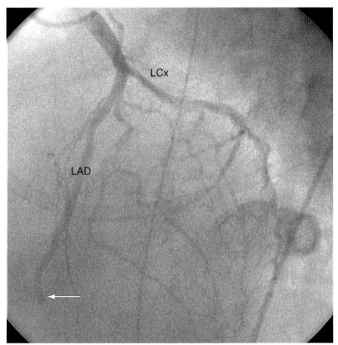

FIGURE 25-11 Coronary embolus during endocarditis. *Arrow* shows the abrupt cutoff of the contrast agent within the left anterior descending artery (LAD). *LCx*, left circumflex artery.

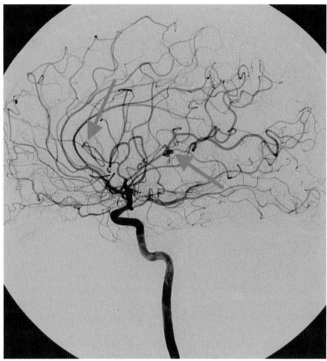

FIGURE 25-12 Angiography of mycotic aneurysm. This cerebral angiogram, of the same patient whose magnetic resonance image is shown in Figure 25-10, clearly delineates the mycotic aneurysms (shown at *arrows*).

of therapy.[138] Pulmonary emboli, usually septic in nature, occur in 66% to 75% of patients with IDU and tricuspid valve endocarditis.[16] Emboli may involve virtually any systemic organ, including the liver, spleen, kidney, and abdominal mesenteric vessels. Renal emboli can cause hematuria and flank pain. Splenic infarction may lead to abscess development and may cause prolonged fevers or left shoulder pain from diaphragmatic irritation. Coronary emboli can result in myocardial infarction (Figure 25-11). Distal emboli can produce peripheral metastatic abscesses, especially of the spine or other bony structure. Muscular and joint pains are not uncommon in IE, but severe osteoarticular pain may indicate a bony embolus.[139]

Mycotic aneurysms result from septic embolization to an arterial intraluminal space or to the vasa vasorum of the cerebral vessels. Vascular branch points are the most common sites of presentation (Figure 25-12). Mycotic aneurysms are uncommon but may be responsible for up to 15% of neurologic complications. The clinical syndrome that results may vary considerably from a slow leak that produces only mild headache and meningeal irritation to sudden intracranial hemorrhage and a major stroke.

Renal Dysfunction

Renal dysfunction is common in patients with endocarditis. Although such dysfunction is often attributed to immune complex glomerulonephritis, a necropsy and biopsy study[140] revealed that localized infarction was present in 31% and acute glomerulonephritis in 26%. The most common type of glomerulonephritis is vasculitic, without deposition of immunoproteins in glomeruli. Of the renal infarcts, more than half are related to septic emboli, primarily in patients infected with *S. aureus*. In patients with renal dysfunction, acute interstitial nephritis, presumably due to antibiotic use, is found in 10%, and renal cortical necrosis is also found in about 10%. Azotemia due to immune complex–mediated glomerulonephritis generally improves with effective antibiotic therapy. The cause of renal dysfunction in many patients is multifactorial, especially when baseline renal function is abnormal or HF is present.

Less Common Complications

Other, less common cardiac complications of IE include the development of pericarditis (either from direct extension of the infection or possibly from embolization to the pericardial vessels) and myocarditis. Invasion of the sinus of Valsalva may result not only in aortic regurgitation but also in pericarditis, hemopericardium, and fistula formation with right heart structures.

Management

Common Features of Management

Once the diagnosis of IE has been established and appropriate treatment initiated, fever should resolve within days, the exception being that in some patients with *S. aureus* infections, it may persist for up to 2 weeks. Recurrent fevers should raise concern that the antimicrobials are ineffective, that there is an abscess or other infection somewhere that is not being resolved, or that there is drug fever. Patients should be monitored daily for new embolic phenomena or signs of worsening hemodynamics. HF should be treated appropriately.

Bacteremia in IE is continuous, so results of each of the set of three recommended blood cultures should be positive. A single positive culture result should raise the suspicion of a contaminant. One should avoid sampling intravascular lines. If the patient is receiving antibiotics and is stable, antibiotic therapy should be discontinued before blood culture specimens are obtained. The 2012 European Society of Cardiology (ESC) guidelines suggest discontinuing antibiotic therapy for 7 to 10 days if necessary.[22]

In most patients, a percutaneous inserted central catheter or similar long-term access line should be placed early for antibiotic administration. Patients should undergo cardiac examination daily and follow-up echocardiography if any sign of a complication from endocarditis becomes evident. If aortic valve involvement is present, the PR interval on the electrocardiogram should be periodically assessed.

Although the erythrocyte sedimentation rate is almost universally elevated in IE, its level does not correlate with the effectiveness of therapy. The CRP level, however, should decline with effective therapy. Periodic measures of renal function as well as complete blood counts and initial hepatic function tests should be performed and a surveillance blood culture specimen should be obtained 72 hours into therapy. For most patients, the minimum inhibitory concentration (MIC) of the antimicrobial being used should help guide therapy. Infectious disease specialists should be involved to help with the antibiotic decision making. It is also prudent to have input from a cardiothoracic surgeon early in the course of IE therapy. Early consultation with a surgeon is particularly important if there is any hemodynamic instability, significant aortic valve disease, or evidence of abscess formation or in the patient with PVE.

Patients requiring anticoagulation present a particular problem. If there is no evidence for stroke, warfarin therapy should be stopped. There are no data that warfarin has any benefit in reducing the incidence of embolic events.[141] When IE is confirmed or suspected, the international normalized ratio value should be allowed to drift down until it is less than 2.0. At that point, unfractionated or low-molecular-weight heparin therapy should be initiated. When it is determined that surgical intervention will not be needed, warfarin therapy may be resumed, usually after about 7 days of antimicrobial therapy.

In patients with mechanical prosthetic valves already in place, the average rate of major thromboembolism is about 8% per year,[142] so a brief stoppage of warfarin is generally safe. The prosthetic valve with the lowest embolic or thrombotic risk is the bileaflet aortic valve. Caged ball valves, mitral mechanical valves, the presence of HF or atrial fibrillation, a prior history of venous thromboembolism within the last 3 months, and a hypercoagulable state all increase the risk of withholding warfarin. If unfractionated heparin is used, the activated partial thromboplastin time should be kept at around 50 to 65 seconds.

A greater dilemma often presents itself when there is evidence of a stroke in someone requiring anticoagulation therapy, usually a patient with a mechanical mitral valve and/or atrial fibrillation. Cerebral hemorrhage is much more likely to be the result of transformation of an ischemic stroke than of a mycotic aneurysm. Patients with *Staphylococcus* spp. endocarditis may be particularly likely to experience embolization to the central nervous system.[143] Stroke in patients with PVE who are undergoing anticoagulation has a much higher chance of being hemorrhagic at the onset (52%) than stroke in patients with NVE who are not undergoing anticoagulation.[143] Although there are no clear guidelines, the investigators in one study suggest that the risk of a hemorrhagic stroke, especially in patients with staphylococcal endocarditis, is greater if the size of the central nervous system infarct is large[144]; one should note, however, that T2-weighted CMR often identifies subacute microbleeds in patients with endocarditis that may be of less concern.[95] In most patients the decision to withhold anticoagulation and for how long is an individual one based on the clinical scenario. In an acute bleed (central nervous system or otherwise), the effects of warfarin should be reversed with vitamin K, and no anticoagulant should be given for at least 72 hours. At that time unfractionated heparin or low-molecular-weight heparin can be started. Warfarin can usually be started at the same time, and the heparin can be discontinued when an international normalized ratio value of at least 2.0 has been documented.

Currently, almost all patients who do not undergo surgical intervention for IE can be treated with an initial 1- to 2-week hospitalization and then with home therapy for the remainder of the antimicrobial course. Patients should be seen in the outpatient setting at the conclusion of therapy, and a second set of laboratory tests, including blood cultures, and an echocardiogram are normally obtained.

In most patients the total duration of intravenous antibiotic treatment is 4 to 6 weeks. Antibiotic therapy for PVE is generally

for at least 6 weeks, and that for NVE, 4 weeks. Patients with IDU and isolated right-sided IE may be eligible for short-course therapy, which generally would not be considered appropriate for left-sided disease.[145] Because these patients are often medically noncompliant, surgery should be offered after considerable discussion with the patients. Several studies have shown that surgical management of patients with IDU and IE can be performed safely with acceptable outcomes.[146,147] In general, the main indications for surgery in patients with IDU are IE due to microorganisms difficult to eradicate (such as fungi), persistent/recurrent bacteremia despite optimal antimicrobial therapy, and tricuspid valve vegetations larger than 2 cm and associated with a dilated right heart and either recurrent pulmonary emboli or right heart failure.[148] Tissue from excised valves should be investigated for the suspected organism.

Mortality, Morbidity, and Role of Surgical Intervention

Medical therapy alone for IE has been reported to be associated with a higher mortality at 6 months than with surgery,[149-153] although most of the demonstrable surgical benefit is seen in patients who have moderate to severe HF (Figure 25-13).[154] The importance of the need for surgery if HF occurs was confirmed in a report from the International Collaboration on Endocarditis Database—Prospective Cohort Study[155] (Figure 25-14). This study also revealed that surgery improved 1-year survival in patients with advanced age, diabetes mellitus, or health care–associated infection, in whom the causative microorganism was *S. aureus* or fungi, or who had the most severe HF (New York Heart Association [NYHA] functional class III or IV), stroke, or paravalvular complications. *S. aureus* infection appears to be associated with poorer surgical survival than other pathogens according to two database reviews.[155,156]

In another study from the International Collaboration on Endocarditis Database—Prospective Cohort Study database, Lalani et al[157] examined which patients might best benefit from early rather than later surgery. They found a mortality benefit in patients with paravalvular complications, systemic embolization, and *S. aureus* infection.

In a 2012 single-institution report[156] of 428 patients, 90% survival was noted after 30 days, although survival at 1 year was only 82% with NVE and even lower, at 77%, with PVE. In a survey from the

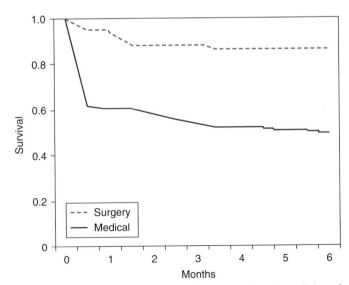

FIGURE 25-13 Six-month survival in patients with endocarditis and moderate to severe heart failure. (*Adapted from Vikram HR, Buenconsejo J, Hasbun R, Quagliarello VJ. Impact of valve surgery on 6-month mortality in adults with complicated, left-sided native valve endocarditis. JAMA 2003;290:3207-3214.*)

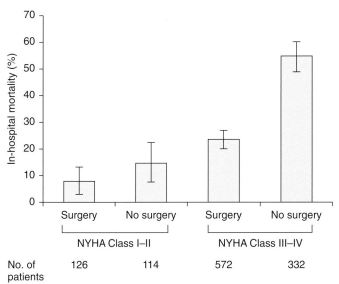

FIGURE 25-14 **Endocarditis surgery and heart failure.** Surgery has a particularly positive mortality advantage in patients as the severity of heart failure increases. NYHA, New York Heart Association. *(From Kiefer T, Park L, Tribouilloy C, et al. Association between valvular surgery and mortality among patients with infective endocarditis complicated by heart failure. JAMA 2011;306:2239-2247.)*

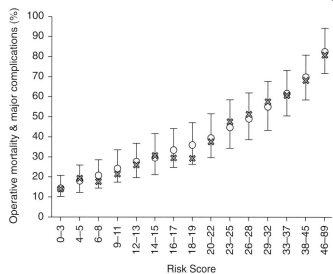

FIGURE 25-15 **Application of the score shown in Table 25-9 to the risk of early mortality and morbidity following surgical intervention.** *(From Gaca JG, Sheng S, Daneshmand MA, et al. Outcomes for endocarditis surgery in North America: a simplified risk scoring system. J Thorac Cardiovasc Surg 2011;141:98-106)*

TABLE 25-9	Risk Scoring System for Operative Mortality and Early Morbidity	
RISK FACTOR	**POINTS FOR MAJOR MORBIDITY AND OPERATIVE MORTALITY**	
Operative status of emergency, salvage, or with cardiogenic shock	17	
Serum creatinine >2.0 mg/dl or renal failure	12	
Intra-aortic balloon pump or inotropes used preoperatively	12	
Surgery on more than one valve	7	
Insulin-dependent diabetes mellitus	7	
Active infective endocarditis	7	
New York Heart Association functional class IV status	6	
Operative status of urgent or emergency without cardiogenic shock	6	
History of prior coronary artery bypass grafting surgery	5	
History of prior valve surgery	5	
Female	5	
Arrhythmia	5	
Age more than 60 years	4	
Body surface area greater than 1.9 cm^2	1	

The variables and the determined risk score with each are shown. See also Figure 25-15.

TABLE 25-10 **Timing of Surgery for Infective Endocarditis**

Emergency Surgery (<24 hours)

NVE (aortic or mitral) or PVE associated with severe or refractory heart failure or cardiogenic shock caused by acute valvular regurgitation or severe prosthetic dysfunction (deshiscence or obstruction)
Fistula into a cardiac chamber or the pericardium

Urgent Surgery (2 to 4 days)

NVE or PVE with persisting heart failure, signs of poor hemodynamic tolerance, or abscess
PVE caused by staphylococci or gram-negative organisms
Large vegetations (>10 mm) with an embolic event despite antimicrobial treatment or other predictors of a complicated course
Very large vegetation (>15 mm) especially if conservative surgery feasible
Large abscess and/or periannular involvement with uncontrolled infection

Early Surgery (4 to 10 Days) During Hospital Stay

Severe aortic or mitral regurgitation with heart failure despite good response to medical therapy
PVE with valvular dehiscence or heart failure despite good response to therapy
Presence of abscess or periannular extension
Persisting infection after extracardiac focus has been excluded
Highly resistant or virulent organism (fungi, *Brucella*, *Pseudomonas*, antibiotic-resistant enterococci, poorly responsive *Staphylococcus aureus*)
Immediate relapse after completion of prior endocarditis treatment

NVE, Native valve endocarditis; *PVE*, prosthetic valve endocarditis.
Modified from Prendergast BD, Tornos P. Surgery for infective endocarditis: who and when? Circulation 2010;121:1141-1152.

Society of Thoracic Surgeons (STS) Adult Cardiac Surgery Database of 19,543 operations for IE performed from 2002 through 2008, operative mortality was 8.2%, although active endocarditis was present in only half of patients (52%) and was associated with a twofold increase in mortality.[158] The investigators reported that the use of a defined scoring system identified those at greatest risk for early death (Table 25-9). With use of the scoring system,

the 30-day combined mortality and morbidity was higher than 50% when more than 28 risk factor points were identified (Figure 25-15).

Table 25-10 outlines a reasonable timetable for cardiac surgical procedures in patients with NVE and PVE.[152] HF is the major reason to proceed with surgical intervention in IE. This concern is especially important in patients with aortic regurgitation, in whom emergency surgery (within 24 hours) should be performed once HF is present. As previously described, the rapid rise in the left ventricular diastolic pressure with acute aortic regurgitation may close the mitral valve prematurely (pre-closure demonstrated by M-mode echocardiography) and is an indication for surgery in acute aortic regurgitation.[135] Emergency surgical intervention should also be performed if there is hemodynamic instability owing to rupture of a sinus of Valsalva into another heart structure or into the pericardium. Urgent surgical intervention (within 2 to 4 days) is indicated if there is any evidence of prosthetic valvular obstruction, paravalvular abscess, prosthetic valve dehiscence, or higher than NYHA functional class II HF. Early surgical intervention (within 4 to 10 days) is also indicated if there is evidence of even moderate (NYHA functional class II, HF), ineffective antimicrobial therapy (persistent fevers, positive surveillance blood culture results, or a highly virulent organism), large (>10 mm) mobile vegetations, recurrence of an embolic event, or endocarditis due to a highly resistant organism or to one for which therapy is not available (fungi, *Brucella*, *Pseudomonas*, or antibiotic-resistant enterococci).

The STS has reported practice guidelines for surgical intervention in IE associated with neurologic events.[150] In patients with neurologic complications, the recommendation is to wait at least 4 weeks (class IIa, level of evidence [LOE] C). If an intracranial bleed or mycotic aneurysm is identified, the recommendation is to withhold heparin for 4 weeks (class I, LOE B). Evidence for an expanding mycotic aneurysm during antibiotic therapy may be considered an indication for surgery (class IIb, LOE C).

Surgical approaches to valvular endocarditis vary widely. An implantable device, such as a pacemaker or implantable defibrillator, almost always needs to be replaced for cure,[38] and this fact should be taken into consideration when surgery is planned (especially if the patient is dependent on the pacemaker). Surgical valve repair rather than replacement has been growing in popularity and is reflected in the STS guideline.[150] For native AVR the valve choice is not dissimilar to that for AVR in general. If a periannular abscess is present, a mechanical or stented valve is recommended (class IIa, LOE B) or, if the destruction is extensive, a homograft (class IIb, LOE B). For aortic PVE, the same recommendations hold. In native mitral endocarditis, mitral valve repair is considered a class I recommendation, with valve replacement class II. For mitral PVE the choice of the replacement prosthetic valve is not unlike the choice in patients without IE. Tricuspid valve excision without replacement continues to have some advocates in patients with IDU who are likely to have recurrent tricuspid valve endocarditis,[149] but severe right heart failure invariably develops. Current guidelines recommend tricuspid valve repair (class I, LOE B) over replacement when possible (class IIa, LOE C). In rare cases cardiac transplantation has been required for survival.[159]

Microbiology and Antimicrobial Treatment

An enormous variety of microorganisms has been implicated in IE, but staphylococci and streptococci account for the majority of all cases. The International Collaboration on Endocarditis–Prospective Cohort Study, identifying the microbiologic agent in 1779 patients from 39 medical centers in 16 countries with definite endocarditis, found that staphylococci were the etiologic agents in 42%, and streptococci in 40%.[160] Table 25-11 outlines the prevalence of the various microorganisms involved in different scenarios.[16,22,25,27,28,161,162] The following presentation is meant to provide an overview but not a comprehensive discussion of the organisms and the principles of antimicrobial therapy for IE.

On the basis of the suspected pathogen, empirical therapy may be initiated during the wait for blood culture and other results. This step is especially important if there is evidence of severe sepsis or shock, in which it may not be possible to obtain the three sets of blood culture specimens. The currently recommended empiric antibiotic treatment is summarized in Table 25-12.[21,22,25]

Culture-Negative Endocarditis

Blood culture results are negative in approximately 5% to 10% of patients with IE in whom the diagnosis is confirmed by strict diagnostic criteria.[163] Most of these causes are attributed to antibiotic use before blood culture specimens are drawn, IE due to fastidious organisms, or IE due to intracellular bacteria such as *C. burnetii*, *T. whippelii* and *Bartonella* spp. Other speculated causes include right-sided endocarditis; culture specimens taken toward the end of a chronic course (longer than 3 months); uremia supervening in a chronic course; mural endocarditis as in ventricular septal defects, infected thrombi after myocardial infarction, or infection related to device implantations; and fungal infections. Viruses and marantic endocarditis may also play some role. Attention to the proper collection of blood culture specimens, care in the performance of serologic tests, and the use of newer diagnostic techniques may reduce the proportion of culture-negative cases. The use of PCR to assist in the diagnosis has been described

TABLE 25-11	Microorganisms Causing Infective Endocarditis in Native Valves, in Injection Drug Users, and with the Early, Mid, and Late (after Placement) Prosthetic Valve Syndromes				
			Prosthetic Valves After Placement (%)		
ORGANISM	NATIVE VALVE (%)	INJECTION DRUG USERS (%)	2 MONTHS	2-12 MONTHS	>12 MONTHS
Staphylococci:					
Staphylococcus aureus	20-48	50-60	22	12	18
Staphylococcus epidermidis	3-5	–	33	32	11
Streptococci:					
Viridans spp.	25-65	1-12	1	9	31
Enterococci	5-17	8-9	8	12	11
Streptococcus bovis	7-10	–	–	–	
β-Hemolytic streptococcus	4-5	10-25	–	–	
Pneumococci	1-3	–	–	–	
Gram-negative bacilli	4-9	5-7	13	3	6
Culture-negative	3-15	3-5	5	2	8
HACEK group (*Haemophilus, Actinobacillus, Cardiobacterium, Eikenella,* and *Kingella*), including fastidious gram-negative organisms	2-5	–	0	0	6
Fungi	1-5	0-4	8	12	3
Polymicrobial	1-2	5-7	3	6	5

TABLE 25-12 Empiric Antibiotic Therapy

ANTIMICROBIAL(S)*	DOSE/ROUTE	COMMENT(S)
Regimen 1: NVE—Intolerant Presentation		
Amoxicillin AND (optional)	2 g q4h IV	If patient is stable, ideally await blood culture results Better activity against enterococci and many HACEK group microorganisms than benzylpenicillin Use Regimen 2 for genuine penicillin allergy
Gentamicin	1 mg per kg actual body weight IV	The role of gentamicin is controversial before culture results are available
Regimen 2: NVE, Severe Sepsis, No Risk Factors for Enterobacteriaceae, *Pseudomonas*		
Vancomycin AND	Dosed according to local guidelines	In severe sepsis, staphylococci (including methicillin-resistant staphylococci) must be covered If patient is allergic to vancomycin, replace with daptomycin, 6 mg/kg q24h IV
Gentamicin	1 mg per kg ideal body weight q12h IV	If there are concerns about nephrotoxicity/acute kidney injury, use ciprofloxacin* in place of gentamicin
Regimen 3: NVE, Severe Sepsis AND Risk Factors for Multiresistant Enterobacteriaceae, *Pseudomonas*		
Vancomycin AND	Dose according to local guidelines, IV	Will provide cover against staphylococci (including methicillin-resistant staphylococci), streptococci, enterococci, HACEK group, Enterobacteriaceae, and *P. aeruginosa*
Meropenem	2 g q8h IV	
Regimen 4: PVE Pending Blood Culture Results or with Negative Blood Culture Results		
Vancomycin AND	1 g q12h IV	
Gentamicin AND	1 mg/kg q12h IV	
Rifampicin	300-600 mg q12h PO/IV	Use lower dose of rifampicin in severe renal impairment

HACEK group, *Haemophilus, Actinobacillus, Cardiobacterium, Eikenella,* and *Kingella; IV,* intravenous; *NVE,* native valve endocarditis; *PO,* orally; *PVE,* prosthetic valve endocarditis; *q_h,* every _ hours.
From Gould FK, Denning DW, Elliott TS, et al. Guidelines for the diagnosis and antibiotic treatment of endocarditis in adults: a report of the Working Party of the British Society for Antimicrobial Chemotherapy. J Antimicrob Chemother 2012;67:269-289.
*Doses require adjustment according to renal function.

earlier. Some clues as to the organism that might be involved on the basis of the clinical scenario may be found in Table 25-11.[21] One diagnostic strategy using PCR data has been suggested by Fournier et al[85] and is shown in Figure 25-16. Based on a series of 740 patients with confirmed culture-negative endocarditis, this strategy is primarily focused on picking up the fastidious and intracellular organisms. No virus or *Chlamydia* species was detected. A diagnosis of *C. burnetii* was found in 37% of the study patients, of *Bartonella* spp. in 12.4%, of a streptococcus in 4.4%, and of *T. whippelii* in 2.8%. Despite these efforts, no etiology could be determined in 36.5% of the patients.

Staphylococcal Endocarditis

NATIVE VALVE ENDOCARDITIS

The 2012 British Society recommendations for antibiotic therapy in staphylococcal endocarditis[22] are summarized in Table 25-13. The recommended first-line therapy for *methicillin-sensitive staphylococci* is now flucloxacillin. Gentamicin adjunctive therapy is no longer recommended, nor is there a perceived advantage for sodium fusidate or rifampin. For *methicillin-resistant staphylococcal IE* or in patients with penicillin allergy, the drug combination of intravenous vancomycin and rifampin is recommended. Because vancomycin and gentamicin have nephrotoxic effects when used together, gentamicin adjunctive therapy is no longer recommended in this situation either. If there is intolerance of or resistance to vancomycin, the antibiotic of choice is daptomycin.

PROSTHETIC VALVE ENDOCARDITIS

For PVE, an aggressive regimen of vancomycin, rifampin, and gentamicin is now recommended, with daptomycin the

alternative if any of the isolates is vancomycin resistant or the patient is intolerant of the first choices.

DURATION OF THERAPY

For NVE, intravenous therapy should be given for 4 weeks in uncomplicated disease, but for at least 6 weeks in PVE or if there is an intracardiac device, lung abscess, or osteomyelitis. No switch to oral antibiotics is recommended.

Streptococcal Endocarditis

Options for the treatment of streptococcal endocarditis should be based on the level of penicillin sensitivity and patient's risk factors. If the MIC is greater than 0.5 mg/L, the guidelines for enterococcal infection should be followed (Table 25-14).

NATIVE VALVE ENDOCARDITIS

Penicillin and ceftriaxone remain the staple of treatment for native valve streptococcal endocarditis. Ceftriaxone should not be used if there is an associated *C. difficile* infection. Adjunctive gentamicin therapy for the first 2 weeks of the course is appropriate if the MIC is greater than 0.125 mg/L or if the patient is a particular risk for *C. difficile* infection. It is not advised if patient has extracardiac foci or indications for surgery. Gentamicin should be used for 4 to 6 weeks to treat nutritionally variant streptococci. If there is a significant penicillin allergy, the combination of vancomycin and gentamicin or teicoplanin and gentamicin is recommended.

PROSTHETIC VALVE ENDOCARDITIS

The basic regimens remain the same for PVE with streptococci, except that gentamicin is not recommended for organisms

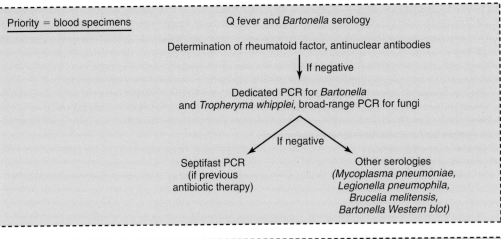

FIGURE 25-16 Evaluation for culture-negative endocarditis. The algorithm recommended as a means to detect the most common organisms that contribute to culture-negative endocarditis. *AIHC,* autoimmunohistochemistry; *PCR,* polymerase chain reaction testing; *PEER,* primer extension enrichment reaction; *rRNA,* ribosomal RNA. *(From Fournier PE, Thuny F, Richet H, et al. Comprehensive diagnostic strategy for blood culture-negative endocarditis: a prospective study of 819 new cases. Clin Infect Dis 2010;51:131-140.)*

TABLE 25-13 Treatment of Staphylococcal Endocarditis

AGENT(S)	DOSE/ROUTE	DURATION (WEEKS)	COMMENT(S)
Native Valve Endocarditis			
***Methicillin-Susceptible** Staphylococcus Spp.*			
Flucloxacillin	2 g every 4-6 hours IV	4	Use q4h regimen if weight >85 kg
Methicillin-Resistant, Vancomycin-Susceptible (MIC ≤1 mg/L), Rifampicin-Susceptible** Staphylococcus Spp. **OR Penicillin Allergy			
Vancomycin AND	1 g q12h IV	4	Or dose according to local guidelines Modify dose according to renal function and maintain pre-dose level 15-20 mg/L
Rifampicin	300-600 mg q12h PO	4	Use lower dose of rifampicin if creatinine clearance <30 mL/min
Methicillin-Resistant, Vancomycin-Susceptible (MIC ≤1 mg/L), Daptomycin-Susceptible (MIC ≤ 1 mg/L)** Staphylococcus Spp. **OR Patient Unable to Tolerate Vancomycin			
Daptomycin AND	6 mg/kg q24h IV	4	Monitor creatinine phosphokinase weekly Adjust dose according to renal function
Rifampicin OR	300-600 mg q12h PO	4	Use lower dose of rifampicin if creatinine clearance <30 mL/min
Gentamicin	1 mg/kg q12h IV	4	
Prosthetic Valve Endocarditis			
***Methicillin, Rifampicin-Susceptible** Staphylococcus Spp.*			
Flucloxacillin AND	2 g every 4-6 hours IV	6	Use q4h regimen if weight >85 kg.
Rifampicin AND	300-600 mg q12h PO	6	Use lower dose of rifampicin if creatinine clearance <30 mL/min.
Gentamicin	1 mg/kg q12h IV	6	
Methicillin-Resistant, Vancomycin-Susceptible (MIC ≤2 mg/L),** Staphylococcus Spp. **OR Penicillin Allergy			
Vancomycin AND	1 g q12h IV	6	Or dose according to local guidelines Modify dose to renal function and maintain pre-dose level 15-20 mg/L
Rifampicin AND	300-600 mg q12h PO	6	Use lower of rifampicin if creatinine clearance <30 mL/min.
Gentamicin	1 mg/kg q12h IV	≥2	Continue gentamicin for the full course if there are no signs or symptoms of toxicity
Methicillin-Resistant, Vancomycin-Resistant (MIC >2 mg/L), Daptomycin-Susceptible (MIC ≤1 mg/L)** Staphylococcus Spp. **OR Patient Unable To Tolerate Vancomycin			
Daptomycin AND	6 mg/kg q24h IV	6	Increase daptomycin dosing interval to every 48 hours if creatinine clearance <30 mL/min
Rifampicin AND	300-600 mg q12h PO	6	Use lower dose of rifampicin if creatinine clearance <30 mL/min
Gentamicin	1 mg/kg q12h IV	≥2	Continue gentamicin for the full course if there are no signs or symptoms of toxicity

IV, intravenously; *PO,* orally; *q_h,* every _ hours.
From Gould FK, Denning DW, Elliott TS, et al. Guidelines for the diagnosis and antibiotic treatment of endocarditis in adults: a report of the Working Party of the British Society for Antimicrobial Chemotherapy. J Antimicrob Chemother 2012;67:269-289.

TABLE 25-14 Therapy for Streptococcal Endocarditis *

REGIMEN	ANTIMICROBIAL(S)	DOSE AND ROUTE	DURATION (WEEKS)	COMMENT(S)
Treatment Options for Streptococci (Penicillin MIC ≤0.125 mg/L)				
1	Benzylpenicllin[†] monotherapy	1.2 g q4h IV	4-6	Preferred narrow-spectrum regimen, particularly for patients at risk of *Clostridium difficile* or high risk of nephrotoxicity
2	Ceftriaxone monotherapy	2 g once a day IV/IM	4-6	Not advised for patients at risk of *C. difficile* infection; suitable for outpatient antimicrobial therapy
3	Benzylpenicllin[†] AND	1.2 g q4h IV	2	Not advised for patients with PVE, extracardiac foci of infection, any indications for surgery, high risk of nephrotoxicity or at risk of *C. difficile*
	Gentamicin	1 mg/kg q12h IV	2	
4	Ceftriaxone AND	2 g once a day IV/IM	2	Not advised for patients with PVE, extracardiac foci of infection, any indications for surgery, high risk of nephrotoxicity, or risk of *C. difficile*
	Gentamicin	1 mg/kg q12h IV	2	
Treatment of Streptococci (Penicillin MIC >0.125 To ≤0.5 mg/L)				
5	Benzylpenicllin[†] AND	2.4 g q4h IV	4-6	Preferred regimen, particularly for patients at risk of *C. difficile*
	Gentamicin	1 mg/kg q12h IV	2	
Treatment of *Abiotrophia* and *Granulicatella* Spp. (Nutritionally Variant Streptococci)				
6	Benzylpenicllin[†] AND	2.4 g q4h IV	4-6	Preferred regimen, particularly for patients at risk of *C. difficile*
	Gentamicin	1 mg/kg q12h IV	4-6	
Treatment of Streptococci Penicillin MIC >0.5 Mg/L[‡]				
Treatment of Streptococci in Patients with Significant Penicillin Allergy				
7	Vancomycin AND	1 g q12h IV	4-6	Or dose according to local guidelines
	Gentamicin	1 mg/kg q12h IV	≥2	
8	Teicoplanin AND	See Table 25-15	4-6	Preferred option in patient at high risk of nephrotoxicity
	Gentamicin	1 mg/kg IV q12h	≥2	

IM, Intramuscularly; *IV*, intraveneously; *PVE*, prosthetic valve endocarditis; *q_h*, every _ hours.
From Gould FK, Denning DW, Elliott TS, et al. Guidelines for the diagnosis and antibiotic treatment of endocarditis in adults: a report of the Working Party of the British Society for Antimicrobial Chemotherapy. J Antimicrob Chemother 2012;67:269-89.
*All drug dosages to be adjusted in renal impariment; gentamicin, vancomycin and teicoplanin levels to be monitored.
[†]Amoxicillin 2 g every 4-6 hours may be used in place of benzylpenicillin 1.2-2.4 g every 4 hours.
[‡]See guidelines for the treatment of enterococci (see Table 25-15).

sensitive to penicillin (MIC ≤0.125 mg/L). Duration of therapy is generally 6 weeks.

Enterococcal Endocarditis

Enterococcal endocarditis is the third most common form of IE, accounting for roughly 10% of cases of the disease. Unlike in therapy for other streptococcal species, gentamicin is considered an important cell wall agent against enterococci, though its nephrotoxicity limits its use. Recommended therapy is outlined in Table 25-15. The ESC guidelines suggest waiting for susceptibility testing results before initiating gentamicin therapy in this situation. The suggested use of ceftriaxone and penicillin as a viable combination has not resulted in better outcomes.[164]

NATIVE AND PROSTHETIC VALVE ENDOCARDITIS

The treatment regimens are similar for NVE and PVE except for duration of therapy. Amoxicillin or high-dose penicillin plus gentamicin is the first option. In penicillin-allergic patients, vancomycin or teicoplanin by be substituted, depending on sensitivity results. The risk of gentamicin nephrotoxicity remains great, however, and the drug should be discontinued at the first sign of deteriorating renal function. Sporadic reports of success of either linezolid[165] or daptomycin[166] therapy against vancomycin-resistant enterococci (VRE) are encouraging, but other reports of long-term failures[167,168] warrant caution in using these agents.

HACEK Endocarditis

Organisms in the HACEK group are fastidious gram-negative bacteria. Current recommendations for treatment are similar for both native and prosthetic valve infections, with the exception of a longer therapeutic duration for PVE. The treatment should include cephalosporin or amoxicillin, depending on susceptibility results, and gentamicin as an adjunct for the first 2 weeks.[22] Oral ciprofloxacin has also been used successfully.[169]

Other Causes of Gram-Negative Endocarditis

A variety of less common organisms have been described as culprits in IE.[170] Many are nosocomial in origin and often resistant to a variety of antibiotics. Combination therapy with a beta-lactam antibiotic (amoxicillin, cephalosporin or carbapenem) and aminoglycoside is recommended. Once-daily gentamicin is acceptable unless sensitivity results are not suggestive of its value or there is concern for nephrotoxicity.

TABLE 25-15 Therapy for Enterococcal Endocarditis

REGIMEN	ANTIMICROBIAL(S)	DOSE AND ROUTE	DURATION (WEEKS)	COMMENT(S)
1	Amoxicillin OR	2 g q4h IV	4-6	For amoxicillin-susceptible (MIC ≤4 mg/L), penicillin-susceptible (MIC ≤4 mg/L) AND gentamicin-susceptible (MIC ≤128 mg/L) isolates Duration 6 weeks for PVE
	Penicillin AND	2.4 g q4h IV	4-6	
	Gentamicin*	1 mg/kg q12h IV	4-6	
2	Vancomycin* AND	1 g q12h IV or dosed according to local guidelines	4-6	For penicillin-allergic patient or amoxicillin- or penicillin-resistant isolate; ensure vancomycin MIC ≤4 mg/L Duration 6 weeks for PVE
	Gentamicin*	1 mg per kg ideal body weight q12h IV	4-6	
3	Teicoplanin* AND	10 mg/kg q24h IV	4-6	Alternative to Regimen 2; see coments for Regimen 2; ensure teicoplanin MIC ≤2 mg/L
	Gentamicin*	1 mg/kg q12h IV	4-6	
4	Amoxicillin*†	2 g q4h IV	≥6	For isolates that are amoxicillin-susceptible (MIC ≤4 mg/L) AND gentamicin-resistant at a high level (MIC >128 mg/L)

IV, Intraveneously; *PVE*, prosthetic valve endocarditis; *q_h*, every _ hours.
From Gould FK, Denning DW, Elliott TS, et al. Guidelines for the diagnosis and antibiotic treatment of endocarditis in adults: a report of the Working Party of the British Society for Antimicrobial Chemotherapy. J Antimicrob Chemother 2012;67:269-89.
*Amend dose according to renal function.
†Streptomycin 7.5 mg/kg every 12 hours intramuscularly can be added if isolate is susceptible.

Q Fever Endocarditis

The pathogen for Q fever is the intracellular *C. burnetii.* Its prevalence is much lower in the United States than in the United Kingdom, where it is the most common cause of culture-negative endocarditis.[171,172] Endocardial lesions are often quite small, and there is a higher incidence of prosthetic than native valve infection. A chronic form appears to develop in some instances.[173] A newer immune-PCR method for detection of the phase II IgM anti–*C. burnetii* antibody has been reported that may improve diagnostic sensitivity.[174] The combination of doxycycline and hydroxychloroquine given orally for 18 months to 4 years is recommended.[22] An alternative is the combination of doxycycline and ciprofloxacin. Therapy should be continued until the phase I IgG antibody level is less than 1:800 and the IgM and IgA antibody levels are less than 1:50.[175]

BARTONELLA ENDOCARDITIS

Bartonella spp. are intracellular gram-negative bacteria that can cause trench fever, cat-scratch disease, and endocarditis.[176] Infection with *Bartonella* is usually associated with poor living conditions, homelessness, and alcoholism and is transmitted by body lice. Treatment should include gentamicin in combination with a beta-lactam antibiotic or doxycycline for a minimum of 4 weeks.[22,177]

Fungal Endocarditis

Fungal infection is a rare cause of infective endocarditis (2% to 4% of all cases).[178] *Candida* spp. are responsible for half of cases, *Aspergillus* spp. for about 25%, and other fungi for the remainder. Fungi are more likely to be etiologic in patients with health care–associated infections, in patients with prosthetic cardiac valves or IDU, and in those who are immunosuppressed.

CANDIDA ENDOCARDITIS

Medical therapy has made major inroads to what has traditionally felt to be a surgical disease. Surgery is still necessary for cure in most cases and is clearly indicated if there are resistant organisms, emboli, HF or other complicating features. Treatment suggestions are outlined in Table 25-16.[22] Initial therapy should be an echinocandin (micafungin, caspofungin, or anidulafungin) or amphotericin B. Intravenous therapy is generally for 4 weeks followed by long term suppressive therapy with oral fluconazole for susceptible organisms. If prosthetic material is involved, lifelong suppressive therapy may be required.

ASPERGILLUS ENDOCARDITIS

Whereas medical therapy may be an option for *Candida* endocarditis, it is not for *Aspergillus* infection. *Aspergillus* endocarditis has particularly been noted as a complication in patients who have undergone lung transplantation.[179] Essentially all infected patients require surgical valve excision for survival.[180] The recommended initial therapy is voriconazole[181] with therapeutic drug monitoring[22] (see Table 25-16). Echinocandins are not fungicidal for *Aspergillus* spp.

ENDOCARDITIS DUE TO OTHER FUNGI

Other fungal organisms are occasionally reported as causes of endocarditis.[182] Therapy is directed toward the individual organism involved because of the high incidence of resistance to antifungal therapy.[22]

TABLE 25-16 Therapy for Fungal Endocarditis

ANTIFUNGAL AGENT	DOSE/ROUTE	SERUM DRUG LEVEL MEASUREMENTS REQUIRED?	ROLE IN TREATING *CANDIDA* ENDOCARDITIS	ROLE IN TREATING *ASPERGILLUS* ENDOCARDITIS
Fluconazole	400 mg daily, only reduced in severe renal failure/dialysis	No	Long-term suppressive therapy	None
Voriconazole	Intravenous therapy prefererd initially, licensed doses	Yes, with dose modification important	Long-term suppressive threapy for fluconazole-resistant, voriconazole-susceptible isolates	First-line therapy with long-term suppression
Amphotericin B	3 mg/kg/24 h (AmBisome) 5mg/kg/day (Abelcet) 1 mg/kg/day (Fungizone)	No	Second-line therapy	Second-line therapy, or first-line if azole resistance; should nto be used for *Aspergillus terreus* or *Aspergillus nidulans* infection
Micafungin	200 mg daily	No	First-line therapy	Third- or fourth-line therapy
Caspofungin	70 mg loading dose, 50-100 mg daily	No	First-line therapy	No role
Anidulafungin	Licensed doses	No	First-line therapy	No role
Posaconazole	400 mg twice daily	Yes	No role	Third- or fourth-line therapy, long-term suppressive therapy
Flucytosine	100 mg/kg/day in three doses, reduced with renal dysfunction	Yes, with dose modification important	As combination threapy with amphotericin B	As combination therapy with amphotericin B
Itraconazole	NA	NA	No role	No role

NA, not applicable.

From Gould FK, Denning DW, Elliott TS, et al. Guidelines for the diagnosis and antibiotic treatment of endocarditis in adults: a report of the Working Party of the British Society for Antimicrobial Chemotherapy. J Antimicrob Chemother 2012;67:269-289.

REFERENCES

1. Levy D. Centenary of William Osler's 1885 gulstonian lectures and their place in the history of bacterial endocarditis. J Royal Soc Med 1985;78:1039–46.
2. Lancisi G. De subitaneis mortibus. Rome: Libri Duo; 1709.
3. Osler W. Gulstonian lectures on malignant endocarditis. Br Med J 1885;i:467–70, 522–6, 577–9.
4. Osler W. Gulstonian lectures on malignant endocarditis. Lecture I. Lancet 1885;1:415–18.
5. Que YA, Moreillon P. Infective endocarditis. Nat Rev Cardiol 2011;8:322–36.
6. Hogevik H, Olaison L, Andersson R, et al. Epidemiologic aspects of infective endocarditis in an urban population: a 5-year prospective study. Medicine (Baltimore) 1995;74:324–39.
7. Berlin JA, Abrutyn E, Strom BL, et al. Incidence of infective endocarditis in the Delaware Valley, 1988-1990. Am J Cardiol 1995;76:933–6.
8. Delahaye F, Goulet V, Lacassin F, et al. Characteristics of infective endocarditis in France 1991: a one year survey. Eur Heart J 1995;16:394–401.
9. Hoen B, Alla F, Selton-Suty C, et al. Changing profile of infective endocarditis: results of a 1-year survey in France. JAMA 2002;288:75–81.
10. Cabell CH, Fowler Jr VG, Engemann JJ, et al. Endocarditis in the elderly: incidence, surgery, and survival in 16,921 patients over 12 years (abstr). Circulation 2002;106:547.
11. Hill EE, Herijgers P, Claus P, et al. Infective endocarditis: changing epidemiology and predictors of 6-month mortality: a prospective cohort study. Eur Heart J 2007;28:196–203.
12. Tleyjeh IM, Abdel-Latif A, Rahbi H, et al. A systematic review of population-based studies of infective endocarditis. Chest 2007;132:1025–35.
13. Pallasch TJ. Antibiotic prophylaxis: problems in paradise. Dent Clin North Am 2003;47:665–79.
14. Lerner PI, Weinstein L. Infective endocarditis in the antibiotic era. N Engl J Med 1966;274:388–93.
15. Johnson CM, Rhodes KH. Pediatric endocarditis. Mayo Clin Proc 1982;57:86–94.
16. Mathew J, Addai T, Anand A, et al. Clinical features, site of involvement, bacteriologic findings, and outcome of infective endocarditis in intravenous drug users. Arch Intern Med 1995;155:1641–8.
17. Griffin MR, Wilson WR, Edwards WD, et al. Infective endocarditis: Olmsted County, Minnesota, 1950 through 1981. JAMA 1985;254:1199–202.
18. McKinsey DS, Ratts TE, Bisno AL. Underlying cardiac lesions in adults with infective endocarditis: the changing spectrum. Am J Med 1987;82:681–8.
19. Cherubin CE, Neu HC. Infective endocarditis at the Presbyterian Hospital in New York City from 1938-1967. Am J Med 1971;51:83–96.
20. Moreillon P, Que Y. Infective endocarditis. Lancet 2004;363:139–49.
21. Baddour LM, Wilson WR, Bayer AS, et al. Infective endocarditis: diagnosis, antimicrobial therapy, and management of complications: a statement for healthcare professionals from the Committee on Rheumatic Fever, Endocarditis, and Kawasaki Disease, Council on Cardiovascular Disease in the Young, and the Councils on Clinical Cardiology, Stroke, and Cardiovascular Surgery and Anesthesia, American Heart Association: endorsed by the Infectious Diseases Society of America. Circulation 2005;111:e394–e434.
22. Gould FK, Denning DW, Elliott TS, et al. Guidelines for the diagnosis and antibiotic treatment of endocarditis in adults: a report of the Working Party of the British Society for Antimicrobial Chemotherapy. J Antimicrob Chemother 2012;67:269–89.
23. Murdoch DR, Corey GR, Hoen B, et al. Clinical presentation, etiology, and outcome of infective endocarditis in the 21st century: the International Collaboration on Endocarditis-Prospective Cohort Study. Arch Intern Med 2009;169:463–73.
24. Tornos P, Iung B, Permanyer-Miralda G, et al. Infective endocarditis in Europe: lessons from the Euro Heart Survey. Heart 2005;91:571–5.
25. Habib G, Hoen B, Tornos P, et al. Guidelines on the prevention, diagnosis, and treatment of infective endocarditis (new version 2009): the Task Force on the Prevention, Diagnosis, and Treatment of Infective Endocarditis of the European Society of Cardiology (ESC). Endorsed by the European Society of Clinical Microbiology and Infectious Diseases (ESCMID) and the International Society of Chemotherapy (ISC) for Infection and Cancer. Eur Heart J 2009;30:2369–413.
26. Stuesse DC, Vlessis AA. Epidemiology of native valve endocarditis. In: Vlessis AA, Bolling SF, editors. Endocarditis: a multidisciplinary approach to modern treatment. Armonk, New York: Futura Publishing Co.; 1999. p. 77–84.
27. Wang A, Athan E, Pappas PA, et al. Contemporary clinical profile and outcome of prosthetic valve endocarditis. JAMA 2007;297:1354–61.
28. Karchmer A. Infective endocarditis. In: Zipes DP, Libby P, Bonow RO, et al, editors. Braunwald's heart disease: a textbook of cardiovascular medicine. Philadelphia: Elsevier Saunders; 2005. p. 1633–56.
29. Grover FL, Cohen DJ, Oprian C, et al. Determinants of the occurrece of and survival from prosthetic valve endocarditis: experience of the VA Cooperative Study on Valve Disease. J Thorac Cardiovasc Surg 1994;108:207–14.
30. Grunkemeier GL, Li H-H. Epidemiology and risk factors for prosthetic valve endocarditis. In: Vlessis AA, Bolling SF, editors. Endocarditis: a multidisciplinary approach to modern treatment. Armonk, NY: Futura Publishing Co.; 1999. p. 85–103.
31. Leontyev S, Borger MA, Modi P, et al. Redo aortic valve surgery: influence of prosthetic valve endocarditis on outcomes. J Thorac Cardiovasc Surg 2011;142:99–105.
32. Miro J, Del Rio A, Mestres C. Infective endocarditis in intravenous drug abusers and HIV-1 infected patients. Infect Dis Clin N Am 2002;16:273–95.
33. Graves MK, Soto L. Left-sided endocarditis in parenteral drug abusers: recent experience at a large community hospital. South Med J 1992;85:378–80.
34. Hecht SR, Berger M. Right-sided endocarditis in intravenous drug users: prognostic features in 102 episodes. Ann Intern Med 1992;117:560–6.
35. Cecchi E, Imazio M, Tidu M, et al. Infective endocarditis in drug addicts: role of HIV infection and the diagnostic accuracy of Duke criteria. J Cardiovasc Med (Hagerstown) 2007;8:169–75.
36. Cabell CH, Heidenreich PA, Chu VH, et al. Increasing rates of cardiac device infections among Medicare beneficiaries: 1990-1999. Am Heart J 2004;147:582–6.
37. Duval X, Selton-Suty C, Alla F, et al. Endocarditis in patients with a permanent pacemaker: a 1-year epidemiological survey on infective endocarditis due to valvular and/or pacemaker infection. Clin Infect Dis 2004;39:68–74.
38. Baddour LM, Epstein AE, Erickson CC, et al. Update on cardiovascular implantable electronic device infections and their management: a scientific statement from the American Heart Association. Circulation 2010;121:458–77.

39. LE KY, Sohail MR, Friedman PA, et al. Clinical predictors of cardiovascular implantable electronic device-related infective endocarditis. Pacing Clin Electrophysiol 2011;34:450–9.

40. Chambers HF, Morris DL, Tauber MG, et al. Cocaine use and the risk for endocarditis in intravenous drug users. Ann Intern Med 1987;106:833–6.

41. Carrel T, Schaffner A, Vogt P, et al. Endocarditis in intravenous drug addicts and HIV infected patients: possibilities and limitations of surgical treatment. J Heart Valve Dis 1993;2:140–7.

42. Greenspon AJ, Prutkin JM, Sohail MR, et al. Timing of the most recent device procedure influences the clinical outcome of lead-associated endocarditis results of the MEDIC (Multicenter Electrophysiologic Device Infection Cohort). J Am Coll Cardiol 2012;59:681–7.

43. Kamalakannan D, Pai RM, Johnson LB, et al. Epidemiology and clinical outcomes of infective endocarditis in hemodialysis patients. Ann Thorac Surg 2007;83:2081–6.

44. Hoen B. Infective endocarditis: a frequent disease in dialysis patients. Nephrol Dial Transplant 2004;19:1360–2.

45. Benito N, Miro JM, de LE, et al. Health care-associated native valve endocarditis: importance of non-nosocomial acquisition. Ann Intern Med 2009;150:586–94.

46. Fowler Jr VG, Miro JM, Hoen B, et al. Staphylococcus aureus endocarditis: a consequence of medical progress. JAMA 2005;293:3012–21.

47. Martin-Davila P, Fortun J, Navas E, et al. Nosocomial endocarditis in a tertiary hospital: an increasing trend in native valve cases. Chest 2005;128:772–9.

48. Finkelstein R, Sobel JD, Nagler A, et al. Staphylococcus aureus bacteremia and endocarditis: comparison of nosocomial and community-acquired infection. J Med 1984;15:193–211.

49. Horstkotte D, Follath F, Gutschik E, et al. Guidelines on prevention, diagnosis and treatment of infective endocarditis executive summary: the task force on infective endocarditis of the European Society of Cardiology. Eur Heart J 2004;25:267–76.

50. Bestetti RB. Cardiac involvement in the acquired immune deficiency syndrome. Int J Cardiol 1989;22:143–6.

51. Nahass RG, Weinstein MP, Bartels J, et al. Infective endocarditis in intravenous drug users: a comparison of human immunodeficiency virus type 1-negative and -positive patients. J Infect Dis 1990;162:967–70.

52. Chu VH, Cabell CH, Benjamin Jr DK, et al. Early predictors of in-hospital death in infective endocarditis. Circulation 2004;109:1745–9.

53. Hasbun R, Vikram HR, Barakat LA, et al. Complicated left-sided native valve endocarditis in adults: risk classification for mortality. JAMA 2003;289:1933–40.

54. Nori US, Manoharan A, Thornby JI, et al. Mortality risk factors in chronic haemodialysis patients with infective endocarditis. Nephrol Dial Transplant 2006;21:2184–90.

55. Jassal DS, Neilan TG, Pradhan AD, et al. Surgical management of infective endocarditis: early predictors of short-term morbidity and mortality. Ann Thorac Surg 2006;82:524–9.

56. Leblebicioglu H, Yilmaz H, Tasova Y, et al. Characteristics and analysis of risk factors for mortality in infective endocarditis. Eur J Epidemiol 2006;21:25–31.

57. Strom BL, Abrutyn E, Berlin JA, et al. Risk factors for infective endocarditis: oral hygiene and nondental exposures. Circulation 2000;102:2842–8.

58. Wilson W, Taubert KA, Gewitz M, et al. Prevention of infective endocarditis: guidelines from the American Heart Association: a guideline from the American Heart Association Rheumatic Fever, Endocarditis and Kawasaki Disease Committee, Council on Cardiovascular Disease in the Young, and the Council on Clinical Cardiology, Council on Cardiovascular Surgery and Anesthesia, and the Quality of Care and Outcomes Research Interdisciplinary Working Group. Circulation 2007;116:1736–54.

59. Gould FK, Elliott TS, Foweraker J, et al. Guidelines for the prevention of endocarditis: report of the Working Party of the British Society for Antimicrobial Chemotherapy. J Antimicrob Chemother 2006;57:1035–42.

60. Warnes CA, Williams RG, Bashore TM, et al. ACC/AHA 2008 Guidelines for the Management of Adults with Congenital Heart Disease: Executive Summary: a report of the American College of Cardiology/American Heart Association Task Force on Practice Guidelines (writing committee to develop guidelines for the management of adults with congenital heart disease). Circulation 2008;118:2395–451.

61. Brooks N. Prophylactic antibiotic treatment to prevent infective endocarditis: new guidance from the National Institute for Health and Clinical Excellence. Heart 2009;95:774–80.

62. Mohindra RK. A case of insufficient evidence equipoise: the NICE guidance on antibiotic prophylaxis for the prevention of infective endocarditis. J Med Ethics 2010;36:567–70.

63. Nishimura RA, Carabello BA, Faxon DP, et al. ACC/AHA 2008 guideline update on valvular heart disease: focused update on infective endocarditis: a report of the American College of Cardiology/American Heart Association Task Force on Practice Guidelines endorsed by the Society of Cardiovascular Anesthesiologists, Society for Cardiovascular Angiography and Interventions, and Society of Thoracic Surgeons. J Am Coll Cardiol 2008;52:676–85.

64. Pharis CS, Conway J, Warren AE, et al. The impact of 2007 infective endocarditis prophylaxis guidelines on the practice of congenital heart disease specialists. Am Heart J 2011;161:123–9.

65. Rahman N, Rogers S, Ryan D, et al. Infective endocarditis prophylaxis and the current AHA, BSAC, NICE and Australian guidelines. J Ir Dent Assoc 2008;54:264–70.

66. Shaw D, Conway DI. Pascal's Wager, infective endocarditis and the "no-lose" philosophy in medicine. Heart 2010;96:15–18.

67. Robard S. Blood velocity and endocarditis. Circulation 1963;27:24–30.

68. Dahl J, Vlessis AA. Pathological and clinical laboratory diagnosis. In: Vlessis AA, Bolling SF, editors. Endocarditis: a multidisciplinary approach to modern treatment. Armonk, NY: Futura Publishing Co.; 1999. p. 19–76.

69. Patti JM, Allen BL, McGavin MJ, et al. MSCRAMM-mediated adherence of microorganisms to host tissues. Ann Rev Microbiol 1994;48:585–617.

70. Heying R, van de Gevel J, Que YA, et al. Contribution of (sub)domains of Staphylococcus aureus fibronectin-binding protein to the proinflammatory and procoagulant response of human vascular endothelial cells. Thromb Haemost 2009;101:495–504.

71. Kreikemeyer B, Klenk M, Podbielski A. The intracellular status of Streptococcus pyogenes: role of extracellular matrix-binding proteins and their regulation. Int J Med Microbiol 2004;294:177–88.

72. Moreillon P, Que YA, Bayer AS. Pathogenesis of streptococcal and staphylococcal endocarditis. Infect Dis Clin North Am 2002;16:297–318.

73. Levine DP, Crane LR, Zervos MJ. Bacteremia in narcotic addicts at the Detroit Medical Center. II: infectious endocarditis: a prospective comparative study. Rev Infect Dis 1986;8:374–96.

74. Grunkemeier GL, Wu Y. The Silzone effect: how to reconcile contradictory reports? Eur J Cardiothorac Surg 2004;25:371–5.

75. McCormick JK, Hirt H, Dunny GM, et al. Pathogenic mechanisms of enterococcal endocarditis. Curr Infect Dis Rep 2000;2:315–21.

76. Paganelli FL, Willems RJ, Leavis HL. Optimizing future treatment of enterococcal infections: attacking the biofilm? Trends Microbiol 2012;20:40–9.

77. Brouqui P, Raoult D. New insight into the diagnosis of fastidious bacterial endocarditis. FEMS Immunol Med Microbiol 2006;47:1–13.

78. Darouiche RO, Hamill RJ. Antibiotic penetration of and bactericidal activity within endothelial cells. Antimicrob Agents Chemother 1994;38:1059–64.

79. Durack DT, Beeson PB. Experimental bacterial endocarditis. I: colonization of a sterile vegetation. Br J Exp Pathol 1972;53:44–9.

80. Roberts GJ. Dentists are innocent! "Everyday" bacteremia is the real culprit: a review and assessment of the evidence that dental surgical procedures are a principal cause of bacterial endocarditis in children. Pediatr Cardiol 1999;20:317–25.

81. Wilson LE, Thomas DL, Astemborski J, et al. Prospective study of infective endocarditis among injection drug users. J Infect Dis 2002;185:1761–6.

82. Dankert J, van der Werff J, Zaat SA, et al. Involvement of bactericidal factors from thrombin-stimulated platelets in clearance of adherent viridans streptococci in experimental infective endocarditis. Infect Immun 1995;63:663–71.

83. Blumental S, Reynders M, Willems A, et al. Enteroviral infection of a cardiac prosthetic device. Clin Infect Dis 2011;52:710–16.

84. Burch GE, Tsui CY. Evolution of coxsackie viral valvular and mural endocarditis in mice. Br J Exp Pathol 1971;53:360.

85. Fournier PE, Thuny F, Richet H, et al. Comprehensive diagnostic strategy for blood culture-negative endocarditis: a prospective study of 819 new cases. Clin Infect Dis 2010;51:131–40.

86. Vuille C, Nidorf M, Weyman AE, et al. Natural history of vegetations during successful medical treatment of endocarditis. Am Heart J 1994;126:1200–9.

87. Osler W. Gulstonian lectures on malignant endocarditis: lecture II. Lancet 1885;1:459–64.

88. Armstrong W, Shea M. Clinical diagnosis of infective endocarditis. In: Vlessis AA, Bolling SF, editors. Endocarditis: a multidisciplinary approach to modern treatment. Armonk, NY: Futura Publishing Co.; 1999. p. 107–34.

89. Alpert JS, Krous HF, Dalen JE, et al. Pathogenesis of Osler's nodes. Ann Intern Med 1976;85:471–3.

90. Falcone PM, Larrison WI. Roth spots seen on ophthalmoscopy: diseases with which they may be associated. Conn Med 1995;59:271–3.

91. Churchill Jr MA, Geraci JE, Hunder GG. Musculoskeletal manifestations of bacterial endocarditis. Ann Intern Med 1977;87:754–9.

92. Hermans PE. The clinical manifestations of infective endocarditis. Mayo Clin Proc 1982;57:15–21.

93. Pruitt AA. Neurologic complications of infective endocarditis. Neurologist 1995;1:20–34.

94. Masuda J, Yutani C, Waki R, et al. Histopathological analysis of the mechanisms of intracranial hemorrhage complicating infective endocarditis. Stroke 1992;23:843–50.

95. Klein I, Iung B, Wolff M, et al. Silent T2* cerebral microbleeds: a potential new imaging clue in infective endocarditis. Neurology 2007;68:2043.

96. Heffner JE. Extracardiac manifestations of bacterial endocarditis. West J Med 1979;131:85–91.

97. Pelletier Jr LL, Petersdorf RG. Infective endocarditis: a review of 125 cases from the University of Washington Hospitals, 1963-72. Medicine 1977;56:287–313.

98. von Reyn CF, Levy BS, Arbeit RD, et al. Infective endocarditis: analysis based on strict definitions. Ann Intern Med 1981;94:505–18.

99. Durack DT, Lukes AS, Bright DK. New criteria for diagnosis of infective endocarditis: utilization of specific echocardiographic findings. Duke Endocarditis Service. Am J Med 1994;96:200–9.

100. Hoen B, Selton-Suty C, Danchin N, et al. Evaluation of the Duke criteria versus the Beth Isreal criteria for the diagnosis of infective endocarditis. Clin Infect Dis 1996;21:905–9.

101. Olaison L, Hogevik H. Comparison of the von Reyn and Duke criteria for the diagnosis of infective endocarditis: a critical analysis of 161 episodes. Scand J Infect Dis 1996;28:399–406.

102. Cecchi E, Trinchero R, Imazio M, et al. Are the Duke criteria really useful for the early bedside diagnosis of infective endocarditis? Results of a prospective multicenter trial. Ital Heart J 2005;6:41–8.

103. Li JS, Sexton DJ, Mick N, et al. Proposed modifications to the Duke criteria for the diagnosis of infective endocarditis. Clin Infect Dis 2000;30:633–8.

104. Palepu A, Cheung SS, Montessori V, et al. Factors other than the Duke criteria associated with infective endocarditis among injection drug users. Clin Invest Med 2002;25:118–25.

105. Heiro M, Helenius H, Sundell J, et al. Utility of serum C-reactive protein in assessing the outcome of infective endocarditis. Eur Heart J 2005;26:1873–81.

106. Verhagen DW, Hermanides J, Korevaar JC, et al. Prognostic value of serial C-reactive protein measurements in left-sided native valve endocarditis. Arch Intern Med 2008;168:302–7.

107. Mueller C, Huber P, Laifer G, et al. Procalcitonin and the early diagnosis of infective endocarditis. Circulation 2004;109:1707–10.

108. Lang S. Getting to the heart of the problem: serological and molecular techniques in the diagnosis of infective endocarditis. Future Microbiol 2008;3:341–9.

109. Stancoven AB, Shiue AB, Khera A, et al. Association of troponin T, detected with highly sensitive assay, and outcomes in infective endocarditis. Am J Cardiol 2011;108:416–20.
110. Shiue AB, Stancoven AB, Purcell JB, et al. Relation of level of B-type natriuretic peptide with outcomes in patients with infective endocarditis. Am J Cardiol 2010;106: 1011–15.
111. Syed FF, Millar BC, Prendergast BD. Molecular technology in context: a current review of diagnosis and management of infective endocarditis. Prog Cardiovasc Dis 2007;50:181–97.
112. Millar BC, Xu J, Moore JE. Risk assessment models and contamination management: implications for broad-range ribosomal DNA PCR as a diagnostic tool in medical bacteriology. J Clin Microbiol 2002;40:1575–80.
113. Voldstedlund M, Norum PL, Baandrup U, et al. Broad-range PCR and sequencing in routine diagnosis of infective endocarditis. APMIS 2008;116:190–8.
114. Cay S. Diagnosis of infective endocarditis: is it always easy? Int J Cardiol 2010;145:226.
115. Cotar AI, Badescu D, Oprea M, et al. Q Fever endocarditis in Romania: the first cases confirmed by direct sequencing. Int J Mol Sci 2011;12:9504–13.
116. Jamil HA, Sandoe JA, Gascoyne-Binzi D, et al. Late-onset prosthetic valve endocarditis caused by *Mycoplasma hominis*, diagnosed using broad-range bacterial PCR. J Med Microbiol 2012;61:300–1.
117. Mencacci A, Leli C, Montagna P, et al. Diagnosis of infective endocarditis: comparison of the LightCycler SeptiFast (Roche Diagnostics) real-time PCR with blood culture. J Med Microbiol 2012;61:881–3.
118. Ruotsalainen E, Karden-Lilja M, Kuusela P, et al. Methicillin-sensitive *Staphylococcus aureus* bacteraemia and endocarditis among injection drug users and nonaddicts: host factors, microbiological and serological characteristics. J Infect 2008;56:249–56.
119. Hill EE, Herijgers P, Claus P, et al. Abscess in infective endocarditis: the value of transesophageal echocardiography and outcome: a 5-year study. Am Heart J 2007;154:923–8.
120. Bayer AS, Bolger AF, Taubert KA, et al. Diagnosis and management of infective endocarditis and its complications. Circulation 1998;98:2936–48.
121. Heidenreich P, Masoudi F, Maini B, et al. Echocardiography in patients with suspected endocarditis: a cost effectiveness analysis. Am J Med 1999;107:198–208.
122. Rosen AB, Fowler VG, Corey GR, et al. Cost-effectiveness of transesophageal echocardiography to determine the duration of therapy for intravascular catheter-associated *Staphylococcus aureus* bacteremia. Ann Intern Med 1999;130:810–20.
123. Vieira ML, Grinberg M, Pomerantzeff PM, et al. Repeated echocardiographic examinations of patients with suspected infective endocarditis. Heart 2004;90:1020–4.
124. Lambl V. Papillare exkreszenzen an der semilunar-klappe der aorta. Wie Med Wochenschr 1856;6:244–7.
125. Sanfilippo AJ, Picard MH, Newell JB, et al. Echocardiographic assessment of patients with infectious endocarditis: prediction of risk for complications. J Am Coll Cardiol 1991;18:1191–9.
126. Tischler MD, Vaitkus PT. The ability of vegetation size on echocardiography to predict clinical complications: a meta-analysis. J Am Soc Echocardiogr 1997;10:562–8.
127. Di Salvo G, Habib G, Pergola V, et al. Echocardiography predicts embolic events in infective endocarditis. J Am Coll Cardiol 2001;37:1069–76.
128. Heinle S, Wilderman N, Harrison JK, et al. Value of transthoracic echocardiography in predicting embolic events in active infective endocarditis. Am J Cardiol 1994;74:799–801.
129. Graupner C, Vilacosta I, SanRoman J, et al. Periannular extension of infective endocarditis. J Am Coll Cardiol 2002;39:1204–11.
130. Sexton DJ, Bashore TM. Infective endocarditis. In: Topol EJ, editor. Textbook of cardiovascular medicine. 2nd ed. Philadelphia: Lippincott Williams & Wilkins; 2002. p. 569–93.
131. Calderwood SB, Swinski LA, Waternaux CM, et al. Risk factors for the development of prosthetic valve endocarditis. Circulation 1985;72:31–7.
132. Gordon SM, Serkey JM, Longworth DL, et al. Early onset prosthetic valve endocarditis: the Cleveland Clinic experience 1992-1997. Ann Thorac Surg 2000;69:1388–92.
133. Hollanders G, De Scheerder I, DeBuyzere M, et al. A six years review of 53 cases of infective endocarditis: clinical, microbiological and therapeutic features. Acta Cardiol 1988;43:121–32.
134. Mills J, Utley J, Abbott J. Heart failure in infective endocarditis: predisposing factors, course and treatment. Chest 1974;66:151–9.
135. Mann T, McLaurin L, Grossman W, et al. Assessing the hemodynamic severity of acute aortic regurgitation due to infective endocarditis. N Engl J Med 1975;293:108–13.
136. Cabell CH, Pond KK, Peterson GE, et al. The risk of stroke and death in patients with aortic and mitral valve endocarditis. Am Heart J 2001;142:75–80.
137. Jones Jr HR, Siekert RG. Neurological manifestations of infective endocarditis. review of clinical and therapeutic challenges. Brain 1989;112:1295–315.
138. Heiro M, Nikoskelainen J, Engblom E, et al. Neurologic manifestations of infective endocarditis: a 17-year experience in a teaching hospital in Finland. Arch Intern Med 2000;160:2781–7.
139. Lamas C, Boia M, Eykyn SJ. Osteoarticular infections complicating infective endocarditis: a study of 30 cases between 1969 and 2002 in a tertiary referral centre. Scand J Infect Dis 2006;38:433–40.
140. Majumdar A, Chowdhary S, Ferreira MA, et al. Renal pathological findings in infective endocarditis. Nephrol Dial Transpl 2000;15:1782–7.
141. Sila C. Anticoagulation should not be used in most patients with stroke with infective endocarditis. Stroke 2011;42:1797–8.
142. Kearon C, Hirsh J. Management of anticoagulation before and after elective surgery. N Engl J Med 1997;336:1506–11.
143. Tornos P, Almirante B, Mirabet S, et al. Infective endocarditis due to *Staphylococcus aureus*: deleterious effect of anticoagulant therapy. Arch Intern Med 1999;159:473–5.
144. Molina CA, Selim MH. Anticoagulation in patients with stroke with infective endocarditis: the sword of Damocles. Stroke 2011;42:1799–800.
145. Fortun J, Navas E, Martinez-Beltran J, et al. Short-course therapy for right-side endocarditis due to *Staphylococcus aureus* in drug abusers: cloxacillin versus glycopeptides in combination with gentamicin. Clin Infect Dis 2003;33:120–5.
146. Mathew J, Abreo G, Namburi K, et al. Results of surgical treatment for infective endocarditis in intravenous drug users. Chest 1995;108:73–7.
147. Mestres CA, Miro JM, Pare JC, et al. Six-year experience with cryopreserved mitral homografts in the treatment of tricuspid valve endocarditis in HIV-infected drug addicts. J Heart Valve Dis 1999;8:575–7.
148. Olaison L, Pettersson G. Current best practices and guidelines: indications for surgical intervention in infective endocarditis. Infect Dis Clin N Am 2002;16:453–75.
149. Ferguson E, Reardon MJ, Letsou GV. The surgical management of bacterial valvular endocarditis. Curr Opin Cardiol 2000;15:82–5.
150. Byrne JG, Rezai K, Sanchez JA, et al. Surgical management of endocarditis: the Society cf Thoracic Surgeons clinical practice guideline. Ann Thorac Surg 2011;91:2012–19.
151. Head SJ, Mokhles MM, Osnabrugge RL, et al. Surgery in current therapy for infective endocarditis. Vasc Health Risk Manag 2011;7:255–63.
152. Prendergast BD, Tornos P. Surgery for infective endocarditis: who and when? Circulation 2010;121:1141–52.
153. Tleyjeh IM, Ghomrawi HM, Steckelberg JM, et al. Conclusion about the association between valve surgery and mortality in an infective endocarditis cohort changed after adjusting for survivor bias. J Clin Epidemiol 2010;63:130–5.
154. Vikram HR, Buenconsejo J, Hasbun R, et al. Impact of valve surgery on 6-month mortality in adults with complicated, left-sided native valve endocarditis. JAMA 2003;290:3207–14.
155. Kiefer T, Park L, Tribouilloy C, et al. Association between valvular surgery and mortality among patients with infective endocarditis complicated by heart failure. JAMA 2011;306:2239–47.
156. Manne MB, Shrestha NK, Lytle BW, et al. Outcomes after surgical treatment of native and prosthetic valve infective endocarditis. Ann Thorac Surg 2012;93:489–93.
157. Lalani T, Cabell CH, Benjamin DK, et al. Analysis of the impact of early surgery on in-hospital mortality of native valve endocarditis: use of propensity score and instrumental variable methods to adjust for treatment-selection bias. Circulation 2010;121:1005–13.
158. Gaca JG, Sheng S, Daneshmand MA, et al. Outcomes for endocarditis surgery in North America: a simplified risk scoring system. J Thorac Cardiovasc Surg 2011;141:98–106.
159. Guerrero ML, Aldamiz G, Bayon J, et al. Long-term survival of salvage cardiac transplantation for infective endocarditis. Ann Thorac Surg 2011;92:e93–e94.
160. Cabell CH, Barsic B, Bayer AS, et al. Clinical findings, complications, and outcomes in a large prospective study of definite endocarditis: the International Collaboration on Endocarditis-Prospective Cohort Study (abstr no. 22). Abstracts of the 7th International Symposium on Modern Concepts in Endocarditis and Cardiovascular Infections, June 26-28, 2003, Chamonix, France.
161. Otto CM. Infective endocarditis. In: Otto CM, editor. Valvular heart disease. Philadelphia: Saunders (Elsevier); 2004. p. 482–521.
162. Nissen H, Nielsen F, Frederiksen M, et al. Native valve infective endocarditis in the general population: a 10-year survey of the clinical picture during the 1980s. Eur Heart J 1992;13:872–7.
163. Tunkel BR, Kaye D. Endocarditis with negative blood cultures. N Engl J Med 1992;326:1215–17.
164. Gavalda J, Len O, Miro JM, et al. Brief communication: treatment of *Enterococcus faecalis* endocarditis with ampicillin plus ceftriaxone. Ann Intern Med 2007;146:574–9.
165. Babcock HM, Ritchie DJ, Christiansen E, et al. Successful treatment of vancomycin-resistant *Enterococcus* endocarditis with oral linezolid. Clin Infect Dis 2001;32:1373–5.
166. Linden PK. Optimizing therapy for vancomycin-resistant enterococci (VRE). Semin Respir Crit Care Med 2007;28:632–45.
167. Berdal JE, Eskesen A. Short-term success, but long-term treatment failure with linezolid for enterococcal endocarditis. Scand J Infect Dis 2008;40:765–6.
168. Hidron AI, Schuetz AN, Nolte FS, et al. Daptomycin resistance in *Enterococcus faecalis* prosthetic valve endocarditis. J Antimicrob Chemother 2008;61:1394–6.
169. Wilson WR, Karchmer A, Dajani AS, et al. Antibiotic treatment of adults with infective endocardits due to streptococci, enterococci, staphylococci, and HACEK microorganisms. JAMA 1995;274:1706–13.
170. Reyes MP, Reyes KC. Gram-negative endocarditis. Curr Infect Dis Rep 2008;10:267–74.
171. Raoult D, Marrie T, Mege J. Natural history and pathophysiology of Q fever. Lancet Infect Dis 2005;5:219–26.
172. Houpikian P, Raoult D. Blood culture-negative endocarditis in a reference center: etiologic diagnosis of 348 cases. Medicine (Baltimore) 2005;84:162–73.
173. Raoult D, Million M, Thuny F, et al. Chronic Q fever detection in the Netherlands. Clin Infect Dis 2011;53:1170–1.
174. Malou N, Renvoise A, Nappez C, et al. Immuno-PCR for the early serological diagnosis of acute infectious diseases: the Q fever paradigm. Eur J Clin Microbiol Infect Dis 2012.
175. Raoult D, Houpikian P, Tissot DH, et al. Treatment of Q fever endocarditis: comparison of 2 regimens containing doxycycline and ofloxacin or hydroxychloroquine. Arch Intern Med 1999;159:167–73.
176. Raoult D, Fournier PE, Drancourt M, et al. Diagnosis of 22 new cases of *Bartonella* endocarditis. Ann Intern Med 1996;125:646–52.
177. Raoult D, Fournier PE, Vandenesch F, et al. Outcome and treatment of *Bartonella* endocarditis. Arch Intern Med 2003;163:226–30.
178. Venditti M. Clinical aspects of invasive candidiasis: endocarditis and other localized infections. Drugs 2009;69(Suppl 1):39–43.
179. Lazaro M, Ramos A, Ussetti P, et al. *Aspergillus* endocarditis in lung transplant recipients: case report and literature review. Transpl Infect Dis 2011;13:186–91.
180. Kalokhe AS, Rouphael N, El Chami MF, et al. *Aspergillus* endocarditis: a review of the literature. Int J Infect Dis 2010;14:e1040–e1047.
181. Herbrecht R, Denning DW, Patterson TF, et al. Voriconazole versus amphotericin B for primary therapy of invasive aspergillosis. N Engl J Med 2002;347:408–15.
182. Varghese GM, Sobel JD. Fungal endocarditis. Curr Infect Dis Rep 2008;10:275–9.

Prosthetic Heart Valves

Patrick T. O'Gara

Key Points

- The need for heart valve replacement surgery marks a major milestone in the natural history of the underlying valve disease. Surgical repair is preferred whenever anatomically feasible and when supported by the experience of the surgeon.
- Valve replacement surgery substitutes a nonimmunogenic foreign body for the native valve. Hemodynamic performance characteristics vary as a function of valve type and size and cardiac output or transvalvular flow. There is a variable degree of stenosis across any mechanical or stented bioprosthetic valve. A small amount of regurgitation is a normal feature of current-generation mechanical valves and of some bioprosthetic valves.
- Mechanical heart valve substitutes are extraordinarily durable but engender an obligate need for lifelong anticoagulation, thus exposing patients to the dual hazards of thromboembolism and bleeding. Bioprosthetic or tissue valves are relatively nonthrombogenic but are susceptible to a predictable rate of structural deterioration over time and the potential need for reoperation. Rates of structural valve deterioration vary as a function of valve type, valve position, and several patient characteristics, such as age at implant, pregnancy, and altered calcium homeostasis. The durability of an aortic homograft does not exceed that of a bovine pericardial valve.
- The novel oral anticoagulants are not approved for use in patients with mechanical heart valves. Management of anticoagulation in pregnant women with mechanical heart valves is very challenging. Choices must be individualized with weekly follow-up during pregnancy.
- The choice of prosthetic heart valve must account for the values and preferences of the individual, informed patient as well as for the trade-offs among durability, anticoagulation, and the aggregate risks of thromboembolism and bleeding. Many patients younger than 60 years now opt to avoid anticoagulation and accept a bioprosthetic valve with an increased likelihood of reoperation. "Valve-in-valve" transcatheter therapies for structural valve deterioration are under investigation.
- Transthoracic echocardiography (TTE) with color-flow Doppler imaging constitutes an integral feature of patient follow-up after valve replacement surgery. In general, there is good correlation between Doppler and catheterization estimates of mean pressure gradients across prosthetic valves, although in certain instances agreement is less robust. The phenomenon of pressure recovery, which may lead to an overestimate of valve gradient, is particularly problematic for bileaflet mechanical valves in the aortic position. Published tables of normal Doppler echocardiographic parameters for prosthetic valves of various makes and sizes should be consulted to help guide management.
- A baseline postoperative TTE is obtained in the first 6 to 12 weeks after operation and serves as a reference against which future comparisons can be made as clinically dictated. Transesophageal echocardiography (TEE) is required for the interrogation of prosthetic valves whenever valve dysfunction, paravalvular leak, or endocarditis is suspected. The frequency with which surveillance TTE is performed depends on the valve type. Routine imaging is not required for mechanical prostheses if there are no symptoms or signs of valve dysfunction. Annual TTE examinations are reasonable after 10 years for bioprosthetic valves. Other imaging modalities may provide corroborative functional information in select circumstances.

- All patients with prosthetic heart valves should receive antibiotic prophylaxis prior to dental procedures that involve manipulation of gingival tissue or the periapical region of teeth or the oral mucosa. Management of prosthetic valve endocarditis requires a multidisciplinary team approach with input from cardiologists, cardiac surgeons, imaging specialists, and infectious disease experts.
- When available, emergency surgery is preferred over fibrinolytic therapy for the management of patients with left-sided prosthetic valve thrombosis (PVT) and shock or New York Heart Association functional class III to IV heart failure. Fibrinolytic therapy is reasonable for patients with small thrombus burden and recent-onset functional class I or II symptoms and for patients with right-sided PVT.
- Severe prosthesis-patient mismatch is an important complication for some patients after valve replacement surgery. Attempts to implant the largest allowable prosthesis are limited by the anatomic constraints posed by the individual patient. Lesser degrees of mismatch are usually well tolerated.

The past six decades have witnessed extraordinary advancements in patient survival and functional outcomes following heart valve replacement surgery. Continued refinements in prosthetic valve design and performance, operative techniques, myocardial preservation, systemic perfusion, cerebral protection, and anesthetic management have enabled the application of surgery to an increasingly wider spectrum of patients. Minimally invasive surgical approaches and the aggressive use of primary valve repair when anatomically appropriate are now the routine in the vast majority of experienced centers. Heart valve teams have been formed to provide multidisciplinary assessment and treatment of patients with complex problems, including the use of transcatheter aortic valve replacement when appropriate.[1] Transcatheter mitral valve techniques remain under active investigation. More than 55,000 aortic or mitral valve replacement operations (with or without coronary artery bypass) were reported to the Society of Thoracic Surgeons' National Adult Cardiac Surgery Database in calendar year 2011.[2] More than 25% of subjects with valvular heart disease in the 2003 Euro Heart Survey had undergone previous heart valve surgery.[3] Familiarity with the specific hemodynamic attributes, durability, thrombogenicity, and inherent limitations of currently available heart valve substitutes, as well as their potential for long-term complications, is critical to appropriate clinical decision making for patients in whom repair is not appropriate or feasible. The choice of valve prosthesis is inherently a trade-off between durability and risk of thromboembolism, with the associated hazards and lifestyle limitations of anticoagulation. The ideal heart valve substitute remains an elusive goal.[4-6] Most surgical centers use a specific type of mechanical or tissue valve for the vast majority of their patients. Although standards have been developed for reporting outcomes after valve surgery,[7] comparisons of prosthetic valve performance are also heavily influenced by patient-, surgeon-, and institutional-related factors.[8]

Mechanical Valves

There are three basic types of mechanical prosthetic valves: bileaflet, tilting disk, and ball-cage (Figure 26-1). The St. Jude bileaflet valve (St. Jude Medical, Inc., St. Paul, Minnesota) was first used in 1977 and is the most frequently implanted mechanical prosthesis worldwide. It consists of two pyrolytic semicircular "leaflets" or disks attached by hinges to a rigid valve ring. The open valve has three orifices: a small, tunnel-like central opening and two larger semi-circular orifies laterally. Its hemodynamic characteristics compare favorably to those of a tilting disk valve (Tables 26-1 and 26-2). Performance indices (the ratio of effective orifice area to the area of the sewing ring) range from 0.40 to 0.70, depending on valve size. Effective orifice areas range from 0.7 cm^2 for a 19-mm valve to 4.2 cm^2 for a 31-mm prosthesis. Average peak velocities are 3.0 ± 0.8 meters per second (m/s) in the aortic position and 1.6 ± 0.3 m/s in the mitral position.[9,10] Peak instantaneous gradients can be estimated using the modified Bernoulli equation, but mean gradient calculations are the more useful clinical parameter. The phenomenon of pressure recovery across bileaflet and ball-cage aortic valves magnifies the estimate of the difference between left ventricular (LV) and aortic pressures (i.e., the systolic gradient), especially when the latter is derived from measurements obtained close to the valve rather than more distally in the ascending aorta[11-13] (Figure 26-2). Additional confounding of the precise measurement occurs from the contribution of flow

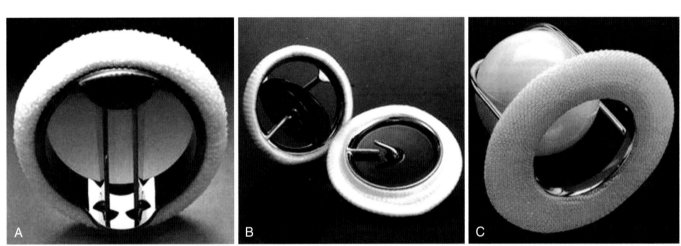

FIGURE 26-1 Mechanical heart valves. A, St. Jude bileaflet valve (St. Jude Medical, Inc., St. Paul, Minnesota). The occluding mechanism consists of two semi-circular leaflets that pivot apart during systole, creating three separate orifices as shown. **B,** Medtronic-Hall tilting disk valve (Medtronic, Inc., Minneapolis, Minnesota). The disk opens to 75 degrees in the aortic model and 70 degrees in the mitral model. It is retained by an S-shaped center guide strut. **C,** Starr-Edwards ball-cage valve (Edwards Lifesciences Corporation, Irvine, California). The poppet is made of siliconized rubber. The sewing ring is more generous than those with bileaflet or tilting disk valves. *(From Antunes MJ, Burke AP, Carabello B, et al. In: Rahimtoola SH, editor. Valvular heart disease. Philadelphia: Current Medicine; 2005. p. 296–7. Braunwald E, series editor. Essential atlas of heart diseases. 3rd ed. vol. XI.)*

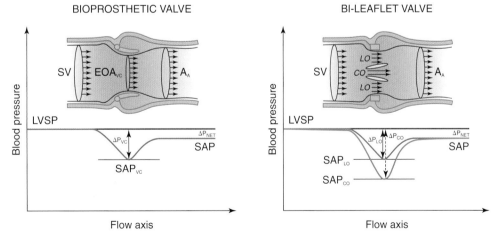

FIGURE 26-2 Pressure recovery. Velocity and pressure changes from the left ventricular (LV) outflow tract to the ascending aorta (A$_A$) in the presence of a stented bioprosthesis *(left)* and a bileaflet mechanical valve *(right)*. Because of pressure recovery, velocities are lower and systolic aortic pressure (SAP) is higher in the distal aorta than at the level of the vena contracta (VC). This phenomenon is more exaggerated in the example of the bileaflet mechanical valve because the velocity is higher in the central orifice (CO), where the pressure drop is higher. Doppler gradients are estimated from the maximal velocity at the level of the vena contracta and represent the maximal pressure drop, whereas catheterization measurements reflect the systolic pressure difference *(ΔP)* between the left ventricle (LV) and the ascending aorta. *EOA,* Effective orifice area; *LO,* lateral orifice; *SP,* systolic pressure; *SV,* stroke volume. *(Adapted from Zoghbi WA, Chambers JB, Dumesnil JG, et al. Recommendations for evaluation of prosthetic valves with echocardiography and Doppler ultrasound. J Am Soc Echocardiogr 2009;22:975–1014.)*

TABLE 26-1   Normal Doppler Echocardiographic Values for Selected Aortic Valve Prostheses

VALVE	TYPE	SIZE	PEAK GRADIENT (mm Hg)	MEAN GRADIENT (mm Hg)	PEAK VELOCITY (m/s)	EFFECTIVE ORIFICE AREA (cm²)
Mechanical						
St. Jude Medical	Bileaflet	19	35.17 ± 11.16	18.96 ± 6.27	2.86 ± 0.48	1.01 ± 0.24
		21	28.34 ± 9.94	15.82 ± 5.67	2.63 ± 0.48	1.33 ± 0.32
		23	25.28 ± 7.89	13.77 ± 5.33	2.57 ± 0.44	1.6 ± 0.43
		25	22.57 ± 7.68	12.65 ± 5.14	2.4 ± 0.45	1.93 ± 0.45
		27	19.85 ± 7.55	11.18 ± 4.82	2.24 ± 0.42	2.35 ± 0.59
		29	17.72 ± 6.42	9.86 ± 2.9	2 ± 0.1	2.81 ± 0.57
		31	16	10 ± 6	2.1 ± 0.6	3.08 ± 1.09
On-X	Bileaflet	19	21.3 ± 10.8	11.8 ± 3.4		1.5 ± 0.2
		21	16.4 ± 5.9	9.9 ± 3.6		1.7 ± 0.4
		23	15.9 ± 6.4	8.5 ± 3.3		2 ± 0.6
		25	16.5 ± 10.2	9 ± 5.3		2.4 ± 0.8
		27-29	11.4 ± 4.6	5.6 ± 2.7		3.2 ± 0.6
Medtronic-Hall	Tilting disk	20	34.37 ± 13.06	17.08 ± 5.28	2.9 ± 0.4	1.21 ± 0.45
		21	26.86 ± 10.54	14.1 ± 5.93	2.42 ± 0.36	1.08 ± 0.17
		23	26.85 ± 8.85	13.5 ± 4.79	2.43 ± 0.59	1.36 ± 0.39
		25	17.13 ± 7.04	9.53 ± 4.26	2.29 ± 0.5	1.9 ± 0.47
		27	18.66 ± 9.71	8.66 ± 5.56	2.07 ± 0.53	1.9 ± 0.16
		29			1.6	
Omniscience	Tilting disk	19	47.5 ± 3.5	28 ± 1.4		0.81 ± 0.01
		21	50.8 ± 2.8	28.2 ± 2.17		0.87 ± 0.13
		23	39.8 ± 8.7	20.1 ± 5.1		0.98 ± 0.07
Starr-Edwards	Ball-and-cage	21	29			1
		22			4 ± 0	
		23	32.6 ± 12.79	21.98 ± 8.8	3.5 ± 0.5	1.1
		24	34.13 ± 10.33	22.09 ± 7.54	3.35 ± 0.48	
		26	31.83 ± 9.01	19.69 ± 6.05	3.18 ± 0.35	
		27	30.82 ± 6.3	18.5 ± 3.7		1.8
		29	29 ± 9.3	16.3 ± 5.5		
Bioprosthetic						
Carpentier-Edwards pericardial	Stented bioprosthesis	19	32.13 ± 3.55	24.19 ± 8.6	24.19 ± 8.6	1.21 ± 0.31
		21	25.69 ± 9.9	20.3 ± 9.08	2.59 ± 0.42	1.47 ± 0.36
		23	21.72 ± 8.57	13.01 ± 5.27	2.29 ± 0.45	1.75 ± 0.28
		25	16.46 ± 5.41	9.04 ± 2.27	2.02 ± 0.31	
		27	19.2 ± 0	5.6	1.6	
		29	17.6 ± 0	11.6	2.1	
Carpentier-Edwards	Stented bioprosthesis	19	43.48 ± 12.72	25.6 ± 8.02		0.85 ± 0.17
		21	27.73 ± 7.6	17.25 ± 6.24	2.37 ± 0.54	1.48 ± 0.3
		23	28.93 ± 7.49	15.92 ± 6.43	2.76 ± 0.4	1.69 ± 0.45
		25	23.94 ± 7.05	12.76 ± 4.43	2.38 ± 0.47	1.94 ± 0.45
		27	22.14 ± 8.24	12.33 ± 5.59	2.31 ± 0.39	2.25 ± 0.55
		29	22	9.92 ± 2.9	2.44 ± 0.43	2.84 ± 0.51
		31			2.41 ± 0.13	
CryoLife-O'Brien stentless	Stentless bioptosthesis	19		12 ± 4.8		1.25 ± 0.1
		21		10.33 ± 2		1.57 ± 0.6
		23		8.5		2.2
		25		7.9		2.3
		27		7.4		2.7
Hancock II	Stented bioprosthesis	21	20 ± 4	14.8 ± 4.1		1.23 ± 0.27
		23	24.72 ±5.73	16.64 ± 6.91		1.39 ± 0.23
		25	20 ± 2	10.7 ± 3		1.47 ± 0.19
		27	14 ± 3			1.55 ± 0.18
		29	15 ± 3			1.6 ± 0.15
Medtronic Mosaic Porcine	Stented bioprosthesis	21		12.43 ± 7.3		1.6 ± 0.7
		23		12.47 ± 7.4		2.1 ± 0.8
		25		10.08 ± 5.1		2.1 ± 1.6
		27		9		
		29		9		
Mitroflow	Stented bioprosthesis	19	18.7 ± 5.1	10.3 ± 3		1.13 ± 0.17
		21	20.2	15.4	2.3	
		23	14.04 ± 4.91	7.56 ± 3.38	1.85 ± 0.34	
		25	17 ± 11.31	10.8 ± 6.51	2 ± 0.71	
		27	13 ± 3	6.57 ± 1.7	1.8 ± 0.2	
Toronto stentless porcine	Stentless bioprosthesis	20	10.9	4.6		1.3
		21	18.64 ± 11.8	7.56 ± 4.4		1.21 ± 0.7
		22	23			1.2
		23	13.55 ± 7.28	7.08 ± 4.33		1.59 ± 0.84
		25	12.17 ± 5.75	6.2 ± 3.05		1.62 ± 0.4
		27	9.96 ± 4.56	4.8 ± 2.33		1.95 ± 0.42
		29	7.91 ± 4.17	3.94 ± 2.15		2.37 ± 0.67

Adapted from Rosenhek R, Binder T, Maurer G, et al. Normal values for Doppler echocardiographic assessment of heart valve prostheses. J Am Soc Echocardiogr 2003;16:1116–27.

TABLE 26-2 Normal Doppler Echocardiographic Values for Selected Mitral Valve Prostheses

VALVE	SIZE	PEAK GRADIENT (mm Hg)	MEAN GRADIENT (mm Hg)	PEAK VELOCITY (m/s)	PRESSURE HALF-TIME (ms)	EFFECTIVE ORIFICE AREA (cm²)
Mechanical						
St. Jude Medical bileaflet	23		4	1.5	160	1
	25		2.5 ± 1	1.34 ± 1.12	75 ± 4	1.35 ± 0.17
	27	11 ± 4	5 ± 1.82	1.61 ± 0.29	75 ± 10	1.67 ± 0.17
	29	10 ± 3	4.15 ± 1.8	1.57 ± 0.29	85 ± 0.29	1.75 ± 0.24
	31	12 ± 6	4.46 ± 2.22	1.59 ± 0.33	74 ± 13	2.03 ± 0.32
On-X bileaflet	25	11.5 ± 3.2	5.3 ± 2.1			1.9 ± 1.1
	27-29	10.3 ± 4.5	4.5 ± 1.6			2.2 ± 0.5
	31-33	9.8 ± 3.8	4.8 ± 2.4			2.5 ± 1.1
Medtronic-Hall tilting disk	27			1.4	78	
	29			1.57 ± 0.1	69 ± 15	
	31			1.45 ± 0.12	77 ± 17	
Bioprosthetic						
Carpentier-Edwards stented bioprosthesis	27		6 ± 2	1.7 ± 0.3	98 ± 28	
	29		4.7 ± 2	1.76 ± 0.27	92 ± 14	
	31		4.4 ± 2	1.54 ± 0.15	92 ± 19	
	33		6 ± 3		93 ± 12	
Hancock II stented bioprosthesis	27					2.21 ± 0.14
	29					2.77 ± 0.11
	31					2.84 ± 0.1
	33					3.15 ± 0.22
Hancock pericardial stented bioprosthesis	29		2.61 ± 1.39	1.42 ± 0.14	105 ± 36	
	31		3.57 ± 1.02	1.51 ± 0.27	81 ± 23	
Mitroflow stented bioprosthesis	25		6.9	2	90	
	27		3.07 ± 0.91	1.5	90 ± 20	
	29		3.5 ± 1.65	1.43 ± 0.29	102 ± 21	
	31		3.85 ± 0.81	1.32 ± 0.26	91 ± 22	

Adapted from Rosenhek R, Binder T, Maurer G, et al. Normal Valves for Doppler echocardiographic assessment of heart valve prostheses. J Am Soc Echocardiogr 2003;16:1116–27.

acceleration through the narrow central orifice of a bileaflet valve.[14] Thus, Doppler velocity determinations can overestimate the transvalvular gradient across bileaflet valves. Published reference tables of expected velocities for the various valve sizes should be consulted, and comparison with baseline postoperative studies made, to avoid misdiagnosis of prosthetic valve stenosis.[15] The Carbomedics valve (Sorin Group, Milan) is a variation of the St. Jude prosthesis that can be rotated to prevent limitation of leaflet excursion by subvalvular tissue. Both types of bileaflet valves have a small amount of normal regurgitation ("washing jet") designed in part to decrease the risk of thrombosis. A small central jet and two converging jets emanating from the hinge points of the disks can be visualized on color-flow Doppler imaging.[16-18]

There are two principal tilting disk valves in clinical use. The Medtronic-Hall valve (Medtronic, Inc., Minneapolis, Minnesota) has a thin, circular disk of tungsten-impregnated graphite with pyrolytic coating, secured at its center by a curved, central guide strut, within titanium housing. The sewing ring is made of polytetrafluoroethylene (Teflon). The disk opens to 75 degrees in the aortic model and to 70 degrees in the mitral model. The Omniscience valve (Medical CV, Inc., Inner Grove Heights, Minnesota) disk is made of pyrolytic carbon and has a seamless polyester knit sewing ring. The disk opens to 80 degrees and closes at an angle of 12 degrees to the annular plane. For both valve types, the major orifice is semicircular in cross-section. Because the disk does not open to 90 degrees, there is slight resistance to flow with estimated pressure gradients of 5 to 25 mm Hg in the aortic position and 5 to 10 mm Hg in the mitral position[19] (see Tables 26-1 and 26-2). Effective orifice areas depend on valve size and range from 1.6 to 3.7 cm², with performance indices of 0.40 to 0.65, similar to those reported for bileaflet mechanical valves.[20] Tilting disk valves also have a small amount of regurgitation, which arises from small gaps at the perimeter of the valve.[16,21] With Medtronic-Hall valves, there is also a small amount of regurgitation around the central guide strut.[19]

The bulky Starr-Edwards ball-cage valve, the oldest commercially available prosthetic heart valve (first used in 1965), is now very rarely implanted. Because of its sheer size, it is not suitable for use in the mitral position in patients with small LV cavities, in the aortic position in patients with small aortic root sizes, or for composite aortic valve-root reconstruction. The poppet is made of silicone rubber, the cage of Stellite alloy, and the sewing ring of Teflon/polypropylene cloth. The aortic cage is formed by three arches located at 120-degree intervals around the sewing ring. The ball-cage valve is more thrombogenic, and has less favorable hemodynamic performance characteristics, than both bileaflet and tilting disk valves. Antegrade flow occurs around the ball and through the struts of the cage. There is a small amount of regurgitant backflow before the ball seats following ejection.[19]

Durability and Long-Term Outcomes

Currently available mechanical valves have excellent long-term durability, with up to 45 years for the Starr-Edwards valve and more than 30 years for the St. Jude valve. In a randomized trial comparing the Starr-Edwards valve with the mechanical St. Jude valve, there were no differences in total or event-free survival rates through 8 years of follow-up for patients receiving either aortic valve replacement (AVR) or mitral valve replacement (MVR).[22] Structural deterioration, exemplified by some older-generation Bjork-Shiley (strut fracture with disk embolization) and Starr-Edwards (ball variance) prostheses, is now extremely rare. Ten-year freedom from valve-related death exceeds 90% for both St. Jude and Carbomedics bileaflet valves.[23] The Medtronic-Hall prosthesis has achieved comparable longevity.[24] Actuarial survival rates—which also depend importantly on several patient factors, such as age, gender, ventricular function, coronary artery disease, functional status, and major comorbidities—range from 94% ± 2% at 10 years for St. Jude valves, to 85% ± 3% at 9 years for

TABLE 26-3   Long-Term Outcome after Mechanical Valve Replacement: Selected Series

| VALVE TYPE | REFERENCE | YEARS IMPLANTED | N | MEAN AGE | SURVIVAL | Complications (%/Patient-Year) | | | |
						THROMBO-EMBOLISM	BLEEDING	PROSTHETIC VALVE ENDOCARDITIS	VALVE THROMBOSIS
Bileaflet									
St. Jude	118	1977-1987	1298	62 ± 13	Event-free: 67 ± 8% at 9 yr	1.5	0.56	0.16	0.09
St. Jude	25	1978-1991	91	39 (range 15-50)	94 ± 2% at 10 yr	0.6	0.8	0.4	—
St. Jude AVR	29	1977-1997	1419	63 ± 14	Actuarial: 82% at 5 yr 51% at 15 yr 45% at 19 yr				
St Jude AVR + coronary artery bypass grafting surgery	29	1977-1997	971	70 ± 10	Actuarial: 72% at 5 yr 45% at 10 yr 15% at 19 yr				
Carbomedics	28	1989-1997	1019	61 ± 10	Event-free: 82% at 7 yr Mortality rate 2.9%/yr	1.0	1.7	0.1	0.1
Tilting Disk									
Medtronic-Hall	24	1977-1987	1104	56	Actuarial: AVR 46 ± 2 % at 15 yr MVR 42 ± 4 % at 15 yr DVR 28 ± 5 % at 15 yr	1.8 1.9 1.9	1.2		0.05 0.19 0.13
Ball-Cage									
Starr-Edwards	26	1963-1977	362	40±10 yr	Event-free: AVR 66.4% at 10 yr MVR 73.4%	1.36% 1.25	1.06 0.56	—	—
Starr-Edwards	27	1969-1991	1100	57 yr	59.6% at 10 yr 31.2% at 20 yr	1.26	0.18	0.39	0.02

AVR, Aortic valve replacement; *DVR*, double valve replacement; *MVR*, mitral valve replacement.

Omniscience valves, and 60% to 70% at 10 years for Starr-Edwards valves[25-31] (Table 26-3). Long-term issues associated with mechanical valves include infective endocarditis, paravalvular leaks, hemolytic anemia, thromboembolism/valve thrombosis, pannus ingrowth, and hemorrhagic complications related to anticoagulation. All patients with mechanical valves require lifelong anticoagulation with a vitamin K antagonist (VKA), the intensity of which varies as a function of prosthesis type, position, and number. Bileaflet and current-generation tilting disk valves are significantly less thrombogenic than the ball-cage valve or older generation Bjork-Shiley valves. Higher-intensity anticoagulation is required for mechanical valves placed in the mitral versus the aortic position, for patients with multiple mechanical prostheses, and often for patients with additional risk factors for thromboembolism, such as atrial fibrillation (AF). Even with appropriately targeted anticoagulation, reported rates of thromboembolism range from 0.6 to 3.3 per 100 patient-years for patients with bileaflet or tilting disk valves.[26,27,30-32] Complications related to anticoagulation in this population occur at rates of 0.9 to 2.3 per 100 patient-years.[33] A thromboembolism rate of 1.4 per 100 patient-years has been reported for the Starr-Edwards 1260 model valve.[29]

Tissue Valves

Tissue valves, or bioprostheses, include stented and stentless heterografts (porcine, bovine), also referred to as "xenografts," homografts (or allografts) from human cadaveric sources, and autografts of pericardial or pulmonic valve origin. They provide an alternative, less thrombogenic heart valve substitute for which long-term anticoagulation in the absence of additional risk factors is not required.

Stented Heterograft Valves

The stented heterograft valve is a trileaflet valve with a circular opening in systole (Figure 26-3). Porcine valves (e.g., Carpentier-Edwards, Hancock) are constructed of glutaraldehyde-fixed porcine aortic leaflets mounted on semisynthetic rigid or flexible stents and the sewing ring. One of the three leaflets of the porcine aortic valve is muscular and is typically replaced during construction with a fibrous leaflet from a second valve.[34,35] There have been several iterative design improvements over time, including glutaraldehyde fixation at low or zero pressure, reconfiguration of the sewing ring, and treatments to retard calcification and reduce leaflet stiffness. The newer bovine pericardial valves (Carpentier-Edwards PERIMOUNT; see Figure 26-3) offer better hemodynamic performance than earlier-generation porcine bioprostheses (see Tables 26-1 and 26-2). In the aortic position, the antegrade velocity varies as a function of valve size but approximates 2.4 m/s, with a mean gradient of 14 mm Hg, and indexed valve area of 1.04 cm^2/m^2.[9] The pericardial aortic valve has a larger effective orifice area at any given valve size between 19 and 29. The average peak gradient in the mitral position is 9 ± 3 mm Hg and effective orifice area 2.5 ± 0.6 cm^2.[36] A small degree of regurgitation can be detected by color-flow Doppler imaging in 10% of normally functioning bioprostheses. In a prospective randomized trial of patients with aortic valve disease, the Carpentier-Edwards

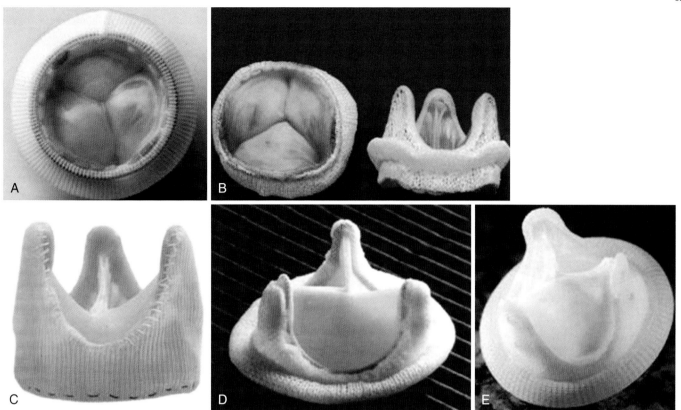

FIGURE 26-3   Bioprosthetic heart valves. A, Hancock modified-orifice (MO) stented valve (Medtronic, Inc., Minneapolis, Minnesota). The MO valve is produced by replacing the muscular right coronary cusp with the noncoronary cusp from another porcine valve. **B,** Carpentier-Edwards stented porcine valve (Edwards Lifesciences Corporation, Irvine, California). The annulus is purposefully asymmetric to obliterate the muscular septal ridge of the porcine right coronary cusp. **C,** St. Jude Medical Toronto SPV stentless valve (St. Jude Medical, Inc., St. Paul, Minnesota). **D,** Carpentier-Edwards pericardial valve (Edwards Lifesciences Corporation). **E,** Autologous pericardial valve. *(From Antunes MJ, Burke AP, Carabello B, et al. In: Rahimtoola SH, editor. Valvular heart disease. Philadelphia: Current Medicine; 2005. p. 296–7. Braunwald E, series editor. Essential atlas of heart diseases, 3rd ed. vol. XI.)*

PERIMOUNT Magna bovine pericardial valve (Edwards Lifesciences Corporation) demonstrated better hemodynamic performance and greater LV mass regression over 5 postoperative years than the newer-generation Medtronic Mosaic porcine valve (Medtronic, Inc.).[37] The major drawback with earlier-generation stented porcine valves was their limited durability, typically beginning within 5 to 7 years after implantation but varying with position and age at implant, with tissue changes characterized by calcification, fibrosis, tears, and perforations (Figure 26-4).[38] Structural valve deterioration (SVD) occurs earlier for mitral than for aortic bioprosthetic valves, perhaps because of exposure of the mitral prosthesis to relatively higher LV closing pressures (Table 26-4). The process of SVD is accelerated in younger patients, in those with disordered calcium metabolism (end-stage renal disease), and, possibly, in pregnant women independent of younger age (Figure 26-5). In several older series, the estimated rate of SVD of porcine valves was 3.3% per patient-year, with freedom from valve failure at 10 years of 78% ± 2% for aortic valves and 69% ± 2% per patient-year for mitral valves.[39-41] The rate of valve failure accelerates further after 10 years, such that the actuarial freedom from porcine bioprosthetic SVD is 49% ± 4% at 15 years for aortic valves and 32% ± 4% for mitral valves.[36] By comparison, the rate of freedom from primary tissue failure with pericardial aortic valves is 86% at 12 years (Figure 26-6; see Table 26-4).[42]

Stentless Heterograft Valves

The rigid sewing ring and stent-based construction of certain bioprostheses allow for easier implantation and maintenance of the three-dimensional relationships of the leaflets. However,

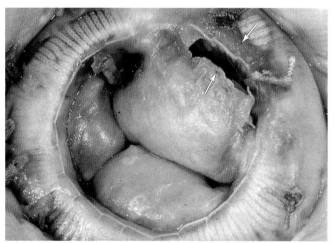

FIGURE 26-4   Bioprosthetic structural valve deterioration. Five-year-old mitral Hancock porcine valve. There is a linear tear at the base of one of the 3 cusps *(white arrows). (From Antunes MJ, Burke AP, Carabello B, et al. In: Rahimtoola SH, editor. Valvular heart disease. Philadelphia: Current Medicine; 2005. p. 296–7. Braunwald E, series editor. Essential atlas of heart diseases. 3rd ed. vol. XI.)*

these features also contribute to impaired hemodynamic performance and accelerated SVD. Stentless porcine valves (Toronto SPV [St. Jude Medical, Inc.], Edwards Prima; see Figure 26-3) were developed in part to address these issues. Their use has been restricted to the aortic position. Implantation is technically more challenging, whether in a subcoronary position or as part

TABLE 26-4 Long-Term Outcome after Tissue Valve Replacement: Selected Series

VALVE TYPE	REFERENCE	YEARS IMPLANTED	N	AGE (YR ± SD)	ACTUARIAL SURVIVAL	FREEDOM FROM OR (ANNUAL RATE) OF THROMBOEMBOLISM	FREEDOM FROM OR (ANNUAL RATE OF) STRUCTURAL VALVE DETERIORATION
Stented Heterografts							
Porcine (Hancock and Carpentier-Edwards)	39	1971-1990	2,879	AVR 60 ± 15	77 ± 1% at 5 yr 54 ± 2% at 10 yr 32 ±3 % at 15 yr	92 ± 1% at 10 yr	78 ± 2% at 10 yr 49 ± 4% at 15 yr
				MVR 58 ± 13	70 ± 1% at 5 yr 50 ± 2% at 10 yr 32 ± 3% at 15 yr	86 ± 1% at 10 yr	69 ± 2% at 10 yr 32 ± 4% at 15 yr
Carpentier-Edwards Porcine	40	1975-1986	1,195	57.3	57.4 ± 1.5% at 10 yr	(1.6%/pt-yr)	(3.3%/pt-year)
Carpentier-Edwards Pericardial	42	1984-1995	254	71 (range 25-87)	80 ± 3% at 5 yr 50 ± 8 at 10 yr 36 ± 9 at 12 yr	67 ± 13% at 12 yr	86 ± 9% at 12 yr
Stentless Heterografts							
Toronto SPV	David et al.*	1987-1993	123	61 ± 12	91 ± 4% at 6 yr	87± 7% at 6 yr	(0%)
Edwards Prima	Dossche et al.*	1991-1993	200	68.5 ± 8	95% at 1 yr	(3% at 1 year)	(AV block requiring pacer 7% at 1 yr, mild AR 27% at 1yr)
Homografts							
Cryopreserved	Kirklin et al.*	1981-1991	18	46	85% at 8 yr		85% at 8 yr
Antibiotic sterilized, subcoronary	Langley et al.*	1973-1983	200	50	81 ± 3% at 10 yr 58 ± 4 % at 20 yr	81 ± 3% at 10 yr 31 ± 5% at 20 yr	
Pulmonic Autografts							
Pulmonic autografts	Elkins et al.*	1986-1995	195	8 mo-62 yr			95 ± 2% at 2 yr 81 ± 5% at 8 yr
Pulmonary autografts	El-Hamamsy et al.*	1994-2001	108	38 (range 19-66)	95% at 5 yr 95% at 10 yr		99% freedom from reoperation at 10 yr

AV, Atrioventricular; *AVR*, aortic valve replacement; *MVR*, mitral valve replacement.

*Data from: David TE, Feindel CM, Bos J, et al. Aortic valve replacement with a stentless porcine aortic valve: a six-year experience. J Thorac Cardiovasc Surg 1994;108:1030-6 ; Yun KL, Sintek CF, Fletcher AD, et al. Aortic valve replacement with the freestyle stentless bioprosthesis: five-year experience. Circulation 1999;100 (19 Suppl): II17-23 ; Dossche K, Vanermen H, Daenen W, et al. Hemodynamic performance of the PRIMA Edwards stentless aortic xenograft: early results of a multicenter clinical trial. Thorac Cardiovasc Surg 1996;44:11-4; Kirklin JK, Smith D, Novick W, et al. Long-term function of cryopreserved aortic homografts: a ten-year study. J Thorac Cardiovasc Surg 1993;106:154-65; Langley SM, McGuirk SP, Chaudhry MA, et al. Twenty-year follow-up of aortic valve replacement with antibiotic sterilized homografts in 200 patients. Semin Thorac Cardiovasc Surg 1999;11(4 Suppl 1):28-34 ; Elkins RC, Lane MM, McCue C. Pulmonary autograft reoperation: incidence and management. Ann Thorac Surg 1996;62:450-5 ; El-Hamamsy I, Eryigit Z, Stevens LM, et al. Long-term outcoms after autograft versus homograft aortic root replacement in adults with aortic valve disease: a randomised controlled trial. Lancet 2010;376:524-31

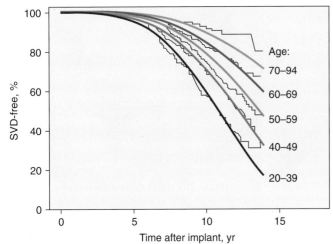

FIGURE 26-5 Freedom from structural valve deterioration (SVD). Actuarial freedom from SVD for 4910 operative survivors of isolated aortic or mitral valve replacement with Hancock (Medtronic, Inc., Minneapolis, Minnesota) or Carpentier-Edwards (Edwards Lifesciences Corporation, Irvine, California) porcine valves. The curves are stratified by age group and show a significantly lower rate of SVD for older than for younger patients. A Weibull regression model based on patient age and valve position (*smooth lines*) was used to fit the actuarial Kaplan-Meier curves (*jagged lines*). (*Adapted from Grunkemeier GL, Jamieson WRE, Miller DC, et al. Actual vs. actuarial risk of structural valve deterioration. J Thorac Cardiovasc Surg 1994;108:709–18.*)

of a mini-root procedure, and hence these valves are preferred by only a minority of surgeons. Early postoperative mean gradients can be lower than 15 mm Hg, with further improvement in valve performance over time as a result of aortic root remodeling, lower peak exercise transvalvular gradients, and more rapid reduction in LV mass.[43-49] There is a low incidence of important aortic regurgitation (AR), although results will vary as a function of technical expertise and appropriate valve sizing at time of implant. David et al[50] reported freedom from SVD with the Toronto SPV at 12 years of 69% ± 4%, 52% ± 8% for patients younger than 65 years, and 85% ± 4% for patients 65 and older.[50] This group has limited the use of this stentless valve to older patients with small aortic annuli. They have also emphasized the marked mortality hazard for reoperation for valve failure within 1 year of implantation.[50]

Homografts

Aortic valve homografts are harvested from human cadavers within 24 hours of death as blocks of tissue comprising the ascending aorta, aortic valve, a portion of the interventricular septum, and the anterior mitral valve leaflet. They are treated with antibiotics and cryopreserved at −196° C.[51] They are now most commonly implanted in the form of a total root replacement with reimplantation of the coronary arteries and trimming of any excess tissue not required for primary valve replacement. Sizing is based on echocardiographic measurement of the dimensions

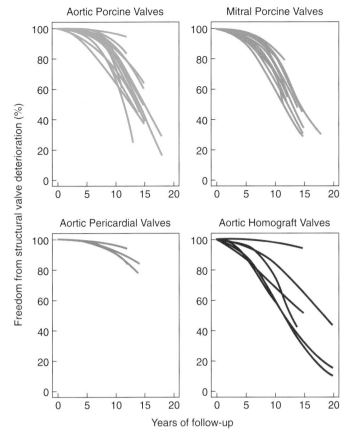

FIGURE 26-6 Freedom from structural valve deterioration (SVD). Weibull distribution curves for freedom from SVD for four types of tissue valves. Note the more gradual rate of SVD for aortic pericardial valves. *(Adapted from Grunkemeier GL, Li H-H, Naftel DC, et al. Long-term performance of heart valve prostheses. Curr Prob Cardiol 2000;25:73–156.)*

appropriate selection of young patients by expert surgeons at experienced centers of excellence, operative mortality rates are less than 1% and freedom from valve–related death is as high as 84% ± 6% at 14 years.[67-70] Advantages of the autograft include the ability to increase in size during childhood growth, excellent hemodynamic performance characteristics, lack of thrombogenicity, and resistance to infection. The hemodynamic performance characteristics of the pulmonary autograft are similar to those of a normal, native aortic valve both at rest and with exercise. However, the homograft in the pulmonic position has a higher mean gradient at rest (9 ±7 mm Hg) and with exercise (21 ± 14 mm Hg) than a normal, native pulmonic valve.[71-73] Early homograft stenosis occurs in 10% to 20% of patients and is due to extrinsic compression from inflammation and adventitial fibrosis.[74,75] The procedure is usually reserved for children and young adults but should be avoided in patients with dilated roots, given the unacceptably high incidence of accelerated degeneration and pulmonary autograft dilation with significant regurgitation. The Ross procedure is not practiced widely, and surgical opinions differ regarding the best approach to the child or young adult with aortic valve disease. The durability of the operation has also been called into question; the rate of SVD at 10 years approximates 30%.[54,61,67-69,76-79] Reoperation can be especially hazardous.[80] The use of pericardial autograft valves for either aortic or mitral replacement, in which the patient's own pericardium is fashioned onto a frame in the operating room, has had very limited support despite excellent hemodynamic performance characteristics and durability in small patient subsets.[81]

Comparison of Mechanical and Tissue Valves

Obvious differences between valve types relate to durability (i.e., indefinite for mechanical versus limited for tissue valves) and need for anticoagulation (i.e., obligatory for mechanical versus none for tissue valves in the absence of other risk factors for thromboembolism). Short- to intermediate-term hemodynamic performance characteristics for low-profile mechanical prostheses (e.g., St. Jude) are comparable to those for stented tissue valves of similar size. There are no important differences in rates of prosthetic valve endocarditis (PVE), although some series have suggested a higher incidence of early (<1 year) infection with mechanical valves than with tissue heterografts.[82] Two earlier randomized trials compared long-term outcomes with a spherical tilting disk valve (Bjork Shiley) and with a stented porcine valve (Hancock or Carpentier-Edwards). In the Veterans Affairs trial, 575 men were randomly assigned to one of the two groups between 1977 and 1982; 394 underwent AVR, and 181 MVR.[83] Among those undergoing AVR, survival at 15 years was better with mechanical AVR (34% ± 3% vs. 21% ± 3%, P = 0.02; Figure 26-7), whereas there was no difference in survival between mechanical and tissue MVR procedures (81% and 79%, respectively). With AVR, the increased mortality among patients allocated a tissue prosthesis was driven largely by the higher rate of SVD and risks associated with reoperation. SVD occurred predominantly in patients younger than 65 years, beginning at 5 to 6 years after MVR and 7 to 8 years after AVR. In patients undergoing AVR, the cumulative incidence of SVD was 23% ± 5% for tissue valves and 0% ± 0% for mechanical valves, and in patients undergoing MVR, 44% ± 8% for tissue valves and 5% ± 4% for mechanical valves. There was an increased risk of bleeding with mechanical valve replacement, but no significant differences were observed for other valve-related complications, such as thromboembolism and PVE. In the Edinburgh Heart Valve Trial, 541 men and women were randomly allocated to treatments between 1975 and 1979 and followed up for a mean of 12 years after AVR (n = 211), MVR (n = 261), or AVR + MVR (n = 61).[84] There was a trend toward improved survival with mechanical valve replacement (P = 0.08) and higher rates of reoperation with tissue valve replacement (AVR 22.6 ± 5.7% vs. 4.2 ± 2.1%, P <0.01; MVR

of the aortic annulus and sinotubular junction. Homograft valves appear resistant to infection and are preferred by many surgeons for management of aortic valve and root endocarditis in the active phase. Neither immunosuppression nor routine anticoagulation is required. Despite earlier expectations, long-term durability of such homografts beyond 10 years is not superior to that for current-generation pericardial valves.[52-54] In an echocardiographic follow-up study of 570 patients with aortic valve homografts, 72% had signs of valve dysfunction at 6.8 ± 4.1 years after implantation, with moderate to severe AR in 15.4 %, moderate aortic stenosis (AS) in 10%, and severe aortic stenosis in 2.5%.[55] Rates of homograft reoperation at 15 years for SVD, which do not account for all cases of SVD, approximate 20% for patients 41 to 60 years of age and 16% for those older than 60 years at time of implantation.[56] Excessive leaflet and root calcification renders reoperation particularly challenging. Mitral homograft valve replacement, a considerably complex technical feat, is not advocated.

Autografts

In the Ross procedure, the patient's own pulmonic valve or autograft is harvested as a small tissue block containing the pulmonic valve, annulus, and proximal pulmonary artery, and is inserted in the aortic position, usually as a complete root replacement with reimplantation of the coronary arteries.[57-66] The pulmonic valve and right ventricular outflow tract are then replaced with either an aortic or pulmonic homograft. Thus, the procedure requires two separate valve operations, a longer time with the patient on cardiopulmonary bypass, and a steep learning curve. With

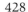

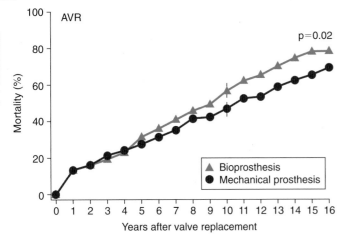

FIGURE 26-7 **Veterans Affairs randomized trial results.** Mortality rates after aortic valve replacement with a mechanical prosthesis (Bjork-Shiley, Pfizer, Inc., New York) and a stented porcine prosthesis (Hancock, (Medtronic, Inc., Minneapolis, Minnesota)). At 15 years, mortality was 66 ± 3% for mechanical valve vs. 79 ± 3% for the porcine valve *P* = 0.02). *(From Hammermeister K, Sethi GK, Henderson WG, et al. Outcomes 15 years after valve replacement with a mechanical versus a bioprosthetic valve: final report of the Veteran Affairs randomized trial. J Am Coll Cardiol 2000;36:1152–8.)*

43.1 ± 6.0% vs. 9.9 ± 3.2%, *P* <0.001). Bleeding rates were higher with mechanical AVR, but there were no differences in rates of thromboembolism or PVE. A meta-analysis found no differences in survival between mechanical and tissue valves when patient age and risk factors were included in the model.[85] A later, smaller randomized trial of 313 patients 55 to 70 years of age with aortic valve disease also found no difference in late survival between newer-generation mechanical and tissue prostheses, with higher rates of SVD and reoperation in patients with tissue valves but no other differences in secondary end points.[86] In an analysis of data from more than 39,000 patients aged 65 to 80 years undergoing AVR reported to the Society of Thoracic Surgeons (STS) Adult Cardiac Surgery Database and linked to Medicare, patients receiving a bioprosthesis had similar adjusted risks for death, higher risks for reoperation and endocarditis, and lower risks for stroke and bleeding in comparison with patients receiving a mechanical valve. Of note, patients aged 65 to 69 years had a substantially elevated 12-year absolute risk of reoperation (10.5%).[87] In a separate analysis of the same database, the proportion of patients older than 70 years who received a tissue prosthesis at the time of valve replacement increased from 87% to 96% between 2004 and 2009 without any associated rise in rates of adverse events.[88]

Choice of Prosthetic Heart Valve

The need for heart valve replacement surgery marks a major milestone in the natural history of the underlying disease and mandates that clinical indications for the procedure are convincingly met and that valve repair by an experienced surgeon is not an option. Because there is no perfect heart valve substitute, judgment and compromise are required. Important factors to consider include patient age, the desire for pregnancy, the anatomic nature of the valve lesion, the presence of infection, the experience of the surgeon, the risks of anticoagulation, the patient's willingness and ability to take anticoagulant medications reliably, the likelihood of reoperation for SVD over 10 to 15 years, and patient preferences and values.[8] There has been a clear trend favoring the use of tissue valves, related to improved durability with current-generation pericardial prostheses, lower rates of mortality and major morbidity with reoperation, and strong patient preferences to avoid the lifestyle limitations and hazards of anticoagulation. The balanced recommendations set

forth by both American College of Cardiology/American Heart Association (ACC/AHA) and European Society of Cardiology/European Association for Cardio-Thoracic Surgery (ESC/EACTS) guideline writing committees for patients with valvular heart disease are a useful reference for clinical decision making.[89,90] A bioprosthesis is recommended for any patient for whom anticoagulation is contraindicated, cannot be managed appropriately, or is not desired (class I recommendation). A bioprosthesis is reasonable for young women contemplating pregnancy (to avoid the hazards of anticoagulation in this setting) and for patients older than 70 years (class IIa). A mechanical prosthesis is reasonable for patients younger than 60 years who can be safely managed with anticoagulants and for patients in whom reoperation would be particularly hazardous (e.g., in the setting of radiation heart disease) (class IIa). Either a bioprosthesis or a mechanical prosthesis is reasonable for patients between ages 60 and 70 years, depending on their preferences and values and the safety of anticoagulation. In younger patients who opt for a bioprosthesis, the anticipated risk of reoperation should be low. Because there may be exceptions to these broad recommendations, shared decision making should be individualized.[89,90]

Medical Management and Surveillance after Valve Replacement

Anticoagulant Therapy

All patients with mechanical heart valves require lifelong anticoagulation with a VKA, the intensity of which varies as a function of valve type or thrombogenicity, valve position and number, and the presence of additional risk factors for thromboembolism, such as AF, LV systolic dysfunction, a history of thromboembolism, and hypercoagulable state. Anticoagulation should be initiated as soon after surgery as is deemed safe, preferably within the first 2 days, beginning with intravenous unfractionated heparin (UFH) and transitioning to a VKA. The risk of thromboembolism is highest in the first postoperative month.

For patients undergoing AVR, a target international normalized ratio (INR) of 2.5 (range 2.0-3.0) is recommended for patients at low-risk of thromboembolism, such as those with either a St. Jude bileaflet or Medtronic-Hall tilting disk AVR in sinus rhythm with normal LV systolic function and no risk factors (Table 26-5). A higher target INR (3.0, range 2.5-3.5) is recommended if additional risk factors for thromboembolism are present or if the mechanical valve used is more thrombogenic (Bjork-Shiley, Omniscience, Starr-Edwards). Patients undergoing MVR with mechanical valves are managed with a target INR of 3.0 (range 2.5-3.5), irrespective of valve type. Those with a bioprosthetic valve and risk factors for thromboembolism are managed with a target INR of 2.5 (range 2.0-3.0). There is general agreement that patients who have bioprosthetic mitral valves and no risk factors should be treated with a VKA for the first three postoperative months to a target INR of 2.5 (range 2.0-3.0) but there is a lack of consensus regarding the need for any VKA therapy over this time for patients who have bioprosthetic aortic valves and no risk factors. These latter patients are most often managed with aspirin alone.[89-91] However, a report from the Danish National Patient Registry has highlighted an association between the discontinuation of warfarin within 6 months of bioprosthetic AVR and an increased risk of cardiovascular death,[92] and thus the use of warfarin in this setting may be considered for 6 months after surgery.

Longer-term treatment of low-risk patients undergoing bioprosthetic AVR or MVR consists of low-dose aspirin, although there are no data to support this practice. The development of thromboembolism at therapeutic levels of anticoagulation is managed by the addition of low-dose aspirin and/or by an increase in the target INR and range. The addition of low-dose aspirin to therapeutic anticoagulation is recommended for all patients with mechanical heart valves (see Table 26-5),[89,91,93] but only if the

TABLE 26-5	Antithrombotic Therapy in Patients with Prosthetic Heart Valves*			
	ASPIRIN (75-100 mg)	Warfarin		NO WARFARIN
		INR 2.0-3.0	INR 2.5-3.5†	
Mechanical Prosthetic Valves				
Aortic valve replacement:				
Low risk:*				
<3 months	Class I	Class I	Class IIa	
>3 months	Class I	Class I		
High risk*	Class I		Class I	
Mitral valve replacement	Class I		Class I	
Biological Prosthetic Valves				
Aortic valve replacement:				
Low risk:				
<3 months	Class I	Class IIa		Class IIb
>3 months	Class I			Class IIa
High risk	Class I	Class I		
Mitral valve replacement:				
Low risk:				
<3 months	Class I	Class IIa		
>3 months	Class I			Class IIa
High risk	Class I	Class I		

Modified from McAnulty J, Rahimtoola SH. Anti-thrombotic therapy in valvular heart disease. In: Schlant R, Alexander RW, editors. Hurst's the Heart. New York: McGraw-Hill; 1988; and from Bonow RO, Carabello BA, de Leon A, et al. ACC/AHA 2006 guidelines for the management of patients with valvular heart disease: a report of the American College of Cardiology/American Heart Association Task Force on Practice Guidelines (Writing Committee to Revise the 1998 Guidelines for the Management of Patients With Valvular Heart Disease) J Am Coll Cardiol 2008;52:e1–142.
*Risk factors: Atrial fibrillation, left ventricular dysfunction, previous thromboembolism, and hypercoagulable condition.
†INR (international normalized ratio) should be maintained between 2.5 and 3.5 for older-generation aortic tilting disk valves (Bjork-Shiley) and Starr-Edwards valves.

increased risk of bleeding with dual antithrombotic therapy is considered low. At this time, the use of novel oral anticoagulants is not recommended for management of patients with prosthetic heart valves.

INTERRUPTION OF ANTICOAGULANT THERAPY

In the planned interruption of VKA therapy for noncardiac surgery, the following factors must be taken into account: the nature of the procedure; the magnitude of risk of thromboembolism based on valve type, position, and number; the underlying patient risk factors; and the competing risk of periprocedural hemorrhage.[94] Low-risk patients with low-profile bileaflet or tilting disk valves in the aortic position can usually stop VKA therapy 3 to 5 days before noncardiac surgery and then resume it postoperatively as soon as it is considered safe, without the need for a heparin "bridge." In all other patients, either low-molecular-weight heparin (LMWH) or intravenous UFH should be given both before and after surgery, as directed by the surgeon. The use of LMWH avoids the need for preoperative hospitalization and has been validated in some settings.[95,96] Randomized trials are lacking, however. A study performed in patients immediately after mechanical heart valve replacement found the use of LMWH to be a safe and effective "bridging" strategy pending achievement of therapeutic levels of oral anticoagulation.[97] Some surgeons prefer intravenous UFH in this setting.

EXCESSIVE ANTICOAGULATION

Correction of a supratherapeutic INR should be considered when the INR exceeds 4.5, especially in the presence of active bleeding. Rapid correction of a therapeutic INR may also be necessary because of bleeding or the need for emergency noncardiac surgery. Any INR value higher than 4.0 obtained with a finger-stick

device should be verified with a laboratory assay performed on a phlebotomized blood specimen. For patients with minimally elevated INR and no active bleeding, VKA therapy is either adjusted or held for one or two doses and the INR measurement repeated. The 2012 American College of Chest Physicians guideline for antithrombotic therapy recommends against the routine use of vitamin K for patients receiving a VKA who have an INR of 4.5 to 10 and no evidence of bleeding (class IIB). Individual patient circumstances may vary. Oral vitamin K is recommended for patients with an INR higher than 10 and no evidence of bleeding (class IIC). When oral vitamin K (5 mg) is given in conjunction with temporary discontinuation of a VKA, 1.4 days are required for an INR between 6 and 10 to decline to less than 4.0. Subcutaneous vitamin K is not recommended. For patients with VKA-related bleeding, prothrombin complex concentrate is preferred over fresh-frozen plasma for rapid reversal (class IIC). The additional use of vitamin K (5 to 10 mg in 50 mL of intravenous fluid delivered over a minimum of 20 minutes to avoid the rare occurrence of an anaphylactoid reaction) may be considered (class 2C).[98]

ANTICOAGULATION IN PREGNANT WOMEN

Management of anticoagulation in the pregnant patient is fraught with hazards for both the mother and fetus. Many authorities consider a mechanical heart valve with the obligate need for anticoagulation to be a contraindication to pregnancy. All treatment choices are associated with an increased risk of spontaneous abortion, and the first principle of management is to engage the mother, her partner, and her family in a discussion of the pitfalls of any approach. The choice must be individualized and guided by the preferences and values of the mother. There are no randomized trial data to guide decision making. Warfarin therapy appears to be the safest anticoagulant strategy for the mother, although it carries a risk of fetal embryopathy, the aggregate incidence of which has been estimated at 6%.[99,100] Exposure during the sixth to twelfth weeks of gestation may be most harmful. There are observational data, however, to suggest that the risk of embryopathy may be dose related and that fetal abnormalities are less common (<3%) with maternal doses of warfarin lower than 5 mg/day.[101-103] There is also a small risk of fetal central nervous system abnormalities with first-trimester use of VKAs.[103] Unfractionated heparin may be advantageous for the fetus, particularly because it does not cross the placenta, yet older studies with relatively thrombogenic valves suggest that it may be less effective than warfarin for the prevention of thromboembolism or prosthetic valve thrombosis in the mother. Long-term use of UFH is associated with risks of thrombocytopenia and osteoporosis. The initial experience with LMWH was characterized by unacceptable rates of maternal complications, possibly related to the lack of dose adjustment to maintain therapeutic anti-Xa levels throughout pregnancy.[104]

The 2011 European Society of Cardiology guidelines on the management of cardiovascular disease in pregnancy generally prefer VKAs over heparin or LMWH for management of mechanical heart valves during pregnancy.[105] In the United States, one approach often used is twice-daily, dose-adjusted LMWH throughout pregnancy, aiming for an anti-Xa level between 0.8 and 1.2 IU/mL, which is assessed 4 hours after a subcutaneous dose. LMWH is not advised if anti-Xa levels cannot be monitored.[89] Testing should be performed every week, given the pharmacokinetic changes that occur with pregnancy. If UFH is provided, the activated partial thromboplastin time (aPTT) should be twice the control value or the anti-Xa level 0.35 to 0.70 IU/mL.[106] For women who choose to use warfarin before 6 and after 12 weeks of gestation, the INR target is 3.0 (range 2.5-3.5). Warfarin is usually discontinued at week 36, or 2 to 3 weeks before anticipated delivery, to avoid traumatic bleeding complications in a fully anticoagulated infant. UFH is given in the weeks leading up to delivery and can be resumed 6 hours postpartum as deemed safe. Therapy with warfarin, which is not excreted in breast milk, is begun the

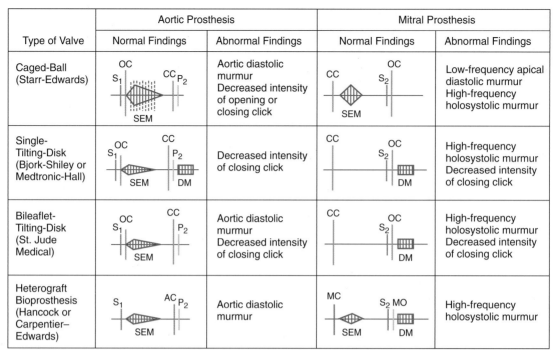

FIGURE 26-8 **Auscultatory characteristics of prosthetic heart valves.** Findings are stratified according to valve type and position. *AC,* Aortic closure; *CC,* closing click; *DM,* diastolic murmur; *MC,* mitral valve closure; *MO,* mitral opening; *OC,* opening click; *SEM,* systolic ejection murmur. *(From Vongpatanasin W, Hillis D, Lange RA. Prosthetic heart valves. N Engl J Med 1996;335:407–16.)*

evening after delivery. For high-risk women (mitral or older, thrombogenic prosthesis, AF, history of thromboembolism), low-dose aspirin can be added to anticoagulant therapy.[89,106]

Antiplatelet Therapy

The addition of low-dose aspirin to VKA therapy in selected subsets of patients, such as those with mechanical valves or following thromboembolic complications despite therapeutic INR values, was discussed previously. Dual antiplatelet therapy with aspirin and clopidogrel or with aspirin and dipyridamole is not a substitute for VKA therapy in patients with mechanical heart valves. Clopidogrel is an appropriate choice for aspirin-allergic patients when antiplatelet therapy is indicated. Bioprosthetic valves implanted by transcatheter techniques (see Chapter 15) are managed with dual antiplatelet therapy with low-dose aspirin (75 to 100 mg) and clopidogrel (75 mg daily) for the first 6 months and with low dose aspirin monotherapy thereafter.[107]

Infective Endocarditis Prophylaxis

Patients with prosthetic heart valves are at high risk for serious complications from infective endocarditis. Antibiotic prophylaxis is reasonable prior to dental procedures that involve manipulation of gingival tissue or the periapical region of teeth or perforation of the oral mucosa (class IIa recommendation).[108] Prophylaxis is not recommended prior to gastrointestinal or genitourinary procedures in the absence of suspected infection. The regimens for dental procedures are provided in Chapter 25. Morbidity and mortality rates with PVE are higher than those associated with native valve endocarditis, especially when the offending organism is *Staphylococcus aureus,* and an aggressive, multidisciplinary approach to diagnosis and treatment is essential.[109]

Clinical Assessment

Postoperative office visits should begin approximately 3 to 4 weeks after the patient has undergone valve implantation. The first visit is focused on ensuring a smooth transition from hospital/

rehabilitation facility to home, reconciling medications, and assessing neurocognitive function, wound healing, volume status, heart rhythm, and the auscultatory characteristics of prosthetic valve function (Figure 26-8). A grade 1 through 3 midsystolic murmur is audible at the base in all patients after AVR. The intensity varies as a function of valve size, cardiac output, and gradient. The closing sound of a mechanical aortic valve (A_2) is often palpable and distinctly loud, even to the extent that it is a nuisance to the patient. Patients who have undergone conduit replacement of the ascending aorta with valve-sparing reconstruction have a grade 2 or 3 systolic murmur below the suprasternal notch and radiating into the carotids and along the course of the clavicles. An aortic diastolic murmur under any circumstances is pathologic. Patients with stented tissue valves in the mitral position have grade 2 or 3 midsystolic murmurs, loudest at the left sternal border and indicative of accelerated flow past the stents, which extend into the LV outflow tract. With a low-profile mechanical mitral valve, an outflow murmur of this type is not present. The S_1 sound is loud and crisp. A soft, grade 1, low-pitched diastolic murmur can sometimes be heard in the left lateral decubitus position with either a tissue or mechanical mitral valve, depending on the cardiac output and the magnitude of the transvalvular diastolic pressure gradient; it need not indicate valve dysfunction.

The history at subsequent visits is tailored to detect symptoms suggestive of heart failure or reduced functional capacity, arrhythmia, thromboembolism, or infection. Adherence to the recommended schedule of INR determinations and the relative time that the INR is in the therapeutic range should be assessed in all patients undergoing anticoagulation. Problems with bleeding should be identified. The interview should include questions regarding other cardiovascular and general health issues as well as a review of medication adherence, drug interactions, and adverse side effects. A focused cardiovascular examination is performed at each visit. Instructions regarding antibiotic prophylaxis are repeated. After the 6-month mark, follow-up visits can be conducted annually unless interim problems arise.

A chest radiograph is obtained by the surgeon at the first visit to assess for residual pleural fluid, pneumothorax, lung aeration, and heart size. An electrocardiogram is routinely performed and should be reviewed for rhythm, conduction, and dynamic repolarization changes. Postoperative baseline values for hemoglobin, hematocrit, lactate dehydrogenase (LDH), and bilirubin should be established for patients with mechanical heart valves, allowing future comparisons should hemolysis be suspected. It is less useful to monitor the serum haptoglobin value. Other laboratory studies are performed as clinically relevant.

Echocardiography

Complete, postoperative baseline transthoracic echocardiogram (TTE) with color-flow Doppler imaging should be performed in all patients after heart valve replacement, typically between 6 weeks and 3 months after surgery. Published tables of transvalvular velocities and prosthetic valve areas, as a function of valve type and size, should be consulted to determine whether valve function is acceptable (see Tables 26-1 and 26-2). Values for these parameters may also be affected by body size and cardiac output. The phenomenon of pressure recovery, especially with mechanical bileaflet aortic valves and in patients with small aortic roots, must be considered in the interpretation, as previously reviewed (see Figure 26-2). The standard TTE examination includes imaging of the valve, measurement of the transvalvular velocity, calculation of instantaneous and mean pressure gradients and valve orifice area, qualitative assessment of the degree of regurgitation, evaluation of LV size and systolic function, and estimation of pulmonary artery systolic pressure. Mean pressure gradients are more useful clinically than instantaneous or maximum pressure gradients, because prosthetic valves have very high velocities at time of valve opening with rapid equilibration thereafter. The baseline, expected degree of regurgitation through a mechanical bileaflet or tilting disk valve should be noted. TTE should be repeated for any relevant change in clinical status or the examination findings. When clinically indicated in cases of suspected valve dysfunction, thrombosis, or infection, transesophageal echocardiogram (TEE) should be performed to obtain higher-quality images with improved spatial resolution (Figures 26-9 and 26-10).

The frequency with which routine, surveillance TTE should be performed in the longitudinal follow-up of patients after prosthetic heart valve replacement has not been established. Annual echocardiographic examinations can be considered after the first 10 years in patients with bioprosthetic valves even in the absence of any clinical change, because of the expected cumulative incidence of SVD after this point. Routine surveillance TTE is generally not necessary after the postoperative baseline evaluation for a normally functioning mechanical prosthesis, although examinations may be reasonable for other indications related to LV function or pulmonary hypertension.[89,90]

The leaflets of a bioprosthesis should appear thin and mobile. The struts of a stented valve are easily identified. The sewing ring/annular interface is thickened and echogenic. Stentless bioprosthetic valves, homografts, and autografts appear very similar to normal, native aortic valves, except for the expected degree of postoperative annular thickening. With time, the homograft root calcifies; the pulmonary autograft may dilate, especially in older patients. The appearance and movement of mechanical bileaflet and tilting disk valves are very difficult to assess with TTE because of the acoustical shadowing and reverberations inherent to these valves. These limitations can be overcome with multiplane TEE when indicated (Figure 26-11). The pattern and degree of valvular regurgitation can be assessed with color-flow Doppler imaging. Because of left atrial shadowing from the prosthesis on TTE, evaluation with TEE is essential in cases of suspected mitral prosthetic valve regurgitation, particularly when it is paravalvular in location. Indirect TTE signs of mitral prosthetic valve regurgitation include an increased early diastolic trans-mitral flow velocity, elevated pulmonary artery pressures, and hyperdynamic LV systolic function. TEE is less useful for the assessment of suspected aortic prosthetic valve regurgitation.

When needed, the echocardiographic data can be supplemented with information obtained from other diagnostic techniques. Fluoroscopy can be very helpful in the evaluation of mechanical leaflet/disk movement, especially in cases of suspected thrombosis. Excessive rocking may indicate dehiscence. Cardiac magnetic resonance (CMR) imaging can provide accurate and quantitative assessment of ventricular volumes and function. Either CMR or computed tomographic (CT) angiography can be used to evaluate the size and contour of the aorta, particularly after root or ascending aortic replacement. These modalities also allow for assessment of at least the proximal portions of the re-implanted coronary arteries. Baseline CMR or CT angiography should be performed 3 months after combined aortic valve/ascending aortic surgery, whether valve-sparing in nature or with a valve-graft conduit, and annually thereafter (Figure 26-12). Surveillance imaging of this type is especially important in patients with an underlying aortopathy, such as that associated with Marfan syndrome or bicuspid aortic valve (BAV) disease. Aneurysmal enlargement may occur in other native aortic locations. False aneurysm development along anastomotic suture lines is uncommon but potentially fatal.

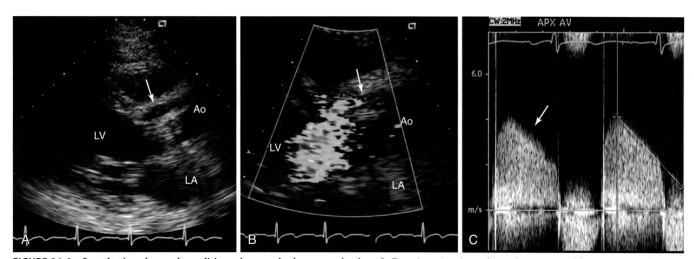

FIGURE 26-9   Prosthetic valve endocarditis and paravalvular regurgitation. A, Transthoracic echocardiography, parasternal long-axis view, shows an echo-free space anterior to a mechanical aortic valve replacement. **B,** Color-flow Doppler imaging shows a diastolic flow disturbance originating in this space with flow into the left ventricular (LV) chamber. **C,** Continuous wave Doppler echocardiography confirms that this flow is aortic regurgitation, showing the typical timing and velocity curve with a density and slope consistent with severe regurgitation. *Ao,* Aorta; *LA,* left atrium. *(From Otto CM. Textbook of echocardiography. 4th ed. Philadelphia: Elsevier Saunders; 2009.)*

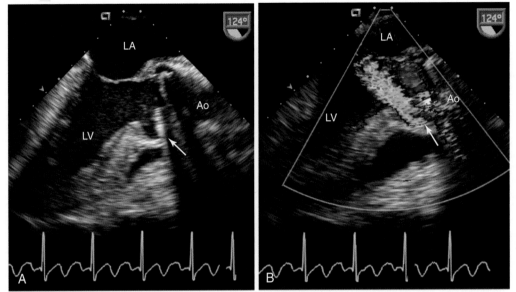

FIGURE 26-10   Prosthetic valve endocarditis and paravalvular regurgitation. Transesophageal echocardiography (TEE) in the same patient as in Figure 26-9. **A,** TEE provides better definition of the area of valve dehiscence adjacent to the septum *(arrow)*. The TEE probe has been positioned so the shadows from the valve prosthesis do not obscure the area of interest. **B,** Color-flow Doppler image shows aortic regurgitation from this site. *Ao,* Aorta; *LA,* left atrium; *LV,* left ventricle. *(From Otto CM. Textbook of echocardiography. 4th ed. Philadelphia: Elsevier Saunders; 2009.)*

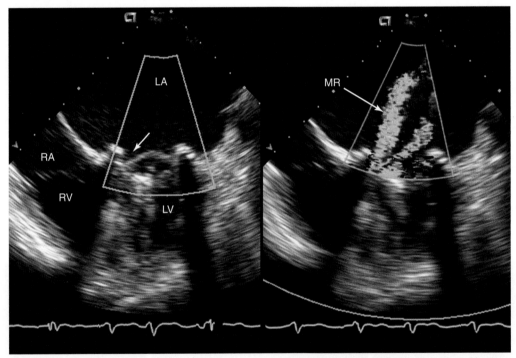

FIGURE 26-11   Prosthetic mitral regurgitation. Prosthetic mitral regurgitation (MR) due to inadequate leaflet closure evaluated by transesophageal echocardiogram. The two-dimensional image *(left)* show incomplete closure of the medial valve disk *(arrow)*, and color-flow imaging *(right)* demonstrates severe prosthetic MR with a wide vena contracta. *LA,* Left atrium; *LV,* left ventricle; *RA,* right atrium; *RV,* right ventricle. *(From Otto CM. Textbook of echocardiography. 4th ed. Philadelphia: Elsevier Saunders; 2009.)*

Evaluation and Treatment of Prosthetic Valve Dysfunction

Structural Valve Deterioration

Primary failure of the components of current-generation mechanical prostheses is extremely rare. Deterioration of tissue heterografts (porcine, bovine) and homografts occurs with predictable frequency as a function of patient age at implantation and prosthesis type (see Figures 26-5 and 26-6). Primary failure is due to leaflet thickening, calcification, perforation, or tearing. Prosthetic valve stenosis may also be due to pannus ingrowth and can often be first suspected on the basis of a change in the physical findings. The severity of stenosis should be characterized with Doppler echocardiography, and the patient instructed to report promptly any change in effort tolerance or new symptoms (Figures 26-13 and 26-14). Echocardiographic follow-up may have to be scheduled more frequently than once yearly, depending on the aggregate findings. Presentation with prosthetic valve

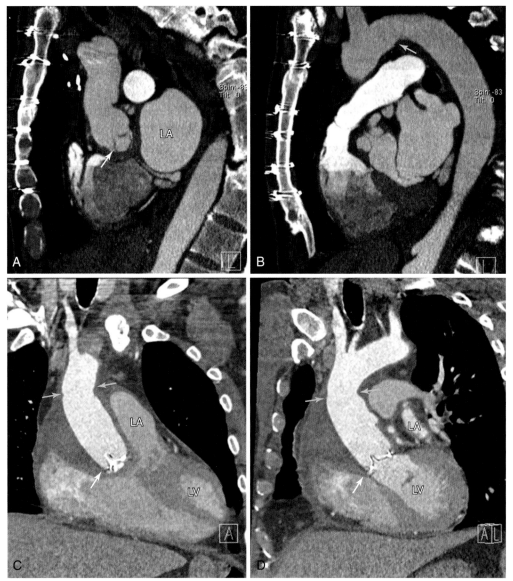

FIGURE 26-12   Computed tomography of surgical replacement of aortic valve and ascending aorta. Cardiac computed tomography evaluation of two patients following surgical replacement of the aortic valve and ascending aorta. **A** and **B,** Lateral views of a 58-year-old man with ankylosing spondylitis after aortic valve replacement with a 29-mm St. Jude Toronto Bioroot (St. Jude Medical, Inc., St. Paul, Minnesota) and ascending aortic replacement with hemiarch reconstruction with a 28-mm Vascutek graft (Vascutek, Ltd., Renfrewshire, Scotland). **A,** aortic valve prosthesis *(white arrow)* and ascending aorta; **B,** aortic arch. **C** and **D,** Anterior and anterolateral views in a 41-year-old man with a bicuspid aortic valve and aortic aneurysm following aortic valve replacement with a 27-mm bovine pericardial valve *(white arrows)* within a 34-mm Dacron graft. *Yellow arrows* indicate the distal anastomoses. *LA,* Left atrium; *LV,* left ventricle.

regurgitation is more common than that with prosthetic valve stenosis. Regurgitant lesions may progress very rapidly, and more often with mitral than with aortic bioprostheses, to the extent that some surgeons advocate early reoperation in this instance, before traditional indications for surgery are met, so as to avoid precipitous clinical decompensation. For most other patients, however, the indications for reoperation are the same as those that pertain to patients with native valve disease, including symptoms, indices of LV size and systolic function, and the development of pulmonary hypertension.

Compared with the initial surgery for native valve disease, reoperation carries an increased risk of mortality and major morbidity, related to older patient age, intrinsic changes in myocardial function, coexistent coronary artery disease, and bleeding. Reoperation is particularly challenging in patients with calcified, homograft aortic root replacements and those with dilated pulmonary autografts after a Ross procedure. On occasion, it is possible to preserve the cylindrical root of a homograft (and its

reimplanted coronary arteries) and to confine reoperation to replacement of the deteriorated valve. The risk of bleeding is increased because of the adhesions and dense scarring that occur after the first operation. Planning for reoperation in patients who have undergone previous coronary artery bypass grafting surgery includes obtaining a chest CT or CMR angiogram to delineate the course of the left internal mammary artery and its anatomic relationship to the sternum and chest wall.

Paravalvular Regurgitation

Paravalvular regurgitation occurs external to the prosthetic valve, at the interface between the sewing ring and the native valve annulus (see Figure 26-10). It can occur as a result of inadequate technique, suture dehiscence, compromised native tissue integrity (dense calcification, extensive myxomatous degeneration), infection, or chronic abrasion of the sewing ring against a calcified or rigid annulus. The magnitude of the regurgitant volume

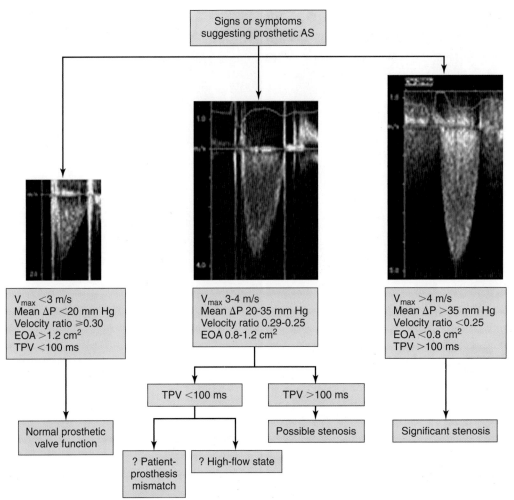

FIGURE 26-13 Evaluation of prosthetic aortic stenosis. A practical approach to evaluation of possible prosthetic aortic stenosis (AS) is to begin with standard measures of stenosis severity, including maximal velocity (V_{max}), mean pressure gradient (ΔP), and effective orifice area (EOA) and the ratio of left ventricular to aortic velocity. Normal values for each valve type and size should be referenced, but simple thresholds of 3 and 4 m/s are a quick first step. For patients with intermediate measures of stenosis severity, the shape of the velocity curve can be helpful, a triangular shape (short time to peak velocity, TPV) suggesting normal valve function and a rounded waveform (longer TPV) suggesting significant stenosis. *(Abstracted from Zoghbi WA, Chambers JB, Dumesnil JG, et al. Recommendations for evaluation of prosthetic valves with echocardiography and Doppler ultrasound. J Am Soc Echocardiogr 2009;22:975–1014.)*

depends on the size of the orifice. A small and clinically inconsequential paravalvular leak is usually discovered incidentally during routine echocardiography with color-flow Doppler imaging. No change in management would be indicated. Small paravalvular leaks may, however, be associated with significant intravascular hemolysis and anemia as red blood cells are forced through a narrow orifice at high velocities. Despite a high clinical index of suspicion in this circumstance, a new, regurgitant murmur may not be audible. TEE may be necessary to visualize the defect appropriately, especially in the patient with a mitral prosthesis. Larger paravalvular leaks may result in significant volume overload and heart failure, to an extent that reoperation might be indicated. There is a growing experience with the use of transcatheter closure devices in patients with clinically important paravalvular regurgitation, although results to date with this technology have been mixed.[110] Management can prove quite challenging, and a compromise approach with medical therapy is often chosen, in part in relation to the risks associated with reoperation in some patients.

Infective Endocarditis

PVE is a life-threatening infection that requires combined medical and surgical management to achieve optimal patient outcomes

(see Chapter 25). The cumulative incidence of PVE is highest within the first few weeks and months after valve implantation, approaching 3% at 1 year and 6% at 5 years.[82] Early infection may be more frequent with mechanical valves, but incidence rates at 1 year and beyond are similar for mechanical and tissue prostheses. From a microbiologic perspective, it is useful to classify PVE into early (within 1 year of valve surgery) and late (>1 year after surgery). Coagulase-negative staphylococci are the predominant cause of early PVE and are almost invariably of nosocomial origin. The majority are due to *Staphylococcus epidermidis* and are resistant to methicillin. Early PVE has also been associated with *S. aureus*, certain gram-negative bacilli, diphtheroids, and fungi. PVE occurring more than 1 year after surgery is more likely related to a community-acquired infection with a pathogen that is more commonly associated with native valve endocarditis (*S. aureus*, streptococci, enterococci).[111] Worldwide, *S. aureus* is the most common cause of endocarditis and is an independent risk factor for in-hospital death among patients with PVE. Infection of a prosthesis is a far more aggressive process than that seen with native valve disease and is characterized pathologically by early peri-annular infection, tissue invasion, abscess formation, and fistulous perforation. PVE involving a bioprosthesis can also result in primary leaflet destruction. TEE is recommended for all patients with suspected PVE. TEE has higher sensitivity and

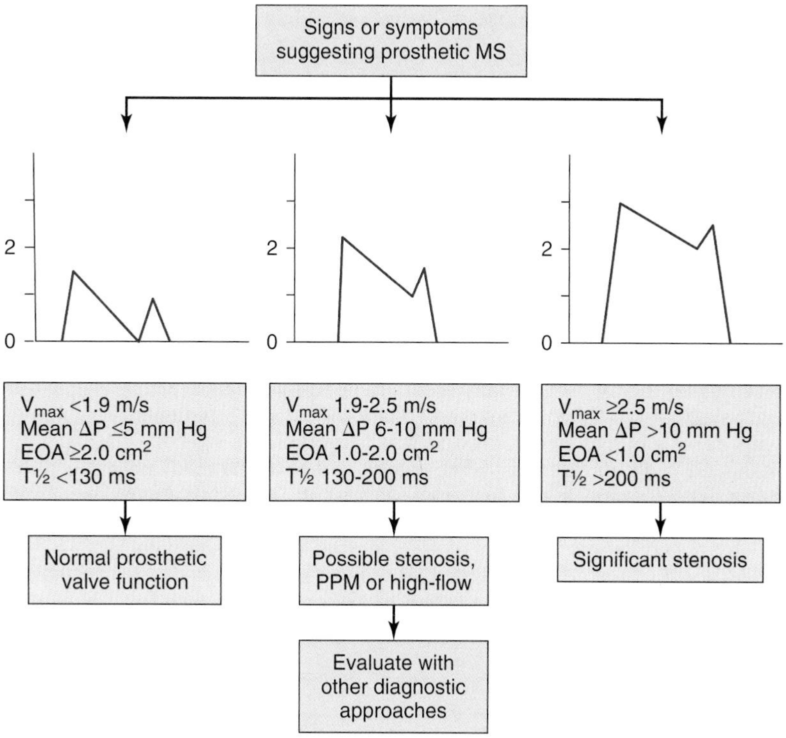

FIGURE 26-14 Evaluation of prosthetic mitral stenosis (MS). The evaluation starts with standard measures of stenosis severity including maximal velocity (V_{max}), effective orifice area (EOA), and pressure half-time (T½). Normal values for each valve type and size should be referenced, but the thresholds shown are a quick first step. In patients with intermediate measures of stenosis severity, the differential diagnosis includes significant stenosis, prosthesis-patient mismatch (PPM), and a high-flow state. Additional imaging or catheterization may be needed. (ΔP), pressure gradient. (*Adapted from Zoghbi WA, Chambers JB, Dumesnil JG, et al. Recommendations for evaluation of prosthetic valves with echocardiography and Doppler ultrasound. J Am Soc Echocardiogr 2009;22:975–1014.*)

specificity for the detection of vegetations and abscess than TTE, though the latter modality provides important supplemental information.[112]

In comparison with treatment outcomes in patients with native valve endocarditis, medical cure with antibiotics is inherently more difficult in patients with PVE, and surgery is more often required. The class I indications for surgery in the active phase of infection, while intravenous antibiotics are being given, include heart failure, abscess formation, valve dehiscence, progressive valve dysfunction, and infection with a resistant or difficult to eradicate microorganism.[89,113] Surgery is also reasonable (class IIa) for patients with persistent bacteremia despite an adequate course of antibiotics when there is no obvious satellite focus of infection and for patients with recurrent emboli and persistent vegetations. Even in surgical centers with an expertise in the management of such patients, perioperative mortality rates for PVE are as high as 25% to 35%.[109,114] Removal of a previously implanted pacemaker or defibrillator system (including the leads and generator) is recommended for patients with PVE even without definite involvement of the leads or device.[115]

Thromboembolism

Thromboemboli are a major source of morbidity in patients with prosthetic heart valves. The incidence of clinically recognizable events ranges from 0.6 to 2.3 per 100 patient-years, an estimate that does not account for any subclinical episodes that might be detected with sensitive imaging techniques.[20-24,94,99-102] Thromboembolic incidence rates are similar for patients with bioprostheses not undergoing anticoagulation and for patients with mechanical valves and appropriate anticoagulation.[7] Risk factors for thromboembolism include the inherent thrombogenicity of the prosthesis, valve position (mitral carries a higher risk than aortic), valve number, time spent out of the therapeutic range of anticoagulation, a history of thromboembolism, hypercoagulable state, AF, left atrial enlargement, and LV systolic dysfunction. The risk of bleeding, estimated at 1 event per 100 patient-years, increases with age and the intensity of anticoagulation.[25-28,84,116,117]

Management of a thromboembolic event in a patient with mechanical valves generally proceeds along one or more of the following lines:[89,91]

- For the patient whose INR is subtherapeutic, the dose of VKA is raised to achieve the intended INR range.
- For the patient whose INR is in the therapeutic range, the dose of the VKA is raised to achieve a higher INR range *and/or* low-dose aspirin is provided if not already used.
- The patient and family are informed about the increased risks of bleeding.
- The potential for drug interactions is reviewed.

Reoperation to implant a less thrombogenic valve is rarely undertaken for the patient with recurrent thromboemboli despite aggressive antithrombotic therapy.

Microcavitary "gas bubbles" are often seen in the left ventricles and left atria of patients with left-sided mechanical prostheses. These phenomena are different in nature from the spontaneous echo contrast observed with stasis of blood in the cardiac chambers. They do not seem to correlate with an increased risk of thromboembolism but may be associated with increased LDH levels and hemolysis.[118]

Prosthetic Valve Thrombosis

Thrombosis of a mechanical heart valve can have devastating consequences. Clinical suspicion should be raised by symptoms of heart failure, thromboembolism, and/or low cardiac output, coupled with a decrease in the intensity of the mechanical valve closure sounds, new and pathologic murmurs, and/or documentation of inadequate anticoagulation. Thrombosis is more common in the mitral and tricuspid positions than in the aortic position. Evaluation with TTE or TEE can help guide management decisions.[90] Confirmation of abnormal leaflet or disk excursion in the presence of an occluding thrombus can also be obtained rapidly with cardiac fluoroscopy. Although differentiation of thrombus from pannus formation can be difficult, the clinical context usually allows accurate diagnosis. Emergency reoperation for prosthetic valve thrombosis (PVT) is associated with high operative mortality rates (17% to 40%).[119] On the other hand,

CH
26

fibrinolytic therapy with either tissue plasminogen activator (10 mg bolus followed by 90 mg over 90 minutes) or streptokinase (500,000 IU over 20 minutes followed by 1,500,000 IU over 10 hours) carries a risk of 15% to 20% for death or cerebral/systemic embolic complications in patients with left-sided PVT. Thus, decisions about clinical management are challenging.[89,90]

Emergency surgery is reasonable for patients with left-sided PVT and shock or New York Heart Association functional class III or IV symptoms and for patients with a large thrombus burden (≥ 0.8 cm^2 on TEE).[120] Fibrinolytic therapy is reasonable for patients with recent-onset functional class I or II symptoms and small thrombus burdens (<0.8 cm^2) (class IIa recommendation) or for sicker patients with larger thrombi when surgery is either not available or inadvisable (class IIb recommendation). Fibrinolytic therapy is generally recommended for patients with right-sided PVT (class IIa recommendation).[89,90] Some patients with no or minimal symptoms and small thrombi can often be managed with intravenous UFH, which can be changed to fibrinolytic therapy if the first approach is unsuccessful. Any course of fibrinolytic therapy is followed at the appropriate interval by a continuous infusion of UFH during the transition to VKA therapy targeted to a higher INR with or without low-dose aspirin. Serial TTE studies are useful to assess the response to treatment.[89,90]

Hemolytic Anemia

The development of a nonimmune hemolytic anemia after valve replacement or repair is usually attributable to a paravalvular leak with intravascular red blood cell destruction. Diagnosis is based on a high index of suspicion coupled with laboratory evidence of hemolysis, including the characteristic changes in red blood cell morphology, elevations of indirect bilirubin value and LDH, a high reticulocyte count, and depressed serum haptoglobin value. Reoperative surgery or catheter closure of the defect is indicated when heart failure, a persistent transfusion requirement, or poor quality of life intervenes. Empirical medical measures include iron and folic acid replacement therapy and beta-adrenoreceptor blockers. It is important to exclude PVE as a cause.

Prosthesis-Patient Mismatch

Prosthesis-patient mismatch (PPM) results when a valve is implanted that is too small for the patient's body size, resulting in a hemodynamic state of functional stenosis. Although PPM is most commonly associated with implantation of small valves (≤ 21 mm) into small-statured older women with small aortic annuli/roots, mitral PPM is also recognized.[121-124] Whereas lesser degrees of PPM can be well tolerated, severe aortic PPM (effective orifice area ≤ 0.65 cm^2/m^2) may lead to less regression of LV hypertrophy, more cardiac events, and reduced survival (Figure 26-15).[123] PPM should not be assumed in the patient with high transvalvular velocities across an aortic bileaflet mechanical prosthesis because of the significant degree of pressure recovery that may be present. Severe, functional mitral stenosis due to mitral PPM (effective orifice area ≤ 0.9 cm^2/m^2) may result in persistent left atrial dilation, AF, pulmonary hypertension, right ventricular dysfunction, and higher long-term mortality.[125,126] It is important to note that the effective orifice area estimated on echocardiography or cardiac catheterization after surgery commonly differs from the preimplantation in vitro area listed by the manufacturer. In addition to selection of a valve with the most favorable hemodynamic characteristics, efforts to reduce the development of significant PPM include choosing the largest valve size believed technically appropriate and enlarging the aortic root. Oversizing a mitral prosthesis increases the risk of disrupting the atrioventricular groove, resulting in false aneurysm formation and posterior wall rupture. Combined aortic root procedures add to the complexity and morbidity of such surgery.

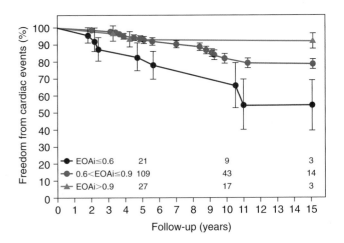

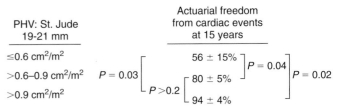

FIGURE 26-15 **Impact of prosthesis-patient mismatch on freedom from cardiac events.** Percentages of patients free from cardiac events over 15 years after implantation of 19- to 21-mm aortic St. Jude prosthetic heart valves (PHV). Outcomes are stratified according to the indexed effective orifice area (EOAi), obtained on predischarge transthoracic echocardiography after valve replacement. *(Adapted from Milano AD, DeCarlo M, Mecozzi G, et al. Clinical outcome in patients with 19 mm and 21 mm St. Jude prostheses: comparison at long-term follow-up. Ann Thorac Surg 2002;73:37–43; and from Rahimtoola SH. Choice of prosthetic heart valve for adult patients. J Am Coll Cardiol 2003;41: 893–904.)*

REFERENCES

1. Holmes DR, Rich JB, Zoghbi WA, et al. The heart team of cardiovascular care. J Am Coll Cardiol 2013;61:903–7.
2. The Society of Thoracic Surgeons. 2011 National Adult Cardiac Surgery Database. Executive Summary. <http://www.sts.org/sts-national-database/database-managers/executive-summaries>.
3. Iung B, Baron G, Butchart EG, et al. A prospective survey of patients with valvular heart disease in Europe: the Euro Heart Survey on Valvular Heart Disease. Eur Heart J 2003;24:1231–43.
4. Stock UA, Vacanti JP, Mayer Jr JE, et al. Tissue engineering of heart valves: current aspects. J Thorac Cardiovasc Surg 2002;50:184–93.
5. Hoerstrup SP, Kadner A, Melnitchouk S, et al. Tissue engineering of functional trileaflet heart valves from human marrow stromal cells. Circulation 2002;106(Suppl I):I143–50.
6. Cebotari S, Mertsching H, Kallenbach K, et al. Construction of autologous human heart valves based on an acellular allograft matrix. Circulation 2002;106(Suppl I):I-63–68.
7. Akins CW, Miller C, Turina MI, et al. Guidelines for reporting mortality and morbidity after cardiac valve interventions. J Thorac Cardiovasc Surg 2008;135:732–8.
8. Rahimtoola S. Choice of prosthetic heart valve in adults. J Am Coll Cardiol 2010;55:2413–26.
9. Zabalgoitia M. Echocardiographic recognition and quantitation of prosthetic valve dysfunction. In: Otto CM, editor. The practice of clinical echocardiography. Philadelphia: WB Saunders, 2002.
10. Rosenhek R, Binder T, Maurer G, et al. Normal values for Doppler echocardiographic assessment of heart valve prostheses. J Am Soc Echocardiogr 2003;16:1116–27.
11. Baumgartner H, Khan S, DeRobertis M, et al. Discrepancies between Doppler and catheter gradients in aortic prosthetic valves in vitro: a manifestation of localized gradients and pressure recovery. Circulation 1990;82:1467–75.
12. Baumgartner H, Schima H, Tulzer G, et al. Effect of stenosis geometry on the Doppler-catheter gradient relation in vitro: a manifestation of pressure recovery. J Am Coll Cardiol 1993;21:1018–25.
13. Zoghbi WA, Chambers JB, Dumesnil JG, et al. Recommendations for evaluation of prosthetic valves with echocardiography and Doppler ultrasound. J Am Soc Echocardiogr 2009;22:975–1014.
14. Baumgartner H, Khan S, DeRobertis M, et al. Effect of prosthetic aortic valve design on the Doppler-catheter gradient correlation: an in vitro study of normal St. Jude, Medtronic-Hall, Starr-Edwards and Hancock valves. J Am Coll Cardiol 1992;19:324–32.
15. Malouf JF, Ballo M, Connolly HM, et al. Doppler echocardiography of 119 normal-functioning St Jude Medical mitral valve prostheses: a comprehensive assessment

including time-velocity integral ratio and prosthesis performance index. J Am Soc Echocardiogr 2005;18:252–6.
16. Hixson CS, Smith MD, Mattson MD, et al. Comparison of transesophageal color flow Doppler imaging of normal mitral regurgitant jets in St. Jude Medical and Medtronic Hall cardiac prostheses. J Am Soc Echocardiogr 1992;5:57–62.
17. Lange HW, Olson JD, Pedersen WR, et al. Transesophageal color Doppler echocardiography of the normal St. Jude Medical mitral valve prosthesis. Am Heart J 1991;122: 489–94.
18. Chambers J, Cross J, Deverall P, et al. Echocardiographic description of the CarboMedics bileaflet prosthetic heart valve. J Am Coll Cardiol 1993;21:398–405.
19. Yoganathan AP, Heinrich RS, Fontaine AA. Fluid dynamics of prosthetic valves. In: Otto CM, editor. The practice of clinical echocardiography. Philadelphia: W.B. Saunders; 2002.
20. Baldwin JT, Deutsch S, Geselowitz DB, et al. LDA measurements of mean velocity and Reynolds stress fields within an artificial heart ventricle. J Biomech Eng 1994;116: 190–200.
21. Kohler J, Wirtz R, Fehske W. In vitro steady leakage jet formation of technical heart valves prostheses: a photo video optical and color Doppler study. In: Liepschs D, editor. 3rd international symposium on biofluid mechanics. Munich, VDI-Verlag gmbH Publishers; 1994. p. 315–23.
22. Murday AJ, Hochstitzky A, Mansfield J, et al. A prospective controlled trial of St. Jude versus Starr Edwards aortic and mitral valve prostheses. Ann Thorac Surg 2003;76: 66–73.
23. Bryan AJ, Rogers CA, Bayliss K, et al. Prospective randomized comparison of CarboMedics and St. Jude Medical bileaflet mechanical heart valve prostheses: ten-year follow-up. J Thorac Cardiovasc Surg 2007;133:614–22.
24. Svennevig JL, Abdelnoor M, Nitter-Hauge S. Twenty-five-year experience with the Medtronic-Hall valve prosthesis in the aortic position: a follow-up cohort study of 816 consecutive patients. Circulation 2007;116:1795–800.
25. Thevenet A, Albat B. Long term follow up of 292 patients after valve replacement with the Omnicarbon prosthetic valve. J Heart Valve Dis 1995;4:634–9.
26. Nitter Hauge S, Abdelnoor M, Svennevig JL. Fifteen-year experience with the Medtronic-Hall valve prosthesis: a follow-up study of 1104 consecutive patients. Circulation 1996;94(Suppl II):II105–8.
27. Tatoulis J, Chaiyaroj S, Smith JA. Aortic valve replacement in patients 50 years old or younger with the St. Jude Medical valve: 14-year experience. J Heart Valve Dis 1996;5: 491–7.
28. Godje OL, Fischlein T, Adelhard K, et al. Thirty-year results of Starr-Edwards prostheses in the aortic and mitral position. Ann Thorac Surg 1997;63:613–9.
29. Orszulak TA, Schaff HV, Puga FJ, et al. Event status of the Starr-Edwards aortic valve to 20 years: a benchmark for comparison. Ann Thorac Surg 1997;63:620–6.
30. Li HH, Hahn J, Urbanski P, et al. Intermediate-term results with 1,019 Carbomedics aortic valves. Ann Thorac Surg 2001;71:1181–7.
31. Emery RW, Arom KV, Kshettry VR, et al. Decision-making in the choice of heart valve for replacement in patients aged 60-70 years: twenty-year follow up of the St. Jude Medical aortic valve prosthesis. J Heart Valve Dis 2002;11(Suppl 1):S37–44.
32. Arom KV, Nicoloff DM, Kersten TE, et al. Ten years' experience with the St. Jude Medical valve prosthesis. Ann Thorac Surg 1989;47:831–7.
33. Akins CW. Results with mechanical cardiac valvular prostheses. Ann Thorac Surg 1995;60:1836–44.
34. Disesa VJ, Allred EN, Kowalker W, et al. Performance of a fabricated trileaflet porcine bioprosthesis: midterm follow-up of the Hancock modified-orifice valve. J Thorac Cardiovasc Surg 1987;94:220–4.
35. Thomson FJ, Barratt Boyes BG. The glutaraldehyde-treated heterograft valve: some engineering observations. J Thorac Cardiovasc Surg 1977;74:317–21.
36. Firstenberg MS, Morehead AJ, Thomas JD, et al. Short-term hemodynamic performance of the mitral Carpentier-Edwards PERIMOUNT pericardial valve. Carpentier-Edwards PERIMOUNT Investigators. Ann Thorac Surg 2001;71(Suppl):S285–8.
37. Dalmau MJ, González-Santos JM, Blázquez JA, et al. Hemodynamic performance of the Medtronic Mosaic and Perimount Magna aortic bioprostheses: five-year results of a prospectively randomized study. Eur J Cardiothorac Surg 2011;39:844–52.
38. Puvimanasinghe JP, Steyerberg EW, Takkenberg JJ, et al. Prognosis after aortic valve replacement with a bioprosthesis: predictions based on meta-analysis and microsimulation. Circulation 2001;103:1535–41.
39. Fann JI, Miller DC, Moore KA, et al. Twenty-year clinical experience with porcine bioprostheses. Ann Thorac Surg 1996;62:1301–11.
40. Jamieson WR, Munro AI, Miyagishima RT, et al. Carpentier-Edwards standard porcine bioprosthesis: clinical performance to seventeen years. Ann Thorac Surg 1995;60: 999–1006.
41. Jones EL, Weintraub WS, Craver JM, et al. Ten-year experience with the porcine bioprosthetic valve: interrelationship of valve survival and patient survival in 1,050 valve replacements. Ann Thorac Surg 1990;49:370–83.
42. Dellgren G, David TE, Raanani E, et al. Late hemodynamic and clinical outcomes of aortic valve replacement with the Carpentier-Edwards Perimount pericardial bioprosthesis. J Thorac Cardiovasc Surg 2002;124:146–54.
43. Mohr FW, Walther T, Baryalei M, et al. The Toronto SPV bioprosthesis: one-year results in 100 patients. Ann Thorac Surg 1995;60:171–5.
44. Vrandecic MP, Gontijo BF, Fantini FA, et al. The new stentless aortic valve: clinical results of the first 100 patients. Cardiovasc Surg 1994;2:407–14.
45. Hofig M, Nellessen U, Mahmoodi M, et al. Performance of a stentless xenograft aortic bioprosthesis up to four years after implantation. J Thorac Cardiovasc Surg 1992;103: 1068–73.
46. Casabona R, De Paulis R, Zattera GF, et al. Stentless porcine and pericardial valve in aortic position. Ann Thorac Surg 1992;54:681–4.
47. Westaby S, Amarasena N, Long V, et al. Time-related hemodynamic changes after aortic replacement with the freestyle stentless xenograft. Ann Thorac Surg 1995;60:1633–8.
48. O'Brien MF. Composite stentless xenograft for aortic valve replacement: clinical evaluation of function. Ann Thorac Surg 1995;60(Suppl):S406–9.
49. Del Rizzo DF, Goldman BS, David TE. Aortic valve replacement with a stentless porcine bioprosthesis: multicentre trial. Canadian Investigators of the Toronto SPV Valve Trial. Can J Cardiol 1995;11:597–603.
50. David TE, Feindel CM, Bos JJ, et al. Aortic valve replacement with Toronto SPV bioprosthesis: optimal patient survival but suboptimal valve durability. J Thorac Cardiovasc Surg 2008;135:19–24.
51. O'Brien MF. Homografts and autografts. In: Baue AE, Geha AS, Hammond GL, et al, editors. Glenn's thoracic and cardiovascular surgery. Stamford, Connecticut: Appleton and Lange; 1996. p. 1981–2004.
52. Pavoni D, Badano LP, Ius F, et al. Limited long-term durability of the Cryolife O'Brien stentless porcine xenograft valve. Circulation 2007;116(Suppl I):I-307–13.
53. Hickey E, Langley SM, Allemby-Smith O, et al. Subcoronary allograft aortic valve replacement: parametric risk-hazard outcome analysis to a minimum of 20 years. Ann Thorac Surg 2007;84:1564–70.
54. Klievenik LMA, Bekkers JA, Roos JW, et al. Autograft or allograft aortic valve replacement in young adult patients with congenital aortic valve disease. Eur Heart J 2008;29: 1446–53.
55. O'Brien MF, McGriffin DC, Stafford EG, et al. Allograft aortic valve replacement: long-term comparative clinical analysis of the viable cryopreserved and antibiotic 40C stored valves. J Cardiac Surg 1991;6(Suppl 4):534–43.
56. O'Brien MF, Hancock S, Stafford EG, et al. The homograft aortic valve: a 29 year, 99.3% follow-up of 1022 valve replacements. J Heart Valve Dis 2001;10:334–44.
57. Ross DN. Replacement of aortic and mitral valves with a pulmonary autograft. Lancet 1967;2:956–8.
58. Somerville J, Saravalli O, Ross D, et al. Long-term results of pulmonary autograft for aortic valve replacement. Br Heart J 1979;42:533–40.
59. Ross D. The versatile homograft and autograft valve. Ann Thorac Surg 1989;48(Suppl) :S69–70.
60. Ross D, Jackson M, Davies J. The pulmonary autograft: a permanent aortic valve. Eur J Cardiothorac Surg 1992;6:113–6.
61. Ross DN. Aortic root replacement with a pulmonary autograft—current trends. J Heart Valve Dis 1994;3:358–60.
62. Stelzer P, Jones DJ, Elkins RC. Aortic root replacement with pulmonary autograft. Circulation 1989;80(Suppl III):III209–13.
63. Oury JH, Angell WW, Eddy AC, et al. Pulmonary autograft: past, present, and future. J Heart Valve Dis 1993;2:365–75.
64. Gerosa G, McKay R, Davies J, et al. Comparison of the aortic homograft and the pulmonary autograft for aortic valve or root replacement in children. J Thorac Cardiovasc Surg 1991;102:51–60.
65. Sievers HH, Leyh R, Loose R, et al. Time course of dimension and function of the autologous pulmonary root in the aortic position. J Thorac Cardiovasc Surg 1993;105: 775–80.
66. Kouchoukos NT, D'avila Roman VG, Spray TL, et al. Replacement of the aortic root with a pulmonary autograft in children and young adults with aortic-valve disease [see comments]. N Engl J Med 1994;330:1–6.
67. Robles A, Vaughan M, Lau JK, et al. Long-term assessment of aortic valve replacement with autologous pulmonary valve. Ann Thorac Surg 1985;39:238–42.
68. Wain WH, Greco R, Ignegeri A, et al. 15 years experience with 615 homograft and autograft aortic valve replacements. Int J Artif Organs 1980;3:169–72.
69. Oury JH, Hiro SP, Maxwell M, et al. The Ross procedure: current registry results. Ann Thorac Surg 1998;66:S162–5.
70. Rubay JE, Buche M, El Khoury GA, et al. The Ross operation: mid-term results. Ann Thorac Surg 1999;67:1355–8.
71. da Costa F, Haggi H, Pinton R, et al. Rest and exercise hemodynamics after the Ross procedure: an echocardiographic study. J Card Surg 1998;13:177–85.
72. Pibarot P, Dumesnil JG, Briand M, et al. Hemodynamic performance during maximum exercise in adult patients with the Ross operation and comparison with normal controls and patients with aortic bioprostheses. Am J Cardiol 2000;86:982–8.
73. Phillips JR, Daniels CJ, Orsinelli DA, et al. Valvular hemodynamics and arrhythmias with exercise following the Ross procedure. Am J Cardiol 2001;87:577–83.
74. Carr-White GS, Kilner PJ, Hon JK, et al. Incidence, location, pathology, and significance of pulmonary homograft stenosis after the Ross operation. Circulation 2001;104(Suppl 1):I16–20.
75. Briand M, Pibarot P, Dumesnil JG, et al. Midterm echocardiographic follow-up after Ross operation. Circulation 2000;102(Suppl 3):III10–14.
76. O'Brien MF. Aortic valve implantation techniques—should they be any different for the pulmonary autograft and the aortic homograft? [editorial; comment]. J Heart Valve Dis 1993;2:385–7.
77. Bodnar E, Wain WH, Martelli V, et al. Long-term performance of homograft and autograft valves. Artif Organs 1980;4:20–3.
78. Takkenberg JJ, Klieverik LM, Schoof PH, et al. The Ross procedure: a systematic review and meta-analysis. Circulation 2009;119:222–8.
79. Klieverik LM, Takkenberg JJ, Bekkers JA, et al. The Ross operation: a Trojan horse? Eur Heart J 2007;28:1993–2000.
80. Yacoub MH, Klieverik LM, Melina GJ, et al. An evaluation of the Ross operation in adults. J Heart Valve Dis 2006;15:531–9.
81. Nunn GR, Bennetts J, Onikul E. Durability of hand-sewn valves in the right ventricular outlet. J Thorac Cardiovasc Surg 2008;136:290–6.
82. Mylonakis E, Calderwood SB. Infective endocarditis in adults. N Engl J Med 2001;345:1318–30.
83. Hammermeister K, Sethi GK, Henderson WG, et al. Outcomes 15 years after valve replacement with a mechanical versus a bioprosthetic valve: final report of the Veterans Affairs randomized trial. J Am Coll Cardiol 2000;36:1152–8.
84. Bloomfield P, Wheatley DJ, Prescott RJ, et al. Twelve-year comparison of a Bjork-Shiley mechanical heart-valve with porcine bioprosthesis. N Engl J Med 1991;324:573–9.
85. Grunkemeier GL, Li H-H, Naftel DC, et al. Long-term performance of heart valve prosthesis. Curr Probl Cardiol 2000;25:73–156.

86. Stassano P, Di Tommaso L, Monaco M, et al. Aortic valve replacement: a prospective randomized evaluation of mechanical versus biological valves in patients ages 55 to 70 years. J Am Coll Cardiol 2009;54:1862–8.

87. Brennan JM, Edwards FH, Zhao Y, et al. Long-term safety and effectiveness of mechanical versus biologic aortic valve prostheses in older patients: results from the Society of Thoracic Surgeons (STS) Adult Cardiac Surgery National Database. Circulation 2013; 127:1647–55.

88. Dunning J, Gao H, Chambers J, et al. Aortic valve surgery: marked increases in volume and significant decreases in mechanical valve use—an analysis of 41,227 patients over 5 years from the Society for Cardiothoracic Surgery in Great Britain and Ireland National database. J Thorac Cardiovasc Surg 2011:142:776–82.

89. Bonow RB, Carabello BA, Chatterjee K, et al. ACC/AHA 2006 practice guidelines for the management of patients with valvular heart disease: executive summary: A report of the American College of Cardiology/American Heart Association Task Force on Practice Guidelines (Writing Committee to Revise the 1998 Guidelines for the Management of Patients With Valvular Heart Disease) developed in collaboration with the Society of Cardiovascular Anesthesiologists endorsed by the Society for Cardiovascular Angiography and Interventions and the Society of Thoracic Surgeons. J Am Coll Cardiol 2006;48:598–675.

90. Vahanian A, Alfieri O, Andreotti F, et al. Guidelines on the management of valvular heart disease (version 2012). The Joint Task Force on the Management of Valvular Heart Disease of the European Society of Cardiology (ESC) and the European Association for Cardio-Thoracic Surgery (EACTS). Eur Heart J 2012;33:2451–96.

91. Whitlock RP, Sun JC, Fremes SE, et al. Antithrombotic and thrombolytic therapy for valvular disease: antithrombotic therapy and prevention of thrombosis, 9th ed. American College of Chest Physicians evidence-based clinical practice guidelines. Chest 2012;141(Suppl):e576S–600S.

92. Merie C, Kober L, Skov Olsen P, et al. Association of warfarin therapy duration after bioprosthetic aortic valve replacement with risk of mortality, thromboembolic complications, and bleeding. JAMA 2012;308:2118–25.

93. Little SH, Massel DR. Antiplatelet and anticoagulation for patients with prosthetic heart valves. Cochrane Database Syst Rev 2003;(4):CD003464.

94. Douketis JD, Berger PB, Dunn AS, et al. The perioperative management of antithrombotic therapy: American College of Chest Physicians evidence-based clinical practice guidelines (8th edition). Chest 2008;133(Suppl):299S–339S.

95. Kovacs MJ, Kearon C, Rodger M, et al. Single-arm study of bridging therapy with low-molecular-weight heparin for patients at risk of arterial embolism who require temporary interruption of warfarin. Circulation 2004;110:1658–63.

96. Dunn AS, Spyropoulos AC, Turpie AG. Bridging therapy in patients on long-term oral anticoagulants who require surgery: the Prospective Peri-operative Enoxaparin Cohort Trial (PROSPECT). J Thromb Haemost 2007;5:2211–8.

97. Meurin P, Tabet JY, Weber H, et al. Low-molecular-weight heparin as a bridging anticoagulant early after mechanical heart valve replacement. Circulation 2006;113:564–9.

98. Ageno W, Gallus AS, Wittkowsky A, et al. Oral anticoagulant therapy: antithrombotic therapy and prevention of thrombosis, 9th ed. American College of Chest Physicians evidence-based clinical practice guidelines. Chest 2012;141(Suppl):e44S–88S.

99. Chan WS, Anand S, Ginsberg JS. Anticoagulation of pregnant women with mechanical heart valves: a systematic review of the literature. Arch Intern Med 2000;160:191–6.

100. Sillesen M, Hjortdal V, Vejlstrup N, et al. Pregnancy with prosthetic heart valves: 30 years' nationwide experience in Denmark. Eur J Cardiothorac Surg 2011;40:448–54.

101. Ansell J, Hirsh J, Hylek E, et al. Pharmacology and management of the vitamin K antagonists: American College of Chest Physicians evidence-based clinical practice guidelines (8th edition). Chest 2008;133(Suppl):160S–98S.

102. Cotrufo M, De Feo M, De Santo LS, et al. Risk of warfarin during pregnancy with mechanical valve prostheses. Obstet Gynecol 2002;99:35–40.

103. van Driel D, Wesseling J, Sauer PJ, et al. Teratogen update: fetal effects after in utero exposure to coumarins: overview of cases, follow-up findings, and pathogenesis. Teratology 2002;66:127–40.

104. Mahesh B, Evans S, Bryan AJ. Failure of low molecular weight heparin in the prevention of prosthetic mitral valve thrombosis during pregnancy: case report and review of options for anticoagulation. J Heart Valve Dis 2002;11:745–50.

105. Regitz-Zagrosek V, Blomstrom Lundqvist C, Borghi C, et al. ESC guidelines on the management of cardiovascular diseases during pregnancy: the Task Force on the Management of Cardiovascular Diseases during Pregnancy of the European Society of Cardiology (ESC). Eur Heart J 2011;32:3147–97.

106. Bates SM, Greer IA, Middeldorp S, et al. VTE, thrombophilia, antithrombotic therapy, and pregnancy: antithrombotic therapy and prevention of thrombosis, 9th ed.

American College of Chest Physicians evidence-based clinical practice guidelines. Chest 2012;141(Suppl):e691S–736S.

107. Leon MB, Smith CR, Mack M, et al. Transcatheter aortic-valve implantation for aortic stenosis in patients who cannot undergo surgery. N Engl J Med 2010;363:1597–607.

108. Bonow RO, Carabello BA, Chatterjee K, et al.: 2008 Focused update incorporated into the ACC/AHA 2006 guidelines for the management of patients with valvular heart disease: a report of the American College of Cardiology/American Heart Association Task Force on Practice Guidelines (Writing Committee to Revise the 1998 Guidelines for the Management of Patients With Valvular Heart Disease) Endorsed by the Society of Cardiovascular Anesthesiologists, Society for Cardiovascular Angiography and Interventions, and Society of Thoracic Surgeons. J Am Coll Cardiol 2008;52:e1–142.

109. Hoen B, Duval X. Infective endocarditis. N Engl J Med 2013;368:1425–33.

110. Pate GE, Al Zubaidi A, Chandavimol M, et al. Percutaneous closure of prosthetic paravalvular leaks: case series and review. Catheter Cardiovasc Interv 2006;68:528–33.

111. Karchmer AW. Infective endocarditis. In: Libby P, Bonow RO, Mann D, et al, editors. Braunwald's heart disease: a textbook of cardiovascular medicine. 8th ed. Philadelphia: Elsevier; 2008. p. 1713–33.

112. Baddour LM, Wilson WR, Bayer AS, et al. Infective endocarditis: diagnosis, antimicrobial therapy, and management of complications: a statement for healthcare professionals from the Committee on Rheumatic Fever, Endocarditis, and Kawasaki Disease, Council on Cardiovascular Disease in the Young, and the Councils on Clinical Cardiology, Stroke, and Cardiovascular Surgery and Anesthesia, American Heart Association. Executive Summary. Endorsed by the Infectious Diseases Society of America. Circulation 2005;111:3167–84.

113. Habib G, Hoen B, Tornos P, et al. Guidelines on the prevention, diagnosis, and treatment of infective endocarditis (new version 2009): the Task Force on the Prevention, Diagnosis, and Treatment of Infective Endocarditis of the European Society of Cardiology (ESC). Endorsed by the European Society of Clinical Microbiology and Infectious Diseases (ESCMID) and the International Society of Chemotherapy (ISC) for Infection and Cancer. Eur Heart J 2009;30:2369–413.

114. Wang A, Athan E, Pappas PA, International Collaboration on Endocarditis-Prospective Cohort Study Investigators. Contemporary clinical profile and outcome of prosthetic valve endocarditis. JAMA 2007;297:1354–61.

115. Baddour LM, Epstein AE, Erickson CC, et al. Update on cardiovascular implantable electronic device infections and their management: a scientific statement from the American Heart Association. Circulation 2010;121:458–77.

116. Cannegieter SC, van der Meer FJ, Briet E, et al. Warfarin and aspirin after heart-valve replacement [letter; comment]. N Engl J Med 1994;330:507–8.

117. Deb'etaz LF, Ruchat P, Hurni M, et al. St. Jude Medical valve prosthesis: an analysis of long-term outcome and prognostic factors. J Thorac Cardiovasc Surg 1997;113: 134–48.

118. Gencbay M, Degertekin M, Basaran Y, et al. Microbubbles associated with mechanical heart valves: their relation with serum lactic dehydrogenase levels. Am Heart J 1999; 137:463–8.

119. Bonow RO, Carabello BA, deLeon AC, et al. ACC/AHA guidelines for the management of patients with valvular heart disease: a report of the American College of Cardiology/American Heart Association Task Force on Practice Guidelines (Committee on Management of Patients With Valvular Heart Disease). J Am Coll Cardiol 1998;32:1486–588.

120. Tong AT, Roudaut R, Ozkan M. Transesophageal echocardiography improves risk assessment of thrombolysis of prosthetic valve thrombosis: results of the international PRO-TEE registry. J Am Coll Cardiol 2004;43:77–84.

121. Rahimtoola SH. The problem of valve prosthesis-patient mismatch. Circulation 1978;58:20–4.

122. Lund O, Emmertsen K, Nielsen TT, et al. Impact of size mismatch and left ventricular function on performance of the St. Jude disc valve after aortic valve replacement. Ann Thorac Surg 1997;63:1227–34.

123. Milano AD, De CM, Mecozzi G, et al. Clinical outcome in patients with 19-mm and 21-mm St. Jude aortic prostheses: comparison at long-term follow-up. Ann Thorac Surg 2002;73:37–43.

124. Pibarot P, Dumesnil JG, Lemieux M, et al. Impact of prosthesis-patient mismatch on hemodynamic and symptomatic status, morbidity and mortality after aortic valve replacement with a bioprosthetic heart valve. J Heart Valve Dis 1998;7:211–8.

125. Magne J, Mathieu P, DUmesnil JG, et al. Impact of patient-prosthesis mismatch on survival after mitral valve replacement. Circulation 2007;115:1417–25.

126. Aziz A, Lawton JS, Maniar HS, et al. Factors affecting survival after mitral valve replacement in patients with prosthesis–patient mismatch Ann Thorac Surg 2010; 90:1202–10.

CHAPTER 27

Valvular Heart Disease in Pregnancy

Karen K. Stout and Eric V. Krieger

Key Points

- Pregnancy increases cardiac output and intravascular volume, which increases gradients across stenotic lesions and can exacerbate heart failure in patients with severe valvular stenosis.
- Intravascular volume increases in the immediate postpartum period, and high-risk patients require 48 to 72 hours of close monitoring following delivery.
- The risk of cardiovascular events ranges between 5% and 70% for women with heart disease. Women with a higher New York Heart Association class, mitral or aortic stenosis, mechanical valves, pulmonary hypertension, or multiple lesions are at highest risk.
- Women at increased risk for adverse maternal or fetal outcomes should be referred to experienced centers.
- A trial of vaginal delivery is safe for the vast majority of cardiac lesions; therefore, in most cases, a cesarean section should be reserved for obstetric indications.
- For women with mechanical valves, meticulous uninterrupted anticoagulation is essential, but morbidity remains elevated in this population. There are various strategies for anticoagulation, and none are perfect. Unfractionated heparin has the highest risk of maternal complications. Warfarin has the lowest risk of maternal complications but can be teratogenic, particularly in the first trimester.

Valvular heart disease in pregnant women includes women with known valve disease who may present to the physician prior to pregnancy for evaluation of potential maternal and fetal risk, women with a known valve disease who present during pregnancy without preconception counseling, and women without known cardiac disease who are diagnosed during pregnancy. In each situation, the normal physiologic changes of pregnancy may exacerbate the hemodynamics of the valve lesion, so that women who are asymptomatic in the nongravid state may decompensate during pregnancy. Management is complicated by the potential effects of medication, radiation, or surgery on the fetus. Despite increased maternal and fetal risks, most women with valvular heart disease can complete a successful pregnancy when carefully managed by a multidisciplinary team at an experienced center.

Physiologic Changes of Pregnancy

Normal Hemodynamic Changes

PREGNANCY

During pregnancy, there is a substantial increase in plasma volume, erythrocyte volume, and cardiac output (Figure 27-1).[1-5] Cardiac output increases by up to 45%, and most of the increase is the result of a 20% to 30% increase in heart rate. There is a smaller increase in stroke volume.[6-9] The increase in cardiac output begins as early as 10 weeks of gestation, with the maximal cardiac output achieved in most by 24 weeks (Figure 27-2).[8,10,11] Pulmonary pressures remain normal during pregnancy because of a decrease in pulmonary vascular resistance through vascular recruitment in the high capacitance pulmonary circulation.[12] Left ventricular (LV) filling pressures remain normal.[13]

During pregnancy, an increase in venous tone augments preload,[14] whereas a decrease in aortic stiffness and alterations in the microcirculation reduce afterload.[6] The decrease in systemic vascular resistance offsets the increase in cardiac output so that blood pressure decreases slightly during pregnancy. LV wall stress decreases by about 30%, which decreases the oxygen demand of the myocardium.[4,15] Paradoxically, several studies suggest that LV contractility may be mildly depressed, although the magnitude of this change is unlikely to be clinically significant.[4,15,16] Stroke volume is maintained in the setting of decreased contractility by the altered loading conditions of pregnancy. At term, the relationship between LV filling pressure and stroke-work index is comparable to the nonpregnant state.[17]

POSITIONAL CHANGES

The effects of positional change on hemodynamics also may be more prominent in women with valve disease. In the supine position, the gravid uterus can compress the inferior vena cava, resulting in decreased preload, stroke volume, and cardiac output. This can be avoided by use of the left lateral decubitus position.[18] Some patients may also need to labor in the left lateral decubitus position to maintain cardiac output.

PERIPARTUM AND POSTPARTUM CHANGES

Peripartum hemodynamics are affected by uterine contractions, the pain of labor and delivery, and blood loss (Figure 27-3). Pain increases heart rate, blood pressure, and stroke volume. Uterine contractions reintroduce blood into the circulating blood pool. The increase in intravascular volume with each contraction is accompanied by an increase in heart rate so that cardiac output is augmented by about 20% with each contraction (Figure 27-4). When valve disease is present, these hemodynamic alterations may result in clinical deterioration.[19,20] Labor and delivery are associated with mild increases in LV diastolic pressure, which, in a patient with decreased LV compliance, may lead to pulmonary edema. Therefore, the increase in intravascular volume that occurs with uterine contraction can increase LV end-diastolic pressure and pulmonary edema.

Blood loss from vaginal delivery partially compensates for the increased blood volume of pregnancy, but acute changes

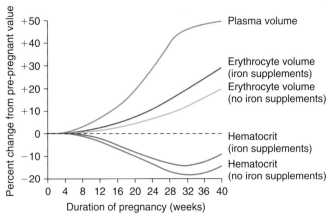

FIGURE 27-1   Plasma and erythrocyte increase during pregnancy. *(From Pitkin PM. Clin Obstet Gynecol 1976;19:489–513, with permissions.)*

may not be well tolerated in women with valvular heart disease. This is particularly true when the LV diastolic pressure-volume relationship is very steep, such as in women with severe aortic stenosis; a small loss of volume and preload may result in a large fall in cardiac output. However, the volume changes with a cesarean section are even greater than with vaginal delivery.[5,21] Therefore, the cesarean section is rarely indicated for cardiac reasons.

After delivery of the placenta, stroke volume and cardiac output rise by about 10% and remain elevated for about 24 hours. Over the next 2 weeks, cardiac output declines by 25% to 30% related to a decrease in heart rate and intravascular volume.[22,23] In some patients, symptoms occur postpartum because of intravascular and extravascular volume shifts that result in spontaneous volume loading.[17,24] Although hemodynamics return toward the baseline by 6 to 12 weeks after delivery, the new postpartum baseline may be different than prepregnancy hemodynamics. For example, both LV and aortic dimensions may remain slightly larger than the baseline.[7,23]

Evaluation by Echocardiography

NORMAL ANATOMIC CHANGES

Echocardiographic findings reflect the normal physiologic changes of pregnancy. LV end-diastolic diameter increases by 2 to 3 mm, with no change in end-systolic dimension, so both fractional shortening and ejection fraction are increased compared to the baseline.[25-31] In addition, both aortic root and LV outflow tract diameters increase by 1 to 2 mm, and this often persists after pregnancy.[32,33] The left atrial area increases by about 2 cm^2,[28] in association with an increase in serum atrial natriuretic peptide levels.[34,35] There is a small increase in mitral annulus diameter and a larger increase in tricuspid annulus diameter.[28] A small pericardial effusion is seen in 25% of healthy women during pregnancy.[35]

DOPPLER CHANGES

The increased cardiac output of pregnancy leads to increased transvalvular flow velocities. Aortic and LV outflow velocities increase by about 0.3 m/s. The transmitral early ventricular filling (E) velocity increases by 0 to 0.1 m/s, with an increase in the late ventricular filling (A) velocity of 0.1 to 0.2 m/s.[8,28] The greater increase in A velocity compared to E velocity results in a shift from the normal E/A ratio seen in young adults to an equalized or reversed E/A ratio. The pulmonary venous flow pattern shows an increase in the velocity, but not duration, of the pulmonary venous A wave.[6] For these reasons, pregnant women can appear to have diastolic dysfunction on echocardiography.

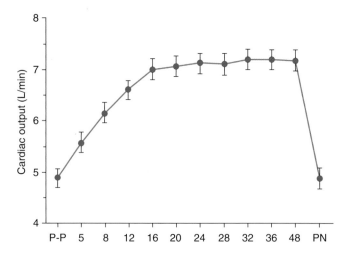

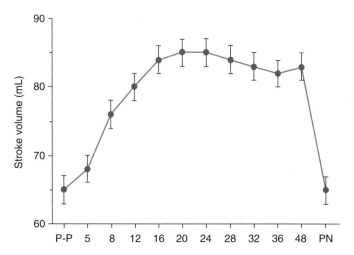

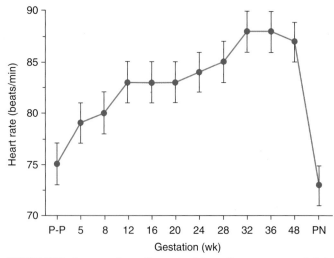

FIGURE 27-2   Increase in cardiac output from the nonpregnant state throughout pregnancy. *P-P*, prepregnancy; *PN*, postnatal. *(From Hunter S, Robson SC. Br Heart J 1992;68:540–3, with permissions.)*

Mild tricuspid and pulmonic regurgitation are usually seen during pregnancy. Physiologic mitral regurgitation is also common, likely a result of annular dilation.[36]

Epidemiology

The incidence of rheumatic heart disease has declined in industrialized nations over the last 40 years.[37,38] During that same time,

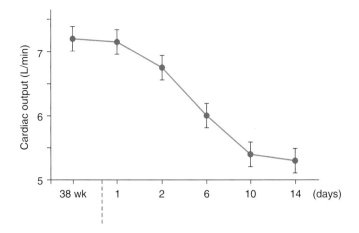

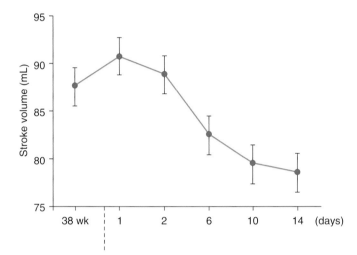

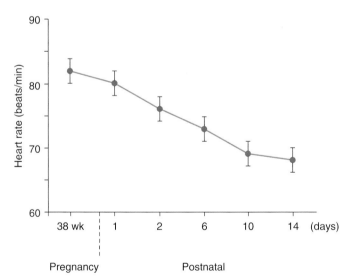

Pregnancy   Postnatal

FIGURE 27-3 **Changes in heart rate and cardiac output after normal delivery.** *(From Hunter S, Robson SC. Br Heart J 1992;68:540–3, with permissions.)*

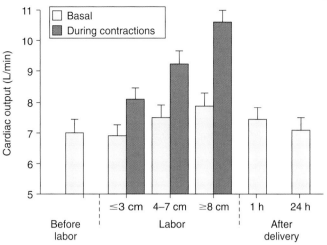

FIGURE 27-4 **Changes in cardiac output and stroke volume during normal labor.** *(From Hunter S, Robson SC. Br Heart J 1992;68:540–3, with permissions.)*

frequently have associated cardiovascular abnormalities beyond the valve disease itself; some patients have a systemic right ventricle or aortic pathology that introduces additive risk. The spectrum of valve disease in pregnancy makes risk assessment somewhat difficult, but there are general risk factors that are identified, as well as risks based upon the specific valvular lesion.

Risk Factors for Adverse Outcomes

The European Society of Cardiology has created the Registry of Pregnancy and Cardiac disease and prospectively enrolled more than 1300 pregnant women with heart disease. In those with valvular heart disease, maternal mortality was 2.1% and hospitalization rate was 38%.[43] However, risk is not increased uniformly in all pregnancy women with valve disease. Accurately identifying risk factors for adverse outcomes is needed for prepregnancy counseling and decisions about appropriate monitoring during pregnancy.

A multicenter Canadian study prospectively enrolled consecutive pregnancies in women with all types of heart disease.[39] Predictors of adverse maternal events were a history of cardiac events prior to pregnancy, New York Heart Association (NYHA) functional class greater than II, cyanosis, and left heart obstruction or systemic ventricular dysfunction. These four predictors allow prediction of the risk of maternal events (Table 27-1 and Figure 27-5). In this series, the live birth rate was 98%. Maternal risk factors for fetal or neonatal death are shown in Table 27-2. Adverse neonatal events occurred in 20% of pregnancies, including premature birth in 18% and small-for-gestational-age birth weight in 4% of pregnancies. In women with congenital heart disease, but not a recognized genetic syndrome, 7% of infants had congenital heart disease.

In this same study population, 302 pregnancies in women with heart disease were compared to 575 pregnancies in women without heart disease. The rate of maternal cardiac complications was 17% in women with heart disease, compared to 0% in the control group. Heart failure and arrhythmias accounted for most of the cardiac complications (94%). There were two postpartum maternal deaths as a result of heart failure or pulmonary hypertension. In addition, the risk of neonatal complications was 2.3 times normal (Figure 27-6). The additive effects of maternal cardiac and obstetric risk factors support referral of these patients to high-risk obstetric clinics (Figure 27-7).[40]

There is an increasing number of women with complex congenital heart disease, which often includes valve dysfunction. In

there has been an increase in the number of adults with congenital heart disease. Additionally, other causes of valve disease, including connective tissue disorders such as Marfan syndrome, are more frequently recognized in pregnancy. Consequently, although rheumatic heart disease remains common in pregnancy in developing countries, in industrialized nations congenital and genetic valvulopathies are more common. This adds further complexity because patients with congenital or genetic valve disease

CH
27

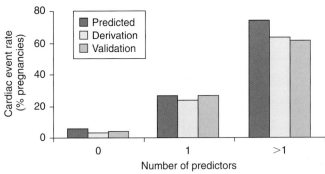

FIGURE 27-5 Frequency of maternal primary cardiac events. Frequencies are shown for derivation and validation groups, expressed as a function of the number of cardiac predictors, as shown in Table 27-1. *(From Siu SC, Sermer M, Colman JM, et al. Circulation 2001;104:515–21, with permissions.)*

TABLE 27-1	Predictors of Primary Adverse Events* in Pregnant Women with Cardiac Disease[39]
PREDICTORS	**DEFINITION**
Cardiac event before pregnancy	Heart failure Transient ischemic attack Stroke
Functional status	Baseline NYHA Class >II Cyanosis
Left heart obstruction	MVA <2 cm² AVA <1.5 cm² LVOT gradient >30 mm Hg
Systemic ventricular systolic dysfunction	EF <40%

Risk Index	
NO. OF PREDICTORS	**RATE OF CARDIAC EVENTS**
0	5%
1	27%
>1	75%

AVA, aortic valve area; *EF*, ejection fraction; *LVOT*, left ventricular outflow tract; *MVA*, mitral valve area.
*Primary adverse events were defined as pulmonary edema, sustained symptomatic arrhythmia requiring treatment, stroke, cardiac arrest, or cardiac death.

TABLE 27-2	Predictors of Neonatal Events in Women with Cardiac Disease[39]

Predictors of Neonatal Events
NYHA class >II or cyanosis at the baseline prenatal visit
Maternal left heart obstruction
Smoking during pregnancy
Multiple gestations
Use of anticoagulants throughout pregnancy

Risk Index	
NO. OF PREDICTORS	**RATE OF FETAL OR NEONATAL DEATH**
0	2%
1 or more	4%

a report of 90 pregnancies in 54 women with various types of congenital heart disease,[41] risk factors for maternal events were NYHA class greater or equal to II, prior history of heart failure, and smoking. Severe pulmonic regurgitation (PR) or subpulmonic ventricular dysfunction also were risk factors for adverse maternal outcomes (Table 27-3). Multivariate analysis identified LV outflow tract obstruction (peak outflow gradient greater than 30 mm Hg) as a risk factor for adverse fetal outcomes (Table 27-4). Based on

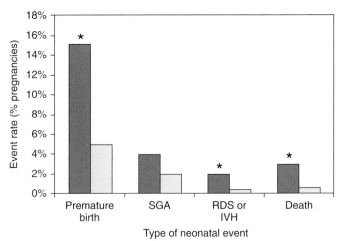

FIGURE 27-6 Neonatal complications in women with and without heart disease. Specific types of neonatal complications in 302 pregnancies in women with heart disease *(purple bars)* are compared to 572 pregnancies in women without heart disease *(light blue bars).* Premature birth indicates delivery at <37 weeks of gestation. *SGA,* small for gestational age birth weight; *RDS or IVH,* respiratory distress syndrome or intraventricular hemorrhage; and death, fetal, or neonatal death. *P <0.005, heart disease versus controls. *(From Siu SC, Colman JM, Sorensen S, et al. Circulation 2002;105:2179–84, with permissions.)*

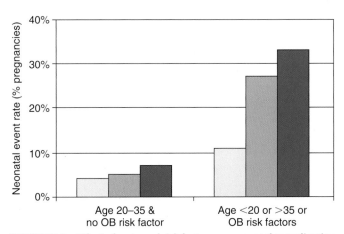

FIGURE 27-7 Effect of maternal risk factors on neonatal complication rates. Frequency of neonatal complications when patients are divided into two groups by the presence or absence of maternal noncardiac risk factors (obstetric high-risk characteristics, including smoking, use of anticoagulation, multiple gestation, maternal age). *Light blue bars* represent control group. *Medium blue bars* represent the heart disease group without left heart obstruction or poor functional class/cyanosis. *Dark blue bars* represent the high-risk cardiac patients, with left heart obstruction or poor functional class/cyanosis. *(From Siu SC, Colman JM, Sorensen S, et al. Circulation 2002;105:2179–84, with permissions.)*

this data, a risk score for pregnant women with complex congenital heart disease was proposed (Figure 27-8) that emphasizes the impact of PR and right ventricular dysfunction.

In another study of 1302 pregnancies in women with congenital heart disease, the overall rate of maternal complications was 7.6%. The strongest predictors of adverse maternal risk were presence of a mechanical valve, mitral or aortic stenosis, NYHA class greater than II, a history of arrhythmia, and the need for cardiac medications prior to pregnancy. Risk factors were additive and women with greater than 1 risk factors had a greater than 18% risk of a maternal complication during pregnancy (see Table 27-3).[42]

Bicuspid aortic valve is associated with an aortopathy that shares many characteristics of Marfan syndrome (see Chapter 13) (Figure 27-9). Congenital abnormalities, such as tetralogy of

TABLE 27-3   Comparison of Risks for Adverse Maternal Outcomes

	ACC/AHA GUIDELINES[44]	SIU 2001[39]	KHAIRY 2006[41]	DRENTHEN 2010[42]
Study group*		599 pregnancies, 224 women with heart disease	90 pregnancies, 54 women with congenital heart disease	1302 women with congenital heart disease
History		Prior cardiac event or arrhythmia	Prior history of heart failure Smoking history Weight	Prior arrhythmia Cardiac medication prior to pregnancy
NYHA class	AR, MS, MR with class NYHA III-IV symptoms	NYHA >II or cyanosis	NYHA ≥II	NYHA >II
Valve lesion	AS with or without symptoms Mechanical prosthesis	Left heart obstruction	Severe PR	≥ moderate MR ≥ moderate TR Left heart obstruction (AVA <1 cm²), pressure gradient >50 mmHg Mechanical prosthesis
Ejection fraction	Aortic or mitral valve disease with EF <40%	Systemic ventricular dysfunction (EF <40%)	Decreased subpulmonic ventricular EF Decreased morphologic right ventricular EF	
Pulmonary pressures	Aortic or mitral valve disease with >75% systemic pulmonary pressures			
Other	Marfan syndrome with or without AR			Cyanotic heart disease (corrected or uncorrected)

AR, aortic regurgitation; *AS,* aortic stenosis; *MS,* mitral stenosis; *MR,* mitral regurgitation; *NYHA,* New York Heart Association class; *EF,* ejection fraction; *AVA,* aortic valve area; *TR,* tricuspid regurgitation.
*The ACC/AHA guidelines are based on synthesis of data from multiple publications.

TABLE 27-4   Comparison of Risk Factors for Fetal Complications

SIU 2001[39]	KHAIRY 2006[41]	DRENTHEN 2010[42]
Cyanosis	Decreased saturation	Cyanosis
NYHA >II	Symptomatic arrhythmia	Cardiac medication prior to pregnancy
Left heart obstruction	Subaortic obstruction >30 mm Hg*	Smoking
Smoking	Smoking	Mechanical valve
Anticoagulation		Multiple gestation
Multiple gestation		

NYHA, New York Heart Association.
*The only risk factor remaining in multivariate analysis.

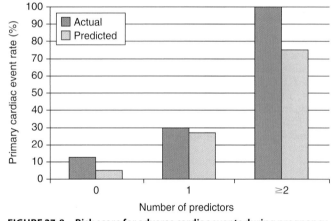

FIGURE 27-8   Risk score for adverse cardiac events during pregnancy. The actual versus the predicted event rates with 0, 1 and ≥2 risk factors. There was no significant difference between the actual and predicted groups. Risk factors in this study are shown in Table 27-4. *(From Khairy P, Ouyang DW, Fernandes SM, et al. Circulation 2006;113:517–24, with permissions.)*

Fallot, transposition of the great vessels, and truncus arteriosus, may have associated aortic dilation. Some surgical repairs of valvular heart disease are associated with the development of aortic dilation, including the Ross repair of aortic stenosis or arterial switch repairs for transposition of the great vessels. The risk of dissection in congenital abnormalities does not appear to be as high as the risk in connective tissue disorders. Although the American College of Cardiology (ACC)/American Heart Association (AHA) guidelines recommend consideration for aortic surgery to repair the aorta in patients with bicuspid valves and aortic diameter greater than 5.0 cm,[44] the aortic diameter that poses increased risk during pregnancy in such patients is not known. In those patients with Marfan syndrome, the risk appears highest for those patients with aortic diameters greater than 4.0 cm.[45-47]

Pregnancy increases the risk of dissection through several mechanisms, including estrogen interference with collagen deposition, elastase accelerating destruction of the elastic lamellae, and relaxin decreasing collagen synthesis.[48,49] Aortic dissection during pregnancy is rare but appears to be more common in women with bicuspid aortic valve.[48,50,51]

These studies emphasize the importance of placing the valvular disease in the context of a patient's other cardiac lesions, as risk factors for adverse outcomes may be additive. Additionally, functional class is important in risk assessment, independent of the underlying hemodynamic abnormality. Table 27-3 compares identified risk factors from the Valvular Heart Disease Guidelines of the ACC/AHA and the studies by Siu, Khairy, and Drenthen.[39,41,42]

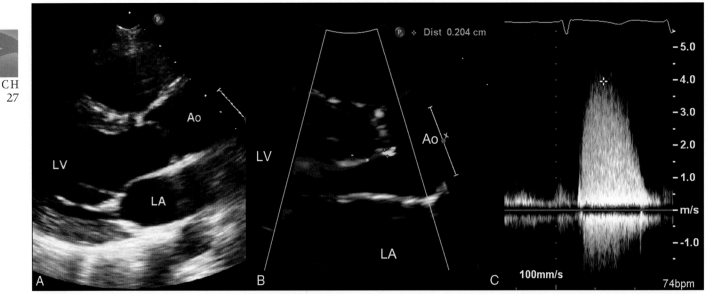

FIGURE 27-9 Aortic dilation. A 29-year-old woman who underwent a Ross repair for congenital aortic stenosis presents for preconceptual counseling. She is asymptomatic, able to keep up with her friends on long hikes and bike rides. Serial echocardiograms have shown progressive stenosis of her pulmonic homograft and enlargement of her proximal aorta (neo-aortic root). **A,** The parasternal long-axis 2D view shows a dilated aorta at the sinuses of Valsalva, with an end-diastolic diameter of 5.2 cm that has increased from 4.7 cm in the last 18 months. **B,** Color Doppler shows mild neo-aortic regurgitation. **C,** Continuous wave Doppler imaging of the pulmonic valve demonstrates severe pulmonic stenosis with a maximum velocity of 4.0 m/s. *LV,* left ventricle; *LA,* left atrium; *Ao,* Aorta.

Basic Clinical Approach

Evaluation of Disease Severity

The first step in evaluation of the pregnant woman with possible valve disease is to establish a specific diagnosis and determine the severity of disease. History and physical examination are important to identify cardiac symptoms or abnormal cardiac findings.

Healthy pregnant women frequently have symptoms or exam findings that may be suggestive of heart disease (Table 27-5). On exam, a systolic murmur is present in 80% of pregnant women and typically represents a benign flow murmur.[52]

In 103 women without a previous cardiac history who were referred for echocardiography for a murmur appreciated during pregnancy, about 80% had a physical examination consistent with a flow murmur; all of these women had a normal echocardiogram.[52] In the 7% with a pansystolic, late systolic, or diastolic murmur, all had abnormal echocardiograms, including three ventricular septal defects, one large atrial septal defect, one atrial septal defect with rheumatic mitral regurgitation, and one nonobstructive hypertrophic cardiomyopathy.

Echocardiography is warranted in pregnant women with a murmur if there is a previous history of cardiac disease, cardiac symptoms, arterial oxygen desaturation, a grade 3/6 or louder systolic murmur, or any diastolic murmur. In these patients, echocardiography allows accurate diagnosis of the location and severity of valve disease, associated hemodynamic abnormalities (such as pulmonary hypertension), and assessment of ventricular function.

Echocardiography is usually adequate to characterize valve and ventricular function. However, in patients with poor acoustic windows or complex anatomy, transthoracic echocardiography may be inadequate. Transesophageal echocardiography may be a useful surrogate, depending on the information needed. Cardiac magnetic resonance imaging appears to be safe in pregnant women, particularly after the first trimester, and can accurately quantify valvular regurgitation, ventricular dimensions, and ventricular function.[53] Gadolinium contrast is not required for the evaluation of ventricular and valvular function. The safety of gadolinium has not been well documented in pregnancy,

TABLE 27-5	Cardiac Findings During a Normal Pregnancy
Symptoms	
Fatigue	
Orthopnea	
Decreased exercise tolerance	
Palpitations	
Lower extremity edema	
Exam	
Mid-systolic murmur at left sternal border (pulmonic flow murmur)	
Split S1	
Continuous murmur (mammary souffle or venous hum)	
Lower extremity edema	
S3	

and, because it crosses the placenta, it is usually avoided in pregnancy.

Functional status plays an important role in risk stratification. Poor functional class is a risk factor for maternal and fetal complications. In addition to a careful symptom history, exercise testing may have a role in preconception counseling. If there is a significant valvular lesion and impaired functional status, valve surgery prior to pregnancy may be considered.

Management During Pregnancy

CLINICAL MONITORING

Once the diagnosis of valve disease is made, the cardiologist should work with a perinatologist to determine the optimal interval for evaluation and whether medical therapy is needed. The cardiologist and obstetrician should determine a plan for labor and delivery and discuss contingencies in the event of deterioration during pregnancy.

Women with valve disease require very close monitoring during pregnancy to prevent maternal and fetal complications. The frequency of evaluation is based on disease severity and clinical course. At each visit, a structured review of symptoms is performed to elicit early evidence of orthopnea, paroxysmal nocturnal dyspnea, a decrease in exercise tolerance, chest pain, dyspnea, or palpitations. Any change in exercise tolerance or subtle symptoms should prompt reevaluation for cardiac deterioration. In addition, long-range planning for interventions postpartum and plans for future pregnancies should be initiated early to ensure that appropriate postpartum cardiac evaluation is not delayed.

MEDICAL THERAPY

Medications need to be carefully reviewed prior to pregnancy to avoid medications that have adverse fetal effects. New medical therapies are used only as needed for symptoms or prevention of adverse events. For example, patients with mechanical prosthetic valves require anticoagulation, despite the risks of this therapy. However, when medical therapy is not essential and may not be safe in pregnancy, it should be discontinued during pregnancy. For example, a woman on an angiotensin-converting enzyme inhibitor for asymptomatic aortic regurgitation (AR) should discontinue this medication during pregnancy. On the other hand, medications that are critical to maintaining clinical stability may need to be continued or changed prior to pregnancy. For those patients in whom teratogenic medications are essential to maintain stability, pregnancy is likely ill-advised. For example, women on angiotensin-converting enzyme inhibitors for severely impaired ventricular function may not tolerate discontinuation or an alternative medication during pregnancy.

Occasionally, nonpharmacologic measures, such as bedrest, oxygen supplementation, avoiding the supine position, and patient education, can be effective at reducing symptoms. Diuretics and beta-blockers have been used extensively in pregnancy. Metoprolol undergoes accelerated metabolism during pregnancy so dose should be titrated to heart rate effect in conjunction with the obstetrics team.[54] Other beta-blockers have similarly accelerated metabolism, and many programs have found atenolol to be most effective, noting, however, that atenolol has a class D pregnancy rating from the U.S. Food and Drug Administration. Loop diuretics should be used to treat pulmonary congestion. However, diuretics can precipitate oligohydramnios so they should be used with caution.[55]

EFFECTS OF INTERCURRENT ILLNESS

Women with valve disease who are initially well compensated during pregnancy may abruptly decompensate with superimposition of another hemodynamic stress such as an intercurrent febrile illness.[56] Infection may lead to cardiac symptoms of angina or heart failure caused by increased metabolic demands associated with fever and tachycardia. Anemia, pulmonary embolus, or infection should be diligently sought in pregnant women with heart disease when decompensation occurs. Vaccination against influenza and pneumococcus is appropriate.

HERITABILITY

Women with congenital heart disease, including congenital valve disease, are more likely to have children with congenital heart disease.[57] Bicuspid aortic valve is heritable in many families, although penetrance is incomplete.[58,59] Children of patients with bicuspid aortic valve are also more likely to have associated conditions such as coarctation of the aorta, aortopathy, or hypoplastic left heart syndrome.[58,60] Fetal echocardiography has advanced substantially over the last 20 years, allowing diagnosis and hemodynamic assessment of fetal congenital heart disease.[61] Some congenital heart disease, such as coarctation of the aorta and patent ductus arteriosus, cannot be accurately detected by fetal echocardiography, however. Fetal echocardiography is appropriate in those women at higher risk, allowing the opportunity to identify significant cardiac defects and plan appropriately for the care of the fetus after delivery. If a significant cardiac abnormality is identified, there is opportunity prior to delivery to meet with the pediatric cardiologists, perinatologists, and cardiac surgeons to discuss management. For those patients considering termination of pregnancy, timing of fetal echo should also take into account the laws regarding elective termination.

Management in the Peripartum Period

Guidelines do not recommend antibiotic prophylaxis for vaginal deliveries in women with valvular heart disease.[62,63]

PERIPARTUM HEMODYNAMIC MONITORING

In patients with severe valve disease, particularly those with severe symptomatic left-sided obstructive lesions, a planned delivery with invasive hemodynamic monitoring can be considered. Placement of a Swan-Ganz catheter and arterial line allows continuous monitoring of hemodynamics and optimization of preload and afterload during labor and delivery and in the early postpartum period. In high-risk patients, monitoring may be continued for 24 to 48 hours postpartum to avoid deterioration caused by the intravascular fluid shifts during this time period.

TYPE OF DELIVERY

Most women with heart disease should undergo vaginal delivery. Cesarean delivery should be reserved for obstetric indications.[63] There is no difference in peripartum complication rates between vaginal delivery and cesarean delivery in women with heart disease.[40] In 599 consecutive pregnancies in women with heart disease, 27% were by cesarean section, with 96% of those for obstetric indications. Maternal cardiac status was the indication for cesarean section in only 4% of these patients.

Many high-risk obstetric centers recommend induction of labor to ensure the availability of an experienced cardiac and obstetric team for patient management. The optimal timing of induction is near term, with a favorable cervix. Prolonged inductions should be avoided. Pain control is especially important in women with heart disease to minimize catecholamine surges and changes in heart rate and systemic vascular resistance. Epidural analgesia can cause hypotension, which is usually easily treated with volume infusion. In addition, if the fetus has a cardiac abnormality, a planned delivery allows prompt care of the newborn infant. Many centers avoid Valsalva maneuver to minimize maternal hemodynamic stress. However, this practice is not evidence-based and may increase the risk of severe lacerations and postpartum hemorrhage.[64] Cesarean delivery is often preferable for women with aortic dimensions greater than 40 mm, chronic aortic dissection, or women who are anticoagulated.[63]

Timing of Surgical Intervention

In women with valve disease who present for evaluation prior to pregnancy, risk assessment can assist in deciding whether surgical intervention before pregnancy is necessary. Most women with mild-to-moderate valve disease tolerate pregnancy well so that valve surgery can be deferred. With severe regurgitation or stenosis, decision making is more difficult. If normal hemodynamics can be restored with retention of the native valve, such as mitral valve repair for mitral regurgitation or balloon valvotomy for mitral stenosis (MS), intervention for correction of the valve lesion prior to pregnancy usually is indicated. If correction requires valve replacement, the advantages of correcting the hemodynamic abnormality must be weighed against the risks of a prosthetic valve during pregnancy. When valve replacement is needed, the decision of whether to use a mechanical valve or tissue valve is difficult. Mechanical valves require anticoagulation, whereas tissue valves have limited durability, although the impact of pregnancy on durability is debated. Some studies suggest that pregnancy hastens valve degeneration, whereas others suggest that the rate of degeneration is related to the young age of the patients not pregnancy. Individualized recommendations are needed, balancing the risk of anticoagulation against the risk of reoperation.[65-67] In all young women undergoing valve replacement surgery, the possibility of a subsequent pregnancy should be also taken into account in deciding on the type of valve prosthesis.

In women with valvular heart disease who are first seen during pregnancy, surgical intervention usually can be deferred until the postpartum period, even when valve disease is severe. However, surgical intervention may rarely be needed in women with valvular heart disease and hemodynamic compromise during pregnancy that does not respond to medical management. Valve surgery during pregnancy has been performed with a maternal mortality of 3%, similar to nonpregnant women, but with a fetal loss rate between 12% and 50%.[68-72] Risk factors for adverse maternal or fetal outcomes include NYHA class greater than III, LV dysfunction, and emergent procedures, particularly aortic dissection. Surgical procedures should be performed by the most adept surgeon available, to minimize cardiopulmonary bypass time because risks to the fetus increase with increasing bypass time.[73] Balloon mitral valvotomy or aortic valvuloplasty can be performed during pregnancy, if needed, with shielding of the abdomen to limit radiation exposure to the fetus. However, complications at the time of valvotomy that require urgent surgical intervention would be expected to have adverse outcomes for the fetus.

Women with severe valve disease who are managed medically during pregnancy should be referred for surgical intervention postpartum using the same criteria as for valve disease in nonpregnant patients (Figure 27-10). However, a postpartum improvement in well-being combined with caring for an infant may result in poor compliance with follow-up visits. Therefore, a reasonable approach is to evaluate the valve disease carefully during pregnancy, to discuss the options with the patient, and, if intervention is indicated, to proceed with valve surgery or balloon valvotomy early postpartum, possibly during the same hospital admission.

Specific Valvular Lesions and Outcomes

Aortic Stenosis

The etiology of aortic stenosis in pregnant women usually is congenital, often a unicuspid valve.[39,74] A substantial number of patients have undergone previous surgical valvotomy as a child; in 20% of patients with unicuspid aortic valve who received valvuloplasty, restenosis requires reoperation at a mean of 13 years after the initial surgery, at the age when pregnancy is most likely.[75] In women with aortic stenosis, the increased stroke volume of pregnancy is associated with an increase in transvalvular velocity and pressure gradient. Valve area calculations are accurate, allowing decision making regarding postpartum management. Many previously asymptomatic women with aortic stenosis have symptom onset during pregnancy caused by increased systemic metabolic demands and a limited ability to increase stroke volume.[74,76] Heart failure symptoms also may be a result of decreased LV compliance. The relative tachycardia of pregnancy limits the time for diastolic coronary blood flow, sometimes leading to angina. Even if pregnancy itself is well tolerated, any superimposed hemodynamic stress, such as infection or anemia, can lead to clinical decompensation.

Aortic stenosis is associated with an increased maternal and fetal risk with the level of risk related to the severity of LV outflow obstruction.[74,76-78] Symptoms typically increase by one NYHA functional class in about one half of patients. Heart failure is the most common complication, occurring in up to 40% of cases.[39,76,79] The risk of neonatal complication is high, occurring in as many as 25% of pregnancies in women with aortic stenosis.[39] The most common neonatal complications are prematurity and being small for gestational age, which may be the result of reduced placental perfusion.[80,81] Most women with mild and moderate stenosis have no events during pregnancy. Conversely, approximately 40% of those with severe stenosis have events, even when asymptomatic prior to pregnancy.[80,82] Clinical deterioration during pregnancy may persist after delivery and increase the probability of late interventions in this population.[83]

Echocardiography allows quantitative evaluation of the severity of aortic stenosis and any associated abnormalities. Peak and mean aortic gradients predictably rise during pregnancy because of increased cardiac output. Aortic valve area, however, should remain unchanged. Although aortic stenosis increases maternal risk, many patients can be managed medically. Even when stenosis is severe, maternal mortality is rare.[76,84] Patient education and frequent monitoring are used in asymptomatic patients. If symptoms occur, treatment options include bed rest, diuretics, oxygen supplement, and use of beta-blockers to increase LV and coronary diastolic filling times. Intercurrent febrile events are

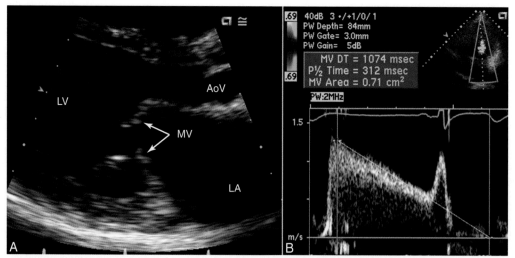

FIGURE 27-10 Severe mitral stenosis. A 39-year-old woman presented in the third trimester of her fifth pregnancy with dyspnea and pulmonary crackles on examination. Echocardiography *(left)* shows rheumatic mitral stenosis with characteristic doming of the mitral leaflets in diastole in a parasternal long-axis view. Pressure half time *(right)* showed a valve area of 0.71 cm². The patient was diuresed and symptomatically improved. The remainder of her pregnancy was spent at bed rest, and she underwent an uncomplicated delivery. Dyspnea and pulmonary edema developed in the first 2 days of postpartum and responded to diuretics. She then underwent balloon valvotomy with a significant improvement in her valve area. *LV,* left ventricle; *LA,* left atrium; *Ao,* aorta; *MV,* mitral valve.

commonly associated with decompensation and often can be managed with fever reduction, beta-blockers, supplemental oxygen, and bed rest. With severe decompensation, hemodynamic monitoring in the intensive care unit with optimization of preload and afterload may be needed. Balloon aortic valvuloplasty and aortic valve replacement (AVR) have been described in patients with severe aortic stenosis who failed medical therapy.[85-87] As transcatheter aortic valve implantation (TAVI) is more widely used, there may be opportunities for use in pregnant women as an alternative to the rare circumstances of valvuloplasty failure or need for traditional surgical AVR. To date, there are no data or case reports of TAVI in pregnant women, and this would be an off-label indication.

Mitral Stenosis

Mitral valve stenosis is most often due to rheumatic valve disease, although congenital mitral stenosis is encountered.[38] The murmur of MS is difficult to appreciate in the pregnant patient. Echocardiography allows evaluation of stenosis severity, associated regurgitation, and estimation of pulmonary systolic pressure.

Previously asymptomatic patients with MS may first experience symptoms during pregnancy because of hemodynamic changes of pregnancy.[39] A mild decrease in functional status is experienced by 43% of patients, with 30% experiencing a more severe reduction in functional status, although it should be noted that even normal women have a fall in functional status with pregnancy.[55] The increased transmitral flow rate and the shortened diastolic filling time lead to an increase in left atrial pressure, which may result in pulmonary edema and an obligatory rise in pulmonary artery pressure. Symptoms most often begin in the second trimester with 43% developing heart failure, 20% arrhythmias, 50% having a change in medication, and 43% requiring hospitalization during pregnancy.[55]

Beta-blockers may be helpful in pregnant women with MS by increasing the diastolic filling time, resulting in both a decrease in left atrial pressure and an increase in forward stroke volume.[88] Diuretics may be used judiciously for volume overload. Diuresis may impair uteroplacental blood flow; therefore, caution must be taken in their use. With rheumatic mitral valve disease, it also is important to continue antibiotic prophylaxis to prevent recurrent rheumatic fever during pregnancy.

Admission to the intensive care unit with placement of a pulmonary artery catheter may be needed to guide medical therapy in severely symptomatic patients. In cases unresponsive to medical therapy, balloon mitral valvotomy can be performed during pregnancy. Abdominal shielding limits radiation exposure. Alternatively, transesophageal echocardiographic guidance can be used to minimize radiation exposure.[89-94] If radiation exposure is kept below 5 rad, the risk of teratogenicity is very low. If there is greater than 10 rad of exposure, the risk of teratogenicity, central nervous system abnormalities, and childhood cancers increases, and consideration should be given to termination.

Immediate and long-term results of balloon valvotomy are good even when performed in pregnancy. In a study of 71 NYHA class III-IV patients who underwent valvotomy, 98% were NYHA class I-II at the end of pregnancy. Event-free survival at 44 months was 54%. The majority of events were initiation of medical therapy, with some patients undergoing repeat valvotomy or mitral valve surgery. The neonates born following valvotomy had normal growth and development and no clinical abnormalities. A 2010 Cochrane review of 68 publications described 1289 women who underwent mitral balloon valvotomy or surgery for MS during pregnancy. There was a 3% incidence of minor adverse events and most events and a 0.7% rate of major complications.[95] This and other data suggest that, in patients failing medical therapy, mitral valvotomy is an acceptable option.[96,97]

Patients at highest risk for significant decompensation are those with moderate or severe mitral stenosis and cardiac symptoms prior to pregnancy.[55,98-100]

Aortic Regurgitation

AR is uncommon in pregnant women. Causes include a bicuspid aortic valve, previous valvuloplasty, endocarditis, rheumatic valve disease, or aortic root dilation (Figure 27-11). When aortic disease is present, such as in Marfan syndrome, the risk of

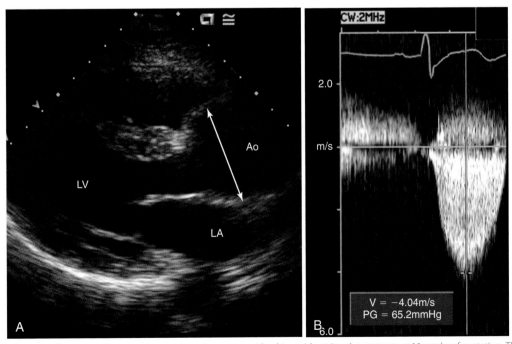

FIGURE 27-11 **Aortic valve disease.** A 20-year-old asymptomatic woman with a bicuspid aortic valve presents at 16 weeks of gestation. The parasternal long-axis view shows a bicuspid aortic valve with a dilated aorta and normal left ventricular size **(A).** Continuous wave Doppler imaging showing significant aortic stenosis with an aortic velocity of 4.0 m/s **(B).** She was cared for and delivered in a center with expertise heart disease during pregnancy and had an uneventful pregnancy and delivery. *LV,* left ventricle; *LA,* left atrium; *Ao,* aorta.

pregnancy is more closely linked to the risk of the aortic dissection than to the AR. In theory, the decrease in systemic vascular resistance and shortened diastole of pregnancy might decrease aortic regurgitant severity. In reality, AR severity is unchanged because the decrease in systemic vascular resistance is counterbalanced by the increased intravascular volume, and slight increase in aortic root dimension is associated with pregnancy. Typically, patients with AR tolerate pregnancy well. If symptoms occur, a careful evaluation to distinguish worsening of valve disease from other causes of symptoms is warranted.

Mitral Regurgitation

Mitral regurgitation (MR) in pregnancy may be a result of mitral valve prolapse, endocarditis, or rheumatic disease. Mild-to-moderate MR is well tolerated. Mitral valve prolapse is not associated with increased maternal risk, unless severe mitral regurgitation is present.[101,102] Even severe mitral regurgitation may be well tolerated unless atrial fibrillation or pulmonary hypertension complicates the presentation. There also have been case reports of clinical deterioration during pregnancy caused by acute severe MR secondary to chordal rupture as a result of endocarditis or myxomatous mitral valve disease.

Management of MR during pregnancy is directed toward careful monitoring during pregnancy and at the time of labor and delivery. There are no data to support the use of vasodilators for MR in pregnancy, and pregnancy itself is a powerful afterload reducer.

Right-Sided Valve Disease

Pulmonic stenosis (PS) in pregnancy is invariably congenital in origin and, if severe, has usually been treated in infancy or childhood. Severe PS is rare in adults because milder forms of PS rarely progress to severe stenosis during adulthood. Cases of severe PS during pregnancy usually are a result of restenosis or prosthetic valve dysfunction in patients with congenital heart disease. Mild-to-moderate PS is well tolerated in pregnancy.[55,103] When using the Doppler tricuspid regurgitant jet velocity to estimate right ventricular systolic pressure, the transpulmonic gradient must then be subtracted to obtain pulmonary pressure when PS is present.

PS accounted for about 10% of all patients in a series of 599 pregnancies in women with heart disease.[39] There were no adverse cardiac events in these 58 pregnancies, and only 1 patient had worsening cardiac symptoms. However, neonatal complications occurred in 17% of these pregnancies.[39] In a systematic review, there were no maternal cardiovalvular events in the 123 women with PS, out of a total of 2491 pregnancies.[104] However, noncardiac complications were common with a higher-than-expected rate of pregnancy-induced hypertension and fetal complications such as prematurity, small for gestational age, and intrauterine growth retardation.[105] However, these findings have not been confirmed in other studies, and the mechanism for increased pregnancy-induced hypertension is not evident. Tricuspid stenosis in pregnancy is rare, but treatment with balloon mitral valvuloplasty has been reported.

Right-sided valve regurgitation is generally well tolerated in pregnancy. PR also is a result of congenital heart disease and is most often a sequelae of a previous surgical procedure, such as repair of tetralogy of Fallot (Figure 27-12). In patients with repaired tetralogy of Fallot, maternal and fetal complication rates are generally low, but severe PR with impaired right ventricular function, LV dysfunction, and severe pulmonary hypertension are risk factors for maternal cardiac events.[106,107] Severe PR combined with another risk factor (such as twin pregnancy, right ventricular dysfunction, or a concomitant right-sided obstructive lesion) may increase the risk of adverse outcomes.[108] Because of the low rate of maternal and fetal complications associated with PR, prophylactic pulmonic valve replacement is not necessarily indicated prior to pregnancy in asymptomatic women.[108] Tricuspid regurgitation may be a result of Ebstein anomaly or previous endocarditis.[39,109]

Prosthetic Valves

In patients with heart valve prostheses, the hemodynamic changes of pregnancy result in increased transvalvular velocities, even with no change in valve function. Valve area should remain stable during pregnancy. A baseline echocardiographic study early in pregnancy is useful if symptoms occur later in pregnancy.

OUTCOMES

The major issues in management of women with heart valve prostheses are anticoagulation for mechanical valves and the risk of valve degeneration with tissue valves.

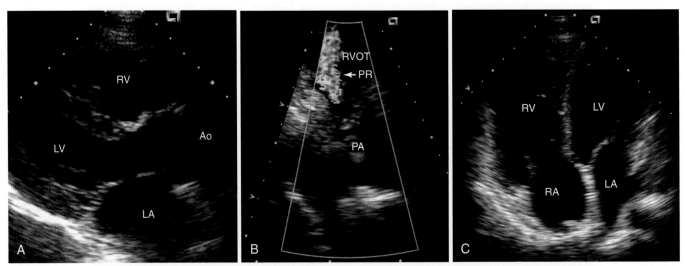

FIGURE 27-12 Tetralogy of Fallot. A 28-year-old G2P1 asymptomatic woman with tetralogy of Fallot is seen in the clinic at 15 weeks of gestation. At age 3, she had surgical repair with closure of the ventricular septal defect (VSD) and a transannular right ventricular outflow patch for relief of pulmonic stenosis. She has been followed for pulmonic regurgitation and RV enlargement. **A,** The parasternal long axis shows an overriding aorta, VSD patch and right ventricular enlargement. **B,** Color Doppler imaging of the pulmonic valve and main pulmonary artery demonstrates pulmonic regurgitation. **C,** The apical four-chamber view shows RV enlargement.

Women with either tissue or mechanical heart valves have significantly worse outcomes with pregnancy than women without valvular disease.[110-112] Older generation mechanical valves appear to have higher complication rates[111-114] than newer generation valves, but little data are available directly comparing the types of valves, and the literature largely reports the experience with older generation valves.[115]

In women with bioprosthetic valves, there are fewer thromboembolic or bleeding complications; however, the incidence of maternal death still ranges from 0% to 5%. Data regarding the outcome of bioprosthetic valves during pregnancy are conflicting. Some series suggest a rapid deterioration during or after pregnancy[65,111-113] and have speculated that high flow and high calcium turnover during pregnancy can precipitate valve degradation.[66,111] Others, however, have suggested that newer generation bioprosthetic valves fare better and have found no impact of pregnancy on valve durability.[65-67,116-119] It remains controversial whether pregnancy accelerates valve degeneration or whether the degeneration seen in pregnant women reflects the relatively rapid valve degeneration seen in younger patients. Pregnancy with a pulmonic autograft (Ross procedure) has been reported, but the experience with pregnancy after this procedure is limited.[120,121]

ANTICOAGULATION

Although the importance of maintaining adequate anticoagulation during pregnancy in women with mechanical prosthetic valves is clear,[113,122] the specific management of anticoagulation remains controversial.[112,123] Each option for anticoagulation during pregnancy carries risks for mother and fetus. Overall, the maternal complication rate is high in women with mechanical valves, and the thromboembolic rate ranges from 2.5% to 11%, depending on the strategy of anticoagulation used.[124] Major society guidelines for anticoagulation during pregnancy are summarized in Table 27-6.

Both unfractionated heparin and low-molecular weight heparin (LMWH) are safe for the fetus, do not cross the placenta, and provide effective anticoagulation when used in therapeutic doses and are meticulously monitored.[125,126] Unfractionated heparin can be given twice daily by subcutaneous injections or by continuous infusion.[125,126] LMWH is dosed according to Xa levels. Weight-based fixed dosing of LMWH is absolutely contraindicated.[127] Valve thrombosis occurs at a rate of 4% to 9% and is more common in women with subtherapeutic Xa levels.[127-129] A disadvantage of heparin therapy is the development of osteoporosis with a small risk (less than 2%) of symptomatic fractures but a higher risk of a detectable decrease in bone density (in one third of women).[130-133] Heparin offers significant challenges in optimal methods of drug administration and monitoring of the anticoagulation effect, and there is frequent need for dose adjustment.[114,134] Overall, the use of heparin during pregnancy has a higher risk of thromboembolic complications than warfarin.[124]

Warfarin provides the lowest risk of thromboembolic complications during pregnancy and is easier to administer, although monitoring remains challenging.[115] The major risks of warfarin during pregnancy are the risk of embryopathy and fetal bleeding. The risks of warfarin therapy during pregnancy include first trimester teratogenicity, particularly between the sixth and twelfth weeks of gestation.[135-137] There also may be an increased

TABLE 27-6	ACC/AHA, ACCP, and ESC Guidelines Regarding Anticoagulation during Pregnancy in Women with Mechanical Valves

ACC/AHA Guidelines

(1) Women who stop warfarin from weeks 6-12 should be anticoagulated with continuous IV UFH, dose adjusted subcutaneous UFH or dose adjusted LMWH.

(2) Up to 36 weeks of gestation, the choice of warfarin, continuous IV UFH, dose adjusted subcutaneous UFH or dose adjusted LMWH should be discussed fully with the patient.
   In patients who receive dose adjusted LMWH, it is administered twice daily, with goal antifactor Xa levels of 0.7-1.2 four hours after administration.
   The target for dose adjusted UFH should be twice control
   Warfarin should be dosed to a goal INR of 3 (range 2.5-3.0).

(3) Warfarin should be stopped 2 weeks prior to planned delivery and replaced with continuous IV UFH.

ACCP Guidelines. The selection of any of the following regiments is acceptable.

(1) Adjusted-dose bid LMWH throughout pregnancy.
   Doses adjusted to achieve the manufacturer's peak anti-Xa LMWH 4 hours post injection.

(2) Adjusted-dose UFH throughout pregnancy.
   Administered subcutaneously every 12 hours in doses adjusted to keep the mid-interval aPTT at least twice control or attain an anti-Xa heparin level of 0.35 to 0.70 units/mL.

(3) UFH or LMWH (as above) until the thirteenth week, with substitution by vitamin K antagonists until close to delivery when UFH or LMWH is resumed.

ESC GUIDELINES	CLASS*
(1) OACs recommended during the second and third trimesters until the week 36.	I
If delivery starts while on OACs, cesarean delivery is indicated.	I
(2) OAC should be discontinued and dose-adjusted UFH** or adjusted-dose LMWH† started at the week 36 of gestation.	I
(3) In pregnant women managed with LMWH, the post-dose anti-Xa level should be assessed weekly. LMWH should be avoided, unless anti-Xa levels are monitored.	I
LMWH should be replaced by intravenous UFH at least 36 hours before planned delivery. UFH should be continued until 4–6 hours before planned delivery and restarted 4–6 hours after delivery if there are no bleeding complications.	I
(4) Continuation of OACs should be considered during the first trimester if the warfarin dose required for therapeutic anticoagulation is <5 mg/day.	IIa
(5) Discontinuation of OAC between weeks 6 and 12 and replacement by adjusted-dose UFH**; in high risk patients applied as intravenous infusion or LMWH twice daily† should be considered in patients with a warfarin dose required of >5 mg/day.	IIa
Discontinuation of OACs between weeks 6 and 12 and replacement by UFH** or LMWH† may be considered on an individual basis in patients with warfarin dose required for therapeutic anticoagulation <5 mg/day.	IIb
Continuation of OACs may be considered between weeks 6 and 12 in patients with a warfarin dose required for therapeutic anticoagulation >5 mg/day.	IIb

ACC/AHA, American College of Cardiology/American Heart Association; *ACCP*, American College of Chest Physicians; *ESC*, European Society of Cardiology; *UFH*, unfractionated heparin; *LMWH*, low-molecular weight heparin; *OACs*, oral anticoagulants.
Adapted from Bonow RO, Carabello BA, Kanu C, et al. Circulation 2006;114(5):e84–231; Bates SM, Greer IA, Middeldorp S, et al. Chest 2012;141:e691S–736S; and Regitz-Zagrosek V, Blomstrom Lundqvist C, Borghi C, et al. Eur Heart J 2011;32(24):3147–97.
*All recommendations are Level of Evidence "C".
**Dose adjusted to aPTT ≥2× control.
†LMWH adjusted to target anti-Xa level 4–6 hours post-dose 0.8-1.2 U/mL.

risk of central nervous system abnormalities with exposure to warfarin at any time during pregnancy.[135] In addition, there is a substantial risk of bleeding in the anticoagulated fetus, especially at the time of delivery, so it is necessary to transition to unfractionated heparin at approximately 35 weeks of gestation.[63,138] The incidence of warfarin embryopathy is reported to be anywhere from less than 5% to well over 10%.[56,111,115,139-141] In an attempt to consolidate disparate data, literature reviews are available. One well-done review found a rate of warfarin embryopathy of 6.4%,[115] whereas another review found a rate of 7.4% of live births.[67] A reasonable estimate is 4% to 10%. This adverse effect of warfarin may be dose-dependent: In one small study, women taking greater than 5 mg/day had a fetal complication rate of 88%, and embryopathy was seen in 8%. Conversely, women taking less than or equal to 5 mg/day had a fetal complication rate of 15% and embryopathy in 0%.[139] Low dose warfarin (less than 5 mg/day, target INR 1.5 to 2.0) for patients with mechanical aortic valves has been attempted. However, valve thrombosis rate was 3.5% and fetal malformation rate was greater than 3%, which suggests that this is not an optimal strategy.[142] Because of the teratogenicity associated with warfarin in the first trimester, most societies recommend the use of adjusted dose heparin (either unfractionated or low-molecular weight) during the first trimester, after which point women can consider transition to warfarin. However, for women at extremely high risk of thrombosis during pregnancy (older style atrioventricular valves, for example), uninterrupted warfarin can be considered after a careful discussion about fetal risks.

Unfortunately, there are no randomized controlled trials comparing options for anticoagulation of mechanical heart valves in pregnancy. A Danish nationwide registry found similar levels of maternal complications among contemporary strategies of anticoagulation.[143] A large meta-analysis demonstrated lowest maternal risk with warfarin and highest maternal risk with unfractionated heparin. Other available data are cohort studies, small case series, or case reports. Therefore, the literature is rife with reviews and opinion, but little contemporary, quality data on which to make recommendations. Accordingly, the AHA and ACC and American College of Chest Physicians recommendations emphasize the importance of *continuous effective anticoagulation with frequent monitoring throughout pregnancy*. The guidelines then discuss several options for achieving continuous effective anticoagulation, and Class I recommendations for anticoagulation during pregnancy in women with mechanical heart valves are listed in Table 27-6. The guidelines state that if antifactor Xa levels cannot be monitored, LMWH should not be used.[44,63] The addition of low dose aspirin (75 to 100 mg daily) is encouraged by most societies.

With any approach to anticoagulation, close monitoring is essential to maintain therapeutic anticoagulation and to avoid bleeding or thrombotic complications. Without meticulous management, the complication rate is high.[111] Many of the hemorrhagic and thromboembolic complications associated with anticoagulation and prosthetic valves during pregnancy can be avoided by a rigorous approach to management and monitoring of anticoagulation.

Acute valve thrombosis during pregnancy is rare and appears to be more common in patients treated with heparin, although data are limited to case reports. Recombinant tissue plasminogen activator (Alteplase) does not cross the placenta and is not known to cause teratogenicity in animals.[144] Thrombolytics can cause placental bleeding, however, and may result in premature labor or placental abruption.[145] Thrombolytics are not absolutely contraindicated in pregnancy, but a careful risk-benefit analysis must be undertaken. The fetal loss rate with thrombolytic therapy is approximately 6%,[146] and maternal hemorrhage is possible if delivery occurs less than 24 hours after thrombolytic therapy.

New anticoagulants, such as oral direct thrombin inhibitors, oral Xa inhibitors, and direct thrombin inhibitors, have not been shown to be safe for patients with mechanical valves and should not be used.

REFERENCES

1. Cole P, St. John Sutton M. Cardiovascular physiology in pregnancy. In: Douglas PS, editor. Cardiovascular health and disease in women. Philadelphia: Saunders; 1993. p. 305–28.
2. Katz VL. Physiologic changes during normal pregnancy. Curr Opin Obstet Gynecol 1991;3:750–8.
3. Capeless EL, Clapp JF. Cardiovascular changes in early phase of pregnancy. Am J Obstet Gynecol 1989;161:1449–53.
4. Gilson GJ, Samaan S, Crawford MH, et al. Changes in hemodynamics, ventricular remodeling, and ventricular contractility during normal pregnancy: a longitudinal study. Obstet Gynecol 1997;89:957–62.
5. Tihtonen K, Koobi T, Yli-Hankala A, et al. Maternal hemodynamics during cesarean delivery assessed by whole-body impedance cardiography. Acta Obstet Gynecol Scand 2005;84:355–61.
6. Mesa A, Jessurun C, Hernandez A, et al. Left ventricular diastolic function in normal human pregnancy. Circulation 1999;99:511–17.
7. Robson SC, Dunlop W. When do cardiovascular parameters return to their preconception values? Am J Obstet Gynecol 1992;167:1479.
8. Mabie WC, DiSessa TG, Crocker LG, et al. A longitudinal study of cardiac output in normal human pregnancy. Am J Obstet Gynecol 1994;170:849–56.
9. Easterling TR, Benedetti TJ. Measurement of cardiac output by impedance technique. Am J Obstet Gynecol 1990;163:1104–6.
10. Easterling TR, Benedetti TJ, Schmucker BC, et al. Maternal hemodynamics in normal and preeclamptic pregnancies: a longitudinal study. Obstet Gynecol 1990;76:1061–9.
11. Hunter S, Robson SC. Adaptation of the maternal heart in pregnancy. Br Heart J 1992;68:540–3.
12. Robson SC, Hunter S, Boys RJ, et al. Serial changes in pulmonary haemodynamics during human pregnancy: a non-invasive study using Doppler echocardiography. Clin Sci (Lond) 1991;80:113–17.
13. Clark SL, Cotton DB, Lee W, et al. Central hemodynamic assessment of normal term pregnancy. Am J Obstet Gynecol 1989;161:1439–42.
14. Edouard DA, Pannier BM, London GM, et al. Venous and arterial behavior during normal pregnancy. Am J Physiol 1998;274:H1605–12.
15. Geva T, Mauer MB, Striker L, et al. Effects of physiologic load of pregnancy on left ventricular contractility and remodeling. Am Heart J 1997;133:53–9.
16. Mone SM, Sanders SP, Colan SD. Control mechanisms for physiological hypertrophy of pregnancy. Circulation 1996;94:667–72.
17. Clark SL. Cardiac disease in pregnancy. Crit Care Clin 1991;7:777–97.
18. McLennan FM, Haites NE, Rawles JM. Stroke and minute distance in pregnancy: a longitudinal study using Doppler ultrasound. Br J Obstet Gynaecol 1987;94:499–506.
19. Robson SC, Dunlop W, Boys RJ, et al. Cardiac output during labour. Br Med J (Clin Res Ed) 1987;295:1169–72.
20. Lee W, Rokey R, Miller J, et al. Maternal hemodynamic effects of uterine contractions by M-mode and pulsed-Doppler echocardiography. Am J Obstet Gynecol 1989;161:974–7.
21. Strickland RA, Oliver Jr WC, Chantigian RC, et al. Anesthesia, cardiopulmonary bypass, and the pregnant patient. Mayo Clin Proc 1991;66:411–29.
22. Robson SC, Hunter S. Haemodynamic changes during the early puerperium. Br Med J (Clin Res Ed) 1987;294:1065.
23. Robson SC, Hunter S, Boys RJ, et al. Hemodynamic changes during twin pregnancy. A Doppler and M-mode echocardiographic study. Am J Obstet Gynecol 1989;161:1273–8.
24. Clark SL, Horenstein JM, Phelan JP, et al. Experience with the pulmonary artery catheter in obstetrics and gynecology. Am J Obstet Gynecol 1985;152:374–8.
25. Easterling TR, Schmucker BC, Benedetti TJ. The hemodynamic effects of orthostatic stress during pregnancy. Obstet Gynecol 1988;72:550–2.
26. Robson SC, Hunter S, Moore M, et al. Haemodynamic changes during the puerperium: a Doppler and M-mode echocardiographic study. Br J Obstet Gynaecol 1987;94:1028–39.
27. Robson SC, Hunter S, Boys RJ, et al. Serial study of factors influencing changes in cardiac output during human pregnancy. Am J Physiol 1989;256:H1060–5.
28. Sadaniantz A, Kocheril AG, Emaus SP, et al. Cardiovascular changes in pregnancy evaluated by two-dimensional and Doppler echocardiography. J Am Soc Echocardiogr 1992;5:253–8.
29. Rubler S, Damani PM, Pinto ER. Cardiac size and performance during pregnancy estimated with echocardiography. Am J Cardiol 1977;40:534–40.
30. Vered Z, Poler SM, Gibson P, et al. Noninvasive detection of the morphologic and hemodynamic changes during normal pregnancy. Clin Cardiol 1991;14:327–34.
31. Laird-Meeter K, van de Ley G, Bom TH, et al. Cardiocirculatory adjustments during pregnancy—an echocardiographic study. Clin Cardiol 1979;2:328–32.
32. Easterling TR, Benedetti TJ, Schmucker BC, et al. Maternal hemodynamics and aortic diameter in normal and hypertensive pregnancies. Obstet Gynecol 1991;78:1073–7.
33. Hart MV, Morton MJ, Hosenpud JD, et al. Aortic function during normal human pregnancy. Am J Obstet Gynecol 1986;154:887–91.
34. Bradley TD, Logan AG, Kimoff RJ, et al. Continuous positive airway pressure for central sleep apnea and heart failure. N Engl J Med 2005;353:2025–33.
35. Pouta AM, Rasanen JP, Airaksinen KE, et al. Changes in maternal heart dimensions and plasma atrial natriuretic peptide levels in the early puerperium of normal and preeclamptic pregnancies. Br J Obstet Gynaecol 1996;103:988–92.
36. Campos O, Andrade JL, Bocanegra J, et al. Physiologic multivalvular regurgitation during pregnancy: a longitudinal Doppler echocardiographic study. Int J Cardiol 1993;40:265–72.
37. Boudoulas H. Etiology of valvular heart disease. Expert Rev Cardiovasc Ther 2003;1:523–32.

38. Soler-Soler J, Galve E. Worldwide perspective of valve disease. Heart 2000;83: 721–5.

39. Siu SC, Sermer M, Colman JM, et al. Prospective multicenter study of pregnancy outcomes in women with heart disease. Circulation 2001;104:515–21.

40. Siu SC, Colman JM, Sorensen S, et al. Adverse neonatal and cardiac outcomes are more common in pregnant women with cardiac disease. Circulation 2002;105:2179–84.

41. Khairy P, Ouyang DW, Fernandes SM, et al. Pregnancy outcomes in women with congenital heart disease. Circulation 2006;113:517–24.

42. Drenthen W, Boersma E, Balci A, et al. Predictors of pregnancy complications in women with congenital heart disease. Eur Heart J 2010;31:2124–32.

43. Roos-Hesselink JW, Ruys TP, Stei JI, et al. Outcome of pregnancy in patients with structural or ischaemic heart disease: results of a registry of the European Society of Cardiology. Eur Heart J 2013 34(9):657–65.

44. Bonow RO, Carabello BA, Kanu C, et al. ACC/AHA 2006 guidelines for the management of patients with valvular heart disease: a report of the American College of Cardiology/American Heart Association Task Force on Practice Guidelines (writing committee to revise the 1998 Guidelines for the Management of Patients With Valvular Heart Disease): developed in collaboration with the Society of Cardiovascular Anesthesiologists: endorsed by the Society for Cardiovascular Angiography and Interventions and the Society of Thoracic Surgeons. Circulation 2006;114:e84–231.

45. Milewicz DM, Dietz HC, Miller DC. Treatment of aortic disease in patients with Marfan syndrome 10.1161/01.CIR.0000155243.70456.F4. Circulation 2005;111:e150–7.

46. Lind J, Wallenburg HC. The Marfan syndrome and pregnancy: a retrospective study in a Dutch population. Eur J Obstet Gynecol Reprod Biol 2001;98:28–35.

47. Meijboom LJ, Vos FE, Timmermans J, et al. Pregnancy and aortic root growth in the Marfan syndrome: a prospective study. Eur Heart J 2005;26:914–20.

48. Immer FF, Bansi AG, Immer-Bansi AS, et al. Aortic dissection in pregnancy: analysis of risk factors and outcome. Ann Thorac Surg 2003;76:309–14.

49. Bryant-Greenwood GD, Schwabe C. Human relaxins: chemistry and biology. Endocr Rev 1994;15:5–26.

50. Nienaber CA, Fattori R, Mehta RH, et al. Gender-related differences in acute aortic dissection. Circulation 2004;109:3014–21.

51. McKellar SH, MacDonald RJ, Michelena HI, et al. Frequency of cardiovascular events in women with a congenitally bicuspid aortic valve in a single community and effect of pregnancy on events. Am J Cardiol 2011;107:96–9.

52. Mishra M, Chambers JB, Jackson G. Murmurs in pregnancy: an audit of echocardiography. BMJ 1992;304:1413–14.

53. De Wilde JP, Rivers AW, Price DL. A review of the current use of magnetic resonance imaging in pregnancy and safety implications for the fetus. Prog Biophys Mol Biol 2005;87:335–53.

54. Wadelius M, Darj E, Frenne G, et al. Induction of CYP2D6 in pregnancy. Clin Pharmacol Ther 1997;62:400–7.

55. Hameed A, Karaalp IS, Tummala PP, et al. The effect of valvular heart disease on maternal and fetal outcome of pregnancy. J Am Coll Cardiol 2001;37:893–9.

56. Elkayam U, Gleicher N. Cardiac problems in pregnancy: diagnosis and management of maternal and fetal disease. 3rd ed. New York: Wiley-Liss; 1998.

57. Siu SC, Colman JM. Heart disease and pregnancy. Heart 2001;85:710–15.

58. Cripe L, Andelfinger G, Martin LJ, et al. Bicuspid aortic valve is heritable. J Am Coll Cardiol 2004;44:138–43.

59. Huntington K, Hunter AG, Chan KL. A prospective study to assess the frequency of familial clustering of congenital bicuspid aortic valve. J Am Coll Cardiol 1997;30:1809–12.

60. Biner S, Rafique AM, Ray I, et al. Aortopathy is prevalent in relatives of bicuspid aortic valve patients. J Am Coll Cardiol 2009;53:2288–95.

61. Gardiner HM. Fetal echocardiography: 20 years of progress. Heart 2001;86(Suppl 2):II12–22.

62. Wilson W, Taubert KA, Gewitz M, et al. Prevention of infective endocarditis: guidelines from the American Heart Association: a guideline from the American Heart Association Rheumatic Fever, Endocarditis, and Kawasaki Disease Committee, Council on Cardiovascular Disease in the Young, and the Council on Clinical Cardiology, Council on Cardiovascular Surgery and Anesthesia, and the Quality of Care and Outcomes Research Interdisciplinary Working Group. Circulation 2007;116:1736–54.

63. Regitz-Zagrosek V, Blomstrom Lundqvist C, Borghi C, et al. ESC Guidelines on the management of cardiovascular diseases during pregnancy: the Task Force on the Management of Cardiovascular Diseases during Pregnancy of the European Society of Cardiology (ESC). Eur Heart J 2011;32:3147–97.

64. Ouyang DW, Khairy P, Fernandes SM, et al. Obstetric outcomes in pregnant women with congenital heart disease. Int J Cardiol 2010;144:195–9.

65. Badduke BR, Jamieson WR, Miyagishima RT, et al. Pregnancy and childbearing in a population with biologic valvular prostheses. J Thorac Cardiovasc Surg 1991;102:179–86.

66. Jamieson WR, Miller DC, Akins CW, et al. Pregnancy and bioprostheses: influence on structural valve deterioration. Ann Thorac Surg 1995;60:S282–6; discussion S7.

67. Hung L, Rahimtoola SH. Prosthetic heart valves and pregnancy. Circulation 2003;107:1240–6.

68. Mahli A, Izdes S, Coskun D. Cardiac operations during pregnancy: review of factors influencing fetal outcome. Ann Thorac Surg 2000;69:1622–6.

69. Pomini F, Mercogliano D, Cavalletti C, et al. Cardiopulmonary bypass in pregnancy. Ann Thorac Surg 1996;61:259–68.

70. Parry AJ, Westaby S. Cardiopulmonary bypass during pregnancy. Ann Thorac Surg 1996;61:1865–9.

71. Avila WS, Gouveia AM, Pomerantzeff P, et al. Maternal-fetal outcome and prognosis of cardiac surgery during pregnancy. Arq Bras Cardiol 2009;93:9–14.

72. John AS, Gurley F, Schaff HV, et al. Cardiopulmonary bypass during pregnancy. Ann Thorac Surg 2011;91:1191–6.

73. Arnoni RT, Arnoni AS, Bonini RC, et al. Risk factors associated with cardiac surgery during pregnancy. Ann Thorac Surg 2003;76:1605–8.

74. Lao TT, Sermer M, MaGee L, et al. Congenital aortic stenosis and pregnancy—a reappraisal. Am J Obstet Gynecol 1993;169:540–5.

75. Horstkotte D, Loogen F. The natural history of aortic valve stenosis. Eur Heart J 1988;9(Suppl E):57–64.

76. Easterling TR, Chadwick HS, Otto CM, et al. Aortic stenosis in pregnancy. Obstet Gynecol 1988;72:113–18.

77. Arias F, Pineda J. Aortic stenosis and pregnancy. J Reprod Med 1978;20:229–32.

78. Shime J, Mocarski EJ, Hastings D, et al. Congenital heart disease in pregnancy: short- and long-term implications. Am J Obstet Gynecol 1987;156:313–22.

79. Hameed A, Karaalp IS, Tummala PP, et al. The effect of valvular heart disease on maternal and fetal outcome of pregnancy. J Am Coll Cardiol 2001;37:893–9.

80. Yap SC, Drenthen W, Pieper PG, et al. Risk of complications during pregnancy in women with congenital aortic stenosis. Int J Cardiol 2008;126:240–6.

81. Roberts JM, Gammill HS. Preeclampsia: recent insights. Hypertension 2005; 46:1243–9.

82. Silversides CK, Colman JM, Sermer M, et al. Early and intermediate-term outcomes of pregnancy with congenital aortic stenosis. Am J Cardiol 2003;91:1386–9.

83. Tzemos N, Silversides CK, Colman JM, et al. Late cardiac outcomes after pregnancy in women with congenital aortic stenosis. Am Heart J 2009;157:474–80.

84. Brian Jr JE, Seifen AB, Clark RB, et al. Aortic stenosis, cesarean delivery, and epidural anesthesia. J Clin Anesth 1993;5:154–7.

85. Lao TT, Adelman AG, Sermer M, et al. Balloon valvuloplasty for congenital aortic stenosis in pregnancy. Br J Obstet Gynecol 1993;100:1141–2.

86. Sreeram N, Kitchiner D, Williams D, et al. Balloon dilatation of the aortic valve after previous surgical valvotomy: immediate and follow up results. Br Heart J 1994; 71:558–60.

87. Banning AP, Pearson JF, Hall RJ. Role of balloon dilatation of the aortic valve in pregnant patients with severe aortic stenosis. Br Heart J 1993;70:544–5.

88. al Kasab SM, Sabag T, al Zaibag M, et al. Beta-adrenergic receptor blockade in the management of pregnant women with mitral stenosis. Am J Obstet Gynecol 1990;163:37–40.

89. Ben Farhat M, Gamra H, Betbout F, et al. Percutaneous balloon mitral commissurotomy during pregnancy. Heart (Br Cardiac Soc) 1997;77:564–7.

90. Gupta A, Lokhandwala YY, Satoskar PR, et al. Balloon mitral valvotomy in pregnancy: maternal and fetal outcomes. J Am Coll Surg 1998;187:409–15.

91. Patel JJ, Mitha AS, Hassen F, et al. Percutaneous balloon mitral valvotomy in pregnant patients with tight pliable mitral stenosis. Am Heart J 1993;125:1106–9.

92. Ribeiro PA, Fawzy ME, Awad M, et al. Balloon valvotomy for pregnant patients with severe pliable mitral stenosis using the Inoue technique with total abdominal and pelvic shielding. Am Heart J 1992;124:e84–231.

93. Ruzyllo W, Dabrowski M, Woroszylska M, et al. Percutaneous mitral commissurotomy with the Inoue balloon for severe mitral stenosis during pregnancy. J Heart Valve Dis 1992;1:209–12.

94. Stoddard MF, Longaker RA, Vuocolo LM, et al. Transesophageal echocardiography in the pregnant patient. Am Heart J 1992;124:785–7.

95. Henriquez DD, Roos-Hesselink JW, Schalij MJ, et al. Treatment of valvular heart disease during pregnancy for improving maternal and neonatal outcome. Cochrane Database Syst Rev (Online) 2011:CD008128.

96. Esteves CA, Munoz JS, Braga S, et al. Immediate and long-term follow-up of percutaneous balloon mitral valvuloplasty in pregnant patients with rheumatic mitral stenosis. Am J Cardiol 2006;98:812–16.

97. Mangione JA, Lourenco RM, dos Santos ES, et al. Long-term follow-up of pregnant women after percutaneous mitral valvuloplasty. Catheter Cardiovasc Interv 2000;50:413–17.

98. Silversides CK, Colman JM, Sermer M, et al. Cardiac risk in pregnant women with rheumatic mitral stenosis. Am J Cardiol 2003;91:1382–5.

99. Reimold SC, Rutherford JD. Clinical practice. Valvular heart disease in pregnancy. N Engl J Med 2003;349:52–9.

100. Elkayam U, Bitar F. Valvular heart disease and pregnancy part I: native valves. J Am Coll Cardiol 2005;46:223–30.

101. Jana N, Vasishta K, Khunnu B, et al. Pregnancy in association with mitral valve prolapse. Asia Oceania J Obstet Gynaecol 1993;19:61–5.

102. Tang LC, Chan SY, Wong VC, et al. Pregnancy in patients with mitral valve prolapse. Int J Gynaecol Obstet 1985;23:217–21.

103. Hameed AB, Goodwin TM, Elkayam U. Effect of pulmonary stenosis on pregnancy outcomes—a case-control study. Am Heart J 2007;154:852–4.

104. Drenthen W, Pieper PG, Roos-Hesselink JW, et al. Outcome of pregnancy in women with congenital heart disease: a literature review. J Am Coll Cardiol 2007;49:2303–11.

105. Drenthen W, Pieper PG, Roos-Hesselink JW, et al. Non-cardiac complications during pregnancy in women with isolated congenital pulmonary valvar stenosis. Heart (Br Cardiac Soc) 2006;92:1838–43.

106. Veldtman GR, Connolly HM, Grogan M, et al. Outcomes of pregnancy in women with tetralogy of fallot. J Am Coll Cardiol 2004;44:174–80.

107. Meijer JM, Pieper PG, Drenthen W, et al. Pregnancy, fertility, and recurrence risk in corrected tetralogy of Fallot 10.1136/hrt.2004.034108. Heart 2005;91:801–5.

108. Greutmann M, Von Klemperer K, Brooks R, et al. Pregnancy outcome in women with congenital heart disease and residual haemodynamic lesions of the right ventricular outflow tract. Eur Heart J 2010;31:1764–70.

109. Connolly HM, Warnes CA. Ebstein's anomaly: outcome of pregnancy. J Am Coll Cardiol 1994;23:1194–8.

110. Pavankumar P, Venugopal P, Kaul U, et al. Pregnancy in patients with prosthetic cardiac valve. A 10-year experience. Scand J Thorac Cardiovasc Surg 1988;22:19–22.

111. Sbarouni E, Oakley CM. Outcome of pregnancy in women with valve prostheses. Br Heart J 1994;71:196–201.

112. Born D, Martinez EE, Almeida PA, et al. Pregnancy in patients with prosthetic heart valves: the effects of anticoagulation on mother, fetus, and neonate. Am Heart J 1992;124:413–17.

113. Hanania G, Thomas D, Michel PL, et al. Pregnancy and prosthetic heart valves: a French cooperative retrospective study of 155 cases. Eur Heart J 1994;15:1651–8.
114. Salazar E, Izaguirre R, Verdejo J, et al. Failure of adjusted doses of subcutaneous heparin to prevent thromboembolic phenomena in pregnant patients with mechanical cardiac valve prostheses. J Am Coll Cardiol 1996;27:1698–703.
115. Chan WS, Anand S, Ginsberg JS. Anticoagulation of pregnant women with mechanical heart valves: a systematic review of the literature. Arch Intern Med 2000;160:191–6.
116. El SF, Hassan W, Latroche B, et al. Pregnancy has no effect on the rate of structural deterioration of bioprosthetic valves: long-term 18-year follow up results. J Heart Valve Dis 2005;14:481–5.
117. Avila WS, Rossi EG, Grinberg M, et al. Influence of pregnancy after bioprosthetic valve replacement in young women: a prospective five-year study. J Heart Valve Dis 2002;11:864–9.
118. Cleuziou J, Horer J, Kaemmerer H, et al. Pregnancy does not accelerate biological valve degeneration. Int J Cardiol 2010;145:418–21.
119. Salazar E, Espinola N, Roman L, et al. Effect of pregnancy on the duration of bovine pericardial bioprostheses. Am Heart J 1999;137:714–20.
120. Dore A, Somerville J. Pregnancy in patients with pulmonary autograft valve replacement. Eur Heart J 1997;18:1659–62.
121. Yap SC, Drenthen W, Pieper PG, et al. Outcome of pregnancy in women after pulmonary autograft valve replacement for congenital aortic valve disease. J Heart Valve Dis 2007;16:398–403.
122. Sareli P, England MJ, Berk MR, et al. Maternal and fetal sequelae of anticoagulation during pregnancy in patients with mechanical heart valve prostheses. Am J Cardiol 1989;63:1462–5.
123. Vongpatanasin W, Hillis LD, Lange RA. Prosthetic heart valves. N Engl J Med 1996;335:407–16.
124. North RA, Sadler L, Stewart AW, et al. Long-term survival and valve-related complications in young women with cardiac valve replacements. Circulation 1999;99:2669–76.
125. Ginsberg JS, Hirsh J, Turner DC, et al. Risks to the fetus of anticoagulant therapy during pregnancy. Thromb Haemost 1989;61:197–203.
126. Ginsberg JS, Kowalchuk G, Hirsh J, et al. Heparin therapy during pregnancy. Risks to the fetus and mother. Arch Intern Med 1989;149:2233–6.
127. Oran B, Lee-Parritz A, Ansell J. Low molecular weight heparin for the prophylaxis of thromboembolism in women with prosthetic mechanical heart valves during pregnancy. Thromb Haemost 2004;92:747–51.
128. Rowan JA, McCowan LM, Raudkivi PJ, et al. Enoxaparin treatment in women with mechanical heart valves during pregnancy. Am J Obstet Gynecol 2001;185:633–7.
129. Yinon Y, Siu SC, Warshafsky C, et al. Use of low molecular weight heparin in pregnant women with mechanical heart valves. Am J Cardiol 2009;104:1259–63.
130. Ginsberg JS, Kowalchuk G, Hirsh J, et al. Heparin effect on bone density. Thromb Haemost 1990;64:286–9.
131. Dahlman T, Lindvall N, Hellgren M. Osteopenia in pregnancy during long-term heparin treatment: a radiological study post partum. Br J Obstet Gynaecol 1990;97:221–8.
132. Barbour LA, Kick SD, Steiner JF, et al. A prospective study of heparin-induced osteoporosis in pregnancy using bone densitometry. Am J Obstet Gynecol 1994;170:862–9.
133. Dahlman TC. Osteoporotic fractures and the recurrence of thromboembolism during pregnancy and the puerperium in 184 women undergoing thromboprophylaxis with heparin. Am J Obstet Gynecol 1993;168:1265–70.
134. Shapiro NL, Kominiarek MA, Nutescu EA, et al. Dosing and monitoring of low-molecular-weight heparin in high-risk pregnancy: single-center experience. Pharmacotherapy 2011;31:678–85.
135. Hall JG, Pauli RM, Wilson KM. Maternal and fetal sequelae of anticoagulation during pregnancy. Am J Med 1980;68:122–40.
136. Becker MH, Genieser NB, Finegold M, et al. Chondrodysplasis punctata: is maternal warfarin therapy a factor? Am J Dis Child 1975;129:356–9.
137. Iturbe-Alessio I, Fonseca MC, Mutchinik O, et al. Risks of anticoagulant therapy in pregnant women with artificial heart valves. N Engl J Med 1986;315:1390–3.
138. Ville Y, Jenkins E, Shearer MJ, et al. Fetal intraventricular haemorrhage and maternal warfarin. Lancet 1993;341:1211.
139. Vitale N, De Feo M, De Santo LS, et al. Dose-dependent fetal complications of warfarin in pregnant women with mechanical heart valves. J Am Coll Cardiol 1999;33:1637–41.
140. Cotrufo M, De Feo M, De Santo LS, et al. Risk of warfarin during pregnancy with mechanical valve prostheses. Obstet Gynecol 2002;99:35–40.
141. Khamooshi AJ, Kashfi F, Hoseini S, et al. Anticoagulation for prosthetic heart valves in pregnancy. Is there an answer? Asian Cardiovasc Thorac Ann 2007;15:493–6.
142. Bian C, Wei Q, Liu X. Influence of heart-valve replacement of warfarin anticoagulant therapy on perinatal outcomes. Arch Gynecol Obstet 2012;285:347–51.
143. Sillesen M, Hjortdal V, Vejlstrup N, et al. Pregnancy with prosthetic heart valves—30 years' nationwide experience in Denmark. Eur J Cardiothorac Surg 2011;40:448–54.
144. Leonhardt G, Gaul C, Nietsch HH, et al. Thrombolytic therapy in pregnancy. J Thromb Thrombol 2006;21:271–6.
145. Keyser DL, Biller J, Coffman TT, et al. Neurologic complications of late prosthetic valve endocarditis. Stroke 1990;21:472–5.
146. Turrentine MA, Braems G, Ramirez MM. Use of thrombolytics for the treatment of thromboembolic disease during pregnancy. Obstet Gynecol Surv 1995;50:534–41.

ACC/AHA Guidelines Classification and Levels of Evidence

"Size of Treatment Effect"

"ESTIMATE OF CERTAINTY (PRECISION) OF TREATMENT EFFECT"	Class I Benefit >>> Risk Procedure/Treatment SHOULD be performed/administered	Class IIa Benefit >> Risk Additional studies with focused objectives needed IT IS REASONABLE to perform procedure/ administer treatment	Class IIb Benefit ≥ Risk Additional studies with broad objectives needed; additional registry data would be helpful Procedure/treatment MAY BE CONSIDERED	Class III Risk ≥ Benefit No additional studies needed Procedure/treatment SHOULD NOT be performed/administered since it is NOT HELPFUL and MAY BE HARMFUL
Level A *Multiple (3-5) population risk strata evaluated** *General consistency of direction and magnitude of effect*	Recommendation that procedure or treatment is useful/effective Sufficient evidence from multiple randomized trials or meta-analyses	Recommendation in favor of treatment or procedure being useful/effective Some conflicting evidence from multiple randomized trials or meta-analyses	Recommendation's usefulness/efficacy less well established Greater conflicting evidence from multiple randomized trials or meta-analyses	Recommendation that procedure or treatment not useful/effective and may be harmful Sufficient evidence from multiple randomized trials or meta-analyses
Level B *Limited (2-3) population risk strata evaluated**	Recommendation that procedure or treatment is useful/effective Limited evidence from single randomized trial or non-randomized studies	Recommendation in favor of treatment or procedure being useful/effective Some conflicting evidence from single randomized trial or non-randomized studies	Recommendation's usefulness/efficacy less well established Greater conflicting evidence from single randomized trial or non-randomized studies	Recommendation that procedure or treatment not useful/effective and may be harmful Limited evidence from single randomized trial or non-randomized studies
Level C *Very limited (1-2) population risk strata evaluated**	Recommendation that procedure or treatment is useful/effective Only expert opinion, case studies, or standard-of-care	Recommendation in favor of treatment or procedure being useful/effective Only diverging expert opinion, case studies, or standard-of-care	Recommendation's usefulness/efficacy less well established Only diverging expert opinion, case studies, or standard-of-care	Recommendation that procedure or treatment not useful/effective and may be harmful Only expert opinion, case studies, or standard-of-care
Suggested phrases for writing recomemndations†	should is recommended is indicated is useful/effective/ beneficial	is reasonable can be is useful/ effective/beneficial is probably recommended or indicated	may/might be considered may/might be reasonable usefulness/effectiveness is unknown/unclear/ uncertain or not well established	is not recommended is not indicated should not is not useful/effective/ beneficial may be harmful

Applying classification of recommendations and level of evidence.

*Data available from clinical trials or registries about the usefulness/efficacy in different subpopulations, such as gender, age, history of diabetes, history of prior myocardial infarction, history of heart failure, and prior aspirin use. A recommendation with Level of Evidence B or C does not imply that the recommendation is weak. Many important clinical questions addressed in the guidelines do not lend themselves to clinical trials. Even though randomized trials are not available, there may be a very clear clinical consensus that a particular test or therapy is useful or effective.

†In 2003 the ACC/AHA Task Force on Practice Guidelines recently provided a list of suggested phrases to use when writing recommendations. All recommendations in this guideline have been written in full sentences that express a complete thought, such that a recommendation, even if separated and presented apart from the rest of the document (including headings above sets of recommendations), would still convey the full intent of the recommendation. It is hoped that this will increase readers' comprehension of the guidelines and will allow queries at the individual recommendation level.

ESC Guidelines Classification and Levels of Evidence

Class I	Class IIa	Class IIb
Evidence and/or general agreement that a given treatment or procedure is beneficial, useful, and effective	Conflicting evidence and/or a divergence of opinion about the usefulness/efficacy of a given treatment or procedure	Conflicting evidence and/or a divergence of opinion about the usefulness/efficacy of a given treatment or procedure
	Weight of evidence/opinion is in favor of usefulness/efficacy	*Usefulness/efficacy is less well established by evidence/opinion*

Level of Evidence A	Level of Evidence B	Level of Evidence C
Data derived from multiple randomized clinical trials or meta-analyses	Data derived from a single randomized clinical trial or large non-randomized studies	Consensus of opinion of the experts and/or small studies, retrospective studies, registries

INDEX

Page numbers followed by "f" indicate figures, "t" indicate tables, and "b" indicate boxes.